Manual of
Cardiovascular Medicine

Manual of
Cardiovascular Medicine

Editors

Steven P. Marso, M.D.
Brian P. Griffin, M.D.
Eric J. Topol, M.D.

The Cleveland Clinic Foundation
Cleveland, Ohio

With 44 contributors

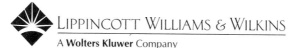

LIPPINCOTT WILLIAMS & WILKINS
A **Wolters Kluwer** Company
Philadelphia · Baltimore · New York · London
Buenos Aires · Hong Kong · Sydney · Tokyo

Acquisitions Editor: Ruth W. Weinberg
Developmental Editor: Delois Patterson
Production Editor: Aureliano Vázquez, Jr.
Manufacturing Manager: Kevin Watt
Cover Designer: Patricia Gast
Compositor: Circle Graphics
Printer: RR Donnelley, Crawfordsville

© 2000 by LIPPINCOTT WILLIAMS & WILKINS
227 East Washington Square
Philadelphia, PA 19106-3780 USA
LWW.com

Printed in the USA

Library of Congress Cataloging-in-Publication Data

Manual of cardiovascular medicine / edited by Steven P. Marso, Brian P. Griffin, Eric J. Topol; with 44 contributors.
    p.   cm.
    Includes bibliographical references and indexes.
    ISBN 0-683-30685-5
    1. Cardiology—Handbooks, manuals, etc. 2. Heart—Diseases—Handbooks, manuals, etc. I. Marso, Steven P. II. Griffin, Brian P., 1956– III. Topol, Eric J., 1954–
    [DNLM: 1. Heart Diseases—diagnosis. 2. Heart Diseases—therapy. WG 210 M294 1999]
RC682.M315   1999
616.1′2 21—dc21
                                    99-042919

10 9 8 7 6 5 4 3 2 1

CONTENTS

Contributing Authors xiii

Preface xvii

Acknowledgments xviii

SECTION I.   ACUTE CORONARY SYNDROMES
Michael A. Lauer and A. Michael Lincoff

1   Acute Myocardial Infarction 3
    Michael A. Lauer

2   Unstable Angina and Non-ST–Segment Elevation MI 25
    Matthew T. Roe

3   Complications of Myocardial Infarction 39
    Debabrata Mukherjee

4   Post–Myocardial Infarction Risk Stratification and Management 56
    Elaine K. Moen

SECTION II. CHRONIC ISCHEMIC SYNDROMES
Samir R. Kapadia and David J. Moliterno

5A Stable Angina 71
    Samir R. Kapadia

5B Silent Ischemia 91
    Stanley Chetcuti and Samir R. Kapadia

6   Syndrome X: Angina with Normal Coronary Arteries 95
    Marc Penn

SECTION III. CHRONIC HEART FAILURE
John G. Peterson and James B. Young

7   Systolic Heart Failure 99
    Eric Bowen

8   Diastolic Heart Failure 115
    John G. Peterson

9   Hypertrophic Cardiomyopathy.................................... 129
    Mark Robbins

10 High-output Heart Failure 142
    John G. Peterson

11 Isolated Right Heart Failure 145
    John G. Peterson

12 Surgical Options in Heart Failure 149
    Leslie Campbell

13 Cardiac Transplantation 154
    Leslie Campbell

SECTION IV. VALVULAR HEART DISEASE
David N. Rubin and Brian P. Griffin

14 Aortic Valve Disease.. 167
    Matthew Deedy

15 Mitral Valve Disease 194
    Maran Thamilarasan

16 Tricuspid Valve Disease 220
    Amy P. Scally

17 Pulmonary Valve Disease....................................... 229
    Marc Penn

18 Prosthetic Heart Valves....................................... 232
    Steve Lin and James Wong

SECTION V. ARRHYTHMIA
Robert A. Schweikert and Gregory Kidwell

19 Tachyarrhythmias 249
    Thomas Dresing

20 Bradyarrhythmias, Atrioventricular Block, Asystole, and Pulseless
    Electrical Activity.. 281
    Christopher Cole

21 Sudden Cardiac Death 301
    Robert A. Schweikert

22 Syncope.. 310
    Vasant B. Patel

23 Long QT Syndrome... 320
   Rodolfo D. Farhy

24 Antiarrhythmic Drugs... 325
   Wakkas Tayara and Robert A. Schweikert

SECTION VI. DISEASES OF THE AORTA AND PERICARDIUM
Steven P. Marso and Richard A. Grimm

25 Aortic Aneurysm and Aortic Dissection........................... 335
   John P. Gassler

26 Acute Pericarditis 354
   Jenny Wu

27 Pericardial Effusion 363
   Stanley Chetcuti

28 Constrictive Pericarditis...................................... 373
   Joel P. Reginelli and Tom A. Grady

SECTION VII. ADULT CONGENITAL HEART DISEASE
J. Donald Moore and Douglas S. Moodie

29 Atrial Septal Defect 387
   J. Donald Moore and Douglas S. Moodie

30 Ventricular Septal Defect 392
   J. Donald Moore and Douglas S. Moodie

31 Patent Ductus Arteriosus 396
   J. Donald Moore and Douglas S. Moodie

32 Coarctation of the Aorta 399
   J. Donald Moore and Douglas S. Moodie

33 Tetralogy of Fallot 402
   J. Donald Moore and Douglas S. Moodie

34 Miscellaneous Defects 407
   J. Donald Moore and Douglas S. Moodie

SECTION VIII. COMMON CARDIOLOGY CONSULTS
Harpreet Bhalla and Brian P. Griffin

35 Assessing and Managing Cardiac Risk in Noncardiac
   Surgical Procedures 421
   Vasant B. Patel

36   Hypertensive Crisis   434
     Harpreet Bhalla

37   Evaluation of Chest Pain in the Emergency Department   446
     Jason B. Wischmeyer and Samir R. Kapadia

SECTION IX. PREVENTIVE CARDIOLOGY
JoAnne Micale Foody and Dennis Sprecher

38   Cardiovascular Risk Factors   455
     JoAnne Micale Foody

39   Coronary Artery Disease and Women   482
     JoAnne Micale Foody

SECTION X. NONINVASIVE ASSESSMENT
Steven P. Marso and Thomas H. Marwick

40   Exercise Electrocardiographic Testing   503
     Christopher Cole

41   Nuclear Imaging   523
     Jeffrey A. Skiles

42   Stress Echocardiography   537
     Matthew Deedy

43   Myocardial Viability   549
     C. Patrick Green

SECTION XI. ELECTROPHYSIOLOGY
Robert A. Schweikert and Patrick Tchou

44   Electrophysiologic Studies   563
     Ayman S. Al-Khadra

45   Cardiac Pacing   588
     Robert A. Schweikert and Navin Gupta

46   Antitachycardia Devices   612
     Ralph S. Augostini

47   Head-upright, Tilt Table Testing   620
     Stavros G. Maragos

SECTION XII. MISCELLANEOUS CONDITIONS
Steven P. Marso

48   Infective Endocarditis   629
Mark Murphy

49   Rheumatic Fever.   644
Simone Nader

SECTION XIII. PROCEDURES
Deepak L. Bhatt and Stephen G. Ellis

50   Right Heart Catheterization.   653
Leslie Cho

51   Temporary Transvenous Pacing.   666
Debabrata Mukherjee

52   Pericardiocentesis.   670
Tom A. Grady and Deepak L. Bhatt

53   Cardioversion   676
JoAnne Micale Foody and Gregory Kidwell

54   Endomyocardial Biopsy.   682
Milind Shah

55   Intraaortic Balloon Counterpulsation.   687
Matthew T. Roe

56   Left Heart Catheterization   700
Deepak L. Bhatt

57   Interventional Cardiology   722
Walter A. Tan and Stephen G. Ellis

58   Transthoracic Echocardiography   744
Steve Lin and Guy Armstrong

59   Transesophageal Echocardiography   758
Maran Thamilarasan

Appendix: Drug Index   775
Michael A. Militello

Subject Index   837

CONTRIBUTING AUTHORS

Unless otherwise noted, the following contributors are affiliated with the Cleveland Clinic Foundation, 9500 Euclid Avenue, F-25, Cleveland, Ohio 44195

Ayman S. Al-Khadra, M.D.
Cardiology Fellow

Guy Armstrong, M.D.
Cardiology Fellow

Ralph S. Augostini, M.D.
Cardiology Fellow

Harpreet Bhalla, M.D.
Cardiology Fellow

Deepak L. Bhatt, M.D.
Cardiology Fellow

Eric Bowen, M.D.
Cardiology Fellow

Leslie Campbell, M.D.
Cardiology Fellow

Stanley Chetcuti, M.D.
Cardiology Fellow

Leslie Cho, M.D.
Cardiology Fellow

Christopher Cole, M.D.
Cardiology Fellow

Matthew Deedy, M.D.
Cardiology Fellow

Thomas Dresing, M.D.
Cardiology Fellow

Stephen G. Ellis, M.D.
Staff

Rodolfo D. Farhy, M.D.
Cardiology Fellow

JoAnne Micale Foody, M.D.
Cardiology Fellow

John P. Gassler, M.D.
Cardiology Fellow

Tom A. Grady, M.D.
Cardiology Fellow

C. Patrick Green, M.D.
Cardiology Fellow, St Luke's Hospital, 4401 Wornall Road, Kansas City, Missouri 64111

Brian P. Griffin, M.D.
Director, Cardiology Fellowship Program

Richard A. Grimm, D.O.
Cardiology Staff

Navin Gupta, M.D.
Cardiology Fellow

Samir R. Kapadia, M.D.
Cardiology Fellow

Gregory Kidwell, M.D.
Staff

Michael A. Lauer, M.D.
Cardiology Fellow

Steve Lin, M.D.
Cardiology Fellow

A. Michael Lincoff, M.D.
Staff

Stavros G. Maragos, M.D.
Chief Cardiology Fellow

Steven P. Marso, M.D.
Chief Cardiology Fellow

Thomas H. Marwick, M.D.
Cardiology Staff

Michael A. Militello, PHARM. D.
Cardiology Clinical Pharmacist

Elaine K. Moen, M.D.
Cardiology Fellow

David J. Moliterno, M.D.
Cardiology Staff

Douglas S. Moodie, M.D.
Staff, Pediatric Cardiology

J. Donald Moore, M.D.
Cardiology Fellow

Debabrata Mukherjee, M.D.
Cardiology Fellow

Mark Murphy, M.D.
Cardiology Fellow

Simone Nader, M.D.
Cardiology Fellow

Vasant B. Patel, M.D.
Cardiology Fellow

Marc Penn, M.D.
Cardiology Fellow

John G. Peterson, M.D.
Cardiology Fellow

Joel P. Reginelli, M.D.
Cardiology Fellow

Mark Robbins, M.D.
Cardiology Fellow

Matthew T. Roe, M.D.
Cardiology Fellow

David N. Rubin, M.D.
Cardiology Fellow

Amy P. Scally, M.D.
Cardiology Fellow

Robert A. Schweikert, M.D.
Cardiology Fellow

Milind Shah, M.D.
Cardiology Fellow

Jeffrey A. Skiles, M.D.
Cardiology Fellow

Dennis Sprecher, M.D.
Cardiology Staff

Walter A. Tan, M.D.
Cardiology Fellow

Wakkas Tayara, M.D.
Cardiology Fellow

Patrick Tchou, M.D.
Staff

Maran Thamilarasan, M.D.
Cardiology Fellow

Eric J. Topol
Chairman, Department of Cardiology

Jason B. Wischmeyer, M.D.
Cardiology Fellow

James Wong, M.D.
Cardiology Fellow

Jenny Wu, M.D.
Cardiology Fellow

James B. Young, M.D.
Cardiology Staff

PREFACE

The *Manual of Cardiovascular Medicine,* written almost exclusively by cardiology fellows and staff at the Cleveland Clinic Foundation, provides a concise and thorough discussion in a readily accessible outline format of cardiovascular diseases commonly encountered in the care of patients. The first part is organized by clinical syndromes. Although there is detailed discussion regarding the clinical presentations of cardiovascular illnesses, the main focus of these chapters is on diagnosis and management strategies. This format allows the reader to rapidly access information, thus facilitating rapid assessment, diagnosis and management of patients with complex diseases.

The remaining chapters focus on reviewing the numerous procedures often required for the complete care of patients with cardiovascular syndromes. These chapters not only cover indications, contraindications, and patient preparation, but also provide a detailed discussion of the technique of each procedure.

The *Manual of Cardiovascular Medicine* is well suited for cardiology fellows, practicing physicians, and house staff who frequently care for patients with advanced cardiovascular diseases. We hope that you will find this Manual both informative and easy to use in your everyday practice of medicine.

Steven P. Marso, M.D.
Brian P. Griffin, M.D.
Eric J. Topol, M.D.

ACKNOWLEDGMENTS

We acknowledge the following people, without whose expertise this project would not have been possible: Lois Adamski, for her editorial assistance; and Suzanne Turner, Charlene Surace, and Mary Ann Citrano, for their graphic design.

SECTION I. ACUTE CORONARY SYNDROMES

Michael A. Lauer and A. Michael Lincoff

1. ACUTE MYOCARDIAL INFARCTION

Michael A. Lauer

I. **Introduction. Acute myocardial infarction (MI) is the leading cause of death in North America and Europe.** Approximately 1 million people each year in the United States are admitted to the hospital because of acute MI. An additional 200,000 to 300,000 are estimated to die of acute MI before reaching the hospital. The overall mortality is approximately 40%. Fortunately, the incidence and mortality have declined over the last 30 years. However, although **thrombolytic therapy has made progress** in lowering mortality, **most patients with acute MI are not eligible for this therapy.** With an increasing proportion of the population being represented by the elderly, who have a high incidence of and mortality from acute MI, it will likely remain the leading cause of death over the next several decades.

II. **Acute MI.** When a patient seeks evaluation because of a clinical history compatible with ongoing or stuttering cardiac ischemia, **an electrocardiogram (ECG)** should be quickly performed and interpreted to determine whether **acute ST segment elevations or new left bundle branch block (LBBB)** is present. If either of these criteria is present, **reperfusion therapy is indicated.** ST-elevation MI and non-ST-elevation MI with unstable angina are part of a continuum of a pathophysiologic syndrome. However, the distinction between these two types of MI is clinically relevant because **management differs in regard to reperfusion therapy.** Non-ST-elevation MI and unstable angina are addressed in Chapter 2.

  A. **Clinical presentation**

    1. **Signs and symptoms**

      a. The classic symptoms are **intense, crushing, left-sided substernal chest pain with radiation to the left arm** and **an impending sense of doom.** The discomfort resembles that of angina pectoris but is typically more severe, of longer duration (generally longer than 20 minutes) and is not relieved with rest or nitroglycerin. Peak intensity usually is not instantaneous, as it would be with pulmonary embolus or aortic dissection.

        (1) In addition to the left arm, the **discomfort may radiate to the neck, jaw, back, shoulder, right arm, or epigastrium.** Pain in any of these locations without chest pain is possible. Acute MI may occur without chest pain, especially among postoperative patients, the elderly, and those with diabetes mellitus or hypertension.

        (2) **If pain radiates to the back, aortic dissection** must be considered.

      b. **Associated symptoms** may include diaphoresis, dyspnea, fatigue, lightheadedness, palpitations, acute confusion, indigestion, nausea, or vomiting. Gastrointestinal symptoms are especially common with inferior infarction.

    2. **Physical examination.** The physical examination generally does not add a great deal to the diagnosis of acute MI. However, the examination is **extremely important in excluding other diagnoses** that may mimic acute MI, in **risk stratification,** in the diagnosis of impending heart failure, and in serving as a **baseline examination** to monitor for mechanical complications of acute MI that may develop.

      a. **Risk stratification,** which aids in treatment decisions and counseling patients and families, is based in part on heart rate, blood pressure, and the presence or absence of pulmonary edema and a third heart sound (S_3).

3

    b. The **mechanical complications** of mitral regurgitation and ventricular septal defect often are heralded by a new systolic murmur (see Chapter 3). Early diagnosis of these complications relies on well-documented examination findings at baseline and frequently during the hospital course.

B. Differential diagnosis

    1. **Pericarditis. Chest pain** that is **worse when the person is lying down and improves when the person is sitting upright or slightly forward** is typical of pericarditis. Care must be taken in excluding acute MI, however, because pericarditis can complicate acute MI. The ECG abnormalities of acute pericarditis can mimic acute MI. Diffuse ST-segment elevation can occur with pericarditis or acute MI that involves the proximal left anterior descending artery or left main coronary artery. PR depression, peaked T waves, or ECG abnormalities out of proportion to the clinical scenario may favor the diagnosis of pericarditis. Reciprocal ST depression does not occur in pericarditis, except in a VR and V1. Echocardiography may be useful, not in evaluating pericardial effusion, which may be variable in either condition, but in documenting the lack of wall motion abnormalities in the setting of ongoing pain and ST elevation.

    2. **Myocarditis.** As with pericarditis, the symptoms and ECG findings of myocarditis can be similar to those of acute MI. Echocardiography is less useful, however, because diffuse left ventricular (LV) dysfunction may be expected with either myocarditis or acute MI associated with left main coronary artery or prior LV dysfunction. **A complete history often reveals a more insidious onset and associated viral syndrome with myocarditis.**

    3. **Acute aortic dissection. Sharp chest pain that bores through to the back** is typical of aortic dissection. This type of radiation pattern should be thoroughly investigated before administration of antithrombotic, antiplatelet, or thrombolytic therapy. Proximal extension of the dissection into either coronary ostium can produce concurrent acute MI. A chest radiograph may reveal a widened mediastinum. Transthoracic echocardiography may reveal a dissection flap in the proximal ascending aorta. If it does not, a more definitive diagnosis should be obtained with transesophageal echocardiography, computed tomography (CT), magnetic resonance (MR) imaging, or aortography if the level of suspicion is high.

    4. **Pulmonary embolism. Shortness of breath** with an onset concurrent with that of chest pain without evidence of pulmonary edema suggests pulmonary embolism. Echocardiography may help to rule out wall motion abnormalities and help to determine the presence of right ventricular strain, which is an indication for lytic therapy in the setting of pulmonary embolism.

    5. **Acute cholecystitis** can mimic the symptoms and ECG findings of inferior acute MI, although the two can coexist. **Tenderness in the right upper quadrant, fever, and an elevated leukocyte count** favor cholecystitis, which can be diagnosed by means of HIDA scanning.

C. Laboratory examination

    1. **Creatine kinase.** An elevated level of creatine kinase (CK) is rarely helpful in making the diagnosis of acute MI for a patient with ST elevation. Because it usually takes 4 to 6 hours to see an appreciable rise in CK, a normal value may simply signify recent complete occlusion. CK and CK MB levels can be elevated in the presence of pericarditis and myocarditis, which may cause diffuse ST elevation. **CK levels are more helpful in gauging the size and timing** of acute MI than in making the diagnosis. The peak CK level is believed to occur earlier among patients who undergo successful reperfusion.

    2. **Troponins.** Although high sensitivity and the availability to perform them rapidly at bedside have made troponin T and troponin I assays

useful in the diagnosis and management of unstable angina and non-ST-elevation MI, the **lag time** (3 to 6 hours) between occlusion and detectable elevations in serum levels, as with CK, **limits their usefulness** in the diagnosis of ST-elevation acute MI.

D. **Diagnostic testing**
   1. **Electrocardiography**
      a. **Definitive ECG diagnosis** of acute MI requires ST elevation of 1 mm or more in two or more contiguous leads, often with reciprocal ST depression in the contralateral leads.
      b. **ECG subsets.** ST-segment elevations can be divided into subgroups that may be correlated with the infarction-related artery and risk for death. These five subgroups are listed in Table 1-1 and illustrated in Fig. 1-1.
      c. **Left bundle branch block (LBBB)**
         (1) **New LBBB in the setting of symptoms consistent with acute MI** may be indicative of large anterior wall acute MI involving the proximal left anterior descending coronary artery and should be managed as ST-elevation acute MI.
         (2) **In the absence of an old ECG or in the presence of LBBB at baseline** the diagnosis of ST-segment elevation acute MI can be made in the presence of LBBB with greater than 90% specificity on the basis of the criteria listed in Table 1–2 and illustrated in Fig. 1-2.
         (3) **Right bundle branch block (RBBB)** complicates interpretation of ST elevation in leads V1 through V3. The diagnosis of anterior acute MI is possible when a patient with RBBB has secondary T-wave changes (opposite to the QRS complex) in leads V1 through V3 or V4 replaced with T waves of concordant polarity with the QRS (pseudonormalization). RBBB does not obscure ST elevation in other leads.
   2. **Echocardiography** maybe helpful in the evaluation of LBBB of undetermined duration in that the lack of regional wall motion abnormality in the presence of continuing symptoms makes the diagnosis of acute MI unlikely.

E. **Risk stratification.** It is possible and useful to estimate the risk for death of a patient with acute MI. The estimate can **aid in making treatment decisions and recommendations and in counseling patients and families.** Five simple baseline parameters have been demonstrated to explain more than 90% of the prognostic information for 30-day mortality. These characteristics are (in descending order of importance): age, systolic blood pressure, Killip classification (Table 1-3), heart rate, and location of MI (see Table 1-1, Fig. 1-1) (1).

F. **Therapy**
   1. **Immediate management and stabilization**
      a. **Aspirin and antiplatelet therapy. Aspirin should be administered immediately to all patients with acute MI,** unless there is a clear history of true aspirin allergy (not intolerance). Aspirin therapy conveys as much mortality benefit as streptokinase, and the combination provides additive benefit (2). The dose should be either four chewable 80-mg tablets (for more rapid absorption) or one 325-mg nonchewable tablet. If oral administration is not possible, a rectal suppository can be given. Other antiplatelet agents such as dipyridamole, ticlopidine (500 mg immediately, followed by 250 mg twice a day) or clopidogrel (300 mg immediately, followed by 75 mg every day) may be substituted if true aspirin allergy is present. Results of pilot studies of the use of glycoprotein IIb/IIIa inhibitors as an adjunct to thrombolysis are encouraging, and randomized trials are underway.
      b. **Oxygen.** Supplemental oxygen via nasal cannula should be given to all patients with suspected MI, with the exception of patients with

Table 1-1. Acute myocardial infarction: ECG subsets and correlated infarct-related artery and mortality

Category	Anatomy of occlusion	ECG findings	30-day mortality rate (%)	1-year mortality rate (%)
1, Proximal LAD	Proximal to first septal perforator	ST↑V_{1-6}, I, aVL and fasicular or bundle branch block	19.6	25.6
2, Mid LAD	Proximal to large diagonal but distal to first septal perforator	ST↑V_{1-6}, I, aVL	9.2	12.4
3, Distal LAD or diagonal	Distal to large diagonal or diagonal itself	ST↑V_{1-4}, or I, aVL, V_{5-6}	6.8	10.2
4, Moderate to large inferior (posterior, lateral, right ventricular)	Proximal RCA or left circumflex	ST↑II, III, aVF and any of the following: a. V_1, V_3R, V_4R b. V_{5-6} c. R > S in V_1, V_2	6.4	8.4
5, Small inferior	Distal RCA or left circumflex branch	ST↑II, III, aVF only	4.5	6.7

Mortality rate based on GUSTO I cohort population in each of the 5-year categories, all receiving reperfusion therapy.
LAD, Left anterior coronary descending; ↑, increased; *RCA*, right coronary artery.
From Topol EJ, Van de Werf FJ. Acute myocardial infarction: early diagnosis and management. In: Topol EJ, ed. *Textbook of cardiovascular medicine.* New York: Lippincott-Raven, 1998, with permission.

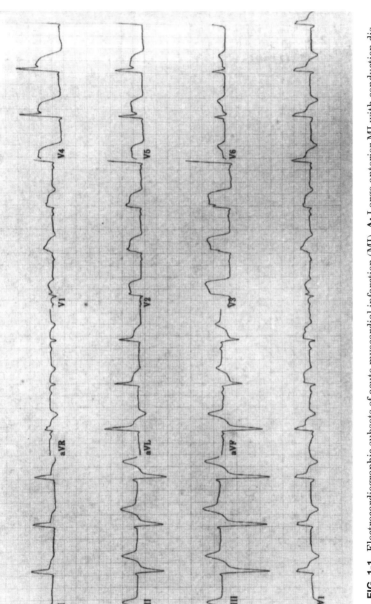

FIG. 1-1. Electrocardiographic subsets of acute myocardial infarction (MI). **A:** Large anterior MI with conduction disturbance (proximal left anterior descending coronary artery [LAD]).

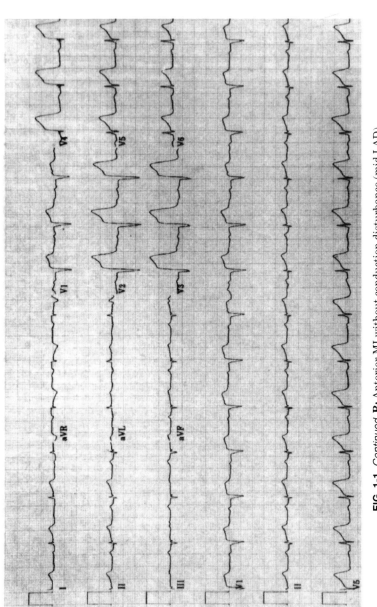

FIG. 1-1. *Continued* **B:** Anterior MI without conduction disturbance (mid LAD).

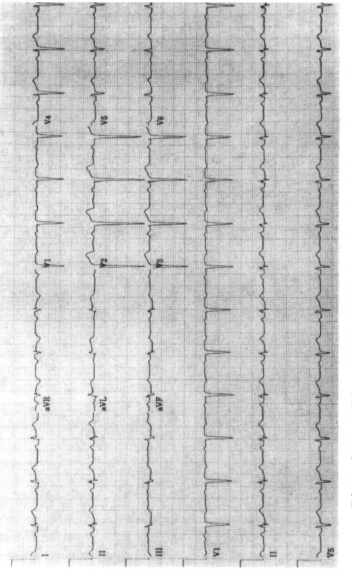

FIG. 1-1. *Continued* **C:** Lateral MI (distal LAD, diagonal branch, or left circumflex branch).

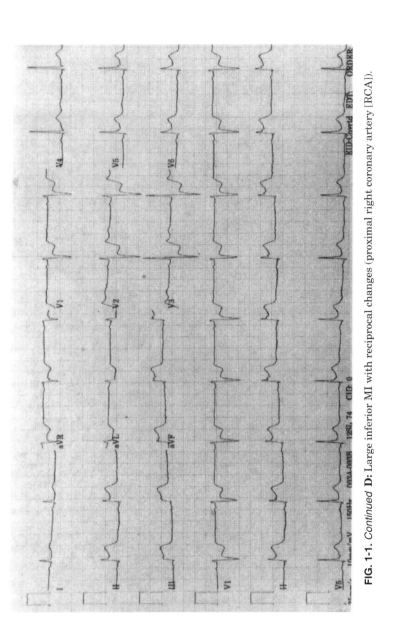

FIG. 1-1. *Continued* **D:** Large inferior MI with reciprocal changes (proximal right coronary artery [RCA]).

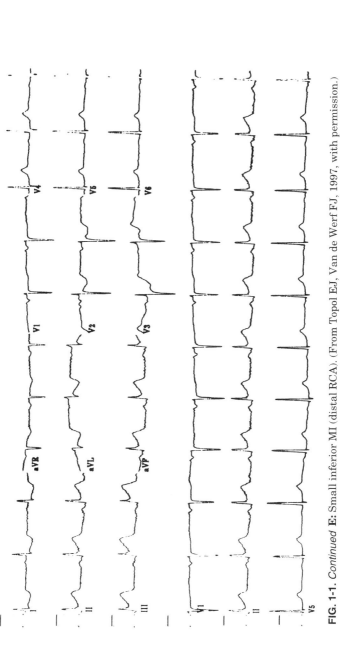

FIG. 1-1. *Continued* **E:** Small inferior MI (distal RCA). (From Topol EJ, Van de Werf FJ, 1997, with permission.)

Table 1-2. ECG criteria for the diagnosis of acute myocardial infarction in the presence of left bundle branch block

Criterion	Score
ST-segment elevation ≥ 1 mm concordant with QRS	5
ST-segment depression ≥ 1 mm in lead V1, V2, or V3	3
ST-segment elevation ≥ 5 mm discordant with QRS	2

Point scores for each criterion met are added. Total point score of 3 yields ≥ 90% specificity and an 88% positive predictive value.
Adapted from Sgarbossa EB, Pinski SL, Barbagelata A, et al. Electrocardiographic diagnosis of evolving acute myocardial infarction in the presence of left bundle branch block. *N Engl J Med* 1996;334:481–487, with permission.

chronic obstructive pulmonary disease who are known to retain carbon dioxide. Administration through a face mask or endotracheal tube may be necessary for patients with severe pulmonary edema or cardiogenic shock.

  c. **Nitroglycerin.** It is worthwhile to give **sublingual nitroglycerin** (0.4 mg) to determine whether the ST elevation represents coronary artery spasm while arrangements for reperfusion therapy are being initiated. Patients should be questioned about recent use of sildenafil (Viagra) because administration of nitroglycerin within 24 hours of sildenafil may cause life-threatening hypotension. A metaanalysis performed before reperfusion was developed suggested a mortality benefit with intravenous (IV) nitroglycerin (3), although this benefit was not confirmed in large randomized trials. Nitroglycerin can be useful in the management of acute MI complicated by congestive heart failure, ongoing symptoms, or hypertension. A 30% reduction in systolic blood pressure can be expected with appropriately aggressive dosing (10 to 20 μg/min with 5 to 10 μg/min increases every 5 to 10 minutes). IV therapy can be continued for 24 to 48 hours, after which time patients with heart failure or residual ischemia can convert to oral or topical therapy with an appropriate nitrate-free interval to avoid tachyphylaxis.

  d. **Reperfusion.** The primary goal in the management of acute MI is to **institute reperfusion therapy as quickly as possible.** All patients with ST-segment elevation or new LBBB MI who seek treatment within 12 hours from onset of continuous symptoms should be considered for reperfusion therapy. Persistent ischemic symptoms after 12 hours have elapsed may indicate a stuttering course of occlusion–spontaneous reperfusion–reocclusion. Patients with these symptoms also should be considered for reperfusion therapy.

    (1) **Benefit.** The benefit of reperfusion therapy has been well documented in the management of acute MI, regardless of age, sex, and most baseline characteristics. However, the **patients who derive the most benefit are those treated earliest and those at highest risk,** such as the elderly and those with anterior MI.

    (2) **Time to treatment is paramount.** Patients treated in the first hour have the highest mortality benefit. It is unclear whether this is due entirely to the prevention of myocardial damage or whether those who seek treatment early have a larger infarction and are preselected to derive pronounced benefit. Regardless, numerous trials support an inverse relation

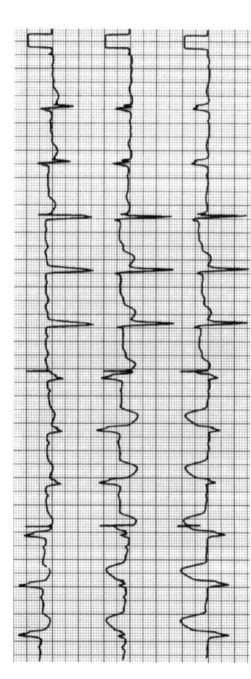

FIG. 1-2. Electrocardiogram displays all of the criteria for the diagnosis of acute MI in the setting of left bundle branch block: ST-segment elevation >1 mm concordant with QRS in lead II (5 points); ST-segment depression >1 mm in lead V2 and V3 (3 points); and ST-segment elevation >5 mm discordant with QRS in leads III and aVF (2 points). A score of 10 points indicates extremely high likelihood of inferior MI. (From Sgarbossa EB, Wagner G, 1997, with permission.)

Table 1-3. 30-Day mortality based on hemodynamic (Killip) class

Killip class	Characteristics	Patients (%)	Mortality rate (%)
I	No evidence of CHF	85	5.1
II	Rales, ↑ JVD, or S3	13	13.6
III	Pulmonary edema	1	32.2
IV	Cardiogenic shock	1	57.8

CHF, Congestive heart failure; ↑, increased; *JVD,* jugular venous distention.
Adapted from reference 1, with permission.

between time to treatment and survival benefit. After 12 hours of continuous symptoms have elapsed there is little benefit to immediate reperfusion.

(3) **Fibrinolysis versus direct percutaneous coronary intervention (PCI).** Once it has been determined that a patient is a candidate for immediate reperfusion therapy, the decision must be made quickly between fibrinolytic and direct PCI therapy.

  (a) If facilities for **immediate catheterization and PCI** are available, this is the preferred therapy. Pooled data from several large trials show a strong trend toward mortality reduction and a significant reduction in the composite rates of death and reinfarction with angioplasty. PCI also is associated with a reduction in the incidence of intracerebral hemorrhage.

  (b) If facilities for **immediate catheterization and revascularization are not immediately available, thrombolytic therapy should be instituted** unless contraindicated (Table 1-4).

  (c) **If a contraindication to thrombolytic therapy exists or if there is some question in the diagnosis,** arrangements should be made for **transfer** to a facility that has the capability for catheterization and mechanical reperfusion.

  (d) Because of the relative lack of efficacy of lytic therapy among patients with **cardiogenic shock or prior bypass operations,** such patients may be especially well-suited for **mechanical reperfusion** rather than thrombolytic therapy. If there is to be a long delay before catheterization, however, thrombolytic therapy should be instituted while arrangements for catheterization are being made.

(4) **Direct PCI.** Once the decision has been made to perform reperfusion with direct PCI, the patient should be moved to the catheterization laboratory and undergo angiography **as rapidly as possible.** Once the culprit lesion has been identified, the lesion should be opened with standard PCI technique (see Chapter 57), usually without ventriculography.

  (a) **Platelet glycoprotein IIb/IIIa inhibitors.** The Evaluation of 7E3 for the Prevention of Ischemic Complications (EPIC) trial demonstrated a 35% reduction in adverse cardiovascular events with abciximab compared with placebo among patients with recent or evolving acute MI, unstable angina, or high-risk angiographic lesions (4). In the Evaluation in PTCA to Improve Long-Term Outcome with Abciximab Glycoprotein IIb/IIIa Blockade (EPILOG) trial, abciximab was given in combination with a lower

Table 1-4. Contraindications and cautions for use of thrombolytic agents to manage myocardial infarction

CONTRAINDICATIONS

Previous hemorrhagic stroke at any time; other strokes or cerebrovascular events within 1 year
Known intracranial neoplasm
Active internal bleeding (does not include menses)
Suspected aortic dissection

RELATIVE CONTRAINDICATIONS

Severe, uncontrolled hypertension at presentation (blood pressure >180/110 mm Hg) or history of chronic severe hypertension
History of cerebrovascular accident or known intracerebral pathologic condition not covered in contraindications
Current use of anticoagulants in therapeutic doses (INR >2); known bleeding diatheses
Recent trauma (within 2–4 wk),including head trauma or traumatic or prolonged (>10 min) CPR or major surgery (<3 wk)
Noncompressible vascular punctures
Recent (within 2–4 wk) internal bleeding
For streptokinase or anistrepeplase: prior exposure (especially with 5 d–2 yr) or prior allergic reaction
Pregnancy
Active peptic ulcer

INR, International normalized ratio: *CPR*, cardiopulmonary resuscitation.
Adapted from Ryan TJ, et al., 1996, with permission.

dose of weight-adjusted heparin to a broad spectrum of patients. There was a more than 30% reduction in death rate and rate of MI compared with results with a placebo. There was no increase in bleeding events as occurred in EPIC (5). Results from the ReoPro and Primary PTCA Organization and Trial (RAPPORT) showed a significant, more than 50%, reduction in events with abciximab compared with placebo among patients undergoing direct percutaneous transluminal coronary angioplasty (PTCA) for acute MI. **Abciximab** (0.25 mg/kg bolus IV followed by 10 µg/min infusion over 12 hours) should be considered in the care of **all patients undergoing coronary intervention for acute MI.**

(b) **Stenting.** The early benefit of angioplasty over thrombolytic therapy is attenuated with more extended follow-up. In the Global Use of Strategies to Open Occluded Coronary Arteries (GUSTO IIb) trial in which use of accelerated tissue plasminogen activator (tPA) was compared with PTCA, the reduction in rates of death and nonfatal MI at 30 days (13.7% for tPA versus 9.6% for PTCA) dwindled so that by 6 months the difference (16.1% for tPA versus 14.1% for PTCA) had lost statistical significance (6). This loss of effect may be at least partially caused by restenosis of the lesion that was managed directly with angioplasty. Stenting in the setting of acute MI has been shown in initial trials to be **associated with a reduced rate of restenosis and reocclusion and may prevent the loss of benefit with primary mechanical revascularization** over time. Although it once was believed that stents should not be placed in thrombus-laden lesions, such as those associated with acute MI, because of risk for in-stent thrombosis, trials with adequate antiplatelet therapy have shown stenting to be safe. Results from the Evaluation of Platelet IIb/IIIa Inhibitor for Stenting (EPISTENT) trial show that there is additive benefit with abciximab and stenting (6B). The objective of the Controlled Abciximab in Device Investigation to Lower Late Angioplasty Complications (CADILLAC) trial is to examine the combined effects of abciximab and stenting in the management of acute MI.

(5) Fibrinolytic therapy. The **life-saving capability** of early fibrinolytic therapy has been well-established, beginning with the Gruppo Italiano per lo Studio dell Streptochi-nasi nell'Inrarto Miocardico (GISSI-1) trial in 1986 (7). Pooled data show a relative reduction in mortality of 18% and an absolute reduction of nearly 2%. Even more dramatic long-term mortality benefit may be the result of preservation of normal cardiac function.

(a) Contraindications. The only absolute contraindications to fibrinolytic therapy are recent or hemorrhagic stroke, intracranial neoplasm, active internal bleeding, or suspected aortic dissection. The presence of one of these or one or more of the relative contraindications listed in Table 1-4 would favor use of direct PCI even if it means a delay in establishing reperfusion.

(b) Choice of agent

(i) tPA. The Global Utilization of Streptokinase and Tissue Plasminogen Activator for Occluded Coronary Arteries (GUSTO I) trial showed that **use of accelerated tPA significantly reduced the 30-day mortality by 15%** relative to streptokinase with subcutaneous or IV heparin or combined with tPA (8). This benefit was challenged because of the high cost of tPA (approximately $2200 per episode of MI) compared with that of streptokinase (approximately $300). For tPA, this corresponds to a cost of $32,678 per year of life saved, less than that of the well-accepted standard of hemodialysis for end-stage renal disease (9). This benefit was consistent across all subgroups, although the patients at highest risk derived the most benefit. The accelerated protocol consisted of a bolus IV dose of 15 mg followed by 0.75 mg/kg (up to 50 mg) over 30 minutes then 0.5 mg/kg over 60 minutes. tPA is considered a fibrin-specific agent because of its relative selectivity for clot-bound fibrin.

(ii) Streptokinase. When tPA is not available or cannot be used because of limited financial resources, streptokinase (1.5 million IU IV over 60 minutes) **is a reasonable alternative.** Because of the possible development of antibodies, **streptokinase should not be administered to a patient who has received it in the past.** Because the overall rate of intracerebral hemorrhage is lower with streptokinase (0.5%) than with tPA (0.7%), some cardiologists advocate its use in the care of patients at high risk for this potentially catastrophic complication, such as elderly patients with a history of a cerebrovascular event or severe hypertension. Streptokinase is a non-fibrin-specific agent capable of lysing both circulating and clot-bound plasminogen to plasmin. This process results in substantial systemic fibrinogenolysis, fibrinogenemia, and elevation in fibrin degradation products.

(iii) **Reteplase.** The first of the third-generation fibrinolytic agents approved for use in the United States, reteplase is a fibrin-specific mutant of the native tPA. Reteplase has a longer half-life than tPA and can be administered in a double bolus (10 mg each, 30 minutes apart). The GUSTO III trial showed no mortality benefit of reteplase over tPA, but its ease of use may help to reduce time to administration. Use of reteplase is becoming more common (10).

(iv) **Anistreplase (anisoylated plasminogen streptokinase activator complex)** is a non-fibrin-specific agent that is inactive and protected from inhibitors until it is activated within the circulation. This prolongs its half-life and allows bolus administration (30 mg IV).

(c) **Bleeding complications of thrombolysis.** The most serious complication of thrombolytic therapy is **intracerebral hemorrhage,** which occurs among approximately 1 in 200 patients (0.5%) receiving streptokinase and 1 in 140 (0.7%) patients receiving tPA. The diagnosis must be considered if a patient has **severe headache, visual disturbance, new neurologic deficit, acute confusional state, or seizure.** When clinical suspicion is high, thrombolytic, antithrombin, and antiplatelet therapy should be interrupted while **emergency CT or MRI** is performed and **neurosurgical consultation** is obtained. Surgical evacuation may be life saving. Even with prompt recognition and treatment, the mortality is higher than 60%. It is more than 90% among patients older than 75 years. **Gastrointestinal, retroperitoneal, and access site bleeding** may complicate thrombolytic therapy but are usually not life threatening if promptly recognized and managed.

(6) **Rescue percutaneous revascularization** is the use of PCI when thrombolytic therapy is unsuccessful. Despite the proved benefit in mortality reduction, at least 30% of patients who receive lytic therapy have Thrombolysis in Myocardial Infarction trial (TIMI) 0 to 1 flow at 90 minutes, and patency at 90 minutes has been shown to correlate with long-term survival (11). **If reperfusion is not clearly evident 90 minutes after initiation of lytic therapy,** particularly among patients with large acute MI, **the decision to perform emergency angiography and possible mechanical reperfusion should be made promptly.** Patients in **cardiogenic shock after lytic therapy** should undergo **immediate catheterization** and should not await clinical assessment of reperfusion.

(a) **Clinical determination of successful reperfusion.** It can be **difficult** to determine clinically whether a patient has had successful reperfusion with lytic therapy. Resolution of chest pain is an inaccurate measure of reperfusion, because the pain may be affected by narcotic analgesia or the partial denervation that has been shown to occur among some patients with MI. Serial assessment of a 12-lead ECG is a more reliable indicator of reperfusion, although it is still suboptimal. Accelerated idioventricular rhythm (AIVR) is fairly specific for reperfusion, but arrhythmias other than AIVR, although frequent with reperfusion, are not reliable indicators because a variety of ventricular and supraventricular arrhythmias can be associated with a nonreperfused infarction-related artery. Complete resolution of chest pain and ECG abnormalities accompanied by a run of AIVR is highly specific for successful reperfusion, but it occurs among less than 10% of patients receiving lytic therapy.

(b) **Benefit.** The only patients who have been shown to derive definite benefit from rescue angioplasty are **patients with anterior MI who have undergone unsuccessful thrombolysis.** These data are from the Randomized Evaluation of Salvage Angioplasty with Combined Utilization of Endpoints (RESCUE) trial, in which patients with TIMI 2 or 3 flow did not undergo revascularization (12). Because other groups of patients have not been the subject of objective investigations, questions remain whether there is a benefit among patients with inferior MI or TIMI 2 flow.

(c) **Routine, immediate angiography and revascularization after successful reperfusion with lytic therapy generally are not performed** because early studies showed an increased incidence of events with this strategy (13–15). These studies were performed in the era before abciximab and stents, however, and this issue may have to be reexamined.

(d) **Routine late angiography** and whether it should be performed are discussed in Chapter 4.

(e) **Recurrent ischemia** after MI is an indication for catheterization and revascularization (see Chapter 3).

(7) **Emergency coronary bypass surgery** is the treatment of choice for patients for whom the intent is to undergo direct or rescue percutaneous mechanical reperfusion but are found to have a critical **left main-stem lesion or severe three-vessel disease** unapproachable with percutaneous revascularization. Limited reports of this strategy are fairly encouraging, especially when patients can be taken to the operating room early in the course of infarction, before severe myocardial necrosis has occurred. **Right ventricular infarction is essentially a contraindication** to bypass surgery because it greatly complicates discontinuation of cardiopulmonary support.

2. Adjuvant therapy
a. Antithrombins
(1) **Heparin without thrombolysis.** Although heparin was never shown to reduce mortality in the era before reperfusion, the trials that examined this were underpowered. One trial (16) and a metaanalysis of three large trials (17) suggested a **mortality benefit with IV heparin.** Reductions in the incidence of LV thrombus and stroke have been especially evident among patients with large anterior MI or documented thrombus.

(2) **Heparin with thrombolysis**
(a) **tPA. As an adjunct to therapy with tPA, heparin has been shown to improve late patency.** Heparin is considered by most cardiologists to be an essential adjunct to tPA to overcome the thrombogenic state induced by systemic fibrinolytic therapy. Although it has not been shown to improve mortality compared with placebo, IV heparin was used in conjunction with accelerated tPA in the GUSTO I trial, in which tPA was shown to be superior to

streptokinase. Another lesson from GUSTO I was that when heparin is used with thrombolytic therapy, there is a relation between activated partial thromboplastic time (aPTT) and 30-day mortality, the optimal range being 50 to 70 seconds. When used in conjunction with thrombolytic therapy, heparin should be administered as a 5,000 U bolus followed by a 10 U/kg per hour infusion (up to 1,000 U/hr). A smaller bolus may be used to treat elderly patients, women, and patients who weigh less than 50 kg. The aPTT should be checked at 6 hours and the infusion titrated to achieve the goal of aPTT of 50 to 70 seconds.

- (b) **Streptokinase.** There are **no data to support the routine use of IV heparin with streptokinase, unless the patient has recurrent ischemia or another indication for heparin therapy.** In the GUSTO I trial, IV heparin was shown not to be superior to subcutaneous heparin when used with streptokinase, which considerably more fibrinogenolytic action than tPA.

- (3) **Heparin with direct angioplasty.** When direct angioplasty is planned, patients will most likely receive a **glycoprotein IIb/IIIa inhibitor such as abciximab.** In this case, an **initial, low-dose, weight-adjusted bolus of heparin** should be given (50 to 70 U/kg up to 7,000 U). This combination was shown to be associated with the lowest rate of death and ischemic complications in the EPILOG trial. If abciximab is not given, standard procedural doses of heparin (100 U/kg, up to 10,000 U) may be administered before percutaneous revascularization.

- (4) **Direct thrombin inhibitors.** Although direct thrombin inhibitors such as hirudin offer several theoretical advantages over heparin, **several large trials have failed to show an advantage of direct thrombin inhibitors over heparin** as an adjunct to either thrombolytic therapy or percutaneous intervention. Analysis of data from GUSTO II, however, showed that among **patients who received streptokinase rather than tPA,** the **death and reinfarction rates were lower with hirudin** then they were with heparin (18). Another possible role for direct thrombin inhibitors in acute MI is treatment of patients with a history of heparin-induced thrombocytopenia. A form of hirudin, lepirudin (0.4 mg/kg bolus up to 44 mg, followed by an infusion of 0.15 mg/kg for 2 to 10 days) has been approved. Argatroban is being studied for this indication.

b. **β-Blockers.** β-Adrenergic blocking agents should be administered **orally to patients with normal or mildly impaired LV function within the first 24 hours of acute MI, unless complicated by hypotension, bradycardia, or symptoms of congestive heart failure.** They are also contraindicated in the care of patients with reactive airway disease that is severe or known to be exacerbated by β-blockade or with "brittle" diabetes accompanied by a history of hypoglycemic episodes.

- (1) **For ischemia or for tachycardia and hypertension,** IV metoprolol can be given (5 mg every 5 minutes for 3 doses). Patients who tolerate the IV loading can be begin moderate oral doses (50 mg metoprolol twice a day). Those with borderline hemodynamic values or mild LV dysfunction should begin with lower doses (12.5 to 25 mg metoprolol twice a day). The dose should be titrated upward over several days to the maximally tolerated dose (for metoprolol up to 100 mg twice a day).

(2) Extensive data from the era before reperfusion established the usefulness of β-blockers in **reducing recurrent ischemia, arrhythmias, and mortality.** Several small randomized trials performed in the reperfusion era have confirmed the anti-ischemia and antiarrhythmic benefits, although data from the GUSTO I trial raise **concern that β-blockade may be associated with worse outcomes among patients with large areas of infarction or marginal LV function.**

c. **Angiotensin-converting enzyme (ACE) inhibitors** can be started orally in the first 24 hours for all patients without hypotension, acute renal failure, or other contraindication. These medications were shown to reduce mortality in the GISSI-3 (19) and International Study of Infarct Survival (ISIS-4) (20) trials. ACE inhibitors should be **continued indefinitely for patients with LV dysfunction or clinical congestive heart failure,** because these patients have been shown to derive a mortality benefit. A graded oral regimen should be used to avoid hypotension. IV formulations should not be used, because they have been shown to have no benefit and may increase mortality.

d. **Calcium channel blockers.** Evidence of the potential increase in mortality risk with calcium channel blockers has limited the use of these agents in the care of patients with acute MI to the very narrow indications of management of **supraventricular tachyarrhythmia, cocaine-induced MI, or relief of postinfarction angina unresponsive to β-blockade.** Otherwise the use of these agents should be avoided. **Nifedipine is contraindicated** because of its reflex sympathetic activation.

e. **Magnesium.** There once was enthusiasm for the use of IV magnesium to treat patients with acute MI. This enthusiasm was based on the findings of the Leicester IV Magnesium Intervention Trial (LIMIT-2) (21) trial, which showed a 24% reduction in mortality compared with placebo. These findings were contradicted by those of the larger ISIS-4 (20) trial, which failed to show a benefit of IV magnesium. Although there was some speculation that the lack of effect during ISIS-4 was the result of late administration or low control-group mortality, **magnesium is not routinely used** other than to replete serum magnesium levels lower than 2.0 μg/dL or for the management of torsades de pointes polymorphic ventricular tachycardia (1 to 2 g over 5 minutes).

f. **Diabetes control.** Preliminary evidence suggests that aggressive control of blood glucose levels within the range of 100 to 200 mg/dL during the early stages of acute MI may reduce morbidity and mortality.

g. **Antiarrhythmics.** The **use of lidocaine or other antiarrhythmic agents is not warranted** for the prophylactic suppression of ventricular tachycardia and fibrillation. Although lidocaine may decrease tachyarrhythmias, there is no survival benefit. There also is evidence to suggest an increase in mortality related to an increased incidence of bradycardia and asystole. The use of antiarrhythmic therapy to manage specific arrhythmias is discussed in Chapters 3 and 44 through 47.

h. **Intraaortic balloon pump (IABP).** In the treatment of patients with **cardiogenic shock** an IABP is the **preferred means of augmenting systolic pressure** because use of an IABP decreases afterload and thus oxygen requirements while increasing diastolic coronary flow. IABP is **contraindicated in the care of patients with marked aortic regurgitation,** because it can worsen the regurgitation and cause rapid hemodynamic deterioration and an increase in myocardial oxygen demand (see Chapters 3 and 59).

      i. **Inotropic agents.** In general these agents should be **avoided whenever possible** because of their effect on increasing myocardial oxygen demand and their promotion of tachycardia and arrhythmias. When use of an IABP is not sufficient or until it can be inserted, IV inotropic support is warranted and should be guided by means of pulmonary arterial catheter monitoring whenever possible.

        (1) Patients with **hypotension accompanied by a pulmonary capillary wedge pressure (PCWP) less than 15 mm Hg** should be managed with **rapid infusion of normal saline solution,** as should patients with inferior MI who are found to have right ventricular infarction.

        (2) If **fluids are insufficient,** PCWP is greater than 15 mm Hg, or overt signs of heart failure accompany hypotension, **dopamine** is used at doses up to 20 µg/kg per minute, with norepinephrine as backup if necessary. The benefit of improving cerebral and systemic perfusion pressure through an increase in inotropism comes at a cost of increased afterload and myocardial oxygen demand from vasoconstriction.

        (3) **Dobutamine** can be useful when **PCWP higher than 18 mm Hg is associated with mild to moderate hypotension** (70 to 90 mm Hg) or inability to use nitroglycerin or nitroprusside because of risk for inducing hypotension. **Use of phosphodiesterase inhibitors such as amrinone or milrinone,** which have combined vasodilating and inotropic action, **is problematic because of renal excretion by patients with low output.** Use of these drugs is viable if the other agents have failed to maintain adequate systemic pressure and forward output. The main goal, however, should be to avoid these agents or reduce the need for them in terms of absolute dose and duration.

III. **Acute MI associated with cocaine abuse.** The pathophysiologic process and management of acute MI associated with the use of cocaine differ from those of classic MI.

  A. **Pathophysiology**

    1. The underlying pathophysiologic factor in acute MI associated with cocaine abuse is believed to be **coronary spasm or thrombus formation** caused by α-adrenergic stimulation by the cocaine. This can occur in a normal segment of artery or be superimposed on mild to moderate atherosclerosis, the development of which can be accelerated by chronic cocaine use.

    2. **Plaque rupture,** as usually occurs with acute MI, generally **does not occur** with acute MI due to cocaine abuse.

    3. **Increased oxygen demand** caused by β-adrenergic stimulation of heart rate and contractility also likely contributes to the scenario.

  B. **Clinical presentation. Chest pain** caused by infarction after cocaine ingestion typically occurs **within 3 hours,** although it can vary from minutes to days, and depends on route of administration (median 30 minutes with IV cocaine, 90 minutes with crack smoking, 135 with nasal inhalation). More than 80% of persons with infarction are also cigarette smokers. Studies with animals have shown a synergistic effect between cigarette smoking and cocaine use. More than 90% of patients with cocaine-related chest pain do not have objective evidence of infarction or ischemia.

  C. **Therapy**

    1. **Initial management** of ST elevation associated with cocaine use includes administration of **aspirin, oxygen, and heparin.** Aggressive use of **sublingual and IV nitroglycerin** and **IV calcium channel blockade** should be instituted in an effort to relieve coronary spasm.

    2. **β-Blockers should not be given to patients with cocaine-induced acute MI.** Although they block undesirable β-adrenergic effects, these agents allow unopposed α-adrenergic stimulation and have been associated with increased mortality.

3. Consideration should be given to **reperfusion therapy if vasodilator therapy is unsuccessful** in relieving symptoms and ST-segment changes.
4. **Immediate angiography and mechanical revascularization as appropriate** may be favored more heavily than in the management of acute MI not associated with cocaine use. Many patients who use cocaine may have contraindications to thrombolysis such as severe hypertension or may have persistent vasospasm without thrombosis, which would not be amenable to thrombolytic therapy.

IV. **Postoperative acute MI**
   A. **Etiology and pathophysiology.** Acute MI following noncardiac operations most commonly occurs on the **third or fourth postoperative day.** Conventional theory was that MI was caused by increased oxygen demand and arterial shear stress associated with the increased adrenergic drive that accompanies pain and ambulation in the postoperative period in combination with rapid intravascular volume shifts caused by redistribution of fluids, IV administration of fluids, and decreased enteral intake. Recent data, however, suggest to implicate marked **hypercoagulability with an increase in fibrinogen and the inflammatory state** associated with the acute-phase response after a surgical procedure.
   B. **Therapy**
      1. Management is complicated by limitations on the use of fibrinolytic agents depending on the extent and type of surgical intervention, Therapy relies more heavily on the use of **IV use of β-blockers and urgent angiography and mechanical revascularization.**
      2. **Close communication with the surgical team** is vital in determining the maximal acceptable use of fibrinolytic, antithrombotic, and antiplatelet therapy.

V. **Controversies.** The **current standard of care** of patients with acute MI lies in rapid and accurate diagnosis based on history and ECG findings, rapid initiation of reperfusion therapy with a thrombolytic agent or direct mechanical reperfusion, and a customized regimen of adjunctive therapies that include antiplatelet, antithrombin, β-blocker, and vasodilator therapies. However, there are several areas of controversy, most of which are being addressed by trials in various stages of development.
   A. The **combined use of glycoprotein IIb/IIIa inhibition and fibrinolysis** has been shown to be efficacious in management of non-ST-elevation MI and is being evaluated in ST-elevation MI. Although lytic therapy followed routinely by catheterization and mechanical reperfusion was shown to increase complications in early trials, recent evidence suggests that a lower dose of fibrinolytic agent en route to the catheterization laboratory may be advantageous.
   B. Early evidence suggested the **percutaneous intervention of non-infarct-related arteries after establishment of reperfusion of the infarct-related artery** was detrimental. With the protection of glycoprotein IIb/IIIa inhibition, however, this strategy may have to be reexamined.

SUGGESTED READINGS
References
1. Lee K, Woodlief L, Topol E, et al. Predictors of 30-day mortality in the era of reperfusion for acute myocardial infarction. *Circulation* 1995;91:1659–1668.
2. Group Ic. Randomised trial of intravenous streptokinase, oral aspirin, both, or neither among 17,187 cases of suspected acute myocardial infarction. *Lancet* 1988;2:349–360.
3. Yusuf S, Collins R, MacMahon S, Peto R. Effect of intravenous nitrates on mortality in acute myocardial. *Lancet* 1988;1:1088–1092.
4. The EPIC Investigators. Use of a monoclonal antibody directed against the platelet glycoprotein IIb/IIIa receptor in high-risk coronary angioplasty. *N Engl J Med* 1994;330:956–961.

5. The EPILOG Investigators. Platelet glycoprotein IIb/IIIa receptor blockade and low-dose heparin during coronary revascularization during percutaneous coronary revascularization. *N Engl J Med* 1997;336:1689–1696.
6. The Global Use of Strategies to Open Occluded Coronary Arteries in Acute Coronary Syndromes (GUSTO IIb) Angioplasty Substudy Investigators. A clinical trial comparing primary coronary angioplasty with tissue plasminogen activator for acute myocardial infarction. *N Engl J Med* 1997;336:1621–1628.
6B. Lincoff AM, Califf RM, Moliterno DM, et al. Complementary clinical benefits of coronary-artery stenting and blockade of platelet glycoprotein IIb/IIIa receptors. *N Engl J Med* 1999;341:319–327.
7. Gruppo Italiano per lo Studio dell Streptochi-nasi nell'Inrarto Miocardico. Long-term effects of intravenous thrombolysis in acute myocardial infarction: final report of the GISSI study. *Lancet* 1987;2:871–874.
8. GUSTO Investigators. An international randomized trial comparing four thrombolytic strategies for acute myocardial infarction. *N Engl J Med* 1993;329: 673–682.
9. Mark D, Hlatky M, Califf R, et al. Cost effectiveness of thrombolytic therapy with tissue plasminogen activator as compared with streptokinase for acute myocardial infarction. *N Engl J Med* 1995;332:1418–1424.
10. The GUSTO III Investigators. A comparison of reteplase with alteplase for acute myocardial infarction. *N Engl J Med* 1997;337:1118–1123.
11. The GUSTO Angiographic Investigators. The effects of tissue plasminogen activator, streptokinase, or both on coronary-artery patency, ventricular function, and survival after acute myocardial infarction. *N Engl J Med* 1993;329:1615–1622.
12. Lincoff A, Topol E, Califf R, et al. Significance of a coronary artery with thrombolysis in myocardial infarction grade 2 flow "patency." *Am J Cardiol* 1995;75: 871–876.
13. Topol E, Califf R, George B, et al. A randomized trial of immediate versus delayed elective angioplasty after intravenous tissue plasminogen activator in acute myocardial infarction. *N Engl J Med* 1987;317:581–588.
14. Simoons M, Arnold A, Betriu A, et al. Thrombolysis with tissue plasminogen activator in acute myocardial infarction: no additional benefit from immediate percutaneous coronary angioplasty. *Lancet* 1988;1:197–203.
15. The TIMI Research Group. Immediate vs delayed catheterization and angioplasty following thrombolytic therapy for acute myocardial infarction. *JAMA* 1988;260: 2849–2858.
16. Report of the Working Party on Anticoagulant Therapy in Coronary Thrombosis to the Medical Research Council. Assessment of short-anticoagulant administration after cardiac infarction. *Br Med J* 1969;1:335–342.
17. Mitchell JR. Anticoagulants in coronary heart disease: retrospect and prospect. *Lancet* 1981;1:257–262.
18. Metz BK, White HD, Granger CB, et al. Randomized comparison of direct thrombin inhibition versus heparin in conjunction with fibrinolytic therapy for acute myocardial infarction: results from the GUSTO-IIb Trial. Global Use of Strategies to Open Occluded Coronary Arteries in Acute Coronary Syndromes (GUSTO-IIb) Investigators. *J Am Coll Cardiol* 1998;31:1493–1498.
19. Gruppo Italiano per lo Studio della Sopravvivenza nell' infarto Miocardico. GISSI-3: effects of lisinopril and transdermal glyceryl trinitrate singly and together on 6-week mortality and ventricular function after acute myocardial infarction. *Lancet* 1994;343:1115–1122.
20. Flather M, Pipilis A, Collins R, et al. Randomized controlled trial of oral captopril, of oral isosorbide mononitrate and of intravenous magnesium sulphate started early in acute myocardial infarction: safety and haemodynamic effects. ISIS-4 (Fourth International Study of Infarct Survival) Pilot Study Investigators. *Eur Heart J* 1994;15:608–619.
21. Woods Kl, Fletcher S. Long-term outcome after intravenous magnesium sulphate in suspected acute myocardial infarction: the second Leicester Intravenous Magnesium Intervention Trial (LIMIT-2). *Lancet* 1994;343:816–819.

Landmark Articles

Flather M, Pipilis A, Collins R, et al. Randomized controlled trial of oral captopril, of oral isosorbide mononitrate and of intravenous magnesium sulphate started early in acute myocardial infarction: safety and haemodynamic effects. ISIS-4 (Fourth International Study of Infarct Survival) Pilot Study Investigators. *Eur Heart J* 1994;15:608–619.

Gruppo Italiano per lo Studio dell Streptochi-nasi nell'Inrarto Miocardico. Long-term effects of intravenous thrombolysis in acute myocardial infarction: final report of the GISSI study. *Lancet* 1987;2:871–874.

Gruppo Italiano per lo Studio dell Streptochi-nasi nell'Inrarto Miocardico. GISSI-3: effects of lisinopril and transdermal glyceryl trinitrate singly and together on 6-week mortality and ventricular function after acute myocardial infarction. *Lancet* 1994;343:1115–1122.

The GUSTO Investigators. An international randomized trial comparing four thrombolytic strategies for acute myocardial infarction. *N Engl J Med* 1993;329:673–682.

GUSTO IIb Angioplasty Substudy Investigators. A clinical trial comparing primary coronary angioplasty with tissue plasminogen activator for acute myocardial infarction. *N Engl J Med* 1997;336:1621–1628.

The GUSTO III Investigators. A comparison of reteplase with alteplase for acute myocardial infarction. *N Engl J Med* 1997;337:1118–1123.

ISIS-2 (Second international study of infarct survival) Collaborative Group. Randomised trial of intravenous streptokinase, oral aspirin, both, or neither among 17,187 cases of suspected acute myocardial infarction. *Lancet* 1988;2:349–360.

Key Reviews

Falk E, Shah PK, Fuster V. Coronary plaque disruption. *Circulation* 1995;92:657–671.

Ryan TJ, Anderson JL, Antman EM, et al. ACC/AHA guidelines for the management of patients with acute myocardial infarction: a report of the American College of Cardiology/American Heart Association Task Force on Practice Guidelines (Committee on Management of Acute Myocardial Infarction). *J Am Coll Cardiol* 1996;28:1328–1428.

White HD, Van de Werf FJ. Thrombolysis for acute myocardial infarction. *Circulation* 1998;97:1632–1646.

Relevant Book Chapters

Sgarbossa EB, Wagner G. Electrocardiography. In: Topol EJ, ed. *Textbook of cardiovascular medicine.* New York: Lippincott-Raven, 1998.

Topol EJ, Van de Werf FJ. Acute myocardial infarction: early diagnosis and management. In: Topol EJ, ed. *Textbook of Cardiovascular Medicine.* New York: Lippincott-Raven, 1998.

2. UNSTABLE ANGINA AND NON-ST-SEGMENT ELEVATION MI

Matthew T. Roe

I. **Introduction. Unstable angina (UA)** is the leading cause of admissions to coronary care units in the United States with 700,000 hospital admissions per year. UA encompasses a wide range of clinical scenarios from **worsening exertional angina** to **postinfarction angina.** Unlike acute ST-segment elevation myocardial infarction (MI), however, the clinical presentation of UA can be insidious with waxing and waning chest pain. Myocardial necrosis often occurs with UA without ST-segment elevation and is thus termed **non-ST-segment-elevation MI.** For example, in the Thrombosis in Myocardial Infarction (TIMI) III trial registry of 3,318 patients with UA, 21% had non-ST-segment-elevation MI (1). Diagnostic techniques have been developed for rapid risk stratification of patients with UA, so the therapeutic approach to UA has changed considerably in the last decade.

II. **Clinical presentation**
   A. **Risk factors**
   1. **Clinical characteristics** that indicate which patients with UA are at high risk include rest angina lasting more than 20 minutes, congestive heart failure, known reduced left ventricular (LV) function, hypotension, or diffuse ST-segment changes on an electrocardiogram (ECG). Patients at intermediate or low risk are in hemodynamically stable condition, have angina of short duration, and have no ischemic ST-segment changes (Table 2-1).
   2. The **Braunwald classification system** of UA can be used to risk stratify patients at presentation (Table 2-2). Braunwald defined UA according to the characteristics of the anginal pain and the underlying cause of angina. Patients with rest angina in the postinfarction setting (class III C) have the highest incidence of recurrent ischemia and death at 6 months. In a group of 282 patients with UA, recurrent ischemia developed in 64% of Braunwald class IIIa patients, 45% of class II patients, and 28% of class I patients. Mortality rates at 6 months were 3% to 4% among class I and II patients as opposed to 6% among class III patients. The rates were 3% in association with primary UA and 11% in association with postinfarction UA (2).
   3. **Non-ST-segment-elevation MI** is a powerful predictor of poor outcome among patients with UA. Multivariate predictors of non-ST-segment-elevation MI among patients with UA include prolonged chest pain (>60 minutes), ST-segment depression or transient ST-segment elevation, and recent onset of angina (within 1 month). **Troponins** are cardiac contractile proteins that are elevated when myocardial necrosis occurs. Troponin I and T are more commonly elevated among patients with UA than are creatine kinase (CK) levels (3). Troponin I or T levels >0.1–0.4 ng/mL are independently predictive of mortality and MI among patients with UA (see later) (4,5).
   4. **ECG.** The initial ECG can be used for risk stratification of patients with UA. Patients with ST-segment deviation (ST depression or transient ST elevation) ≥0.5 mm or with preexisting left bundle branch block (LBBB) are at increased risk for death or MI 1 year after the initial incident. T-wave inversions are not predictive of adverse ischemic events.
   B. **Demographics.** Compared with patients with ST-segment-elevation MI, patients with UA are older and have a higher incidence of diabetes, hypertension, and hypercholesterolemia. Patients with UA are more likely to have had prior MI and revascularization procedures (angioplasty and coronary artery bypass grafting). In a 1996 registry of almost 3,000 consecutively hospitalized patients with UA in the United States, 61% of the patients were

Table 2-1. Risk stratification of patients with unstable angina

High risk	Intermediate risk	Low risk
One of the following must be present:	No high-risk feature but must have one of the following:	No high- or intermediate-risk features present
Prolonged ongoing rest pain (>20 min): Moderate or high likelihood of CAD	Prolonged rest pain (>20 min) that resolves	Increased frequency or duration of angina
Pulmonary edema: Most likely caused by ischemia	Rest angina (>20 min or relieved with rest or sublingual NTG)	Angina provoked by less exertion
Rest angina with dynamic ST changes ≥1 mm	Nocturnal angina	New-onset angina (within 2 wk–2 mo)
Angina with new or worsening rales, S3, or MR murmur	Angina with dynamic T-wave changes	Normal or unchanged ECG
Angina with hypotension	New-onset, severe angina within 2 wk with moderate or high likelihood of CAD Pathologic Q waves or resting ST depression in multiple lead groups Age older than 65 years	

Risk stratification involves considering clinical characteristics and ECG findings to make early triage decisions.
CAD, Coronary artery disease; *NTG*, nitroglycerin; *ECG*, electrocardiogram; *MR*, mitral regurgitation.

men, 61% had hypertension, 26% had diabetes, 43% had hypercholesterolemia, 36% had prior MI, 22% had undergone angioplasty, and 21% had undergone coronary artery bypass grafting (6).

- C. **Signs and symptoms.** Patients with ongoing chest pain without ST-segment elevation on an ECG may have either UA or non-ST-segment-elevation MI. The distinction cannot be made without cardiac enzyme analysis. Anginal pain among patients with UA can be of new onset, can occur at rest or with minimal exertion, or can occur with less exertion or with an increased frequency as compared to prior anginal episodes. Compared with stable angina, **chest pain with UA** is typically more **severe and prolonged.** Multiple administrations of nitroglycerin or prolonged periods of rest often are needed for relief of chest pain.
- D. **Physical findings.** A physical examination alone provides insufficient evidence for diagnosis of UA. It is important, however, to exclude other diagnoses that may mimic angina such as costochondritis, pneumonia, or pericarditis. **Signs of volume overload** (jugular venous distention or an S_3 on cardiac examination) and **bruits** indicate **congestive heart failure** and **peripheral vascular disease.** The presence of heart failure or peripheral vascular disease predicts a higher likelihood of serious coronary artery disease.

III. **Laboratory examination**
- A. **ECG.** Common ECG findings in UA and non-ST-segment-elevation MI include **ST-segment depression, T-wave inversion, and transient ST-segment elevation.** However, approximately 20% of patients with UA who have non-ST-segment-elevation MI confirmed with cardiac enzyme eleva-

Table 2-2. Braunwald classification of unstable angina

Class	Characteristics
I	**Exertional angina** New onset, severe, or accelerated Angina of less than 2 mo duration More frequent angina Angina precipitated by less exertion No rest angina in the last 2 mo
II	**Rest angina, subacute** Rest angina within the last month but none within 48 h of presentation
III	**Rest angina, acute** Rest angina within 48 h of presentation
CLINICAL CIRCUMSTANCES	
A	**Secondary unstable angina** Caused by a noncardiac condition, such as anemia, infection, thyrotoxicosis, or hypoxemia
B	**Primary unstable angina**
C	**Postinfarction unstable angina** Within 2 wk of documented myocardial infarction

This classification can be used for risk stratification. Clinical characteristics at presentation and severity of angina are considered.

tions have no ischemic ECG changes. Persistent ST-segment elevation of more than 1 mm in two or more contiguous leads or new LBBB indicates acute transmural injury, and the patients should be promptly treated with reperfusion therapy (see Chapter 1).

1. Older classification systems recognized non-ST-segment-elevation MI as **non-Q-wave MI** because myocardial necrosis occurs without ECG evidence of transmural injury. However, because the transmural extent of myocardial injury cannot be determined on the basis of the presence or absence of ST-segment elevation, *non-ST-segment-elevation MI* has become the favored term.

2. In the **TIMI III trial** with 1,473 patients with UA or non-ST-segment-elevation MI, 10% of the patients had transient ST-segment elevation, 33% had ST-segment depression, 46% had T-wave inversion, and 9% had no ECG changes of ischemia (7).

B. **Cardiac enzymes**

1. **Creatine kinase.** Standard laboratory analysis of patients with suspected acute coronary syndromes includes serial CK and CK MB isoenzyme evaluations every 6 to 8 hours after admission for the first 24 hours. Total CK level peaks 12 to 24 hours after the onset of symptoms, whereas the more sensitive and specific CK MB levels peak 10 to 18 hours after the onset of symptoms. Total CK and CK MB levels above the normal values of a given laboratory indicate that myocardial necrosis has occurred. Total CK elevation without an increase in CK MB can occur with many nonischemic conditions, such as pericarditis, skeletal muscle injury, and renal failure.

2. **Troponins.** Specific serologic analysis in the management of acute coronary syndromes has focused on cardiac contractile proteins called troponins. Serum levels of troponins I and T increase 3 to 12 hours after myocardial necrosis occurs, remain elevated afterward, and have not been shown to correlate with the extent of myocardial damage. Troponins

are useful for determining whether ischemia has occurred and have important prognostic significance.

  a. In the **GUSTO IIb** trial, the 30-day mortality rate among patients with UA who had a troponin T level >0.1 ng/mL was 11.8% compared with 3.9% among patients who had normal troponin levels (4).

  b. Troponin I levels >0.4 ng/mL also were associated with a higher 42-day mortality rate in the **TIMI IIIb** trial (3.7% versus 1.0%) (5).

  c. **Bedside tests** for troponins I and T have been developed. When the bedside troponin assay was tested in the care of a cohort of patients with UA, levels of troponins were found to be elevated more frequently than those of CK MB isoenzymes. Elevated troponin levels were strongly predictive of mortality and MI, whereas normal troponin levels were associated with low risk for cardiac events (3).

3. Recommendations. Because troponin levels provide more useful, immediate prognostic information than CK levels, all patients with UA should undergo troponin level measurement at presentation (see earlier), and have serial CK and CK MB levels obtained.

IV. Etiology

  A. Plaque rupture. UA, non-ST-segment-elevation MI, and ST-segment-elevation MI share a common initiation when an atheromatous plaque in a coronary artery ruptures or fissures. Plaque rupture causes platelet deposition at the site of injury followed by thrombus formation. There is pathophysiologic continuity of plaque rupture between the acute coronary syndromes because once intracoronary thrombus in a patient with UA becomes transiently or persistently occlusive, myocardial necrosis and non-ST-segment-elevation or ST-segment-elevation MI occurs. Factors thought to be involved in plaque rupture include increased inflammatory activity at the plaque site through lymphocytes or macrophages and possibly infection of the vessel wall with *Chlamydia pneumoniae.*

  B. Thrombus formation. When subendothelial components are exposed to platelets, thrombus formation occurs. Platelets are activated, and the glycoprotein IIb/IIIa receptor on the platelet surface is made functional to mediate platelet aggregation. Platelet aggregation markedly increases thrombin production, which expands and stabilizes the developing thrombus. Coronary vasospasm frequently occurs at sites of unstable plaque and is thought to contribute to thrombus formation.

  C. Secondary causes. UA can be caused by excess demand or inadequate supply of oxygen to the myocardium. With stable obstructive coronary lesions the following conditions can precipitate UA: increased myocardial oxygen demand caused by fever, severe hypertension, cocaine use, hyperthyroidism, or tachycardia. Oxygen supply to the myocardial tissue can be decreased when anemia or hypoxemia is present.

V. Diagnostic testing. UA is a clinical diagnosis made when a patient presents with unstable chest pain. Diagnostic testing can confirm or disprove the initial clinical suspicion of UA through documentation of myocardial ischemia, myocardial damage manifested as LV wall motion abnormalities, or substantial coronary arterial plaques. Noninvasive testing is generally reserved for patients with UA who are at low risk (see earlier). Cardiac catheterization is often undertaken when definite ischemia is demonstrated.

  A. Echocardiography. In the acute phase of UA, echocardiography can be useful to evaluate wall motion abnormalities that might confirm ischemia. However, because of poor acoustic windows in many patients and uncertainty about the duration of wall motion abnormalities (if they do exist), echocardiography usually does not contribute a great deal to the diagnosis of UA. Echocardiography can be useful in the evaluation of **resting LV function of patients with congestive heart failure or definitive signs of ischemia** who do not undergo early cardiac catheterization.

  B. Noninvasive stress testing. Because UA is a diverse diagnosis, some patients at low risk can undergo stress testing. Stress testing traditionally has been discouraged in the management of UA because the presence of unstable plaques was thought to be associated with high risk for acute occlusion with increased myocardial workloads. Patients with UA at low risk are those without symptoms for 24 to 48 hours after admission, those with normal or nondiagnostic ECG findings, those with atypical symptoms, or those with few cardiac risk factors. Patients with accelerated or new-onset exertional angina are considered to be at low risk compared with patients who have rest angina or postinfarction angina.

    1. Patients with **abnormal findings on thallium scans** should be considered for **cardiac catheterization** because they are at risk for adverse ischemic events. Patients with **normal findings on thallium scans** can be **discharged** safely and treated on an outpatient basis.

    2. For patients unable to exercise, **pharmacologic stress testing** with dobutamine or dipyridamole can be performed, but no large-scale studies have evaluated these forms of stress testing among patients with UA.

C. Diagnostic cardiac catheterization

    1. Results of cardiac catheterization in the management of UA show normal coronary arteries or mild disease (all lesions < 50%) among 10% to 20% of patients, single-vessel disease among 30% to 35%, two-vessel disease among 25% to 30%, three-vessel disease among 20% to 25%, and left main disease among 5% to 10%.

    2. The Agency for Health Care Policy and Research (ACHPR) developed **clinical practice guidelines** for UA in 1994. The guidelines recommend **routine catheterization** for all patients with **high-risk clinical characteristics,** medically refractory symptoms, congestive heart failure, malignant ventricular arrhythmias, depressed LV function (LV ejection fraction <50%), a large perfusion defect on noninvasive stress or pharmacologic testing, or significant valvular heart disease (mitral regurgitation or aortic stenosis) (Table 2–3). Patients who have undergone percutaneous transluminal coronary angioplasty (**PTCA**) or coronary artery bypass grafting (**CABG**) should undergo **catheterization** unless previous angiographic data indicate that further revascularization would be technically impossible.

D. Key suggestions

    1. **Stress testing** should be performed in all patients who do not undergo cardiac catheterization. Patients with an ischemic perfusion defect should undergo cardiac catheterization.

    2. An aggressive approach to performing **cardiac catheterization** on all hospitalized patients with UA is justified but is not clearly superior to a conservative approach.

VI. Therapy. The goals of medical treatment of patients with UA are **rapid initiation of antiplatelet and antithrombotic therapies** and **relief of anginal**

Table 2-3. Indications for cardiac catheterization in unstable angina

Prior revascularization (PTCA or CABG)
Congestive heart failure
Depressed left ventricular function (EF <50%)
Malignant ventricular arrhythmias
Persistent or recurrent angina or ischemia
Large perfusion defect on noninvasive functional test
Significant valvular heart disease (MR or AS)

It is generally recommended that patients with these risk factors undergo early cardiac catheterization regardless of response to medical therapy.
PTCA, Percutaneous transluminal coronary angioplasty; *CABG,* coronary artery bypass graft; *EF,* ejection fraction; *MR,* mitral regurgitation; *AS,* aortic stenosis.

pain with antianginal therapy. Patients whose condition is refractory to medical treatment can be triaged to urgent cardiac catheterization and percutaneous revascularization. Patients whose condition has been medically stabilized can undergo catheterization on an elective basis. Decisions about surgical revascularization are based on the results of cardiac catheterization.

A. Priority of Therapy
   1. Aspirin
   2. Antianginal therapy with nitrates and β-blockers
   3. Antithrombotic therapy with heparin or low-molecular-weight heparin
   4. Glycoprotein IIb/IIIa inhibitor
B. Antiplatelet Agents
   1. **Aspirin.** Aspirin has a substantial effect on mortality in UA even though it is a relatively weak inhibitor of platelet aggregation. Aspirin blocks only thromboxane A_2-induced platelet activation while many other stimuli to platelet activation remain unchecked. Five trials have studied aspirin therapy for UA at doses of 75 mg to 325 mg per day. The collective incidence of death or nonfatal MI was reduced by 50% with aspirin.
      a. **Kinetics.** Aspirin almost completely inhibits platelet thromboxane A_2 production within 15 minutes, so it should be given **as soon as the patient arrives for treatment.**
      b. **Dosing.** Unless there is active bleeding or documented hypersensitivity to aspirin, 325 mg of aspirin should be given initially to all patients with suspected UA. Subsequent daily aspirin doses can be reduced, but the first aspirin dose should be at least 325 mg because low-dose aspirin requires several days to achieve a full antiplatelet effect.
   2. **Ticlopidine** and **clopidogrel.** Ticlopidine and clopidogrel are more potent inhibitors of platelet aggregation than aspirin because they selectively antagonize adenosine diphosphate (ADP)–induced platelet aggregation. Compared with no antiplatelet treatment, ticlopidine reduces mortality and MI rates at 6 months among patients with UA by a magnitude similar to that of aspirin. Clopidogrel, compared with aspirin, slightly reduces the rate of ischemic events among patients with recent MI.
      a. **Kinetics.** Ticlopidine has a delayed onset of clinical action (2 to 3 days for maximum antiplatelet effect). Clopidogrel has a shorter onset of action.
      b. **Side effects.** Ticlopidine causes neutropenia among 1% to 5% of patients and is associated with the development of thrombotic thrombocytopenic purpura. No serious side effects of clopidogrel have been reported.
      c. **Dosing.** Ticlopidine is given as a loading dose of 500 mg followed by 250 mg twice per day. Clopidogrel is started at 150 mg for the loading dose and is given 75 mg per day thereafter.
      d. **Recommendations.** Because of cost and potential side effects, ticlopidine or clopidogrel is recommended only in the care of patients with UA who have a contraindication to use of aspirin or of patients who undergo stent placement, in which case it should be given in addition to aspirin.
C. Antithrombins
   1. **Heparin.** Unfractionated heparin reduces the rate of ischemic events among patients with UA when used in combination with aspirin during the period of drug infusion. A metaanalysis of six trials involving patients with UA showed that aspirin plus heparin reduced the rate of death and MI by 33% compared with those associated with aspirin alone (8).
      a. **Duration of therapy.** The optimal length of heparin therapy is not known, but studies have suggested that to achieve beneficial effects, heparin therapy must be continued for 3 to 7 days. A shorter duration of heparin therapy (2 days) showed no effect on rates of death or MI (8). A longer duration of heparin therapy (>7 days) has not been studied.

b. **Rebound ischemia.** After heparin therapy is stopped, there may be a rebound in ischemic events related to accumulation of thrombin, which stimulates platelet aggregation. Concomitant use of aspirin may attenuate this response.

c. **Recommendations.** Patients with intermediate- or high-risk UA should be treated with intravenous (IV) unfractionated heparin unless there is a contraindication to its use (active bleeding, known hypersensitivity, history of heparin-associated thrombocytopenia).

d. **Dosing.** An initial weight-adjusted heparin bolus of 60 U/kg should be given and be followed by an infusion of 15 U/kg per hour. Partial thromboplastin time (PTT) should be checked every 6 hours until it is stabilized between 50 and 70 seconds and then checked every 12 to 24 hours thereafter. Standardized heparin nomograms have simplified heparin dosing and the monitoring of PTT levels.

2. **Low-molecular-weight heparin.** The advantages of low-molecular-weight heparin over unfractionated heparin include a predictable anticoagulant effect caused by increased bioavailability, fixed dosing by means of subcutaneous injections, more effective thrombin inhibition because of increased anti–factor IIa and anti–factor Xa activity, lower rates of thrombocytopenia, and cost savings because activated PTT levels do not have to be followed to monitor anticoagulant activity.

a. **Comparison with heparin.** A pooled analysis of three trials that compared use of unfractionated heparin and aspirin with use of low-molecular-weight heparin and aspirin in the care of almost 4,800 patients with UA demonstrated that the incidence of death and MI was reduced by 17% with low-molecular-weight heparin. However, only enoxaparin was shown to be superior to unfractionated heparin in the ESSENCE trial (9).

b. **Dosing.** There are many low-molecular-weight heparin analogues, including **enoxaparin,** which is administered 1 mg/kg every 12 hours, and **dalteparin,** which is administered 120 units/kg every 12 hours.

3. **Direct antithrombins.** Direct antithrombin agents are more potent inhibitors of clot-bound thrombin than heparin and are not inactivated by plasma proteins and platelet factor 4 as is heparin. However, direct antithrombins have not been widely accepted as replacement therapy for heparin. They may, however, have a role in the treatment of patients with heparin-associated thrombocytopenia.

a. **Hirudin** is a direct antithrombin isolated from leech saliva. Hirudin was compared with unfractionated heparin in the care of more than 8,000 patients with UA in the **GUSTO IIb** trial. It was found to be equivalent to heparin in preventing adverse ischemic events (10).

b. **Hirulog** is a hirudin derivative with a shorter half-life than hirudin. Patients with UA treated with hirulog had a trend toward better outcomes after angioplasty compared with patients treated with unfractionated heparin (11,12).

c. A new agent, **argatroban,** is a synthetic thrombin inhibitor that is being evaluated in clinical trials.

D. **Platelet glycoprotein IIb/IIIa antagonists**

1. **Background.** Platelet aggregation involves activation of the glycoprotein IIb/IIIa receptor on the surface of platelets. The IIb/IIIa receptors of adjacent platelets bind fibrinogen molecules to cross link platelets, and the cross linking initiates thrombus formation. Antagonism of the IIb/IIIa receptor inhibits platelet aggregation and retards thrombus formation at sites of plaque rupture.

2. **IV glycoprotein IIb/IIIa inhibitors. Abciximab** is a monoclonal antibody to the IIb/IIIa receptor. It tightly binds to the receptor to inhibit platelet aggregation for days after drug infusion is completed. **Eptifibatide** is a cyclic peptide inhibitor of the IIb/IIIa receptor that

acts rapidly and has a short half-life. Continuous drug infusion is required for maximal platelet aggregation inhibition. **Tirofiban** and **lamifiban** are nonpeptide antagonists of the IIb/IIIa receptor that have half-lives of 4 to 6 hours.

   a. **Use during percutaneous coronary intervention.** Abciximab, eptifibatide, and tirofiban have been approved for use during percutaneous coronary intervention (PCI).

   (1) **Abciximab** was first evaluated in the care of patients undergoing high-risk PTCA in the Evaluation of 7E3 for the Prevention of Ischemic Complications (EPIC) trial. Among nearly 500 patients with UA in the EPIC trial, rates of death and MI were reduced 90% at 30 days and mortality decreased 60% at 3 years (13,14). Subsequent studies showed similar results with abciximab in the care of patients with UA at low and intermediate risk who underwent PCI (15). Abciximab is now commonly used during PCI to treat patients with acute coronary syndromes. A bolus of 0.25 mg/kg abciximab is followed by infusion of 10 µg/min for 12 hours.

   (2) Both **tirofiban** and **eptifibatide** were evaluated in the care of patients with acute coronary syndromes undergoing PCI. Although there was an early treatment benefit for both drugs, adverse ischemic events were not significantly reduced at 30 days compared with results with a placebo (16,17). Abciximab is therefore preferred for use during PCI in the care of patients with acute coronary syndromes.

   b. **Use before percutaneous coronary intervention.** Only abciximab has been evaluated for use before planned PCI in the care of patients with medically refractory UA. In the c7E3 Fab Antiplatelet Therapy for Unstable Refractory Angina (CAPTURE) study, abciximab given 18 to 24 hours before PCI reduced the rate of pre-PCI MI, death, MI, and urgent revascularization 29% at 30 days (18). Whether abciximab or another glycoprotein IIb/IIIa inhibitor is the best agent to use before planned PCI in the care of patients with acute coronary syndromes requires further study.

   c. **Use independently of PCI.** Eptifibatide and tirofiban have been approved for use in the care of patients with UA as a primary medical therapy whether or not PCI is performed.

   (1) In the Platelet Glycoprotein IIb/IIIa in Unstable Angina: Receptor Suppression Using Integrilin Therapy (PURSUIT) trial, **eptifibatide** was tested in close to 11,000 patients with UA or non-ST-segment-elevation MI treated with aspirin and heparin in a 180 µg/kg bolus followed by an infusion of 1.3 or 2.0 µg/kg per minute (19). Eptifibatide reduced the 30-day rate of death or nonfatal MI 10%.

   (2) In the Platelet Receptor Inhibition for Ischemic Syndrome Management (PRISM) trial, **tirofiban** reduced the 7-day rate of death, MI, and refractory ischemia 41% compared with heparin in the care of patients with UA at intermediate risk (the dose used was a 0.6 µg/kg per minute bolus for 30 minutes followed by an infusion of 0.15 µg/kg per minute) (20). In the Platelet Receptor Inhibition for Ischemic Syndrome Management in Patients Limited to Very Unstable Signs and Symptoms (PRISM-PLUS) trial, patients with UA at higher risk were treated with a similar dose of tirofiban plus heparin or heparin alone. Tirofiban and heparin reduced the 30-day rate of death, MI, and refractory ischemia 17% (21).

3. **Lamifiban** was tested in patients with UA in the Platelet IIb/IIIa Antagonism for the Reduction of Acute Coronary Syndrome Events in a Global Organization Network (PARAGON) trial and was used with and

without heparin. PARAGON was a dose-finding study, and lamifiban was found to reduce the rate of long-term adverse ischemic cardiac events when used at a low dose (0.1 µg/kg per minute infusion) with heparin (22). High-dose lamifiban (0.5 µg/kg minute infusion) with heparin showed no treatment benefit.

E. **Nitrates.** There have been no randomized trials of use of nitrates to manage UA, but nitrates are a mainstay to relieve anginal pain. **Dosing:** Sublingual nitroglycerin (0.4 mg) should be administered immediately to relieve anginal discomfort. If angina persists, IV nitroglycerin should be started at 10–20 µg/min. IV nitroglycerin can then be rapidly titrated (5–10 µg/min increases every 5 to 10 minutes) to relieve angina, but it can cause hypotension, and tachyphylaxis can develop within 24 hours. Topical or oral nitrates are used to prevent recurrent angina for patients who do not need IV nitroglycerin for relief of chest pain.

F. **β-Blockers.** β-Blockers relieve ischemia by lowering myocardial oxygen demand, blood pressure, and heart rate. A pooled analysis involving 4,700 patients with UA and impending MI showed that β-blockers reduced risk for MI, but no clear effect on mortality was seen.

   1. **Indications.** All patients with UA should be given β-blockers to relieve ischemia. The target resting heart rate is 50 to 60 beats/min. Cardio-selective β-blockers such as metoprolol or atenolol are typically used to prevent side effects.

   2. **Contraindications.** Contraindications to β-blocker therapy include advanced atrioventricular block, active bronchospasm, cardiogenic shock, hypotension, baseline sinus bradycardia, and congestive heart failure.

   3. **Dosing.** Patients with ongoing chest pain or persistent hypertension can be initially treated with IV β-blockers. IV metoprolol usually is given in 5-mg increments every 5 to 10 minutes until the desired heart response is seen or systemic blood pressure is sufficiently lowered. Oral metopro-lol therapy is started at a dose of 25 to 50 mg every 6 to 12 hours and is titrated to achieve the desired heart rate and blood pressure response.

G. **Calcium-channel blockers.** Calcium-channel blockers have diverse effects, including vasodilatation, slowing of atrioventricular conduction, and negative ionotropic and chronotropic properties. A metaanalysis of trials of calcium-channel blockers in the management of UA showed no effect on death or MI. However, short-acting nifedipine increased risk for MI or recurrent angina compared with metoprolol. Diltiazem was shown to reduce adverse events among patients with UA, except for patients with LV dysfunction, who had worse outcomes with diltiazem.

   1. **Indications.** Calcium channel blockers are recommended for patients with UA only when β-blockers and nitrates fail to relieve symptoms of ischemia. If coronary artery spasm with variant angina is present, how-ever, calcium-channel blockers are recommended, and β-blockers are contraindicated.

   2. **Contraindications.** Common contraindications to using calcium-channel blockers include LV dysfunction, hypotension, or atrioventric-ular conduction abnormalities.

H. **Angiotensin-converting enzyme (ACE) inhibitors.** ACE inhibitors re-duce the death rate and ameliorate ventricular remodeling when used after ST-elevation MI in the care of patients with LV dysfunction. The effects of ACE inhibitors in the care of patients with UA or non-ST-elevation MI have not been studied. However, **if patients have LV dysfunction, ACE inhibitors should be added to existing medical therapy** if the blood pressure is sufficient.

I. **Lipid-lowering therapy.** 3-Hydroxy-3-methylglutaryl coenzyme A (**HMG CoA**) reductase inhibitors (also known as **statins**) have been shown to have an important benefit in primary and secondary prevention of coronary artery disease through reduction in the rate of death and MI. Statins have not been investigated specifically in the care of patients with UA. However, any patient with an **elevated low-density cholesterol** (LDL) (>100 mg/dL) or **total cholesterol** (>200 mg/dL) level who has symptoms of UA should be treated with lipid-lowering therapy if there is at least reasonable suspicion of coronary artery disease. Trials are currently underway to evaluate the use of statins during acute ischemic events.

J. **Antibiotics.** Serologic evidence of an association between the presence of bacteria such as *C. pneumoniae* and *Helicobacter pylori* and coronary disease has been suggested. The ROXIS trial involving 200 patients with UA demonstrated a reduction in rates of death, MI, and recurrent ischemia among patients treated with roxithromycin for 30 days to eradicate *C. pneumoniae* (23). **Routine treatment of patients with UA with antibiotics is not recommended** until more data become available.

K. **Antiarrhythmic agents.** Hemodynamically significant ventricular arrhythmias should be managed with appropriate medications such as lidocaine or amiodarone. Prophylactic use of antiarrhythmic agents (flecainide and encainide) for increased ventricular ectopy has been associated with increased mortality.

L. **Thrombolytic agents.** Although thrombolytic therapy has clearly been shown to decrease mortality and to preserve LV function among patients with ST-segment-elevation MI, use of thrombolytic agents is associated with worse overall outcomes among patients with UA and non-ST-segment-elevation MI. More than 3,500 patients with ST-segment depression were enrolled in four major thrombolysis trials, and mortality was increased with use of thrombolytic agents. A metaanalysis of trials of thrombolysis in the management of UA revealed that the rate of death or nonfatal MI was 9.8% among patients treated with thrombolytic agents compared with 6.9% among the placebo-treated group. **Pathophysiology:** The lack of efficacy of thrombolytic agents in the management of UA may be related to a pro-thrombotic state caused by exposure of clot-bound thrombin when fibrin is cleaved within a coronary thrombus. Plasmin generation increases, and platelets are activated. Because thrombi in UA are mainly nonocclusive, thrombolytic agents would not be expected to dramatically improve coronary blood flow as they do in ST-segment-elevation MI.

M. **Percutaneous revascularization.** The goals of percutaneous revascularization in the care of patients with UA are to relieve angina and to prevent death, infarction, and recurrent ischemia.

1. **PTCA.** Registries of patients treated with PTCA have shown a higher incidence of complications among patients with UA treated with PCI compared with patients with chronic stable angina, but adverse event rates are still acceptably low. In the TIMI IIIb trial of patients with UA treated with PTCA, the incidence of periprocedural MI was 2.7%, emergency CABG was 1.4%, and death was 0.5% (24). Although the initial success rate of PTCA among this cohort of patients was 96%, 28% of patients needed repeat revascularization 1 year after the procedure.

2. **Coronary stents.** Coronary stents reduce the rate of restenosis after PCI and are widely used during contemporary percutaneous revascularization procedures. Data are limited from studies comparing stents and PTCA in the care of patients with UA undergoing PCI. Outcomes after PCI among patients with UA may be improved with stents because patients with stable angina and those with UA have had similar outcomes with the use of coronary stents during intervention.

3. **Adjunctive therapies.** Adjunctive pharmacologic agents such as glycoprotein IIb/IIIa receptor inhibitors reduce ischemic complications during PCI and improve outcomes after percutaneous revascularization (see earlier). Results from the Evaluation of Platelet IIb/IIIa Inhibitor for Stenting (EPISTENT) trial demonstrated that when **stents and abciximab** are used together, the rate of adverse ischemic events is lower than that with stents alone (25).

N. **Surgical revascularization.** Percutaneous revascularization is used extensively to treat patients with UA, but the decision to refer a patient for CABG involves multiple factors including age, coexisting medical conditions, severity of coronary disease, prior revascularization procedures, and the technical feasibility of percutaneous revascularization.

O. **Intraaortic balloon counterpulsation.** For patients with UA who have medically refractory angina, placement of an intraaortic balloon pump (IABP) should be considered when emergency cardiac catheterization cannot be performed. In consecutive series of patients with UA, about 1% of patients need an IABP to relieve ischemia. By reducing myocardial oxygen demand and increasing coronary perfusion pressure, the IABP produces almost immediate relief of angina and ischemic ECG changes. **Recommendations:** Placement of an IABP is a short-term strategy for relieving ischemia because there is a limited duration of IABP support. Patients with medically refractory UA should undergo IABP placement only as a bridge to revascularization.

VII. CONTROVERSIES

A. **Cardiac catheterization.** There is considerable controversy regarding whether to proceed directly with cardiac catheterization in the care of all hospitalized patients with UA or to medically stabilize the patient's condition and proceed with catheterization only when angina is medically refractory or the patient is at high risk. Data from clinical trials are controversial about which strategy is preferred.

1. **Early invasive strategy.** The rationale behind the early invasive strategy of cardiac catheterization is that early determination of coronary anatomy helps ascertain which patients with three-vessel or left main coronary disease can be most appropriately treated with surgical revascularization. Early determination also reduces the length and cost of the hospital stay by means of accelerating revascularization decisions.

2. **Early conservative strategy.** The goal of medical therapy for UA is to "pacify" the unstable plaque and convert a platelet-active surface to a platelet-inactive surface. Successful medical treatment of patients with UA usually necessitates a longer hospital stay but can reduce the need for cardiac catheterization among patients who do not have high-risk clinical characteristics. Patients with angina refractory to medical therapy or who have an ischemic perfusion defect found at noninvasive stress testing are referred for cardiac catheterization when this strategy is used.

3. **Randomized trials**

a. The **TIMI IIIb trial** randomized more than 1,400 patients with non-Q-wave MI or UA to undergo medical therapy or routine cardiac catheterization and revascularization of all severe lesions 1 to 2 days after admission (7). Patients in the conservative therapy group underwent catheterization and revascularization only if they had recurrent ischemia or if they failed a predischarge stress thallium test. The rates of death or nonfatal MI at 1 year were similar in both groups (10.8% in the early conservative therapy group versus 12.2% in the early invasive therapy group) (7,26). In the early conservative therapy group, 64% of the patients eventually underwent catheterization, but patients in the early invasive therapy group had fewer rehospitalizations and less recurrent angina. Patients older than 65 years had a dramatic reduction in death and MI rate at 6 weeks with the invasive strategy (7.9% versus 14.8%).

b. The Veterans Affairs Non-Q-Wave Infarction Strategies in Hospital (**VANQWISH**) trial compared catheterization and revascularization strategies in the care of 920 patients with non-Q-wave MI at Veterans Affairs medical centers (27). An increase in early mortality among the invasive therapy group was entirely caused by an unacceptably high perioperative mortality (11.6%) among patients who underwent CABG. In the early conservative therapy group, 29% of the patients eventually underwent cardiac catheterization.

After an average of 23 months of follow-up study, there was no significant difference in death and MI rates between the groups.

   c. **Criticisms.** Both the TIMI IIIb and VANQWISH trials have been criticized because contemporary methods of percutaneous revascularization (coronary stents and glycoprotein IIb/IIIa inhibitors) were not used and because many patients assigned to the early conservative strategy crossed over to undergo cardiac catheterization.

B. **Glycoprotein IIb/IIIa inhibitors.** Whether all hospitalized patients with UA should be treated with an IV IIb/IIIa inhibitor is debatable. All four IV IIb/IIIa inhibitors have been shown modestly to reduce ischemic complications among patients hospitalized with UA. Which patients at high risk have a greater benefit from treatment with IIb/IIIa inhibitors remains unclear. High-risk characteristics among patients with UA that may help determine which patients are more likely to benefit from use of a IIb/IIIa inhibitor include positive troponin levels, ischemic ST-segment changes, and hemodynamic instability. Determining the cost effectiveness of routine treatment with IIb/IIIa inhibitors requires further study.

C. **Heparin versus low-molecular-weight heparin.** Certain low-molecular-weight heparins such as enoxaparin are superior to unfractionated heparin when used to treat patients with UA. Low-molecular-weight heparins are easier to administer than IV unfractionated heparin and may be more cost effective because serial activated PTT levels do not have to be monitored. Low-molecular-weight heparins thus appear to be a better choice for treating patients with UA, but it is not clear how to continue low-molecular-weight heparin therapy when patients undergo PCI or CABG. Therefore unfractionated heparin is still used to treat most patients with UA.

VIII. **Future therapies: oral glycoprotein IIb/IIIa inhibitors.** Although no phase III clinical trials evaluating oral glycoprotein IIb/IIIa inhibitors have been completed, the TIMI-12 trial demonstrated that sibrafiban (an oral glycoprotein IIb/IIIa inhibitor) produced a rapid and sustained inhibition of platelet aggregation at the expense of an increase in minor bleeding (28). Ongoing phase III clinical trials are enrolling patients with acute coronary syndromes to determine the effects of extended platelet blockade with orally active glycoprotein IIb/IIIa inhibitors.

IX. **Follow-up.** Patients with UA usually receive definitive therapy during hospitalization, but close follow-up care after hospital discharge is needed to monitor for recurrent ischemia. There are no guidelines regarding noninvasive stress testing of patients without symptoms who have undergone percutaneous or surgical revascularization for UA. Many clinicians perform yearly stress tests on these patients to monitor for silent ischemia. If anginal symptoms recur after hospital discharge, stress testing or cardiac catheterization can be performed depending on the clinical presentation.

SUGGESTED READINGS

References
 1. Stone PH, Thompson B, Anderson HV, et al. Influence of race, sex, and age on management of unstable angina and non-Q-wave myocardial infarction: the TIMI III registry. *JAMA* 1996;275:1104–1112.
 2. Van Miltenburg AJ, Simoons ML, Veerhoek RJ, et al. Incidence and follow-up of Braunwald subgroups in unstable angina. *J Am Coll Cardiol* 1995;25:1286–1292.
 3. Hamm CW, Goldmann BU, Heeschen C, et al. Emergency room triage of patients with acute chest pain by means of rapid testing for cardiac troponin T or I. *N Engl J Med* 1997;337:1648–1653.
 4. Ohman EM, Armstrong PW, Christenson RH, et al. Cardiac troponin T levels for risk stratification in acute myocardial ischemia. *N Engl J Med* 1996;335:1333–1341.
 5. Antman EM, Tanasijevic MJ, Thompson B, et al. Cardiac-specific troponin I levels to predict the risk of mortality in patients with acute coronary syndromes. *N Engl J Med* 1996;335:1342–1349.

6. Moliterno DJ, Granger CB. Differences between unstable angina and acute myocardial infarction: the pathophysiological and clinical spectrum. In: Topol EJ, ed. *Acute coronary syndromes,* 1st ed. New York: Marcel Dekker, 1998:67–104.
7. TIMI IIIB Investigators. Effects of tissue plasminogen activator and a comparison of early invasive and conservative strategies in unstable angina and non-Q-wave myocardial infarction. *Circulation* 1994;89:1545–1556.
8. Oler A, Whooley MA, Oler J, et al. Adding heparin to aspirin reduces the incidence of myocardial infarction and death in patients with unstable angina: a meta-analysis. *JAMA* 1996;276:811–815.
9. Cohen M, Demers C, Garfinkel EP, et al. Low-molecular-weight heparins in non-ST-segment elevation ischemia: the ESSENCE trial. *Am J Cardiol* 1998;82:196–246.
10. GUSTO IIB Investigators. A comparison of recombinant hirudin with heparin for the treatment of acute coronary syndromes. *N Engl J Med.* 1996;335:775–782.
11. Serruys PW, Herman JP, Simon R, et al. A comparison of hirudin with heparin in the prevention of restenosis after coronary angioplasty. *N Engl J Med* 1995;333: 757–763.
12. Bittl JA, Strony J, Brinker JA, et al. Treatment with bivalirudin (Hirulog) as compared with heparin during coronary angioplasty for unstable or postinfarction angina. *N Engl J Med* 1995;333:764–769.
13. Lincoff AM, Califf RM, Anderson KM, et al. Evidence for prevention of death and myocardial infarction with platelet membrane glycoprotein IIb/IIIa receptor blockade by abciximab (c7E3 Fab) among patients with unstable angina undergoing percutaneous coronary revascularization. *J Am Coll Cardiol* 1997;30:149–156.
14. Topol EJ, Ferguson JJ, Weisman HF, et al. Long-term protection from myocardial ischemic events in a randomized trial of brief integrin beta 3 blockade with percutaneous coronary intervention. *JAMA* 1997;278:479–484.
15. EPILOG Investigators. Platelet glycoprotein IIb/IIIa receptor blockade and low-dose heparin during percutaneous coronary revascularization. *N Engl J Med* 1997; 336:1689–1696.
16. RESTORE Investigators. Effects of platelet glycoprotein IIb/IIIa blockade with tirofiban on adverse cardiac events in patients with unstable angina or acute myocardial infarction undergoing coronary angioplasty. *Circulation* 1997;96:1445–1453.
17. IMPACT-II Investigators. Randomised placebo-controlled trial of effect of eptifibatide on complications of percutaneous coronary intervention. *Lancet* 1997;349: 1422–1428.
18. CAPTURE Investigators. Randomised placebo-controlled trial of abciximab before and during coronary intervention in refractory unstable angina. *Lancet* 1997;349: 1429–1435.
19. PURSUIT Investigators. Inhibition of platelet glycoprotein IIb/IIIa with eptifibatide in patients with acute coronary syndromes. *N Engl J Med* 1998;339:436–443.
20. PRISM Investigators. A comparison of aspirin plus tirofiban with aspirin plus heparin for unstable angina. *N Engl J Med* 1998;338:1498–505.
21. PRISM-PLUS Investigators. Inhibition of the platelet glycoprotein IIb/IIIa receptor with tirofiban in unstable angina and non-Q-wave myocardial infarction. *N Engl J Med* 1998;338:1488–1497.
22. PARAGON Investigators. An international, randomized, controlled trial of lamifiban, a platelet glycoprotein IIb/IIIa inhibitor, heparin, or both in unstable angina. *Circulation* 1998;97:2386–2395.
23. Gurfinkel E, Bozovich G, Daroca A, et al. Randomised trial of roxithromycin in non-Q-wave coronary syndromes: ROXIS pilot study. *Lancet* 1997;350:404–407.
24. Williams DO, Braunwald E, Thompson B, et al. Results of percutaneous transluminal coronary angioplasty in unstable angina and non-Q-wave myocardial infarction: observations from the TIMI IIIB trial. *Circulation* 1996;94:2749–2755.
25. Lincoff AM, Califf RM, Moliterno DM, et al. Complementary clinical benefits of coronary-artery stenting and blockade of platelet glycoprotein IIb/IIIa receptors. *N Engl J Med* 1999;341:319–327.
26. Anderson HV, Cannon CP, Stone PH, et al. One-year results of the thrombolysis in myocardial infarction (TIMI) IIIB clinical trial. *J Am Coll Cardiol* 1995;26: 1643–1650.

27. Boden WE, O'Rourke RA, Crawford MH, et al. Outcomes in patients with acute non-Q-wave myocardial infarction randomly assigned to an invasive as compared with a conservative management strategy. *N Engl J Med* 1998;338:1785–1792.

28. Cannon CP, McCabe CH, Borzak S, et al. Randomized trial of an oral platelet glycoprotein IIb/IIIa antagonist, sibrafiban, in patients after an acute coronary syndrome: results of the TIMI 12 trial. *Circulation* 1998;97:340–349.

Landmark Articles

Braunwald EG, Mark DB, Jones RH et. al. Unstable angina: diagnosis and management. Clinical Practice Guideline Number 10. AHCPR Publication No. 94-0602. Rockville, MD: Agency for Health Care Policy Research and the National Heart, Lung, and Blood Institute, Public Health Service, U.S. Department of Health and Human Services, 1994.

Fuster V, Badimon L, Badimon JJ, et. al. The pathogenesis of coronary artery disease and the acute coronary syndromes. *N Engl J Med* 1992;326:242–250.

Global Use of Strategies to Open Occluded Arteries (GUSTO) IIb Investigators. A comparison of recombinant hirudin with heparin for the treatment of acute coronary syndromes. *N Engl J Med* 1996;335:775–782.

Theroux P, Ouimet H, McCans J, et. al. Aspirin, heparin, or both to treat acute UA. *N Engl J Med* 1988;319:1105–1111.

TIMI IIIB Investigators. Effects of tissue plasminogen activator and a comparison of early invasive and conservative strategies in unstable angina and non-Q-wave myocardial infarction: results of the TIMI IIIB trial. *Circulation* 1994;89:1545–1556.

Relevant Book Chapters

Gersh BJ, Braunwald EG, Rutherford JD. Chronic coronary artery disease: unstable angina. In: Braunwald EG, ed. *Heart disease: a textbook of cardiovascular medicine,* 5th ed. Philadelphia: WB Saunders, 1997:1331–1339.

Granger CB, Califf RM. Stabilizing the unstable artery. In: Califf RM, Mark DB, Wagner GS, eds. *Acute coronary care,* 2nd ed. St. Louis: Mosby, 1995:525–541.

Moliterno DJ, Granger CB. Differences between unstable angina and acute myocardial infarction: the pathophysiological and clinical spectrum. In: Topol EJ, ed. *Acute Coronary Syndromes,* 1st ed. New York: Marcel Dekker, 1998:67–104.

White HD. Unstable angina: ischemic syndromes. In: Topol EJ, ed. *Textbook of cardiovascular medicine.* 1st ed. Philadelphia: Lippincott–Raven, 1998:365–393.

3. COMPLICATIONS OF MYOCARDIAL INFARCTION

Debabrata Mukherjee

I. **Introduction.** In-hospital mortality among patients with acute myocardial infarction (MI) is primarily caused by circulatory failure from either severe left ventricular (LV) dysfunction or one of the mechanical complications of MI. The complications of MI may be broadly classified as **mechanical, electrical or arrhythmic, ischemic, embolic, and inflammatory** (pericarditis).

II. **Mechanical complications.** Serious life-threatening mechanical complications of acute MI include ventricular septal defect (VSD), papillary muscle rupture, cardiac free-wall rupture, large ventricular aneurysms, LV pump failure, cardiogenic shock, and right ventricular (RV) failure.

   A. **Ventricular septal defect**
   1. **Clinical presentation.** VSD occurs among 0.5% to 2% of patients after acute MI (1). The incidence is similar for anterior, inferior, and posterior MI. VSD typically occurs among patients with large infarcts, single-vessel disease, and poorly developed collateral vessels to the occluded vessel. VSD may develop as early as 24 hours after MI but is commonly seen 3 to 7 days after MI.
      a. **Signs and symptoms.** Patients with post-MI development of VSD may appear relatively comfortable early in the disease course and have no clinically significant orthopnea or pulmonary edema. Recurrence of angina, pulmonary edema, hypotension, and shock may suddenly develop later in the course.
      b. **Physical findings.** The diagnosis should be suspected when a **pansystolic murmur** develops that was not present initially. For this reason, it is important that **all patients with MI have a well-documented cardiac examination** at presentation and frequent evaluations thereafter.
         (1) The murmur is usually best heard in the lower left sternal area; it is accompanied by a thrill in 50% of cases. In patients with a large VSD and severe heart failure or shock, the murmur may be of low intensity or inaudible, thus the **absence of a murmur does not rule out VSD.**
         (2) Several features differentiate the murmur of VSD from that of mitral regurgitation (MR) caused by rupture of the papillary muscle (Table 3-1). The murmur may radiate to the base and the apex of the heart. A third heart sound, loud P_2, and signs of tricuspid regurgitation may be present.
   2. **Histopathology.** The defect usually occurs at the border of nonnecrotic and infarcted myocardium in the **apical septum with anterior MI** and in the **basal posterior septum with inferior MI.** The defect may not always be a single large defect; it can be a meshwork of serpiginous channels.
   3. **Laboratory examination and diagnostic testing**
      a. **An electrocardiogram (ECG)** may show AV node and infranodal conduction abnormalities in approximately 40% of patients.
      b. **Echocardiography**
         (1) Echocardiography with color flow imaging is the **test of choice** for diagnosis the of VSD.
            (a) **Basal VSD** is best visualized in the parasternal long axis with medial angulation, apical long axis, and subcostal long axis.
            (b) **Apical VSD** is best visualized in the apical four-chamber view.

Table 3-1. Differential diagnosis of new systolic murmur after acute myocardial infarction

Differentiating features	Ventricular septal defect	Papillary muscle rupture
Location of MI	Anterior > inferoposterior	Inferoposterior then anterior
Location of murmur	Lower left sternal area	Cardiac apex
Intensity	Loud	Variable; may be faint
Thrill	50% of patients	Rare
V waves in PCWP	Present or absent	Almost always present
V waves in PA tracing	Absent	Present
O_2 step-up in PA	Almost always present	Present or absent

MI, Myocardial infarction; *PA*, pulmonary artery; *PCWP*, pulmonary capillary wedge pressure.

    (2) In some cases, **transesophageal echocardiography** may help in determining the extent of the defect.

    (3) Echocardiography can help determine the size of the defect and the magnitude of the left-to-right shunt by means of comparison of flow through the pulmonary valve with flow through the aortic valve.

    (4) Echocardiography also is useful in defining LV and RV function, which are important determinants of mortality.

  c. Right heart catheterization. Pulmonary artery catheterization with oximetry is a useful diagnostic aid. It involves fluoroscopically guided measurement of oxygen saturation in the superior and inferior vena cava, right atrium, right ventricle, and pulmonary artery.

    (1) Normal saturations for these chambers are: superior vena cava 64% to 66%; inferior vena cava 69% to 71%; right atrium 64% to 67%; right ventricle 64% to 67%; and pulmonary artery 64% to 67%.

    (2) A greater than 8% increase in oxygen saturation occurs between the right atrium and the right ventricle and pulmonary artery with a left-to-right shunt across the ventricular septum.

    (3) Shunt fraction can be calculated as follows:

$$\frac{Q_p}{Q_s} = \frac{SaO_2 - MvO_2}{PvO_2 - PaO_2}$$

where Q_p = pulmonary flow; Q_s = systemic flow; SaO_2 = arterial oxygen saturation; MvO_2 = mixed venous oxygen saturation; PvO_2 = pulmonary venous oxygen saturation; and PaO_2 = pulmonary arterial oxygen saturation. $Q_p/Q_s \geq 2$ suggests a considerable shunt, which is likely to be poorly tolerated by the patient.

    (4) For a patient with an intracardiac shunt, cardiac output measured by means of the thermodilution technique is inaccurate; the Fick method should be used. The **key to measurement of accurate systemic flow** in the presence of a shunt is that the mixed venous oxygen content must be measured in the chamber immediately proximal to the shunt.

  4. Therapy

    a. Priority of therapy. **Early surgical closure** is the treatment of choice, even if the patient's condition is stable.

b. Medical therapy

(1) The mortality rate among patients with VSD treated medically is 24% at 24 hours, 46% at 1 week, and 67% to 82% at 2 months. Therefore patients should be considered for urgent surgical repair.

(2) Vasodilators can decrease left-to-right shunt and increase systemic flow by means of reducing systemic vascular resistance (SVR); however, a greater decrease in pulmonary vascular resistance may actually increase shunting. The vasodilator of choice is intravenous (IV) **nitroprusside,** which is started at 5 to 10 μg/kg per minute and titrated to a mean arterial pressure (MAP) of 70 to 80 mm Hg.

c. Percutaneous therapy. An **intraaortic balloon pump (IABP)** should be inserted as early as possible as a bridge to a surgical procedure, unless there is marked aortic regurgitation. The IABP decreases SVR, decreases shunt fraction, increases coronary perfusion, and maintains blood pressure. After insertion of an IABP, vasodilators can be used with close hemodynamic monitoring.

d. Surgical therapy. Surgical closure is the treatment of choice even if the patient's condition is stable.

(1) Cardiogenic shock and multisystem failure are associated with high surgical mortality, further supporting earlier operations on these patients before complications develop.

(2) Surgical mortality is high among patients with **basal septal rupture associated with inferior MI** because of greater technical difficulty and the need for a mitral valve operation on these patients, who often have coexisting MR. However, surgical **repair should be considered** in the care of patients with cardiogenic shock and basal septal rupture with MR because medical therapy alone almost always results in death.

(3) Earlier surgical intervention in the care of patients in hemodynamically stable condition is associated with lower mortality than watchful waiting and delayed surgical treatment.

B. Papillary muscle rupture. MR was shown to be a predictor of poor prognosis in the trial of Global Utilization of Streptokinase and Tissue Plasminogen Activator for Occluded Coronary Arteries (GUSTO I). MR of mild-to-moderate severity is common among patients with acute MI, and most MR is transient, asymptomatic, and benign. However, severe MR caused by papillary muscle rupture is a life-threatening and manageable complication of acute MI. Papillary muscle rupture, typically seen between day 2 and day 7, contributes to 5% of the mortality after acute MI. The overall incidence is 1%.

1. Clinical presentation. Papillary muscle rupture is **more likely to occur with inferior MI.** Thrombolytic agents decrease the incidence, but rupture may occur earlier in the post-MI period. In some instances the hemodynamic stress imposed by acute MI causes rupture of a chord in patients who are predisposed to this problem.

a. Signs and symptoms. Complete transection of the papillary muscles is rare and usually results in immediate shock and death. Patients with rupture of one or more heads of the muscle typically have **sudden severe respiratory distress** from development of pulmonary edema and may rapidly experience **cardiogenic shock.**

b. Physical findings. A new **pansystolic murmur** is audible at the cardiac apex with radiation to the axilla or the base of the heart. In posterior papillary muscle rupture, the murmur radiates to the left sternal border and may be confused with the murmur of VSD or aortic stenosis. (Intensity of the murmur does not predict the severity of MR). The murmur may be quiet, soft, or absent in patients with severe failure with poor cardiac output and persons with elevated left atrial pressures.

2. **Pathophysiology.** Papillary muscle rupture is more common with an inferior MI. It involves the posteromedial papillary muscle because of its single blood supply through the posterior descending coronary artery. The anterolateral papillary muscle is perfused through the left anterior descending (LAD) and left circumflex coronary arteries. In 50% of patients, the infarct is relatively small with single-vessel disease.

3. **Laboratory examination**
   a. An ECG usually shows evidence of recent inferior or posterior MI.
   b. A **chest radiograph** shows evidence of pulmonary edema. In some patients, focal pulmonary edema may be seen in the right upper lobe because of flow directed at the right pulmonary veins.

4. **Diagnostic testing**
   a. **Two-dimensional echocardiography** with Doppler and color flow imaging is the **diagnostic modality of choice.**
      (1) The **mitral valve leaflet is usually flail** with severe MR.
      (2) Color-flow imaging is useful in differentiating papillary muscle rupture with severe MR from VSD after MI.
      (3) In some patients with posteriorly directed jets, the amount of MR may not be fully appreciated with transthoracic echocardiography, and transesophageal echocardiography may be particularly useful.
   b. **Pulmonary artery (PA) catheterization.** Hemodynamic monitoring with a PA catheter may reveal large V waves in the pulmonary capillary wedge pressure (PCWP). However, patients with VSD also may have large V waves because of increased pulmonary venous return in a normal-size and normally compliant left atrium. Among patients with severe MR and reflected V waves in the PA tracing, oxygen saturation in the PA may be higher than that in the right atrial blood, complicating differentiation from VSD. Two means by which to **differentiate MR from VSD** are:
      (1) **Prominent V waves** in the PA tracing before the incisura almost always are associated with acute severe MR (Fig. 3-1).
      (2) Blood for oximetry is obtained with fluoroscopy to ensure sampling from the main PA rather than distal branches.

5. **Therapy**
   a. **Priority of therapy.** Papillary muscle rupture should be identified early. Patients should receive **aggressive medical therapy** and be considered for an **emergency cardiac operation.**
   b. **Medical therapy**
      (1) **Vasodilator therapy** is very useful in the treatment of patients with acute MR. Nitroprusside decreases SVR, reduces regurgitant fraction, and increases stroke volume and cardiac output. Nitroprusside is started at 5 to 10 µg/kg per minute and is titrated to a MAP of 70 to 80 mm Hg.
      (2) **Vasodilators cannot be used** as the first line of treatment of patients with **hypotension,** and an IABP should be inserted promptly. An IABP decreases LV afterload, improves coronary perfusion, and increases forward cardiac output. Patients with hypotension can be given vasodilators after insertion of an IABP to improve hemodynamic values. Patients with moderate MR after MI benefit from vasodilators.
   c. **Percutaneous therapy.** Improvement in hemodynamic values and reduction in MR has been reported after percutaneous intervention in the care of patients with severe MR caused by papillary muscle ischemia rather than rupture. Percutaneous interventions have **no role in true papillary muscle rupture.**
   d. **Surgical therapy** should be considered immediately for patients with papillary muscle rupture.

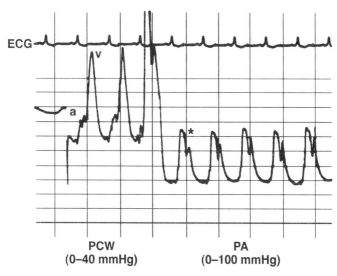

FIG. 3-1. Giant V waves on the pulmonary capillary wedge (*PCW*) tracing can be transmitted to the pulmonary artery (*PA*) pressure, producing a notch (*asterisk*) on the pulmonary artery downslope. (Adapted from Kern M. *The cardiac catheterization handbook,* 2nd ed. St. Louis: Mosby–Year Book, 1991, with permission.)

      (1) The prognosis is very poor among patients treated medically. Even though perioperative mortality (20% to 25%) is higher than it is for elective surgical treatment, surgical repair should be considered for every patient.

      (2) **Coronary angiography** should be performed before a surgical procedure.

      (3) Patients with moderate MR who do not improve with afterload reduction may benefit from mitral valve repair. Many of these valves can be repaired and may not have to be replaced.

C. Cardiac rupture

  1. Clinical presentation. Cardiac free-wall rupture occurs among 3% of patients. It accounts for approximately 10% of mortality after MI. Rupture occurs in the first 5 days among 50% of patients and within 2 weeks among 90% of patients. Free-wall rupture occurs only among patients with transmural MI. Risk factors include advanced age, female sex, hypertension, first MI, and poor coronary collateral vessels.

    a. Signs and symptoms

      (1) **Acute course.** With acute rupture, patients have electromechanical dissociation and sudden death. Sudden onset of chest pain with straining or coughing may suggest the onset of myocardial rupture.

      (2) **Subacute course.** Some patients may have a subacute course as a result of a contained rupture with pain suggestive of pericarditis, nausea, and hypotension. Immediate bedside echocardiography may reveal localized pericardial effusion or pseudoaneurysm.

    b. Physical findings. Jugular venous distention, pulsus paradoxus, diminished heart sounds, and a pericardial rub suggest subacute rupture. New to-and-fro murmurs may be heard in patients with subacute rupture.

2. **Pathophysiology.** Free-wall rupture constitutes part of the **early hazard function** among patients treated with thrombolytic agents. (Mortality among patients who receive thrombolytic agents is higher for the first 24 hours and is partially attributable to cardiac rupture.) Rupture most commonly occurs at the lateral wall, although any wall may be involved.

3. **Laboratory examination.** An **ECG** in addition to evidence of a new MI may show junctional or idioventricular rhythm, low-voltage complexes, and tall precordial T waves. A large number of patients have transient bradycardia just before rupture.

4. **Diagnostic testing.** There **may not be time** for diagnostic testing in the treatment of patients with acute rupture.

   a. **Echocardiography** reveals findings of cardiac tamponade among patients with a subacute course: right atrium and RV diastolic collapse, dilated inferior vena cava, and marked respiratory variation in mitral and tricuspid inflow.

   b. **Cardiac catheterization.** Hemodynamic evaluation with a PA catheter may reveal equalization of pressures in the right atrium, RV diastolic pressure, and PCWP consistent with pericardial tamponade.

5. **Therapy.** Reperfusion therapy has reduced the overall incidence of cardiac rupture and shifted its occurrence to earlier after acute MI.

   a. **Priority of therapy.** The goal is to identify the problem rapidly and perform emergency surgical treatment.

   b. **Medical therapy has little role** in the treatment of these patients except for use of vasopressors to temporarily maintain blood pressure as the patient is taken to the operating room.

   c. **Percutaneous therapy**

      (1) **Immediate pericardiocentesis** should be performed on patients with tamponade as soon as the diagnosis is made and while arrangements are being made for transport to the operating room.

      (2) If the index of suspicion is high, and if the patient's condition is unstable, pericardiocentesis should be attempted without waiting for diagnostic tests.

      (3) An indwelling catheter should be left in the pericardial cavity and connected to a drainage bag during transfer to the operating room.

   d. **Surgical therapy. Emergency thoracotomy** with surgical repair is the definitive therapy and is the only chance for survival among patients with cardiac rupture.

D. **Pseudoaneurysm (contained rupture)**

   1. **Clinical presentation**

      a. **Signs and symptoms.** Pseudoaneurysms may remain **clinically silent** and be discovered during routine investigations. However, some patients may have recurrent tachyarrhythmia and heart failure.

      b. **Physical findings.** Some patients may have systolic, diastolic, or to-and-fro murmurs related to flow of blood across the narrow neck of the pseudoaneurysm during LV systole and diastole.

   2. **Pathophysiology.** Pseudoaneurysm is caused by contained rupture of the LV free wall.

      a. The aneurysm may remain small or undergo progressive enlargement. The outer walls are formed by the pericardium and mural thrombus.

      b. Pseudoaneurysms communicate with the body of the left ventricle through a narrow neck, the diameter of which is less than 50% of the diameter of the fundus.

   3. **Laboratory examination and diagnostic testing**

      a. A **chest radiograph** may show cardiomegaly with an abnormal bulge on the cardiac border.

       b. An **ECG** may have persistent ST elevation as with true aneurysms.

       c. Echocardiography, magnetic resonance imaging, or computed tomography is used to **confirm the diagnosis.**

   4. Therapy. Spontaneous rupture occurs without warning among approximately one third of patients with a pseudoaneurysm, thus **surgical resection is recommended for patients with and for those without symptoms** regardless of the size of the aneurysm to prevent death with rupture.

E. LV pump failure and cardiogenic shock. LV dysfunction is inevitable after acute MI. The severity of dysfunction correlates with the extent of myocardial injury. Patients with small infarcts may have regional wall motion abnormalities with overall normal LV function because of compensatory hyperkinesia of the unaffected segments. Prior MI, older age, female sex, diabetes, and anterior infarction are risk factors for development of cardiogenic shock.

   1. Classification

       a. Killip and Kimball (2) classified four subsets of patients on the basis of clinical presentation and physical findings at the onset of MI (Table 3-2). Killip and Kimball (2) reported an 81% mortality rate. The 30-day mortality rate among the 0.8% of GUSTO I patients with cardiogenic shock treated with thrombolytic agents was 58% (3).

       b. Four hemodynamic subsets (4) are based on PCWP and cardiac index (Table 3-3). The hemodynamic subsets correlate well with mortality rate. There is approximately 50% mortality in subset IV; however, these data precede the reperfusion era.

   2. Clinical presentation

       a. Signs and symptoms. Patients may have respiratory distress, diaphoresis, and cool, clammy extremities in addition to the typical signs and symptoms of acute MI. Patients in cardiogenic shock may have severe orthopnea, dyspnea, and oliguria and may have altered mental status from cerebral hypoperfusion.

       b. Physical findings frequently include an S_3 gallop, pulmonary rales, hypotension, tachycardia, and pulsus alternans. Patients in cardiogenic shock are prone to supraventricular and ventricular arrhythmias.

   3. Etiology. Table 3-4 lists the causes of cardiogenic shock. Patients with acute MI and cardiogenic shock typically have **severe three-vessel disease** and commonly have substantial involvement of the LAD. Autopsy studies have demonstrated that at least 40% of the left ventricle is affected in patients with cardiogenic shock. Prior MI is present among 40% of patients. If the previous MI was large, even a small acute MI may cause shock.

   4. Laboratory examination

       a. Lactic acidosis, elevated creatinine levels, and **arterial hypoxemia** are common.

       b. A **chest radiograph** reveals pulmonary congestion.

Table 3-2. 30-Day mortality based on hemodynamic (Killip) class

Killip class	Characteristics	Patients (%)	Mortality rate (%)
I	No evidence of CHF	85	5.1
II	Rales, ↑ JVD, or S3	13	13.6
III	Pulmonary edema	1	32.2
IV	Cardiogenic shock	1	57.8

CHF, Congestive heart failure; ↑ , increased; *JVD,* jugular venous distention.
Adapted from reference 1, with permission.

Table 3-3. Forrester classification

Subset	PCWP (mm Hg)	Cardiac index	Mortality rate (%)
I	<18	>2.2	3
II	>18	>2.2	9
III	<18	<2.2	23
IV	>18	<2.2	51

PCWP, Pulmonary capillary wedge pressure.

    c. Patients with cardiogenic shock due to LV failure usually have extensive **ECG abnormalities** consistent with massive infarction, severe diffuse ischemia, or evidence of large prior MI.

    d. Extensive ST-segment depressions are common.

    e. An unremarkable ECG in the presence of shock suggests another cause of shock such as aortic dissection or mechanical complications of acute MI (free-wall rupture, ventricular septal rupture, papillary muscle rupture).

5. Diagnostic testing

    a. Cardiac catheterization. Hemodynamic monitoring with an arterial line and PA catheter is crucial. It is of diagnostic value and helps in minute-to-minute care. Hemodynamic data help identify RV infarction, acute MR, and ventricular septal rupture that contribute to the shock state.

    b. Echocardiography helps determine the extent of myocardial necrosis and identify complications of MI that contribute to cardiogenic shock.

6. Therapy

    a. Priority of therapy. An **IABP** should be inserted as soon as possible in a patient with cardiogenic shock.

    b. Medical therapy

        (1) Vasodilators play an important role in the management of post-MI heart failure by means of afterload reduction. The main determinants of myocardial oxygen consumption are heart rate, contractility, and wall stress. Wall stress depends on peak LV pressure, volume, and wall thickening. Vasodilators reduce wall stress and decrease oxygen requirements;

Table 3-4. Causes of cardiogenic shock

COMPLICATIONS OF ACUTE MYOCARDIAL INFARCTION

Extensive left ventricular infarction
Extensive right ventricular infarction
Ventricular septal rupture
Acute severe mitral regurgitation
Cardiac tamponade with or without free-wall rupture

OTHER CONDITIONS

Aortic dissection
Myocarditis
Massive pulmonary embolism
Critical valvular stenosis
Acute mitral or aortic regurgitation
Calcium channel blocker or β-blocker overdose

they also improve cardiac output by means of decreasing SVR. Vasodilators are indicated **only to treat patients with adequate arterial pressure.**

(a) **Nitroglycerin.** IV nitroglycerin is the drug of choice among vasodilators because it is less likely to produce coronary steal and is antiischemic. The starting dose is 10 to 20 mg/min and is increased 10 mg/min every few minutes. Nitroglycerin is titrated to achieve an MAP of approximately 70 mm Hg.

(b) **Nitroprusside.** IV nitroprusside may be added if further reduction in afterload is warranted because nitroglycerin is predominantly a venodilator. Nitroprusside is started at 5 to 10 mg/kg per minute and is titrated to an MAP of approximately 70 mm Hg.

(2) **Angiotensin-converting enzyme (ACE) inhibitors** improve LV performance by means of reducing the cardiac preload and afterload of patients with heart failure and acute MI. ACE inhibitors should be instituted early in the care of patients with pulmonary congestion, particularly in those with hypertension. On the basis of the beneficial effects on infarct expansion in the International Study of Infarct Survival (ISIS-4) and Gruppo Italiano per lo Studio dell Streptochi-nasi nell'Inrarto Miocardico (GISSI-30) trials, early (<12 hours) initiation of captopril at 6.25 mg three times a day is recommended. The amount may be doubled with each subsequent dosage as tolerated, up to 50 mg every 8 hours. ACE inhibitors should not be given to patients with cardiogenic shock.

(3) **Diuretics.** Patients with mild pulmonary edema MI can be treated with diuretics such as furosemide. Furosemide is administered initially 20 mg IV for patients with normal creatinine levels. This can be followed with higher and repeated doses as needed.

(4) **Cardiac glycosides.** The use of digitalis glycosides in the setting of an acute MI should be **restricted** to treatment of patients with atrial fibrillation or atrial flutter or treatment of patients with heart failure that persists after appropriate therapy.

(5) **β-Adrenergic agonists.** Patients with severe heart failure and cardiogenic shock may need dopamine and dobutamine.

(a) **Dopamine** is started at a dose of 3 mg/kg per minute and increased gradually to a maximal dose of 20 mg/kg per minute.

(b) **Dobutamine** has positive inotropic action comparable with that of dopamine but is less chronotropic and may decrease afterload. Dobutamine is started at a dose of 2.5 mg/kg per minute and increased to a maximal dose of 30 mg/kg per minute.

(6) **Phosphodiesterase inhibitors. Milrinone,** a phosphodiesterase inhibitor with inotropic and vasodilator action, may be beneficial to some patients. Milrinone is given as a 50 mg/kg bolus over 10 minutes followed by an infusion of 0.375 to 0.75 mg/ kg per minute infusion. The bolus may be omitted in the care of patients with marginal blood pressures. Table 3-5 lists the hemodynamic effects of medications used to manage heart failure. Patients without adequate MAP may not tolerate milrinone.

(7) **Vasopressors.** Some patients may need norepinephrine to maintain arterial pressure. Norepinephrine is started at 2 mg/min and titrated to 20 mg/min to maintain an MAP of 70 to 75 mm Mg.

Table 3-5. Hemodynamic effects of medications used to manage heart failure

Medication	Preload ↓	Afterload ↓	Contractility	Vasoconstriction
Dopamine (medium dose)	–	–	+ +	–
Dopamine (high dose)	–	–	+ +	+ +
Dobutamine	+	+ +	+ + +	–
Milrinone	+ +	+ +	+ + +	–
Nitroglycerin	+ + +	+	–	–
Nitroprusside	+ + +	+ + +	–	–

Decrease; –, no effect; +, little effect; + +, moderate effect; + + +, great effect.

    c. Percutaneous therapy
        (1) IABP. An IABP should be inserted as soon as possible in a patient with cardiogenic shock. It reduces afterload, improves cardiac output, and decreases the myocardial oxygen requirement by means of reduction in wall stress.
        (2) Percutaneous transluminal coronary angioplasty (PTCA). Percutaneous intervention of the infarction-related artery has been associated with a good prognosis among patients with cardiogenic shock; the approximate reduction in the mortality rate is from 80% to 50%. In most studies, investigators performed PTCA on the infarction-related artery only. Some investigators, however, reported multivessel PTCA with more complete revascularization. Considering the dismal prognosis among patients with acute MI and cardiogenic shock, immediate percutaneous revascularization should be considered.
    d. Surgical therapy
        (1) Emergency surgical revascularization is indicated in the care of patients with severe multivessel disease or substantial left main coronary artery stenosis.
        (2) Other surgical modalities that may be used include use of LV or biventricular assist devices or extracorporeal membrane oxygenation as a bridge to heart transplantation. Some patients may gradually discontinue use of assist devices after recovery of the stunned portion of myocardium.
  F. RV pump failure. Mild RV dysfunction is common after MI of the inferior wall; however, hemodynamically significant RV impairment occurs among only 10% of patients with inferior wall MI.
    1. Clinical presentation
        a. Signs and symptoms. The triad of hypotension, jugular venous distention with clear lungs, and absence of dyspnea is highly specific but has poor sensitivity for RV infarction. Patients with severe RV failure have symptoms of a **low cardiac output state,** which includes diaphoresis, cool, clammy extremities, and altered mental status. Patients often have oliguria and hypotension. Table 3-6 lists the causes of hypotension among patients with inferior wall MI.
        b. Physical findings. Patients with RV failure without concomitant LV failure have elevated jugular venous pressure and RV S_3, with clear lungs. The presence of **jugular venous pressure >8 cm water and Kussmaul's sign** (inspiratory increase in jugular venous pressure) is sensitive and specific for severe RV failure.
    2. Pathophysiology. RV involvement depends on the location of the right coronary artery occlusion. Marked dysfunction occurs only if occlusion

Table 3-6. Causes of hypotension among patients with inferior myocardial infarction

Severe right ventricular infarction
Bradyarrythmia
Acute severe mitral regurgitation
Prior myocardial infarction
Left ventricular subacute rupture
Ventricular septal rupture
Bezold-Jarisch reflex

is proximal to the acute marginal branch. The degree of RV involvement also depends on whether collateral flow from the LAD is present and the extent of blood flow through the thebesian veins. The right ventricle is a thin-walled chamber that has low oxygen demand with coronary perfusion during the entire cardiac cycle; therefore extensive irreversible infarction is rare.

3. **Laboratory examination**
   a. An **ECG** usually shows inferior MI. ST elevation in V_4R in the setting of suspected RV infarction has a positive predictive value of 80%. ST-segment elevation exceeding 1 mm may be seen in V_1 and occasionally in V_2 and V_3 (Fig. 3-2).
   b. A chest radiograph usually is normal; there is no evidence of pulmonary congestion.
4. **Diagnostic testing**
   a. Echocardiography is the diagnostic **study of choice** for RV infarction. It shows RV dilatation, severe RV dysfunction, and usually LV inferior wall dysfunction. It is also helpful in excluding cardiac tamponade, which may mimic RV infarction.
   b. Cardiac catheterization. Hemodynamic monitoring with a PA catheter usually reveals high right atrial pressures with low PCWP. Acute RV failure results in underfilling of the left ventricle and a low cardiac output state. The PCWP usually is low unless severe LV dysfunction is present. In some patients, RV dilatation can cause decreased LV performance on the basis of poor filling. As the right ventricle dilates, flattening or bowing of the septum into the left ventricle develops and restricts ventricular filling and elevation of PCWP. A right arterial pressure greater than 10 mm Hg and right arterial pressure to PCWP ratio of 0.8 or more strongly suggest RV infarction (5).
5. **Therapy**
   a. Medical therapy
      (1) Fluid administration. Management of RV infarction involves volume loading to increase preload and cardiac output. Some patients may need as mush as several liters in 1 hour. **Hemodynamic monitoring is crucial** because overzealous fluid administration to a patient with severe RV dilatation can further decrease LV preload and cardiac output. (The septum shifts toward the left ventricle and intrapericardial pressure shifts substantially.) The target central venous pressure for fluid administration is approximately 15 mm Hg.
      (2) Inotropes. When volume loading fails to increase cardiac output, use of inotropes is indicated. Administration of **dobutamine markedly increases cardiac index** and RV ejection fraction and is superior to afterload reduction with nitroprusside.
   b. Percutaneous therapy
      (1) Patients who undergo successful reperfusion of RV branches have improved RV function and decreased 30-day mortality (6).
      (2) AV sequential pacing may markedly improve the condition of a patient with RV infarction, bradyarrhythmias, or loss of

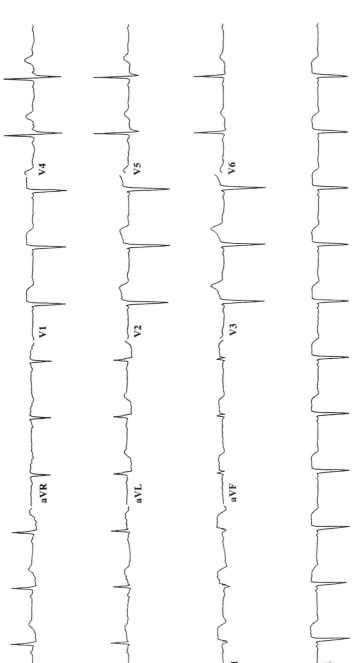

FIG. 3-2. Electrocardiogram shows acute inferior myocardial infarction with right ventricular involvement.

sinus rhythm. A longer AV delay of approximately 200 msec and a heart rate of 80 to 90 beats per minute is usually optimal for these patients.

    (3) An **IABP** may be useful even though it acts primarily on the left ventricle.

    (4) Most patients with RV infarction spontaneously improve after 48 to 72 hours if they survive the acute phase.

  c. Surgical therapy

    (1) Pericardiectomy may be considered in the care of patients with refractory shock.

    (2) An **RV assist device** is indicated in the care of patients who remain in cardiogenic shock in spite of the foregoing measures.

G. Ventricular aneurysm

  1. Clinical presentation

    a. Signs and symptoms

      (1) Acute aneurysms. Acute development of a large LV aneurysm can result in severe congestive heart failure and even cardiogenic shock. Patients with an acute MI that involves the apex of the left ventricle, particularly those with transmural anteroapical infarcts, are at greatest risk. Acute aneurysms expand during systole. The expansion wastes contractile energy generated by normal myocardium and puts the entire ventricle at a mechanical disadvantage.

      (2) Chronic aneurysms, which persist more than 6 weeks after the MI, are less compliant than acute aneurysms and rarely expand during systole. They occur among 10% to 30% of patients after MI, especially MI involving the anterior wall. Patients with chronic aneurysms may have heart failure, ventricular arrhythmias, and systemic embolism, or they may have no symptoms.

    b. Physical findings. A **dyskinetic segment of the ventricle** may be apparent during inspection or may be felt during palpation. S_3 **gallop sounds** may be heard in patients with poor ventricular function.

  2. Pathophysiology. Expansion of infarction and progressive LV dilatation are associated with occlusion of an infarction-related artery, and inhibition of LV dilatation is associated with an open infarction-related artery. The **early open artery hypothesis** is that early reperfusion results in myocardial salvage and inhibits infarct expansion. Late reperfusion limits infarct expansion through multiple mechanisms, including immediate change in infarction characteristics, preservation of small amounts of residual myofibrils and interstitial collagen, accelerated healing, and the scaffold effect of a blood-filled vasculature.

  3. Diagnostic testing

    a. ECG

      (1) Acute aneurysms. ECG reveals evidence of ST-elevation MI, which may persist despite evidence of reperfusion.

      (2) Chronic aneurysms. ST elevation that persists longer than 6 weeks occurs among patients with chronic ventricular aneurysms.

    b. A **chest radiograph** may reveal a localized bulge in the cardiac silhouette.

    c. Echocardiography is the diagnostic test of choice and accurately depicts the aneurysmal segment. It also shows the presence of a mural thrombus. Echocardiography is useful in differentiating true aneurysms and pseudoaneurysm. True aneurysms have a wide neck, whereas pseudoaneurysms have a narrow neck in relation to the diameter of the aneurysm.

    d. Cardiac **magnetic resonance imaging** also depicts the aneurysm.

4. **Therapy**
    a. **Medical therapy**
        (1). **Acute aneurysm.** Heart failure with acute aneurysms is managed with IV vasodilators and an IABP. ACE inhibitors have been shown to reduce infarct expansion and progressive LV remodeling. Because infarct expansion starts early, ACE inhibitors should be started within the first 24 hours of the onset of acute MI.
        (2) **Chronic aneurysm.** Heart failure with chronic aneurysms is managed with ACE inhibitors, digoxin, and diuretics.
        (3) **Anticoagulation**
            (a) Anticoagulation with **warfarin sodium** is indicated for patients with a mural thrombus. Patients are initially treated with IV heparin with a target partial thromboplastin time (PTT) of 50 to 65 seconds. Warfarin is started simultaneously. Patients should be treated with warfarin with a target international normalized ratio of 2 to 3 for 3 to 6 months.
            (b) It is **controversial whether patients with large aneurysms without thrombus should receive anticoagulants.** Many clinicians prescribe anticoagulants for 6 to 12 weeks after the acute phase.
            (c) Patients with LV aneurysms and a low global ejection fraction (<40%) have a higher stroke rate and should take anticoagulants for at least 3 months after the acute event. They may be subsequently observed with echocardiography. Anticoagulation is reinitiated if a thrombus develops.
    b. **Percutaneous therapy**
        (1) A patent infarction-related artery has beneficial effects on LV remodeling that are independent of myocardial salvage (decreased 1-year mortality, decreased LV dilatation, and expansion). These patients may be candidates for **late reperfusion with percutaneous intervention** (>12 hours but <24 hours). There are no data to suggest benefit with percutaneous intervention after 24 hours.
        (2) **Implantation** of an implantable cardioverter defibrillator is indicated in the care of patients with chronic aneurysms and intractable ventricular arrhythmias that cannot be controlled with medication.
    c. **Surgical therapy.** Patients with refractory heart failure and refractory ventricular arrhythmias should be considered for surgical resection. Surgical resection may be followed by either conventional closure or newer techniques (inverted T closure, endocardial patch) to maintain LV geometry. Revascularization is beneficial to patients with a large amount of viable myocardium in the aneurysmal segment.

III. **Complications of arrhythmia.** Arrhythmias are the most common complications after acute MI. They affect approximately 90% of patients who have had an MI (see Chapters 19 through 24).

IV. **Ischemic complications**
    A. **Clinical presentation**
        1. **Infarct extension** is a progressive increase in the amount of myocardial necrosis within the same arterial territory as the original MI. This may manifest itself as subendocardial MI that extends to transmural MI or as MI that extends and involves the adjacent myocardium.
            a. Patients usually have continuous or recurrent **chest pain,** new **ECG changes,** and prolonged elevations in creatine kinase (CK) level.
            b. **Echocardiography** or **nuclear imaging** helps confirm the diagnosis by showing a larger infarct than was seen immediately after the MI.

     c. Reinfarction occurs more frequently when the infarction-related artery reoccludes than when it remains patent; however, reocclusion of the infarction-related artery does not always cause reinfarction. After thrombolytic therapy, reocclusion is found on angiograms of 5% to 30% of patients and is associated with a poor outcome.

2. Postinfarction angina

     a. Recurrent angina within a few hours to 30 days after acute MI is defined as postinfarction angina. The incidence is between 23% and 60%. The frequency of postinfarction angina is higher after non-Q-wave MI and after administration of thrombolytic agents than after PTCA.

     b. Patients with postinfarction angina have a worse prognosis in regard to sudden death, reinfarction, and acute cardiac events.

     c. The pathophysiologic mechanism of postinfarction angina is similar to that of unstable angina and should be managed as such.

3. Reinfarction

     a. Infarction in a separate territory (recurrent infarction) may be difficult to diagnose in the first 24 to 48 hours after the initial event. Infarct extension and infarction in a separate territory may be difficult to differentiate.

       (1) It may be very difficult to delineate the ECG changes of reinfarction from the evolving ECG changes of the index MI.

       (2) Rapidly rising and falling markers of MI such as **CK** are more useful in diagnosing reinfarction than are troponins. Recurrent elevations in CK MB after its normalization or to greater than 50% of the prior value are regarded as the standard for reinfarction.

       (3) **Echocardiography** reveals a wall motion abnormality in a new area.

B. Therapy

     1. Medical therapy. Aggressive medical therapy with aspirin, heparin, nitrates, and β-blockers is indicated in the care of patients who have had MI and have ongoing ischemia.

     2. Percutaneous therapy

       a. An **IABP** should be promptly inserted in patients with hypotension and those with severe LV systolic dysfunction.

       b. Urgent **coronary angiography** with percutaneous intervention is indicated after stabilization with medical therapy or as an emergency if the patient's condition is unstable or the patient has refractory chest pain. Percutaneous or surgical revascularization improves the prognosis among these patients.

V. Embolic complications. The incidence of clinically evident systemic embolism after MI is approximately 2%. The incidence is higher among patients with anterior wall MI. The overall incidence of mural thrombus after MI is approximately 20%. Large anterior MI may be accompanied by mural thrombus among 60% of patients.

A. Clinical presentation

     1. Signs and symptoms. The most common clinical presentation of embolic complications is **stroke,** although patients may have limb ischemia, renal infarction, and intestinal ischemia. Most episodes of systemic emboli occur in the first 10 days after acute MI.

     2. Physical findings. The physical findings depend on the site of embolism.

       a. Patients with stroke have a neurologic deficit.

       b. Embolism to the peripheral circulation causes limb ischemia, which makes the extremity cold, pulseless, and painful.

       c. Renal infarctions may cause hematuria and flank pain.

       d. Mesenteric ischemia causes abdominal pain and bloody diarrhea.

B. Therapy

     1. IV heparin is administered for 3 or 4 days to a target PTT of 50 to 65 seconds to patients with large anterior MI or mural thrombi.

2. **Oral warfarin sodium therapy** should be continued for at least 3 months for patients with mural thrombi and those with large akinetic areas detected at echocardiography.
3. In one study patients with a large MI treated with **heparin followed by oral anticoagulation** (international normalized ratio 2 to 3) for 1 month had a decrease from 3% to 1% in the incidence of cerebral emboli.

VI. Pericarditis

A. **Early pericarditis.** The incidence of early pericarditis after acute MI is approximately 10%. The inflammation usually develops 24 to 96 hours after MI (7).

1. **Clinical presentation.** Early pericarditis occurs among patients with transmural MI. Most of these patients have no symptoms, although transient pericardial friction rubs may be audible in some patients.

   a. **Signs and symptoms**
      (1) Patients report progressive, severe chest pain that lasts for hours. The **pain is postural,** worse when the patient is supine, and is alleviated if the patient sits up and leans forward. The pain usually is pleuritic in nature and is worsened with deep inspiration, coughing, and swallowing.
      (2) **Radiation of pain to the trapezius ridge is nearly pathognomonic** for acute pericarditis and does not occur among patients with ischemic pain. The pain also may radiate to the neck and less frequently to the arm or back.

   b. **Physical findings.** The presence of a **pericardial friction rub is pathognomonic** for acute pericarditis; however, it can be evanescent.
      (1) The rub is best heard at the **left lower sternal edge** with the diaphragm of the stethoscope.
      (2) The **rub has three components,** a component each in atrial systole, ventricular systole, and ventricular diastole. In about 30% of patients, the rub is biphasic, and in 10% it is uniphasic.
      (3) The development of pericardial effusion may cause fluctuation in the intensity of the rub, although the rub may still be heard in spite of substantial pericardial effusion.

2. **Etiology and pathophysiology.** Pericarditis is caused by an area of localized pericardial inflammation overlying the infarcted myocardium. The inflammation is fibrinous in nature. The development of an evanescent pericardial rub correlates with a larger infarct and hemodynamic derangements.

3. **Laboratory examination and diagnostic testing**
   a. An **ECG** is the most useful test in the diagnosis of pericarditis; however, evolving ECG changes may make the diagnosis difficult among patients who have had MI. Unlike ischemia, in which the changes are limited to a particular territory, pericarditis produces generalized ECG changes.
      (1) The ST-segment elevation seen with pericarditis is concave upward or saddle-shaped.
      (2) In pericarditis, T waves become inverted after the ST segment becomes isoelectric, whereas in acute MI, T waves may become inverted when the ST segment is still elevated.
      (3) Four phases of ECG abnormality have been described in association with pericarditis (Table 3-7).
   b. Chest radiography is of limited value in the diagnosis of pericarditis.
   c. **Echocardiography** may reveal pericardial effusion, which is strongly suggestive of pericarditis, although the absence of effusion does not rule out the diagnosis.

4. **Therapy**
   a. **Aspirin** is used to manage post-MI pericarditis in doses of 650 mg every 4 to 6 hours.

Table 3-7. ECG changes of pericarditis

Stage I	ST elevation, upright T waves
Stage II	ST elevation resolves, upright to flat T waves
Stage III	ST isoelectric, inverted T waves
Stage IV	ST isoelectric, upright T waves

      b. Nonsteroidal antiinflammatory agents and corticosteroids should not be used to treat these patients. These agents may interfere with myocardial healing and contribute to infarct expansion (8).

      c. Colchicine may be beneficial to patients with recurrent pericarditis.

B. Late pericarditis (Dressler's syndrome). The incidence of Dressler's syndrome is between 1% and 3%. The syndrome occurs 1 to 8 weeks after MI. The pathogenesis is not known, but an autoimmune mechanism has been suggested.

    1. Clinical presentation. Patients have chest discomfort that suggests pericarditis, pleuritic chest pain, fever, arthralgia, malaise, an elevated leukocyte count, and an elevated sedimentation rate. Echocardiography may reveal pericardial effusion.

    2. Therapy is similar to that for early post-MI pericarditis: **aspirin and avoidance of nonsteroidal antiinflammatory drugs and corticosteroids.** However, if more than 4 weeks have elapsed since the MI, nonsteroidal agents, and even steroids, may be indicated for severe symptoms.

SUGGESTED READINGS

References
1. Fox AC, Glassman E, Isom OW. Surgically remediable complications of myocardial infarction. *Prog Cardiovasc Dis* 1979;21:4612–4615.
2. Killip T, Kimball JT. Treatment of myocardial infarction in a coronary care unit: a two year experience with 250 patients. *Am J Cardiol* 1967;20:457–461.
3. Holmes DR Jr, Bates ER, Kleiman NS, et al. for the GUSTO-I investigators. Contemporary reperfusion therapy for cardiogenic shock: the GUSTO-I trial experience. *J Am Coll Cardiol* 1995;26:668–674.
4. Forrester JS, Diamond GA, Chatterjee K. Medical therapy of acute myocardial infarction by application of hemodynamic subsets. *N Engl J Med* 1976;295:1356–1361.
5. Dell'Italia LJ, Starling MR. Right ventricular infarction: an important clinical entity. *Curr Probl Cardiol* 1984;9:1–58.
6. Bowers TR. Effect of reperfusion on biventricular function and survival after right ventricular infarction. *N Engl J Med* 1998;338:933–940.
7. Lichstein E. Early post-myocardial infarction pericarditis. *Pract Cardiol* 1982:8:60–66.
8. Berman J, Haffajee CI, Alpert JS. Therapy of symptomatic pericarditis after myocardial infarction: retrospective and prospective studies of aspirin, indomethacin, prednisone and spontaneous resolution. *Am Heart J* 1981;101:750–753.

Landmark Article
Chatterjee K. Complications of acute myocardial infarction. *Curr Probl Cardiol* 1993;18:1–79.

Key Reviews
O'Donnell L. Complications of MI beyond the acute stage. *Am J Nurs* 1996;96:25–31.
Reeder GS. Identification and treatment of complications of myocardial infarction. *Mayo Clin Proc* 1995;70:880–884.
Subramaniam PN. Complications of acute myocardial infarction. *Postgrad Med* 1994;95:143–148.

Relevant Book Chapter
Topol EJ, ed. *Textbook of cardiovascular medicine.* Philadelphia: Lippincott—Raven, 1997.

4. POST–MYOCARDIAL INFARCTION RISK STRATIFICATION AND MANAGEMENT

Elaine K. Moen

I. **Introduction.** More than 1 million myocardial infarctions (MIs) occur in the United States every year. Although the mortality following acute MI has decreased, morbidity remains considerable. The task of the physician is to initiate **risk factor modification, lipid-lowering therapy, smoking cessation,** and other interventions during the hospitalization phase of recovery after MI. Some therapies, such as **β-blockade,** are still widely underprescribed, whereas others, such as cardiac catheterization for otherwise healthy patients with small infarctions, are relatively overprescribed. **No trials have defined what the ideal post-MI regimen should be** or the length of time that patients should be treated. Some subsets of the population may not benefit from a given therapy.

II. **Risk stratification.** Post-MI risk stratification is used to ascertain which patients are at high **risk for subsequent cardiovascular events and who will benefit from revascularization.** All patients who have had an MI should **undertake aggressive modification of their risk factors.** The guidelines for therapy that has been shown to be of benefit are presented herein; however, therapy must be individualized and polypharmacy avoided. Fig. 4-1. provides algorithms that summarize the risk stratification process. The main goal of risk stratification is **ascertaining whether a patient is at risk for subsequent events,** because the patient may benefit from revascularization and other interventions.

   A. The **age** of the patient is the most important predictor of mortality after MI. Many studies have shown that a more aggressive approach is taken in the care of younger patients who have a very low mortality overall (less than 4% in some studies). Older patients, however, are at greater risk and may gain the most benefit from interventions.

   B. **Assessment of left ventricular (LV) function**
      1. LV function is the second most important predictor of mortality after MI. Studies have shown an inverse relation between LV ejection fraction (LVEF) and mortality. Patients with an LVEF less than 40% have a substantially greater mortality than patients with a higher LVEF.
      2. Assessment of LV function is indicated for all patients who have had an MI.
         a. Patients are considered at high risk if they have marked LV dysfunction after MI (LVEF less than 40%) or multiple wall motion abnormalities. **Cardiac catheterization** should be performed to ascertain whether the patient might benefit from revascularization.
         b. Radionuclide angiography, echocardiography, or left ventriculography during cardiac catheterization is useful in evaluating LV function. **No imaging method has been shown to be superior** to the others. Cost, availability, and expertise are considered when choosing which procedure to use.
         c. LV dysfunction is an indication for initiation of **angiotensin converting enzyme (ACE) inhibitor** therapy after MI.

   C. **Assessment of residual ischemia.** The extent of coronary artery disease and the presence of recurrent or residual ischemia are two other strong predictors of mortality among patients who have had an MI. Predischarge **stress testing** can be used for noninvasive assessment of the degree of exercise-induced ischemia.
      1. **The optimal test for risk stratification is an exercise stress test,** because it provides considerable prognostic information. Exercise testing

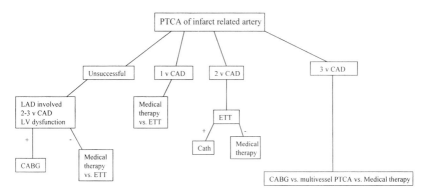

FIG. 4-1. A: Suggested algorithm for post–myocardial infarction (MI) risk stratification for patients undergoing percutaneous transluminal coronary angioplasty, excluding patients with cardiogenic shock or mechanical complications. *CAD,* Coronary artery disease; *v,* vessel; *CABG,* coronary artery bypass grafting; *LV,* left ventricle; *LAD,* left anterior descending artery; Cath, catheterization; *ETT,* exercise treadmill test.

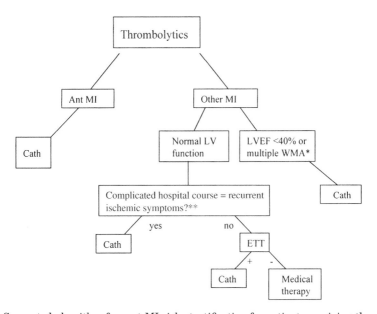

B: Suggested algorithm for post-MI risk stratification for patients receiving thrombolytic agents, excluding patients with cardiogenic shock or mechanical complications. *Ant MI,* Anterior myocardial infarction; LV, left ventricle; *Cath,* catheterization; *LVEF,* left ventricular ejection fraction; *WMA,* wall motion abnormalities.

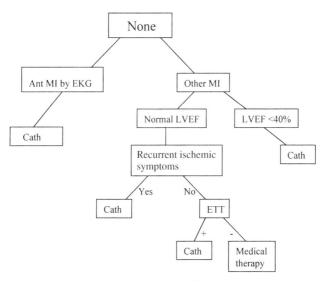

FIG. 1. *Continued* **C:** Suggested algorithm for post-MI risk stratification for patients not receiving primary revascularization therapy, excluding patients with cardiogenic shock or mechanical complications. *Ant MI,* Anterior myocardial infarction; *EKG,* electrocardiogram; *Cath,* catheterization; *LVEF,* left ventricular ejection fraction.

also is useful for assessment of functional capacity, and the results can guide postdischarge activity level. (Before thrombolytic agents became available, exercise stress testing was recommended before discharge for all patients with uncomplicated MI. Coronary angiography now is so widely used that exercise stress testing today is seldom performed in many hospitals. The mortality among patients treated with thrombolytic therapy is low, 1% to 2% in the first year; therefore the positive predictive value of stress testing is low.)

2. The addition of **echocardiography** or **radionuclide imaging** is required for risk stratification of patients who cannot exercise or who have uninterpretable electrocardiograms (ECGs) because of LV hypertrophy, intraventricular conduction delays, or digoxin-induced ST-T wave changes. Stress echocardiography and radionuclide imaging increase the sensitivity and specificity for detection of coronary disease for these two groups of patients. Dobutamine, adenosine, and dipyridamole have been used with either echocardiography or radionuclide imaging, and all have been demonstrated to be safe for use after MI.

3. **American College of Cardiology and American Heart Association (ACC/AHA) guidelines** recommend either a submaximal exercise stress test for all patients with uncomplicated MI who have not undergone coronary angiography before discharge or a symptom-limited stress test 3 weeks after discharge. The timing of the stress test is somewhat controversial. Some cardiologists recommend symptom-limited stress testing as early as the first week after MI. Others wait until 3 weeks after MI. Both approaches have been found to be safe for patients who have had an MI. Patients who achieve at least 3 MET have a good prognosis. Inability to achieve 3 MET, hypotension during exercise, or marked ST-segment depression or elevation is an indication for coronary angiography.

III. **Therapy after MI**
   A. **Coronary angiography** and late **percutaneous transluminal coronary angioplasty (PTCA)**
      1. **Indications**
         a. Clear indications for coronary angiography among patients who have had an MI are postinfarction angina or recurrent infarction; failed thrombolysis; and congestive heart failure, mechanical complications, or hemodynamic instability.
         b. Whether patients should undergo routine cardiac catheterization after thrombosis in uncomplicated cases has been evaluated in many trails (Table 4-1).
         c. Results of nonrandomized studies have demonstrated that **coronary patency after MI is an important predictor of subsequent mortality** (also known as the **open-artery hypothesis**). Patients who have had an MI with an occluded artery have increased LV dilatation, more spontaneous and induced arrhythmias, and a worse prognosis than patients who have had an MI but have patent infarction-related arteries. All the factors may be related to adverse LV remodeling after MI. No randomized, controlled clinical trials of late PTCA after MI have been conducted to firmly established the benefit of this approach.
         d. Patients who have **evidence of ischemia** on noninvasive stress testing are at increased **risk for reinfarction or death.** All such patients should undergo **coronary angiography and revascularization** of the arteries that supply the ischemic bed if they are suitable candidates for coronary artery bypass grafting (CABG) or PTCA. LV function is a powerful predictor of outcome after MI. Patients with impaired LV function (LVEF less than 40%) are more likely to have multivessel disease and would likely derive a survival benefit from coronary revascularization. All such patients should undergo coronary angiography.
         e. Coronary angiography is recommended **before surgical intervention to correct mechanical complications of MI,** such as acute mitral regurgitation caused by papillary muscle rupture, ventricular septal defect, or LV aneurysm. Angiography is used to define any potential areas for revascularization and to further assess the mechanical problem, if necessary. In rare instances, hemodynamic instability precludes coronary angiography before an operation, and the surgeon may use saphenous vein grafts to bypass all or selective coronary arteries.
      2. **Contraindication.** Catheterization should not be performed on patients who are not candidates for surgical or percutaneous revascularization because of severe comorbid conditions or personal preference.
      3. **Controversy.** There is substantial evidence that **not all patients who have sustained acute MI need to undergo coronary angiography.** Most post-MI angiography procedures are performed on patients without symptoms who have sustained an uncomplicated MI. These patients generally have a good long-term prognosis. Many cardiologists, however, advocate catheterization for all patients after MI. Catheterization and primary catheter-based reperfusion are discussed in Chapter 1.
   B. **CABG after MI.** CABG after MI can be divided into two categories: emergency and elective.
      1. **Emergency CABG.** The indications and management considerations for emergency CABG are discussed in Chapter 1.
      2. **Elective CABG.** Studies have clearly demonstrated a survival benefit for CABG among patients with left main or severe three-vessel coronary artery disease, especially among patients with decreased LV function. Patients with proximal stenosis of the left anterior descending coronary artery and two-vessel coronary disease or two-vessel disease with

Table 4-1. Analysis of trials of conservative versus routine invasive strategies 48 hours after thrombolytic therapy

Study	Time to angioplasty (hr)	No. of patients enrolled	Mortality rate (%) Conservative	Mortality rate (%) Invasive	Bleeding rate (%) Conservative	Bleeding rate (%) Invasive
TIMI IIB	18–48	3,162	7.4	6.9	12.7 (transfusions)	15.5
European Cooperative	Immediate	367	8.9	10.5	23.0	41.0
SWIFT	3–48	800	5.0	5.8	16.1	19.9
TAMI	Immediate	386	1.0	4.0	— (all patients)	42

TIMI, Thrombolysis in Myocardial Infarction; *SWIFT*, Should We Intervene Following Thrombolysis?; *TAMI*, **Thrombolysis and Angioplasty in Myocardial Infarction.**

From Stempien-Otero A, Weaver DW. Post-myocardial infarction management. In Topol EJ, ed: *Textbook of cardiovascular medicine.* Philadelphia: Lippincott-Raven, 1998:481–502.

decreased LVEF may benefit from elective CABG. No prospective, randomized trials have been performed to determine the optimal timing of elective CABG after MI. Results of most studies, however, suggest that **CABG 3 to 7 days after MI is associated with a low operative mortality** (similar to that for elective CABG among patients without recent infarction).

3. **Operative risk** increases among patients with low LVEF, advanced age, or multiple comorbid conditions and those undergoing an emergency operation. Reoperations on patients who have undergone bypass surgery are associated with a higher operative mortality.

IV. Secondary prevention

A. **Smoking cessation is mandatory** for all patients who have had an MI. Smoking doubles the rate of reinfarction and death after MI, causes coronary artery spasm, and reduces the effectiveness of β-blocker therapy after MI. The reduction in risk after smoking cessation is rapid. Within 3 years it approaches that among survivors of MI who never smoked. One third to one half of all patients who stop smoking after MI start smoking again 6 to 12 months after MI. Many approaches to smoking cessation have been attempted, including pharmacologic therapy, formal smoking cessation programs, hypnosis, and abstinence.

1. **Nicotine substitutes,** such as patches, chewing gum, nasal spray, or inhalers, can deliver 30% to 60% of the nicotine of cigarettes. Although it is not recommended for the acute phase of MI, use of these agents is safe in later phases. Patients who start smoking again should discontinue use of nicotine substitutes.

2. Other agents, such as **clonidine** and **bupropion,** have been shown to increase the number of patients who abstain from smoking. Bupropion appears to be an effective agent to aid in smoking cessation. The initial dosage is 150 mg by mouth every day for 3 days then 150 mg by mouth twice a day for 7 to 12 weeks. Patients should aim to stop smoking 1 to 2 weeks into therapy.

3. **Recommendations.** Physicians can aid patients in the effort to stop smoking by using a stepped approach with education and a firm recommendation to quit smoking, devising a plan, and reinforcement of efforts to quit. Patients likely to relapse are older, less educated, or heavy smokers. Formal smoking cessation programs have been shown to have high rates of patient abstinence.

B. **Lipid management**

1. **Low-density lipoprotein (LDL).** Most patients with acute MI have abnormal lipid profiles. Several large secondary prevention trials have demonstrated that **lowering of lipids can reduce the incidence of future mortality and reinfarction** (1–3).

   a. **Diagnostic testing.** All patients who have had an MI should have a complete lipid panel (total cholesterol, LDL cholesterol, high-density lipoprotein [HDL] cholesterol, and triglycerides) determined within 24 hours of admission. If this is not possible, a random cholesterol level can be measured immediately and a complete lipid profile determined 4 weeks after MI.

   b. **Therapy.** Current ACC/AHA guidelines recommend that **all patients should start the AHA step II diet** (less than 7% of total calories as saturated fat and less than 200 mg/d cholesterol). If LDL cholesterol levels remain higher than 125 mg/dL, **drug therapy should be instituted with the goal of achieving a LDL cholesterol level less than 100 mg/dL.** Given that adherence to the step II diet is low and that repeat cardiac events occur frequently, **all patients should start drug therapy immediately.** Drug therapy usually is initiated with a 3-hydroxy-3-methylglutaryl coenzyme A (HMG-CoA) reductase inhibitor. Other agents that can be used include bile-acid sequestrants or niacin. In view of the Helsinki

Primary Prevention Trial results that showed a trend toward more clinical events among patients receiving gemfibrozil than among those in the placebo group, **gemfibrozil should be avoided** (4). Other therapies, including stress reduction classes, moderate alcohol consumption (particularly red wine), and exercise, have been shown to decrease LDL cholesterol levels.

2. **HDL.** About 25% of patients with acute MI have low HDL levels and normal cholesterol levels. The finding of **a low HDL level on a lipid panel is an independent risk factor for MI.** Consideration can be given to **exercise, niacin, or estrogen therapy** (for women) in an effort to raise HDL levels.

3. **Triglycerides.** Hypertriglyceridemia alone has not been shown to be an independent risk factor for coronary artery disease; however, it usually is accompanied by low HDL levels or diabetes. **Therapy:** There are **few data to support drug therapy** to manage hypertriglyceridemia, and the results are confounded by low HDL levels. **Niacin and atorvastatin can lower elevated triglycerides.**

C. **Antiplatelet therapy**

1. All patients who have had an MI should continue to take **aspirin** unless there are absolute contraindications. The use of aspirin after MI has resulted in a reduction in mortality of 25 lives per 1000 patients treated. Aspirin therapy after MI has been shown to reduce the rates of vascular mortality, nonfatal stroke, and nonfatal MI. **Patients who take ticlopidine or clopidogrel after stent implantation should continue taking aspirin,** because there is evidence that the benefit of aspirin may be based on an antiinflammatory effect in addition to the effect on platelet function and adhesion.

2. **Other medications.** Sulfinpyrazone and dipyridamole are not recommended for use by patients who have had an MI. They have been tested in clinical trials but have not been found to be more efficacious than aspirin alone. **Ticlopidine** (250 mg by mouth twice a day) and **clopidogrel** (75 mg/d) are reasonable alternatives for patients who have true aspirin allergies. Clopidogrel is favored for long-term administration because of the greater incidence of hematologic dyscrasia associated with ticlopidine.

D. **Warfarin sodium** is recommended for use by patients who have had an MI who are **unable to take aspirin,** have chronic or **persistent atrial fibrillation,** or have **LV thrombosis.**

1. Patients with a large anterior infarction and LV thrombosis treated with warfarin sodium are at decreased risk for embolic stroke. Randomized trials of this approach have not been done; however, many physicians recommend 6 weeks of warfarin sodium therapy for patients with evidence of LV thrombus on two-dimensional echocardiograms to assist in stabilization and endothelialization of the thrombus.

2. **Controversy.** The use of warfarin sodium as opposed to aspirin for secondary prevention of reinfarction is controversial. The lower cost and more favorable side-effect profile make **aspirin alone the recommended antithrombotic regimen.**

E. **β-Blockers**

1. **Indications.** β-Blockers reduce mortality by means of reducing risk for both sudden and nonsudden cardiac death and reducing risk for nonfatal infarction. β-Blockers are antiischemic and antihypertensive and reduce LV wall stress. There is approximately 20% relative risk reduction in post-MI events with use of β-Blockers.

a. The **beneficial effects of β-blockers are greatest among patients who are at high risk,** such as patients with anterior infarction, previous infarction, complex ventricular ectopy, advanced age, and LV dysfunction. The mortality benefit seems to extend to patients who have undergone reperfusion with thrombolytic therapy or primary angioplasty. Several studies have found that only 50% of patients who have had an MI actually receive β-blockers, despite the proved benefits. **β-Blockers should be started within 24 hours in the care of all patients who have had an MI** who are in hemodynamically stable condition and should be continued indefinitely. Moderate LV dysfunction and compensated congestive heart failure are not contraindications to β-treatment.

    b. β-Blockers without intrinsic sympathomimetic activity, such as metoprolol, propranolol, timolol, and atenolol, appear to have the greatest benefit. Reduction in heart rate seems to be important in achieving a mortality benefit.

  2. Contraindications. Relative contraindications include second- or third-degree heart block, severe asthma, severe chronic obstructive pulmonary disease, severe congestive heart failure, a heart rate less than 60 beats/min, and severe peripheral vascular disease. Diabetes is not an absolute contraindication; however, patients with diabetes who have frequent or severe hypoglycemic episodes may have to discontinue or reduce the dosage of the β-blocker.

F. ACE inhibitors

  1. Indications. The process of ventricular remodeling can be attenuated through the use of ACE inhibitors, which hinder ventricular dilatation and development of congestive heart failure. During infarction, the expression of ACE increases within the myocardium. Several large, randomized clinical trials have demonstrated that ACE inhibitors reduce mortality. These trails include Survival and Ventricular Enlargement (SAVE) (5), Acute Infarction Ramipril Efficacy (AIRE) (6), Trandolapril Cardiac Evaluation (TRACE) (7), and Cooperative New Scandinavian Enalapril Survival Study (CONSENSUS II) (8). With the exception of CONSENSUS II, these trails demonstrated a consistent benefit for ACE inhibition among patients who had had an MI. The greatest benefit was found among patients with large areas of infarction, anterior infarction, and infarction that impaired LV function. The current recommendation is that **ACE inhibitor therapy be started for all patients with marked LV dysfunction** (EF less than 40%) as soon as their condition is stable with titration to full dose as tolerated.

  2. Side effects include cough, worsening renal function, hypotension, and angioedema.

G. Calcium channel blockers. The preferred agent after MI is a β-blocker unless there are true contraindications. Calcium channel blockers should be reserved for patients with **refractory angina,** if necessary, and the longer-acting preparations should be used. **ACC/AHA guidelines do not recommend** the use of calcium channel blockers after MI.

  1. Indications. The use of calcium channel blockers should be **limited to patients with ongoing ischemia or with rapid atrial arrhythmias and patients with clear contraindications to use of β-blockers,** such as severe asthma or chronic obstructive pulmonary disease.

  2. Contraindications. Calcium channel blockers should not be used to treat any patient who has had an MI and has evidence of congestive heart failure or atrioventricular block. There is evidence that the short-acting dihydropyridines, such as nifedipine, may increase the risk for death or reinfarction after MI. This finding is true for all patients, regardless of type of infarction (Q wave or non–Q wave) and whether or not thrombolytic therapy was given. Short-acting nifedipine may be especially harmful to patients with hypotension or tachycardia. It can induce coronary steal or reflex sympathetic activation and thereby increase myocardial oxygen demand.Verapamil and diltiazem are contraindicated in the care of patients with **LV dysfunction or congestive heart failure after MI.** Some trials have shown that these drugs may be useful to patients with non-Q-wave MI; however, the results are questionable in view of the increase in aspirin and β-blocker therapy. No data are available about the effect of the newer second-generation agents, amlodipine and felodipine on survival after MI.

H. Estrogen replacement therapy. The role of estrogen therapy after MI is controversial. Estrogen replacement therapy has beneficial effects on osteoporosis, skin tone, and sexuality, and it might reduce risk for development of Alzheimer's disease. Given the results of the Heart and Estrogen/progestin Replacement Study (HERS), it is not clear that there is any role for adding estrogen to a post-MI medical regimen (see Chapter 39). Concern has been raised regarding whether there is an increase in the incidence of breast cancer among patients undergoing estrogen replacement therapy. Because of this concern, many patients and physicians are reluctant to undertake hormone replacement therapy. Estrogens probably **should not be used by women with a personal or family history of breast cancer.**

I. Antioxidants. Previous epidemiologic studies have suggested that intake of vitamin E and β-carotene is associated with a lower incidence of coronary artery disease and acute MI. **Current guidelines do not support use of vitamins C or E or β-carotene for primary or secondary prevention.** Large, ongoing trials may provide answers.

V. Prevention of sudden cardiac death after MI (see also Chapter 21).

  A. Diagnosis

    1. The risk for sudden cardiac death after MI is greatest during the **first year.**

    2. **Reduced LV function** (less than 40%) remains the best predictor of mortality, even in the era of thrombolytic therapy.

    3. Several studies have suggested that patients with an **occluded infarction-related artery** have a markedly worse mortality than patients with a patent artery.

    4. Many studies have found that patients who have more than six **premature ventricular contractions** per hour have 60% increased risk for sudden cardiac death. Patients with ventricular fibrillation or sustained ventricular tachycardia more than 48 hours after MI also are at increased risk.

    5. Various techniques have been tested to ascertain which patients are at risk for sudden cardiac death; however, none is sensitive enough to be recommended for routine use. Signal-averaged ECG, heart rate variability, and baroreflex sensitivity are noninvasive, and all have low (less than 30%) positive predictive values. In the absence of proved treatment options, these modalities are not recommended for routine post-MI risk stratification. Invasive electrophysiologic testing has been used, but it also has a low predictive value for future cardiac events.

  B. Therapy

    1. The only drugs that have been proved to reduce risk for sudden cardiac death are β-blockers. There is an approximately 20% reduction in mortality with the use of β-blockers after MI. They should be prescribed to **all patients who have had an MI** in the absence of clear contraindications.

    2. **Other medications.** The use of type IC antiarrhythmic agents (encainide, flecainide, and propafenone) essentially has been eliminated after MI (9). Amiodarone has multiple antiarrhythmic effects but is primarily classified as a Class III agent. Trials of amiodarone in the care of patients who have had an MI and have an LVEF of 40% or less have shown conflicting results. This drug has not been shown to reduce all causes of death among patients who have had MI.

VI. Therapy and prevention after hospital treatment

  A. Achievement of treatment goals of exercise, weight loss, proper diet, and smoking cessation is supported by a **cardiac rehabilitation program.**

    1. Formal rehabilitation programs use **exercise and patient education** to help patients modify their lifestyles. The benefits of cardiac rehabilitation include improvement in commitment to treatment, increased

functional capacity, and reduced likelihood of readmission for recurrent ischemia. The **social support** offered is valuable; subsequent cardiac and all-cause mortality have been shown to be as much as 20% to 25% lower among patients with good social support than among other patients. Depression is common after MI and is an independent risk factor for mortality, possibly by decreasing commitment to therapy and exercise. Physicians should look for depression during follow-up visits.

2. **Home programs and family care.** Even though cardiac rehabilitation has been shown to have many benefits, less than half of patients who have had an MI participate in formal programs. Home programs may be helpful, but they do not provide the social network found in group rehabilitation programs. Because most cardiac arrests after MI occur within 18 months after discharge, family members should be encouraged to learn basic cardiopulmonary resuscitation (CPR).

B. Soon after receiving the diagnosis of MI, patients should be counseled regarding **lifestyle modification** to improve their risk factors. Areas that need improvement include weight control, diet, lipid control, exercise, and smoking cessation.

1. Optimum control of **hypertension and diabetes** should be achieved. The Diabetes Control and Complication Trial (DCCT) (10) and the United Kingdom Prospective Diabetes Study (UKPDS) (11) determined the need for strict glucose control of both type 1 and type II diabetes. Improvement in serum glucose levels decreases the progression of microvascular complications. In both trials there was a trend toward decreased microvascular events among the groups that received aggressive treatment.

2. **Weight reduction.** Among adults in the United States, one third of the population, or nearly 34 million persons, is overweight (defined as body mass index greater than 25 kg/m^2). Patients should be encouraged to achieve (or maintain) an ideal body weight. All patients should begin an AHA step I diet (8% to 10% of total calories from saturated fat, 30% or less of calories from total fat, less than 300 mg of cholesterol intake per day). The goal is achieving a LDL cholesterol level less than 100 mg/dL. Less than 50% of patients are able to comply with the step I diet, and many patients need pharmacologic therapy to manage hyperlipidemia (see earlier).

3. **Resumption of daily activities**

   a. At discharge, all patients who have had an MI should receive information regarding resumption of sexual activity, driving, return to work, and exercise.

   b. **Sexual activity** can be resumed within a week for most patients, as can **driving.** Most patients who have had an MI who do not have symptoms can **return to work** within 2 weeks.

   c. A patient's performance on an **exercise test** can be used to generate an activity prescription. Patients who can perform at least 5 MET on a submaximal exercise test without marked ST-segment depression or development of angina have a good long-term prognosis.

   d. Because of the lowered oxygen tension in most commercial aircraft (pressurized to 7500 to 8000 feet), only patients in stable condition should **travel by plane** within the first 2 weeks after MI. They should carry sublingual nitroglycerin and request wheelchair or cart transportation. For patients whose condition is complicated or unstable, air travel and driving should be delayed until symptoms resolve.

SUGGESTED READINGS

References
1. Scandinavian Simvastatin Survival Study Group. Randomized trial of cholesterol lowering in 4444 patients with coronary heart disease: the Scandinavian Simvastatin Survival Study (4S). *Lancet* 1994;344:1383–1389.

2. Sacks FM, Pfeffer MA, Moye LA, et al. for Cholesterol and Recurrent Events Trial Investigators. The effect of pravastatin on coronary events after myocardial infarction in patients with average cholesterol levels. *N Engl J Med* 1996;335:1001–1009.

3. Tonkin AM. Management of the long-term intervention with pravastatin in ischaemic disease (LIPID) study after the Scandinavian Simvastatin Survival Study (4S). *Am J Cardiol* 1995;76:107C–112C.

4. Frick MH, Elo O, Haapa K, et al. Helsinki Heart Study: primary prevention trial with gemfibrozil in middle-aged men with dyslipidemia—safety of treatment, changes in risk factors, and incidence of coronary heart disease. *N Engl J Med* 1987;317:1237–1245.

5. Pfeffer MA, Braunwald E, Moye LA, et al. Effect of captopril on mortality and morbidity in patients with left ventricular dysfunction after myocardial infarction: results of the Survival and Ventricular Enlargement trial the SAVE Investigators. *N Engl J Med* 1992;327:669–677.

6. The Acute Infarction Ramipril Efficacy (AIRE) Study Investigators. Effect of ramipril on mortality and morbidity of survivors of acute myocardial infarction with clinical evidence of heart failure. *Lancet* 1993;342:821–828.

7. Kober L, Torp-Pedersen C, Carlsen JE, et al. A clinical trial of the angiotensin-converting-enzyme inhibitor trandolapril in patients with left ventricular dysfunction after myocardial infarction. Trandolapril Cardiac Evaluation (TRACE) Study Group. *N Engl J Med* 1995;333:1670–1676.

8. Sigurdsson A, Swedberg K. Left ventricular remodeling, neurohormonal activation and early treatment with enalapril (CONSENSUS II) following myocardial infarction. *Eur Heart J* 1994;15[Suppl B]:14–19.

9. The Cardiac Arrhythmia Suppression Trial (CAST) Investigators. Preliminary report: effect of encainide and flecainide on mortality in a randomized trial of arrhythmia suppression after myocardial infarction. *N Engl J Med* 1989:321: 406–412.

10. The Diabetes Control and Complication Trial Research Group. The effect of intensive treatment of diabetes on the development and progression of long-term complications in insulin-dependent diabetes mellitus. *N Engl J Med* 1993;329: 977–986.

11. UKPDS Investigators. Intensive blood-glucose control with sulphonyl ureas or insulin compared with treatment and risk of complications in patients with type 2 diabetes (UKPO33). UK Prospective Diabetes Study (UKPDS). *Lancet* 1998; 352:873–853.

Landmark Articles

Bates ER, Califf RM, Stack RS, et al. Thrombolysis and Angioplasty in Myocardial Infarction (TAMI-I) trial: influence of infarct location on arterial patency, left ventricular function and mortality. *J Am Coll Cardiol* 1989;13:12–18.

CAPRIE Steering Committee. A randomized, blinded, trial of clopidogrel versus aspirin in patients at risk of ischaemic events (CAPRIE). *Lancet* 1996;348: 1329–1339.

First International Study of Infarct Survival Collaborative Group. Randomized trial of intravenous atenolol among 16,027 cases of suspected acute myocardial infarction—ISIS-I. *Lancet* 1986;2:57–65.

Pfeffer MA, Braunwald E, Moy LA, et al. Effect of captopril on mortality and morbidity in patients with left ventricular dysfunction after myocardial infarction. *N Engl J Med* 1992;327:669–677.

Scandinavian Simvastatin Survival Study Group. Randomized trial of cholesterol lowering in 4444 patients with coronary heart disease: the Scandinavian Simvastatin Survival Study (4S). *Lancet* 1994;344:1383–1389.

Stephens NG, Parsons A, Schofield PM, Kelly F, Cheeseman K, Mitchinson MJ. Randomized controlled trial of vitamin E in patients with coronary disease: Cambridge Heart Antioxidant Study (CHAOS). *Lancet* 1996;347:781–786.

Sullivan JM, Vander Zwaag R, Hughes JP, et al. Estrogen replacement and coronary artery disease: effect on survival in postmenopausal women. *Arch Inter Med* 1990; 150:2557–2562.

The TIMI Research Group. Immediate vs. delayed catheterization and angioplasty following thrombolytic therapy for acute myocardial infarction: TIMI IIA results. *JAMA* 1988;260:2849–2858.

TIMI Study Group. Comparison of invasive and conservative strategies after treatment with intravenous tissue plasminogen activator in acute myocardial infarction (TIMI) phase II trial. *N Engl J Med* 1989;320:618–627.

Key Reviews

Deedwania PC, Amsterdam EA, Vagelos RH. Evidence-based, cost-effective risk stratification and management after myocardial infarction. *Arch Intern Med* 1997;157: 273–280.

Guidelines and indications for coronary artery bypass graft surgery: A report of the ACC/AHA Task Force of Assessment of Diagnostic and Therapeutic Cardiovascular Procedures. J *Am Coll Cardiol* 1991;17:543–589.

Peterson ED, Shaw LJ, Califf RM. Risk stratification after myocardial infarction. *Ann Intern Med* 1997;126:561–582.

Ryan TJ, Anderson JL, Antman EM, et al. ACC/AHA guidelines for the management of patients with acute myocardial infarction. *J Am Coll Cardiol* 1996;28:1328–428.

Relevant Book Chapters

Antman EM, Braunwald E. Acute myocardial infarction. In: *Heart disease: a textbook of cardiovascular medicine,* 5th ed. Philadelphia: WB Saunders, 1997:1184–1288.

Stempien-Otero A, Weaver WD. Post–myocardial infarction management. In: Topol EJ, ed. *Textbook of cardiovascular medicine.* Philadelphia: Lippincott–Raven, 1998: 511–532.

SECTION II. CHRONIC ISCHEMIC SYNDROMES

Samir R. Kapadia and David J. Moliterno

5A. STABLE ANGINA

Samir R. Kapadia

I. **Introduction. Angina pectoris** is the term used to describe a syndrome resulting from myocardial ischemia. Angina is considered **stable** or **unstable** on the basis of symptom pattern.

   A. Anginal symptoms are defined as **stable** if there is **no substantial deterioration** in symptoms over several weeks. Symptoms of stable angina can fluctuate from time to time, however, depending on myocardial oxygen consumption, emotional stress, and change in ambient temperature. For most patients, the clinical definition of stable angina pectoris closely correlates with the stability or quiescence of an **atherosclerotic plaque.**

   B. Angina is said to be **unstable** when the symptom pattern **worsens abruptly** (increase in frequency and duration) without an obvious cause of increased myocardial oxygen consumption.

   C. For some patients with new-onset angina that has been stable over a few weeks, clear distinction between stable and unstable angina is not possible. These patients can be considered to be in an **intermediate stage** between unstable and stable angina.

II. **Clinical presentation.** For most patients with chest pain, the diagnosis of angina pectoris can be made with careful history taking. The presence of **risk factors** for coronary artery disease (CAD) such as hypertension, diabetes mellitus, smoking, family history, hyperlipidemia, and advanced age, increases the likelihood that the chest pain is being caused by myocardial ischemia.

   A. **Signs and symptoms.** The constellation of symptoms characteristic of angina pectoris include the following four cardinal features:

      1. **Location.** Discomfort is commonly located in the **retrosternal area** with radiation to the neck, shoulders, arms, jaws, epigastrium, or back. In some instances it involves these areas without affecting the retrosternal area.

      2. **Relation to a trigger.** Symptoms typically are triggered by physical activity, emotional stress, exposure to cold, consuming a heavy meal, or smoking.

         a. About 20% of patients have **second-wind angina,** in which the second physical exertion occurs 2 to 5 minutes after the first and is predictably longer than the first. This effect can last as long as 30 minutes. Some patients have resolution of symptoms despite continuing physical activity. These patients usually can maintain or even increase their level of physical exertion without symptoms.

         b. Less common presentations include **decubitus angina,** which occurs with change in posture and is believed to be caused by a shift in blood volume; **nocturnal angina,** which occurs at night and frequently is associated with nightmares; or **angina associated with tachyarrhythmia.**

      3. **Character.** Most patients describe angina as **vague chest discomfort.** They describe squeezing, burning, tightness, choking, heaviness, and occasionally a hot or cold sensation. Many patients do not perceive angina as pain. Some patients have dyspnea, profound fatigue, weakness, lightheadedness, nausea, diaphoresis, altered mental sensorium, or syncope in the absence of any chest discomfort. These symptoms often are referred to as **angina equivalents.**

      4. **Duration.** The symptoms associated with ischemia typically last 3 to 5 minutes. Ischemic pain usually does not last more than 30 minutes without causing myocardial infarction (MI). Chest pain triggered by emotional distress tends to last longer than that triggered by exercise.

Chest pain that lasts less than 1 minute is unlikely to be of cardiac origin, especially when it is not associated with other typical symptoms or findings.

5. **Classification.** Various classifications are available to assess severity and to predict outcome among patients with angina. The Canadian Cardiovascular Society classification is the most popular (Table 5A-1). Other classification systems include the Specific Activity Scale and the Duke Activity Status Index.

B. **Physical findings.** For patients with history of chest pain, physical examination helps to identify **risk factors for CAD** and **occult cardiac abnormalities.**

1. The signs associated with **high risk for CAD** include elevated blood pressure, corneal arcus, xanthelasma, retinal arteriolar changes, diagonal earlobe crease, and evidence of carotid or other peripheral vascular disease. Aortic stenosis and hypertrophic cardiomyopathy can be ruled out with a careful physical examination.

2. Physical examination performed **during an episode of chest pain** may reveal rales, S_3, S_4, systolic murmur from ischemic mitral regurgitation, decreased intensity of S_1, or paradoxic splitting of S_2 from mitral regurgitation, all of which generally disappear with resolution of symptoms.

C. **Baseline electrocardiogram (ECG)**

1. A baseline ECG is useful for the **initial screening for CAD,** although about 60% of patients with chest pain have a normal ECG. Presence of a Q wave or persistent ST depression is associated with an unfavorable outcome. The ECG also can demonstrate other abnormalities, such as left ventricular (LV) hypertrophy, bundle branch block, and preexcitation.

2. Information obtained from the ECG is useful in the assessment of **chest pain** and helps to stratify patients who are at **risk for an adverse event.**

3. ECG at the time of chest pain can also help to identify the **cause of the chest pain.** Transient changes in T-wave, ST-segment, or conduction patterns point toward a cardiac source of the chest pain. **A normal ECG does not exclude ischemia** as being the cause of chest pain.

III. **Diagnostic testing.** For a patient with stable CAD, investigations are aimed at **risk stratification and management.**

A. **Stress testing.** The basic principle of stress testing is to provoke ischemia or produce coronary vasodilatation followed by functional assessment with different monitoring systems. Stress tests can be categorized according to the methods used to provoke and detect myocardial ischemia. The sensitivity and specificity of each test to identify coronary stenosis vary according to

Table 5A-1. Classification of angina

Canadian class	Definition	Comment
I	Ordinary physical activity does not cause angina	Angina only with extraordinary exertion at work or recreation
II	Slight limitation of ordinary activity	Angina with walking more than 2 blocks on a level surface or climbing more than 1 flight of stairs at a normal pace
III	Marked limitation of ordinary physical activity	Walking 1 to 2 blocks on a level surface or climbing 1 flight of stairs at a normal pace
IV	Inability to carry on any activity without discomfort	Angina at rest or with minimal activity or stress

the study population, definition of disease, definition of a positive test result, protocol used for the stress testing, and experience of the interpreter.

1. **Methods to induce ischemia.** Exercise is the most physiologically sound and useful method for inducing ischemia. Pharmacologic testing can be used for patients who cannot exercise adequately.

    a. **Exercise**

    (1) **Mechanism.** Exercise increases myocardial contractility, preload, and afterload, causing an increase in myocardial oxygen demand. The increase in oxygen demand is proportional to the rate-pressure product, that is, the product of heart rate and systolic blood pressure. Because the increased heart rate is primarily responsible for the increased oxygen demand, **adequacy of exercise response is judged on the basis of heart rate achieved during exercise.** An exercise test is considered adequate if 85% or more of age-adjusted maximum heart rate (220 minus age) is achieved.

    (2) **Strengths.** Exercise can be used for objective assessment of functional capacity which provides useful prognostic information.

      (a) The **prognosis** of a patient with stable angina largely depends on the **exercise capacity** and the **stage at which ischemia is induced.**

      (b) **Chronotropic incompetence,** defined as inability to attain 85% of maximum predicted heart rate with maximum effort among patients who have not been treated with negative chronotropic agents, is a marker for poor prognosis.

    (3) **Limitations.** Exercise testing is not useful for patients with claudication, severe lung problems, arthritis, poor physical fitness, or other conditions that limit the ability to exercise.

    b. **Pharmacologic testing with adenosine and dipyridamole**

    (1) **Mechanism**

      (a) **Adenosine.** Acting through a specific adenosine receptor to cause coronary microvascular vasodilatation, adenosine helps to detect coronary stenosis by causing a discrepancy in myocardial blood flow. The stenosed artery is not able to increase blood flow the way a normal artery does. In severe epicardial stenosis this leads to **coronary steal,** in which blood is diverted to normal vessels from the stenosed vessels and ischemia occurs.

      (b) **Dipyridamole.** By inhibiting cellular uptake of adenosine, dipyridamole leads to similar biologic effects as adenosine but with slower onset, longer duration of action, and higher patient-to-patient variability.

    (2) **Strengths.** Pharmacologic testing, which depends on coronary flow reserve rather than increasing myocardial oxygen demand, may be a better way of assessing coronary perfusion because changes in flow reserve may precede development of ischemia. Because discrepancy in flow pattern is easily detected with radionuclide tracers, adenosine and dipyridamole are ideal for use in a nuclear stress laboratory.

    (3) **Limitations**

      (a) **Heart block** (first and second degree) commonly develops with infusion of adenosine. Hemodynamically significant heart block, however, is rare. Because of the short half-life of adenosine, reversal with aminophylline is rarely needed.

      (b) Dipyridamole can cause bronchospasm, hypotension, chest pain, flushing, dizziness, and dyspnea, which may necessitate reversal with aminophylline.

(c) ECG changes and wall motion abnormalities are less likely to occur with these agents, so they are not ideal for stress echocardiography.

(d) The significance of increased lung uptake of the radio-nuclide tracer with dipyridamole is unclear.

(e) Results of tests involving use of these agents have lower negative predictive value compared with results of exercise stress tests.

c. **Pharmacologic testing with dobutamine or arbutamine**

(1) **Mechanism. Dobutamine** and **arbutamine** (β_1 agonists) increase the rate-pressure product, causing an increase in myocardial oxygen demand. For adequate stress, patients should achieve 85% or more of maximum predicted heart rate. **Atropine and handgrip** can be used as **adjuncts** to achieve an adequate heart rate.

(2) **Strengths.** This pharmacologic stress mimics physiologic changes during exercise, but the **rate-pressure product usually is lower than that from exercise testing.** There is evidence that chronotropic incompetence with dobutamine infusion is associated with poor outcome. ECG changes with dobutamine infusion have a predictive value similar to ECG changes associated with exercise.

(3) **Limitations.** Atrial fibrillation, ventricular tachycardia, and hypotension can be precipitated among some patients, leading to premature termination of the test. β-adrenergic blockers may interfere with use of this method of stress testing.

2. **Methods to assess ischemia**

a. **Stress ECG**

(1) **Strengths.** Exercise ECG provides useful information about patients with normal baseline ECGs who are at high risk for CAD. It is less useful when the pretest probability of CAD is low.

(a) Stress ECG helps to **ascertain whether a patient is at high risk for future adverse events.** Patients with results indicative of high risk (Table 5A-2) have an annual mortality of which exceeds 5%.

(b) Stress ECG is used to **identify a safe limit for exercise** in patients with stable angina.

(c) For some patients, exercise testing is used to **evaluate the response to antianginal therapy.** These patients continue to receive medications, and a maximum capacity stress test is performed to determine the functional benefit of the therapy.

(2) **Limitations**

(a) The sensitivity and specificity of stress ECG are poor among patients with an abnormal baseline ECG, LV

Table 5A-2. High risk predicted with exercise electrocardiogram

---

Inability to complete 6 minutes of Bruce protocol
Early positive test result (≤3 min)
Strongly positive test result (≥2 min ST depression)
Sustained ST depression ≥3 minutes after cessation of exercise
Down-sloping ST depression
Ischemia at low (≤120 beats/min) heart rate
Flat or lowered blood pressure response
Serious ventricular arrhythmia at heart rate ≤120 beats/min

---

hypertrophy, ventricular pacing, left bundle branch block, or intraventricular conduction disturbance and among patients taking digitalis or other medications that affect conduction and depolarization.

   (b) Stress ECG is not indicated for judging the functional significance of stenosis because it does not localize ischemia.

   (c) The viability of myocardium cannot be determined with stress ECG.

(3) **Sensitivity and specificity.** For exercise ECG testing, **sensitivity** ranges from 48% to 94% (mean 65%) and **specificity** ranges from 58% to 98% (mean 70%). Specificity of the test is poor for assessing restenosis. ECG changes during **dipyridamole or adenosine infusion** have high specificity but poor sensitivity. ECG changes during **dobutamine and arbutamine infusion** have sensitivity and specificity similar to those of exercise ECG.

b. **Echocardiographic imaging**

   (1) **Strengths.** Stress echocardiography is an economical test with good specificity for identifying ischemic territories. It also can be used to assess the severity and significance of valvular dysfunction.

   (a) **Exercise stress echocardiography** should be performed for patients who can exercise. There has been increasing interest in a **supine bicycle test,** because it allows for imaging at peak exercise rather than immediately after peak exercise. Exercise-induced wall motion abnormalities help to identify and localize ischemic myocardium.

   (b) If the patient is unable to exercise, a **dobutamine or arbutamine stress test** can be performed. A **biphasic response with dobutamine,** in which contractility initially increases with lower doses of dobutamine and then decreases with higher doses, is **diagnostic of ischemia.** Dobutamine stress testing also is useful to assess the viability of the myocardium.

   (c) At some medical centers, **dipyridamole and adenosine stress tests** are performed with echocardiographic imaging. Compared with stress echocardiography with exercise or dobutamine or arbutamine, this method is less sensitive in detecting underlying CAD.

   (2) **Limitations.** Results of stress echocardiography are difficult to interpret in some patients with a hypertensive response to exercise and in some patients with severe mitral or aortic regurgitation. Image quality and experience of the interpreter greatly influence the accuracy of this test.

   (3) **Sensitivity and specificity.** Sensitivity to identify coronary stenosis with exercise echocardiography varies from 70% to 90% (mean about 75%) and **specificity** ranges from 85% to 95% (mean about 85%). Dobutamine echocardiography has similar sensitivity and specificity. The sensitivity and specificity of stress echocardiography decrease with poor image quality and among patients with left bundle branch block, small LV cavity, substantial valvular heart disease, hypertensive response to exercise, and dilated cardiomyopathy.

c. **Radionuclide imaging**

   (1) **Radiopharmaceuticals.** Radionuclide imaging can be performed with thallium 201 or technetium 99m–labeled radiopharmaceuticals (^{99m}Tc-sestamibi or ^{99m}Tc-tetrafosmin).

(a) The initial distribution of **thallium** is directly proportional to coronary blood flow, but because thallium quickly redistributes, images have to be acquired soon after peak exercise. With ^{99m}**Tc isotopes** repeat injection is necessary to visualize blood flow at rest, but the images do not have to be acquired immediately after exercise.

(b) The ^{99m}Tc-labeled isotopes have a shorter half-life and higher energy than thallium. Five to ten times higher doses can be safely given to patients. This higher dosage improves images for obese patients and women with large breast tissue.

(2) **Strengths.** Radionuclide stress testing provides useful information regarding prognosis for patients with stable angina.

(a) An **abnormal perfusion scan** is associated with **15-fold higher cardiovascular mortality** than with patients with a normal scan. The mortality is higher with increasing number of segments with abnormal perfusion. The **most important** segment that determines prognosis is the **proximal septum,** which corresponds to proximal left anterior descending coronary artery (LAD) distribution.

(b) Exercise-induced dilatation of the left ventricle and increased lung uptake also are predictive of poor outcome. If the **scan is normal,** there is less than a 1% risk for nonfatal MI or death in the subsequent year.

(3) **Limitations.** The sensitivity of radionuclide imaging is higher than that of stress echocardiography, but the specificity is lower. Attenuation or artifact from adjoining tissue can decrease the sensitivity and specificity of radionuclide imaging.

(4) **Sensitivity and specificity.** The **sensitivity** to identify coronary stenosis varies from 75% to 90% (mean about 80%); **specificity** ranges from 65% to 90% (mean about 70%). The sensitivity and specificity are **decreased** among patients with severe obesity, three-vessel disease, and left bundle branch block.

B. **Echocardiography** is a noninvasive method for analyzing the **anatomic structure and function of the heart.** It provides useful information in the overall assessment of suspected stable angina.

1. **Regional wall motion abnormalities involving the left ventricle** are commonly caused by CAD. Moderate impairment in LV systolic function, LV hypertrophy, and presence of substantial mitral regurgitation are associated with poor outcome. LV systolic function frequently guides the choice of medical therapy.

2. Echocardiography is the test of choice to **rule out aortic stenosis** or **hypertrophic cardiomyopathy.** Dobutamine stress echocardiography and positron emission tomography can be used to assess **myocardial viability** for patients with angina and considerable LV dysfunction (see Chapter 14).

C. **Coronary angiography**

1. **Strengths.** Coronary angiography is the standard for anatomic assessment of coronary arterial stenosis and provides important prognostic information.

a. **Risk for MI increases with incremental stenosis.** Patients with more than 75% stenosis involving at least one coronary artery have a worse survival rate than patients with 25% to 50% or less than 25% stenosis. Even for mild (less than 25%) stenosis, risk for MI is markedly higher than for no stenosis.

b. The severity of lesions demonstrated with angiography is not predictive of plaque stability; two thirds of patients with acute MI have less than 50% diameter stenosis at the site of plaque rupture before MI. It is possible, however, to **assess plaque instability** on the basis of angiographic characteristics or morphologic features of the lesion.

    (1) Eccentric lesions with narrow necks, overhanging edges, or scalloped borders (type II plaques) are more unstable than concentric lesions with smooth borders (type I lesions).

    (2) Lesion roughness (irregular borders) has been shown to be predictive of future infarction.

    (3) The morphologic characteristics of the plaque help to judge the feasibility and risk of percutaneous or surgical intervention.

  c. Ventriculography performed at the time of selective coronary angiography adds an important dimension to risk stratification.

2. Indications. In the management of stable angina, use of angiography is variable. An American College of Cardiology–American Heart Association task force classified the indications for coronary angiography into three categories. The relevant indications in the context of stable angina are presented in Table 5A-3.

3. Limitations. Coronary angiography **underestimates plaque burden,** possibly because of vascular remodeling and the diffuse nature of the disease. Coronary angiography **does not depict intraluminal plaque burden** and **does not show coronary flow reserve.** Adjunctive use of intravascular ultrasonography greatly facilitates investigation of hazy areas on coronary angiograms, which may be caused by calcium, thrombus, severe eccentric lesion, or dissection.

D. Intravascular ultrasonography allows visualization of the cross-sectional image of coronary arteries. This modality helps to quantitate plaque area, artery size, and luminal stenosis; assess hazy areas on coronary angiograms, questionable areas of stenosis, and extent of stenosis; and, at times, determine calcium content of a plaque. Hypodense areas in a plaque may correlate with high lipid content, which may indicate fast growing or potentially unstable plaque. This information can help to assess the need and options for therapy. This modality does not, however, have a role in routine evaluation of patients with stable angina.

E. Invasive functional assessment. Invasive assessment of the functional significance of stenosis can be made by means of **coronary blood flow measurement with intracoronary Doppler ultrasound** and **direct measurement of a pressure gradient** across a stenosis.

  1. With the help of a small transducer mounted on a guidewire, coronary blood flow can be measured by means of a **fixed sample volume and pulsed Doppler.**

Table 5A-3. Indications for coronary angiography in stable angina

CLASS I (GENERAL AGREEMENT AMONG CARDIOLOGISTS IS PRESENT)

Inadequate control of symptoms with optimal medical therapy
Patient at high risk as determined with stress testing
Evidence of moderate left ventricular dysfunction
Preparation for major vascular operation
Occupation or lifestyle that involves unusual risk

CLASS II (FREQUENTLY USED BUT CONTROVERSIAL)

Young patient with evidence of ischemia on stress test or history of previous myocardial infarction
Evidence of worsening ischemia on serial stress testing

CLASS III (GENERAL AGREEMENT THAT ANGIOGRAPHY IS NOT JUSTIFIED)

Patient has mild (Canadian Class I or II) symptoms with no impairment of left ventricular systolic function and no signs at stress test that suggest high risk

     a. In the left coronary artery, most coronary flow occurs during diastole. In the presence of coronary stenosis, coronary blood flow becomes mainly systolic because the diastolic component of the flow is jeopardized first.

     b. Three indices to help identify physiologically important stenoses are as follows:

        (1) Diastolic to systolic average peak velocity in a ratio of less than 1.8 distal to the obstruction

        (2) A proximal to distal average peak velocity ratio more than 1.7

        (3) Coronary flow reserve (defined as an increase in coronary flow with adenosine, which is administered after intracoronary nitroglycerin) with a less than twofold increase in peak velocity.

  2. Direct measurement of pressure gradients can be accomplished with a transducer mounted on a catheter. Translesion gradients more than 20 mm Hg indicate considerable stenosis. These techniques supplement angiography in determining severity of stenosis. The importance of this invasive assessment in predicting the a patient's overall risk for future cardiac events remains controversial.

F. Holter monitoring

  1. After MI, increased ventricular ectopy is predictive of increased cardiovascular morbidity and mortality. This association is less important among patients with stable angina without prior MI. Therefore routine Holter testing for risk stratification is not indicated.

  2. When **silent ischemia is suspected,** there is likely a role for Holter monitoring to identify these clinically asymptomatic events. A high number of episodes of silent ischemia recorded with Holter monitoring are associated with worse outcome and may call for more aggressive evaluation and treatment.

IV. Therapy. The goals of therapy are to **prevent cardiovascular morbidity and mortality** and to **improve quality of life.**

A. Priority of therapy. Medical therapy, percutaneous transluminal coronary angioplasty (PTCA), and coronary artery bypass grafting (CABG) have been shown to control symptoms and improve exercise time to ischemia, but effectiveness varies. Medical therapy and CABG improve cardiovascular mortality and morbidity and quality of life. PTCA has been shown to improve anginal symptoms but has not yet been shown to decrease mortality.

B. Pharmacologic therapy

  1. Platelet inhibitors

     a. Aspirin was shown in the Swedish Angina Pectoris Aspirin Trial (SAPAT) to reduce the rate of vascular events, including MI and vascular deaths by 33% among patients with stable angina (1). Results of smaller randomized trial confirmed the beneficial role of a 325 mg alternate-day regimen of aspirin among patients with chronic stable angina without prior MI. Some information suggests efficacy of 75 to 160 mg aspirin and current recommendations are for 81-325 mg daily.

     b. Among patients with true allergy or intolerance to aspirin, **ticlopidine** and **clopidogrel** have been shown to decrease the frequency of nonfatal vascular events in peripheral, cerebral, and coronary vessel disease.

        (1) Ticlopidine has been associated with **side effects** such as neutropenia, thrombocytopenia, and pancytopenia and with the development of thrombotic thrombocytopenic purpura. Blood count monitoring is necessary.

        (2) These **side effects do not occur with clopidogrel.** Therefore, considering the safety profile, clopidogrel is a better alternative to aspirin than is ticlopidine.

     c. Other antiplatelet agents. Oral glycoprotein IIb/IIIa antagonists may prove useful in the management of stable angina, although no trials to determine efficacy have been completed. **Warfarin**

sodium may be beneficial to a certain group of patients with stable angina, although this subgroup is not well defined. Therefore routine use of warfarin for all patients is not recommended.

2. **Lipid-lowering agents.** Aggressive control of hyperlipidemia has been shown to be beneficial in primary and secondary prevention of CAD. Among patients with established CAD, lipid-lowering therapy has demonstrated marked reduction in disease progression and risk for subsequent cardiovascular events.

   a. **Indications.** The Scandinavian Simvastatin Survival Study (4S) trial provided convincing evidence that for patients with **hyperlipidemia** (cholesterol 212 to 308 mg/dL) and a history of angina or previous MI, lipid lowering with simvastatin reduces mortality, rate of MI, and need for CABG (2). Patients who have undergone **bypass operations also** should be treated with cholesterol-lowering medications to retard atherosclerosis in the venous grafts.

   b. **Effectiveness.** Angiographic trials studying the effects of lipid lowering have demonstrated that the reduction in clinical events is substantially greater than the minor decrease in coronary stenosis progression. The mechanism of action and individual differences in 3-hydroxy-3-methylglutaryl coenzyme A (HMG-CoA) inhibitors in this regard remain unclear.

   c. **Choice of agents.** Because the benefits of lipid-lowering medication appear to be due to a class effect of HMG-CoA inhibitors, any statin that is effective and economical can be used. The quantification of lipoprotein(a) [Lp(a)], fibrinogen, apolipoprotein (apo) A, and apo B100 is investigational.

      (1) The suggested goal is to lower low-density lipoprotein (LDL) cholesterol level to less than 100 mg/dL among patients with known CAD.

      (2) It is important to measure liver enzymes and creatine kinase 6 weeks after starting therapy with a lipid-lowering agent and every 6 months thereafter.

3. **Nitrates** (Table 5A–4)

   a. **Mechanism of action.** Nitrates decrease cardiac workload and oxygen demand by means of **reducing preload and afterload** of the left ventricle. They also redistribute blood flow to the ischemic subendocardium by means of **decreasing LV end diastolic pressure** and **vasodilatation of epicardial vessels.** Nitrates may even **inhibit platelet aggregation.**

   b. **Evidence for effectiveness.** Nitrates can decrease exercise-induced myocardial ischemia, alleviate symptoms, and increase exercise tolerance among patients with stable angina.

      (1) Adding nitrates to an optimal β-blocker regimen does not improve frequency of anginal episodes, glyceryl trinitrate consumption, exercise duration, or duration of silent ischemia.

      (2) In some small studies, the efficacy of nitrates in reducing anginal episodes was increased with concomitant use of angiotensin-converting enzyme (ACE) inhibitors.

      (3) No study has shown survival benefit with the use of nitrates to treat patients with chronic stable angina.

   c. **Selection of preparations.** Because nitrates have a fast onset of action, a sublingual tablet or oral spray offers immediate relief of an anginal episode.

      (1) For **short-term prophylaxis** (up to 30 minutes), nitroglycerin tablets can be used when activities known to precipitate angina are anticipated. Timing and frequency of the doses can be individualized according to the diurnal rhythm of anginal episodes. A **nitrate-free interval** of about 8 hours is adequate for preventing tolerance.

Table 5A-4. Nitrates

Medication	Route of administration	Each dose	Frequency
Nitroglycerin	Sublingual tablet	0.15–0.6 mg	As needed
(Glyceryl trinitrate,	Sublingual spray	0.4 mg	As needed
Nitro-bid,	Sustained release capsule	2.5–9.0 mg	Every 6–12 hr
Nitrostat,			
Nitro-dur)	Ointment (topical)	0.5–2 inches (1.25–5 cm)	Every 4–8 hr
	Disk (patch)	1 disk (2.5–15 mg)	Every 24 hr
	Intravenous	5–400 microgram/min	continuous
	Buccal tablet	1 mg	Every 3–5 hr
Isosorbide dinitrate	Sublingual tablet	2.5–10 mg	Every 2–3 hr
(Isordil, Sorbitrate,	Chewable tablet	5–10 mg	Every 2–3 hr
Dilatrate)	Oral tablet	10–40 mg	Every 6 hr
	Sustained release tablet	40–80 mg	Every 8–12 hr
Isosorbide-5-mononitrate	Sublingual tablet	10–40 mg	Every 12 hr
(Imdur, Ismo)	Sustained release	60 mg	Every 24 hr
Erythrityl tetranitrate	Sublingual tablet	5–10 mg	As needed
(Cardilate)	Tablet	10 mg	Every 8 hr

(2) Use of **long-acting** medications and **transcutaneous** delivery systems improve compliance but still necessitate a nitrate-free interval.

   d. **Side effects.** Oral nitrates should be taken with meals to prevent heartburn.

(1) **Headache** is common and can be severe. Severity usually decreases with continued use and often can be controlled by decreasing the dose.

(2) Transient episodes of **flushing, dizziness, weakness,** and **postural hypotension** can occur, but these effects usually are abrogated by positioning and other procedures that facilitate venous return.

(3) Glaucoma is not precipitated by the use of nitrates.

   e. **Drug interactions**

(1) Hypotension can occur with the use of **other vasodilators,** such as ACE inhibitors, hydralazine, or calcium channel blockers. Concurrent use of **sildenafil and nitrates** can lead to severe hypotension and therefore is contraindicated.

(2) Extremely high intravenous doses (more than 200 (microgram/min) of nitrates can displace heparin from antithrombin III and cause relative **heparin resistance.** Frequent measurement of partial thromboplastin time is necessary when the nitroglycerin infusion rate is high and frequently changed.

   f. **Controversies**

(1) **Tolerance.** Sustained therapy attenuates the vascular and antiplatelet effects of nitrates. Although the basis for this phenomenon of nitrate tolerance is not completely understood, sulfhydryl depletion, neurohormonal activation, and increased plasma volume are likely involved. Administration of N-acetyl-cysteine, ACE inhibitors, or diuretics does not consistently pre-

vent nitrate tolerance. **Intermittent nitrate therapy is the only way to avoid nitrate tolerance.**

(2) **Rebound.** Intermittent use of nitrates is not associated with serious rebound of angina among patients taking maintenance therapy with β-blockers. Dosing to allow for a longer nitrate-free interval also is not associated with rebound.

4. **β-Blockers** (Table 5A–5).

a. **Mechanism of action.** Blocking the β_1-adrenergic receptors in the heart **decreases the rate-pressure product and oxygen demand.** Decreased tension in the LV wall allows **favorable redistribution of blood flow** from epicardium to endocardium.

(1) Coronary vasospasm is rare from β_2-receptor–blocking effect, but use of β-blockers should be avoided among patients with known, active vasospasm.

(2) β-Blockers have a variable degree of membrane-stabilizing effect.

b. **Evidence of effectiveness.** β-Blockers decrease mortality after MI. The mortality benefit is not proved among patients with stable angina without prior MI, although symptomatic improvement is well documented.

c. **Side effects.** The most important **side effects** are related to blockade of β_2 receptors.

(1) **Bronchoconstriction, masking of symptoms due to hypoglycemic reaction** among patients with diabetes, exacerbation of symptoms of **peripheral vascular disease,** and **central nervous system** side effects such as somnolence, lethargy, depression, and vivid dreaming are well documented. The CNS side effects are thought to be related to the lipid solubility of these compounds.

(2) Symptomatic **bradycardia** and **precipitation of heart failure** are concerns among patients with a diseased conduction system or preexisting heart failure, respectively.

(3) Decreased libido, impotence, and reversible alopecia can be a problem for some patients.

(4) β-Blockers adversely alter lipid profile by increasing LDL cholesterol and decreasing high-density lipoprotein (HDL) cholesterol.

d. **Drug interactions.** Severe bradycardia and hypotension can occur with concomitant use of some **calcium channel blockers.**

e. **Selection of preparations.** Cardioselectivity, lipid solubility, mode of excretion, and frequency of dosing are the main considerations when selecting a particular agent. Intrinsic sympathomimetic activity is not a clinically important factor in the choice of a medication.

f. **Controversies.** The importance of increased lipid levels with β-blockers is unclear. β-Blockers can improve survival among patients with New York Heart Association (NYHA) class 1 or 2 heart failure and angina. The condition of a patient with NYHA class 3 or 4 disease should be stabilized before β-blocker therapy is instituted.

5. **Calcium channel blockers** (Table 5A-6)

a. **Mechanism of action.** These agents block calcium entry into vascular smooth muscle cells and cardiac cells by inhibiting calcium channels, but they do not affect the regulation of intracellular calcium release. The result is decreased contraction of muscle cells.

(1) The four **types** of calcium channels are L, T, N, and P.

(a) The **T-type** calcium channels are located in the atria and sinoatrial node and affect the phase I of depolarization.

(b) **L-type** channels contribute to entrance of calcium into the cell during phase III of the action potential.

Table 5A-5. β-Blockers

Compound	Daily dose (mg)	Frequency	Excretion	Lipid solubility	Intrinsic sympathomimetic activity	Membrane stabilization
SELECTIVE β_1 BLOCKERS						
Metoprolol						
Lopressor	50–400	Every 12 hr	Liver	Moderate		
Long-acting		Every 24 hr			None	Possible
Atenolol	25–200	Every 24 hr	Kidney	None	None	None
Acebutolol	200–600	Every 12 hr	Kidney	Moderate	Low	Low
Betaxolol	20–40	Every 24 hr	Kidney		Low	
NONSELECTIVE β ($\beta_1 + \beta_2$) BLOCKERS						
Propranolol	80–320	Every 4–6 hr	Liver	High		
Long-acting		Every 12 hr		Low	None	Moderate
Nadolol	80–240	Every 24 hr	Kidney	Moderate	None	None
Timolol	15–45	Every 12 hr	Liver	Moderate	None	None
Pindolol	15–45	Every 8–12 hr	Kidney	Moderate	Moderate	Possible
Labetalol[a]	600–2400	Every 6–8 hr	Liver	None	None	Possible

[a]Labetalol is also a potent α_1 antagonist.

Table 5A-6. Calcium channel blockers

Compound	Each dose (mg)	Frequency	Vasodilation	Sinoatrial node inhibition	Atrioventricular node inhibition	Negative inotrope
Nifedipine	30–120	Every 8 hr	5	1	0	1
Nifedipine XL (Procardia)	30–180	Every 24 hr				
Diltiazem	30–90	Every 6–8 hr	3	5	4	2
Diltiazem CD (Cardizem)	120–300	Every 24 hr				
Verapamil	40–120	Every 6–8 hr	4	5	5	4
Verapamil SR (Calan, Isoptin)	120–240	Every 12 hr				
Amlodipine (Norvasc)	2.5–10	Every 24 hr	4	1	0	1
Felodipine (Plendil)	5–20	Every 24 hr	5	1	0	0
Bepridil (Vascor)	200–400	Every 24 hr	4	4	4	5
Isradipine (DynaCirc)	2.5–10	Every 24 hr	4	4	0	0
Nicardipine (Cardene)	10–20	Every 8 hr	5	1	0	0

0, No activity; 5, most potent effect. Intermediate numbers suggest intermediate potency of effects.

            (c) The **N** and **P types** of channels are present mainly in the nervous system.

       (2) The three main **groups** of calcium channel blockers are dihydropyridines (e.g., nifedipine), benzothiazipines (e.g., diltiazem), and phenylalkylamines (e.g., verapamil).

            (a) The **dihydropyridines** bind to the extracellular portion of the L channels at a specific site. They do not bind to the T channels and do not have a negative chronotropic effect. Because of their extracellular site of action, dihydropyridines do not inhibit receptor-induced intracellular calcium increase.

            (b) **Verapamil** binds to the intracellular part of the L channel and inhibits the T channel. Intracellular calcium release is inhibited by verapamil because of its intracellular binding site, so **reflex sympathetic activation is less effective.** Use dependence occurs with verapamil because open channels are needed for transport of the drug into the intracellular binding site. In stable angina, verapamil helps by improving rate-pressure product and increasing oxygen delivery from coronary vasodilatation.

  b. Evidence of effectiveness. Numerous placebo-controlled, double-blind trials have shown that calcium channel blockers **decrease the number of anginal attacks** and **attenuate exercise-induced depression of ST segments.**

       (1) Studies comparing the efficacy of β-blockers and calcium channel blockers in the management of stable angina in which death, infarction, and unstable angina were used as end points showed calcium channel blockers to be as effective as β-blockers.

       (2) Use of a short-acting nifedipine preparation without β-blockers can be potentially harmful, as pointed out in a recent meta-analysis (3).

  c. Side effects. The **most common side effects** are hypotension, flushing, dizziness, and headache. A negative inotropic effect can precipitate heart failure, so **use of calcium channel blockers to treat patients with impaired LV function is relatively contraindicated.** Conduction disturbances and symptomatic bradycardia occur with use of compounds that have a marked inhibitory effect on the sinoatrial and atrioventricular nodes. Bepridil is known to prolong QTc, so QT monitoring is necessary when this medication is used.

  d. Drug interactions. Digitalis levels are increased by calcium channel blockers. Therefore use of these drugs is contraindicated in the presence of digitalis toxicity.

  e. Selection of preparations. Calcium channel blockers have a variable negative inotropic effect.

       (1) **Amlodipine** is most likely to be tolerated by patients with compensated heart failure. In **decompensated heart failure, all calcium channel blockers should be avoided.**

       (2) Patients with conduction disturbances should take agents with minimal effects on the conduction system. Longer-acting preparations minimize risk for precipitation of angina caused by reflex tachycardia.

       (3) **Mibefradil** acts on T channels. In clinical trials, its effectiveness was comparable with that of sustained-release diltiazem in the treatment of patients with chronic stable angina pectoris. Mibefradil, however, provides greater reduction in heart rate and cardiac workload.

  f. Controversies

       (1) Increased mortality caused by short-acting nifedipine among patients with CAD was demonstrated in a retrospective study

and metaanalysis (3). If the use of nifedipine is contemplated, a long-acting preparation in conjunction with β-blocker therapy is the safer approach. The mechanism of increased mortality is unclear, but reflex tachycardia and coronary steal phenomenon are potential explanations.

(2) The initial enthusiasm for regression of atherosclerosis with calcium channel blockers has not been validated.

6. **ACE inhibitors.** The rationale for use of ACE inhibitors to manage chronic stable angina comes from post-MI and heart failure trials that demonstrated a **significant reduction in ischemic events** with use of ACE inhibitors.

   a. It is possible that ACE inhibitors, by decreasing mainly the preload and to some extent afterload, decrease myocardial oxygen demand and help in the management of chronic stable angina. No large trial has evaluated the outcome benefit of ACE inhibitors in the management of chronic stable angina. If there are any other indications for use of these agents, such as decreased LV systolic function or hypertension, they should be added to the antiischemia regimen.

   b. The relative efficacy of different ACE inhibitors for relieving ischemia has not been well studied.

   c. Serious side effects of ACE inhibitors include cough, hyperkalemia, and decreased glomerular filtration rate. They are **contraindicated** in the care of patients with hereditary angioedema or patients with bilateral renal artery stenosis.

7. **Hormone replacement.** The lipid profiles of women change unfavorably after menopause. LDL, total cholesterol, and triglycerides increase and HDL decreases. All these changes have an adverse effect on cardiovascular morbidity and mortality. Several large cross-sectional studies and a randomized study showed that postmenopausal use of **estrogen** alone or in combination with medroxyprogesterone acetate **has a favorable effect on lipid profile and cardiovascular events** (4). It is also clear that this strategy is distinctly beneficial to women with established CAD.

   a. **Benefits of use.** The beneficial effects of estrogen cannot be entirely explained by changes in lipid profile. Other positive effects of use of estrogen, such as maintenance of normal endothelial function, reduction in levels of oxidized LDL, alteration in vascular tone, and maintenance of normal hemostatic profile, may play a role.

   b. **Dosage.** The usual dose is 0.625 mg of conjugated estrogen per day. Except when hot flashes preclude intermittent use, therapy for 25 days followed by 5 days drug free interval is recommended. For women with an intact uterus, some experts prescribe estrogen alone for 15 days, estrogen plus progesterone for an additional 10 to 13 days, and nothing for 7 days in repeated cycles.

   c. **Side effects** include bleeding, nausea, and water retention. Because doses of estrogen are small, these side effects are not frequent. For patients with an intact uterus, routine gynecologic examination is mandatory for cancer surveillance.

8. **Antioxidants.** In large epidemiologic studies, the use of vitamin E and to a lesser extent vitamins A and C has been associated with lower rates of coronary atherosclerosis.

   a. There is evidence that 400 to 800 IU **vitamin E** supplement every day can decrease risk for cardiovascular events among patients with proved atherosclerotic heart disease. This benefit is thought to be the result of decreased oxidation of LDL cholesterol, although other mechanisms have been proposed.

   b. Data are lacking about vitamins A and C. Most of the available information suggests no benefit of taking these vitamin supplements. **Vitamin A** does not prevent LDL oxidation even though it binds to LDL molecules. Because it is water soluble, **vitamin C** does not bind to the LDL molecule. Thus **these two vitamins are not recommended** for prevention of progression of atherosclerosis.

   c. The role of **probucol,** a lipid-lowering medication with antioxidant properties, is under investigation.

9. **Newer pharmacologic approaches**

   a. Therapy with direct infusion of **vascular endothelial growth factor** (VEGF) and basic fibroblast growth factor (bFGF) proteins have been shown to increase collateral blood flow in animal models. Studies are underway to investigate the role of these agents in improving collateral blood flow to the ischemic myocardium of patients with angina. Although early results are encouraging, long-term risks and benefits of such therapy remain largely unknown.

   b. Approaches involving the use of **gene therapy** to overexpress these endogenous growth factors to improve development of collateral blood vessels have been proposed. These approaches have to be perfected before they become clinically useful.

C. **PTCA.** The effectiveness of PTCA to control symptoms in chronic stable angina and to prevent death or MI has been compared with medical management and CABG (5).

1. **Comparative studies**

   a. The **Angioplasty Compared to Medicine (ACME)** study showed better symptomatic relief at 6 months but no difference in mortality or MI among patients with single-vessel CAD managed initially with PTCA compared with initial medical management.

   b. The **Medicine, Angioplasty or Surgery Study (MASS)** demonstrated no difference in primary end point (death, MI, refractory angina necessitating revascularization) among patients with proximal LAD stenosis. These results were consistent and demonstrated that patients with stable angina and single-vessel CAD do well with either appropriate medical management or PTCA.

   c. The **Randomized Intervention Treatment of Angina trial (RITA-2)** showed symptomatic improvement with **PTCA compared with medical management.** In that study, however, results showed a higher incidence of death, MI, and repeat CABG or PTCA among patients initially randomized to undergo PTCA compared with those who underwent medical therapy. When considering PTCA for symptomatic relief for patients with stable angina, the small excess hazard from procedural complications of PTCA should be taken into account.

   d. A small nonrandomized study in which **PTCA was compared to surgery with left internal mammary artery bypass graft** for a proximal LAD stenosis showed that the rate of death and MI were comparable between the two treatment groups during a mean follow-up period of 66 months. Even in this study, the rate of repeat procedure was higher in the PTCA group. In multivessel disease, the long-term (up to 5 years) risk of death and MI is similar for PTCA and CABG, but patients treated with PTCA have a higher need for repeat procedures.

   e. The **Bypass Angioplasty Revascularization Investigators (BARI)** conducted the largest trial comparing PTCA with CABG in the management of multivessel disease. In this trial, there was no difference in survival benefit between patients randomized to PTCA or CABG, although patients with diabetes and multivessel disease had a better 5-year survival rate with CABG than with PTCA (80.6% versus 65.5%). Whether this finding will be validated in a prospective trial remains to be seen.

2. **Revascularization methods.** Many different percutaneous methods such as balloon angioplasty, stents, atherectomy (rotablation, directional, laser), and transluminal extraction catheterization are used in conjunc-

tion with various antiplatelet and anticoagulant drug regimens. The rapidly evolving mechanical and pharmacologic approach to revascularization makes it difficult to fully apply the results of previous studies in contemporary practice. Furthermore, most clinical trials include highly selected patients with lesions suitable for percutaneous intervention. This definition is in evolution because of advances in percutaneous techniques. These points should be kept in mind while recommending one therapy versus the other on the basis of evidence.

D. CABG

1. **Compared with medical treatment.** Compared with medical treatment CABG improves survival rate among patients at high risk with stable angina. Population groups at high risk include patients with three-vessel CAD, impaired LV function, or substantial left main coronary artery stenosis.

    a. This information is derived from the Coronary Artery Surgery Study (CASS), European Coronary Surgery Study (ECSS), and Veterans Administration Cooperative Study (VACS) studies (7–9). These trials were completed before generalized awareness grew regarding the benefits of medical treatment with β-blockers, ACE inhibitors, antiplatelet agents, or lipid-lowering medications.

    b. **Surgical techniques** have also changed significantly, with greater use of **arterial conduits** including internal mammary artery grafts, minimally invasive surgery, and improved techniques of cardiac tissue preservation and anesthesia.

2. **Venous or arterial grafts.** There are different techniques of CABG. The role of minimally invasive bypass surgery in the management of LAD stenosis or bifurcation lesions involving the LAD and diagonal branch is under investigation. At least compared with open thoracotomy, in which the use of the left internal mammary artery is well studied, mammary arterial grafting has better long-term outcome compared with vein-graft conduits.

    a. Twenty percent of venous grafts are nonfunctional after 5 years and 40% to 60% are nonfunctional after 10 years. In contrast, 90% to 95% of the mammary artery grafts are patent 10 years after the operation.

    b. Internal mammary artery grafts have a better patency rate at 10 years when used for LAD lesions (95%) than for circumflex (88%) or right coronary artery (76%) lesions. The patency rates are higher for left internal mammary compared with right internal mammary and for in situ grafts compared with free grafts.

    c. Patient survival is better with an internal mammary artery graft than when only saphenous venous grafts are used. This survival benefit persists for up to 20 years. The use of bilateral internal mammary artery grafts is under investigation and appears promising.

    d. The use of grafts composed of artery alone has been suggested. Data are available only on the early postoperative period, in which the patency rate has been high.

3. **Previous CABG.** Little information is available on treatment of patients who have already undergone bypass surgery and have stable angina. Although another bypass operation is offered to these patients, head-to-head comparison with medical treatment of this patient population has not been made.

4. **Compared with PTCA.** The rate of symptom recurrence after CABG is lower, as is the need for repeat procedures compared with PTCA, but the incidence of death and MI is similar. These data are from 5-year follow-up studies after initial randomization. This time period is important because recurrence of stenosis necessitating repeat intervention is likely to occur in the first year after the percutaneous procedure, whereas graft attrition occurs much later. It remains to be proved whether there will

be catching up of repeat procedures with longer follow-up evaluation of patients who have undergone CABG.

E. **Myocardial laser revascularization.** Percutaneous and intraoperative transmyocardial revascularization are potential treatments for patients with coronary disease not amenable to PTCA or CABG. Reports suggest improvement in symptoms, a decrease in perfusion defects, and improvement in contractile function after these procedures. This procedure should be reserved for patients with medically refractory angina and no other revascularization option.

F. **Lifestyle modification**

   1. **Exercise**

      a. **Rationale.** Exercise **conditions the skeletal muscles,** which decreases total body oxygen consumption for the same amount of workload. Exercise training also **lowers heart rate** for any level of exertion, which decreases the oxygen demand on the myocardium for any workload. Some evidence shows that higher physical activity and exercise can decrease cardiovascular morbidity and mortality.

      b. **Recommendation.** For secondary prevention, **aerobic, isotonic exercises** with a goal of achieving a sustained heart rate of approximately 85% of the maximum predicted heart rate for 20 to 30 minutes is useful. This type of exercise should be done at least 3 to 4 times per week. For beginners, a supervised exercise or rehabilitative program is helpful. **Isometric exercises are not recommended** because they increase myocardial oxygen demand substantially.

   2. **Diet.** A strict vegetarian diet with less than 10% fat and no dairy products has shown to be beneficial, although few patients can follow these recommendations. For all patients, individualization of approach according to personal and cultural needs can help to decrease fat and calorie intake.

   3. **Smoking cessation.** Cigarette smoking is associated with progression of atherosclerosis, increase in myocardial demand due to an α-adrenergic increase in coronary tone, and adverse effects on hemostatic values, all of which can lead to worsening of stable angina. Smoking cessation decreases cardiovascular risk among patients with established CAD, including patients who have undergone CABG. Physician **counseling** is the best approach to achieve this goal. For some patients, **transdermal nicotine patches** or similar therapies may help to minimize withdrawal symptoms (see Chapter 38).

   4. **Psychologic factors.** Anger, hostility, and stress are shown to adversely affect CAD. Results of small, nonrandomized trials show that biofeedback and various relaxation techniques can help to modify these factors.

V. **Controversies and approach to stable angina**. The approach to management of stable angina remains highly controversial. Data from clinical trials evaluating the diagnostic and therapeutic strategies lag behind technical advances.

A. **Controversial findings**

   1. Because the ideal cost-effective **methods for risk stratification** are debatable, individualized approaches based on the availability of technology and expertise are commonly used.

   2. **The relative roles of medical therapy, PTCA, and CABG** are controversial, especially for patients with proximal LAD stenosis, two-vessel disease, or silent ischemia. Heterogeneity in the response to different medications makes generalized recommendations ineffective. Drug therapy tailored according to the genetic makeup of a patient may prove to be the optimal method (e.g., platelet glycoprotein IIIa gene polymorphism and antiplatelet therapy) to select appropriate pharmacotherapy for an individual patient.

   3. The long-term **effectiveness of different surgical and percutaneous therapies** in the management of stable angina also remains controversial.

B. Recommended approach. Despite the controversies, the following approach is suggested for the treatment of patients with stable angina.

1. It is reasonable to **risk stratify** patients with stable angina using **stress testing with imaging,** such as nuclear isotope imaging or echocardiography.

   a. **LV systolic function** should be assessed with **echocardiography** to guide therapy and to identify patients with moderate LV systolic dysfunction.

   b. Patients with small perfusion defects or small wall motion abnormalities, high threshold for ischemia, normal LV systolic function, and clear symptoms should be treated with **medication.**

2. If **symptoms continue** after medical therapy is maximized, **angiography** should be planned. **Coronary angiography** should be performed for patients with evidence of impaired perfusion involving multiple territories, a low threshold for ischemia, and moderate LV systolic dysfunction. For patients with vague and atypical symptoms, it may be useful to perform **Holter monitoring** for 24 hours to assess the contribution of silent ischemia.

3. **Single-vessel disease.** If a patient has a single-vessel CAD that does not involve the proximal LAD or supply a large myocardial territory, **medical management with risk factor modification** is the appropriate first step.

   a. If patients cannot tolerate medical treatment or have symptoms despite maximum medical therapy, **percutaneous revascularization** should be offered.

   b. For patients with **proximal LAD lesions**, the decision is more complex. PTCA and bypass surgery are more likely to be successful than initial medical management. The relative roles are evolving with the option of minimally invasive surgery and development of intracoronary stents.

4. Among patients with **multivessel CAD,** medical treatment remains as an alternative for patients who have normal LV systolic function, mild symptoms, and relatively smaller areas of myocardium at risk.

   a. **Surgical revascularization** is indicated in the care of patients with left main coronary artery stenosis or patients with three-vessel disease and impaired LV systolic function.

   b. For the other patients with multivessel CAD, **CABG** or **PTCA** is a reasonable options, provided coronary anatomy is suitable.

      (1) Because the likelihood for a repeat revascularization procedure within 1 to 3 years is higher with PTCA as an initial strategy, the patient's personal preference should be a strong factor in the decision.

      (2) Any doubt regarding viability of the myocardium at risk should be addressed with appropriate diagnostic studies before revascularization.

5. Regardless of treatment strategy, **aggressive risk factor modification,** including use of lipid-lowering medications, lifestyle modification, and aspirin therapy are essential components of management.

SUGGESTED READINGS

References
1. Armstrong PW. Stable ischemic syndromes. In: Topol EJ, ed. *Textbook of cardiovascular medicine.* Philadelphia: Lippincott—Raven, 1998:333–365.
2. The Scandinavian Simvastatin Survival Study Group. Randomised trial of cholesterol lowering in 4444 patients with coronary heart disease: The Scandinavian Simvastatin Survival Study (4S). *Lancet* 1994;344:1383–1389.
3. Furberg CD, Psaty BM, Meyer JV. Nifedipine: dose related increase in mortality in patients with coronary heart disease. *Circulation* 1995;92:1326–1331.

4. Grady D, Rubin SM, Petitti DB, et al. Hormone therapy to prevent disease and prolong life in post menopausal women. *Ann Intern Med* 1992;117:1016–1037.
5. Solomon AJ, Gersh BJ. Management of chronic stable angina: medical therapy, percutaneous transluminal coronary angioplasty, and coronary artery bypass graft surgery, lessons from randomized trials. *Ann Intern Med* 1998;128:216–223.
6. The Bypass Angioplasty Revascularization (BARI) Investigators. Comparison of coronary bypass surgery with angioplasty in patients with multivessel disease. *N Engl J Med* 1996;335:217–225.
7. Alderman EL, Bourassa MG, Cohen LS, et al. Ten-year follow-up of survival and myocardial infarction in the randomized coronary artery surgery study. *Circulation* 1990;82:1629–1646.
8. Eleven-year survival in the Veterans Administration Randomized Trial of Coronary Bypass Surgery for Stable Angina. The Veterans Administration Coronary Artery Bypass Surgery Cooperative Study Group. *N Engl J Med* 1984;311: 1333–1339.
9. Varmauskas E. Twelve-year follow-up of survival in the Randomized European Coronary Artery Surgery Study. *N Engl J Med* 1988;319:332–337.

Landmark articles

CAPRIE Steering Committee. A randomized, blinded trial of clopidogrel versus aspirin in patients at risk of ischemic events (CAPRIE). *Lancet* 1996;348:1329–1339.
Juul-Moller S, Edvardsson N, Jahnmatz B, et al. Double blind trial of aspirin in primary prevention of myocardial infarction in patients with stable chronic angina pectoris. *Lancet* 1992;114:1421–1425.
Mark DB, Shaw L, Harrell FE, et al. Prognostic value of a treadmill exercise score in outpatients with suspected coronary artery disease. *N Engl J Med* 1991;325: 849–853.
Passamani E, Davis KB, Gilepsi MJ, et al. A randomized trial of coronary artery bypass surgery. *N Engl J Med* 1985;312:1665–1671.

Key Review

Diaz MN, Frei B, Vita JA, Keaney JF Jr. Mechanism of disease: antioxidants and atherosclerotic heart disease. *N Engl J Med* 1997;337:408–416.
Ferrari R. Major differences among the three classes of calcium antagonists. *Eur Heart J* 1997;18:A56–A70.
Guidelines and management of stable angina pectoris: recommendations of the Task Force of the European Society of Cardiology. *Eur Heart J* 1997;18:394–413.
Mark DB, Nelson CL, Califf RM, et al. Continuing evolution of therapy for coronary artery disease. *Circulation* 1994;89:2015–2125.
Parker JD, Parker JO. Drug therapy: nitrate therapy for stable angina pectoris. *N Engl J Med* 1998;338:520–531.
Wilson RF. Assessing the severity of coronary artery stenosis [Editorial]. *N Engl J Med* 1996;334:1735–1737.

Relevant Book Chapter

Gersh BJ, Braunwald E, Rutherford JD. Chronic coronary artery disease. In: Braunwald E, ed. *Heart disease: a textbook of cardiovascular medicine,* 5th ed. Philadelphia: WB Saunders, 1997:1289–1366.

5B. SILENT ISCHEMIA

Stanley Chetcuti and Samir R. Kapadia

I. **Introduction.** Silent ischemia is defined as documented episodes of ischemia not associated with any typical or atypical symptoms that occur among patients with obstructive coronary artery disease.

II. **Clinical presentation.** Three distinct groups of patients are frequently encountered in clinical practice (Table 5B-1). Prognostic significance and the treatment of these groups of patients are different.

   A. **Group 1** patients have **documented ischemia** from obstructive coronary artery disease **but never have symptoms of ischemia.** It is not uncommon to experience asymptomatic ischemia, even with myocardial infarction (MI). In the Farmingham Study, 25% of patients who had MI had unrecognized infarction, and approximately half of the infarctions were truly silent. Group 1 patients **come to medical attention** when they undergo routine electrocardiography (ECG) or stress testing or experience arrhythmia. This group also includes patients who present with sudden cardiac death as the first manifestation of coronary artery disease (CAD).

   B. **Group 2** constitutes patients who have had a symptomatic or asymptomatic **MI** and have **asymptomatic angina** without concomitant symptomatic angina.

   C. **Group 3** patients are most frequently encountered in clinical practice. **Some episodes of ischemia** are associated with **chest discomfort** and **other episodes** are **asymptomatic.** *Total ischemic burden* is a term used to describe the total period of ischemia, both symptomatic and asymptomatic.

III. **Diagnostic testing**

   A. **Group 1.** Ischemia is identified with any **stress test** in which ischemia is induced without symptoms. The indication for stress testing of these patients usually is abnormal findings on a resting ECG or the presence of a risk factor for CAD.

   B. **Group 2.** Patients with documented MI at **ambulatory ECG** may have episodes of asymptomatic angina. Ambulatory ECG monitoring is the most important diagnostic tool for the study of silent ischemia. However, ischemia can occur, as documented by evidence of left ventricular functional abnormalities, without a significant ST-segment shift, so-called supersilent ischemia during stress imaging. These functional tests are still investigational and are not commonly used for clinical decision making.

   C. **Group 3.** With the extensive use of ambulatory ECG monitoring, it has become evident that **anginal pain is a poor indicator of ischemia.** Approximately one half of patients with symptomatic angina have episodes of asymptomatic angina. These asymptomatic episodes may be even more frequent among persons with diabetes. Transient ST-segment depression of 0.1 mV or more that lasts for more than 30 to 60 seconds is a rare finding

Table 5B-1. Classification of patients with silent ischemia

Group	Clinical presentation
1	Patients with no symptomatic ischemia
2	Patients with silent ischemia who have had myocardial infarction
3	Patients with symptomatic angina who have episodes of silent ischemia

among healthy persons. Rubidium 82 **positron emission tomography** shows that patients with known CAD have a strong correlation between transient ST-segment depression and independent measurements of impaired myocardial perfusion and ischemia. The perfusion defects occur in the same myocardial regions during symptomatic and asymptomatic episodes of ST-segment depression.

IV. **Mechanisms**

A. The **exact explanation** for a lack of symptoms in the face of unequivocal ischemia remains **unknown.** It is likely to be determined by means of modulation of cardiac **pain perception at different levels in the afferent pathway from the heart** (Table 5B-2). The afferent impulses from chemoreceptors and mechanoreceptors in the pericardium, connective tissue, adventitia, and walls of the heart pass by peripheral sensory axons through symptomatic plexuses and the lower two cervical and upper four thoracic sympathetic ganglia to the thoracic dorsal ganglia, where the cell bodies of the neurons are located. The impulses are carried by the central axons of these neurons through the dorsal roots of the posterior gray column of the spinal cord, where fibers synapse with second-order neurons. From these neurons, the fibers of the median plane ascend in the ventral spinothalamic tract and terminate in the posteroventral nucleus of the thalamus. From both thalami the impulses activate basal frontal, anterior, and ventral cingulate cortices and the left temporal pole.

B. The **association between diabetes and both silent ischemia and painless infarction** has been attributed to autonomic neuropathy (1,2). A higher threshold for pain has been related to increased baseline β-endorphin plasma levels and increased age. A potential connection exists between baroreceptor function and pain perception. This explains the relation between increased systolic blood pressure, reduced sensitivity to ischemic pain, and the demonstration that carotid sinus stimulation relieves angina. Results of one study (2) suggested the gating of the afferent signals at the thalamic level as a possible mechanism for silent ischemia. In that study, patients with symptoms had activation of basal frontal, anterior, and ventral cingulate cortices and the left temporal pole. In patients with silent ischemia, cortical activation was limited to the right frontal region. It also has been proposed that among group 3 patients asymptomatic ischemia may represent shorter and less severe episodes compared with symptomatic episodes (3,4).

V. **Management**

A. **Medications** effective in preventing episodes of symptomatic ischemia (nitrates, calcium antagonists, and β-blockers) are effective in reducing or eliminating episodes of silent ischemia. In one randomized study (5), metoprolol was better than diltiazem in reducing the mean number and duration of ischemic episodes. However, the combination of calcium antagonists and β-blockers is more effective than either agent alone.

B. The **goal** of therapy is still **controversial.** It is not clear whether the therapy should be ischemia guided or angina guided. The Asymptomatic Cardiac Ischemia Pilot study (ACIP) showed no difference in benefit from either of these approaches. However, the 2-year follow-up data from this study demonstrated that a strategy of initial revascularization appears to improve the prognosis among this population compared with angina- or ischemia-guided

Table 5B-2. Putative mechanisms of silent ischemia

Autonomic dysfunction and evidence of sympathetic cardiac denervation
Higher threshold for pain
Linkage between baroreceptor function and pain perception
Dynamic gating in pain perception within the cerebral cortex and spinal tract
Effect of duration and severity of ischemia

medical therapy (5). A larger long-term study is needed to confirm this benefit of revascularization therapy, especially with recently available more aggressive medical therapy, including 3-hydroxy-3-methylglutaryl coenzyme A inhibitors.

VI. Prognosis. Myocardial ischemia, whether it is symptomatic or asymptomatic, is associated with poor outcome among patients with CAD. Patients with frequent and accelerating episodes of ST-segment depression at ambulatory ECG monitoring are at higher risk for subsequent cardiac events than patients with fewer or no such episodes. Although suggested by many studies, it has not been proved conclusively that detection of silent ischemia is an independent risk factor for future cardiac events (6–9).

VII. Controversies

    A. The **mechanism through which ischemia detected** at ambulatory ECG monitoring is linked to adverse outcomes remains unclear. Silent ischemia might be a marker of unstable, complex coronary plaque. Results of the angiographic part of the ACIP study suggested that most patients with silent ischemia have proximal coronary lesions or complex coronary plaques (10). This hypothesis has not been tested in a larger population in a rigorous investigation.

    B. The potential role of **ambulatory ECG monitoring** for ischemia should be studied to investigate the usefulness of this test in relation to the more commonly used tests, such as exercise testing and thallium scanning, to establish a prognosis. Different populations at specific times after their events should be carefully examined to answer these questions.

    C. It appears that **some therapy** should be used to decrease or eliminate ischemia; however, the relative role of medical therapy compared with revascularization therapy remains unclear.

SUGGESTED READINGS

References

1. Chiariello M, Indolfi C. Silent myocardial ischemia in patients with diabetes mellitus. *Circulation* 1996;93: 2081–2091.
2. Ahluwalia G, Jain P, Chugh SK, Wasir HS, Kaul U. Silent myocardial ischemia in diabetes with normal autonomic function. *Int J Cardiol* 1995;48: 147–153.
3. Nihoyannopoulos P, Marsonis A, Joshi J, Athanassopoulos G, Oakley CM. Magnitude of myocardial dysfunction is greater in painful than in painless myocardial ischemia: an exercise echocardiographic study. *J Am Coll Cardiol* 1995;25: 1507–1512.
4. Narins CR, Zareba W, Moss AJ, Goldstein RE, Hall WJ. Clinical implications of silent versus symptomatic exercise-induced myocardial ischemia in patients with stable coronary disease. *J Am Coll Cardiol* 1997;29;756–763.
5. Davies RF, Goldberg AD, Forman S, et al. Asymptomatic Cardiac Ischemia Pilot (ACIP) study 2 year follow-up: outcomes of patients randomized to initial strategies of medical therapy versus revascularization. *Circulation* 1997;95:2037–2043.
6. Leroy F, McFadden EP, Lablanche JM, Bauters C, Quandalle P, Bertrand ME. Prognostic significance of silent myocardial ischaemia during maximal exercise testing after a first acute myocardial infarction. *Eur Heart J* 1993;14;1471–1475.
7. Mickley H, Nielson JR, Berning J, Junker A, Moller M. Prognostic significance of transient myocardial ischaemic after first acute myocardial infarction: five year follow-up study. *Br Heart J* 1995;73:320–326.
8. Detry JM, Robert A, Luwaert RJ, Melin JA. Prognostic significance of silent exertional myocardial ischaemia in symptomatic men without previous myocardial infarction. *Eur Heart J* 1992;13:183–187
9. Stone PH, Chaitman BR, Forman S, et al. Prognostic significance of myocardial ischemia detected by ambulatory electrocardiography, exercise treadmill testing, and electrocardiogram at rest to predict cardiac events by one year (the Asymptomatic Cardiac Ischemia Pilot [ACIP] study). *Am J Cardiol* 1997;80:1395–1401.
10. Sharaf BL, Bourassa MG, McMahon RP, et al. Clinical and detailed angiographic findings in patients with ambulatory electrocardiographic ischemia without critical

coronary narrowing: results from the Asymptomatic Cardiac Ischemia Pilot (ACIP) study. *Clin Cardiol* 1998;21:86–92.

Landmark Articles
Conti CR. Silent myocardial ischemia: prognostic significance and therapeutic implications. *Clin Cardiol* 1998;11: 807–811.
Weiner DA, Ryan TJ, McCabe CH, et al for the CASS. Results from the Asymptomatic Cardiac Ischemia Pilot (ACIP) Study. *Clin Cardiol* 1998; 21:86–92

6. SYNDROME X: ANGINA WITH NORMAL CORONARY ARTERIES

Marc Penn

I. **Introduction. Syndrome X is typical angina** with **normal coronary arteries** as determined at cardiac catheterization. Although this definition is the most inclusive description of syndrome X, many cardiologists believe that patients also should have **abnormal results of an exercise stress test.**

II. **Clinical presentation.** Approximately 10% to 30% of patients who undergo cardiac catheterization for anginal chest pain have normal coronary arteries. In syndrome X there is a preponderance of women (3:1), approximately 50% to 70% of whom are postmenopausal and have a mean age at presentation of 50 years (1).

III. **Etiology and pathophysiology.** The exact **cause of syndrome X is unknown,** and the population with the syndrome is believed to be heterogenous. It is believed that the **chest pain is a result of small-vessel disease** (thus the term **microvascular angina**) that decreases coronary reserve. Increased lactate production and decreased oxygen content have been measured in the coronary sinus during cardiac stress among patients with syndrome X. This suggests at least an **ischemic component.** Twenty percent to 80% of patients with syndrome X have abnormal thallium 201 perfusion scans (1). Possible causes of the small-vessel dysfunction proposed with syndrome X include increased release of endothelin (2) by endothelial cells or abnormal adrenergic nerve function with increased release of norepinephrine (3).

IV. **Diagnostic testing.** Syndrome X is a clinical syndrome and is a diagnosis of exclusion; several entities must be ruled out (Table 6-1).

V. **Therapy.** The primary goal should be **aggressive management of hypertension** (4), although the **ideal treatment regimen is unknown.** The pain syndrome typically responds better to **calcium channel blockers** than to β-blockers. Nitroglycerin is effective among less than 50% of patients and has been shown to decrease exercise tolerance during stress testing (1,5). Other treatments that have shown some improvement are estrogen treatment of postmenopausal women (6) and oral aminophylline (7).

VI. **Prognosis.** The prognosis of syndrome X is that of the general population and is significantly better than the prognosis among patients with coronary artery disease. There usually is no decrement in left ventricular function during the follow-up period (1). However, the following three subsets of patients with syndrome X may be at increased **risk for cardiomyopathy:**

   A. Patients with **left bundle branch block** (LBBB) at rest or with a rate-dependent LBBB evident on a stress test (4).

   B. Patients who, during an exercise stress test, demonstrate **increased sympathetic tone,** defined as either an increase of more than 20 mm Hg during the first stage of the modified Bruce protocol or a rate pressure product greater than 1050 (4).

   C. Patients who later have **hypertension** (4).

Table 6-1. Differential diagnosis of syndrome X

Syndrome	Diagnostic tool
Left ventricular hypertrophy	Echocardiography, electrocardiography
Coronary artery disease	Coronary angiography
Coronary artery spasm	Ergotamine infusion
Anomalous coronary anatomy	Coronary angiography
Esophogeal dysmotility	Manometry
Gastroesophageal regurgitation	pH monitoring

SUGGESTED READINGS

References

1. Kaski JC, Rosano GMC, Collins P, Nihoyannopoulos P, Maseri A, Poole-Wilson PA. Cardiac syndrome X: clinical characteristics and left ventricular function—long term follow-up study. *J Am Coll Cardiol* 1995;25:807–814.

2. Kaski JC, Elliott PM, Salomone O, et al. Concentration of circulating plasma endothelin in patients with angina and normal coronary angiograms. *Br Heart J* 1995;74:620–624.

3. Lanza GA, Giordano A, Pristpino C, et al. Abnormal cardiac adrenergic nerve function in patients with syndrome X detected by 123I-metaiodobenzylguandine myocardial scintigraphy. *Circulation* 1997;96:821–826.

4. Romeo F, Rosano GMC, Martuscelli E, Lombardo L, Valente A. Long-term follow-up of patients initially diagnosed with syndrome X. *Am J Cardiol* 1993;71:669–673.

5. Lanza GA, Manzoli A, Bia E, Crea F, Maseri A. Acute effects of nitrates on exercise testing in patients with syndrome X: clinical and pathophysiological implications. *Circulation* 1994;90:2695–2700.

6. Rosano GMC, Peters NS, Lefroy D, et al. 17-Beta-estradiol therapy lessens angina in postmenopausal women with syndrome X. *J Am Coll Cardiol* 1996;28:1500–1505.

7. Elliott PM, Dickinson KK, Calvino R, Hann C, Kaski JC. Effect of oral aminophylline in patients with angina and normal coronary arteriograms (cardiac syndrome X). *Heart* 1997;77:523–526.

Relevant Book Chapters

Armstrong PW. Stable ischemic syndromes. In: Topol EJ, ed. *Textbook of cardiovascular medicine.* Philadelphia: Lippincott–Raven, 1998:339–340.

Gersh BJ, Braunwald E, Rutherford JD. Chronic coronary artery disease: other manifestations of coronary artery disease. In: Braunwald E, ed. *Heart disease: a textbook of cardiovascular medicine.* Philadelphia: WB Saunders, 1997:1343–1344.

SECTION III. CHRONIC HEART FAILURE

John G. Peterson and James B. Young

7. SYSTOLIC HEART FAILURE

Eric Bowen

I. **Introduction**
   A. **Systolic heart failure** is a complex clinical syndrome characterized by **circulatory congestion, impaired left ventricular (LV) systolic function, and progressive activation of the neuroendocrine systems.** In the U.S. more than three million people have heart failure, and approximately 200,000 each year die of this disease. Heart failure is the leading indication for hospitalization in the United States among patients older than 65 years. Treatment cost exceeds that for both coronary artery disease and cancer. Approximately 35% of patients each year who receive the diagnosis of heart failure are treated in a hospital. As many as 47% need readmission to the hospital within 3 months. With the increasing age of the population, improved survival of patients with acute myocardial infarction (MI), and reduced mortality from other diseases, the incidence of congestive heart failure (CHF) is expected to continue to increase.
   B. **CHF** is associated with a high mortality, similar to that of many malignant diseases. A patient with New York Heart Association Class 4 disease has a 1-year survival rate between 30% and 50%. In the Framingham study, patients with heart failure had a mortality four to eight times higher than that of the general population of the same age. In the care of a patient with heart failure it is important to identify classes or groups of patients who may be at a higher risk because of coexisting morbidity (Table 7-1).

II. **Signs and symptoms**
   A. The spectrum of signs and symptoms in LV systolic failure varies markedly among patients.
      1. Some patients with severe LV systolic dysfunction have **no symptoms** and have normal exercise capacity.
      2. Among patients with symptoms, the **most common and earliest presenting symptom is dyspnea,** usually with exertion. The threshold for dyspnea to occur defines New York Heart Association (NYHA) functional class (Table 7-2). **Orthopnea** is typical with more advanced cases of LV dysfunction or in decompensated CHF. As further decompensation occurs, paroxysmal nocturnal dyspnea, nocturnal cough, and Cheyne-Stokes respiratory patterns may occur.
      3. **Fatigue, anorexia, and abdominal pain** are frequent symptoms of advanced CHF.
      4. Physical signs and symptoms commonly seen in the **heart failure syndrome** (Table 7-3) vary according to the degree of compensation, the chronicity of heart failure, and chamber involvement.
   B. **Physical examination** of a patient with appreciable but well-compensated systolic heart failure may reveal no abnormalities. A high index of suspicion based on symptoms must be maintained. However, patients in decompensated CHF typically have **pulmonary rales, jugular venous distention, edema, hepatomegaly, a murmur of mitral regurgitation (MR), and an S_3 gallop.** A pulsus alternans or low-amplitude pulse is associated with advanced heart failure. An S_3 is best heard with the bell of the stethoscope in the left lateral position and signifies increased LV end-diastolic pressure in patients with decreased LV function.

III. **Laboratory evaluation**
   A. **Serum studies**
      1. Although CHF is a clinical diagnosis, a thorough evaluation of patients with new-onset disease is warranted. **Electrolyte abnormalities** are common among patients with CHF and may be caused by the disease itself or by the treatment (e.g. administration of diuretics). Hyponatremia

Table 7-1. Factors adversely affecting prognosis in heart failure

Diabetes mellitus
Hypertension
Tobacco use
ECG abnormalities: left ventricular hypertrophy
Ejection fraction <25%
Exercise capacity (peak VO$_2$ <14 mL/kg per min)
Hemodynamics (PCWP >18 mm Hg)
Race (1.5–2.0 times higher mortality among African-Americans)
Age older than 65 y
Male sex
Serum sodium level <135 mmol/L
Arrhythmias (left ventricular conduction delay, NSVT)
Neurohormonal plasma levels (norepinephrine >400 ng/mL)

PCWP, Pulmonary capillary wedge pressure; NSVT, nonsustained ventricular tachycardia.

typically signifies decompensated CHF. Serum **hemoglobin** level should
be reviewed to rule out anemia as a contributing factor in heart failure
syndrome.

2. Elevation of **liver function test results** can occur when right-sided failure is predominant. This may be reflected in an elevation in transaminase level or coagulation factors. Patients at risk for thyroid abnormalities (those with atrial fibrillation, those who use amiodarone, and those older than 65 years) and patients with past or current thyroid abnormalities should have their **thyroid status** evaluated with serum thyroxine (T$_4$) and thyroid-stimulating hormone (TSH) measurements.

B. An **electrocardiogram (ECG)** may provide information about or help confirm the diagnosis that may be causing heart failure. It is important to look for signs of previous infarction, LV hypertrophy, arrhythmias, pericardial effusion (voltage less than 5 mm in frontal leads and less than 10 mm in precordial leads), and cardiac amyloidosis (low voltage and a pseudoinfarction pattern in anterior leads).

C. Examination of a **chest radiograph** should include heart size and the condition of the pulmonary parenchyma. Enlargement of the heart silhouette implies LV or biventricular failure. It is not unusual for patients with severe systolic dysfunction to have a nearly normal chest radiography is the dysfunction is compensated. A **normal-size cardiac silhouette does not rule out systolic or diastolic dysfunction.** The lung fields may range from mild engorgement of the perihilar vessels to bilateral pleural effusions, Kerley B lines, and frank pulmonary edema.

IV. **Diagnostic testing.** The evaluation for heart failure must be individualized.
The following studies should be considered.

A. **Echocardiography** is useful in evaluating LV function and identifying possible causes of CHF. The assessment of LV function may be qualitative (normal function, mild, moderate, or severely impaired function) or quanti-

Table 7-2. New York Heart Association classification

Class 1	No symptoms with ordinary physical activity
Class 2	Symptoms with ordinary activity Slight limitation of activity
Class 3	Symptoms with less than ordinary activity Marked limitation of activity
Class 4	Symptoms with any physical activity or at rest

Table 7-3. Signs and symptoms of heart failure

Symptoms	Physical findings
Dyspnea	Jugular venous distention
Orthopnea	Gallop rhythm
Paroxysmal nocturnal dyspnea	Pulmonary rales or wheezes
Cough	Hepatomegaly
Fatigue	Hepatojugular reflux
Nocturia	Ascities
Anorexia	Peripheral edema

tative. Quantitative measures of left ventricular ejection fraction (LVEF) can be made with newer machines with reasonable accuracy.

1. **Assessment of LV function**

   a. **Fractional shortening** was one of the earliest attempts to estimate LV function using M-mode technology. It is calculated by the following equation:

   $$\text{Fractional shortening} = \frac{(\text{LVED} - \text{LVES}) \times 100}{(\text{LVED})}$$

   where *LVED* is LV end-diastolic internal dimension and *LVES* is LV end-systolic internal dimension. A normal value for fractional shortening is 25% to 45%.

   b. **LVEF** can be estimated with LV volume calculations based on geometric assumptions about the shape of the left ventricle. Tomographic measurements are used in these calculations and are measured by means of two-dimensional echocardiography. The most common geometric assumption is that the LV cavity approximates a series of stacked disks. The modified Simpson rule is used to predict LV volume as follows:

   $$V = \frac{(\text{Am})\text{L}}{3} + \frac{(\text{Am} + \text{Ap})}{2} + \frac{\text{L}}{3} + \left(\frac{\text{Ap}}{3} \times \frac{\text{L}}{3}\right)$$

   where *Am* is LV cavity area at the mitral area, *Ap* is LV cavity area at the papillary muscle, *L* is length of the LV cavity, and *V* is ventricular volume. Once the end-systolic and end-diastolic volumes (ESV and EDV) are calculated, ejection fraction is found as follows:

   $$\frac{\text{EDV} - \text{ESV} \times 100}{\text{EDV}} = \text{ejection franction}$$

   c. With **Doppler** techniques, **cardiac output** can be estimated by means of measurement of the time velocity integral (TVI) and cross-sectional area (CSA) in the ascending aorta or in the LV outflow track. The equation for cardiac output (CO) is as follows:

   CO = Stroke volume × heart rate

   Stroke volume = CSA × TVI at site of CSA measurement

   The limitations of this calculation are that that laminar flow is assumed and that small deviations in CSA measurements lead to large errors in stoke volume.

    d. Ratio of change of ventricular pressure to change in volume (dP/dT). Among patients with MR, one can obtain an indirect measure of LV contractility by means of measuring the slope of the MR Doppler jet. Among patients with poor LV contractility, one would expect a slow increase in MR velocity as the failing LV pressure slowly overcomes left atrial pressure. Mathematical manipulations of the Bernoulli equation allow calculation of dP/dT as follows:

    dP/dT = 32,000/time (msec) for MR velocity to rise from 1 m/sec to 3 m/sec

    A **normal dP/dT is greater than 1200** and implies normal contractility. A dP/dT less than 1000 implies abnormal function.

  2. Other echocardiographic findings. Patients with systolic LV dysfunction invariably have diastolic dysfunction. They often have right ventricular dysfunction, segmental wall motion abnormalities, and marked valvular disease. One must also rule out an infiltrative myocardial process, constriction, and pericardial effusion.

B. Right heart catheterization (see Chapter 50). Invasive hemodynamic monitoring is invaluable in the diagnosis and management of CHF. It allows one to observe the response to intravenous (IV) therapy on a minute-to-minute basis. Right heart catheterization can be combined with exercise testing to study effects on hemodynamics.

  1. Cardiac index is one of the important measurements provided by right heart catheterization. This can be calculated by means of thermodilution dilution technique or the Fick method.

  2. Some methods of right heart catheterization allow continuous monitoring of cardiac output. Routine **determination of cardiac output** for patients with decompensated heart failure is critical to pharmacotherapy. It also provides early indication that medication is not effective and a more aggressive approach is warranted (intraaortic balloon pump, ventricular assist device).

  3. Other key information includes filling pressures, pulmonary arterial pressure, pulmonary capillary wedge pressure, systemic vascular resistance, pulmonary vascular resistance, pulmonary artery to pulmonary artery wedge gradient, and shunt calculation.

C. Left heart catheterization. In the care of patients with a **history of coronary artery disease,** evaluation of the coronary anatomy may be warranted. It is important to identify the cause of decompensation to guide therapy. The role of catheterization is to identify whether decompensation is caused by ischemia and whether revascularization (percutaneous or surgical) is indicated. Patients with CHF should undergo evaluation to rule out ischemic heart disease. Whether the evaluation is invasive or noninvasive depends on patient and physician preference.

D. Endomyocardial biopsy is indicated when myocardial disease is suspected and other causes of decompensation have been ruled out (coronary artery disease, valvular disease, drugs, endocrine disorders, for example). Biopsy should be considered if one suspects myocarditis, infiltrative or inflammatory disorders, arrhythmogenic right ventricular dysplasia, posttransplantation rejection, or cardiotoxicity by chemotherapeutic agents (anthracycline-induced cardiomyopathy).

E. Viability assessment for patients known to have had ischemia is important to determine the amount of ischemia and hibernation (see Chapter 43). This can be facilitated by dobutamine echocardiography, [18F] fluorodeoxyglucose positron emission tomography, and thallium 201 single-photon emission computed tomography. Once the ischemic and viability burden have been identified, the choice between revascularization and evaluation for transplantation can be made.

F. Metabolic stress testing. Patients who are considered for heart transplantation usually undergo risk stratification with a metabolic stress test.

Patients with a peak oxygen consumption less than 14 mL/kg per minute or exercise tolerance less than 50% predicted for age have a poor prognosis and may benefit from transplantation. This examination also is beneficial in differentiating the effects of respiratory versus cardiac dysfunction on patients with dyspnea during exertion.

G. **Other considerations.** Radionuclide ventriculography and echocardiography are acceptable for the evaluation of LV function. For patients who need very accurate measurements of LVEF (patients undergoing chemotherapy and receiving doxorubicin hydrochloride [Adriamycin]), radionuclide ventriculography is the better test. For patients believed to have valvular or congenital heart disease, echocardiography is preferred. The choice of test usually is based on the availability and accuracy of the test equipment within the local medical community.

V. **Etiology.** Table 7-4. is a partial list of causes of heart failure. It is important to identify the cause if possible to tailor therapy. Identification of an offending agent or reversible course is important.

A. **Peripartum cardiomyopathy** is LV dysfunction that occurs during the third trimester of pregnancy and up to 6 months post partum without a definitive cause. It most commonly occurs within 2 months after delivery. The incidence has been reported to be approximately 1:1,300 to 1:15,000 births. **Risk factors** include twin pregnancy, age older than 30 years, African descent, family history of peripartum cardiomyopathy, prolonged use of tocolytic agents, and multiparity. Approximately 50% of patients recover spontaneously within the first 6 months, after which time recovery is unlikely. Patients who do not recover eventually die of the disease or undergo cardiac transplantation. This diagnosis can be missed because many of the signs and symptoms can be confused with the normal physiologic changes of pregnancy during the third trimester. If symptoms persist after delivery, this condition should be suspected, and further investigation pursued.

B. **Dilated cardiomyopathy** is a condition in which the mass of the heart increases and systolic function of the left or both ventricles is impaired in the absence of coronary artery disease. Dilated cardiomyopathy is the most common type of cardiomyopathy among young persons, accounting for approximately 25% of cases. Approximately 10% to 20% of the cases of dilated cardiomyopathy are thought to be familial. Idiopathic cardiomyopathy is the most common cause of dilated cardiomyopathy; other causes are familial, alcohol-related, and viral.

Table 7-4. Causes of heart failure

Hypertensive heart disease
Cardiomyopathy
  Ischemic
  Dilated
  Restrictive
  Inflammatory
    Autoimmune
    Infectious
  Peripartum
  Tachycardia induced
Valvular heart disease
Congenital heart disease
Pericardial disease
Drugs and toxins
  Alcohol
  Cocaine
  Anthracyclines
Endocrine disorders

C. **Ischemic cardiomyopathy** is a condition caused by disease of the coronary arteries with resultant wall motion abnormalities and impaired LV function. It is the most common cardiomyopathy in the United States. The degree of atherosclerosis may involve the epicardial coronary arteries or smaller subendocardial vessels, as occurs among persons with diabetes. Ischemic cardiomyopathy may be associated with ventricular aneurysm, MR from papillary muscle dysfunction, ventricular septal defect, or arrhythmia. It is important to define this condition because treatment differs from that of nonischemic cardiomyopathy. Coronary anatomy should be defined, and myocardial viability should be assessed. Revascularization may slow the progression of heart failure syndrome. Ischemic cardiomyopathy usually has a worse long-term prognosis than dilated cardiomyopathy.

D. **Toxins.** The list of toxins that can produce cardiomyopathy is extensive. A list is provided in Table 7-5. Identification of the toxin and removal of the offending agent may halt progression of heart failure and in some instances lead to improvement. Most of the agents known are drugs used to manage malignant tumors, but other classes of drugs can cause cardiomyopathy. **Anthracycline** toxicity can cause myocyte destruction and cardiomyopathy. Patients who receive a cumulative dose of **doxorubicin hydrochloride** of less than 400 mg/m^2 are at low risk for this syndrome, whereas those who receive a cumulative dose exposure greater than 700 mg/m^2 have nearly a 20% likelihood of development of cardiomyopathy. **Alcohol** consumption is a common cause of toxin-mediated cardiomyopathy. It accounts for 30% of all cases of nonischemic cardiomyopathy. Total abstinence from alcohol may completely reverse this disease in its early stages. The continued use of alcohol is associated with high mortality (50% at 3 to 6 years).

E. **Valvular disorders** that produce chronic volume overload (MR and aortic regurgitation) are most commonly responsible for valve-related systolic heart failure. Differentiating primary from secondary MR can be difficult. A long-standing history of cardiac murmur favors the diagnosis of primary MR, whereas a centrally directed MR jet without leaflet abnormalities at echocardiography favors secondary MR. Appropriate follow-up and surgical management of MR and aortic regurgitation are discussed in Chapters 14 and 15. Severe aortic stenosis can lead to progressive LV dysfunction.

F. **Thyroid disorders.** Although uncommon, severe hypothyroidism may cause decreased cardiac output and heart failure. Bradycardia and pericardial effusion can develop in extreme cases of hypothyroidism. The diagnosis is confirmed with an elevated TSH and a reduced T$_4$ level. Treatment consists of thyroid replacement beginning at 25 to 50 μg/day levothyroxine for elderly patients or 100 μg/day for young, otherwise healthy patients.

G. **Duchenne's muscular dystrophy,** limb girdle dystrophy, and myotonic dystrophy are genetic diseases associated with dilated cardiomyopathy. Friedreich's ataxia is commonly associated with hypertrophic cardiomyopathy but in rare instances can cause dilated cardiomyopathy.

VI. **Treatment**

A. **Acute heart failure** consists of development of symptoms of severe CHF over a period of minutes to hours. It may be caused by cardiac ischemia, acute valvular dysfunction, or uncontrolled hypertension. A **hemodynamics-**

Table 7-5. Drugs and toxins associated with cardiomyopathy

Antibiotics	Antipsychotics	Chemotherapeutics	Other agents
Choloroquine	Phenothiazines	Doxorubicin	Alcohol
Didanosine	Lithium	Busulfan	Cocaine
Zidovudine		Bleomycin	Irradiation
		Cisplatin	
		Methotrexate	
		Vincristine	

directed protocol for decompensated heart failure is shown in Table 7-6. Rapid diagnosis and treatment of this syndrome are needed to prevent progressive deterioration. All patients should receive supplemental oxygen as needed. The underlying cause of the syndrome should be aggressively pursued and managed.

    1. Acute pulmonary edema. The development of high left atrial pressures caused by systolic or diastolic dysfunction results in accumulation

Table 7-6. Hemodynamics-directed protocol for therapy for decompensated heart failure

---

I. GENERAL HEMODYNAMIC GOALS

RAP 7 mm Hg
PCWP 15 mm Hg
SVR 1000–1200 dyne/sec per cm^5
CI >2.5 L/min per m^2
Optimum systolic or mean BP[a]

II. PATIENT-SPECIFIC HEMODYNAMIC GOALS

Optimum filling pressure (PCWP)[b]
Optimum afterload (SVR)[c]

III. SPECIFIC INTRAVENOUS PHARMACOLOGIC THERAPY

Nitroprusside: begin when combined pre- and afterload reduction is most important hemodynamic goal
Start at 0.1 to 0.2 µg/kg per min
Titrate upward by 0.2 µg/kg per min at 3- to 5-min intervals
Target hemodynamics (section I)
Hemodynamic effects resolve rapidly when infusion stopped

Nitroglycerin: begin when preload reduction is primarily desired
Start at 0.2 to 0.3 µg/kg per min
Titrate at 3- to 5-min intervals
Be aware of tolerance
Target hemodynamics (section I)
Effects resolve rapidly when infusion is stopped

Dobutamine: begin when both inotropic and vasodilating effects are desired but inotropic effects are most important
Start at 2.5 µg/kg per min
Attempt to keep dose <15 µg/kg per min; avoid marked tachycardia
Consider adding low-dose dopamine or milrinone to assist with augmenting renal perfusion or achieving hemodynamic end points
Hemodynamic effects resolve over minutes to hours when infusion is stopped, but benefits occasionally persist longer

Milrinone: begin when both vasodilating and inotropic effects are desired
Dose range is 0.375 to 0.75 µg/kg per min (usual is 0.5 µg/kg per min)
Target hemodynamics (section I)
Excessive hypotension with loading dose; avoid loading in acute heart failure
Prolonged hemodynamic effects after drug is stopped

---

[a]"Optimum" systolic or mean BP is the lowest pressure that adequately supports renal function and central nervous system activity without significant orthostatic symptoms (systolic BP generally 80 to 90 mm Hg).
[b]Optimum filling pressure (PCWP): lowest PCWP that can be maintained without preload-related decline in systolic BP or CI. A higher PCWP (18 to 20 mm Hg) is usually required in acute myocardial injury.
[c]Optimum afterload (SVR): lowest SVR that leads to reasonable CI while maintaining adequate systolic BP (generally 80 mm Hg) and renal perfusion (urine output >0.5 mL/kg per hour).
RAP, Right atrial pressure; PCWP, pulmonary capillary wedge pressure; SVR, systemic vascular resistance; CI, cardiac index; BP, blood pressure.

of fluid in the pulmonary interstitium and alveoli. When perfusion pressure is adequate and oxygenation pharmacotherapy is being maintained, treatment is as follows (Table 7-7).

   a. **Nitroglycerin.** Because of its ability immediately to lower preload and afterload, nitroglycerin is the first-line drug for the management of acute pulmonary edema among patients who are not in cardiogenic shock. Nitroglycerin may be given **rapidly by the sublingual approach in the emergency setting** (0.4 to 0.8 mg sublingually every 3 to 5 minutes) and by means of **IV drip in the subacute setting** (starting dosage 0.2 to 0.4 µg/kg per minute) and **titration every 5 minutes** on the basis of symptoms or mean arterial pressure (MAP). Increasing to more than 300 to 400 µg/min will likely not provide additional benefit, and another vasodilating agent usually is needed.

   b. **Sodium nitroprusside.** This potent vasodilator is a **second-line agent** when nitroglycerin is not effective in resolving pulmonary congestion. It requires careful hemodynamic monitoring, usually by means of continuous intraarterial catheterization. A starting dosage of 0.1 to 0.2 µ/kg per minute is used and titrated every 5 minutes to achieve a clinical response or until hypotension develops. Thiocyanate toxicity is rare in management of acute heart failure. However, nitroprusside should be **used with caution** in the care of patients with severe liver dysfunction and those who need long-term, high-dose infusions. For patients with suspected ischemia, initiation of IV nitroglycerin before nitroprusside is warranted to prevent coronary steal.

   c. **Diuretics.** Although most useful in the management of volume overload in chronic heart failure, IV diuretics may be useful in the immediate management of pulmonary edema. In addition to the ability to gradually reduce intravascular volume, diuretics have an immediate vasodilator effect, which may be responsible for the immediate beneficial effect. Because more potent vasodilators are available and many patients with acute pulmonary edema do not have whole-body salt and water excess, the **judicious use of diuretics** is recommended. Patients without chronic exposure to loop diuretics usually respond to 20 to 40 mg furosemide IV.

Table 7-7. Initial management of acute cardiogenic pulmonary edema

1. Sublingual nitroglycerin
   0.4 mg every 5 min
2. Intravenous nitroglycerin
   Start at 0.2 to 0.4 µg/kg per min
3. Intravenous furosemide
   20 to 40 mg
   Follow volume status closely
4. Nitroprusside
   Use if further afterload reduction is needed
5. Supplemental oxygen/mechanical ventilation
   Follow arterial blood gases and oxygen saturation
6. Intravenous morphine
   2 to 6 mg if no contraindications
7. Search for underlying cause when condition is stable
   Careful physical examination
   Electrocardiogram
   Cardiac enzyme analysis
   Echocardiography

Patients undergoing long-term furosemide therapy usually need an IV bolus dose at least equivalent to their oral dose.

  d. Inotropic therapy. When pulmonary edema persists despite administration of vasodilators and diuretics, aggressive hemodynamic monitoring is needed with right heart catheterization and inotropic therapy. For patients without hypotension **dobutamine or milrinone** can be used to augment cardiac output. Both drugs are associated with increased oxygen demand and cardiac arrhythmias and should be **used with extreme caution** to treat patients with ischemia and preexisting arrhythmias. Both drugs may cause hypotension, although this is more common with loading doses of milrinone. Dobutamine has a shorter half-life than milrinone and usually is the drug of choice in the acute setting. Dobutamine infusions act rapidly and are usually begun at 2.5 to 5.0 µg/kg per minute. On the basis of hemodynamic response, it may be titrated by 1 to 2 µg/kg per minute every 30 minutes until the desired effect is reached or until dosage reaches 15 to 20 µg/kg per minute. Milrinone is a vasodilator and an inotropic agent and should be used cautiously to treat patients with borderline hypotension. For patients who need an immediate inotropic response, a loading dose of 50 µg/kg is followed by an infusion of 0.375 to 0.75 µg/kg per minute.

2. Cardiogenic shock. Hypotension, tachycardia, low cardiac output, and organ hypoperfusion are the clinical manifestations of cardiogenic shock. It is usually caused by large MI, acute valvular insufficiency, or acute development of an intracardiac shunt. **Hemodynamic monitoring** is essential in diagnosing the cause of shock and in guiding therapy. Bedside **echocardiography** should be performed to evaluate for valvular insufficiency, intracardiac shunt, ventricular function, and cardiac tamponade. An algorithm for treatment of these patients is given in Fig. 7-1. If ischemia is suspected, urgent catheterization and revascularization should be performed if the anatomic features are suitable.

  a. Inotropic agents are essential for short-term use to treat patients with cardiogenic shock caused by poor LV or right ventricular function. For patients with hypotension (systolic blood pressure less than 80 to 85 mm Hg or MAP less than 60 mm Hg), pure inotropic agents (dobutamine and milrinone) can rarely be used alone. A combination vasopressor and inotropic agent, such as dopamine (5 to 15 µg/kg per minute), often is required. In some instances more potent vasopressor agents, such as norepinephrine (0.02 to 0.04 µg/kg per minute) must be used in combination with inotropic agents to maintain acceptable arterial pressure.

  b. Intraaortic balloon counterpulsation has the benefit of increasing MAP, cardiac output (10% to 20%), and coronary perfusion and reducing afterload. Insertion of the pump, complications, and benefits are discussed in Chapter 55. This device may serve as a bridge to coronary revascularization, surgical repair of MR, cardiac shunts, or transplantation. It is absolutely **contraindicated in the care of patients with severe aortic insufficiency or aortic dissection.**

  c. Vasodilators. Patients with arterial hypotension are not candidates for use of vasodilators. However, as ventricular performance improves with use of inotropic agents or balloon counterpulsation, patients may benefit from the use of vasodilators.

  d. Diuretics. Diuretics usually are **not indicated** in the management of acute cardiogenic shock caused by LV or right ventricular dysfunction. These drugs worsen organ hypoperfusion and hypotension. After appropriate therapy, diuretics may be useful to decrease pulmonary edema and salt and water retention.

  e. Ventricular assist devices (see also Chapter 12). When aggressive medical management of cardiogenic shock fails, long-term or

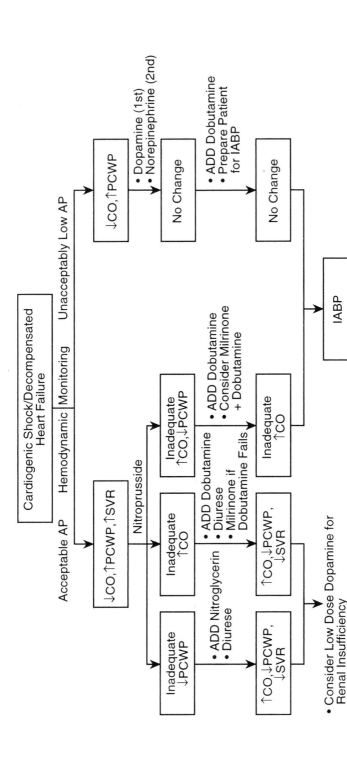

FIG. 7-1. Algorithm for heart failure.

short-term use of a ventricular assist device may be helpful. These devices supply adequate cardiac output in the setting of severe LV dysfunction and minimal native cardiac output. Patients with a reasonable chance for ventricular recovery are usually given short-term, nonimplantable devices. Patients for whom chronic ventricular dysfunction is expected and who are candidates for transplantation are usually given long-term, implantable ventricular assist devices.

B. Acute decompensation of chronic heart failure. Patients with chronic stable CHF often have episodes of acute or subacute decompensation in clinical status. Precipitating causes of acute decompensation include ischemia, high blood pressure, atrial fibrillation, alcohol consumption, endocrine abnormalities, use of negative inotropic drugs or nonsteroidal antiinflammatory drugs (NSAIDs), and lack of compliance with medical or dietary therapy.

   1. **Atrial fibrillation.** About 15% to 20% of patients with chronic heart failure have atrial fibrillation. New-onset atrial fibrillation can cause decompensation among patients with heart failure, presumably because of loss of the atrial contribution and lack of control of ventricular rate, which causes a decrease in cardiac output. Attempts should be made with either pharmacologic therapy or electrical cardioversion to restore sinus rhythm quickly to avoid chronic anticoagulation.

   2. **Alcohol** is a myocardial toxin. Excessive alcohol consumption is associated with depressed systolic and diastolic function, atrial and ventricular arrhythmias, hypertension, and sudden death. Patients with CHF should stop drinking alcohol.

   3. One of the most common causes of decompensation is **lack of compliance** with the medical regimen. Patients with chronic heart failure often have many other comorbid conditions. They have extensive lists of medications and may miss doses. **A physician responsible for treating a patient with heart failure must be aware of all medications the patient is taking.** The patient may have other physicians prescribing medications unknown to the primary provider. Patients should be asked about certain offenders: eye drops (β-blockers for glaucoma), negative chronotropic agents (verapamil, diltiazem), thyroid supplements, and NSAIDs (sodium and water retention).

   4. **Dietary indiscretions** commonly occur. Resistance to diuretics may be caused by excessive sodium intake. Patients should receive dietary instruction and constant reinforcement regarding the importance of a low-sodium diet.

   5. In many cases, patients do not need aggressive hemodynamic monitoring and IV vasodilators or inotropic agents. Administration of IV diuretics and oxygen, continuation of angiotensin-converting enzyme (ACE) inhibitors and digoxin, and identification of precipitating factors usually are the standard of care. Patients who do not respond to the foregoing measures or who have severe renal or hemodynamic compromise with diuresis are candidates for more aggressive care. The algorithm in Fig. 7-1 is a guide to the treatment of these patients.

C. Long-term therapy

   1. The goals of medical therapy are to **relieve vascular congestion and improve symptoms and functional status.** There are differences between the initial medical management of acute heart failure and therapy for chronic heart failure. In an **acute** exacerbation or decompensated state, IV inotropic agents, vasodilators, and pressors may be needed to support the patient. Management of **chronic** heart failure focuses on a medical regimen tailored to the patient to optimize hemodynamic values and fluid balance. Although the list of medications in the management of heart failure is extensive, it is imperative that the patient receive the medications to reduce morbidity and mortality.

      a. **ACE inhibitors** have been clearly established to reduce morbidity and mortality among patients with depressed LV function. Although these drugs are vasodilators, the mechanism of long-term benefit is most likely related to attenuation of the neurohormonal response to heart failure. Most clinical trials involving patients who have had an MI and have symptomatic CHF or asymptomatic LV dysfunction (LVEF less than 35% to 40%) have shown approximately 20% to 25% reduction in mortality in more than 2 years of follow-up study.

(1) Use of ACE inhibitors is considered **first-line therapy** for symptomatic CHF due to LV dysfunction or asymptomatic LV dysfunction. Patients should increase the dose of ACE inhibitor as tolerated.

(2) Unique **side effects** of ACE inhibitors are cough and angioedema. The **cough** associated with use of ACE inhibitors is believed to be related to increased levels of bradykinin. The cough tends to be dry, nonproductive, and involuntary. No particular ACE inhibitor has been proved more likely than others to cause a cough. A true ACE-inhibitor cough rarely resolves with changing the dosage or the type of ACE inhibitor. All attempts should be made to identify an alternative cause of the cough before discontinuing ACE inhibitors, because ACE inhibitor therapy is clearly efficacious.

(3) **Angioedema** is a rare complication of use of ACE inhibitors (0.4%). It involves soft-tissue edema of the lips, face, tongue, and occasionally the oropharynx and epiglottis. Angioedema usually begins within 2 weeks of initiation of ACE inhibitor therapy, but some patients manifest this complication months to years after starting therapy. **Angioedema is an absolute contraindication** to the use of any type of ACE inhibitor. There are no data regarding the safety of angiotensin receptor blockers in this setting.

b. **Digoxin** is both a positive and negative chronotropic drug. It is the drug of choice to treat patients with CHF and atrial fibrillation. Large clinical trials have demonstrated that digoxin is safe and significantly reduces hospitalization for CHF.

(1) Questions remain regarding appropriate **dosing** of digoxin. Serum digoxin levels likely have no correlation with clinical response. The use of 0.125 to 0.25 mg/day of digoxin to treat patients with normal renal function is recommended. For patients with normal renal function, digoxin levels need not be monitored unless toxicity is expected. For patients with renal insufficiency, digoxin level should be checked after 1 to 2 weeks of therapy to screen for accumulation of the drug. Levels can be helpful to see whether the drug is being absorbed. Levels beyond the therapeutic range may cause arrhythmia, atrioventricular block, nausea, and visual disturbances.

(2) The **side effects** of digoxin may be more pronounced in the setting of hypokalemia. Whether digoxin should be added to an initial medical regimen is unknown. Digoxin should not be withdrawn from patients with CHF who are tolerating the medication.

c. The combination of **hydralazine and isosorbide dinitrate** is effective alternative therapy for patients with CHF who cannot tolerate ACE inhibitors. It has been associated with a reduction in mortality among patients with CHF compared with treatment with prazosin and placebo.

(1) **Treatment** typically begins with 25 mg hydralazine three times a day and 10 mg isosorbide dinitrate three times a day with titration to a maximal dosage of 75 mg hydralazine three times a day and 40 mg isosorbide dinitrate three times a day as tolerated.

      (2) **Side effects** of hydralazine may include reflex tachycardia and a lupus-like syndrome. Nitrates can cause headaches and tolerance.

d. Diuretics are an important part of the therapeutic regimen for chronic CHF. They are classified according to their site of action and are effective in reducing salt and water retention and therefore symptoms of CHF. Overuse of these drugs, however, may cause worsening organ perfusion, weakness, and electrolyte abnormalities.

      (1) The **lowest possible dose** of diuretic needed to prevent substantial volume overload should be used. A patient often must tolerate some degree of peripheral edema if right heart failure is present. For patients with chronic, stable CHF, an effective and inexpensive initial regimen includes 20 mg to 120 mg furosemide once a day as needed to maintain a constant body weight. If dosages higher than 120 mg/day are needed, a second evening dose usually is prescribed. If this regimen fails, a daily dose of a thiazide diuretic, such as metolazone, often is added.

      (2) More expensive loop diuretics (torsemide, bumetanide) were not shown to be clinically superior to furosemide in large clinical trials.

e. β-Blockers. CHF activates the sympathetic nervous system. This is manifested by elevated plasma levels of norepinephrine often before appreciable symptoms occur. Elevated levels of plasma norepinephrine may be toxic to the myocardium. β-Blocker therapy may modulate this neuroendocrine axis.

      (1) Several trials have evaluated use of β-blockers by patients with heart failure. They include the Cardiac Insufficiency Bisoprolol Study (CIBIS) (1), the carvedilol trial (2), and Multicenter Oral Carvedilol Heart Failure Assessment (MOCHA) (3). Although the end point of the carvedilol trial (2) was not mortality, a reduction in mortality occurred among the group of subjects who received carvedilol. CIBIS (1) evaluated the use of bisoprolol and found a trend toward a reduction in morbidity but not in mortality. A trial is underway to compare the use of carvedilol with use of metoprolol to determine whether there is a class difference effect (selective versus nonselective) regarding sudden death and overall mortality. It remains to be seen whether there is definitive evidence for the use of β-blockers to manage heart failure. Early evidence appears to show that some patients may derive benefit from the use of these drugs.

      (2) Current recommendations are to start carvedilol to treat patients with symptomatic CHF who are not decompensated (NYHA class 2 to 3). It is unknown whether patients without symptoms or in decompensated class 4 will derive benefit from β-blockers. The initial dosage of carvedilol is 3.125 mg twice a day. The dosage is slowly titrated over 3 to 4 months to a target dosage of either 25 mg or 50 mg twice a day depending on the patient's weight. It is imperative to maintain contact and to see the patient frequently when increasing the dose, which is typically every 2 weeks until the target dose is reached.

f. Although useful in the management of acute or decompensated CHF, **inotropic agents** other than digoxin are considered **second-line therapy** for chronic CHF. Although low-output symptoms usually improve with chronic dobutamine or milrinone therapy, this is at the expense of higher risk for sudden death. Use of oral inotropic agents, such as vesnarinone, has been associated with improvement in symptoms but **increased mortality.** Patients who despite aggressive medical therapy have intractable chronic CHF may undergo long-term outpatient therapy with continuous IV infusion of inotropic agents on a compassionate basis. However, patients who are on a list for heart transplantation should stay in the hospital and undergo continuous telemetric monitoring for rapid management of arrhythmias should they occur. Although some cardiologists advocate intermittent outpatient dobutamine infusion, there has been no scientific evidence of improvement in morbidity or mortality with this regimen.

   g. **Angiotensin II receptor blockers** are a direct competitive antagonist to the angiotensin II type 1 receptor. These drugs do not appear to block the angiotensin type 2 receptor, which may be responsible for ventricular remodeling. These drugs are not currently first-line therapy and are **not to be used in place of ACE inhibitors.** They are appropriate for patients who do not tolerate ACE inhibitors. Whether angiotensin II receptor blockers are as efficacious as ACE inhibitors in the management of CHF remains to be seen.

VII. Controversies in CHF

   A. **Anticoagulation** in the setting of CHF is controversial. Heart failure predisposes a patient to increased risk for thromboembolism. This is manifested by altered endothelial function, increased coagulation factors, and increased plasma viscosity. Results of clinical trials implied that cerebrovascular events were a common cause of death among patients with heart failure. More recent clinical trials have shown that the incidence of fatal events may not be as common as once thought. This may reflect better management of atrial fibrillation. The potential for ventricular or atrial thrombus to embolize peripherally remains controversial.

   1. The general rule in regard to anticoagulation of patients with CHF is to use **warfarin sodium** in the following settings:
      a. Ventricular thrombi documented at echocardiography
      b. Atrial fibrillation
      c. Pulmonary embolism or chronic deep venous thrombosis
      d. After anterior wall MI

   2. Most patients with CHF are on an extensive regimen of medications, and care should be used when adding any medication because of the possible side effect and drug interaction profile of the new medication. Whether use of warfarin sodium lowers mortality among patients with decreased LVEF (less than 35%) without other indications for anticoagulants is unknown. Use of warfarin certainly complicates the medical regimen and increases risk for bleeding complications.

   B. The role of **calcium channel blockers** in CHF remains controversial. The new dihydropyridines have less negative inotropic and more potent vasodilatory properties. However, most trials have demonstrated increased morbidity and mortality among patients with CHF. Two newer agents, amlodipine and felodipine, may not have increased rates of adverse events among patients with CHF. In the Prospective Randomized Amlodipine Survival Evaluation Study (PRAISE) (4), amlodipine had no adverse influence on rates of death or serious cardiac events associated with ischemic cardiomyopathy. Amlodipine treatment reduced by 31% the rate of fatal and nonfatal events associated with nonischemic heart failure (4). PRAISE II will give additional information on amlodipine and nonischemic heart failure.

   C. **Antiarrhythmic therapy in CHF.** Sudden cardiac death is unpredictable and accounts for nearly half of all deaths among patients with CHF. Although frequent premature ventricular contractions (PVCs) are a marker of increased mortality among these patients, studies involving patients who have had an MI revealed that the use of conventional antiarrhythmic agents to suppress PVCs leads to higher mortality.

1. **Amiodarone** has been extensively studied in the care of patients with CHF because of its low incidence of proarrhythmia and its favorable hemodynamic effects. Data from four large randomized trials (5–8) involving patients with CHF but without previous sustained ventricular tachyarrhythmia or ventricular fibrillation revealed the following:
   a. Amiodarone appears not to be harmful to patients with CHF and frequent PVCs.
   b. Amiodarone reduces the incidence of arrhythmic death among these patients.
   c. Although trends toward reduced overall mortality with amiodarone were found in a large metaanalysis, no single study has shown a reduction in death rate with this drug.
   d. Retrospective analysis of the trials suggested that patients with nonischemic LV dysfunction derive more benefit from amiodarone. The overall neutral effect on mortality, however, makes the use of this drug to treat supraventricular arrhythmias and symptomatic PVCs more reassuring.
2. Patients with CHF who have had definite sustained ventricular tachycardia or ventricular fibrillation are more likely to benefit from use of an **implantable cardiac defibrillator** (ICD) than from drug therapy, including use of amiodarone. However, for patients who are not candidates for ICD therapy and patients who receive multiple ICD discharges, amiodarone therapy is the drug of choice to manage CHF.

D. **Immunosuppressive therapy for myocarditis.** Myocarditis with dilated cardiomyopathy can be a precursor to the development of heart failure. The Myocarditis Treatment Trial was designed to determine whether immunosuppressive therapy with methylprednisolone sodium succinate (Solu-Medrol) improves LV function among patients with myocarditis. Immunosuppression did not have a beneficial effect on the primary end point, a change in LVEF, and did not improve survival. However, this trial did not examine all forms of myocarditis, and the subjects may not have been representative of all patients with myocarditis. The **IMAC** trial is evaluating the role of immunoglobulin in the management of dilated cardiomyopathy from presumed myocarditis.

VIII. **Clinical predictors of LV function after MI.** The Silver criteria allow one to predict which patients will have an LVEF greater than 40% after MI with a high positive predictive value. Patients who meet the following criteria are highly likely to have an LVEF greater than 40%:
A. An interpretable ECG (no left bundle branch block, ventricular pacing, or left ventricular hypertrophy)
B. No previous Q-wave MI
C. No history of CHF
D. An index MI that is not a Q-wave anterior infarction.

SUGGESTED READINGS
References
1. CIBIS Investigators and Committees. A randomized trial of beta-blockade in heart failure: the Cardiac Insufficiency Bisoprolol Study (CIBIS). *Circulation* 1994;90: 1765–1773.
2. Packer M, Bristow MR, Cohn JN, et al. for the U.S. Carvedilol Heart Failure Study Group. The effect of carvedilol on morbidity and mortality in patients with chronic heart failure. *N Engl J Med* 1996;334:1349–1355.
3. Bristow MR, Gilbert EM, Abraham WT, et al. for the MOCHA Investigators. Carvedilol produces dose-related improvements in left ventricular function and survival in subjects with chronic heart failure. *Circulation* 1996; 94:2807–2816.
4. Packer M, O'Conner CM, Ghali JK, et al. for the Prospective Randomized Amlodipine Survival Evaluation Study Group (PRAISE). Effect of amlodipine on morbidity and mortality in severe chronic heart failure. *N Engl J Med* 1996;335: 1107–1114.

5. Doval HC, Nul DR, Grancelli HO, et al., For Gruppo de Estudio de la Insuficiencia Cardiaca en Argentina. Randomized trial of low dose amiodarone in severe congestive heart failure (GESICA). *Lancet* 1994;344:493–498.
6. Moss AJ, Hall AJ, Cannom DS, et al. for the Multicenter Automatic Defibrillator Implantation Trial Investigators (MADIT). Improved survival with an implanted defibrillator in patients with coronary disease at high risk for ventricular arrhythmias. *N Engl J Med* 1996;335:1933–1940.
7. Cairns JA, Connolly SJ, Roberts RS, Gent M. Canadian Amiodarone Myocardial Infarction Arrhythmia Trial (CAMIAT): rationale and protocol. *Am J Cardiol* 1993;72:87F–94F.
8. The Antiarrhythmics versus Implantable Defibrillators (AVID) Investigators. A comparison of antiarrhythmic-drug therapy with implantable defibrillators in patients resuscitated from near-fatal ventricular arrhythmias. *N Engl J Med* 1997; 337:1576–1583.

Landmark Articles
CAST Investigators. Preliminary report: effect of encainide and flecainide on mortality in a randomized trial of arrhythmia suppression after myocardial infarction. *N Engl J Med* 1989;321:406–412.
Cohn JN, Archibald DG, Ziesche S, et al. Effect of vasodilator therapy on mortality in chronic congestive heart failure: results of a Veterans Administration Cooperative Study (V-Heft I). *N Engl J Med* 1986;314:1547–1552.
CONSENSUS Trial Study Group. Effects of enalapril on mortality in severe congestive heart failure: results of the Cooperative North Scandinavian Enalapril Survival Study (CONSENSUS). *N Engl J Med* 1987;316:1429–1435.
Packer M, Gheorghiade M, Young JB, et al. for the RADIENCE Study. Withdrawal of digoxin from patients with chronic heart failure treated with angiotensin-converting-enzyme inhibitors. *N Engl J Med* 1993;329:1–7.
Pitt B, Segal R, Martinez FA, et al. Randomized trial of losarten versus captopril in patients over 65 with heart failure (Evaluation of Losarten in the Elderly Study, ELITE). *Lancet* 1997;349:747–752.
Singh SN, Fletcher RD, Gross Fischer S, et al. for the Survival Trial of Antiarrhythmic Therapy in Congestive Heart Failure. Veterans Affairs Anti-arrhythmia in Heart Failure Trial. *N Engl J Med* 1995;333:77–82.
SOLVD Investigators. Effect of enalapril on survival in patients with reduced left ventricular ejection fractions and congestive heart failure. *N Engl J Med* 1991;325: 293–302.
Uretsky BF, Young JB, Shahidi FE, Yellen LG, Harrison MC, Jolly MK. Randomized study assessing the effect of digoxin withdrawal in patients with mild to moderate congestive heart failure: results of the PROVED trial. PROVED Investigative Group. *J Am Coll Cardiol* 1993;22:955–962.

Key Reviews
Chatterjee K. Heart failure therapy in evolution. *Circulation* 1996;94:2689–2693.
Cohn JN. The management of chronic heart failure. *N Engl J Med* 1996;335:490–498.
Young JB. Contemporary management of patients with heart failure. *Med Clin North Am* 1995;79:1171–1191.

Relevant Book Chapters
Hosenpud JD, Greenberg BH. In: Hosenpud J, ed. *Congestive heart failure.* New York: Springer-Verlag, 1994.
Poole-Wilson PA, Massie BM, Yamani MH. In: Poole-Wilson P, ed. *Heart failure.* New York: Churchill Livingstone, 1997. Chapters 19 and 37.
Young JB, Haas GA, Rodkey SR. In: Topol E, ed. *Textbook of cardiovascular medicine.* Philadelphia: Lippincott–Raven, 1997. Chapters 81–83.

8. DIASTOLIC HEART FAILURE

John G. Peterson

I. **Introduction.** The function of the heart relies on its ability to receive low-pressure blood during diastole and eject blood at higher pressure during systole into the great vessels to produce cardiac output to meet the metabolic demands of the body. The ability of the ventricles to fill with blood under low pressure is a complex process that depends on many factors, including blood volume, blood pressure, heart rate, age, and intrinsic properties of the ventricle.

   A. **Three mechanisms govern the intrinsic ability of the ventricle to fill:** (1) relaxation of the ventricle after systole (in early diastole); (2) ventricular compliance (in mid-to-late diastole); and (3) pericardial restraint. Diseases that affect any of these mechanisms may cause diastolic heart failure. Therefore **diastolic dysfunction can be the result of impaired relaxation, myocardial restriction, or pericardial constriction** (restriction and constriction are differentiated in section VII of this chapter).

   B. **Diastole can be defined** by several methods.

      1. On an **electrocardiogram (ECG),** diastole is the period between the end of the T wave and the beginning of the QRS complex.

      2. At **physical examination,** S_2 marks the beginning of diastole and S_1 its end.

      3. The **hemodynamic** definition of diastole is the period from the onset of isovolumic relaxation to the onset of isovolumic contraction (Fig. 8-1).

   C. **Patients with congestive heart failure (CHF) usually have a combination of both systolic and diastolic dysfunction.** However, some patients have normal systolic function and no appreciable valvular heart disease but still have signs and symptoms of CHF. These patients usually have isolated diastolic dysfunction. This chapter concentrates on finding and treating such patients.

II. **Clinical presentation.** Among patients with CHF, 30% to 40% have normal or near-normal left ventricular (LV) systolic function and are presumed to have mainly diastolic heart failure. The prevalence of diastolic dysfunction in various populations depends on patient age and the presence of other diseases. At highest risk are elderly patients with hypertension. Because diastolic heart failure has multiple causes, ranging from systemic disorders to primary myocardial disorders, a single prognosis that can be generalized to all patients is not possible. However, the yearly mortality among patients with mostly diastolic dysfunction has been shown to be approximately 50% of that of patients with systolic dysfunction. **Poor prognostic signs** include severely reduced exercise tolerance and ventricular tachycardia on Holter monitoring. Recurrent hospitalizations for pulmonary congestion are common. Specific causes of diastolic dysfunction, such as endomyocardial fibrosis, amyloidosis, and hemochromatosis carry a particularly poor prognosis. A restrictive filling pattern at echocardiography is independently associated with high mortality.

   A. **Signs and symptoms.** Patients with diastolic dysfunction have symptoms indistinguishable from those associated with systolic dysfunction.

      1. **Dyspnea on exertion** and **reduced exercise tolerance** are the earliest symptoms of diastolic dysfunction and should make one suspect this diagnosis if LV systolic function and valvular anatomy are known to be normal.

      2. As the disease progresses, **dyspnea at rest, paroxysmal nocturnal dyspnea,** and **orthopnea** can occur.

      3. Patients with some types of **diastolic dysfunction, such as restrictive myocardial disease or constrictive pericardial disease, may have predominantly right-sided heart failure symptoms,** such as edema, anorexia, right upper quadrant pain, and abdominal bloating.

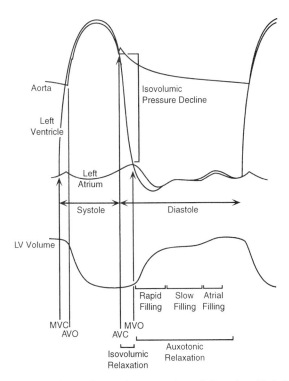

FIG. 8-1. Schematic of the cardiac cycle in systole and diastole with left ventricular and left atrial pressures and left ventricular volumes. Diastole is divided into two phases. The first is an isovolumic relaxation period from aortic valve closure (*AVC*) to mitral valve opening (*MVO*) when left ventricular pressure falls with no change in volume. The second phase is an auxotoric period (from mitral valve opening to mitral valve closure) when left ventricular volume increases with a variable increase in pressure. The second phase includes a rapid filling phase, slow filling, and atrial filling. (From Zile MR. Diastolic dysfunction: detection, consequences, and treatment, 1: definition and determinants of diastolic function. *Mod Concepts Cardiovasc Dis* 1989;58:67, with permission.)

   B. Physical findings vary considerably depending on causation and cardiac chamber involvement.
      1. Patients often have **hypertension.**
      2. Typical findings at physical examination include **pulmonary rales, edema, venous distention,** and **audible S_3 and S_4 gallops.** These findings are useful in diagnosing CHF but not in differentiating systolic from diastolic heart failure.
         a. In early stages of diastolic heart failure, a preserved S_1 and an S_4 gallop alone tend to be more prevalent.
         b. In diastolic heart failure caused by myocardial restriction or pericardial constriction, jugular venous waveforms characteristically show preserved *x* **descents** and steep *y* **descents** (the exaggerated *m* or *w* configuration) because of abnormal ventricular filling. **Kussmaul's sign** (paradoxic elevation of jugular venous pressure with inspiration) may occur among these patients.

3. Certain **systemic disorders,** such as amyloidosis and hemochroma-tosis, have classic physical examination findings and are discussed separately.

III. **Laboratory examination**

A. **ECG.** The most common ECG abnormality in diastolic dysfunction is **LV hypertrophy.** However, because neither the sensitivity nor the specificity of ECG criteria for LV hypertrophy is high, the predictive value of this sign in the diagnosis of diastolic dysfunction is poor. ECG evidence of a left atrial abnormality due to elevated left atrial pressures sometimes can be seen. Specific causes, such as amyloidosis and hypertrophic cardiomyopathy, also have their own ECG manifestations: (see **IV.C.2.a** and Chapter 9).

B. **Chest radiograph.** There are no specific chest radiographic findings in diastolic dysfunction. In general, patients tend to have normal chest ra-diographs early in the course of the disease. The first manifestation of dias-tolic heart failure on a chest radiograph is **pulmonary venous hyperten-sion with a normal-sized cardiac silhouette.** Left atrial enlargement, although difficult to differentiate on a routine chest radiograph and not spe-cific for diastolic dysfunction, may be seen with this disorder. Evidence of LV enlargement tends to occur in later stages of the disease.

IV. **Etiology.** Many disorders can affect the ability of heart to fill normally. This chapter focuses on those primarily caused by diseases of the myocardium and endocardium. Pericardial diseases are discussed in Chapters 26 through 28 and are mentioned herein only to differentiate them from myocardial restriction.

A. **Myocardial ischemia.** The early phase of diastole, the **isovolumic relax-ation period,** is an active, energy-consuming process much like systole. It requires adenosine triphosphate (ATP) and therefore depends on adequate oxygen supply and is affected by ischemia. Experiments in cardiac catheter-ization laboratories have confirmed the development of diastolic dysfunction with balloon occlusion of coronary arteries. This event occurs before chest pain, systolic dysfunction, or ECG changes. Therefore symptoms of heart fail-ure caused by diastolic dysfunction may be one of the earliest manifestations of coronary ischemia.

B. **LV hypertrophy.** Most commonly caused by long-standing hypertension, LV hypertrophy affects both the passive elastic properties of the ventricle and ventricular relaxation. Some studies have shown abnormalities in intra-cellular calcium handling among patients with LV hypertrophy with resul-tant depressed active relaxation. Increased wall thickness also impairs the passive filling phase of diastole. Hypertension itself, even in the absence of LV hypertrophy, has been shown to be associated with impaired diastolic filling. Hypertrophic cardiomyopathy resulting in diastolic dysfunction is discussed in Chapter 9.

C. **Restrictive cardiomyopathies** are a group of diseases characterized by CHF, restrictive filling function, and normal LV contractility. Myocardial constriction can be primary or secondary (Fig. 8-2).

1. **Primary restrictive cardiomyopathy**

a. **Idiopathic restrictive cardiomyopathy,** sometimes familial and associated with distal skeletal myopathy, is a diagnosis of exclusion when no other cause of myocardial restriction can be found. It typi-cally causes **symptoms** of right or left heart failure. **Echocardio-graphic** findings are biatrial enlargement, normal LV thickness, and normal systolic function. Heart block caused by fibrosis of the sino-atrial or atrioventricular node can be seen. Postmortem microscopic examination shows patchy areas of interstitial fibrosis.

b. **Endomyocardial fibrosis (Davies' disease)** is a common cause of CHF and death in equatorial Africa. Affecting mainly children and young adults, this disease leads to fibrosis and obliteration of the ventricular apices. Thromboembolism is common. Endomyocardial fibrosis appears to be mediated by tissue eosinophils that are directly toxic to the endomyocardium. Treatment is mainly symptomatic;

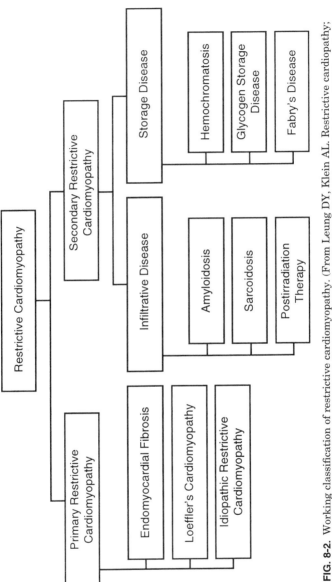

FIG. 8-2. Working classification of restrictive cardiomyopathy. (From Leung DY, Klein AL. Restrictive cardiopathy; diagnosis and prognostic implications. In: Otto CM, *Practice of clinical echocardiography.* Philadelphia: WB Saunders, 1997:474, with permission.)

however, a surgical procedure sometimes is performed to remove the fibrotic material in the ventricular apices; the surgical mortality rate is 15% to 25%.

c. **Eosinophilic cardiomyopathy (Löffler's disease)** occurs mainly in temperate climates and is associated with the hypereosinophilic syndrome (eosinophilia, arteritis, and thromboembolism in the absence of an underlying cause). As with endomyocardial fibrosis, there is endocardial thickening and obliteration of the cardiac apex; thromboembolism is common. If the disease is managed early with corticosteroids, progression may be delayed.

2. **Secondary restrictive cardiomyopathy**

   a. **Amyloidosis**

   (1) Amyloidosis is a group of diseases caused by the **deposition of pathologic insoluble fibrillar proteins in organs and tissues.** The **clinical features** of cardiac amyloidosis are biventricular heart failure (usually right-sided failure exceeds left), atrial fibrillation, and low voltage on an ECG with a pseudo-infarction pattern (anteroseptal Q waves). The diagnosis of cardiac amyloidosis can be made by means of **endomyocardial biopsy** or **echocardiography.** Echocardiography typically reveals concentrically thickened ventricles, a bright and speckled myocardium, and Doppler evidence of restricted filling. Low voltage on an ECG may help differentiate amyloidosis from hypertrophic cardiomyopathy, although biopsy occasionally is needed to confirm the diagnosis.

   (a) The **most common form** of amyloidosis that affects the heart is **AL,** or **primary, amyloidosis.** It is caused by the inappropriate production of immunoglobulins by clonal plasma cells in bone marrow. AL amyloidosis often occurs with multiple myeloma. It also is associated with the nephrotic syndrome caused by light-chain deposition in the kidneys. Autonomic and sensory neuropathies are common, although motor neuropathy is rare. Liver infiltration may cause hepatomegaly, and Howell-Jolly bodies can be seen on peripheral blood smears, indicating hyposplenism. Vascular infiltration can lead to easy bruising, and macroglossia occurs among about 20% of patients.

   (b) **Familial amyloidosis,** or **ATTR type,** is caused by one of the many mutations of the transthyretin gene. This differs clinically from AL amyloidosis; in ATTR amyloidosis there is less renal disease, no macroglossia, and less serious heart involvement. It does, however, tend to affect the cardiac conduction system more frequently. Because ATTR amyloidosis is caused by production of a mutant prealbumin protein by the liver, transplantation of the liver may be beneficial.

   (c) **Senile cardiac amyloidosis** occurs among elderly people and is caused by deposition of a normal transthyretin protein in the myocardium. Myocardial biopsy usually is needed for diagnosis because the amyloidosis may be localized strictly to the myocardium.

   (2) Patients with amyloidosis are sensitive to the proarrhythmic effects of digoxin; therefore this drug should be used with caution. Symptoms also may worsen with the addition of calcium channel blockers. **Chemotherapy** (generally with melphalan and prednisone) has been used in the management of AL amyloidosis with varying success. Otherwise healthy persons with ATTR amyloidosis have been treated with liver transplanta-

tion. Symptomatic treatment is discussed in Section VI of this chapter.

  b. Hemochromatosis

    (1) Primary hemochromatosis is a recessive genetic disease that causes inappropriate absorption of iron from the gastrointestinal tract and subsequent deposition of iron into tissues, including the heart. It can lead to both systolic and diastolic myocardial dysfunction. It is frequently associated with hypogonadism, skin discoloration, diabetes, arthropathy, and liver failure. **Phlebotomy** may improve cardiac symptoms, but if severe systolic impairment develops, the prognosis is poor.

    (2) Secondary hemochromatosis is iron overload of other causes, usually multiple blood transfusions. Because many patients acquire this disease from treatment for chronic anemia or hemoglobinopathy, phlebotomy is not an option for treatment. **Chelation** of iron with deferoxamime, although not as efficacious in removing iron as phlebotomy, can be used to treat these patients.

  c. Storage disorders. Numerous genetic disorders, usually enzymatic defects, can cause accumulation of inappropriate lipids or polysaccharides within the myocardium. Gaucher's disease, Hurler's disease, and Fabry's disease are examples of these disorders.

  d. Sarcoidosis is a noncaseating granulomatous disorder that affects the heart in about 5% of cases. It causes myocardial restriction by means of scar formation around infiltrating granulomas in the myocardium. It also is associated with ventricular arrhythmias, heart block, and wall motion abnormalities. Diagnosing this disorder by means of endomyocardial biopsy can be difficult because of the patchy nature of myocardial involvement. Treatment with corticosteroids is indicated when substantial cardiac involvement is present.

  e. Miscellaneous causes. Use of anthracycline and radiation therapy can cause endocardial fibrosis that leads to restrictive cardiomyopathy. Radiation therapy also may be complicated by pericardial constriction, which also impairs ventricular filling.

V. Diagnostic testing. Diastolic heart failure is a clinical syndrome and must be supported by both clinical criteria and results of laboratory studies. The diagnosis should be considered for patients with signs and symptoms of left or right heart failure and normal left and right ventricular (RV) systolic function.

  A. Echocardiography has long been considered the best modality to assess diastolic dysfunction. It is used to detect LV hypertrophy and evaluate systolic function. It also is used to measure relaxation intervals and Doppler flow to detect filling abnormalities consistent with diastolic dysfunction (Table 8-1). However, these measurements can vary substantially depending on loading conditions and heart rate. Aging also causes changes in Doppler filling patterns that are difficult to differentiate from impaired relaxation caused by specific diseases. With these limitations in mind, the following measurements are helpful.

    1. The isovolumic relaxation time (IVRT) is the interval between aortic valve closure and mitral valve opening. A prolonged IVRT (>100 msec) is consistent with impaired ventricular relaxation (see Fig. 8-3).

    2. Ventricular inflow. During sinus rhythm there are two periods of inflow across the mitral valve: the early transmitral flow **(E wave)** and late flow consistent with atrial contraction **(A wave)**.

      a. The time from the peak filling velocity of the E wave to baseline is called the **deceleration time** (Fig. 8-3). Among healthy young adults, the ratio of peak E to peak A (E/A) velocities is about 2:1. This declines to about 1:1 among healthy persons older than 50 years.

Table 8-1. Filling patterns in diastolic dysfunction

Pattern	E/A ratio	Deceleration time (msec)	IVRT (msec)	S/D	AR (cm/sec)
Normal	2.1	180	76	1.0	19
Age older than 50 y	1.0	210	90	1.7	23
Impaired relaxation	<1.0	>220	>100	>1.0	<35
Pseudonormal	1.0–2.0	150–220	60–100	<1.0	>35
Restriction	>2.0	<150	60	<1.0	>35

E/A ratio, Peak early mitral inflow/peak late mitral inflow; *IVRT,* isovolumic relaxation time; *S/D,* peak systolic pulmonary vein inflow/peak diastolic pulmonary vein inflow; *AR,* velocity of atrial reversal of pulmonary venous flow.

      (1) A **low E/A ratio** combined with a long deceleration time and long IVRT is consistent with impaired relaxation of the ventricle.

      (2) A **high E/A ratio,** short deceleration time, and short IVRT are consistent with a restrictive filling pattern (Fig. 8-4).

   b. Because many patients with diastolic dysfunction progress from a physiologic state of impaired relaxation to one of restrictive filling as the disease progresses, they pass through a period E/A ratio, deceleration time, and IVRT are normal despite the presence of marked diastolic impairment (the **pseudonormal pattern**).

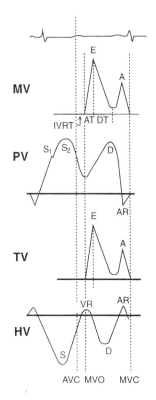

FIG. 8-3. Diastole using Doppler echocardiography. Combined schematic displays left atrial (*L*) and left ventricular (*LV*) and aortic (*Ao*) pressure during diastole (*PRESSURE*). The equation shows how instantaneous LV pressure (*Pv*) falls exponentially through the isovolumic relaxation period (*IVRT*) from *Po* (LV pressure at aortic valve closure [*AVC*]) to *Pa* (LV pressure at mitral valve opening [*MVO*]). Transmitral (*MV*) Doppler scan demonstrates an early rapid filling wave (*E*) broken into an acceleration time (*AT*) and a deceleration time (*DT*); a diastasis period with very little inflow; and an atrial contraction wave (*A*) associated with an elevation of left atrial pressure above LV pressure until mitral valve closure (*MCV*) is induced by the onset of ventricular systole. The pulmonary vein (*PV*) demonstrates a systolic wave (*S1*) related to atrial relaxation and mitral annular descent (*S2*), a diastolic wave (*D*) associated with atrial emptying through an open mitral valve, and an atrial reversal wave (*AR*) associated with atrial systole causing regurgitation of flow back up the pulmonary veins. Trans-tricuspid (*TV*) inflow has a similar pattern velocity to transmitral flow. Hepatic vein (*HV*) flow is similar to pulmonary vein flow with a more prominent reversal of flow between the S and D waves associated with ventricular systole (*VR*).

Natural History of LV Filling

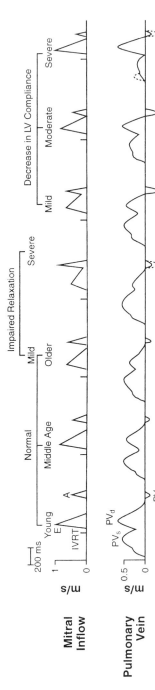

FIG. 8-4. Schematic of transmitral and pulmonary venous Doppler scans demonstrates the progression of patterns with normal aging and with diseases of diastolic function that cause impaired relaxation and a decrease in LV compliance. Isovolumic relaxation time (*IVRT*), E-wave (*E*) and A-wave (*A*) filling, and pulmonary venous systolic (*Pvs*), diastolic (*Pvd*) and atrial reversal waves (*Pva*) are shown. *Left*, In a healthy person, the E/A ratio is greater than 1, deceleration time and isovolumic relaxation period (*IVRT*) are short, and there is mild blunting of pulmonary venous systolic flow. With age, ventricular relaxation becomes impaired, the E/A ratio reverses, the A wave increases, mitral deceleration time and IVRT lengthen, and pulmonary venous systolic flow increases. *Center*, With diseases that impair relaxation, there may be similar findings with a further decrease in E/A ratio. *Right*, Severe derangement of diastolic function causes chamber compliance to decrease. Left atrial pressure rises, deceleration time decreases, E/A ratio increases, and IVRT becomes shorter (restrictive physiologic state). Pulmonary venous systolic flow (*Pvs*) becomes progressively blunted as mean left atrial pressure and the atrial reversal (*Pva*) increase. This helps to differentiate the pseudonormal pattern from normal. (From Appleton CP, Hatle LK. The natural history of left ventricular filling abnormalities: assessment by two dimensional and Doppler echocardiography. *Echocardiography* 1992;9:453, with permission.)

(1) Repeating mitral valve inflow measurements during a Valsalva maneuver or after administration of nitroglycerin to decrease preload often reverts a pseudonormal pattern to one of impaired relaxation (E < A). A patient with a truly normal pattern has a reduction in both E and A velocities, but the E/A ratio should not change.

(2) Measurement of atrial inflow also is helpful in resolving the issue of a pseudonormal filling pattern.

3. Atrial inflow

   a. Atrial inflow through the pulmonary or hepatic vein can be measured by means of pulse wave Doppler ultrasound.

     (1) During ventricular systole, descent of the cardiac apex and relaxation of the atria result in atrial inflow, called the **S wave** (the x descent on venous pressure tracings).

     (2) When the mitral and tricuspid valves open, another period of inflow occurs, the **D wave** (the y descent).

     (3) At the end of diastole, atrial contraction causes venous flow reversal, the **AR wave** (see Fig. 8-3).

   b. The S and D waves in general are equal among healthy young patients. Among patients with impaired ventricular relaxation, **S/D ratio increases.** Among patients with myocardial restriction or pericardial constriction, the **S/D ratio decreases.** Restrictive filling leads to increased amplitude (>35 cm/sec) and duration (more than 20 msec longer than the A wave) of venous flow reversal (see Fig. 8-4).

B. The hemodynamic abnormalities associated with diastolic dysfunction are most precisely evaluated by means of **cardiac catheterization.** Both left and right heart catheterizations usually are performed to assess for pericardial constriction and myocardial restriction as causes of diastolic abnormalities. The following measurements often are helpful in this evaluation.

   1. Both right and left **atrial pressures** typically are increased among patients with marked diastolic dysfunction. Preserved x descent and steep y descent on atrial tracings caused by rapid early filling are seen with myocardial restriction or pericardial constriction (Fig. 8-5). Pulmonary capillary wedge pressure, an estimate of left atrial pressure, also is elevated.

   2. Ventricular pressures. Diastolic heart failure, like systolic heart failure, causes elevated RV systolic and LV end-diastolic pressures. Diastolic heart failure caused by restrictive myocardial or constrictive pericardial disease shows unique pressure recordings from the ventricles. The classic RV and LV tracings in these disorders show a brisk pressure descent early in diastole followed immediately by a rapid rise and early plateau of the pressure waveform, the **square-root sign** (see Fig. 8-5). This pattern represents the early rapid filling and poor late-diastolic filling that occur with constriction and restriction.

   3. Time constant of relaxation (τ). One of the problems with noninvasive measurement of diastolic values is dependence on loading conditions that can change the values from moment to moment. The LV pressure decay constant, τ, which can be measured with a high-fidelity manometer, reflects energy-dependent LV relaxation that occurs during isovolumic relaxation and is **relatively unaffected by changes in loading conditions.** The time constant τ tends to decrease with increased heart rate, reflecting improved relaxation to accommodate faster filling. Because of the expense of the equipment needed to measure this variable, and unclear clinical relevance, τ is not routinely measured during cardiac catheterization.

C. Radionuclide techniques. The utility of radionuclide ventriculography in reproducible and accurate assessment of systolic function is unquestioned. The ability to detect diastolic dysfunction in individual patients is

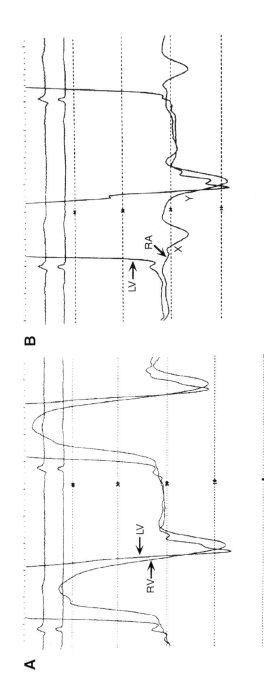

FIG. 8-5. A,B: Simultaneous right ventricular (*RV*) and left ventricular (*LV*) pressure recordings demonstrate equalization of diastolic pressure and a dip and plateau physiologic state. Simultaneous right atrial (*RA*) and LV pressure recordings demonstrate equalization during diastolic and prominent *x* and *y* descents in the RA tracing. (From Vaitkus PV, et al. Constrictive pericarditis. *Circulation* 1996;93:834–835, with permission.)

less certain. Diastolic filling values that can be measured with sophisticated analysis include peak filling rate and filling fraction. Neither measurement is widely used, and accuracy among individual patients has yet
to be determined. However, accurate assessment of ejection fraction is
valuable in assessing symptoms of CHF and can help confirm suspicion of
diastolic dysfunction.

D. **Endomyocardial biopsy** (see Chapter 54) is an invasive technique that may
be helpful in establishing the cause of isolated diastolic dysfunction. If there
is high suspicion of infiltrative myocardial diseases, endomyocardial biopsy
may provide a tissue diagnosis that can affect therapy. However, many of the
infiltrative diseases, especially sarcoidosis, can be patchy in distribution
within the myocardium, and the biopsy may yield a false-negative result. The
presence of several systemic diseases, such as hemochromatosis and systemic
amyloidosis, can be confirmed on the basis of clinical manifestations and
biopsy of other, more easily accessible tissues.

VI. **Therapy.** Because there are myriad causes of diastolic dysfunction, the primary therapy is **management of the underlying pathologic condition.**
General concepts are as follows.

A. **Decrease central blood volume.** The judicious use of diuretics and nitrates
to reduce intravascular volume can be helpful in alleviating symptoms of vascular congestion. There is a narrow therapeutic window for these medications,
however, because reductions in preload may lead to inadequate ventricular
filling, resulting in reduced cardiac output. Angiotensin-converting enzyme
(ACE) inhibitors are good venodilating agents. Use of these agents decreases
central blood volume. These drugs may be appropriate when hypertension is
difficult to control.

B. **Improve ventricular relaxation. β-Adrenergic agonists,** such as dobutamine, exert a **lusitropic** effect, or enhancement of relaxation, in addition
to their effects on systolic dysfunction. They are best reserved for patients
with a **combination of systolic and diastolic heart failure and severe
symptoms not responsive to usual therapy.** Although studies have
shown improvement in measurements of relaxation with the use of these
drugs to treat patients with primarily systolic dysfunction, their use in isolated diastolic dysfunction is untested and discouraged because of their side
effects.

C. **Manage hypertension.** Several antihypertensive agents have been shown
to reduce LV mass. These include ACE inhibitors, calcium channel blockers,
β-blockers, and central-acting sympatholytic agents. Proof of effectiveness
in regression of LV hypertrophy to improve diastolic filling is clouded by the
fact that all antihypertensive agents change loading conditions, which
affects noninvasive measurements of filling. Adequate control of blood pressure is a reasonable goal because of its beneficial effects on cardiovascular
and cerebrovascular disease.

D. **Control arrhythmias.** Even common cardiac arrhythmias, such as atrial
fibrillation or flutter, are poorly tolerated by patients with diastolic dysfunction. As resistance to filling increases, the dependence of cardiac output
on atrial contribution and adequate filling time increases. All steps should
be taken to restore and maintain the sinus rhythm of these patients.

E. **Control ischemia.** Revascularization or antianginal medications should be
used to treat patients whose diastolic dysfunction is caused by reduced coronary blood flow. β-Blocking agents, although they have no direct beneficial
effects on relaxation, are excellent antiischemic drugs. Aspirin, nitrates, and
calcium channel blockers may also be useful to these patients.

F. **Reduce heart rate.** Neither β-blockers nor calcium channel blockers have
been proved to reduce LV filling pressure or improve morbidity or mortality in CHF caused by diastolic dysfunction. In theory, reduction of heart
rate should improve ventricular filling among patients whose main problem is **impaired relaxation** of the ventricle because diastole would be
prolonged and allow more time for filling. However, as patients progress to

a **restrictive filling** physiologic state, ventricular filling occurs mainly in early and late diastole only, and this filling takes place rapidly. Thus prolonged diastole does not lead to more ventricular filling, and cardiac output is reduced because of the reduction in heart rate. Therefore the **use of β-blockers and calcium channel blockers** to treat patients with moderate to severe diastolic dysfunction should be **undertaken with extreme caution.**

VII. **Clinical Controversies: restriction versus constriction.** Differentiation of **restrictive myocardial disease** from **constrictive pericardial disease** among patients with diastolic dysfunction is difficult but **extremely important.** Therapy for constrictive disease is surgical pericardial stripping. Symptomatic therapy is used to manage restriction unless a treatable cause can be found.

A. The **history** can occasionally be helpful in this distinction. Previous cardiac operations, pericarditis, or irradiation to the mantle favor a diagnosis of constriction. In rare instances a paradoxic pulse occurs with constrictive pericarditis. Myocardial restriction is more often associated with regurgitant valve murmurs.

B. **Clinical suspicion is confirmed** by means of hemodynamic, anatomic, and echocardiographic analysis.

1. The **hemodynamic pressure tracings** obtained at right and left heart catheterization are **similar in constrictive and restrictive disease.** Traditional teaching is that minor differences in the relations between various left and right heart catheterization data can be used to differentiate pericardial constriction from myocardial restriction (Table 8-2).

2. New data suggest that the **only reliable discriminators are the hemodynamic changes that accompany respiration.** Among patients with pericardial **constriction,** the changes in RV and LV peak systolic pressures with inspiration or expiration occur in **opposite directions.** In **restrictive** cardiomyopathy, this change occurs in the **same direction.** This invasive method of **differentiating restriction and constriction** may be helpful in the care of patients with technically difficult echocardiograms or irregular heart rhythms.

3. **Echocardiography** using two-dimensional and Doppler recordings has proved to be a valuable tool in differentiating constriction and restriction.

a. The most sensitive value to examine is the variation in mitral valve inflow velocities with respiration (Fig. 8-6). Healthy persons and patients with a **restrictive** condition have **less than 10%** variability in mitral valve inflows with respiration. Patients with **constrictive** pericardial disease, because of cardiac chamber interdependence, usually have **greater than 25%** variation in mitral valve inflows with respiration. Pulmonary venous flow varies with respiration in constriction but not with restriction.

b. **Cardiac tamponade** is associated with similar changes in mitral inflow patterns, but clinical characteristics, the presence of pericardial effusion, and differences in atrial inflows make differentiation

Table 8-2. Conventional hemodynamic parameters: constriction versus restriction

Myocardial restriction	Pericardial constriction
LVEDP – RVEDP > 5 mm Hg	LVEDP – RVEDP ≤ 5 mm Hg
RVEDP < ⅓ RVSP	RVEDP ≥ ⅓ RVSP
RVSP > 55 mm Hg	RVSP < 55 mm Hg

LVEDP, left ventricular end-diastolic pressure; *RVEDP,* right ventricular end-diastolic pressure; *RVSP,* right ventricular systolic pressure.

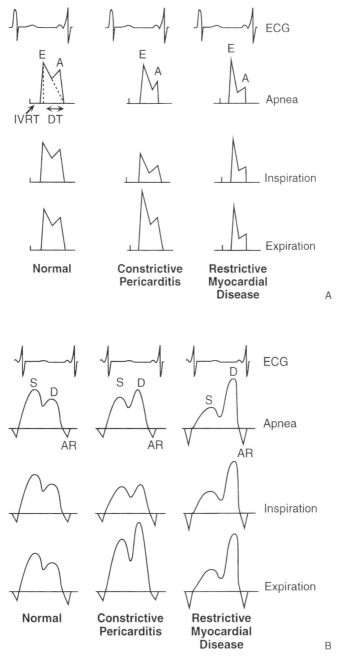

FIG. 8-6. A,B: Left ventricular inflow velocities and pulmonary venous flow during different phases of respiration. (From Klein Al, Cohen GI. Doppler echocardiographic assessment of constrictive pericarditis, cardiac amyloidosis, and cardiac tamponade. *Cleve Clin J Med* 1992;59:278–290, with permission.)

relatively easy. Newer techniques using Doppler tissue imaging of the mitral annulus have been used to differentiate constriction and restriction.

  c. **Two-dimensional echocardiography** can give clues in differentiating constriction and restriction. A **septal bounce** in early diastole is a clue that **constriction** is present. A thickened pericardium sometimes occurs with constriction, but this finding is not highly sensitive. Although magnetic resonance imaging is the most sensitive method for measuring pericardial thickness, the presence or absence of a thickened pericardium alone is neither sensitive nor specific for the diagnosis of constrictive pericarditis.

SUGGESTED READINGS

Landmark Articles

Bonow RO, Udelson JE. Left ventricular diastolic dysfunction as a cause of congestive heart failure. *Ann Intern Med* 1992;117:502–510.

Hurrell DG, Nishamura RA, Higano ST, et al. Value of dynamic respiratory changes in left and right ventricular pressures for the diagnosis of constrictive pericarditis. *Circulation* 1996;93:2007–2013.

Key Reviews

Cohen GI, Pietrolungo JF, Thomas JD, Klein AL. A practical guide to the assessment of ventricular diastolic dysfunction using Doppler echocardiography. *J Am Coll Cardiol* 1996;27:1753–1760.

Kushwala SS, Fallon JT, Fuster V. Restrictive cardiomyopathy. *N Engl J Med* 1997; 336:267–275.

Lenihan DJ, Gerson MC, Hoit BD, Walsh, RA. Mechanisms, diagnosis, and treatment of diastolic heart failure. *Am Heart J* 1995;130:153–166.

Nishimura RA, Tajik AJ, Evaluation of diastolic dysfunction in health and disease: Doppler echocardiography is the clinician's Rosetta stone. *J Am Coll Cardiol* 1997; 30:8–18.

9. HYPERTROPHIC CARDIOMYOPATHY

Mark Robbins

I. **Introduction.** Hypertrophic cardiomyopathy (HCM) is most commonly defined as myocardial hypertrophy in the absence of an identifiable cause. It is now the preferred term because it does not connote that obstruction (present in only approximately 25% of cases) is an invariable component of the disease, as did *idiopathic hypertrophic subaortic stenosis, hypertrophic obstructive cardiomyopathy,* and *muscular subaortic stenosis.*

II. **Clinical Presentation**

   A. **Natural history**

   1. The **histologic features** of HCM are disarray of cell to cell arrangement, disorganization of cellular architecture, and fibrosis. The most common sites of ventricular involvement are the septum, apex, and midventricle in decreasing order. These morphologic and histologic features, which vary in phenotypic and clinical expression, give rise to the characteristic unpredictable natural history of HCM.

   2. The **prevalence** of HCM is approximately 1 in 500. This makes HCM probably the most common genetically transmitted cardiovascular disease. It is found among 0.5% of unselected patients referred for echocardiographic examination and is the leading cause of sudden death among athletes younger than 35 years.

   B. **Signs and symptoms**

   1. **Heart failure.** Symptoms that include dyspnea, dyspnea on exertion, paroxysmal nocturnal dyspnea, and fatigue are largely a consequence of elevated left ventricular (LV) diastolic pressure caused by lack of compliance of the ventricle.

      a. Events that accelerate heart rate, shorten diastolic filling time, and increase LV outflow obstruction (exercise and tachyarrhythmias) or worsen compliance (ischemia), exacerbate these symptoms.

      b. Severe LV systolic dysfunction has been reported among patients with end-stage disease. It is characterized by progressive LV wall thinning and cavity enlargement but is extremely rare.

   2. **Myocardial ischemia.** Myocardial ischemia is known to occur in both obstructive and nonobstructive cardiomyopathy.

      a. The **clinical** and **electrocardiographic (ECG)** presentation is similar to that of ischemic syndromes among persons without HCM. Ischemia has been demonstrated with thallium perfusion studies, elevated myocardial lactate levels during rapid atrial pacing, and positron emission tomography (PET).

      b. Although the exact mechanism of ischemia is in question, the physiologic process likely is a **supply and demand mismatch.** Contributing factors include the following:

         (1) Small-vessel coronary disease with decreased vasodilator capacity

         (2) Elevated myocardial wall tension as a consequence of delayed diastolic relaxation time and obstruction to LV outflow

         (3) Decreased capillary to myocardial fiber ratio

         (4) Decreased coronary perfusion pressure

   3. **Syncope and presyncope.** Syncope and presyncope usually are a consequence of diminished cerebral perfusion caused by inadequate cardiac output. These episodes are commonly associated with exertion or cardiac arrhythmia. Syncope among adult patients with HCM is not necessarily associated with a poor clinical outcome. Among children and adolescents it is associated with increased risk for sudden death.

4. **Sudden death.** The annual mortality for HCM ranges from 1% to 6%. Most deaths are sudden or unexpected.

   a. Not all patients with HCM are at equal **risk for sudden death.** As many as 22% of patients may have no symptoms. Sudden death appears to be most common among older children and young adults; it is rare in the first decade of life. Approximately 60% of deaths occur during periods of inactivity; the remaining deaths occur after vigorous physical exertion.

   b. Both **arrhythmogenic and ischemic mechanisms** can initiate a clinical spiral of hypotension, decreased diastolic filling time, and increased outflow obstruction that often culminates in death.

III. **Physical examination**

A. **Inspection** of the jugular venous system might reveal a prominent *a* wave that indicates hypertrophy and lack of compliance of the right ventricle. A precordial heave, representing right ventricular (RV) strain, can be found in persons with concomitant pulmonary hypertension.

B. **Palpation**

   1. The **apical precordial pulse usually is laterally displaced and diffuse.** LV hypertrophy may cause a presystolic apical impulse or palpable S_4. A three-component apical impulse may occur, the third impulse resulting from a late systolic bulge of the left ventricle.

   2. The carotid pulse has been classically described as being bifid, and so has been named **pulsus biferiens.** This **rapid carotid upstroke followed by a second peak** is caused by a hyperdynamic left ventricle.

C. **Auscultation**

   1. S_1 usually is normal and is preceded by S_4.

   2. S_2 can be normal or paradoxically split as the result of the prolonged ejection time of patients with severe outflow obstruction.

   3. The **harsh, crescendo-decrescendo systolic murmur** associated with HCM is heard best at the left sternal border. It radiates to the lower sternal border but not to the neck vessels or axilla.

      a. An important aspect of the murmur is its **variation in intensity and duration** with ventricular loading conditions. During periods of increased venous return, the murmur is of shorter duration and is less intense. In the underfilled ventricle and during periods of increased contractility, the murmur is harsh and of longer duration.

      b. **Maneuvers that affect preload and afterload** can be helpful in diagnosing HCM and differentiating it from other systolic murmurs (Table 9-1).

         (1) The **concomitant murmur of mitral insufficiency** can be differentiated because of its holosystolic, blowing quality that radiates to the axilla.

         (2) A soft, early, decrescendo, **diastolic murmur of aortic insufficiency** is found among approximately 10% of patients with HCM.

IV. **Genetic aspects of HCM.** Familial HCM is inherited as an autosomal dominant trait and is caused by missense mutations involving a single amino acid substitution on one of several sarcomeric genes (Table 9-2). These genetic alterations that encompass familial HCM should be differentiated from those of other diseases with similar phenotypic expression, such as apical hypertrophic cardiomyopathy, hypertrophic cardiomyopathy of the elderly, and from myocyte disarray and systolic dysfunction that occurs in a family without hypertrophy.

A. A **poor prognosis and a higher risk for sudden death** are associated with certain mutations within the β-myosin heavy chain (Arg403Gln, Arg453Cys, and Arg719Trp) and cardiac troponin T mutations. Almost all malignant mutations result from an amino acid substitution that changes the net charge (usually to a negative charge) of the encoded residue.

B. A **relatively benign prognosis and near-normal survival** are associated with Val606Met, Leu908Val, and Phe513Cys mutations on the β-myosin

Table 9-1. Effects of maneuvers or pharmacologic intervention to differentiate hypertrophic cardiomyopathy from aortic stenosis

Maneuver	Physiologic effect	Hypertrophic cardiomyopathy	Aortic stenosis	Mitral regurgitation
Valsalva and standing	Decreases VR, SVR, CO	↑	↓	↓
Squat and handgrip	Increases VR, SVR, CO	↓	↑	↑
Amyl nitrite	Increases VR Decreases SVR, LV volume	↑	↑	↓
Phenylephrine	Increases SVR, VR	↓	↑	↑
Extrasystole	Decreased LV volume	↑	↓	No change
Post-Valsalva release	Increased LV volume	↓	↑	No change

VR, Venous return; SVR, systemic vascular resistence; CO, cardiac output; LV, left ventricular; ↑, increase; ↓, decrease.

heavy chain gene, and mutations involving the α-tropomyosin gene, which have no change in net charge.
- **C.** Genetic analyses that lead to a preclinical diagnosis of familial HCM may offer a survival advantage to persons who can be determined to be at increased risk for sudden death on the basis of the specific mutation.
- **V. Diagnostic testing**
    - **A. ECG.** Although most patients have ECG evidence of disease, no changes are pathognomonic for HCM. Common ECG findings in HCM are listed in Table 9-3.
    - **B. Echocardiography** is the preferred diagnostic method because of its high sensitivity and low risk profile.
        - **1. M-mode and two-dimensional** echocardiographic criteria for the diagnosis of HCM are listed in Table 9-4. Some cardiologists have used two-dimensional imaging to include all patterns of RV and LV hypertrophy in establishing the diagnosis of HCM (Table 9-5).
        - **2. Doppler echocardiography** enables recognition and quantification of the consequences of **systolic anterior motion of the mitral valve (SAM).**
            - **a.** Approximately one fourth of patients with HCM have a resting pressure gradient between the body and outflow tract of the left ventricle; others have only provocable gradients.

Table 9-2. Location of genetic alterations and their relative frequency of occurrence in familial hypertrophic cardiomyopathy

Gene	Chromosome	Frequency (%)
β-Myosin heavy chain	14q1	35–45
Cardiac troponin T	1q31	15
α-Tropomyosin	15q2	5
Myosin binding protein C	11p13-q13	10
Ventricular myosin regulatory light chain	12q2	Rare
Ventricular myosin essential light chain	3p	Rare

Table 9-3. ECG findings in hypertrophic cardiomyopathy

Evidence of right and left atrial enlargement
Q waves in the inferiolateral leads
Voltage criteria for large negative precordial T waves[a]
Left axis deviation
Short PR interval with slurred upstroke

[a]Associated with Japanese variant.

  b. The **diagnosis of HCM with obstruction** is based on resting gradients greater than 30 mm Hg or provocable gradients greater than 50 mm Hg. These gradients correlate directly with the time of onset and duration of contact between the mitral leaflet and the septum. The earlier and longer the contact, the higher is the pressure gradient.
    (1) Inducing obstruction and therefore gradients in patients believed to have latent obstruction can be accomplished with substances or maneuvers that either decrease LV preload or increase contractility, such as amyl nitrite, isoproterenol, dobutamine, Valsalva maneuver, or exercise.
    (2) The most accepted explanation of SAM is that the high flow velocity caused by the narrowed outflow tract draws the mitral valve anteriorly toward the septum, resulting in subaortic obstruction and flow gradients. This suctioning effect on the mitral leaflet has been called the **Venturi effect.**
    (3) Although the clinical relevance of outflow obstruction has been debated, relief by means of surgical or pharmacologic technique is associated with clinical improvement among many patients. Therefore echocardiographic recognition of not only HCM but also HCM with outflow obstruction is important.
  c. **Recognition of mitral regurgitation (MR).** Echocardiographic evaluation of MR and the detection of valve anomalies may have a considerable effect on medical and surgical strategies in the care of patients with HCM.
    (1) Approximately 60% of patients with HCM have structural abnormalities of the mitral valve, including increased leaflet area, elongation of leaflets, and anomalous insertion of papillary muscles directly into the anterior mitral leaflet.
    (2) When there is no leaflet abnormality, the degree of MR is directly related to the severity of obstruction and lack of leaflet coaptation.

Table 9-4. Two-dimensional, M-mode, and Doppler echocardiographic criteria for diagnosis of hypertrophic cardiomyopathy

Asymmetric septal hypertrophy (>13 mm)
Systolic anterior motion of the mitral valve
Small left ventricular cavity
Septal immobility
Premature closure of the aortic valve
Resting gradients >30 mm Hg
Provocable gradients >50 mm Hg
Normal or increased motion of the posterior wall
Reduced rate of closure of the mitral valve in middiastole
Mitral valve prolapse with regurgitation
Maximal left ventricular diastolic wall thickness >15 mm

Table 9-5. Echocardiographic classification of left ventricular hypertrophy in hypertrophic cardiomyopathy

Type	Location	Frequency (%)
1	Anterior septum	10
2	Anterior and posterior septum	20
3	Anterior and posterior septum including the lateral free wall	52
4	Regions other than the anterior septum and posterior free wall	18

C. **Magnetic resonance imaging (MRI).** Advantages of MRI in the evaluation of HCM include excellent resolution, lack of radiation, inherent contrast, three-dimensional imaging, and tissue characterization. Disadvantages are cost, length of study, and exclusion of patients with contraindications to exposure to magnetism, such as patients with implantable cardioversion devices (ICDs) or pacemakers.
   1. Use of **cine MRI** allows morphologic evaluation of the cardiac apex, the right ventricle, and intraventricular function.
   2. **Myocardial tagging,** a relatively new development with which specific myocardial points can be traced from end diastole to end systole, allows evaluation of regional myocardial strain. This technique may help ascertain whether a patient with HCM has only focal areas of myocardial involvement.
   3. Although still in its infancy, **magnetic resonance spectroscopy** may one day be used to evaluate tissue metabolism and ischemia.
   4. It is possible that in the near future a single MRI study can be used to assess ventricular structure, function, and tissue metabolism.
D. **Cardiac catheterization** has a role in the evaluation of coronary anatomic features before myectomy or a mitral valve operation and evaluation of ischemic symptoms. Characteristic findings of HCM during hemodynamic assessment are listed in Table 9-6 and illustrated in Fig. 9-1.
   1. Patients with normal coronary arteries may have **typical ischemic symptoms.** These symptoms may indicate myocardial bridges, phasic narrowing during systole, reduced coronary flow reserve, or systolic reversal of flow in the epicardial vessels.
   2. **Left ventriculography** usually reveals a hypertrophied ventricle, prominent septal bulge, nearly complete obliteration of the ventricular cavity during systole, SAM, and MR. The spade-like appearance of the ventricular cavity is confined ventricles with apical involvement.
   3. **Simultaneous right and left ventriculography** in a left anterior oblique cranial projection facilitates assessment of the intraventricular septum.

Table 9-6. Hemodynamic findings during cardiac catheterization

Subaortic or midventricular outflow gradient on catheter pullback
Spike-and-dome pattern of aortic pressure tracing[a]
Elevated right and left ventricular end diastolic pressures
Elevated pulmonary capillary wedge pressure
Increased V wave on wedge tracing[b]
Elevated pulmonary arterial pressure

[a]A consequence of outlet obstruction.
[b]May result from either mitral regurgitation or elevated left atrial pressure.

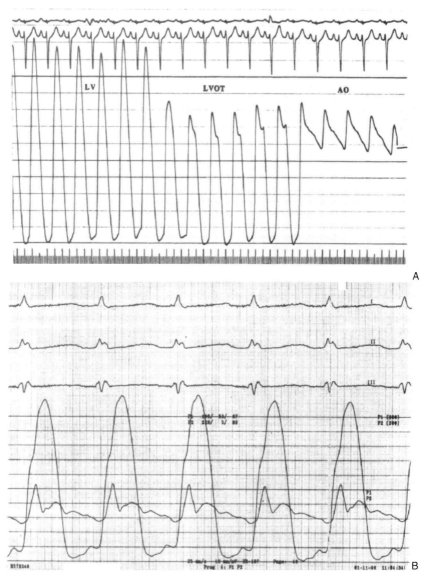

FIG. 9-1. Hemodynamic tracings. **A:** Pressure difference in left ventricular outflow tract and left ventricle. **B:** Spike and dome of left ventricular pressure.

    E. Radionuclide scanning and PET. The role of **radionuclide scanning** for assessment of ischemia is similar for patients with or without HCM with some distinctions. **Fixed defects** that represent scar and presumed myocardial infarction usually are associated with reduced ventricular function and exercise capacity. **Reversible defects** may reflect ischemia caused by atherosclerotic disease or reduced coronary reserve in disease-free arteries.

Although often clinically silent, these reversible defects are likely to be associated with increased risk for sudden death, especially among younger patients with HCM.

1. The characteristic **radionuclide ventriculographic findings** of HCM include abnormal diastolic filling, delayed peak filling, and prolonged isovolumic relaxation.

2. **PET** has higher sensitivity than conventional radionuclide scanning, and attenuation can be corrected during PET. [^{18}F] Fluorodeoxyglucose (FDG) PET studies have corroborated the clinical features of ischemia with pronounced impairment of coronary vasodilator reserve and resultant subendocardial underperfusion.

VI. Management strategies

A. **Priority of therapy.** Effective therapy must include pathways for the **management of heart failure** caused by diastolic and systolic dysfunction, arrhythmias, ischemia, failed medical therapy, and the **prevention of sudden death** (Fig. 9-2). The specific strategies for patients with HCM can be as heterogeneous as the clinical presentation and evolution.

B. **Medical therapy.** Although never proved to reduce mortality in clinical trails, **β-blockers are first-line therapy** for HCM regardless of the presence of LV outflow obstruction.

1. **β-Blockers** are effective in relieving angina, dyspnea, and syncope among as many as 70% of patients in some studies. It is reasonable to assume that there is a class effect and that any of the commonly prescribed will be effective (Table 9-7).

    a. The mechanism of action of β-blockers is inhibition of sympathetic stimulation brought about by the negative inotropic and chronotropic properties of the drugs. β-blockers diminish myocardial oxygen requirements and augment diastolic filling, which mitigate angina and the detrimental effects of LV outflow obstruction, respectively.

    b. **Contraindications** to the use of β-blockers are the presence of bronchospastic lung disease, a high degree heart block in the absence of a pacer, and decompensated LV systolic dysfunction.

2. **Calcium channel blockers** are effective in reducing the common symptoms of HCM among patients who are intolerant of or have undergone unsuccessful treatment with β-blockers.

    a. **Calcium channel blockers** have a negative inotropic effect, reduce heart rate, and blood pressure. They may also have beneficial effects on diastolic function by improving rapid diastolic filling, although possibly at the expense of higher LV end-diastolic pressures. The beneficial effects seem to be limited to the nondihydroperidines **verapamil** and **diltiazem** (see Table 9-7).

    b. Because of the unpredictable hemodynamic effects of their vasodilatory properties, calcium channel blockers should be administered cautiously to patients with considerable outlet obstruction and elevated pulmonary pressures. **Contraindications** to use of calcium channel blockers include evidence of conduction system abnormalities in the absence of a pacer or in the presence of systolic dysfunction.

3. **Disopyramide,** a class 1A antiarrhythmic agent, may be an effective alternative or adjunct to β-blocker and calcium channel blocker therapy. Its strong negative inotropic qualities coupled with its ability to suppress both ventricular and supraventricular arrhythmias make it an effective treatment when marked outflow obstruction or arrhythmias are manifested. Potential disadvantages are anticholinergic properties, accumulation in patients with hepatic or renal dysfunction, the possibility of augmenting atrioventricular (AV) nodal conduction in the presence of atrial fibrillation (AF), and waning hemodynamic effects with time.

C. **Nonpharmacologic treatment.** Transplantation is the only option for patients with severely symptomatic nonobstructive HCM. However, persons

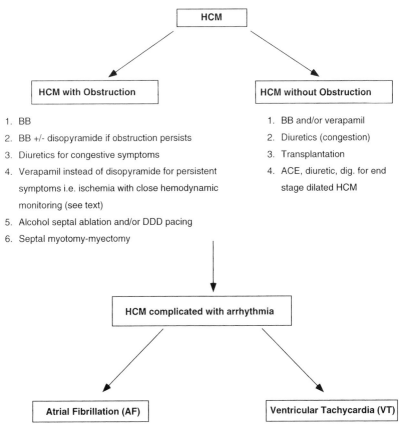

FIG. 9-2. Management algorithm for hypertrophy cardiomyopathy. BB, Beta-blocker; ACE, Angiotensin-Converting Enzyme Inhibitor; HCM, Hypertrophic Cardiomyopathy; DDD, dual chamber; Dig, Digoxin; DCC, Direct Current Cardioversion; AF, atrial fibrillation; AICD, Automatic Implantable Cardiac Defibrillator; NSVT, Non-sustained ventricular tachycardia; VT, ventricular tachycardia.

with obstruction who continue to have symptoms despite optimal medical treatment are candidates for dual-chamber pacing, septal myotomy-myectomy with or without mitral valve replacement, and alcohol septal ablation.

1. **Dual-chamber pacing.** Initial reports of symptom relief and decreased LV outflow obstruction with dual-chamber pacing have been questioned. Pacing may have deleterious effects on ventricular filling and cardiac

Table 9-7. Pharmacologic therapy for hypertrophic cardiomyopathy

Drug	Standard Dose[a] (mg/day)
β-BLOCKERS	
Propanolol	80–240
Metoprolol	50–200
Atenolol	50–100
CALCIUM CHANNEL ANTAGONISTS	
Verapamil	120–360
Diltiazem	120–360
ANTIARRYTHMICS	
Disopyramide	400–1200
Amiodarone	200–400
Sotalol	160–320

[a]Doses can be increased to treat patients with persistent symptoms who have no evidence of an adverse response.

output. Because of the lack of large, prospective, placebo-controlled trials, the use of pacing in the management of HCM remains controversial.

    a. Paradoxic motion of the septum (moving away from the outflow tract during ventricular systole) by means of pacing the right ventricular apex is the proposed mechanism by which **pacing reduces SAM** and therefore LV outflow obstruction. The success of dual-chamber pacing relies on the precise timing of AV delay, which should be short enough to prevent intrinsic LV depolarization but long enough to avoid interfering with atrial emptying.

    b. The American Heart Association and American College of Cardiology find the use of dual-chamber pacing in the management of HCM is beneficial, useful, and effective (class I recommendation) only for patients with sinus or AV node dysfunction. Pacing also may benefit patients with symptomatic, refractory AF for whom AV nodal ablation is considered (see later).

2. Alcohol septal ablation is undergoing study as a possible alternative to myotomy-myectomy. Continued study and follow-up evaluation are needed to further elucidate and perfect this new technique.

    a. Technique. In the cardiac catheterization laboratory, a guidewire is advanced through the left main trunk to probe the first or second septal perforator or both. An angioplasty catheter is placed in the proximal portion of the septal branch for vessel isolation. Ultrasonic contrast agents are infused in the cannulated perforator to define the area at risk for infarction. Infusion of alcohol causes infarction in the zone of septal myocardium served by the cannulated septal branch.

    b. Results. The akinesis and thinning that occur reduce if not abolish the outflow obstruction. Like surgical removal of myocardium, alcohol ablation has been associated with heart block and persistence of provocable gradients.

3. Surgical management of HCM has been relegated to use only in the care of patients with evidence of resting obstruction and persistent symptoms despite adequate medical therapy.

    a. When performed by an experienced surgeon, **septal myotomy-myectomy** is associated with a mortality of less than 1% to 2%. It is effective in abolishing resting gradients in more than 90% of patients, and most patients have long-lasting symptomatic relief. Enlargement of the LV outflow tract has been found to reduce SAM, MR, LV systolic and end-diastolic pressures, left atrial pressure, and resting gradients.

    b. Mitral valve replacement with a low-profile prosthesis abrogates outflow obstruction, but it is considered mainly for patients with mild septal thickening, failed myotomy-myectomy, or intrinsic abnormalities of the mitral apparatus.

4. Special management considerations

    a. Atrial fibrillation, which occurs among approximately 10% of patients with HCM, can have devastating consequences. AF decreases diastolic filling time, and loss of atrial systole can lead to acute hemodynamic decompensation and pulmonary edema. Because of the increased risk for thromboembolism, all patients with HCM-associated AF should be considered for long-term anticoagulation.

        (1) Acute paroxysms of AF are best managed with cardioversion. The treatment of choice for the prevention of recurrence is disopyramide or sotalol; low-dose amiodarone is reserved for refractory cases. When considerable obstruction is present, the combination of a β-blocker and disopyramide or sotalol is an alternative.

        (2) Chronic AF may be well tolerated if heart rate is controlled with β-blockers or calcium channel antagonists. For patients who do not tolerate AF and cannot be maintained in sinus rhythm, AV nodal ablation and implantation of a dual-chamber pacemaker may be an option.

    b. Risk stratification for sudden death. Ascertaining whether a patient is at high risk for sudden death requires establishing risk factors with sufficient sensitivity, specificity, and positive predictive value to prompt implementation of preventive therapy, such as placement of an ICD or permanent pacemaker and administration of amiodarone, the long-term efficacy of which has not been established.

        (1) Although no conclusive data exist on the relative value of the markers associated with sudden death, accepted **risk factors** include the following:

            (a) Previous cardiac arrest

            (b) Sustained ventricular tachycardia

            (c) Adverse genotype

                (i) β-myosin heavy chain

                (ii) Cardiac troponin T

            (d) Family history of sudden death

            (e) Nonsustained ventricular tachycardia during ambulatory monitoring

            (f) Recurrent syncope

            (g) Abnormal decrease in exercise blood pressure

            (h) Massive LV wall thickness (>35 mm)

        (2) The role of **electrophysiologic (EP) testing** in the management of HCM is uncertain. Evidence that EP testing helps to ascertain whether a patients is at increased risk for sudden death is inconclusive. EP studies have been unable to consistently induce ventricular arrhythmias with standard stimulation protocols in cardiac arrest survivors. In other EP studies, however, investigators have been able to induce nonspecific ventricular arrhythmias with unconventional stimulation protocols in patients believed to be at low risk for sudden death.

        (3) Until ongoing studies of HCM and ICD implantation yield solid recommendations, implantation of an ICD seems prudent in the care of patients who survive an episode that might have ended in sudden death, have sustained ventricular arrhythmias, or have multiple risk factors for sudden death.

VII. Key Suggestions
 A. Athlete's heart
  1. Differentiating HCM from hypertrophy of athletes. Failure to diagnose HCM places an athlete at undue risk for sudden death, although incorrect labeling of HCM often leads to irrational treatments, unnecessary fears, and inappropriate recommendations concerning exercise. Diagnostic uncertainty is greatest when maximal diastolic LV wall thickness exceeds the upper limit of normal (12 mm) but is less than the defined lower limit of normal (15 mm) for HCM in the absence of SAM and LV outflow obstruction.
   a. Characteristics that **substantiate the diagnosis of HCM** include unusual patterns of hypertrophy; LV end-diastolic diameter less than 45 mm; left atrial enlargement; female sex; family history of HCM; and abnormal left ventricular filling.
   b. Characteristics more consistent with the **hypertrophied heart of an athlete** are LV end-diastolic diameter greater than 55 mm and a decrease in LV thickness with deconditioning.
  2. Participation in sports. Recommendations hold true after medical or surgical intervention.
   a. Athletes with HCM younger than 30 years of age with or without obstruction should not participate in competitive, aerobically demanding sports.
   b. Individual judgment is used for athletes older than 30 years (because of the possible reduction in sudden death with age) who lack any of the following criteria that would place them at high risk: ventricular tachycardia at ambulatory monitoring; sudden death among family members with HCM; syncope; outflow gradient greater than 50 mm Hg; exercise-induced hypotension; myocardial ischemia; left atrium larger than 5 cm; severe MR; paroxysmal AF.
 B. Subacute bacterial endocarditis
  1. Incidence and mortality. Seven percent to 9% of patients with HCM contract bacterial endocarditis. The associated mortality is 39%.
  2. Predisposing factors. Dental, intestinal, and prostate surgical procedures place patients at increased risk for bacteremia.
  3. Pathophysiology. Bacterial seeding of endomyocardial lesions is caused by repeated trauma associated with hemodynamic and intrinsic valvular abnormalities.
  4. Prophylaxis. All patients with HCM with or without obstruction should be treated with prophylactic antibiotics before any procedure that might be associated with high risk for bacterial seeding of the bloodstream.
 C. Yamaguchi's apical hypertrophic cardiomyopathy
  1. Clinical presentation. Patients experience chest pain, dyspnea, fatigue, and in rare instances sudden death.
  2. Prevalence. Within Japan, apical hypertrophic cardiomyopathy constitutes 25% of all cases of HCM. Outside Japan, only 1% to 2% of cases are associated with isolated apical hypertrophy.
  3. Diagnostic testing
   a. An **ECG** reveals giant negative T waves in the precordial leads and LV hypertrophy.
   b. Echocardiographic findings include the following:
    (1) Localized hypertrophy in the distal left ventricle beyond the origin of the chordae tendineae
    (2) Wall thickness in the apical region of at least 15 mm or a ratio of maximal apical to posterobasal thickness greater than 1.5
    (3) Exclusion of hypertrophy and other parts of the ventricular wall
    (4) No LV outflow tract obstruction or gradient
   c. MRI demonstrates localized hypertrophy to the cardiac apex. MRI is useful in the care of patients with poor echocardiographic windows.

         d. Cardiac catheterization reveals a spade-like configuration of the LV cavity at end diastole and apical end-systolic LV cavity obliteration.

    4. Prognosis is favorable compared with that associated with other forms of HCM.

    5. Therapy. Therapeutic efforts are limited to management of diastolic dysfunction with β-blockers and calcium channel antagonists.

D. HCM among the elderly

    1. Clinical presentation. In addition to the signs and symptoms of other forms of HCM, hypertension is more common with HCM among the elderly population.

    2. Incidence. Although the incidence is unknown, HCM among the elderly is likely more common than expected.

    3. Genetic aspects. Reports have suggested that the delayed expression of mutations in the gene for cardiac myosin-binding protein C may play an important role in HCM among the elderly.

    4. Echocardiographic findings for elderly patients (65 years and older) are compared with findings for young patients (40 years and younger) as follows:

        a. Common findings

            (1) LV outflow tract gradient both provocable and at rest

            (2) Asymmetric hypertrophy

            (3) Systolic anterior motion of the mitral valve

        b. Differences pertaining to the elderly

            (1) Less hypertrophy

            (2) Less RV involvement

            (3) Ovoid versus crescentic left ventricle

            (4) Prominent septal bulge (sigmoid septum)

            (5) More acute angle between the aorta and septum as the aorta uncoils with age

    5. Management of HCM among the elderly is similar to that of other forms of HCM.

    6. The **prognosis** is favorable compared with that for forms of HCM that occur at a younger age.

SUGGESTED READINGS

Landmark Articles

Maron JM. Hypertrophic cardiomyopathy. *Lancet* 1997;350:127–133.

Maron JM, Bonow RG, Cannon RB, et al. Hypertrophic cardiomyopathy: interrelations of clinical manifestations, pathophysiology, and therapy, part 2. *N Engl J Med* 1987;316:844–852.

Spirito P, Seidman CE, McKenna WS, et al. The management of hypertrophic cardiomyopathy. *N Engl J Med* 1997;336:775–784.

Wigle D, Rakowski H, Kimball B. Hypertrophic cardiomyopathy: clinical spectrum and treatment. *Circulation* 1995;92:1680–1692.

Key Reviews

Alessandri N, Pannarale G, Del Monte F, et al. Hypertrophic obstructive cardiomyopathy and infective endocarditis: a report of seven cases and a review of the literature. *Eur Heart J* 1990;11: 1041–1048.

Almendral JM, Ormastre J, Martinez-Abby JD, et al. Treatment of ventricular arrhythmias in patients with hypertrophic cardiomyopathy. *Eur Heart J* 1993;14: 71–72.

Fananapazir L, Epstein ND. Prevalence of hypertrophic cardiomyopathy and limitations of screening methods. *Circulation* 1995;92:700–704.

Lakkis N, Kleinman N, Killip D, et al. Hypertrophic obstructive cardiomyopathy: alternative therapeutic options. *Clin Cardiol* 1997;20:417–418.

Lever HM, Karam RF, Currie PS, et al. Hypertrophic cardiomyopathy in the elderly: distinctions from the young based on cardiac shape. *Circulation* 1989;79:580–589.

Maron JM, Cerchi F, McKenna WS, et al. Risk factors and stratification for sudden death in patients with hypertrophic cardiomyopathy. *Br Heart J* 1994;72 [Suppl]: S13–S18.

Maron JM, Isner JM, McKenna WS, et al. Task Force 3: hypertrophic cardiomyopathy, myocarditis, and other myopericardial diseases and mitral valve prolapse. *J Am Coll Cardiol* 1994;24: 880–885.

Maron JM, Gardin JM, Flack JM, et al. Prevalence of hypertrophic cardiomyopathy in a general population of young adults. *Circulation* 1995;92:785–789.

Maron JM, Pelliccia A, Spirito P. Cardiac disease in young trained athletes: insights methods for distinguishing athlete's heart from structural heart disease, with particular emphasis on hypertrophic cardiomyopathy. *Circulation* 1995;91:1596–1601.

Morten ET. Hypertrophic obstructive cardiomyopathy: problems in management. *Chest* 1997;112:262–264.

Nishimura RA. Dual-chamber pacing for cardiomyopathies: a 1996 perspective. *Mayo Clin Proc* 1996;71:1077–1087.

Posma JL, van de Wall EE, Blauksma P. New diagnostic options in hypertrophic cardiomyopathy. *Am Heart J* 1996;132:1031–1041.

Slade A, Sadoul N, Shapiro L. DDD pacing in hypertrophic cardiomyopathy: a multicenter clinical experience. *Heart* 1996;75:44–49.

Smolders W, Redemakers F, Conraads V, et al. Apical hypertrophic cardiomyopathy. *Acta Cardiol* 1993;48: 369–383.

Watkins H. Multiple disease genes cause hypertrophic cardiomyopathy. *Br Heart J* 1994;72:S4–S9.

Relevant Book Chapters

Topol EJ, ed. *Textbook of cardiovascular medicine.* Philadelphia: Lippincott–Raven, 1998:745–768.

Braunwald E, ed. *Heart disease: a textbook of cardiovascular medicine,* 5th ed. Philadelphia: WB Saunders, 1997, 1414–1426.

Schlant RC, Alexander RW, eds. Hurst's The Heart, 8th ed. New York: McGraw-Hill, 1621–1635.

10. HIGH-OUTPUT HEART FAILURE

John G. Peterson

I. **Introduction.** High-output heart failure is an uncommon clinical syndrome. In response to exercise, a normal heart increases its cardiac output four- to sixfold without evidence of pulmonary venous congestion. However, hearts affected by serious myocardial, valvular, or pericardial disease may be unable to compensate for an increase in demand for cardiac output. Conditions that exert a **constant** increased need for supranormal cardiac output can lead to symptoms of congestive heart failure (CHF) among patients who would otherwise be without symptoms. Patients with symptoms of CHF but who have normal or increased cardiac output at hemodynamic evaluation may have high-output CHF.

II. **Clinical presentation**
   A. **Symptoms.** High-output heart failure usually manifests itself as **fatigue, edema, dyspnea on exertion, and palpitations.** Because these symptoms are common in other forms of heart failure, they alone cannot be used to differentiate syndromes. **Differentiating etiologic features** of high-output heart failure include **tremor** among patients with hyperthyroidism and **neuropathy** with thiamine deficiency.
   B. **Physical findings.** Each cause of a high-output state has its own unique findings at physical examination. However, the following signs and symptoms are common to all of them.
      1. **Increased heart rate and pulse pressure**
      2. **Hyperdynamic impulse,** a snapping, crisp first heart sound, and a midsystolic flow murmur over the aortic and pulmonary area revealed on cardiac examination
      3. **Diastolic low-pitch murmur at the apex and left lower sternal border** indicative of increased flow across the arteriovenous valves can occasionally be heard
      4. **Warm hands and feet**

III. **Diagnosis.** Confirmation of high-output heart failure requires right heart catheterization, which typically reveals normal to mildly elevated right-sided pressures at rest, elevated pulmonary capillary wedge pressure, high cardiac output, low systemic vascular resistance, and resting tachycardia. This syndrome can be differentiated from sepsis because in high-output heart failure there is no arterial hypotension, fever, or source of infection.

IV. **Etiology and treatment**
   A. **Anemia.** Acute anemia due to rapid blood loss is associated with depressed cardiac output caused by hypovolemia. Chronic anemia, however, causes symptoms of CHF due to compensatory mechanisms. Most healthy persons tolerate moderate degrees of chronic anemia (hemoglobin less than 9 g/dL) without symptoms of CHF, but persons with baseline heart disease have symptoms early. However, even normal hearts experience CHF with chronic anemia of severe proportions (hemoglobin less than 4 g/dL). The **main compensatory mechanisms** are decreased vascular resistance, increased 2,3-diphosphoglycerate (DPG), which shifts the hemoglobin-oxygen dissociation curve to the right, fluid retention, and increased cardiac output caused by resting tachycardia. Management of the cause of anemia and blood transfusion with diuresis improve clinical symptoms. Patients with CHF should be given transfusions slowly (1 to 2 units over 24 hours) and undergo diuresis.
   B. Connections between arteries and veins without intervening capillary beds are called **arteriovenous fistulas.** These fistulas can be the result of inva-

sive procedures (e.g., dialysis fistula), trauma (e.g., gunshot wound, arterial puncture), or congenital anomalies (e.g., Osler-Weber-Rendu syndrome).

1. If these fistulas carry enough blood flow, typically at least 1.5 L/min, the resulting demand on myocardial reserve can lead to LV dilatation and symptoms of CHF. A healthy heart can tolerate even large fistula flows, up to 10 L/min, quite well.

2. An arteriovenous fistula usually is easily identified with a **thrill and bruit.** Elevated pulse pressure is common. If the fistula can be compressed manually, hemodynamic studies can be performed with the fistula open and with the fistula occluded to determine its contribution to cardiac function. A reduction in heart rate with compression of the fistula is an indication that the shunt is substantial. This knowledge is especially helpful in evaluation of the effect of a dialysis fistula.

3. **Surgical** revision of a dialysis fistula sometimes is needed to correct the abnormality. Other fistulas are repaired surgically, such as an arteriovenous fistula that develops after arterial puncture, or by means of occlusion with intravascular coils.

C. **Hyperthyroidism.** Severe manifestations of hyperthyroidism may include CHF, especially among the elderly and patients with low ventricular reserve. Atrial fibrillation is a common accompanying arrhythmia, occurring among 9% to 22% of patients with thyrotoxicosis. Angina pectoris that had previously been stable may become unstable.

1. **Clinical diagnosis** is very difficult for older patients because nonpalpable toxic nodular goiter is a more common cause of hyperthyroidism, and nonspecific symptoms such as fatigue, weight loss, and insomnia predominate. High clinical suspicion also is necessary in the care of patients with inappropriate tachycardia or atrial fibrillation, especially if atrial fibrillation is resistant to digoxin. Patients treated with amiodarone are at increased risk for hyperthyroidism.

2. Therapy with **β-blockers,** normally used in the immediate management of hyperthyroid symptoms and atrial fibrillation, must be administered with close monitoring if the patient has CHF.

3. Routine **cardioversion for atrial fibrillation is not recommended** until hyperthyroidism is controlled because of the high recurrence rate. Spontaneous conversion to sinus rhythm is expected among 50% of patients within 6 weeks of start of treatment if no preexisting heart disease is present. Thromboembolism risk among patients with thyrotoxicosis and atrial fibrillation is high, so **anticoagulation with heparin or warfarin sodium** is recommended.

4. Standard therapy with **anti-thyroid drugs** (propylthiouracil, methimazole, or inorganic iodine) is first-line therapy; **diuretics** are used for symptomatic therapy. If CHF develops during thyrotoxicosis the patient is a candidate for eventual **radioactive thyroid ablation** because return of CHF with recurrence of thyrotoxicosis is common.

D. **Thiamine deficiency (beriberi).** Though rare in the western world, thiamine deficiency is still common in developing countries. It also occurs among persons who observe fad diets for long periods of time and among persons with alcoholism. **Wet beriberi** includes the features of high-output cardiac failure such as marked edema, peripheral vasodilatation, and pulmonary congestion. The signs and symptoms of **dry beriberi** include glossitis, hyperkeratosis, and peripheral neuropathy. **Laboratory evaluation** may show metabolic acidosis caused by lactic acid and depressed red blood cell ketolase levels. Intravenous therapy with 100 mg thiamine followed by daily oral dietary replacement can lead to dramatic improvement in clinical symptoms.

E. **Other causes** include Paget's disease, Albright's syndrome, pregnancy, and multiple myeloma. The treatment is individualized on the basis of the underlying disorder.

SUGGESTED READINGS
Key Reviews
Engelberts I, Tordoir JHM, Boon ES, Schreij, G. High output cardiac failure due to excessive shunting in a hemodialysis access fistula: an easily overlooked diagnosis. *Am J Nephrol* 1995;15:323–326.
Polikar R, Burger AG, Scherrer U, Nicod P. The thyroid and the heart. *Circulation* 1993;87:1435–1441.
Woeber KA. Thyrotoxicosis and the heart. *N Engl J Med* 1992;327: 94–98.

11. ISOLATED RIGHT HEART FAILURE

John G. Peterson

I. **Introduction.** Right heart failure is a clinical syndrome consisting of elevated venous pressure and inadequate cardiac output that may be independent of left ventricular (LV) failure. It is commonly associated with right ventricular (RV) dilatation and decreased RV systolic function. Although the most common cause of right heart failure is chronic left heart failure, isolated right heart failure does occur in certain clinical states, and these are the focus of this chapter. Many of the causes of right heart failure are discussed in greater detail in other chapters; only a brief description of their clinical characteristics is presented here.

II. **Clinical presentation**

   A. **Signs and symptoms** (Table 11-1).

   1. Predominant symptoms are lethargy, weight gain, abdominal bloating, early satiety, and shortness of breath.

   2. Chest pain and palpitations also are common.

   B. **Physical findings**

   1. Physical findings include edema, jugular venous distention with large V waves, ascites, hepatomegaly with a pulsatile liver, a loud pulmonic valve closure sound, a murmur of tricuspid regurgitation, and RV lift or S_3 (see Table 11-1).

   2. These signs and symptoms are not specific to right heart failure, because pericardial constriction may present similarly.

III. **Etiology.** Because of the complexity and diverse causes of right heart failure, a full discussion of the etiologic factors is beyond the scope of this chapter. The following are the **common causes** of isolated right heart failure.

   A. **Congenital heart disease.** Several congenital diseases can cause isolated right heart failure, some of which do not present themselves until adulthood. These can be divided into left-to-right shunts and valvular abnormalities.

   1. **Left-to-right shunts.** Because of recirculation of blood into the right heart, the shunts are associated with increased pulmonary flow and a pattern of overcirculation on chest radiographs (although not necessarily cephalization of flow).

   a. **Isolated secundum atrial septal defect** is the most common left-to-right shunt that presents itself in adulthood.

   b. A **sinus venosus atrial septal defect** with anomalous pulmonary venous return may have a similar presentation.

   2. **Valvular abnormalities**

   a. Right-sided valvular heart disease (e.g., pulmonary stenosis, Ebstein's anomaly) is demonstrated by decreased pulmonary flow and a pattern of undercirculation on chest radiographs.

   b. Ebstein's anomaly, pulmonic stenosis or regurgitation, tetralogy of Fallot, and pulmonary atresia are less common causes of isolated right heart failure but should be considered in the differential diagnosis.

   B. **RV infarction.** Approximately one-third of inferior myocardial infarctions are complicated by RV involvement. Clinically significant RV infarction is much less common, however, because the right ventricle usually has sufficient collateral vascularization, and maintaining flow in the branches that feed this area of the heart requires low perfusion pressures. RV free-wall infarction usually is needed for development of the syndrome of RV infarction. A very proximal occlusion of a dominant right coronary artery usually is the cause of this complication. In a small portion of cases, RV infarction may occur alone, usually caused by proximal occlusion of a nondominant right coronary artery. Because the right ventricle acutely dilates in response

Table 11-1. Signs and symptoms of right heart failure

Signs	Symptoms
Edema	Fatigue
Jugular venouse distention	Weight gain
Ascites	Anorexia, early satiety, nausea
Loud P_2	Dyspnea
Right ventricular lift or S_3	Chest pain
Jaundice	Abdominal pain
Hepatomegaly	Palpitations

to this event, evidence of chronic right heart failure (edema, ascites, and hepatomegaly) usually is not seen.

1. The triad of **hypotension, jugular vein distention, and clear lung fields** is typical of the syndrome of RV infarction; however, these signs also may occur with acute pulmonary embolus and cardiac tamponade.

2. An **electrocardiogram (ECG)** and the clinical history may be helpful in differentiating these syndromes. Kussmaul's sign may occur as a result of RV dilatation, which causes functional pericardial constraint. Several ECG criteria for acute RV infarction exist and may be helpful in diagnosing difficult cases.

   a. The most commonly used ECG criterion is **1-mm ST elevation in the right precordial lead signal** (V_4R [right chest, midclavicular line, fifth interspace]), which has been shown to be highly sensitive and specific.

   b. ST elevation in V_1 alone or in conjunction with ST depression or elevation in V_2 also is indicative of RV infarction.

3. **Hemodynamic clues** to substantial RV infarction include a right atrial pressure greater than 10 mm Hg, with a ratio of right atrial pressure to pulmonary capillary wedge pressure (PCWP) greater than 0.8.

C. **Pulmonary vascular and parenchymal disease**

   1. Chronic severe lung disease, such as chronic obstructive pulmonary disease, interstitial lung disease, and chronic bronchitis, causes pulmonary vasculature damage and ventilation-perfusion ($\dot{V}/\dot{Q}$) mismatch in addition to parenchymal effects. This results in increased pulmonary resistance, right heart strain, and, eventually, right heart failure. Primary pulmonary hypertension and chronic pulmonary emboli also can cause this syndrome.

   2. A **screening $\dot{V}/\dot{Q}$ scan** usually is recommended in the care of patients with pulmonary hypertension of unexplained causation. High-resolution **computed tomography (CT)** of the chest to evaluate the pulmonary parenchyma often is obtained if the chest radiograph or pulmonary function tests suggest interstitial lung disease.

D. **Arrhythmogenic RV dysplasia (ARVD) and Uhl's anomaly** are primary myocardial diseases that mainly affect the right ventricle alone and are thought by some cardiologists to be different manifestations of the same disorder.

   1. **ARVD** usually presents itself among young persons as syncope, sudden death due to ventricular arrhythmias, or, more rarely, right heart failure. There is a male predominance, and the condition often is diagnosed after syncope or sudden death occurs during exercise. There is histologically evidence of patchy programmed cell death (apoptosis) of cardiac myocytes, and myocytes are replaced with adipose tissue. The diagnosis of ARVD is difficult to make with endomyocardial biopsy because of the patchy nature of the disease. Magnetic resonance imaging sometimes helps in identifying fatty infiltration of the right ventricle. Diagnostic criteria have been established (see Suggested Readings).

    2. Uhl's anomaly is also known as **parchment heart** because of the paper-thin RV wall characteristic of this disease. This disease more often presents itself in early childhood with signs of right heart failure. The disease involves death of myocytes throughout the right ventricle.

IV. Laboratory examination

    A. ECG. There may be many ECG findings associated with right heart failure. In general, however, long-standing right heart failure produces evidence of RV hypertrophy, with a tall R wave in V_1 and R greater than S in V_6. Acute right heart failure may reveal a right heart strain pattern with a deep S wave in lead I, a Q wave and T-wave inversion in lead III, and tachycardia ($S_1Q_3T_3$ pattern).

    B. Chemistry. Elevated liver function test results and prolonged prothrombin time occur with chronic, severe right heart failure.

    C. Chest radiographic findings vary depending on the cause of right heart failure; however, increased pulmonary vascular markings without cephalization of flow are characteristic of increased right heart blood flow. RV enlargement can be best appreciated on lateral chest radiographs, which show loss of the anterior free space.

V. Diagnosis. Although the history and physical examination findings establish a tentative diagnosis of right heart failure, confirmation of the diagnosis and determination of causation necessitate imaging studies, hemodynamic studies, or both.

    A. Echocardiography is valuable in evaluating LV and RV function, valvular abnormalities, and intracardiac shunts. All patients with isolated right heart failure of unknown causation should be evaluated for intracardiac shunting by means of echocardiography. They also should undergo an oxygen saturation study at the time of right heart catheterization.

    B. Right heart catheterization reveals elevated right atrial pressures in all patients with right heart failure.

        1. If right heart failure is caused by intracardiac shunt, LV failure, mitral stenosis, or a pulmonary disorder, RV systolic and pulmonary arterial pressures also are elevated.

Table 11-2. Right heart filling parameters in right ventricular failure

Cause	Right atrial pressure	Pulmonary artery pressure	PCWP	Left ventricular end-diastolic pressure
Left ventricular failure	Increased	Increased	Increased	Increased
Mitral stenosis	Increased	Increased	Increased	Decreased or normal
Pulmonary disorders	Increased	Increased	Normal	Normal
Pulmonary valve stenosis	Increased	Normal or decreased	Normal	Normal
Tricuspid valve regurgitation	Increased	Normal or decreased	Normal	Normal
Right ventricular infarct, Uhl's anomaly, ARVD	Increased	Normal or decreased	Normal or decreased	Normal
Left-to-right intracardiac shunt	Increased	Increased	Normal or decreased	Normal

PCWP, Pulmonary capillary wedge pressure; *ARVD,* arrhythmogenic right ventricular dysplasia.

    2. If RV infarction or RV myocardial disease is the cause, RV systolic and pulmonary arterial pressures are expected to be near normal. In all cases of isolated RV failure, the **PCWP is normal** (Table 11-2).

VI. Therapy. Management of right heart failure depends on the cause.

  A. Congenital heart disease. In the absence of the Eisenmenger complex, **surgical repair** of congenital abnormalities usually is recommended as primary therapy.

  B. RV infarction. Management of RV infarction involves restoration of blood flow to the RV wall through the use of **pharmacologic or catheter-based reperfusion.** The injured right ventricle usually begins to recover within 3 days after infarction. Return of adequate RV function may take up to several weeks and necessitate long-term hemodynamic monitoring, use of inotropic agents, and occasionally sequential atrioventricular pacing.

  C. Pulmonary vascular and parenchymal disease. Because many pulmonary vascular and parenchymal diseases are irreversible, lung or heart-lung (if RV dysfunction is severe) **transplantation** should be considered for eligible patients.

  D. ARVD and Uhl's anomaly

    1. Management of ARVD includes antiarrhythmic drugs and devices, diuretics, digoxin, and sodium restriction.

    2. Uhl's anomaly is more refractory to treatment than is ARVD and can be an indication for heart transplantation.

SUGGESTED READING

Key Review
Setaro JF, Cabin HS. Right ventricular infarction. *Cardiol Clin* 1992;10:68–69.

Relevant Book Chapter
Hochman JS, Gersh BJ. Acute myocardial infarction: complications. In: Topol EJ, ed. *Textbook of cardiovascular medicine.* Philadelphia: Lippincott–Raven, 1998:462–464.

12. SURGICAL OPTIONS IN HEART FAILURE

Leslie Campbell

I. **Introduction.** More than 4,000 patients are listed for transplantation in the United States; 30% of them will die before a suitable donor is found. Because the donor population is not expanding, there has been a need for the development and use of innovative surgical procedures and mechanical assist devices to prolong survival during the wait for heart transplantation.

II. **Ventricular assist devices (VADs)**

A. **Indications and contraindications.** VADs are used primarily as a bridge to transplantation; therefore potential recipients must meet heart transplantation criteria (see Chapter 13). Candidates for VAD typically have a cardiac index less than 2 L/min per square meter, systolic blood pressure less than 90 mm Hg, atrial pressures greater than 20 mm Hg, pulmonary capillary wedge pressure greater than 12 to 18 mm Hg, systemic vascular resistance greater than 2,100 dynes-sec/cm^2, and oliguria with urine output less than 20 mL/hr despite aggressive medical therapy. **Contraindications** to VAD placement include any disease that precludes cardiac transplantation (in the absence of participation in a clinical trial), including active malignant disease, infection, peripheral vascular disease, hepatic dysfunction, and chronic renal failure.

B. **Devices.** A number of VADs are available, and the decision on which device to use is based on duration of predicted use, reversibility of the underlying cause of cardiogenic shock, need for left-chamber versus dual-chamber support, and patient size. The seven available systems can be considered in the following general categories.

1. **Hemopumps.** A hemopump is indicated only for short-term use (several days) and is similar to an intraaortic balloon pump except that it completely unloads the ventricular work rather than simply augmenting it. Inserted through the femoral artery, the system is designed on a catheter that crosses the aortic valve into the left ventricle. The catheter is available in 14F, 21F, and 24F and contains a flow pump the output of which can reach 3.5 to 5.7 L/min. The system requires anticoagulation with heparin and has allowed a 38% survival rate at 30 days. The **disadvantages** are prolonged supervision, bed rest because of the femoral artery approach, and lack of right ventricular support. A hemopump cannot be used by patients with aortic or aortic valve disease. The most common complications are hemolysis and ventricular arrhythmia caused by catheter position.

2. **External devices** are most commonly used for biventricular support. Device selection is based on likelihood of recovery and the nature of heart failure. The two major **indications** are postcardiotomy cardiogenic shock (inability to function without the cardiopulmonary bypass pump) and acute myocardial infarction with shock. If the patient is small (body surface area less than 1.3 m^2), the only choice is a centrifugal external device. Otherwise the choice can be made between a centrifugal or pulsatile (pneumatic drive) device. There are two of each.

a. **Centrifugal devices** are simple and versatile (can be used with extracorporeal membrane oxygenation [ECMO]) but lines are typically left between an unclosed sternum with only skin closure. This necessitates continuous supervision by trained staff and limits the devices to short-term use only. Heparin anticoagulation is needed. The most troublesome **complication** is systemic interstitial edema, which compounds mechanical difficulty in this preload-dependent machine. The two devices available for use are the Biomedicus Bio-

Pump (20% to 40% survival at 30 days) and the Sarns/3M system (50% survival at 30 days). Survival is best if the systems are used for less than a week.

   b. Pulsatile devices. Pulsatile pneumatic drive pumps also are extracorporeal. The advantage over centrifugal systems is that subcostal lines allow sternal closure and there is a lower rate of thromboembolism, although heparin anticoagulation still is used. Less interstitial edema is thought to be related to the pulsatile manner of blood flow. The Abiomed BVS-5000 device has been most successful when used for an average of 3.5 days. It can generate stroke volumes of 80 mL and flows of 5.5 L/min. Anticoagulation is achieved with heparin to an activated clotting time of 180 seconds. The Thoratec device has been used up to 75 days as bridge to transplantation and can generate stroke volumes of 65 mL and flows of 7.0 L/min. Anticoagulation is recommended with heparin, warfarin sodium, or dipyridamole to lower the rate of thromboembolism.

 3. Implantable devices. Two implantable devices are available for long-term use: the Novacor and the Heartmate. The Novacor has an electromagnetic converter and the blood pump is inserted. The device is synchronized to pump systole at the end of native systole. It has a maximum stroke volume of 70 mL and flows up to 10 L/min. Thromboembolism rate is 10%, so patients need heparin or warfarin after implantation of the device. The **Heartmate** device also has an implanted pump that is pneumatically driven and electrically powered. It can generate volumes of 85 mL and 11 L/min. The interior surfaces of the Heartmate are designed to allow pseudointimal layering, which reduces risk for thromboembolism. In theory, no anticoagulation is needed, but some patients receive antiplatelet agents.

C. Choosing the device. Indications for short-term devices are postcardiotomy cardiogenic shock, acute myocardial infarction, acute cardiomyopathy, or cardiac arrest as a complication of interventional cardiologic procedures. Preimplantation cardiac arrest is associated with high mortality and poor survival rates. If recovery is anticipated, the best device is the least traumatic, least complicated for the individual patient. If the patient is small (body surface area less than 1.3 m²), the only choice is a centrifugal external device. If recovery of ventricular function is not expected, patients should be considered for use of a long-term implantable device.

D. Surgical approach
 1. Left ventricular assist device (LVAD)
   a. The surgical approach differs between short- and long-term devices. Both connect the device outflow tract to the aorta. The device inflow of short-term devices is connected to the left atrial appendage or the right superior pulmonary vein. This keeps the myocardium intact for removal. Long-term devices receive inflow from the ventricular apex (aortic valve competency is required for optimal function) and necessitate additional incisions in the abdomen for pumps and drive lines.
   b. Decisions for right ventricular assist device (RVAD) support (needed by 20% of patients) are based on hemodynamics after LVAD placement. Because the short-term device operation is less complicated and can better tolerate additional cardiopulmonary bypass time, there is a lower threshold to place biventricular systems to ensure early hemodynamic stability. However, implantation of long-term RVAD devices is more labor intensive and requires long bypass times for placement, which carries higher morbidity.
   c. Once a device is in place, transesophageal echocardiography is used to monitor left heart filling. The skin is closed around the cannulas with persistent sternotomy in extracorporeal pumps (to facilitate reexploration for bleeding and tamponade) or sternal closure for implantable devices.

      d. When postoperative bleeding subsides, heparin is used with all devices except the Heartmate to achieve an activated clotting time of 160 to 200 seconds. The femoral approach to cannulation is avoided if future transplantation is expected.

    2. RVAD. Inotropic agents, volume infusions, and vasodilators are used to optimize pulmonary pressures and LVAD flows with right heart hemodynamic values as a guide. If VAD flow remains less than 2 L/min per square meter, an RVAD system may be placed with the inflow from the right atrium and outflow to the pulmonary artery. Inhaled nitric oxide has gained popularity as a potential alternative to RVAD implantation. With nasal cannula delivery, dosing begins at 20 ppm and is advanced to a maximum of 80 ppm or reduced pulmonary pressure. In one center, it has reduced the need for RVAD support from 7% to zero.

E. Postimplantation management. Early evaluation after VAD implantation includes assessment of hemodynamics, echocardiographic assessment of pressures and volumes, measurement of cardiac isoenzymes, and electrocardiographic (ECG) monitoring. Patients should continue aggressive heart failure medical regimens with the goal of removal of the device if ventricular function returns. Patients with RVADs will likely need aggressive diuresis.

F. Complications

    1. Perioperative **bleeding** increases with prolonged cardiopulmonary bypass times and causes excess fibrinolysis and platelet consumption. The degree of bleeding is intimately associated with right ventricular failure and thus RVAD support. In lengthy procedures, aprotinin is used to reduce perioperative bleeding. This bovine protease inhibitor acts on plasmin, kallikrein, and several other coagulation cascade sites with a net effect of inhibition of fibrinolysis and decreased bleeding. It has reduced postoperative thoracostomy drainage, the need for postoperative transfusions, and the need for RVADs. Transfusion is associated with infection and HLA immunization, which can increase risk for hyperacute humoral rejection for a patient who goes on to transplantation. The use of LVADs, because of the need for perioperative transfusions, increases this risk from 4% to 25%. Leukocyte-poor blood products should be used to minimize this risk as much as possible.

    2. Malignant arrhythmias. There is a high incidence of malignant cardiac arrhythmia after device implantation. Causes include cardiomyopathy, ischemia, chamber dilatation, use of inotropic agents, and focal abnormalities at the sewing ring. Each should be treated appropriately.

    3. Infection. Antibiotic prophylaxis should be administered to prevent infection. Standard therapy for 3 days after the operation is vancomycin, aztreonam, and fluconazole. If there is proved fungal infection, fluconazole should be used for a full 10-day course. In the long term there is a 25% to 45% rate of infection, which temporarily removes 20% of patients from the active transplantation list. The most serious infection is VAD endocarditis, which carries a 50% mortality and necessitates removal or replacement of the device.

    4. Embolic complications. Thromboembolism still occurs at a high rate despite proper use of anticoagulation. The Thoratec device carries a 22% risk for cerebrovascular embolic events, the Novacor 10%, and the Heartmate 3% to 5%. Immediate diagnosis and management of embolic complications is indicated, even thrombolysis if appropriate.

III. ECMO

    A. Design. Current ECMO systems have a centrifugal pump to drive blood from the patient to a membrane for carbon dioxide and oxygen exchange similar to that provided with cardiopulmonary bypass systems in open heart procedures. The insertion site is extrathoracic, however, with arterial and venous cannulation typically at the femoral vessels. Once in place, the device requires systemic anticoagulation and may cause substantial trauma to blood components.

B. Indications and use. ECMO is considered only as a short-term device (1 to 2 weeks) for patients with acute ventricular failure. If the cause of the failure is reversible, the device can be removed without further surgical therapy. This is best done in an intensive care unit with observation of ventricular function by means of transesophageal echocardiography as use of the system is discontinued. If the attempt at removal fails, or if the cause of ventricular dysfunction is not reversible, the options for longer-term management include exchange to a long-term VAD or cardiac transplantation.

C. Contraindications. The same indications for and contraindications to LVAD apply to ECMO regarding cardiac and noncardiac comorbidities. Because the device usually is inserted peripherally, patients must be free of severe peripheral vascular disease for safe insertion of this device.

IV. Dynamic cardiomyoplasty has been in use more than 12 years. The basic principle involves wrapping the latissimus dorsi muscle around the apex of the ventricle. A myostimulator, often a dual-chamber pacemaker, is implanted. Candidates for the procedure have an ejection fraction of 20% or less, a left ventricular end-diastolic diameter greater than 75 mm and an absence of RV failure. Data have shown an operative mortality of 6% to 15% and a 1-year mortality of 30%, most often from arrhythmia (60% to 70%). A 1-year benefit with increased cardiac indices, increased ejection fraction, decreased end-diastolic diameter, and decreased length of hospitalizations has been shown. Long-term results, however, have been disappointing.

V. Partial left ventriculectomy. Ventricular reduction is an experimental procedure first performed by Batista in Brazil in 1994. The procedure has been performed in several centers in the United States. The mathematical theory that formed the basis of Batista's approach centered on the return of the dilated ventricular chamber to a more normal volume-mass-diameter relation. Laplace's law describes wall stress as proportional to pressure and radius and inversely proportional to wall thickness. Reduction in diameter should decrease wall stress and allow improved function.

A. The basic **surgical approach** involves resection of the lateral wall from the apex to the atrioventricular groove between the anterior and posterior papillary muscles. This often includes resection of the left posterolateral coronary artery. Although Batista's approach to the mitral valve has varied, the current approach is to combine the myocardial resection with mitral valve repair using a suture between the anterior and posterior leaflets (Alfieri technique). This is done to insure valvular competency in the new setting of juxtaposed papillary muscles.

B. Postoperative medical management includes afterload reduction, digoxin, and diuretics. Because there have been several arrhythmic deaths, amiodarone or internal cardiac defibrillators are becoming standard empiric therapy.

C. Each center has had different **patient selection** criteria. Some perform the procedure only on patients not candidates for transplantation and without other options. Others perform the procedure only on transplantation candidates to provide backup options in the event of failure. Patient groups have had diverse causes of illness, and selection criteria and prognostic information are yet to be established. Evidence has shown that patients with ischemic cardiomyopathy are poor candidates for this procedure.

D. Echocardiographic findings have shown preoperative ejection fractions of 16% improving to 27% in the early postoperative period and remaining 30% after 3 months of follow-up study. The average preoperative left ventricular end-diastolic diameter of 7.9 cm has decreased to 6.1 cm postoperatively.

E. Published data from Brazil, the United Kingdom, Buffalo, and Cleveland have shown 67% to 90% 6-month survival as New York Heart Association functional class 1 to 2 and a 1-year survival rate of 63% to 87%. Another set of data on 120 combined patients from Buffalo and Brazil showed a 78% survival rate at 30 days and 55% at 2 years. The most common complication was congestive heart failure (18%). Other complications included surgical bleeding and suture dehiscence, renal failure, ventricular arrhythmia, and sudden death.

    F. The procedure remains experimental. It is unknown whether the improvement among some patients is caused by reduced diameter of the chamber or resolution of mitral regurgitation (MR) from the valvular repair. Much more information is needed to establish appropriate patient selection criteria and prognostic information. Future data analysis will help to sort out the many questions that surround this new procedure and help establish where it might fit into the current treatment options for patients with severe heart failure.

VI. Mitral annuloplasty. Secondary MR from ventricular dilatation is common in severe congestive heart failure. This phenomenon can lead to further depression of forward cardiac output, volume overload, and progressive MR. A preliminary study has revealed an improvement in functional class, ejection fraction, and ventricular dilatation among patients treated primarily with mitral annuloplasty for severe secondary MR. In a nonrandomized, historically controlled trial involving 48 patients with functional class 3 to 4 heart failure, patients with severe MR, actuarial survival at 1 and 2 years after mitral annuloplasty was 82% and 71%, respectively. This outcome compares favorably with that for historical controls. The future use of this procedure to manage severe congestive heart failure with secondary MR requires further investigation.

SUGGESTED READINGS

Key Reviews

Argenziano M, Oz M, Rose E. The continuing evolution of mechanical ventricular assistance. *Curr Probl Surg* 1997;34:328–386.

Bocchi E, Bellotti G, Vilella de Koraes A, et al. Clinical outcome after left ventricular surgical remodeling in patients with idiopathic dilated cardiomyopathy referred for heart transplantation. *Circulation* 1997;96 [Suppl II]:II-165–II-172.

Hunt S, Fraizer OH. Mechanical circulatory support and cardiac transplantation. *Circulation* 1998;97:2079–2090.

Relevant Book Chapters

Braunwald E. *Heart disease: a textbook of cardiovascular medicine,* 4th ed. Philadelphia: WB Saunders, 1992:535–550.

Topol EJ, ed. *Textbook of cardiovascular medicine.* Philadelphia: Lippincott–Raven, 1998:2273–2307.

13. CARDIAC TRANSPLANTATION

Leslie Campbell

I. **Introduction.** More than 4,000 patients in the United States are registered with the United Network Organ Sharing (UNOS) for cardiac transplantation. There are only about 2,500 heart donors yearly. Scarcity of donors is complicated by the use of single organs, heart injury with common brain-death injuries, difficulty with ex vivo preservation, heart disease among donors, and the complexity of the operation.

II. **Indications for heart transplantation**

   A. Indications for heart transplantation are as follows:
   1. Cardiogenic shock requiring mechanical assistance
   2. Refractory heart failure with continuous inotropic infusion
   3. New York Heart Association functional class 3 to 4 with a poor 12-month prognosis
   4. Progressive symptoms with maximal therapy
   5. Severe symptomatic hypertrophic or restrictive cardiomyopathy
   6. Medically refractory angina with unsuitable anatomy for revascularization
   7. Life-threatening ventricular arrhythmias despite aggressive medical and device interventions
   8. Cardiac tumors with low likelihood for metastasis
   9. Hypoplastic left heart and complex congenital heart disease.

   B. Patients should receive maximal medical therapy before being consideration for transplantation. They should also be appropriately considered for alternative surgical treatments such as coronary artery bypass surgery, valve repair or replacement, aneurysmectomy, cardiomyoplasty or partial ventriculectomy. A peak exercise oxygen consumption ($\dot{V}o_2$max) less than 14 mL oxygen per kilogram per minute or marked serial decline in $\dot{V}o_2$max warrants consideration for transplantation.

   C. Reversible causes of decompensation should be addressed. These include ischemia, atrial arrhythmia, atrioventricular (AV) block, alcohol use, thyroid disorders, uncontrolled diabetes mellitus, hypertension, ineffective diuretic therapy, use of negative inotropic agents, use of nonsteroidal anti-inflammatory agents, sodium and water restriction, obesity, obstructive sleep apnea, and cardiovascular deconditioning.

   D. If cardiac decompensation persists and indications for transplantation are met but no organ is available, use of mechanical circulatory devices should be considered (see Chapter 12). Ventricular assist devices can allow rehabilitation to increase physical condition and thus improve posttransplantation rehabilitation.

   E. Once accepted for transplantation, a patient is entered on the list and given a status based on severity of illness. Descriptions of each status are shown in Table 13-1. If status changes, time accrual starts over. Status I heart recipients are given priority over heart-lung transplantation candidates, who have priority over status II heart recipients. Zones are established to give local priority to recipients within a 500- to 1,000-mile radius centered on the donor site.

III. **Cardiac donor**

   A. **Criteria. Brain death** is necessary for any cadaveric organ donor. This is defined as absent cerebral function and brainstem reflexes with apnea during hypercapnia in the absence of any central nervous system depressant. There should be no hypothermia, hypotension, metabolic abnormalities, or drug intoxication. If brain death is uncertain, confirmatory tests including electroencephalography, cerebral flow imaging, or cerebral angi-

Table 13-1. Descriptions of transplantation status listings

STATUS I

1. Cardiac assistance
   Total artificial heart
   Ventricular assist device (inpatient or outpatient)
   Intraaortic balloon pump
   Ventilator
2. Inotrope dependent for maintaining cardiac output and in hospital intensive care unit
3. Younger than 6 mo.

STATUS II

Patients not status I according to criteria

STATUS VII

Patients improved and not in immediate need of transplantation or with new complications making transplantation contraindicated

---

ography may be indicated. Further criteria for cardiac donors are listed in Table 13-2.

B. Matching of donor and recipient

1. Because ischemic time during cardiac transplantation is crucial, donor-recipient matching is based primarily not on HLA typing but on the severity of the recipient's illness, ABO blood type (match or compatible), response to a panel of reactive antibodies (PRA), donor weight to recipient weight ratio (index 75% to 125%), geographic location relative to the donor, and length of time at current status. If the donor is small, heterotopic transplantation can be considered.

2. The PRA is a rapid measurement of preformed reactive anti-HLA antibodies in the transplant recipient. In general, if the PRA is less than 10% to 20%, no prospective crossmatch is needed. If the PRA is greater, a T- and B-cell crossmatch should be performed. If a more compatible donor cannot be found, the recipient may need plasmapheresis, immunoglobulins, or immunosuppressive agents to lower the PRA. Treatment with plasmapheresis, immunoglobulins, or immunosuppressants may lower the PRA activity.

C. Care of donor before transplantation

1. If a likely donor is found, the following things should be done.

Table 13-2. Cardiac donor exclusion criteria

Age older than 55 yr (with some exceptions)
Positive serologic results for HIV and acute hepatitis (some donors with hepatitis B or C can be accepted)
Systemic infection
Malignant tumors with metastatic potential (except primary brain tumors)
Systemic comorbidity (diabetes mellitus, collagen vascular disease)
Cardiac disease or trauma
Coronary artery disease
Allograft ischemic time estimated to be less than 4–5 hr
LVH at echocardiography
Death of carbon monoxide poisoning
Intravenous drug abuse
Left ventricular dysfunction

HIV, Human immunodeficiency virus; *LVH*, left ventricular hypertrophy.

    a. Contact local organ procurement organization (OPO).

    b. Obtain patient's height and weight.

    c. Collect blood for blood cell counts, metabolic profile, ABO typing, and testing for human immunodeficiency virus, hepatitis virus, and cytomegalovirus (CMV).

    d. Obtain an electrocardiogram.

    e. Obtain an echocardiogram early.

    f. Consider cardiac catheterization for coronary angiography if donor is a man older than 40 to 45 years or a woman older than 45 to 50 years.

    g. Optimize medical management for perfusion of potentially transplantable organs.

    h. Insert an arterial line and a right heart catheter for monitoring.

2. The OPO will handle all laboratory tests needed, the medical treatment of the donor, and organization of surgical harvesting teams. The OPO also is responsible for obtaining consent for use of organs for transplantation.

3. Donors with beating heart often are volume depleted because of therapy to reduce cerebral edema. **Volume resuscitation** should begin with normal saline solution or, sparingly, blood.

    a. A central venous pressure (**CVP**) of 5 to 10 cm water, a pulmonary capillary wedge pressure (**PCWP**) of 10 to 16 mm Hg, and a minimal arterial systolic blood pressure of 100 mm Hg are recommended. If the CVP and PCWP are adequate but hypotension persists inotropic support (5 to 15 µg/kg per minute dobutamine or 5 to 10 µg/kg per minute dopamine) should be initiated.

    b. **Diabetes insipidus** should be suspected if urine output is greater than 300 mL/hr or if hypernatremia develops. In this case vasopressin and hypotonic fluids may be needed.

    c. **Electrolytes** should be measured and abnormalities corrected hourly. Hypertension as a result of sympathetic discharge, fluid resuscitation, and vasopressin administration should be managed with intravenous (IV) nitroglycerin or nitroprusside.

    d. **Hypoxemia** often responds to inspired oxygen and additional positive end-expiratory pressure.

    e. **Hyperpyrexia** or **hypothermia** should be addressed with surveillance cultures followed by empirical administration of broad-spectrum antibiotics and use of cooling blankets.

    f. **Metabolic acidosis** from the loss of adrenal axis and thyroid hormone secretion of brain death can depress myocardial contractility, cause hypotension from vasodilatation, and attenuate the response to inotropic agents.

    g. **Ventricular dysfunction** sometimes responds to levothyroxine (2 to 4 µg/kg per hour) and methylprednisolone (100 mg IV per hour) in addition to inotropic agents; prophylactic administration of these two agents has been suggested.

D. Procedures and investigations

    1. Echocardiography should be performed on the donor heart as early as possible for assessment of ventricular function. If unexpected dysfunction is found in a young person, left ventricular end-diastolic diameter (LVEDD) and wall thickness should be measured. If dimensions are normal, thyroid and corticosteroid replacement should be initiated with correction of acidosis. Wall motion abnormalities, aortic stenosis, and mitral valvular disorders should be excluded, especially among older patients. If the electrocardiogram, cardiac history, and physical examination findings are normal, the donor heart may still be adequate.

    2. Coronary angiography should be performed on men older than 45 years and women older than 50 years. Precise definition of coronary anatomy is not the goal; **quick exclusion of severe lesions** is. Fluoroscopy is efficient in exclusion of pneumothorax or effusion after line placement. The femoral approach should be used in anticipation of coagulopathy, and the sheath should be sutured in place for intensive care unit monitoring and blood sampling. Risk to potential donor kidneys necessitates limiting use of contrast material as much as possible (approximately 25 mL). Ventriculography is not recommended, but if it is needed, a nonionic contrast agent should be used.

IV. **Surgical transplantation techniques**
   A. **Orthotopic implantation** is most common; it involves complete explantation of the native heart. This approach can be performed with either biatrial or bicaval anastomosis.
      1. **Biatrial anastomosis** is most common because the ischemic time is shorter. Complications include atrial dysfunction due to size mismatch of atrial remnants and arrhythmias (sinus node dysfunction, bradyarrhythmias, and AV conduction disturbances) that necessitate permanent use of a pacemaker by 10% to 20% of patients.
      2. **Bicaval anastomosis** decreases the incidence of arrhythmias, the need for a pacemaker, and risk for mitral or tricuspid regurgitation. However, narrowing of the superior vena cava and inferior vena cava make biopsy surveillance difficult, ischemic times can be prolonged, and there is no survival benefit with this approach.
   B. **Heterotopic implantation** is an alternative in which the donor heart functions in parallel with the recipient's heart. It accounts for less than 0.3% of transplants. This procedure can be considered only if the donor heart is small enough to fit into the mediastinum without physical restriction of function. Heterotopic transplantation is beneficial if the patient has pulmonary hypertension that would exclude orthotopic transplantation or has heart failure that is potentially reversible (e.g., myocarditis), allowing future removal of the transplant. The negative aspects of this approach are that the operation is difficult, provides no anginal relief, and necessitates anticoagulation because the native heart can potentially cease to function and become completely thrombosed. The heterotopic approach also cannot be used if the native heart has considerable mitral or tricuspid regurgitation.

V. **Physiologic concerns of the transplant recipient.** Biatrial connection means less atrial contribution to stroke volume. Resting heart rate is faster (95 to 110 beats/min) because of denervation, and acceleration of heart rate is slower during exercise. Diurnal changes in blood pressure are abolished. Diastolic dysfunction is expected because the myocardium is stiff from rejection and possibly from denervation.

VI. **Complications in the immediately postoperative period**
   A. Postoperative complications are listed in Table 13-3. Treatment is basically directed at maintaining organ perfusion, oxygenation, and acid-base balance, avoiding right ventricular failure, and managing arrhythmias. If needed, drugs used to maintain perfusion include α- and β-agonists, dopamine, phosphodiesterase inhibitors (milrinone), and vasodilators (nitroglycerin or nitroprusside). Isoproterenol can increase heart rate with peripheral vasodilatation.
   B. Management of right ventricular failure after transplantation is difficult. Improving hypoxemia, acidosis, uremia, and electrolyte imbalances often improves right ventricular function. The goal is to achieve a transpulmonary gradient of 5 to 10 mm Hg (mean pulmonary arterial pressure to mean PCWP) and pulmonary vascular resistance less than 6 Wood units (transpulmonary gradient to cardiac output). If vasodilators, volume reduction with diuretics or ultrafiltration, and inotropic agents fail to improve right ventricular function, then use of a right ventricular assist device or extracorporeal membrane oxygenation should be considered.
   C. **Arrhythmias.** Bradyarrhythmias should be managed with 0.01 to 0.02 μg/kg per minute IV isoproterenol or AV sequential pacing. Terbutaline and theophylline can be useful but are less desired because of limiting side effects. Most bradyarrhythmias improve 1 to 2 weeks after transplantation. AV disturbances in the early postoperative period may indicate incomplete

Table 13-3. Postoperative Complications of transplantation

SURGICAL

Aortic pseudoaneurysm or rupture at cannulation site
Hemorrhage
Pericardial effusion due to bleeding or coagulopathy

MEDICAL

Tricuspid regurgitation, severe
Right ventricular failure due to
  Pulmonary arterial compression
  Pulmonary hypertension
Left ventricular failure due to
  Ischemia
  Operative injury
  Acute rejection
Rhythm disturbances
  Asystole
  Complete heart block
  Sinus node dysfunction with bradyarrhythmia (resolution expected in 2 wk, as
    many as 25% permanent)
  Atrial fibrillation
  Ventricular tachycardia
Coagulopathy induced by cardiopulmonary bypass
Respiratory failure due to
  Cardiogenic pulmonary edema
  Noncardiogenic pulmonary edema
  Infection
Renal or hepatic insufficiency due to
  Congestive heart failure
  Drugs

myocardial preservation, pulmonary hypertension, acute rejection, or cardiac edema. Twenty-five percent of patients who undergo transplantation have postoperative sinus node dysfunction. The onset of atrial or ventricular arrhythmias may signify acute rejection.

VII. Postoperative management

  A. Initiation of medications, particularly immunosuppressive agents, begins on the day of the operation. Each center has its own immunosuppressive protocol, but a typical regimen includes 0.5 mg/kg cyclosporine IV at 2 mg/min, 2 mg/kg azathioprine IV every day, and 125 mg methylprednisolone IV every 8 hours for three doses.

    1. Cyclosporine usually is continued IV until the second or third postoperative day when an oral form can be initiated (e.g., Neoral 1 mg/kg every 12 hours with strict dosing times). Cyclosporine trough levels are measured beginning on postoperative day 2. Target levels for the first month are 150 to 250 ng/dL.

    2. Azathioprine usually is continued parenterally until about day 3; then an oral form is used (e.g., Immuran).

    3. Parental **steroids** can be converted quickly to prednisone (0.6 mg/kg per day) when the patient can take oral medication.

    4. If muromonab-CD3 (**OKT3**) is used, it is usually started on the first postoperative day at 5 mg IV.

  B. *Pneumocystis carinii* pneumonia prophylaxis is started within the first week after transplantation. If the patient or donor has positive serologic results for CMV, ganciclovir is necessary (see **VI.B**), often started on day 2.

  C. Endomyocardial biopsy is performed on about the fourth day and steroids can be tapered if no rejection above grade 2b is detected.

    D. Anticoagulation is needed if heterotopic transplantation is performed.

    E. Amylase and lipase are measured on day 3 to detect occult pancreatitis.

    F. Daily measurements of blood pressure, urine output volume status, electrolytes with magnesium and hematocrit are followed. Electrocardiograms are obtained on day 1, 2, 3, 5, 7, and 9.

    G. Tissue typing is performed twice a week for comparison and detection of rejection in the event of hypotension in the early postoperative period.

VIII. Long-term management. A typical posttransplantation regimen is shown in Table 13-4.

    A. Endomyocardial biopsy is performed once a week for the first month then can be performed less frequently depending on the presence or absence of rejection.

    B. If the **donor was CMV positive,** a Hickman or peripherally inserted central catheter is placed for long-term IV ganciclovir therapy (5 mg/kg twice a day for 14 days then 6 mg/kg daily for 14 days). If the **recipient is CMV negative** then oral acyclovir is administered daily. If the **recipient is CMV seropositive** the antiviral agent can be discontinued. CMV titers are measured at 1, 2, 3, and 6 months. If seroconversion occurs, ganciclovir is initiated for at least another 2-week period.

    C. Cyclosporine levels are measured periodically by individual center protocol.

    D. Echocardiography in the post transplant patient is useful for suspected pathology, and sometimes used to supplement endomyocardial biopsy findings.

    E. Cardiac catheterization is performed annually for early detection of allograft vasculopathy.

    F. There is probably no need for routine exercise testing or nuclear scans.

IX. Immunosuppressive agents.

    A. Azathioprine is purine analogue. The mechanism of action is nonspecific suppression of T- and B-cell lymphocyte proliferation.

        1. Typical dosage is 1 to 2 mg/kg per day by mouth. Because of steroid-induced elevation of white blood cell counts, long-term dosage decisions should be made after prednisone doses are less than 30 mg/d.

        2. Side effects are primarily bone marrow suppression (dose related). Use of azathioprine also is associated with skin cancer (limit sun exposure), warts, cutaneous fungal infections, and rarely liver failure or pancreatitis.

        3. Drug interactions include allopurinol (requires 75% reduction in azathioprine dose) and trimethoprim-sulfamethoxazole (worsened thrombocytopenia).

    B. Cyclosporine inhibits T-cell lymphokine production. It is highly lipophilic, and absorption is varied and influenced by gastrointestinal motility disorders. Neoral is a new microemulsion form of cyclosporine designed for more consistent absorption and blood levels.

        1. The **oral dosage** of cyclosporine is usually 8 to 10 mg/kg per day in two divided doses every 12 hours. IV doses are one-third the oral dose usually in continuous infusion. Serum drug levels are frequently measured for dosage and toxicity, but the level is not highly predictive of the actual immunosuppressive effect. Therapeutic ranges vary depending on the assay, and target levels vary depending on the time after transplantation and the degree of rejection detected by means of endomyocardial biopsy. Dosages should not be changed more than 20% at one time. Drug levels are reflected for 5 to 10 days because of the half life.

        2. The most common and troublesome **side effect** of cyclosporine is nephrotoxicity caused by afferent arteriolar constriction and manifested by oliguria. Loop diuretics may exacerbate this side effect. Mild elevation in creatinine level should be expected, and dosage adjustments should be made only if creatinine level is 3.0 mg/dL or more. Other side effects include hypertension, hypertrichosis, tremor, hyperkalemia, hyperlipidemia, and hyperuricemia (if allopurinol is initiated, reduction of azathioprine doses is necessary).

Table 13-4. Basic drug regimens

1. Immunosuppressive agents
   Uncertain mechanisms
     Corticosteroids
       Prednisone
       Cortisol
       Methylprednisolone
       Dexamethasone
   Inhibition of T-cell lymphokine production
   Cyclosporine
   FK506, tacrolimus
   Inhibition of lymphocyte proliferation
     Nonselective
       Azathioprine
     Selective
       Mycophenolate mofetil
   Antibodies to T-cell surface antigens
     Polyclonal
       Antilymphocyte globulin
     Monoclonal
       Muromonab-CD3
   Inhibition of nonimmune cell proliferation (endothelial, fibroblasts, smooth
     muscle)
   Rapamycin
2. Antibiotic prophylaxis
   Pneumocystis carinii pneumonia
     Trimethoprim sulfamethoxazole
       or dapsone
       or pentamidine aerosols
   Cytomegalovirus infection
     Ganciclovir, acyclovir
   Fungal infection
     Nystatin liquid *or* clotrimazole troches
3. Antihypertensives
   Nifedipine
4. Diuretics only as needed for edema
5. Potassium and Magnesium supplements (because of cyclosporine electrolyte
   wasting)
6. Lipid-lowering agents
7. Glucose-lowering agents (because of steroids or prior diabetes mellitus)
8. Cyclosporine dose–lowering agents
   Theophylline, diltiazem
9. Anticoagulation if transplant is heterotopic

---

    3. Drug interactions are numerous (Table 13-5).
  C. **Corticosteroids** act as immunosuppressive agents by means of uncertain
    mechanisms. They are used for maintenance immunosuppression and to
    manage acute rejection.
      1. Initially high **dosages usually** are tapered over the first 6 months to
      maintenance dosages of 5 to 15 mg/d (prednisone). Alternate-day regi-
      mens may decrease related complications.
      2. Short-term **side effects** include mood and sleep disturbances, acne, and
      weight gain. Long-term side effects include obesity, hypertension, osteo-
      penia, aseptic necrosis of the femoral head, and hyperglycemia.

Table 13-5. Drug-cyclosporine interaction

Increased levels	Decreased levels
Acetazolamide	Carbamazepine
Cimetidine	Cholestyramine
Ciprofloxacin	Phenobarbital
Diltiazem	Phenytoin
Erythromycin	Rifampin
Grapefruit	Warfarin sodium
Ketoconazole	
Nicardipine	
Verapamil	

D. **Mycophenolate mofetil** is a relatively new drug that selectively inhibits lymphocyte proliferation. It has performed favorably in the care of patients who have undergone renal transplantation.
   1. The recommended **dosage** is 2.0 g/d by mouth.
   2. The main **side effects** are gastrointestinal disturbances. Mycophenolate mofetil does not cause substantial bone marrow suppression; 2.5 to 4.5 µg/mL is therapeutic, but the assay is not generally available.
E. **FK-506 (tacrolimus)** is a relatively new lipophilic macrolide that inhibits lymphokine production in a manner similar to that of cyclosporine. In liver transplantation, FK-506 is successful in preventing rejection but more toxic than cyclosporine. The primary **side effects** are nephrotoxicity and neurotoxicity.
F. **Antilymphocyte globulin** is a horse polyclonal antibody designed to inhibit T cells by binding to surface antigens. It is generally used for induction of immunosuppression at the time of transplantation or to manage acute rejection.
   1. Typical **dosage** is 10 to 15 mg/kg per day through a central venous catheter. T-cell lymphocyte counts are monitored and kept at 200 cells/µL.
   2. **Side effects** include fevers and chills, urticaria, serum sickness, and thrombocytopenia.
G. **Muromonab-CD3 (OKT3)** is a murine monoclonal antibody to the CD3 complex on the T-cell lymphocyte designed for selective T-cell depletion.
   1. The usual **dosage** is 5 mg/d IV bolus injection over 10 to 14 days. CD3 cells are monitored with the goal of less than 25 cells/mL.
   2. The most common **side effect** is cytokine release syndrome, which consists of fever, chills, nausea, emesis, myalgia, diarrhea, weakness, and occasionally bronchospasm and hypotension. Acute pulmonary edema can develop if a patient experiences volume overload. Development of antibody to mouse protein makes retreatment in future rejection episodes contraindicated. This drug should be considered to treat patients with baseline renal dysfunction.
H. **Rapamycin** is relatively new and not routinely used. Its structure and mechanism of action are similar to those of FK-506 except that it antagonizes the proliferation of nonimmune cells such as endothelial cells, fibroblasts, and smooth muscle cells. This action makes it attractive for the prevention of immunologically mediated coronary allograft vasculopathy.
X. **Complications**
   A. **Rejection.** Preoperative therapy with cyclosporine, corticosteroids, and azathioprine is commonly used to prevent rejection. Investigation of suspected acute rejection should include measurement of cyclosporine and creatine kinase MB levels, two-dimensional echocardiography for left ventricular function, and endomyocardial biopsy. Overt signs and symptoms of

cardiac rejection are manifested only if rejection is in the end stage, which results in heart failure. Risk for rejection decreases with time.

1. Rejection is classified as hyperacute, acute cellular, or acute vascular (humoral). The term *chronic rejection* refers to allograft vasculopathy and is not in common use.

   a. **Hyperacute rejection** is always caused by preformed antibodies against the donor in the recipient. It occurs within minutes to hours and is uniformly fatal. PRA screening is the best method of avoiding hyperacute rejection.

   b. **Acute cellular rejection** is the most common form and occurs at least once among more than 50% of transplant recipients. Half of the episodes occur in the first 2 to 3 months, and the propensity decreases over time. Early rejection carries a worse prognosis than late rejection.

   c. **Vascular (humoral) rejection** is not well defined. It is characterized by immunoglobulin and complement in the microvasculature with little cellular infiltrate. It is associated with positive cross match, sensitization to OKT3, female sex, and younger recipient age. It is more difficult to treat than acute cellular rejection, is associated with hemodynamic instability, and carries a worse prognosis.

2. **Endomyocardial biopsy** findings of rejection are graded according to the degree of myocardial necrosis and lymphocyte infiltration and categorized 0 through 4. Treatment should be aggressive in the first 6 months after transplantation. In general, grades 0 and 1 do not necessitate therapy, grades 2 and 3 necessitate pulsed administration of high-dose steroids, and grade 4 necessitates T-cell antibody therapy.

B. **Infection.** There are two peak infectious periods after transplantation. During the first 30 days postoperatively, nosocomial infection related to indwelling catheters and wounds is most common. The second peak is 2 to 6 months postoperatively, and opportunistic immunosuppression-related infections predominate. There is considerable overlap, however, because fungi and toxoplasmosis both can be seen during the first month. It is important to remember that immunosuppressed transplant recipients can have severe infections but remain afebrile and that infections may develop in unusual locations.

   1. **CMV** is the most common infection transmitted by donor to recipient. If the donor is CMV positive and the recipient is CMV negative, prophylactic IV ganciclovir or foscarnet is given for 6 weeks and followed by long-term oral prophylaxis. If the recipient is CMV positive, a less potent regimen is used. The most common indication of infection is fever, malaise, and anorexia. However, severe infection can affect the lungs, gastrointestinal tract, and retina. Bone marrow toxicity can occur and confuse azathioprine treatment.

   2. ***Toxoplasma gondii.*** Primary infection can be serious while reactivation is rarely a serious clinical problem. Primary disease is manifest as encephalitis, myocarditis, or pneumonitis and should be treated with pyrimethamine and sulfadiazine.

   3. ***Pneumocystis carinii.*** Prophylactic therapy with trimethoprim-sulfamethoxazole is highly effective in preventing progressive bilateral interstitial pneumonia caused by this protozoan. Dapsone (requires glucose-6-phosphate dehydrogenase testing) and pentamidine aerosols (do not protect lung apex) are quite effective for patients who cannot take sulfa drugs.

   4. *Aspergillus* organisms. Invasive *Aspergillus* infection, typically of the lung or upper respiratory tract, is extremely difficult to manage. It is, fortunately, rare and usually occurs among patients who are severely immunocompromised from use of antilymphocyte antibodies. Standard treatment is IV amphotericin.

C. **Allograft vasculopathy,** or transplant coronary artery disease, is the leading cause of death more than 1 year after transplantation. This disease is likely the result of a proliferative response to immunologically mediated endothelial injury (chronic humoral rejection). It differs from native coronary disease in its concentric stenosis, subendocardial location, lack of calcification, and lack of angina pectoris. The use of angioplasty or bypass surgery is limited in this disease. **Risk factors** for this complication include the degree of histocompatibility, hypertension, hypertriglyceridemia, obesity, and CMV infection. The use of newer immunosuppressive agents that inhibit smooth muscle cell migration (e.g., rapamycin) may be associated with a lower incidence of allograft arteriopathy.

D. **Malignant disease.** Transplant recipients have a 100-fold increase in prevalence of malignant tumors compared with age-controlled cohorts.

1. The predominant tumor is **posttransplantation lymphoproliferative disorder** (PTLD), a type of non-Hodgkin's lymphoma believed to be related to Epstein-Barr virus (EBV). The incidence of PTLD may be as high as 50% in EBV-negative recipients of EBV-positive hearts. Treatment involves reduction of immunosuppressive agents, administration of acyclovir, and chemotherapy for widespread disease.

2. **Skin cancer** is common with the use of azathioprine.

3. **Any malignant tumor** present before transplantation carries risk for rapid growth once immunosuppression is initiated because of the negative effects on the function of T cells.

E. **Hypertension.** As many as 75% of transplant recipients treated with cyclosporine or corticosteroids eventually have hypertension. Treatment is largely empiric with a diuretic added to a calcium channel blocker, β-blocker, or angiotensin-converting enzyme inhibitor. If either diltiazem or verapamil is used, the dosage of cyclosporine should be reduced.

F. **Dyslipidemia.** As many as 80% of transplant recipients eventually have lipid abnormalities related to immunosuppressive medications. These dyslipidemias have been linked to accelerated allograft arteriopathy. Although well-designed studies are lacking, most centers now manage lipid abnormalities aggressively in the hope of alleviating transplant coronary vasculopathy.

G. **Tricuspid regurgitation.** A rare complication is tricuspid regurgitation caused by bioptome-induced trauma to the valvular apparatus.

XI. **Hospitalization of a transplant recipient**

A. If **nausea and vomiting** prevent administration of oral medication, the regimen should be changed to IV cyclosporine (one-third the oral dose) and IV methylprednisolone 1.0 g IV for 3 days.

B. If **fever** develops, the following procedures should be performed: survey cultures; complete blood cell count with differential; basic metabolic measurements; liver function tests; chest radiography; and two-dimensional echocardiography for function and effusion. Infectious causes should be aggressively sought, after which drug fever should be considered.

C. **Abnormal biopsy result.** If biopsy reveals grade 3b or 4 rejection, antithymocyte globulin or OKT3 should be administered for 7 to 10 days. Most other medications can be held until oral medications can be resumed. Drug regimens are as follows:

Grade 0_1, 1A, 1B: No treatment
Grade 2: Optional, consider prednisone 50 mg by mouth for 3 days
Grade 3A: Prednisone 100 mg by mouth for 3 days
Grade 3B: Consider methylprednisolone sodium succinate 1 mg IV for 3 days or antithymocyte globulin or OKT3
Grade 4: Antithymocyte globulin or OKT3

XII. **Outcomes**

A. According to the 1995 annual report of the United States Scientific Registry for Organ Transplantation, the 1-year **survival rate** was 82% and the 3-year survival rate 74%. The most common cause of mortality was cardiac allograft vasculopathy. UNOS data suggested some group differences. There were racial differences with a 3-year survival rate of 75% among white persons, 71% among Hispanic persons, and 68% among black persons. Sex differences were small. The 3-year survival rate among men was 75% and that among women was 72%. After 65 years of age, the survival rate was 66% at 3 years. Among recipients younger than 1 year, the 3-year survival rate was 60%. The highest survival in the UNOS database, 77%, was among recipients 35 to 49 years of age.

B. Typical **causes of death** in the first year are rejection or infection, both of which are linked with immunosuppression. After the first year, the primary cause of death is vasculopathy. In later stages after transplantation, atrial and ventricular rhythm disturbances may be signs of acute rejection or of allograft vasculopathy and dysfunction.

C. **Risk factors** for poor outcome include extreme age (less than 1 year or more than 65 years), ventilator use at the time of transplantation, elevated pulmonary vascular resistance, pulmonary disease, and diffuse atherosclerotic vascular disease. If the recipient has amyloidosis or sarcoidosis, the process can recur in the transplanted heart. Donor characteristics associated with a bad outcome include small body surface area, the need for inotropic agents, diabetes mellitus, ischemic time more than 4 hours, and echocardiographic diffuse wall motion abnormalities (this carries the worst prognosis regarding the donor).

SUGGESTED READING

References

1. Renlund DG. Cardiac transplantation. In: Topol EJ, ed. *Textbook of cardiovascular medicine.* Philadelphia: Lippincott–Raven, 1998:2327–2352.
2. Norman, Suki. *Primer on transplantation.* Thorofare, N.J.: American Society of Transplant Physicians, 1998:46–56.
3. Hosenpud JD, Cobanoglu A, Norman DJ, Starr A. *Cardiac transplantation: a manual for health care professionals.* New York: Springer-Verlag, 1991.

Key Reviews

Costanzo M, Augustine S, Bourge R, et al. Selection and treatment of candidates for heart transplantation. *Circulation* 1995;92:3593–3612.

Hunt S. Bethesda Conference: cardiac transplantation. *J Am Coll Cardiol* 1993;22:1–64.

Kirklin J, Bourge R, McGriffin D. Recurrent or persistent cardiac allograft rejection: therapeutic options and recommendations. *Transplant Proc* 1997;29[Suppl 8A]: 40S–44S.

Rabinovitch M. New insights and therapeutic strategies for postcardiac transplantation coronary artery disease. *Transplant Proc* 1997;29:2585–2586.

Valantine H. Individualizing immunosuppression for heart transplantation: strategies for the next decade. *Transplant Proc* 1997;29[Suppl 8A]:5S–8S.

Relevant Book Chapters

Braunwald E, ed. *Heart disease: a textbook of cardiovascular medicine,* 5th ed. Philadelphia: WB Saunders, 1997:515–533.

Topol EJ, ed. *Textbook of cardiovascular medicine.* Philadelphia: Lippincott–Raven, 1998:2327–2352.

SECTION IV. VALVULAR HEART DISEASE

David N. Rubin and Brian P. Griffin

14. AORTIC VALVE DISEASE

Matthew Deedy

I. **Aortic stenosis**

   A. **Introduction.** Valvular aortic stenosis (AS) is the most common cause of left ventricular outflow tract (LVOT) obstruction. Other causes of LVOT obstruction include subvalvular AS caused by a fixed membrane or fibromuscular tunnel, dynamic subvalvular obstruction caused by hypertrophic cardiomyopathy, and supravalvular AS.

   B. **Clinical presentation.** AS should be suspected when any patient has a **systolic ejection murmur at the right upper sternal border that radiates to the carotid arteries.** Most patients have no symptoms at presentation. A careful **review of systems** is necessary to establish any history of chest pain, lightheadedness, syncope, or symptoms suggestive of heart failure. A **history** of coarctation of the aorta may indicate the presence of a bicuspid aortic valve. A history of rheumatic fever may suggest a rheumatic cause of AS.

   1. **Signs and symptoms.** The presence of symptoms usually indicates severe AS.

      a. **Angina** usually is related to an increase in myocardial oxygen demand and a decrease in myocardial oxygen supply or to coronary atherosclerosis. As many as 25% of patients without angina may have coronary artery disease (CAD), and 40% to 80% of those with angina and AS have CAD.

      b. **Syncope.** Because of the fixed LVOT and a limited ability to augment cardiac output, patients with AS may have severe hypotension in conditions that decrease total peripheral resistance with resultant presyncope or syncope.

      c. **Heart failure** may be caused by either diastolic or systolic dysfunction. Over the course of the disease, myocardial fibrosis impairs contractility. Compensatory mechanisms that increase intravascular volume may increase left ventricular end diastolic pressure (LVEDP) and pulmonary capillary wedge pressure (PCWP), resulting in pulmonary congestion. Conditions that impair filling of the left ventricle, such as atrial fibrillation or tachycardia alone, may cause heart failure.

   2. **Physical findings**

      a. **Arterial examination.** A hallmark finding in AS is a diminished and delayed carotid upstroke, **pulsus parvus et tardus.** This is the best estimate of the severity of stenosis at bedside. A **systolic thrill** over the carotid arteries may be palpable in severe AS. Among some elderly patients with noncompliant vessels, the carotid pulsation may seem normal, which may lead the clinician to underestimate the severity of stenosis. All peripheral pulses may be diminished in severe AS.

      b. **Palpation.** With left ventricular (LV) hypertrophy but no enlargement of the left ventricle, the **apical impulse** usually is **nondisplaced, diffuse, and sustained.** A double apical impulse usually represents a palpable *a* wave, or S_4, caused by a noncompliant left ventricle. A systolic thrill may be palpable in the second right intercostal space in AS.

      c. **Auscultation.** The main auscultatory findings are shown in Fig. 14-1.

         (1) The typical murmur of AS is a systolic ejection murmur heard at the right upper sternal border that radiates to the neck.

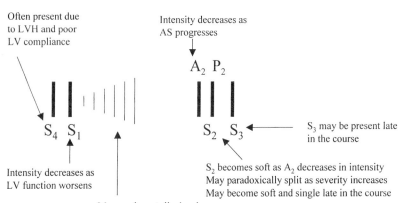

Often present due to LVH and poor LV compliance

Intensity decreases as AS progresses

A_2 P_2

S_4 S_1

S_2 S_3

S_3 may be present late in the course

Intensity decreases as LV function worsens

S_2 becomes soft as A_2 decreases in intensity
May paradoxically split as severity increases
May become soft and single late in the course

Murmur is systolic, harsh
Heard best at right upper sternal border
Radiates to carotids
Peaks in early to mid-systole until late in the course when it peaks later and is more intense

FIG. 14-1. Physical findings in aortic stenosis.

With a mobile bicuspid valve, an aortic opening sound may precede the murmur. As the severity of stenosis increases, the murmur becomes longer and more intense and peaks later in systole. However, if cardiac output is severely reduced, the murmur may become less intense. Thus **murmur intensity does not necessarily relate to the severity of stenosis.**

(2) S_1 usually is normal in AS; however, if severe systolic dysfunction and an elevated LVEDP are present, S_1 may be diminished because of premature closure and decreased force of closure of the mitral valve. The aortic component of S_2 decreases with more severe stenosis, and S_2 becomes soft and single, because only the pulmonary valve component is audible. Among some patients with severe AS, S_2 is paradoxically split because of the prolonged LV systolic ejection period through the severely narrowed valve. A paradoxically split S_2 may be heard in other forms of LVOT obstruction and left bundle branch block. S_3 when present suggests poor systolic function in the left ventricle. S_4 when present represents left atrial contraction into a poorly compliant left ventricle and strongly suggests severe AS.

(3) Careful examination for **other murmurs** should be performed. AS often is accompanied by aortic regurgitation (AR). Maneuvers during the physical examination may help clarify the cause of a systolic ejection murmur (see Chapter 9). The **Gallavardin's phenomenon** occurs in severe calcific AS when high-frequency components of the typical murmur selectively radiate to the apex. This sound may be confused with that of coexisting mitral regurgitation (MR).

C. **Etiology**
  1. **Congenital AS**
    a. The most common congenital abnormality associated with AS among adults is a bicuspid aortic valve. Abnormal flow characteristics of a

bicuspid valve are likely to lead to premature degeneration and calcification. About 1% to 2% of Americans, with a male predominance, are born with a bicuspid aortic valve. The murmur typically is found during childhood, but the patient may not need surgical intervention until much later, in the fifth or sixth decade of life.

   b. Other congenital causes of AS usually present themselves in childhood. They include abnormal trileaflet valve with leaflet fusion, unicuspid valve, and a commissural valve.

2. Acquired AS

   a. Degenerative calcific AS is the most common cause in developed countries. This is caused by abnormal calcification of a trileaflet aortic valve. This condition typically becomes apparent in the seventh or eighth decades of life. Processes that cause abnormal calcium metabolism may cause accelerated calcification; examples are Paget's disease of bone and end-stage renal disease. Risk factors for coronary atherosclerosis also predispose patients to degenerative aortic valve calcification.

   b. Rheumatic AS is uncommon without coexisting mitral valve disease. When present, rheumatic AS typically manifests itself as fibrosis, calcification, and fusion of the aortic valve cusps and commissures, with leaflet thickening, particularly at the edges.

D. Pathophysiology

1. AS is a condition characterized by progressive narrowing of the aortic valve orifice over time. As the aortic valve area gradually decreases, the left ventricle faces increasing afterload.

2. To **maintain cardiac output, the left ventricle must develop higher systolic pressures,** which increase wall stress. This leads to compensatory, concentric hypertrophy of the left ventricle, which allows the wall stress to normalize according to Laplace's law [wall stress = (pressure × radius) ÷ (2 × thickness)]; however, LV compliance (change in volume with change in pressure [dV/dP]) decreases.

3. With a **less compliant left ventricle,** less filling occurs passively in the early phase of diastole. **Left atrial contraction becomes more important** in maintaining adequate LV preload.

4. The greater LV muscle mass, the elevated systolic pressure required and the prolongation of ventricular systole **increase myocardial oxygen demand.**

5. The elevation in LVEDP decreases the perfusion pressure across the coronary vascular bed and may cause endocardial compression of small intramyocardial arteries and a reduction in myocardial oxygen supply.

E. Natural history

1. **Patients without symptoms.** In general patients with pure AS do not have symptoms until the aortic valve area is less than 1.0 cm².

   a. The disease process of AS is characterized by a long latent phase during which the patient has no symptoms. During this time, there is marked individual variability in the rate of progression of stenosis.

   b. In general the rate of increase in the mean aortic valve gradient is about 7 mm Hg per year among patients without symptoms, and the aortic valve area decreases by about 0.12 to 0.19 cm²/year (1). Because the rate of progression varies, **all patients with AS should be instructed about the signs and symptoms that indicate progression** of AS.

   c. Patients without symptoms have near-normal survival rate. The risk for sudden death among patients with asymptomatic severe AS is less than 2% per year.

2. **Patients with symptoms.** Once symptoms of AS develop, the survival rate decreases markedly.

   a. Patients with **angina** have a 50% 5-year survival rate without surgical intervention. Those with **syncope** have a 50% 3-year survival rate without surgical intervention. Patients with **heart failure** have a mean survival time of less than 2 years if treated medically (2).

b. Sudden death may occur among patients with symptomatic AS. This may be caused by primary ventricular arrhythmias among patients with LV hypertrophy and ventricular dysfunction or by arrhythmias due to myocardial ischemia.

F. Laboratory examination

1. The typical **electrocardiogram (ECG)** of a patient with isolated severe AS usually demonstrates **left atrial abnormality** (80%) and **LV hypertrophy** (85%). **Arrhythmias are rare until late in the course of AS.** The most common arrhythmia is **atrial fibrillation;** this is even more common if there is coexisting mitral valve disease. Because of its proximity to the atrioventricular node and His's bundle, high-degree heart block can occur if an aortic valve ring abscess forms as a complication of infectious endocarditis.

2. **Chest radiography** is not useful in the diagnosis of AS; the findings may be entirely normal. The cardiac silhouette may become boot-shaped because of concentric LV hypertrophy. Cardiomegaly may be present if there is LV dysfunction or coexisting AR. Aortic valve calcification may occur among adults with severe AS and is best appreciated in a lateral view. Poststenotic dilatation of the ascending aorta may be evident.

G. Diagnostic testing. The goal of diagnostic testing is to determine the presence, severity, and cause of AS. Provocative testing with dobutamine or nitroprusside occasionally is helpful in assessing the severity of stenosis.

1. **Echocardiography.** Doppler echocardiography is the **method of choice** for establishing the diagnosis of AS and assessing its severity. Parasternal two-dimensional and M-mode views are the best for determining the precise mechanism and for measurements of chamber dimensions and wall thickness.

   a. Echocardiographic technique

   (1) Parasternal long-axis view

   (a) The location of the **coaptation line of the aortic valve** within the LVOT should be documented. A normal, trileaflet valve coapts in the center of the LVOT. The leaflets of a bicuspid valve often have an eccentric closure line, typically posterior to the midline.

   (b) Leaflet thickening may be seen, and **systolic leaflet doming,** which is associated with congenital and rheumatic AS, may be apparent. The pattern of leaflet thickening may help **differentiate rheumatic AS from congenital or degenerative calcific AS.** In **rheumatic AS,** there is focal thickening of the free edges of the domed leaflets compared with the body of the leaflet. The presence of mitral stenosis with characteristic doming of the mitral leaflets supports a rheumatic cause of AS when present. In **degenerative calcific AS,** the calcification typically progresses from the base of the leaflets to the tips. As calcification progresses, leaflet mobility decreases to the point where the leaflets appear fixed.

   (c) The presence of LV hypertrophy, LV enlargement, or left atrial enlargement may be established in the parasternal long axis with two-dimensional and M-mode imaging. The LV cavity typically is small in pure AS, and there is hypertrophy of the left ventricle. The LVOT dimension for the continuity equation is measured in the parasternal long-axis view.

   (d) Color Doppler imaging is helpful to visualize flow acceleration proximal to the aortic valve and to visualize coexisting AR in this view. Because the transducer is perpendicular to the direction of flow through the LVOT, spectral Doppler data to assess transvalvular and LVOT velocities are not usually obtained in the parasternal windows.

(2) The **parasternal short-axis view** is the **most useful** view in establishing the cause of congenital AS. The aortic valve should be examined during both systole and diastole. The number of commissures and the shape of the valve orifice should be assessed (Fig. 14-2). A single coaptation line in diastole and an elliptical orifice suggest a bicuspid valve. A single commissure with a coaptation line extending from the vessel wall to an elliptic orifice suggests a unicommissural, unicuspid valve. A bicuspid aortic valve in diastole may appear trileaflet because of the presence of a raphe (an underdeveloped aortic cusp). Once the aortic valve is severely calcified, it becomes much more difficult to establish the cause of AS.

(3) **Apical two- and four-chamber views** are used to assess overall ventricular function and wall motion with two-dimensional imaging.

(4) The **apical five-chamber view** is well-aligned with flow through the aortic valve. Aortic valve motion can be assessed in this view. Color flow Doppler imaging is useful in this view to detect AR and acceleration of flow proximal to the aortic

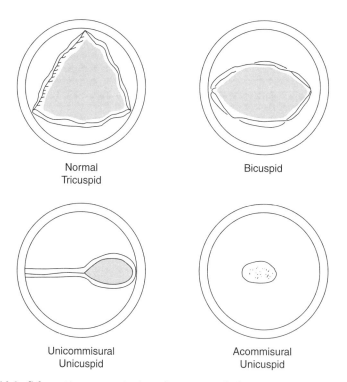

Normal
Tricuspid

Bicuspid

Unicommisural
Unicuspid

Acommisural
Unicuspid

FIG. 14-2. Schematic representation of parasternal short axis of a congenitally abnormal aortic valve.

valve. Continuous wave Doppler recordings across the aortic valve are obtained in this view. Pulsed wave Doppler flow in the LVOT proximal to the aortic valve is recorded here for the continuity equation.

(5) The **apical long-axis view** is useful for establishing the presence of AR with color Doppler ultrasound. Continuous wave Doppler imaging can be performed in this view if the alignment is adequate.

b. **Hemodynamic calculations**

(1) Doppler echocardiography is the standard for assessment of the **transvalvular pressure gradient** and **aortic valve area.** The **modified Bernoulli equation** ($P = 4v^2$ where P is pressure and v is peak velocity of flow across the aortic valve) allows estimation of the peak instantaneous gradient and mean gradient across the aortic valve. Sampling with continuous wave Doppler ultrasound should be performed from the apex of the left ventricle, right sternal border in the second intercostal space, and suprasternal notch to estimate most accurately the peak velocity of flow across the aortic valve. A typical continuous wave Doppler recording of a patient with combined AS and AR is shown in Fig. 14-3. The modified Bernoulli equation is generally accurate for determining the mean gradient and peak instantaneous gradient across the aortic valve. Situations in which errors in estimation of the aortic valve gradient may occur are listed in Table 14-1.

(2) Calculation of **aortic valve area** with Doppler data is based on the **continuity principle,** which states that the flow of an incompressible fluid in a closed system must remain constant. Because flow (Q) at a given point equals velocity (v) of

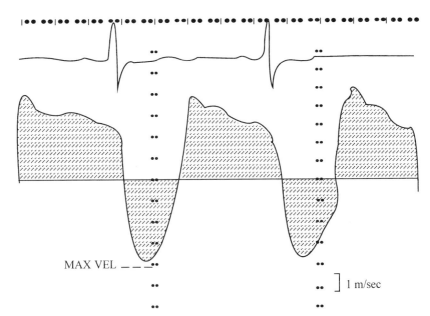

MAX VEL

] 1 m/sec

FIG. 14-3. Continuous wave Doppler recording of combined AS and AR.

Table 14-1. Sources of error in Doppler-derived aortic valve pressure gradients

Causes of gradient overestimation	Causes of gradient underestimation
Coexisting aortic regurgitation	Poor Doppler signals
Subaortic membrane	Inappropriate recording angle or eccentric jet
Inadvertent measurement of mitral regurgitation velocity	Use of proximal velocity in the continuity equation
High output states	Lack of technical expertise
Measurement of velocity of post-extrasystolic beat	
Nonrepresentative sampling among patients with atrial fibrillation	

flow at the given point multiplied by the cross-sectional area (A) at that point, and flow (Q) is constant at points 1 and 2, the following is true:

$$Q_1 = Q_2 = v_1 \times A_1 = v_2 \times A_2$$

A schematic representation of the variables for calculating aortic valve area is shown in Fig. 14-4.

(a) The most common method of calculating aortic valve area is to calculate the area of the LVOT (A_1) just proximal to the aortic valve and the velocity of flow at the same point (v_1). The calculation of LVOT area is based on the assumption that the area is circular in cross section ($A = \pi r^2$). The diameter ($2 \times$ radius) of the LVOT is measured just proximal to the aortic valve in the parasternal long-axis view, usually with a zoom feature in place to allow more accurate measurement.

(b) To determine v_1, the velocity of flow just below the aortic valve is measured from the apical five-chamber view with pulsed wave Doppler. The sample volume is placed in the LVOT and advanced up the LVOT until flow begins to accelerate. Then the sample volume is withdrawn slightly

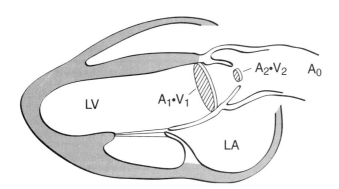

FIG. 14-4. Schematic representation of parasternal long-axis view and the continuity principle.

to the point where the actual velocity measurement is made (usually about 0.5 cm to 1.5 cm below the valve).

(c) To **minimize error** in calculating flow, it is **critical to make a precise perpendicular measurement of the LVOT diameter** and to make every effort to **record the velocity at the identical spot.** It is important to measure peak velocity across the aortic valve (v_2) from several windows. Care should be taken to avoid measuring postextrasystolic beats. If the patient is in atrial fibrillation, ten consecutive beats should be measured and averaged for both velocity measurements.

(d) Once the measurements have been made, aortic valve area may be calculated as follows:

$$A_2 = v_1 \times A_1 / v_2$$

(3) Special care must be taken when measuring the peak aortic velocity to **avoid confusion with MR.** MR is of longer duration than AS and by definition there is no flow through the aortic valve during isovolumic contraction or isovolumic relaxation. The velocity of MR is typically higher because of the greater pressure gradient between the left ventricle and left atrium compared with the left ventricle and aorta.

(4) In assessment of an **aortic valve prosthesis,** the standard continuity equation does not apply because of the irregular shape of the prosthetic orifice. Instead, the **velocity ratio,** or **dimensionless index,** is used to estimate the severity of stenosis. This is calculated by means of dividing the peak velocity in the LVOT by the peak velocity through the aortic valve. A dimensionless index of less than 0.25 is generally accepted to represent severe stenosis. This method also is helpful in difficult clinical situations (e.g., severe AS and severe LV dysfunction in which the gradient may appear less than expected for valve appearance on two-dimensional or M-mode echocardiography).

(5) Doppler-derived gradients and valve area calculations from transthoracic echocardiography correlate well with catheter-derived measurements. A normal aortic valve has an effective orifice area of 2.0 to 4.0 cm² depending on the size of the patient.

(a) **Mild AS** is considered to be from the point of initial narrowing of the LVOT to an aortic valve area of 1.5 cm² or a mean transvalvular gradient of 0 to 20 mm Hg.

(b) **Moderate AS** is defined as an aortic valve area of 1.0 cm² to 1.5 cm² or a mean gradient of 20 to 40 mm Hg.

(c) **Severe AS** is defined as less than 1.0 cm² or a mean gradient of greater than 40 mm Hg. Critical AS is defined as an aortic valve area of less than 0.75 cm² or less than 0.5 cm²/m².

2. **Transesophageal echocardiography (TEE). Planimetry of the aortic valve often is** possible with TEE. Doppler-derived gradients may be difficult to obtain because of problems in aligning the Doppler signal with the AS jet. TEE is particularly useful for **determining morphologic features of the valve in congenital AS.**

3. **Stress echocardiography**

a. Patients with severe LV systolic dysfunction and AS may have low transvalvular gradients; however, patients with primary myocardial dysfunction and mild AS also may have severe LV systolic dysfunction and low transvalvular gradients, so-called **aortic pseudostenosis.** In this situation, **provocative testing may help differentiate** true AS and aortic pseudostenosis. Differentiation is important because patients with pseudostenosis are unlikely to benefit from surgical therapy for AS.

b. Dobutamine infusion may be performed either in the echocardiography laboratory or in the cardiac catheterization laboratory. With this technique, an intravenous dobutamine infusion is given with incrementally higher doses from 5 µg/kg per minute up to 20 µg/kg per minute, according to the standard dobutamine echocardiographic protocol. The goal is increasing cardiac output.

c. The aortic valve area is calculated at each dose. The infusion is stopped immediately if the patient experiences hypotension, angina, or arrhythmia. Interpretation of the test results is outlined in **I.I.2.a.**

4. Cardiac catheterization. Catheter-derived data once were considered the standard for quantification of AS; echocardiography, however, has become widely accepted for the evaluation of AS. **Patients with severe AS are at a higher risk for complications of cardiac catheterization** than are patients without AS; therefore the **benefits of the information obtained must outweigh the risks of the procedure.** The risk for death after cardiac catheterization among patients with severe valvular heart disease has been reported to be 0.2%.

a. Men older than 40 years, women older than 50 years, and patients with angina should undergo coronary cineangiography before aortic valve operations. If there is a question about the severity of AS, invasive hemodynamic data also should be obtained. **Catheter-derived hemodynamic data often are used to confirm the diagnosis when the severity of AS is in doubt after echocardiography.** The mean gradient obtained at catheterization correlates well with simultaneously obtained mean echo gradients. The peak gradient measured with catheterization is the peak-to-peak gradient and usually is lower than the peak instantaneous gradient obtained with echocardiography (Fig. 14-5).

b. Catheterization technique

(1) The catheterization protocol for a patient with AS includes both left and right heart catheterization. The **first priority** is obtaining **simultaneous recordings of cardiac output and transaortic gradient.** This requires separate transducers for the LV and aortic pressures. It is important to make hemodynamic measurements with the patient in a steady state, before any intervention that may alter hemodynamic values. All measurements, therefore, should be made before any injections of contrast material and, if possible, before any pharmacologic sedation of the patient. Cardiac output measurements should be made at the same time as the transvalvular gradient measurements to minimize error.

(2) The most precise **measurement of transaortic valvular gradient** is made with two different catheters, one pigtail in the LV cavity and the other in the ascending aorta. This requires cannulation of both femoral arteries and is uncomfortable for the patient. Other acceptable methods of measuring transvalvular gradient include using a double-lumen pigtail catheter, obtaining simultaneous pressures of the left ventricle and femoral artery, and left ventricle to ascending aorta pullback. If simultaneous pressures of the left ventricle and femoral artery are used to determine the aortic valve gradient, an initial simultaneous measurement of ascending aorta and femoral artery pressures should be performed to rule out an additional gradient that might cause overestimation of the aortic valve gradient. A typical pressure tracing, with simultaneous recording of LV and aortic pressures with a double-lumen pigtail catheter, is shown in Fig. 14-5.

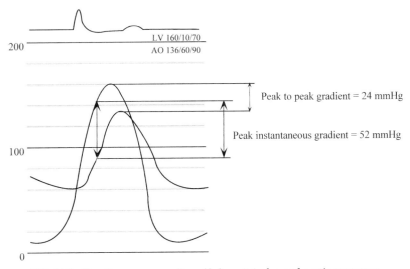

LV 160/10/70
AO 136/60/90

200

Peak to peak gradient = 24 mmHg

Peak instantaneous gradient = 52 mmHg

100

0

FIG. 14-5. Simultaneous recording of left ventricular and aortic pressures.

    (3) Provocative testing to differentiate true AS and aortic pseudostenosis may be performed with nitroprusside in the cardiac catheterization laboratory. The goal is to measure transvalvular gradients and aortic valve area at different cardiac outputs. Nitroprusside infusion is most safely performed in the cardiac catheterization laboratory because of its propensity to induce hypotension. An intravenous infusion beginning at 3 µg/minute is started with continuous monitoring of blood pressure and frequent measurements of cardiac output. The infusion rate is slowly titrated up until a marked change in cardiac output is measured, at which time transvalvular gradients are measured and aortic valve area is calculated again. Interpretation of the findings is discussed in **I.I.2.a.**

    (4) Severe AS is an indication for using lower osmolar, nonionic contrast agents that result in less hypotension from peripheral arterial vasodilation, less bradycardia, less transient myocardial dysfunction, and less osmotic diuresis after the procedure. Each of these features may lower the risk of the procedure. Left ventriculography should be avoided in the care of patients with critical AS.

    (5) Coronary cineangiography may be performed in the usual manner. The left coronary artery may be difficult to engage because of poststenotic dilatation of the ascending aorta. A catheter with a longer distance between the primary and secondary curves, that is, JL5 or JL6 instead of JL4, may be needed. Positioning the right coronary catheter may be difficult because of the high-velocity jet of blood flow through the stenotic aortic valve that hits the tip of the catheter. As always, care should be taken to minimize the contrast load.

  c. Hemodynamic findings and calculations

    (1) Patients with noncritical AS typically have a normal ejection fraction, normal resting cardiac output, normal right heart pressures, and normal mean PCWP. The LVEDP usually is elevated, because of the noncompliant nature of the hypertrophied left ventricle. The *a* wave in the PCWP, left atrial, and LVEDP tracings usually is prominent. As the severity of stenosis increases, LVEDP rises, as do right heart and pulmonary arterial pressures. Cardiac output and ejection fraction decline in the later stages of AS. Among patients with end-stage, critical AS, the transvalvular gradient decreases because of LV systolic dysfunction. It is therefore critical to consider LV function when estimating the severity of AS by means of pressure gradients alone.

(2) The **Gorlin formula** is used to estimate aortic valve area, as follows:

$$AVA(cm^2) = \frac{Cardiac\ Output}{44.3 \times SEP \times \sqrt{MVG}}$$

In this equation, SEP is the systolic ejection period measured in seconds per minute and MVG is the mean valvular gradient in millimeters of mercury. SEP is defined as the time from aortic valve opening to closing. Measurement of SEP and MVG and the calculation of aortic valve area are outlined in Fig. 14-6.

H. Therapy

1. **Priority of therapy.** The mainstay of therapy for severe AS is **surgical replacement of the aortic valve.** Surgical intervention generally is restricted to patients with symptoms because aortic valve replacement carries considerable risk and the survival benefit is apparent only after symptoms occur. There is increasing evidence that once severe AS is present, the likelihood of progression to symptoms and aortic valve replacement in less than 3 years is high. Older patients with asymptomatic, critical AS may benefit from elective surgical treatment rather than waiting until symptoms develop. Younger patients with very high gradients are at higher risk for sudden death and may also benefit from

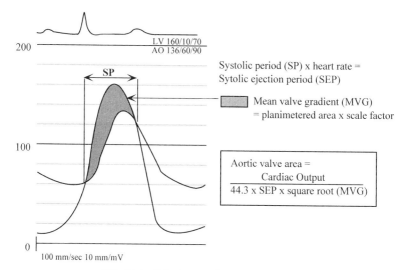

FIG. 14-6. Calculation of aortic valve area.

earlier surgical treatment. Likewise, patients with an aortic valve area of 1.0 cm² or less and considerable obstructive coronary atherosclerosis that necessitates coronary artery bypass grafting should be considered for aortic valve replacement.

2. **Medical therapy**
   a. **Antibiotic prophylaxis.** Once the diagnosis of AS is made, all patients must be instructed on the use of antibiotic prophylaxis (see Chapter 48).
   b. **Treatment of patients without symptoms.** Patients with pure AS often do not have symptoms until the aortic valve area is less than 1.0 cm². During the asymptomatic phase, therapy is directed at **primary prevention of CAD, maintenance of sinus rhythm,** and **blood pressure control.** All **patients must be instructed** at each clinic visit about the signs and symptoms of angina, syncope, or heart failure. They also should be instructed to **notify their physicians immediately** once symptoms develop. At that point, the risk of surgery is usually less than the risk of continued medical therapy.
   c. Therapy for heart failure is directed at **volume control for relief of pulmonary congestion.** This usually is achieved with diuretics. However, because the cardiac output of patients with severe AS depends on adequate preload, **attempts at diuresis should be cautious** because overdiuresis may cause hypotension from decreased cardiac output and cause poor peripheral perfusion. **Nitrates should be avoided by patients with heart failure and severe AS** because they may cause cerebral underperfusion and syncope. Digoxin often is used by patients with heart failure and AS, particularly if atrial fibrillation develops. This therapy has no effect on long-term survival.
   d. **Vasodilators should be avoided** by patients with AS
      (1) Indications. In certain situations, such as mixed AS and AR, AS and MR, or CAD and AS, use of these agents may be considered but only in an intensive care unit with invasive hemodynamic monitoring. Patients with a predominant regurgitant lesion theoretically benefit from use of vasodilators. Patients with coexisting CAD improve because of decreased LV systolic pressures with less peripheral resistance and therefore less oxygen demand. This therapy is **used only as a bridge to definitive surgical therapy.**
      (2) Dosing. Because of the potential for profound hypotension with vasodilators, therapy usually is instituted with low-dose nitroprusside. Once a safe dosage of vasodilator is established in the intensive care unit, patients may be switched to oral therapy with angiotensin converting enzyme (ACE) inhibitors or direct vasodilators such as hydralazine.
   e. **Atrial fibrillation** usually is poorly tolerated by a patient with severe AS because of the importance of the atrial component of diastolic filling in achieving adequate preload. Cardiac output is compromised, and pulmonary vascular congestion may rapidly follow. Myocardial oxygen demand also rises because of tachycardia. For these reasons, **new-onset atrial fibrillation should be rapidly and aggressively managed** for a patient with severe AS with the goal of restoring sinus rhythm if possible.

3. **Percutaneous therapy**
   a. **Intraaortic balloon pump (IABP).** Insertion of an IABP has been reported to be effective in stabilizing the conditions of a small number of patients with severe AS and decompensated heart failure as a bridge to surgical treatment. The effectiveness was postulated to be derived from diastolic augmentation of coronary perfusion, which suggests that global ischemia may play an impor-

tant role in the decompensation of patients with critical AS. This therapy, however, has not been evaluated in a large population of patients. Institution of **IABP should be considered only with invasive hemodynamic monitoring** instruments in place.

    b. **Percutaneous aortic balloon valvuloplasty (PABV)** has not proved to be a definitive therapy for acquired AS, but it does have a role in **pediatric congenital AS.** Although this technique initially carried great promise for improving survival among patients with symptomatic AS, it has not proved to be effective compared with surgical therapy. PABV typically results in 50% improvement in aortic valve area after the procedure; after 6 months, however, nearly 50% of patients have recurrent AS. For this reason, PABV is used in selected cases only. This is a useful technique for **patients who are not candidates for surgical treatment because of comorbidities or advanced age** or perhaps as a bridge to nonelective surgical treatment. The procedure is associated with a mortality rate of 2% to 5%. Patients who are not candidates for surgical treatment because of a concurrent curable illness may undergo PABV to allow definitive therapy for the other illness with the intent to perform elective aortic valve replacement later. PABV also may be considered to treat patients with severe LV systolic dysfunction as a trial to identify patients who may benefit from aortic valve replacement.

4. **Surgical therapy. Replacement** of the aortic valve usually is preferred **over repair** because débridement of aortic valve calcification has been found to result in early postoperative regurgitation from leaflet fibrosis and retraction, which progresses over time. For patients with **AS and noncalcified valves,** however, **repair may be possible.** Surgical mortality rates range from 2% to 3% among patients with pure AS without CAD or other significant comorbid conditions. Ten-year survival rates of 85% have been reported among these patients. The type of aortic valve prosthesis used depends on many factors, including the patient's age, risk of anticoagulation, anatomic features, ventricular function, activity level, and fear of reoperation. Surgical options include pulmonary valve autograft (Ross procedure), aortic valve homograft conduit, a pericardial or porcine bioprosthesis, or a mechanical valve. The relative advantages, disadvantages, and indications for use of the different prostheses are outlined in Chapter 18. The indications for surgical treatment are outlined in Table 14-2.

    a. **Valve replacement procedures**

        (1) **Ross procedure.** The pulmonary valve and main pulmonary artery are removed as a unit and placed in the aortic position with reimplantation of the coronary arteries. A pulmonary homograft is placed in the pulmonic position as a miniature

Table 14-2. Indications for surgical treatment of patients with severe aortic stenosis

PATIENTS WITH SYMPTOMS

Angina
Syncope
Heart failure

PATIENTS WITHOUT SYMPTOMS

Young age and >100 mm Hg gradient
Need for high-risk operation
Severe coronary atherosclerosis that necessitates coronary artery bypass grafting
Left ventricular systolic dysfunction

root. Pulmonary valve autografts have very good hemodynamic function, do not necessitate anticoagulation, and have less long-term calcification than other tissue valves. The procedure, however, is long and technically demanding and results in two valves with potential for postoperative dysfunction. This procedure is best suited for **pediatric and adolescent patients with growth potential, because the autograft is capable of growth.** Long-term follow-up data are not available for a large population of patients who have undergone this procedure. Some surgeons have abandoned this procedure because of concerns about aortic valve regurgitation and late pulmonic insufficiency and stenosis.

(2) **Homografts.** Aortic valve homografts are being used commonly to treat younger patients. Like autografts, homografts in the aortic position have good hemodynamic function, and do not necessitate anticoagulation. These valves, however, do not grow with the patient and tend to become calcified over time and develop regurgitation. The procedure itself is technically difficult, because it usually is performed as a miniroot replacement that necessitates reimplantation of the coronary arteries. It is less complex, however, than the Ross procedure. The useful life of a homograft has been estimated to be about 15 years. This procedure has the lowest rate of reinfection when performed in the setting of endocarditis and is the **procedure of choice for prosthetic valve endocarditis.**

(3) **Bioprostheses** are used most often to treat patients older than 70 years. In 10 years, 80% to 90% of these valves show marked structural deterioration, including stenosis or regurgitation because of leaflet perforation, immobility, or perivalvular leak. These valves do not necessitate anticoagulation, because the risk for thromboembolism is low. Because of the sewing ring and struts, all prostheses have some gradient across them immediately after the operation. This is a greater problem for bioprostheses than for mechanical prostheses. Therefore the largest possible valve should be used to minimize the intrinsic gradient.

(4) **Mechanical valves.** The most commonly used mechanical prostheses today include the St. Jude, Medtronic-Hall, and Carbomedics prostheses. These all necessitate anticoagulation to minimize risk for thromboembolism and valve thrombosis. These valves are **durable if anticoagulation is maintained and careful antibiotic prophylaxis** is used over the years.

b. **Complications.** Potential complications of surgical valve replacement include structural deterioration of the valve, hemodynamic valvular dysfunction, valvular thrombosis, thromboembolism, anticoagulant-related bleeding, prosthetic valve endocarditis, hemolysis, and heart block. Careful anticoagulation for patients who need it and antibiotic prophylaxis in all patients prolong the lives of all prostheses. Patients with low activity levels have less hemodynamic stress on the valve and typically have slower structural deterioration of the valve.

5. **Follow-up care**
   a. Patients **without symptoms** with severe AS should be observed closely and instructed to seek medical attention should any symptoms develop.
   b. After surgical treatment patients usually undergo a **baseline echocardiogram 3 to 4 days to 6 weeks after the operation** to check valve function and baseline gradients. After this point, patients may undergo echocardiography once or twice a year.

     c. A system for **checking the level of anticoagulation** must be in place with **one physician** designated to make all adjustments in dosing of anticoagulants.

I. **Controversies**

  1. **Patients without symptoms.** The role of surgical treatment of patients with severe AS but without symptoms is not clear. As surgical techniques improve and operative mortality declines, the risk-benefit analysis may begin to fall on the side of surgical treatment of patients without symptoms with severe AS and high transvalvular gradients. At this time, surgical therapy generally is reserved for patients with symptoms of angina, syncope, or heart failure. However, patients with asymptomatic severe AS who need high-risk operations, surgery such as repair of an abdominal aortic aneurysm, may benefit from elective replacement of the aortic valve. Consideration also may be given to elective aortic valve replacement in the care of young patients without symptoms who have very high transvalvular gradients.

  2. Treatment of **patients with poor LV function and AS.** Surgical repair improves symptoms for only about 50% of patients with suspected severe AS and severe LV dysfunction with a low transvalvular gradient. The other 50% have no improvement in symptoms or die in the perioperative period. This is partially because a certain percentage of these patients have primary myocardial dysfunction and aortic pseudostenosis caused by a low-output state. For these patients, correction of the AS does not result in marked improvement in LV function.

    a. **Preoperative testing** is performed for these patients to identify true AS with resulting LV dysfunction. Provocative testing with nitroprusside or dobutamine infusion (see **I.G.3** and **I.G.4**) can be used. The goal is to measure the aortic valve area at a higher cardiac output. If there is a **marked increase in cardiac output with little change in transvalvular gradient, the patient is unlikely to have true AS** because the aortic valve area increases with a higher cardiac output. If cardiac output increases and the transvalvular gradient increases, the patient most likely has true AS because the aortic valve area remains fixed with a higher cardiac output.

    b. **Percutaneous aortic valvuloplasty.** Another option is a trial of percutaneous aortic valvuloplasty to see whether the symptoms of heart failure or cardiac output improve. If the patient does not improve considerably with valvuloplasty, the likelihood of improvement after aortic valve replacement may be lower.

J. **Key Suggestions**

  1. For a young patient with a newly diagnosed **bicuspid aortic valve, blood pressure** should be checked in the **upper and lower extremities** to rule out coarctation of the aorta.

  2. **Gradients should never be used alone** to estimate the severity of AS. Poor ventricular function and coexisting MR may cause underestimation of valve stenosis. Coexisting AR may cause higher transvalvular gradients.

  3. **Aggressive medical treatment** of patients with severe AS and ventricular dysfunction may be **dangerous.** Nitrates and diuretics may reduce preload excessively, and vasodilators may cause profound hypotension. Calcium channel blockers and β-blockers may worsen heart failure caused by negative inotropic effects.

  4. As the severity of stenosis increases, **tachycardia** is one means by which cardiac output may be increased; therefore, resting tachycardia in a patient with severe AS may be one of the first signs of low cardiac output.

II. **Aortic regurgitation.**

A. **Introduction.** AR is best classified as being the result of an acute or a chronic process. **Chronic AR** is the result of failure of coaptation of the aortic valve leaflets caused by diseased valve cusps, dilatation of the aortic root, or both. **Acute AR** usually is associated with blunt chest trauma, endocarditis, or aortic dissection and is a surgical emergency in most situations. The regurgitation may be caused by leaflet perforation, prolapse, or acute dilatation of the aortic root, as with aortic dissection.

B. **Clinical presentation**

1. **Signs and symptoms**

   a. **Chronic AR** usually is **asymptomatic for a long time.** When **symptoms do develop,** they are typically related to **pulmonary congestion,** including increased dyspnea with exertion. Later in the course of the disease, patients may experience orthopnea, paroxysmal nocturnal dyspnea, and signs of right heart failure, including anorexia and peripheral edema. **Angina** may develop among patients with severe AR. With the rapid decline of diastolic pressure in the ascending aorta that occurs with severe AR, the driving force for coronary blood flow, which occurs mainly in diastole, is reduced. Late in the course of AR, patients have an elevated LVEDP because of a large regurgitant fraction. This, combined with the low diastolic pressure at the coronary ostia, lowers the pressure gradient across the coronary bed. Patients with coexisting fixed coronary artery obstruction may have dramatic reductions in flow to the myocardium, resulting in typical angina.

   b. **Acute AR.** Patients with acute, severe AR develop **pulmonary edema.** If the AR is caused by endocarditis, the initial degree of regurgitation may be mild. As the infectious process continues, AR may worsen dramatically. These patients should be examined closely every day for signs of AR and heart failure.

2. **Physical findings**

   a. Patients with **chronic AR** typically **do not have symptoms until late in the disease process** when significant LV dysfunction is present. Because patients often have no symptoms, AR usually is **first found at physical examination** as a decrescendo and blowing diastolic murmur at the left sternal border when the patient is sitting in the upright position. A careful review of systems and a detailed history of the patient's exercise capacity help to define the symptom status of a patient with AR. Careful examination for AR should be performed for patients with Marfan syndrome or an ascending aortic aneurysm.

   b. **Severe, acute AR constitutes a surgical emergency.** Any patient with new AR and chest pain should be considered to have aortic dissection until proved otherwise. Patients with blunt trauma to the chest should be examined for AR. A history or presentation consistent with bacterial endocarditis should prompt the physician to rule out AR and other valvular lesions.

   c. **General examination**

      (1) One should examine for **marfanoid characteristics among young patients** with AR, including ectopia lentis, a high arched palate, pectus deformity, and arachnodactyly.

      (2) Peripheral **signs of bacterial endocarditis** may accompany AR caused by infectious valvular destruction.

      (3) Inspection of the **precordium** for visible LV heave or prominent apical impulse is helpful.

      (4) **Blood pressure** is normal early in the course of AR. As the LV chamber enlarges and AR worsens, pulse pressure widens and causes hyperdynamic circulation with an elevated systolic pressure and an abnormally low diastolic pressure. Several physical findings related to this hyperdynamic state are outlined in Table 14-3. As heart failure progresses, there may be peripheral vasoconstriction with elevation of diastolic blood

Table 14-3. Physical findings in aortic regurgitation

Sign	Physical finding
Musset's sign	Head bobbing with each heartbeat
Müller's sign	Systolic pulsation of the uvula
Hill's sign	Popliteal cuff pressure more than 60 mm Hg above brachial cuff pressure
Corrigan's pulse (water-hammer pulse)	Rapid distention and collapse of arterial pulse
Quincke's pulse	Capillary pulsation visible in the fingernail beds or lip
Duroziez's sign	To-and-fro murmur over the femoral artery with the artery compressed
Traube's sign (pistol-shot sounds)	Prominent systolic and diastolic sounds over the femoral arteries

pressure. Systolic blood pressure may fall because of severe systolic dysfunction. Pulsus paradoxus may be present among patients with AR because of aortic dissection and coexisting pericardial effusion.

    d. Arterial examination. Careful attention to arterial pulse intensity and duration helps to establish the severity of AR. The classic pulse is described as a water-hammer pulse, or Corrigan's pulse, with rapid distention and collapse of the pulse. A bifid pulse, or pulsus bisferiens, may be appreciated in the brachial or femoral arteries when both AS and AR are present.

    e. Palpation. With severe AR, the apical impulse is typically enlarged and displaced lateral to the midclavicular line in the fifth intercostal space because of LV enlargement. The impulse may be sustained and hyperdynamic. A triple impulse typically represents a palpable, rapid, filling spike, or S_3, in addition to a palpable a wave. A diastolic thrill may be palpable in the second left intercostal space, as may a systolic thrill caused by increased aortic flow.

    f. Auscultation. The main auscultatory findings are outlined in Fig. 14-7.

        (1) Diastolic murmur. The hallmark murmur of AR is a blowing, diastolic, decrescendo murmur best heard in the left upper sternal border with the patient sitting up and leaning forward slightly in full expiration. The murmur starts immediately after A_2. In general, the severity of AR is related more closely to the duration of the murmur than to its intensity. Early in the course of disease, the murmur is typically short. As the disease progresses the murmur may become pandiastolic. In the end stages of AR, the murmur may shorten again because of rapid equilibration of pressures in the aorta and left ventricle from an elevated LVEDP. In this situation, other signs of severe AR usually are present.

        (2) A systolic murmur heard at the base of the heart that radiates to the carotid arteries may be present because of the increased antegrade flow across the aortic valve.

        (3) A second diastolic murmur may be audible at the apex in severe AR. The Austin Flint murmur is a mitral diastolic rumble believed to be caused by vibration of the anterior mitral leaflet struck by the regurgitant jet or by turbulence in the mitral inflow from partial closure of the mitral valve by the regurgitant jet. No effective mitral stenosis is believed to exist

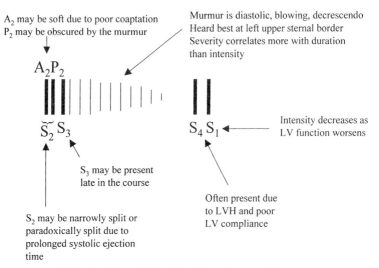

FIG. 14-7. Physical findings in aortic regurgitation.

in this situation; however, coexisting mitral stenosis must be ruled out.

(4) Maneuvers during the physical examination designed to help **define the murmur** are listed in Table 14-4.

(5) **Valve sounds** may be helpful in establishing the severity of regurgitation.

(a) Early in the course of AR, S_1 typically is normal. If severe systolic dysfunction and elevation of LVEDP are present, S_1 may be diminished because of premature closure and decreased force of closure of the mitral valve.

(b) The aortic component of S_2 usually is soft because of poor leaflet coaptation, and the pulmonic component of S_2 may be obscured by the diastolic murmur. If A_2 is audible, S_2 may be narrowly split or paradoxically split because of prolonged LV systolic ejection from increased stroke volume.

(c) S_3 when present suggests poor LV systolic function.

(d) S_4 often is present and represents left atrial contraction into a poorly compliant left ventricle.

C. **Etiology.** Causes of aortic regurgitation are listed in Table 14-5.

D. **Pathophysiology**

1. **Chronic AR** causes volume overload state in the left ventricle that leads to eccentric LV hypertrophy, LV cavity dilatation, and increased LV end-diastolic volume (LVEDV). With the increased LVEDV in com-

Table 14-4. Physical examination maneuvers in aortic regurgitation

Increase murmur	Decrease murmur
Isometric exercise (e.g., handgrip)	Standing from a squatting position
Squatting	Strain of Valsalva maneuver
Inotrope infusion	Inhalation of amyl nitrite

Table 14-5. Causes of aortic regurgitation

Type of abnormality	Acute aortic regurgitation	Chronic aortic regurgitation
Abnormalities of the aortic root resulting in distorted cusp suspension	Aortic dissection Traumatic dissection	Marfan syndrome Aortic aneurysm Annuloaortic ectasia Syphilitic aortitis Systemic lupus erythematosus Pseudoxanthoma elasticum Osteogenesis imperfecta Ehlers-Danlos syndrome Mucopolysaccharidosis Ankylosing spondylitis Reiter's syndrome Giant-cell arteritis Takayasu's arteritis
Abnormalities of the aortic valve cusps	Infectious endocarditis Traumatic leaflet inversion or prolapse	Bicuspid valve Rheumatic heart disease Calcific degeneration Sinus of Valsalva aneurysm Myxomatous degeneration Methysergide therapy Quadricuspid valve Unicuspid valve

pensated AR, overall stroke volume is markedly elevated. The effective forward stroke volume is normal, and the dilated left ventricle can accommodate the regurgitant flow without increasing LVEDP. Patients usually have no symptoms at this time in the disease course.

2. **LV systolic dysfunction** eventually develops in severe AR. As this occurs, there is progressive dilatation and impaired emptying of the left ventricle, which results in a lower LV ejection fraction (LVEF), higher LVEDV, reduced stroke volume, and higher LVEDP. The combined pressure and volume overload of the left ventricle eventually causes concentric and eccentric hypertrophy. Symptoms typically develop at this point.

3. **Acute AR** causes a rapid increase in LVEDV in a ventricle that has not had time to develop compensatory hypertrophy, and LVEDP increases rapidly. LVEDP may exceed the left atrial pressure with resulting premature closure of the mitral valve and diastolic MR. This causes rapid progression to pulmonary edema and necessitates prompt surgical repair. If LVEDP is greater than aortic pressure, premature opening of the aortic valve may occur.

E. **Natural history**

1. Once symptoms develop in a patient with chronic AR, there is relatively **rapid progression and decline in functional status.** Overall **LVEF is the most important** determinant of survival among patients with AR. Patients with AR and normal LV systolic function have a good prognosis; 90% of patients continue to have no symptoms 3 years, 81% 5 years, and 75% 7 years after the diagnosis is made. Patients with mild to moderate AR have reported 10-year survival rates of 85% to 95%. Patients with moderate to severe AR treated with medical therapy have 5-year survival rates of 75% and 10-year survival rates of 50%. Once anginal symptoms develop, the average survival time is 5 years with medical therapy.

2. **Role of therapy.** Survival rates have been improved with the aggressive use of vasodilator therapy including nifedipine, ACE inhibitors, and hydralazine, with improved timing of surgical treatment, with advances in surgical techniques. Although medical therapy may improve survival somewhat, the main effect has been in delaying the need for surgical treatment.

3. **Sudden death** may occur among patients with severe, symptomatic AR. Death may be caused by primary ventricular arrhythmias among patients with LV hypertrophy and ventricular dysfunction, or arrhythmias may be secondary because of myocardial ischemia.

F. **Laboratory testing**

1. The typical **ECG** shows **LV hypertrophy with upright T waves and left atrial abnormality.** The most common arrhythmia is atrial fibrillation; this is more common if there is coexisting mitral valve disease. Because of the proximity of the aortic valve ring, the atrioventricular node, and His's bundle, high-degree heart block can occur if an aortic valve ring abscess forms as a complication of aortic valve endocarditis.

2. **Chest radiography.** Patients with chronic, severe AR may have impressive radiographic findings, including dramatic cardiomegaly termed *cor bovinum*. Left atrial enlargement may be evident. Careful attention should be paid to the ascending aorta, which may be dilated in patients with AR because of aortic abnormalities.

G. **Diagnostic testing**

1. **Echocardiography.** Two-dimensional echocardiography is useful for determining the cause of AR, evaluating the aortic root, and assessing overall LV size and function. Doppler echocardiography is useful for detecting AR and estimating severity. There are several different methods of estimating the severity of AR with color Doppler, pulsed wave Doppler, and continuous wave Doppler ultrasound.

a. **Echocardiographic techniques**

(1) **Parasternal long-axis view**

(a) **The anatomic basis for the presence of AR may be established** in this view. Prolapse of the aortic valve cusps should by carefully sought. Reversed doming of the anterior mitral leaflet generally indicates grade 3+ to 4+ AR and is caused by the impact of the regurgitant flow on the leaflet. This may be caused by a very broad jet with severe AR or an eccentric posteriorly directed jet from prolapse of the right coronary cusp or the anterior cusp of a bicuspid valve. Overall systolic function should be documented.

(b) **M-mode echocardiography** through the LVOT and left atrium is useful for assessing aortic valve leaflet excursion or prolapse and for establishing the presence of left atrial enlargement. Typically the LV cavity is large, and the left ventricle is hypertrophied and hyperdynamic. An end-systolic LV internal diameter of 55 mm or more is an indication for aortic valve replacement or repair. M-mode imaging through the mitral leaflets is helpful for establishing the presence of mitral valve fluttering and preclosure.

(c) In the parasternal long axis, the **transducer should be moved up one interspace to assess the ascending aorta.** Measurements of the diameter may be made with M-mode echocardiography in this position or on line with two-dimensional images. Measurements should be taken at the aortic valve annulus, sinuses of Valsalva, sinotubular junction, and the ascending aorta.

      (d) Continuous and pulsed wave Doppler data are not obtained in the parasternal windows. **Color Doppler** imaging may confirm the presence of AR.

(2) **Parasternal short-axis view.** The aortic valve should be examined during both systole and diastole. The number of commissures and the shape of the valve orifice should be assessed as described in **I.G.1.a(2)** and Fig. 14-2.

(3) **Apical two- and four-chamber views.** Pulsed wave Doppler echocardiography of the mitral inflow typically reveals impaired early diastolic filling caused by LV hypertrophy. Deceleration time usually is less than 200 msec with severe AR. In the end stages, when markedly elevated LV diastolic pressures are invariably present, there may be pseudonormalization of the mitral inflow pattern. Pulmonary venous systolic flows usually are blunted in the later stages of AR.

(4) **Apical five-chamber view.** Aortic valve motion can be assessed in this view. Color flow Doppler imaging is useful in this view for detecting AR and flow acceleration of the regurgitant jet. Continuous wave Doppler recordings across the aortic valve are obtained in this view.

(5) The **apical long-axis view** is good for establishing the presence of AR with color Doppler imaging, but the severity of AR usually is overestimated with color Doppler from the apical views. Continuous wave Doppler can be performed in this view if the alignment is adequate.

(6) **Suprasternal notch and subcostal views.** Attempts should be made to image the aortic arch and descending thoracic aorta from the sternal notch and the abdominal aorta from the subcostal view. The diameters of the aortic arch and abdominal aorta should be measured if the images are adequate.

b. **Estimating AR severity.** The severity of AR may be estimated with color Doppler and continuous wave Doppler. Several methods are presented in Table 14-6. **None of these methods is accepted as the standard** for assessing AR. There may be tremendous variability in the Doppler measurements; they are affected by LV compliance, aortic compliance, and changes in systemic vascular resistance. The **goal** of echocardiographic examination of a patient with AR is to use each parameter to **derive an overall estimation of severity.** If the degree of AR is either mild or severe, there is generally good correlation of severity with each of these techniques. In the moderate range, there may be discrepancy between the different markers of severity, and the clinical presentation becomes important.

(1) **Color Doppler echocardiography**

      (a) **Jet height to LVOT height ratio** represents the percentage of LVOT diameter occupied by the regurgitant jet. This is easily calculated with color Doppler or color Doppler M-mode images through the LVOT at the junction of the LVOT and aortic annulus.

      (b) **Jet area to LVOT area ratio.** The regurgitant jet cross-sectional area relative to the LVOT cross-sectional area may be used to estimate the severity of AR. Two-dimensional images with color Doppler ultrasound at the base of the aortic valve are obtained, and the areas are traced on line.

      (c) If **proximal flow convergence** is seen in the ascending aorta, the AR usually is 3+ or 4+.

      (d) The **depth of penetration of the AR jet into the LV cavity and regurgitant jet area** have been used to esti-

Table 14-6. Echocardiographic grading of aortic regurgitation

degree of AR	AR jet height/ LVOT height (%)	AR jet area/ LVOT area (%)	Continuous wave Doppler spectral tracing intensity	Pressure half-time (m/sec)	Continuous wave Doppler slope (m/sec)
Mild (1+)	<25	<4	Faint, incomplete tracing	≥400	≤2
Moderate (2+)	25–45	4–25	Faint, complete tracing	300–400	2–3
Moderate to severe (3+)	46–64	25–59	Complete, less intense than antegrade flow	300–400	2–3
Severe (4+)	≥65	≥60	Same intensity as antegrade flow	≤300	≥3

AR, Aortic regurgitation, *LVOT*, left ventricular outflow tract.

mate severity; these findings vary greatly, however, depending on loading conditions and the direction of the jet. The AR jet often merges with the mitral inflow jet to give the impression of more severe AR than is actually present. Even with these imperfections, mild AR in general does not penetrate deeply into the LV cavity; severe AR does.

(2) Continuous wave Doppler techniques

   (a) Relative intensity. The continuous wave spectral tracing of the regurgitant jet is useful for characterizing the severity of AR. Comparing the intensity of the regurgitant jet relative to the antegrade flow is one method. This grading method is outlined in Table 14-6.

   (b) Slope and pressure half-time. The slope of the continuous wave spectral tracing correlates with the severity of AR. The slope is measured by means of placing one cursor at the peak velocity of the continuous wave spectral tracing and placing a second cursor at end diastole. The pressure half-time represents the **time it takes the pressure differential between the aorta and left ventricle cavity to decrease by one-half of its initial peak.** It usually is calculated by the software program in the ultrasound machine when the slope is measured. In general, a steeper slope and shorter half-time correspond to more severe AR. If LV pressures are high or if there is a large regurgitant volume, the aortic and LV pressures equilibrate more rapidly, resulting in a brief but steeply sloped regurgitant jet tracing (see Table 14-6).

   (c) Diastolic flow reversal. Continuous wave Doppler echocardiography should be performed in the proximal descending aorta to establish the presence of diastolic flow reversal. If there is reversal of flow in this area throughout diastole, AR is severe.

 c. Hemodynamic calculations. Estimation of the regurgitant fraction may be calculated by means of comparing flow across the pulmonic valve with antegrade flow across the aortic valve. The flow across the pulmonic valve equals the forward cardiac output in the steady state in the absence of intracardiac shunts.

$$\text{Regurgitant fraction} \times 100 = \frac{Qa - Qp}{Qa}$$

where Qa is LVOT$vti \times (0.785 \times Da)$; vti is velocity time integral; Da is diameter of LVOT measured at base of aortic valve; Qp is RVOT$vti \times (0.785 \times Dp)$; Dp is the diameter of the RVOT measured at base of pulmonary valve; and RVOT is right ventricular outflow tract. The echocardiographic features of severe, chronic AR are summarized in Table 14-7.

2. **Transesophageal echocardiography (TEE)**

   a. TEE is most useful to patients who may have **bacterial endo-carditis** to rule out vegetation or aortic valve ring abscess. In pure AR, vegetation typically occurs on the LV side of the aortic valve. Infectious endocarditis usually involves the leaflets and may involve supporting aortic root structures. Acute or rapidly progressive AR may occur with endocarditis because of cusp perforation or disruption of valve suspension.

   b. TEE also is used to assess the **cause of AR** with two-dimensional imaging. With the improved resolution over transthoracic echocardiography, TEE may be helpful in determining the presence of a congenital valvular abnormality and in excluding aortic dissection.

3. **Stress echocardiography** is useful for assessing LV response to exercise. Patients with normal LVEF at rest but who do not have improvement in LV function with stress are believed to have occult LV systolic dysfunction. These patients will likely benefit from aortic valve replacement or repair.

4. **Radionuclide imaging.** Multiple-gated acquisition (MUGA) imaging may be used to assess LVEF and to calculate regurgitant fraction and volume.

5. **Cardiac catheterizationn**

   a. **Men older than 40 years with severe AR and women older than 50 years with severe AR** should undergo coronary cineangiography before any definitive surgical procedure to rule out coexisting CAD. The decision to perform cardiac catheterization on younger patients should be made on an individual basis by taking the patient's risk factors into consideration.

   b. **Catheterization technique**

      (1) A **right heart** catheterization may be helpful in certain circumstances such as new-onset heart failure or combined AR and AS. Coronary cineangiography may be performed in the usual manner with a few special considerations. Catheter manipulation in patients with AR may be difficult because of dilatation of

Table 14-7. Echocardiographic features of severe, chronic aortic regurgitation

Jet diameter/LVOT diameter ≥ 65%
Jet area/LVOT area ≥ 60%
Continuous wave Doppler slope ≥ 3 m/sec
Pressure half-time ≤ 300 m/sec
Pandiastolic flow reversal in the proximal descending aorta
Proximal flow acceleration of aortic regurgitation jet by color Doppler
CW Doppler of aortic regurgitation jet same density as antegrade flow
Restricted mitral inflow pattern
Regurgitant fraction > 50%
Regurgitant volume > 60 mL
Left ventricular internal diameter (diastole) > 6.5 cm

LVOT, left ventricular outflow tract.

the ascending aorta. Among some patients with Marfan syndrome or cystic medial necrosis particularly, the aortic wall may be very thin. **Extreme caution should be exercised when manipulating catheters** to minimize the risk for trauma to the aorta. In addition to difficulty in engaging the coronary ostia, some patients with chronic severe aortitis may have ostial stenoses. Pressure waveforms should be carefully observed for any signs of damping with selective engagement.

   (2) **Aortography.** In addition to conventional coronary cineangiography, **cardiac catheterization of patients with AR should include aortography** to evaluate the degree of regurgitation. This usually is performed in the left anterior oblique cranial projection with the tip of the pigtail catheter about 1 cm above the aortic valve. The size of the aortic root should help guide the amount of contrast agent to use. The grading of AR at angiography is shown in Table 14-8.

c. **Hemodynamic findings**

   (1) Patients with chronic, compensated AR may have an **elevated aortic systolic pressure and depressed aortic diastolic pressure.** Right heart pressure measurements usually are normal. LVEDP is elevated in patients with severe AR. Patients with severe AR eventually have elevated PCWP and pulmonary arterial pressure depending on the degree of heart failure and other comorbid conditions.

   (2) Some attempt at **measurement of a gradient across the aortic valve** should be made to rule out coexisting AS. If a gradient is detected, formal evaluation may be helpful.

H. **Therapy**

1. **Priorities of therapy.** The priorities in the care of a patient with AR are to **establish the cause, ensure that the patient's condition is hemodynamically stable, and determine the need for and timing of surgical intervention.** The method of achieving this differs depending on whether the patient has acute AR, chronic decompensated AR, or chronic compensated AR. **Surgical treatment is definitive therapy** for acute, severe AR of any cause, particularly if the patient has heart failure. Indications for surgical management of AR are outlined in Table 14-9.

2. **Medical therapy**
   a. **Chronic AR**
      (1) **Antibiotic prophylaxis.** Once the diagnosis of AR is made, all patients must be instructed on the use of antibiotic prophylaxis (see Chapter 51).
      (2) The primary **goal** of medical therapy for AR is to **slow the progression of LV systolic dysfunction.** The mainstays of therapy for chronic AR are vasodilators and watchful waiting. **Nifedipine,** compared with digoxin, slows the progression of

Table 14-8. Angiographic grading of aortic regurgitation

Degree of aortic regurgitation	Left ventricular opacification	Rate of clearing
Mild (1+)	Faint, incomplete	Rapid
Moderate (2+)	Faint, complete	Rapid
Moderate to severe (3+)	Equal to aortic opacification	Intermediate
Severe (4+)	Greater than aortic opacification	Slow

Table 14-9. Indications for surgical management of aortic regurgitation

Acute aortic regurgitation
Chronic aortic regurgitation with:
  Symptoms of New York Heart Association class II congestive heart failure
  Ejection fraction ≤50%
  End-systolic left ventricular internal diameter ≥55 mm
  Decreased ejection fraction with exercise

LV dysfunction and delays the time to surgical treatment. ACE inhibitors and hydralazine slow the progression of LV dysfunction and delay the time to surgical treatment. Nifedipine may delay the need for an operation about 2 years; however, many patients are wary of using calcium channel blockers. Although ACE inhibitors may be less effective, they are tolerated better. As always, modification of risk factors is important in the treatment of patients with chronic AR.

  b. Acute AR

    (1) β-blockade. If AR is caused by acute aortic dissection and the patient's condition is hemodynamically stable, it is important to institute aggressive β-blockade for blood pressure control. This should be done before starting vasodilators, which may increase shear forces in the aorta if started alone without β-blocker therapy.

    (2) A **surgical evaluation** should be performed **immediately** for a patient ascertained to have AR caused by aortic dissection or chest trauma. The goal of medical therapy in this setting is to maximize forward cardiac output and minimize propagation of aortic dissection if present.

      (a) For critically ill patients the medical goal usually is achieved with **β-blockade and parenteral vasodilators** such as nitroprusside if tolerated. This therapy should be administered only in an intensive care unit with invasive monitoring in place.

      (b) If AR is associated with **endocarditis, antibiotic therapy** should be instituted as soon as all culture specimens are obtained.

      (c) If AR is caused by **endocarditis or trauma,** consideration may be given to **rapid atrial or ventricular pacing,** which shortens the diastolic filling period and may improve cardiac output.

    (3) If the patient is **not critically ill,** consideration may be given to initiation of **oral vasodilators** such as nifedipine, ACE inhibitors, and hydralazine to decrease afterload and improve forward cardiac output.

  3. Percutaneous therapy. Insertion of an IABP in patients with more than moderate AR or in the presence of aortic dissection is **contraindicated.** Patients with combined AS and AR are poor candidates for percutaneous balloon aortic valvuloplasty because the degree of AR is likely to increase after the procedure.

  4. Surgical therapy

    a. The **timing** of surgical intervention is based on several factors, including symptom status and ventricular size and function.

      (1) Most patients with **symptomatic AR,** regardless of ventricular function, benefit from surgical treatment with regard to survival, functional capacity, and overall LV function.

> > **(2) Asymptomatic AR.**
> >
> > > **(a)** Patients without symptoms who have **LV dysfunction at rest** are at high risk for development of symptoms of heart failure within 2 to 3 years and should be considered for **elective surgical intervention.**
> > >
> > > **(b)** Patients without symptoms with **normal LV size and function and normal exercise tolerance** (able to achieve 8 MET on a standard graded exercise test) may be **observed** closely for the development of symptoms of ventricular dysfunction. **Vasodilators** may be used at the patient's preference.
> > >
> > > **(c)** Patients without symptoms with **abnormal exercise tolerance or an increased LV end-systolic dimension** (more than 55 mm) are likely to have LV dysfunction soon and should be referred for **elective surgical repair.**
> >
> > **b.** The **surgical alternatives** are discussed in **I.H.4.**
> >
> > **c.** Many patients with **prolapse of bicuspid or tricuspid valves** as the cause of AR may be candidates for **surgical repair of the aortic valve.** Some patients with leaflet perforation caused by infectious endocarditis may be candidates for repair in which a pericardial patch is sewn over the defect.
>
> **5. Follow-up care.** Patients with chronic AR should be observed closely for the development of LV systolic dysfunction. Follow-up evaluation typically is conducted with **serial echocardiography.** Once signs of LV systolic dysfunction are manifest, consideration should be given to surgical therapy even if the patient has no symptoms. Routine postoperative care is appropriate once aortic valve replacement or repair is completed.

I. Controversies. The **timing of surgical treatment of patients** with no or minimal symptoms who have normal LV function is somewhat controversial. The response to exercise in the left ventricle has been used to help determine who may have occult LV systolic dysfunction; however, this criterion is not widely accepted. The feasibility of aortic valve repair as opposed to aortic valve replacement may lead to earlier surgical therapy.

J. Key Suggestions

> **1. Acute, severe AR is generally a surgical emergency.** Signs of congestive heart failure and mitral valve preclosure are ominous in acute AR.
>
> **2.** Valve replacement can be performed without infection of the prosthesis in active endocarditis, even when antibiotics have only recently been started. An **aortic valve homograft** is the preferred prosthesis in the setting of endocarditis.
>
> **3. Aortic dissection** should be suspected in any patient with chest pain and AR.
>
> **4.** If **LV systolic dysfunction** is present for less than 18 months, LV function is likely to improve postoperatively.
>
> **5.** Heart rate usually is **normal until late** in the course of disease, when a low effective stroke volume is compensated with tachycardia to maintain cardiac output.
>
> **6. Rapid atrial or ventricular pacing** may be used as a temporary measure to manage acute AR caused by endocarditis or trauma to improve cardiac output. The diastolic filling phase is shorter at higher heart rates; therefore, there is less time for valvular regurgitation.

SUGGESTED READINGS

References
1. Ross J Jr, Braunwald E. Aortic stenosis. *Circulation* 1968;37 [Suppl V]:V-61–V-67.
2. Otto CM, Burwash IG, Legget ME, et al. Prospective study of asymptomatic valvular aortic stenosis: clini-cal, echocardiographic, and exercise predictors of outcome. *Circulation* 1997;95:2262–2270.

Landmark Articles
Borer JS, Hochreiter C, Herrold EM, et al. Prediction of indications for valve replacement among asymptomatic or minimally symptomatic patients with chronic aortic regurgitation and normal left ventricular performance. *Circulation* 1998;97:525–534.
Brener SJ, Duffy CI, Thomas JD, Stewert WJ. Progression of aortic stenosis in 394 patients: relation to changes in myocardial and mitral valve dysfunction. *J Am Coll Cardiol* 1995;25:305–310.
Kelly TA, Rothbart RM, Cooper CM, Kaiser DL, Smucker ML, Gibson RS. Comparison of outcome of asymptomatic to symptomatic patients older than 20 years of age with valvular aortic stenosis. *Am J Cardiol* 1988;61:123–130.
Pellikka PA, Nishimura RA, Bailey KR, Tajik AJ. The natural history of adults with asymptomatic, hemodynamically significant aortic stenosis. *J Am Coll Cardiol* 1990;15:1012–1017.

Key Reviews
Braunwald E. On the natural history of severe aortic stenosis [Editorial]. *J Am Coll Cardiol* 1990;15:1018–1020.
Carabello BA. Timing of valve replacement in aortic stenosis: moving closer to perfection [Editorial]. *Circulation* 1997;95:2241–2243.
Carabello BA, Crawford FA. Valvular heart disease. *N Engl J Med* 1997;337:32–41.
Gaasch WH, Sundaram M, Meyer TE. Managing asymptomatic patients with chronic aortic regurgitation. *Chest* 1997;111:1702–1709.

Relevant Book Chapters
Carabello BA, Stewart WJ, Crawford FA. Aortic valve disease. In: Topol EJ, ed. *Comprehensive cardiovascular medicine.* Philadelphia: Lippincott–Raven, 1998: 563–585.
Donovan CL, Starling MR. Role of echocardiography in the timing of surgical intervention for chronic mitral and aortic regurgitation. In: Otto CM, ed. *The practice of clinical echocardiography.* Philadelphia: WB Saunders, 1997:327–354.
Otto CM. Aortic stenosis: echocardiographic evaluation of disease severity, disease progression, and the role of echocardiography in clinical decision making. In: Otto CM, ed. *The practice of clinical echocardiography.* Philadelphia: WB Saunders, 1997: 405–432.
Weyman AE, Griffin BP. Left ventricular outflow tract: the aortic valve, aorta, and subvalvular outflow tract. In: Weyman AE, ed. *Principles and practice of echocardiography,* 2nd ed. Philadelphia: Lea & Febiger, 1994:498–574.

15. MITRAL VALVE DISEASE

Maran Thamilarasan

I. **Introduction**
 A. The mitral valvular apparatus consists of the anterior and posterior leaflets, the mitral annulus, the chordae tendineae, and the papillary muscles.
 B. **Mitral regurgitation (MR)** can occur as a result of malfunction of any of these components.
 C. **Mitral stenosis** usually is valvular and more rarely is caused by fusion of subvalvular components.
II. **Mitral regurgitation**
 A. **Clinical presentation**
  1. **Signs and symptoms**
   a. With **acute, severe de novo MR,** the symptoms are caused by pulmonary congestion. The symptoms include rest dyspnea, orthopnea, and possibly signs of diminished forward flow, including cardiogenic shock.
   b. **Chronic MR** can be **asymptomatic** for years. The most common presentation is an asymptomatic murmur. **When symptoms do develop,** exercise intolerance and exertional dyspnea usually occur first. Orthopnea and paroxysmal nocturnal dyspnea can develop as MR progresses. Fatigue can be caused by diminished forward cardiac output. With development of left ventricular (LV) dysfunction, further symptoms of congestive heart failure (CHF) are manifest. **Long-standing MR** can cause **pulmonary hypertension** with symptoms of right ventricular (RV) failure. Atrial fibrillation can occur as a consequence of left atrial dilatation.
  2. **Physical findings**
   a. **Palpation.** When LV function is preserved, carotid upstrokes are sharp, and the cardiac apical impulse is brisk and hyperdynamic. An early diastolic LV filling wave may be palpable because of the large volume of blood traversing from left atrium to left ventricle. A late systolic thrust may be present in the parasternal location because of systolic expansion of the left atrium (it may be difficult to differentiate this from a RV lift). With the development of LV dilatation, the apical impulse is displaced laterally. An RV heave and palpable P_2 are present if pulmonary hypertension has developed.
   b. **Auscultation.** The main auscultatory findings are summarized in Fig. 15-1. A loud S_4 (not illustrated) sometimes can be heard, particularly with acute MR. An early and short systolic murmur may be heard with acute severe MR and reflects increased left atrial pressure. If left atrial pressure is markedly elevated, the murmur of acute MR may be inaudible.
   c. With advanced LV dysfunction, the typical **findings of pulmonary congestion** may be manifest. If secondary RV dysfunction develops, an elevated jugular venous pulse, hepatomegaly, ascites, and peripheral edema are present.
  3. The **differential diagnosis of** holosystolic **murmurs** includes MR, tricuspid regurgitation, and ventricular septal defect (VSD). All are high pitched, but the murmur of a VSD is often harsh in quality, unlike the blowing murmurs of MR and tricuspid regurgitation.
   a. The murmur of **MR** is best heard in the apical position and often radiates to the axilla (although possibly to the base with anteriorly directed jets); those of tricuspid regurgitation and VSD typically do not.

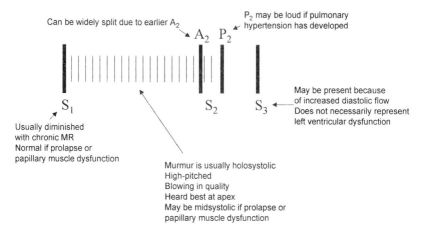

FIG. 15-1. Auscultatory findings in mitral regurgitation.

   b. Tricuspid regurgitation is heard best in the lower left sternal border and radiates to the right of the sternum and left midclavicular line. Tricuspid regurgitation is accentuated by inspiration.

   c. A **VSD** murmur also may be heard in the left sternal border and may radiate over the precordium.

B. Etiology and pathophysiology. MR usually has a myxomatous or ischemic rather than a rheumatic cause. Table 15-1 summarizes the causes of MR.

   1. In **acute MR,** the regurgitant volume that returns from the left atrium causes a **sudden increase in LV end-diastolic volume.** The left ventricle compensates for this by means of the Frank-Starling mechanism: increased sarcomere length (preload) enhances LV contraction (inotropy). This occurs at the cost of increasing LV filling pressure and may cause symptoms of pulmonary congestion. LV wall stress (afterload) is reduced, because blood can be ejected into the lower-pressure left atrium. Increased inotropy and reduced afterload cause more complete LV emptying and hyperdynamic function. Forward cardiac output declines, however, because much of the flow is directed toward the left atrium. If the acute hemodynamic insult is tolerated, the patient's condition **may progress to a chronic compensated state.**

   2. In **chronic compensated MR,** there is **dilatation of the left ventricle with eccentric hypertrophy.**

   a. Wall stress is normalized with the development of hypertrophy. Afterload reduction by the low-resistance left atrium is not as great as it is in the acute phase. Preload remains elevated by the same mechanism as in acute MR. Left atrial dilatation helps to accommodate the increased preload at lower filling pressures. LV function is not as hyperdynamic as in the acute state but is in the high-normal range.

   b. Patients may stay in this asymptomatic or minimally symptomatic phase for years; however, **contractile dysfunction can develop insidiously** during this phase. This may not be apparent with traditional ejection phase indices (such as ejection fraction), which often appear normal because of the effect of increased preload and normal or decreased afterload.

   3. In **chronic decompensated MR,** there is LV dysfunction, along with progressive enlargement of the LV chamber with increased wall stress.

Table 15-1. Causes of mitral regurgitation

LEAFLET ABNORMALITIES

Myxomatous degeneration of leaflets with excessive motion (most common)
Rheumatic disease: scarring and contraction lead to loss of leaflet tissue
Endocarditis: can cause leaflet perforations and retraction in healing phase
Aneurysms: usually from aortic valve endocarditis; aortic insufficiency produces jet
  lesion on mitral valve
Congenital
  Cleft mitral valve: isolated or with ostium primum atrial septal defect
  Double-orifice mitral valve
Hypertrophic cardiomyopathy: systolic anterior motion of the mitral valve

MITRAL ANNULAR ABNORMALITIES

Annular dilatation
  From left ventricular dilatation: dilated cardiomyopathy, ischemic disease,
    hypertension
  Normal 10 cm in circumference
  With sufficient dilatation, loss of adequate leaflet coaptation
  Tethering of leaflet and chordae can occur and produce relative restriction of
    leaflet motion
Mitral annular calcification
  Degenerative disorder, most commonly seen in the elderly
  Accelerated by hypertension or diabetes
  Also seen in renal failure with dystrophic calcification
  Also seen with rheumatic heart disease
  Marfan syndrome, Hurler's syndrome
  Mitral regurgitation results from immobility of the annulus, loss of sphincter
    activity

CHORDAL ABNORMALITIES

Chordal rupture (most severe form is flail leaflet) results in loss of leaflet support
  usually with myxomatous degeneration
Rheumatic heart disease (chordal fibrosis and calcification)

PAPILLARY MUSCLE ABNORMALITIES

Rupture with myocardial infarction
  Complete rupture typically not survived
  Partial rupture more typically encountered
Dysfunctional papillary muscle
  Ischemia
    Posteromedial papillary muscle, single blood supply through posterior descend-
      ing artery
    Anterolateral papillary muscle, supplied by left anterior descending artery and
      left circumflex artery
  Infiltrative processes: amyloid, sarcoid
Congenital: malposition, parachute mitral valve

LV dysfunction and enlargement increase the severity of MR, further
contributing to the cycle of decline in LV function. Irreversible LV
contractile dysfunction may be present by the time overt symptoms
develop. Irreversible contractile dysfunction results in postoperative
CHF and increased morbidity and mortality.

  C. **Laboratory examination**
      1. The **electrocardiographic (ECG)** findings are **nonspecific.** Left
          atrial enlargement, LV hypertrophy, and atrial fibrillation can be seen
          at various stages of the disease.

2. **Chest radiography.** Left atrial and LV enlargement can be seen in chronic MR. Interstitial edema and alveolar edema can be seen in acute cases or with LV failure.

D. **Diagnostic testing**

1. **Echocardiography** plays a pivotal role in the evaluation of MR. It is useful in **diagnosing MR and in determining its severity and cause.** MR is given **four grades of severity,** 1+ for mild, 2+ for moderate, 3+ for moderately severe, and 4+ for severe regurgitation.

   a. **Color Doppler** echocardiography allows diagnosis of MR by means of visualization of the regurgitant jet or jets entering the left atrium and allows assessment of severity.

      (1) **Jet length and area** are used in this assessment (Table 15-2). These measurements are **reliable with central jets,** but underestimation of MR can occur with eccentric jets. With such jets or wall-hugging jets, it is common practice to upgrade the estimated severity of MR by at least one grade. The direction of the MR jet also can aid in assessing the cause of MR (see **II.E.2.c**)

         (a) **Caveats**

            (i) MR assessed with **transesophageal echocardiography (TEE).** Patients often receive sedation before TEE, and the sedation can reduce systemic blood pressure (afterload). This can make the MR appear less severe than it is under normal physiologic circumstances.

            (ii) In evaluation of MR in the **intraoperative setting,** there can be fluctuations in afterload and preload.

         (b) Multiple factors, such as hemodynamic considerations, geometric factors (constraints imposed by left atrial wall), and instrumentation, can affect color Doppler measurements. This has led to the development of other measurements to quantify MR.

      (2) **Width of the vena contracta,** which is the narrowest portion of the proximal regurgitant jet, is a **reliable indicator of the severity of MR** (1). A width greater than 0.50 cm suggests severe MR. High-resolution and zoom images must be used for accurate assessment of the vena contracta, or TEE may be needed. There is some tendency for overestimation with use of width of the vena contracta because of limited lateral resolution.

      (3) **Proximal isovelocity surface area.** A relatively recent assessment has been **flow velocity acceleration,** seen with color Doppler echocardiography, on the LV side of the mitral annulus. Acceleration of blood flow occurs proximal to the regurgitant orifice. This occurs in a predictable manner, isovelocity contours forming hemispheric shells. With adjustment of the Nyquist limit (the color Doppler velocity scale) on the echocardiography machine to obtain a measurable radius at the point of aliasing, the velocity and radius of a single shell can be measured. From this, the orifice flow rate and effective

Table 15-2. Color Doppler assessment of severity of mitral regurgitation

Severity of mitral regurgitation	Jet length (cm)	Jet area (% of left atrium area)
Mild	<1.5	<20
Moderate	1.5–2.9	20–40
Moderate to severe	3.0–4.4	—
Severe	>4.4	>40

regurgitant orifice (ERO) area can be calculated (Fig. 15-2). A larger radius is associated with more severe MR.

Regurgitant flow rate $(Q) = 2\pi r^2 V$

where r is the radius of the shell, and V is the aliasing velocity at that shell.

$$ERO = \frac{Q}{Vmr}$$

where Vmr is the maximum velocity of MR as determined with continuous wave Doppler ultrasound.

ERO $\times$ VTImr = Regurgitant volume

where VTImr is the time velocity integral of the regurgitant jet.

The larger the ERO, the more severe is the MR (1 to 10 mm^2 suggests mild MR, 10 to 25 mm^2 moderate MR, 25 to 50 mm^2 moderately severe MR, and more than 50 mm^2 severe MR). **Pitfalls** with this method include the presence of a nonspherical orifice, multiple jets, and geometric constraints to the flow convergence zone with eccentric jets, in which regurgitant flow and ERO are typically overestimated. Angle correction formulas improve reliability of the calculations in the presence of geometric constraints.

b. **Pulsed wave Doppler** ultrasound can be useful in the assessment of the severity of MR, particularly pulmonary venous flow (Fig. 15-3). **Blunting of the systolic component** of pulmonary venous flow in the presence of normal LV function suggests at least moderately severe MR. **Systolic flow reversal** suggests severe MR. Blunted pulmonary venous flow is a less reliable indicator of substantial MR in the setting of atrial fibrillation or severe LV dysfunction because these conditions also can cause systolic blunting.

c. With **pulsed wave Doppler echocardiography of mitral inflow,** stroke volume across the regurgitant mitral valve can be calculated and compared with the stroke volume derived from pulsed wave Doppler imaging across a competent valve (such as the aortic or pulmonary valve). This can provide an **estimate of the regurgitant volume.**

Apical 4-chamber view

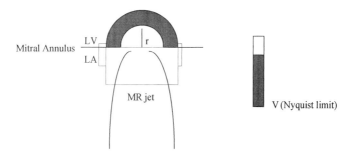

FIG. 15-2. The proximal isovelocity surface area method for determining severity of mitral regurgitation.

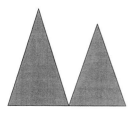
Normal S: D

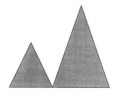
Systolic blunting

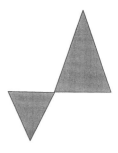
Systolic flow reversal

FIG. 15-3. Patterns of pulmonary venous flow. *First triangle* in each panel represents flow during systole. *Second triangle* represents flow during diastole. The three potential patterns are displayed: normal flow ratio, blunted systolic flow, and reversed systolic flow.

2. Cardiac catheterization

    a. The **amplitude of the v waves** on hemodynamic tracings (which are a reflection of left atrial filling from the pulmonary veins during ventricular systole) can provide clues to the severity of MR, particularly in acute MR.

        (1) Amplitudes of v wave more than two to three times mean left atrial pressure suggest the presence of severe MR. In slowly developing MR, however, an abnormal v wave may not be seen (as the left atrium slowly dilates, it is more compliant toward the increased volume). The v waves also are diminished by means of lowering afterload (which is often the case in the catheterization laboratory, where patients receive sedative agents). When present (particularly with acute MR), v waves can be useful in assessing MR. However, absence of v waves does not exclude severe MR.

        (2) Other conditions that can produce prominent v waves are LV dysfunction with a dilated noncompliant left atrium, postinfarction VSD, and other situations in which there is increased pulmonary blood flow.

    b. **Left ventriculography** allows visual assessment of the severity of MR. The grading system is as follows:

        1+ **(mild)**—clears with each beat; entire left atrium is never opacified

        2+ **(moderate)**—does not clear with one beat; may faintly opacify the entire left atrium

        3+ **(moderate to severe)**—complete opacification of the left atrium, equal in intensity to the left ventricle

        4+ **(severe)**—complete opacification of the left atrium in one beat; contrast material refluxes into the pulmonary veins

    c. Catheterization helps ascertain the **presence of concomitant coronary artery disease** in these patients. Men older than 40 years and women older than 50 years even in the absence of symptoms or risk factors for coronary artery disease should probably undergo coronary angiography before any surgical intervention.

E. Therapy. An understanding of pathophysiologic mechanism of MR is essential to management.

1. **Acute MR**
    a. **Medical therapy.** If there is adequate mean arterial pressure, pharmacologic therapy with afterload-reducing agents may temporize the acute MR. Intravenous nitroprusside and nitroglycerin can reduce pulmonary pressures and maximize forward flow. If an operation is not needed immediately, a change to oral agents can be made. Afterload reducing agents, especially angiotensin-converting enzyme inhibitors and direct-acting vasodilators (such as hydralazine), help to maximize forward output and reduce regurgitant fraction.
    b. **Percutaneous therapy.** The large sudden volume overload on a left ventricle that is not dilated or hypertrophied can cause symptoms of pulmonary congestion and even cardiogenic shock. For such patients with acute hemodynamically significant MR, especially from postinfarction papillary muscle rupture, placement of an intraaortic balloon pump can serve as a temporary stabilizing measure until surgical repair can be undertaken.
    c. **Surgical therapy.** Patients with acute, severe MR often need urgent surgical intervention.
2. **Chronic MR**
    a. **Choosing the appropriate therapy**
        (1) Most patients who have **moderately severe to severe MR** and are **symptomatic** should be considered for elective surgical treatment.
        (2) Treatment of patients with **minimal or no symptoms but severe MR** is more complex. The key is to identify patients before contractile dysfunction of the left ventricle becomes irreversible. Watchful waiting until serious symptoms develop carries risk for development of severe LV dysfunction and a poor prognosis. The feasibility of mitral valve repair with improved postoperative survival and ejection fraction (see later) has been another incentive in the push for earlier surgical intervention. If valve repair is not feasible, one may choose to wait longer before proceeding to surgical treatment.
        (3) A variety of clinical, echocardiographic, and invasively derived values appear to be predictive of the development of postoperative LV dysfunction, CHF, and death among patients with significant MR. Integrating clinical, echocardiographic, and catheterization data can help in determining the timing of a surgical procedure for MR, a decision that must be individualized.
            (a) **Clinical parameters.** Patients older than 75 years, those with concomitant coronary artery disease, or those with renal dysfunction have worse outcomes after surgical treatment (2). Referral for surgical therapy before comorbid conditions become serious may be prudent. The occurrence of **atrial fibrillation** may be a consideration in the recommendation for surgical correction. Atrial fibrillation itself is a potential source of cardiovascular morbidity and appears to correlate with worse outcomes after surgical treatment (2).
            (b) **Echocardiographic parameters** can be useful in ascertaining whether a patient needs a referral for surgical treatment. Given the altered preload and afterload conditions (see **II.C.**), the traditional ejection phase indices should be above normal. Thus an ejection fraction less than 50% (3) implies marked LV contractile dysfunction in the absence of other causes of LV dysfunction). Such patients should be referred for surgical treatment even if no symptoms can be elicited. In one study (3), patients with ejection fractions of 50% to 60% were at increased risk for post-

operative heart failure and excess mortality. Other predictive indices include an LV end-systolic diameter greater than 45 mm (3), LV fractional shortening less than 31% (4), and a ratio of change in pressure to change in time (dp/dt) less than 1,343 (5). The presence or absence of one or more of these parameters can serve as a valuable adjunct in decisions about the timing of surgical treatment.

    (i) When clinical features and resting echocardiographic parameters are equivocal, **exercise echocardiography** can be useful in management decisions. Poor functional capacity may indicate an adaptive response to MR (the patient was not truly asymptomatic) and may influence the decision to proceed with surgical treatment. A decreased response to stress reflects diminished contractile reserve, a sign of latent contractile dysfunction and an indication for surgical intervention. A failure to increase LV ejection fraction with stress is associated with postoperative LV dysfunction. An exercise end-systolic volume index greater than 25 cm^3/m^2 is an excellent predictor of postoperative LV dysfunction (8).

    (ii) The presence of a **flail leaflet implies severe MR** and a large volume overload on the left ventricle. In a study with a 10-year follow-up period (10), all such patients who survived needed surgical treatment. There was a high cardiovascular morbidity and mortality, suggesting that earlier intervention for such patients with severe MR (even with mild or no symptoms) may be indicated.

(c) Similar information can be gained from **invasively derived measurements.**

    (i) Mean pulmonary artery pressure greater than 20 mm Hg (6), cardiac index less than 2 L/min (7), or LV end-diastolic pressure greater than 12 mm Hg (7) have been associated with **poorer outcomes** after surgical treatment.

    (ii) Dynamic exercise in the catheterization laboratory likewise provides useful information in the assessment of MR. Failure of cardiac output to increase appropriately with stress or an increase in pulmonary capillary wedge pressure (PCWP) with stress suggests the presence of occult LV dysfunction.

    (iii) **Elastance** (the slope of the pressure volume relation derived in the catheterization laboratory) is the **best measure of LV contractile function.** Impaired elastance in the setting of normal ejection fraction confirms reversible contractile dysfunction (9), and the patient should be referred for surgical treatment. Although a sensitive measure, elastance is not routinely measured clinically. The measurement requires extensive afterload manipulation with nitroprusside and phenylephrine and the use of special catheters.

b. Medical therapy

    (1) MR caused by LV dysfunction (with annular dilatation) is managed with the agents used to manage heart failure.

        (a) Afterload-reducing agents, particularly angiotensin-converting enzyme inhibitors, minimize regurgitant volumes and maximize forward flow. These agents are also useful in managing MR from primary valvular disease in patients with symptoms who are awaiting surgical treatment.

   (b) **Diuretics and nitrates** can play a role in the management of pulmonary congestion.

   (c) **Ventricular rate–controlling agents and antiarrhythmics** are used for atrial fibrillation. **Digitalis and β-blockers** are the mainstay of therapy for rate control.

   (2) The role of medical therapy for **asymptomatic, chronic MR caused by primary valve disease** is not well established. There is no evidence that pharmacologic agents can delay progression of the disease or prevent ventricular dysfunction. Randomized clinical trials are needed to address this very important question.

   (3) **Endocarditis prophylaxis** is warranted in cases of MR caused by valvular disease. An exception is MR caused by LV dilatation with an otherwise normal valve.

c. **Surgical therapy**

   (1) **Mitral valve replacement** with transection of the subvalvular apparatus once was the only approach used in the surgical management of MR. Postoperative reduction of LV function and CHF were common sequelae. The newer technique of leaving the subvalvular structures intact has been shown to reduce LV volumes and wall stress postoperatively (11). A more ellipsoid ventricular geometry results in improved ejection fraction.

   (2) The increasing success of **mitral valve repair** has greatly reduced the morbidity and mortality associated with severe MR. Five-year survival rates greater than 85% have been reported, and approximately 10% of patients need a reoperation during that time frame (12,13). The increased feasibility of minimally invasive approaches is likely to further reduce morbidity.

   (3) Although no randomized trials have compared repair with replacement, **comparative data suggest better function and survival with repair** (which in part reflects the selection of patients who are able to undergo repair).

      (a) Comparative data suggest a mortality rate in the range of 2% for mitral valve repair compared with 5% to 8% for replacement (depending on the series) (14,15).

      (b) Postoperative ejection fraction is better preserved among patients for whom repair is feasible (16).

      (c) Postoperative risk for thromboembolism is lower among patients undergoing repair (5% incidence of embolic events at 5 to 10 years versus 10% to 35% in the same time frame, depending on series, among those undergoing valve replacement) (12,17). The risk for endocarditis may likewise be lower with repair (0.4% per year versus 2.2%) (14).

      (d) Valves that have been repaired do not need anticoagulation, so the accompanying risks can be avoided.

      (e) The **need for repeat operation appears comparable** between repaired and replaced valves.

      (f) Selected patients with severe LV dysfunction and secondary severe MR have undergone **an LV remodeling procedure with mitral valve repair (the Batista procedure).** Some surgeons advocate mitral valve repair alone for such patients; excellent symptomatic results have been demonstrated in small series (18). The long-term results of these procedures remain to be seen.

(4) Preoperative evaluation helps in assessment of the feasibility of repair, which depends on the cause of MR. The data in Table 15-3 represent the experience at the Cleveland Clinic Foundation for the feasibility of repair according to mechanism of MR (19). The general cause of MR usually is assessed by means of transthoracic echocardiography. However, TEE often is needed to define the mechanism of MR and to help the surgeon plan the repair. When leaflet motion and direction of the color jet are determined, the mechanism of MR can usually be determined. A summary of likely mechanisms according to direction of jet is presented in Table 15-4, as are general methods involved in surgical repair.

(5) Intraoperative echocardiography helps in **assessment of complications** of valve repair or replacement.

   (a) Residual MR is the most common problem after a pump run. If further repair is feasible, a second pump run should be considered to correct residual MR (if 2+ or greater). If further repair is not possible, valve replacement may be needed. A second pump run does not appear to increase in-hospital mortality.

   (b) A postprocedural complication that needs to be sought is development of **dynamic LV outflow obstruction.** This appears to be caused by anterior displacement of the leaflet coaptation point from a redundant posterior leaflet, typically greater than 1.5 cm in height. The result is systolic motion of the mitral leaflet into the outflow tract. This complication typically develops in patients with redundant leaflets and a small, hyperdynamic ventricle. A sliding leaflet technique in which the posterior leaflet is reduced in height reduces the incidence of this complication. When there is severe postoperative dynamic LV outflow obstruction **valve replacement may be necessary.**

Table 15-3. Feasibility of repair of mitral regurgitation at the Cleveland Clinic Foundation

Mechanism causing mitral regurgitation	Repair success rate (%)
Myxomatous degeneration (overall)	75–80
Myxomatous degeneration with posterior chordal rupture	90.9
Myxomatous degeneration with elongated chordae	81.8
Myxomatous degeneration with dilated annulus	67.7
Myxomatous degeneration with anterior chordal rupture	63.3
Myxomatous degeneration with anterior and posterior chordal rupture	40.7
Ischemic mitral regurgitation	65–70
Congenital abnormality	50–55
Rheumatic mitral regurgitation	45–50
Endocarditis	45–50

From ref. 19, with permission.

Table 15-4. Mechanisms, direction of color jet, and surgical management of mitral regurgitation

Jet direction	Leaflet motion	Likely cause	Surgical method
Anterior	Excessive	Posterior leaflet prolapse	Quadrilateral resection Annuloplasty Chordal shortening Shortening of papillary muscle
	Restricted	Anterior leaflet restriction	Débridement
Posterior	Excessive	Anterior leaflet prolapse	Chordal transfer or shortening Posterior leaflet resection to move coaptation apically
	Restricted	Posterior leaflet restriction	Débridement, annuloplasty
	Normal	Ventricular dilatation	Annuloplasty
Central	Excessive	Bileaflet prolapse	Resection, chordal transfer
	Restricted	Bileaflet restriction	Débridement
	Normal	Ventricular dilatation	Annuloplasty
Commissural		Papillary muscle dysfunction	Reattach or fold papillary muscle
Eccentric		Perforation or cleft	Pericardial patch

(From, Stewart WJ. Intraoperative Echocardiography. In Topol EJ, 1998. With permission.)

  d. **Postsurgical follow-up care**
    (1) **Baseline echocardiography** should be performed postoperatively. This is ideally done 4 to 6 weeks after the operation but for the sake of convenience is often done before hospital discharge (within 3 to 4 days).
    (2) **MR can recur** because of failure of the repair or because of progression of the disease that caused MR. Patients should undergo clinical evaluations at least once a year. **Follow-up echocardiography** 1 year after the operation to assess the repair and LV function is reasonable. Starting 5 years after the repair, yearly echocardiograms are obtained. If MR is detected at physical examination, the studies should be performed sooner to define the mechanism and to assess severity. Follow-up echocardiography can be useful to assess symptoms of heart failure, thromboembolism, and suspected endocarditis. Periodic echocardiographic follow-up studies of prosthetic valves is recommended (see Chapter 18).
F. **Controversies**
  1. The **role of afterload reduction therapy** in the care of patients with asymptomatic isolated MR and preserved LV function has not been clearly defined. Reducing regurgitant fraction and the volume overload on the left ventricle would be appear to be beneficial, but there is **no evidence to date that afterload agents can delay the progression of**

the disease or improve postoperative LV function. Aggressive afterload reduction therapy may mask symptoms, perhaps leading to inappropriate deferral of definitive surgical repair.

2. An increasing body of information suggests that an early valve operation, particularly repair, is beneficial to patients with severe MR. However, early referral for surgical treatment among patients without symptoms remains controversial.

III. Mitral valve prolapse

A. Clinical presentation. Mitral valve prolapse is also known as the systolic click murmur syndrome, myxomatous mitral valve, floppy valve syndrome, redundant cusp syndrome, and Barlow's syndrome. Prolapse exists when the mitral leaflets protrude into the left atrium during systole and the coaptation point of the leaflets becomes superior to the plane of the annulus. A wide spectrum of pathologic changes and clinical symptoms occur, from mild degrees of prolapse diagnosed with echocardiography only to clinically evident severe MR. Mitral valve prolapse is the most common form of valvular heart disease in the United States. It affects 3% to 5% of the population with a 2 to 1 female preponderance (20).

1. **Signs and symptoms**

   a. Most patients with mitral valve prolapse have **no symptoms,** and the diagnosis is made by means of routine examination or echocardiography performed for other indications.

   b. Symptoms that do occur include **chest pain** atypical of angina. Abnormal tension on the papillary muscles and autonomic dysfunction have been postulated as mechanisms for the chest discomfort.

   c. Other symptoms include palpitations, easy fatigability, and postural lightheadedness.

   d. A variety of arrhythmias have been reported with mitral valve prolapse. These include **supraventricular tachyarrhythmias, ventricular tachyarrhythmias, and bradyarrhythmias.** There is thought to be an increased incidence of accessory bypass tracks in patients with prolapse. Sudden death has been reported, especially among patients with severe MR or markedly abnormal leaflets.

   e. Transient ischemic attacks have been reported with this syndrome and are thought to be caused by platelet-fibrin emboli from the valve surface (21).

   f. Some authors have reported an increased incidence of anxiety disorders among patients with prolapse, but this finding has not been substantiated.

   g. If prolapse causes MR, symptoms referable to the valvular insufficiency are present.

2. **Physical findings**

   a. Inspection. There is a higher than expected incidence of pectus excavatum among patients with mitral valve prolapse. Straight back and scoliosis also are found. Patients often have low body weight and relative hypotension.

   b. The main **auscultatory** findings are summarized in Fig. 15-4. The **midsystolic click** is the classic finding in prolapse. A systolic murmur is heard if MR is present.

   c. Dynamic changes are elicited by **conditions that decrease LV size** (decreased venous return, increased contractility, or decreased systemic volume), which lead to earlier occurrence of prolapse, an earlier click, and increased duration of the murmur. These conditions include standing, the Valsalva maneuver, dehydration, and exposure to amyl nitrite.

   d. Maneuvers that **increase LV size** by increasing venous return, decreasing contractility, or increasing systemic volume) move the click and murmur later into systole. Examples include squatting and infusion of phenylephrine. The presence of a **click that**

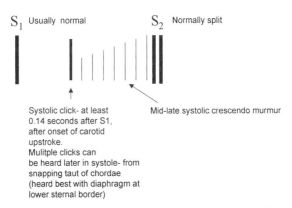

FIG. 15-4. Auscultatory findings in mitral valve prolapse.

responds to provocative maneuvers is **sufficient for the diagnosis of prolapse,** even if an echocardiogram is not diagnostic (see **III.D.1**).

 e. The **intensity of the murmur typically decreases with conditions that result in a later click and murmur.** An exception is exposure to amyl nitrite, which also reduces LV systolic pressure and the gradient that drives regurgitant flow. As such, the murmur is of lower intensity, although it occurs earlier in systole.

 f. **Aortic and pulmonic ejection sounds can produce systolic clicks.** These occur earlier in systole than the click of mitral prolapse and can be differentiated on the basis of timing in conjunction with the carotid upstroke. Other causes of midsystolic clicks include septal and free wall aneurysms and mobile tumors such as myxoma. Clicks produced by these conditions do not change with maneuvers that alter LV volume.

B. Etiology and pathology. Prolapse can exist as a result of valvular abnormalities, deemed primary prolapse, or can occur in the setting of normal leaflets (secondary prolapse).

 1. **Primary prolapse** results from **myxomatous proliferation of the leaflets.** The middle layer of leaflet, the spongiosa, is unusually prominent. This produces redundant leaflets. The chordae usually are thickened and elongated. The annulus can be dilated.

  a. Primary prolapse can be **hereditary,** transmitted as an autosomal dominant trait with variable penetrance. It can occur in isolation or as part of a syndrome in a variety of connective tissue disorders, such as Marfan syndrome, Ehlers-Danlos syndrome, pseudoxanthoma elasticum, and myotonic dystrophy.

  b. Most **complications** of prolapse, particularly severe MR, are associated with primary prolapse. Men in their sixth decade of life represent the most common demographic group with this presentation of prolapse (22).

 2. In **secondary prolapse,** there is relatively **normal valvular structure.** A disproportion between leaflet size and LV cavity size produces mechanical forces that can lead to prolapse. Younger women are particularly affected by this form of prolapse. It also can occur with atrial septal defect, hyperthyroidism, emphysema, and hypertrophic cardiomyopathy. Normalization of the relative disproportion between leaflet size and cavity size often occurs with aging among women, so incidence decreases with age.

C. Laboratory examination and diagnostic testing
    1. Echocardiography. Prolapse is defined as greater than 2 mm displacement of one or both mitral leaflets into the left atrium during systole in the parasternal or apical long axis views. Caution must be used in making the diagnosis with the apical four-chamber view, because normal valve leaflets may appear to prolapse in this view because of the saddle shape of the mitral annulus. With myxomatous degeneration, increased leaflet thickness (more than 5 mm) and redundant leaflets and chordae are seen. The presence of and severity of MR also can be assessed with echocardiography.
    2. ECG. If there is severe MR, the findings described earlier are present. Otherwise, the ECG usually is normal or has nonspecific ST-T changes.
    3. Chest radiography. Pectus excavatum or scoliosis if present is manifest. If severe MR is present, the typical findings described earlier are seen. Otherwise, the **chest radiograph usually is normal.**
D. Therapy. For most patients, mitral valve prolapse carries a benign prognosis and **periodic clinical follow-up examinations and reassurance** are all that is needed.
    1. Endocarditis prophylaxis is indicated if MR is present or if there are thickened leaflets.
    2. Approximately 10% to 15% of patients, particularly those with redundant and thickened leaflets, eventually have progressive MR (23,24). Chordal rupture is a contributing factor among these patients. **Management of MR** is outlined in II.E.
    3. For patients with a history of **transient ischemic attacks, anticoagulant therapy with aspirin** is indicated.
    4. Palpitations should be evaluated with **ambulatory ECG monitoring.** β-Blockers are useful in the management of premature atrial or ventricular contractions. For other documented rhythm disturbances, antiarrhythmic therapy is used as indicated. Ventricular tachycardia, a rare finding, is an indication for **electrophysiologic testing,** to assess risk for sudden death. Patients with abnormal results of electrophysiologic tests may be considered for **implantation of a defibrillator device.**
IV. Mitral stenosis. Although declining in incidence in the United States, rheumatic mitral stenosis is a worldwide public health concern.
  A. Clinical presentation
    1. Signs and symptoms
      a. There is often a **long asymptomatic course.**
      b. When symptoms do develop, **dyspnea** is common. Predominant symptoms are exertional dyspnea initially, then paroxysmal nocturnal dyspnea and orthopnea, which reflect elevated pulmonary venous pressure.
      c. Precipitating factors can induce or dramatically worsen symptoms by means of generating increased transvalvular gradients and left atrial pressure. **Atrial fibrillation with rapid ventricular response is a classic exacerbating factor** and produces pulmonary edema. Left atrial dilatation is a predisposing factor to the development of atrial fibrillation. Women often first have symptoms with **pregnancy** as a result of increased circulatory volume and flow across the valve.
      d. Hemoptysis can occur and likely represents rupture of small bronchial veins from elevated left atrial pressure.
      e. Hoarseness can occur when the dilated left atrium impinges on the recurrent laryngeal nerve (Ortner's syndrome).
      f. Left atrial dilatation and stasis, particularly in the context of atrial fibrillation (persistent or paroxysmal), can cause thrombus formation and embolic events. **Cerebrovascular events, coronary embolization, and renal emboli and infarction** are all possible sequelae. The malformed valve is predisposed to the development of **endocarditis.**

g. **Fatigue** can be caused by low cardiac output.

h. With long-standing mitral stenosis and elevated pulmonary pressure, symptoms of **RV failure** may develop.

i. Patients with elevated pulmonary pressures may have **angina-like chest pain,** which may reflect increased RV oxygen demand.

2. **Physical findings**

a. **Inspection and palpation.** Patients may have a **malar facial flush.** The jugular venous pulse demonstrates a **prominent *a* wave** if there is elevated pulmonary vascular resistance and the patient is still in sinus rhythm. **Jugular venous pressure is elevated with RV failure.** In advanced cases with low cardiac output, **peripheral cyanosis** occurs. The **carotid upstrokes usually are normal** but can be of low amplitude if there is diminished cardiac output. The **apical impulse is not enlarged or forceful.** A **thrill** may be present in the lateral decubitus position. If there is pulmonary hypertension, a **parasternal RV lift with a palpable P_2 is present.**

b. **Auscultation.** The main auscultatory findings are summarized in Fig. 15-5.

   (1) The **opening snap** is the most characteristic auscultatory hallmark of mitral stenosis. However, as the mitral valve becomes more calcified and immobile, the opening snap may be lost (just as S_1 can become softer). An opening snap also can be heard in other conditions, such as MR, VSD, and tricuspid atresia with atrial septal defect.

   (2) Auscultation after a **brief period of exercise may accentuate the murmur** of mitral stenosis as the increased output and heart rate increase the transvalvular gradient. Administration of amyl nitrate also augments the murmur.

   (3) Concomitant **conditions that result in decreased flow across the valve,** such as CHF, pulmonary hypertension, aortic stenosis, may **obliterate the diastolic murmur.** The presence of a loud S_1 may be the only clue to the presence of mitral stenosis in these cases, particularly if pulmonary hypertension exists.

   (4) Other **conditions that can mimic** the clinical presentation of mitral stenosis include left atrial myxoma and cor triatriatum. The tumor plop of myxoma can be mistaken for an opening snap. The diastolic murmurs can be caused by impedance to

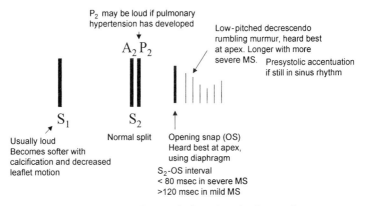

FIG. 15-5. Auscultatory findings in mitral stenosis.

flow. If a patient has a fever and a diastolic rumble is heard, atrial myxoma should be considered strongly in the differential diagnosis. Other conditions in which a diastolic rumble may be present include atrial septal defect or VSD, the Austin-Flint murmur of aortic regurgitation (the murmur lessens with decreased afterload), and tricuspid stenosis (the murmur is heard at the left sternal border and typically increases with inspiration).

B. Etiology

1. Most cases of mitral stenosis are caused by **rheumatic heart disease,** although as many as 50% of patients are not aware of a history of rheumatic fever.

   a. In the **acute phase,** rheumatic fever can cause MR. However, stenosis may develop from 2 years to decades later, although symptoms may not develop for many years thereafter.

   b. **Thickening of leaflets** with **fibrous obliteration** is a characteristic finding. Commissural fusion and chordal fusion and shortening contribute to the development of stenosis. Calcium deposition can occur on leaflets, chordae, and the annulus, further restricting normal valvular function. These changes produce a funnel-shaped mitral valve with a fish-mouth orifice.

2. Other less common causes of mitral stenosis are summarized in Table 15-5.

C. Pathophysiology

1. The normal area of the mitral orifice is 4 to 6 cm^2. When the valve area is less than 2 cm^2, LV inflow is impaired in such a way that a **pressure gradient develops between the left atrium and the left ventricle in diastole.** This gradient and left atrial pressure increases with decreasing orifice area and with increased flow across the valve. The **severity of stenosis is defined by the orifice area** as follows: severe stenosis is associated with a valve area less than 1.0 cm^2, moderate stenosis with a valve area of 1.0 to 1.4 cm^2, and mild stenosis with a valve area 1.4 to 2.0 cm^2.

2. **Increased flow across the valve results in higher gradients in an exponential manner** because the gradient is a function of the square of the flow. Thus exercise and pregnancy (because of increased blood volume) can cause significantly higher left atrial pressures. A decreased diastolic filling period with tachycardia (decreased time for left atrial emptying) also increases gradients and left atrial pressure.

3. The **increased left atrial pressure is transmitted to the pulmonary vasculature** resulting in symptoms of pulmonary congestion. The passive increase in pulmonary venous pressure can elevate pulmonary vascular resistance (reactive pulmonary hypertension). This condition usually is

Table 15-5. Causes of mitral stenosis

Rheumatic: most common cause

Congenital
　Parachute mitral valve: single papillary muscle to which chordae to both leaflets attach; results in mitral stenosis or mitral regurgitation
　Supravalvular mitral ring

Systemic diseases: can cause valvular fibrosis
　Carcinoid
　Systemic lupus erythematosus
　Rheumatoid arthritis
　Mucopolysaccharidosis
　Healed endocarditis

---

reversible if the stenosis is relieved. However, in long-standing, severe mitral stenosis, obliterative changes in pulmonary vasculature may occur.

4. Although the left ventricle is not typically affected by these processes, 25% to 30% of patients have a **depressed ejection fraction.** This appears to result from decreased preload from decreased inflow into the left ventricle.

5. **In severe mitral stenosis,** there may be sufficiently low cardiac output to cause **symptoms of poor perfusion.** Chronically depressed cardiac output causes a reflex increase in systemic vascular resistance and increased afterload. This can further diminish LV performance. Ejection fraction typically returns to normal with correction of mitral stenosis (with restoration of normal preload and then afterload). Some patients may have **persistent myocardial dysfunction** even after correction of stenosis. Smoldering rheumatic myocarditis has been postulated as the cause.

D. **Laboratory examination and diagnostic testing**

1. **Echocardiography** plays a critical role in the evaluation of mitral stenosis.

   a. M-mode findings include dense echoes on the mitral valve and decreased excursion of the mitral valve. **Poor leaflet separation in diastole, anterior motion of the posterior leaflet, and decreased E-F slope on the anterior leaflet** are M-mode hallmarks of mitral stenosis.

   b. **Two-dimensional** findings include restricted motion of the leaflet and diastolic doming of leaflets (hockey-stick sign) (Fig. 15-6). Valvular calcification can also be identified.

   c. **Doppler** echocardiography is **essential** in the assessment of stenosis severity.

      (1) A **transmitral peak velocity** greater than 1 m/sec suggests mitral stenosis. This is not specific, however, because tachycardia, increased inotropy, MR, and VSD can cause increased flow in the absence of mitral stenosis.

      (2) The **transvalvular mean gradient** (assessed by means of tracing mitral inflow) provides an estimate of the severity of

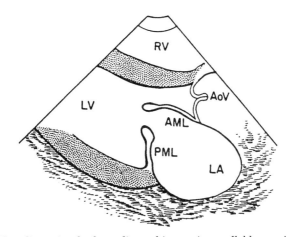

FIG. 15-6. Two-dimensional echocardiographic scan in parallel long-axis view shows findings of mitral stenosis. Doming of leaflets is present. *LV,* Left ventricle; *RV,* right ventricle; *AML,* anterior mitral leaflet; *PML,* posterior mitral leaflet; *LE,* left atrium; *AoV,* aortic valve. (Reprinted from (30), with permission.)

stenosis. A mean gradient less than 5 mm Hg is typical in mild stenosis. Moderate stenosis is associated with a mean gradient between 5 and 12 mm Hg. A gradient higher than 12 mm Hg suggests severe mitral stenosis.

  d. **Echocardiography** is used to estimate **mitral valve area.**
    (1) **Direct planimetry** of the orifice can be performed in the parasternal short axis view.
      (a) **Optimal positioning** is done by first obtaining a parasternal long-axis view and placing the mitral valve orifice in the center of the scan plane. The transducer is then rotated 90 degrees to obtain the short-axis view. Measurements are obtained at the tips of the mitral leaflets.
      (b) **Poor-quality** two-dimensional images and a thick, calcified subvalvular apparatus can make it difficult to obtain accurate measurements. Improper orientation of the scanning plane can produce oblique cuts across the valve and overestimation of valve area. Scanning up and down until the typical fish-mouth appearance is seen helps in this regard. Dense fibrosis or calcification at the margins of the valve orifice can lead to under-estimation of valve area. Low gain settings can cause dropout at the edges of the valve and overestimation of the valve area. High gain settings can lead to underestimation. Planimetry is more difficult if commissurotomy has been performed. Despite the potential problems, planimetry is the preferred method to assess mitral valve area by means of echocardiography.
    (2) **Pressure half-time method.** Impedance to left atrial emptying prolongs the decline in transvalvular pressure gradient. This prolongs pressure half-time (pressure to fall to one-half the starting value), which equates with the time for the velocity to decrease to 70% of peak velocity). The mitral inflow E wave is used in the calculation.
      (a) Empiric pressure half-time has been shown to correlate with valve area (25):

      Mitral valve area (in cm^2) = 220/pressure half-time

      (b) If a software package to perform the calculations is not available, pressure half-time can be found by means of measuring deceleration time and multiplying by 0.29. If diastolic flow is nonlinear, middiastolic flow is used to extrapolate to obtain initial maximal velocity. If atrial fibrillation is present, 5 to 10 consecutive beats are obtained and averaged.
      (c) It is important to have the **Doppler beam parallel to the direction of blood flow.**
      (d) The pressure half-time method **cannot be used if there are rapid changes in left atrial hemodynamics,** such as immediately after balloon valvuloplasty.
      (e) Obtaining a pressure half-time can be very difficult if sinus tachycardia is present (E-A fusion). Aortic insufficiency, which also fills the left ventricle, decreases pressure half-time and leads to overestimation of mitral valve area.

  e. **Stress echocardiography** can be useful in the evaluation of patients with symptoms when the **resting study does not indicate severe mitral stenosis.** Gradients can be assessed during (supine bicycle) or immediately after (treadmill) exercise. Measurement of tricuspid regurgitation velocity, pulmonary insufficiency velocity, or pulmonary flow acceleration time is used to estimate pulmonary pressures with stress.

2. **Cardiac catheterization.** Hemodynamic measurements obtained in a cardiac catheterization laboratory are used to **assess severity of stenosis.** Simultaneous measurement of LV end-diastolic pressure, left atrial pressure (either directly or more commonly with PCWP as a surrogate), cardiac output (Fick method or thermodilution), heart rate, and diastolic filling period (seconds per beat) is required. LV pressure and PCWP (or left atrial pressure) tracings are made simultaneously (Fig. 15-7). A mean transmitral gradient is derived from above (planimeter area between the left ventricle and pulmonary capillary wedge tracings during diastole; this area is multiplied by the scale factor of the tracing in millimeters of mercury per centimeter to obtain the gradient). The PCWP tracing ideally should be realigned by 50 to 70 msec to the left (with tracing paper) to account for the time delay in transmission of left atrial pressure to the pulmonary venous beds.

   a. The **Gorlin formula** is as follows:

$$\text{Area} = \frac{\text{cardiac output/diastolic filling period} \times \text{heart rate}}{3.77 \times \sqrt{(\text{mean transmitral pressure gradient})}}$$

The empirical constant 37.7 was derived by Gorlin. It is the Gorlin constant (44.3) multiplied by 0.85, the correction factor for the mitral valve) (26,27).

   b. A **simplified version of the Gorlin formula** proposed by Hakki et al. (28) has been shown to provide a reasonable approximation of valve area, as follows:

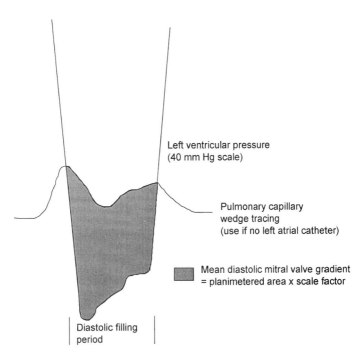

Left ventricular pressure
(40 mm Hg scale)

Pulmonary capillary
wedge tracing
(use if no left atrial catheter)

Mean diastolic mitral valve gradient
= planimetered area x scale factor

Diastolic filling
period

FIG. 15-7. Simultaneous left ventricular and pulmonary capillary wedge pressure tracings used to measure mean gradient across mitral valve during diastole.

$$MVA = \frac{\text{Cardiac Output}}{\sqrt{(\text{mean mitral gradient})}}$$

   c. **Pitfalls. PCWP cannot be used** if the patient has pulmonary venous occlusive disease or cor triatriatum. The catheter must be properly wedged. In addition, **thermodilution cardiac output is less accurate** if there is tricuspid regurgitation or low cardiac output. **Immediately after valvuloplasty** MR or atrial septal defect flow may cause inaccurate estimations of mitral flow.
3. **ECG.** Left atrial enlargement (P-mitrale) is usually present when sinus rhythm persists. Signs of RV hypertrophy are seen with pulmonary hypertension. Atrial fibrillation is common.
4. **Chest radiography.** Left atrial enlargement is apparent with a double density along the right heart border. A convexity can be apparent below the pulmonary artery, representing the left atrial appendage. Elevation of the left main bronchus and posterior displacement of esophagus at barium swallow examination reflect left atrial enlargement. Kerley B lines may be present from increased pulmonary venous pressure. RV enlargement (decreased retrosternal air space on the lateral radiograph) may be present. Evidence of mitral valve calcification may be present. In rare instances evidence of left atrial calcification can be seen.
E. **Therapy**
   1. **Medical therapy**
      a. Patients **without symptoms** need only **endocarditis prophylaxis.**
      b. Patients with only **mild symptoms with exertional dyspnea** can be treated with **diuretics** to lower left atrial pressure. β-**Blockers** blunt the chronotropic response to exercise and may improve exercise capacity. **Arterial vasodilators should be avoided.**
      c. **Atrial fibrillation** can clearly exacerbate symptoms, and **rate control measures** are clearly important to increase diastolic filling time.
         (1) **Digitalis** and β-**blockers** are the preferred agents to achieve rate control.
         (2) **Anticoagulation** with warfarin is imperative for patients with atrial fibrillation and mitral stenosis because they are at risk for thromboembolism. The targeted international normalized ratio in these situations is typically between 2.0 and 3.0.
         (3) **Antiarrhythmic drug therapy** can be used in an attempt to restore sinus rhythm in patients with atrial fibrillation, but long-term efficacy may depend on correction of the mitral stenosis.
   2. **Percutaneous or surgical therapy.** If **more than mild symptoms** (New York Heart Association class 2 or greater) are present, the patient should be **referred for surgical or percutaneous therapy.** Mortality increases once more than mild symptoms develop. Results of natural history studies conducted before valvotomy procedures were developed indicate that young patients have nearly 40% mortality 10 years after diagnosis and almost double that after 20 years. Older patients, who have more symptoms at the time of diagnosis, have 60% to 70% mortality at 10 years (29). Some experts have suggested that the occurrence of **atrial fibrillation** is an indication for surgical treatment or valvuloplasty. Marked **pulmonary hypertension** (pulmonary arterial systolic pressure greater than 55 mm Hg) also is an indication for treatment.
      a. **Percutaneous balloon mitral valvuloplasty** is often the treatment of first choice for mitral stenosis. The technique involves placement of a balloon-tipped catheter into the left atrium through a transseptal puncture and then across the mitral valve. The balloon is inflated and deflated to increasingly larger diameters until the desired result is obtained.

(1) Typically there is an increase in valve area of 1–2 cm², with the primary mechanism for this being splitting of the fused commissures. This procedure is **generally contraindicated in patients with more than mild MR or in whom there is a left atrial or appendage thrombus.**

(2) An **echocardiographic score** has been developed to help select patients who may be candidates for percutaneous valvuloplasty (30). There are four parts to the assessment (mobility, leaflet thickening, subvalvular thickening, and calcification) (Table 15-6). In general, extensive subvalvular disease results in a poorer outcome with valvuloplasty. Patients with extensive fluoroscopically visible mitral valve calcification also have a worse outcome after percutaneous therapy (31).

(a) A total echocardiographic score (adding the four components) **higher than 11** is associated with a poorer outcome and a suboptimal increase in valve area, a higher incidence of heart failure and restenosis, and higher mortality. Patients with high scores **should not undergo valvuloplasty** unless surgical treatment is impossible.

(b) Echocardiographic scores of **9 to 11** represent a **gray zone** in which some patients have good results with valvuloplasty. Others have suboptimal results.

(c) **Optimal** results of balloon valvuloplasty are usually achieved when the echocardiographic score is **8 or less.**

(3) TEE plays a critical role during valvuloplasty. The most immediate concern is to **rule out left atrial and appendage thrombi.** If thrombosis is present, anticoagulation for at least 1 month is undertaken before valvuloplasty. TEE can help to guide balloon positioning; after each inflation, the degree of MR and the gradient can be assessed. The degree of residual mitral

Table 15-6. Echo score assessment for percutaneous valvuloplasty in the management of mitral stenosis

MOBILITY (GRADE 0–4, 0 BEING NORMAL)

1. Highly mobile with only leaflet tips restricted
2. Mild leaflet restriction; base portions have normal mobility
3. Valve moves forward in diastole, mainly from base
4. No or minimal diastolic movement of valve

SUBVALVULAR THICKENING (GRADE 0–4, 0 BEING NORMAL)

1. Minimal thickening below leaflets
2. Chordal thickening up to one-third chordal length
3. Thickening extending to distal one-third of chords
4. Extensive thickening to papillary muscles

THICKENING OF LEAFLETS (GRADE 0–4, 0 BEING NORMAL)

1. Near normal (4–5 mm)
2. Marginal thickening (5–8 mm) with normal thickness of midleaflets
3. Thickening of entire leaflet (5–8 mm)
4. Extensive thickening of all leaflet tissue (>8–10 mm)

CALCIFICATION (GRADE 0–4, 0 BEING NORMAL)

1. Single area of echo brightness
2. Scattered areas of increased brightness along leaflet margins
3. Brightness extending to midportion of leaflets
4. Extensive brightness throughout leaflet tissue

From ref. 30, with permission.

stenosis can be estimated with planimetry of the valve orifice before and after inflation. The pressure half-time method is unreliable (it is inaccurate when hemodynamics change rapidly, such as after valvuloplasty) until 24 to 48 hours after the procedure.

(4) Echocardiography is useful in the determination of immediate **postprocedural complications** (Table 15-7). Among these is MR with an incidence estimated at 3% to 8% depending on series (32). The echocardiographic score is less predictive of the severity of postprocedural MR. **Pre-existent MR is likely to worsen after the procedure.** This is why any more than mild regurgitation (higher than 2+) is a relative contraindication to the procedure. **Injury** to the subvalvular apparatus or leaflets or poor leaflet coaptation can cause MR. If there is only a mild increase in MR, the regurgitant jet likely originates from the commissures. Severe postprocedural MR usually is caused by leaflet tearing or damage to the chordal structures.

(5) The frequency of **restenosis of the valve** ranges from 6% to 21%, depending on series (32,33). Data from the National Heart, Lung, and Blood Institute registry of all functional classes of patients show an 84% survival rate 4 years after treatment (33). Advanced age, high New York Heart Association functional class, presence of atrial fibrillation, lower initial mitral valve area, higher pulmonary arterial pressure, and substantial tricuspid regurgitation are **associated with poorer long-term results.** These variables identify a population with more serious illness that necessitates intervention and should not preclude valvuloplasty.

(6) More postprocedural MR and lower postprocedural mitral valve area are associated with poorer long-term results.

b. **Surgical treatment.** Closed **commissurotomy** was the earliest surgical approach used. This was performed through a thoracotomy (without a cardiopulmonary bypass) and atriotomy with a valve dilator. This procedure has been rarely used in the United States since the development of the percutaneous approach and improvements in open heart surgery. **Open mitral valvotomy** involves direct visualization of the mitral valve (with cardiopulmonary bypass), débridement of calcium, and splitting of fused commissures and chordae. This approach is not used to treat patients who have more than mild MR.

(1) Severe subvalvular disease often leads to the choice of **surgical intervention over valvuloplasty.** Coexistent disease in other valves (e.g., aortic stenosis or aortic regurgitation) that necessitates treatment also leads to the choice of surgical treatment over balloon valvuloplasty. For patients with pulmonary hypertension and secondary severe tricuspid regurgitation (tricuspid regurgitation), valvuloplasty alone and a

---

Table 15-7. Complications of balloon valvuloplasty

Mitral regurgitation
Cardiac perforation: incidence as high as 2%–4%
Embolization: incidence 2% in the National Heart, Lung, and Blood Institute registry
Residual atrial septal defect: most close within 6 mo; can persist long term among as many as 10% of patients; generally small and well tolerated

reduction in pulmonary pressure may not be sufficient to reduce tricuspid regurgitation. This is particularly true among elderly patients. A mitral valve operation with concomitant tricuspid annuloplasty may be the preferred strategy.

   (2) **Mitral valve replacement**

   (a) Mitral valve replacement is often needed, particularly when there is extensive fibrosis and calcification or concomitant MR.

   (b) The choice of **mechanical or bioprosthetic** valve replacement depends on weighing the risk of chronic anticoagulation associated with mechanical valves against the reduced longevity of the bioprosthetic valves. Five-year survival rates of 80% to 85% have been reported among patients undergoing valve replacement (15).

   (3) **Mitral valve repair** is more difficult but can be performed in selected cases. Ten-year survival rates greater than 95% have been reported among patients who have undergone repair (15). The need for reoperation for recurrent stenosis appears to be less than 20% 10 years after the operation (15).

   (4) The **caveats** regarding preservation of the subvalvular apparatus apply to operations on stenotic valves, as they do to operations on regurgitant valves. **Pulmonary hypertension** increases the risk of surgical treatment, but patients fare better with surgical therapy than with continued medical treatment.

   (5) For patients with long-standing **atrial fibrillation,** a combined Maze procedure has been used in conjunction with the valve operation.

   c. **Postprocedural follow-up care.** As with operations for MR, patients who have undergone balloon valvuloplasty or operations for mitral stenosis should undergo **baseline echocardiography. Clinical follow-up examinations** should be performed at least once a year, more often if symptoms develop. It has become common practice at many centers for patients to undergo **follow-up echocardiography on a once a year basis,** although no firm guidelines have been developed for this. Echocardiography is useful when there are symptoms or when clinical examination findings suggest recurrent stenosis or development of MR. Follow-up care of patients with prosthetic valves is discussed in Chapter 18.

F. **Controversies**

   1. The development of **atrial fibrillation has been viewed by some as an indication for surgical or percutaneous treatment,** even in the absence of other symptoms. Those favoring this approach believe that better long-term control of atrial fibrillation and its associated thromboembolic and other risks can be achieved with earlier intervention for mitral stenosis. Additional long-term studies are needed to address the success of such an approach.

   2. There is still some debate over the **role of anticoagulation in mitral stenosis.** Atrial fibrillation is an agreed-upon indication for the initiation of oral anticoagulant therapy. Anticoagulation also has been advocated to manage marked left atrial dilatation. Still others advocate such therapy for all patients with more than mild mitral stenosis, regardless of left atrial size or rhythm. The risk-to-benefit ratio of this approach needs further elucidation.

   3. Although **percutaneous balloon valvuloplasty** has become the treatment of first choice for many patients, long-term (more than 10 years) follow-up data on patients who have undergone this procedure are only now becoming available. Results from additional studies have to be evaluated, as do results of studies that compare percutaneous and open surgical approaches. Two relatively small studies (each with 30 patients

undergoing each treatment) have demonstrated comparable long-term results between the catheter and surgical approaches (34,35). However, in these studies the patients were typically young and had pliable valves that were not heavily calcified. The percutaneous approach may not be as successful among older populations.

SUGGESTED READINGS

References

1. Hall SA, Brickner E, Willett DL, Irani WN, Afridi I, Grayburn PA. Assessment of mitral regurgitation severity by Doppler color flow of the vena contracta. *Circulation* 1997;95:636–642.

2. Enriquez-Sarano M, Tajik AJ, Schaff HV, Orszulak TA, Bailey KR, Frye RL. Echocardiographic prediction of survival after surgical correction of organic mitral regurgitation. *Circulation* 1994;90:830–837.

3. Enriquez-Sarano M, Tajik AJ, Schaff HV, et al. Echocardiographic prediction of left ventricular function after correction of mitral regurgitation: results and clinical implications. *J Am Coll Cardiol* 1994;24:1536–1543.

4. Zik MR, Gaasch WH, Carol JD. Chronic mitral regurgitation: predictive value of pre-operative echocardiographic indexes of left ventricular function and wall stress. *J Am Coll Cardiol* 1984;3:235–242.

5. Pai RG, Bansal RC, Shah PM. Doppler-derived rate of left ventricular pressure rise and its correlation with the postoperative left ventricular function in mitral regurgitation. *Circulation* 1990;82:514–520.

6. Crawford MH, Souchek J, Oprian CA. Determinants of survival and left ventricular performance after mitral valve replacement. *Circulation* 1990;81:1173–1181.

7. Saloman NW, Stinson EB, Griepp RB. Patient-related risk factors as predictors of results following isolated mitral valve replacement. *Ann Thorac Surg* 1977;24: 519–530.

8. Leung DY, Griffin BP, Stewart WJ, Cosgrove DM, Thomas JD, Marwick TH. Left ventricular function after valve repair for chronic mitral regurgitation: predictive value of preoperative assessment of contractile reserve by exercise echocardiography. *J Am Coll Cardiol* 1996;28:1198–1205.

9. Starling MR, Kirsh MM, Montgomery DG, Gross MD. Impaired left ventricular contractile function in patients with long-term mitral regurgitation and normal ejection fraction. *J Am Coll Cardiol* 1993;22:239–250.

10. Ling LH, Enriquez-Sarano M, Seward JB, et al. Clinical outcome of mitral regurgitation due to flail leaflet. *N Engl J Med* 1996;335:1417–1423.

11. Rozich JDE, Carabello BA, Usher BW, Kratz JM, Bell AF, Zile MR. Mitral valve replacement with and without chordal preservation in patients with chronic mitral regurgitation: mechanisms for differences in post-operative ejection performance. *Circulation* 1992;86: 1718–1726.

12. Cohn LH, Couper GS, Aranki SF. Long-term results of mitral valve reconstruction for regurgitation of the myxomatous mitral valve. *J Thorac Cardiovasc Surg* 1994;107:1453–151

13. Cosgrove DM, Stewart WJ. Mitral valve repair. *Curr Probl Cardiol* 1989;14: 359–415.

14. Duran CG, Pomar JL, Revuelta JM. Conservative operation for mitral insufficiency: critical analysis supported by postoperative hemodynamic studies of 72 patients. *J Thorac Cardiovasc Surg* 1980;79:326–337.

15. Alpert JS, Sabik J, Cosgrove DM III. Mitral valve disease. In: Topol EJ, ed. *Textbook of Cardiovascular Medicine*. Philadelphia: Lippincott–Raven, 1998:503–532.

16. Enriquez-Sarano M, Schaff HV, Orszulak TA, Tajik AJ, Bailey KR, Frye RL. Valve repair improves the outcome of surgery for mitral regurgitation: a multivariate analysis. *Circulation* 1995;91:1022–1028.

17. Edmunds LH. Thromboembolic and bleeding complications of prosthetic heart valves. *Ann Thorac Surg* 1987;44:430–445.

18. Bach DS, Bolling SF. Improvement following correction of secondary mitral regurgitation in end-stage cardiomyopathy with mitral annuloplasty. *Am J Cardiol* 1996;78:966–969.

19. Stewart WJ. ACC Heart House Learning Center Highlights. American College of Cardiology, Bethesda, Maryland, 1995;10:2–7.
20. Levy D, Savage DD. Prevalence and clinical features of mitral valve prolapse. *Am Heart J* 1987;113:1281–1290.
21. Barletta GA, Gagliardi R, Benvenuti L, Fantini F. Cerebral ischemic attacks as a complication of aortic and mitral valve prolapse. *Stroke* 1985;16:219–223.
22. Devereax RB, Hawkins I, Kramer-Fox R. Complications of mitral valve prolapse: disproportionate occurrence in men and older patients. *Am J Med* 1986;81:751–758.
23. Wilcken DE, Hickey AJ. Lifetime risk for patients with mitral prolapse of developing severe valve regurgitation requiring surgery. *Circulation* 1988;78:10–14.
24. Zuppiroli A, Rinaldi M, Kramer-Fox R. Natural history of mitral valve prolapse. *Am J Cardiol* 1995;75:1028–1032.
25. Hatle L, Brubakk A, Tronsdal A, Angelsen B. Noninvasive assessment of pressure drop in mitral stenosis by doppler ultrasound. *Br Heart J* 1978;40:131–140.
26. Gorlin R, Gorlin G. Hydraulic formula for calculation of area of stenotic mitral valve, other cardiac values and central circulatory shunts. *Am Heart J* 1951;41:1
27. Cohen MV, Gorlin R. Modified orifice equation for the calculation of mitral valve area. *Am Heart J* 1972;84:839–840.
28. Hakki AM. A simplified valve formula for the calculation of stenotic cardiac valve areas. *Circulation* 1981;63:1050.
29. Olesen KH. The natural history of 271 patients with mitral stenosis under medical treatment. *Br Heart J* 1962;24:349–357.
30. Wilkins GT, Weyman AE, Abascal VM, Block PC, Palacios IM. Percutaneous balloon dilatation of the mitral valve: an analysis of echocardiographic variables related to outcome and the mechanism of dilatation. *Br Heart J* 1988;60:299–308.
31. Tuzcu EM, Block PC, Griffin B, Dinsmore R, Newell JB, Palacios IF. Percutaneous mitral balloon valvotomy in patients with calcific mitral stenosis: immediate and long-term outcome. *J Am Coll Cardiol* 1994;23:1604–1609.
32. Glazier JJ, Turi ZG. Percutaneous balloon mitral valvuloplasty. *Prog Cardiovasc Dis* 1997;40:5–26.
33. Dean LS, Mickel M, Bonan R, et al. Four-year follow-up of patients undergoing percutaneous balloon mitral commissurotomy: a report from the National Heart, Lung, and Blood Institute balloon valvuloplasty registry. *J Am Coll Cardiol* 1996;28:1452–1457.
34. Reyes VP, Raju BS, Wynee J, et al. Percutaneous balloon valvuloplasty compared with open surgical commissurotomy for mitral stenosis. *N Engl J Med* 1994;331:961–967.
35. Farhat MB, Ayari M, Maatouk F, et al. Percutaneous balloon versus surgical closed and open mitral commissurotomy: seven year follow-up results of a randomized trial. *Circulation* 1998;97:245–250.

Landmark Articles

Duran CG, Pomar JL, Revuelta JM. Conservative operation for mitral insufficiency: critical analysis supported by postoperative hemodynamic studies of 72 patients. *J Thorac Cardiovasc Surg* 1980;79:326–337.
Enriquez-Sarano M, Schaff HV, Orszulak TA, Tajik AJ, Bailey KR, Frye RL. Valve repair improves the outcome of surgery for mitral regurgitation: a multivariate analysis. *Circulation* 1995;91:1022–1028.
Enriquez-Sarano M, Tajik AJ, Schaff HV, Orszulak TA, Bailey KR, Frye RL. Echocardiographic prediction of survival after surgical correction of organic mitral regurgitation. *Circulation* 1994;90:830–837.
Enriquez-Sarano M, Tajik AJ, Schaff HV, et al. Echocardiographic prediction of left ventricular function after correction of mitral regurgitation: results and clinical implications. *J Am Coll Cardiol* 1994;24:1536–1543.
Leung DY, Griffin BP, Stewart WJ, Cosgrove DM, Thomas JD, Marwick TH. Left ventricular function after valve repair for chronic mitral regurgitation: predictive value of preoperative assessment of contractile reserve by exercise echocardiography. *J Am Coll Cardiol* 1996;28:1198–1205.

Ling LH, Enriquez-Sarano M, Seward JB, et al. Clinical outcome of mitral regurgitation due to flail leaflet. *N Engl J Med* 1996;335:1417–1423.

Reyes VP, Raju BS, Wynee J, et al. Percutaneous balloon valvuloplasty compared with open surgical commissurotomy for mitral stenosis. *N Engl J Med* 1994;331:961–967.

Wilkins GT, Weyman AE, Abascal VM, Block PC, Palacios IM. Percutaneous balloon dilatation of the mitral valve: an analysis of echocardiographic variables related to outcome and the mechanism of dilatation. *Br Heart J* 1988;60:299–308.

Zuppiroli A, Rinaldi M, Kramer-Fox R. Natural history of mitral valve prolapse. *Am J Cardiol* 1995;75:1028–1032.

Key Reviews

Carabello BA. Mitral valve disease. *Curr Probl Cardiol* 1993;18:426–478.

Carabello BA, Crawford FA. Valvular heart disease. *N Engl J Med* 1997;337:32–41.

Stewart WJ. Choosing the golden moment for mitral valve repair. *J Am Coll Cardiol* 1994;24:1544–1546.

Thomas JD. How leaky is that mitral valve? simplified Doppler methods to measure regurgitant orifice area. *Circulation* 1997;95:548–550.

Relevant Book Chapters

Alpert JS, Sabik J, Cosgrove DM III. Mitral valve disease. In: Topol EJ, ed. *Textbook of cardiovascular medicine.* Philadelphia: Lippincott–Raven, 1998:503–532.

Braunwald E. Valvular heart disease. In: Braunwald E, ed. *Heart disease: a textbook of cardiovascular medicine,* 5th ed. Philadelphia: WB Saunders, 1997:1007–1076.

Carabello B, Grossman W. Calculation of stenotic valve orifice area. In: Baim DS, Grossman W, eds. *Cardiac catheterization, angiography and intervention,* 5th ed. Baltimore: Williams & Wilkins, 1996:151–166.

Donovan CL, Starling MR. Role of echocardiography in the timing of surgical intervention for chronic mitral and aortic regurgitation. In: Otto CM, ed. *The practice of clinical echocardiography.* Philadelphia: WB Saunders, 1997:327–354.

Griffin BP, Stewart WJ. Echocardiography in patient selection, operative planning, and intraoperative evaluation of mitral valve repair. In: Otto CM, ed. *The practice of clinical echocardiography.* Philadelphia: WB Saunders, 1997:355–372.

Grossman W. Profiles in valvular heart disease. In: Baim DS, Grossman W, eds. *Cardiac catheterization, angiography and intervention,* 5th ed. Baltimore: Williams & Wilkins, 1996:735–756.

Reid CL. Echocardiography in the patient undergoing catheter balloon mitral commissurotomy. In: Otto CM, ed. *The practice of clinical echocardiography.* Philadelphia: WB Saunders, 1997:373–388.

Stewart WJ: Intraoperative echocardiography. In Topol EJ, ed. *Textbook of cardiovascular medicine.* Philadelphia: Lippincott–Raven, 1998: 1492–1525.

Weyman AE. Left ventricular inflow tract I: The mitral valve. In: Weyman AE, ed. *Principles and practice of echocardiography,* 2nd ed. Philadelphia: Lea & Febiger, 1994:391–470.

16. TRICUSPID VALVE DISEASE

Amy P. Scally

I. **Introduction.** The trileaflet tricuspid valve has an estimated valve area of 7 cm² and a fibrous annulus with a 10- to 12.5-cm circumference. The anterior leaflet receives chordae from anterior and conal (septal) papillary muscles, the posterior leaflet from anterior and posterior papillary muscles, and the septal leaflet from posterior and conal papillary muscles. Acquired disease of the tricuspid valve is much less common than that of the mitral or aortic valves; this is in part due to the lower pressures on the right side of the heart, which pose less stress on the tricuspid valve.

II. **Tricuspid stenosis**
   A. **Clinical presentation.** Any mean diastolic pressure gradient above 4 mm Hg often raises the right atrial pressure to the point of causing systemic venous congestion.
      1. **Signs and symptoms.** Variables affecting the presentation of tricuspid stenosis are **severity of stenosis,** symptoms associated with the **underlying etiology,** and **concomitant cardiac lesions.**
         a. **Easy fatigability and edema,** related to the low cardiac output state, are common complaints.
         b. The patient may experience a **fluttering sensation** in the neck due to giant A waves in the jugular venous pulse, and **right upper quadrant pain** (from stretching of the liver capsule).
      2. **Physical findings.** The diagnosis of tricuspid stenosis is often missed without a high index of suspicion and careful consideration during the examination. Clues that should raise suspicion of tricuspid stenosis include the presence of **elevated jugular venous pressure** and **accentuation of a diastolic murmur along the left sternal border with inspiration** (not present in mitral stenosis).
         a. **Elevated central venous pressure** leads to marked hepatomegaly, ascites, and refractory edema. In sinus rhythm a giant A wave in the jugular venous pulse at S_1 results from right atrial contraction against the stenotic tricuspid valve.
         b. **Diastolic murmur.** The murmur of tricuspid stenosis is **low pitched,** diastolic, and best heard along the left lower sternal border in the third to fourth intercostal space or over the xiphoid process. If the rhythm is normal sinus, the murmur is prominent at end diastole (presystole); in atrial fibrillation the prominence of the murmur is found in early to mid-diastole. Murmur **intensity increases with inspiration** (Rivero-Carvallo sign) and with any maneuver that increases the volume delivered to the right atrium.
         c. An **opening snap** can be heard at the left sternal border of a stenotic valve that remains flexible.
         d. **Marked hepatic congestion** with resultant cirrhosis, jaundice, malnutrition, anasarca, and cites can be observed in severe tricuspid stenosis.
   B. **Etiology and pathophysiology**
      1. Cases of tricuspid stenosis are **most likely to be rheumatic in origin** (over 90%); almost uniformly the mitral valve is also stenotic. In those patients with severe rheumatic mitral stenosis, 5% to 10% have hemodynamically significant tricuspid stenosis.
      2. **Carcinoid syndrome,** representing the second most common cause of tricuspid stenosis, involves the heart tissues in 10% to 50% of cases. The tricuspid valve diseased by a carcinoid process is more likely to manifest with combined stenosis and regurgitation. Table 16-1 lists the various etiologies.

Table 16-1. Etiologies of tricuspid stenosis

Disease entity	Examples and/or comments
Congenital	Tricuspid atresia
Rheumatic	Most cases of TS are rheumatic in origin Relatively uncommon in Europe and North America. More common in women than men. Pathology like that in rheumatic MS. Only 3% of rheumatic TS cases are isolated; the remainder are accompanied by MS. At least 50% of TS cases have functionally significant TR.
Infective endocarditis	TV vegetation
Prosthetic valve failure	Thrombosis, calcification, or degeneration
Right atrial abnormality	Clot or tumor
Extracardiac tumor	
Whipple's disease	Infectious malabsorptive disease
Fabry's disease	X-Linked accumulation of trihexoside
Trauma	Pacemaker lead, transvenous catheters
Acquired deposition disorders	Deposition of material on endocardium and/or valvular surfaces
1. Eosinophilic endomyo cardial fibrosis (Loeffler's myocarditis)	Eosinophilic infiltration of endocardium (occasionally chordae and valves)
2. Endomyocardial fibroelastosis	
3. Malignant carcinoid	TS of carcinoid etiology is almost always accompanied by TR; valve structure is not damaged, but is altered and rendered dysfunctional. Vasoactive amines, produced by the carcinoid tumor, result in fibrous plaque formation on both sides of the TV, pulmonic valve, and on the endocardium; serotonin is the proposed toxic agent.
Drugs that may lead to deposition-like disorder:	Usually are serotonin-like substances
1. Methysergide	
2. Ergotamine	
3. Fenfluramine with or without phenteramine	

TS, Tricuspid stenosis; MS, mitral stenosis; TR, tricuspid regurgitation; TV, tricuspid valve.

    3. Commissural fusion and fibrosis, calcification, and vegetative masses are the main processes that render the tricuspid valve stenotic.
    4. Given the large fibrous annulus of the tricuspid valve, it is associated with **very few acquired obstructive pathologies.**
  C. Laboratory examination and diagnostic testing. The hemodynamic expression of tricuspid stenosis is a pressure gradient across the tricuspid valve in diastole. A mean diastolic pressure gradient of 2 mm Hg across the tricuspid valve establishes the diagnosis of tricuspid stenosis during catheterization; however, in practice, tricuspid stenosis is assessed by Doppler echocardiography; a **mean Doppler gradient greater than 5 mm Hg across the valve is generally associated with clinically significant tricuspid stenosis.** Tricuspid regurgitation (TR) and increased cardiac output can falsely elevate the gradient.

1. **Echocardiography.** The **echocardiogram is the most useful tool** in distinguishing tricuspid stenosis.
   a. **Two-dimensional findings. Right atrial enlargement, thickening and diastolic doming of the tricuspid leaflets, and a dilated inferior vena cava** are usually seen. The area of a normal right atrium measures less than 20 cm^2, and the diameter of a normal inferior vena cava measures 1.2 to 2.3 cm.
   b. **Doppler analysis.** Reduced diastolic slope and increased velocity are the principal Doppler signs of tricuspid stenosis.
      (1) **Color Doppler.** Turbulent flow is seen across the stenosed tricuspid valve.
      (2) **Calculation of the tricuspid valve area (TVA).** The TVA is estimated by dividing the PHT by 220, as described in Chapter 15. Severe tricuspid valve stenosis would apply to any area less than 2 cm^2.
      (3) **Continuous wave Doppler** cursor array is placed across the tricuspid valve in the four chamber or in the right ventricular two chamber. In tricuspid stenosis this reveals an elevated transvalvular gradient (greater than 2 mm Hg).
      (4) **Estimation of the tricuspid valve area by direct short axis measurement or by Doppler calculation correlates poorly** with hemodynamic measurements; for this reason, **pressure gradients alone are used to assess severity in most instances.**
2. **Cardiac catheterization is usually not necessary** since the diagnosis is made by physical examination and confirmed by echocardiography. The right heart catheterization in tricuspid stenosis reveals a low cardiac output. The right atrial pressure is elevated and the A wave can be very tall, even approaching that of the right ventricular systolic pressure. Simultaneous measurement of the right atrial and right ventricular pressures with dual catheters enables calculation of a diastolic pressure gradient (Fig. 16-1); the pressures are very much dependent on cardiac output and pressure gradients can be as low as 3 to 5 mm Hg. Maneuvers such as lifting the legs (increased cardiac output) can accentuate the gradient as does the administration of atropine (increased heart rate and decreased filling time). The pull-back method using a single catheter across the tricuspid valve is unreliable because the pressures are so low.

D. **Key Suggestions**
   1. **Diagnosing Tricuspid Stenosis.** A high index of suspicion is needed to diagnose tricuspid stenosis. For example, in a patient with right heart failure without evidence for right ventricular hypertrophy (RVH) or mitral stenosis, one should suspect tricuspid stenosis. Elevated jugular venous pressure out of proportion to signs of pulmonary congestion should also raise the suspicion for tricuspid stenosis. Considering that the symptoms of mitral stenosis often precede those of tricuspid stenosis in rheumatic heart disease, any unexpected amelioration of symptoms of mitral stenosis in a patient with rheumatic heart disease should raise suspicion for concomitant tricuspid stenosis.

E. **Therapy**
   1. The patient with tricuspid stenosis often has other valvular disease, and **the treatment of all the valvular abnormalities and their interactions need to be considered.**
   2. **In the early phases of tricuspid stenosis, diuretics and sodium restriction** are often helpful in reducing signs of peripheral edema.
   3. **Severe stenosis often requires balloon valvuloplasty, or tricuspid valve replacement.** The indications for surgery or balloon valvuloplasty are usually determined by the severity of concomitant mitral or aortic valve disease. The contraindications to tricuspid balloon valvuloplasty are similar to those of mitral valvuloplasty (see Chapter 15).

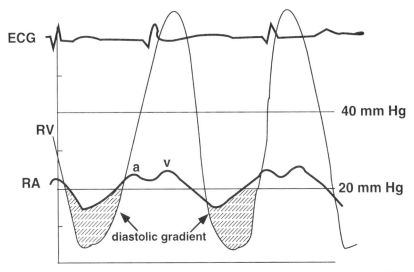

FIG. 16-1. Tracings of simultaneous right atrial (RA) and right ventricular (RV) pressure waveforms in a patient with tricuspid stenosis.

4. **Bioprostheses** are often favored in carcinoid tricuspid stenosis for many reasons, but especially because they have a lower complication rate and no need for systemic anticoagulation.

III. **Tricuspid regurgitation.** A minor degree of TR is common and is detected by echocardiography in more than 70% of normal patients.

A. **Clinical presentation**

1. **Signs and symptoms.** The spectrum of symptoms of TR is wide and depends on its etiology and chronicity.

   Tricuspid regurgitation alone is usually well tolerated. Patients might notice **pulsations in their neck** due to the prominent V wave in the jugular venous pulse, or they may present with **hepatic congestion and peripheral edema. Fatigue** from reduced cardiac output is another common presentation.

2. **Physical findings**

   a. The characteristics of the large V wave in the jugular venous pulse are dependent on TR severity and on the compliance of the system into which the TR flows (Fig. 16-2), a comparison of right atrial pressure tracings in the patients with and without TR. With significant TR the prominent V wave has maximal height at S_2, and the rapid Y descent is most prominent on inspiration.

   b. Tricuspid regurgitation typically produces a **pansystolic murmur** at the third to fourth intercostal space along the left sternal border. Tricuspid regurgitation **murmurs increase with inspiration** (Rivero-Carvallo sign). Other maneuvers that increase venous return and the murmur of TR are raising of the legs, application of abdominal pressure, exercise, inhalation of amyl nitrite, and a postextrasystole. When the right ventricle fails and can no longer respond with a forceful contraction, the murmur does not augment with with these maneuvers. The murmur has a reduced intensity and duration during Valsalva and in the standing position.

   c. A TR murmur that develops **in the presence of pulmonary hypertension is usually high pitched** and pansystolic, whereas a TR **murmur of primary etiology** (from endocarditis or trauma) is **short** (limited to first half of systole) **and low pitched**.

    d. Tricuspid regurgitation causes an increase in diastolic flow across the tricuspid valve. This may be heard as an **early diastolic rumble** (short and low pitched) along the left sternal border.

    e. **Mild** TR produces a **short and barely audible** murmur.

    f. With **severe TR** there is **ventricularization of the right atrium** (the pressure gradient across the tricuspid valve is minimized), and the TR **may be barely audible or absent.**

    g. **Other findings.** A **right-sided S$_3$ or S$_4$ is often present along the left sternal border which augments with inspiration. If pulmonary hypertension coexists, P$_2$ is accentuated. Systolic pulsation** of the liver is often an associated physical finding.

B. Etiology and pathophysiology. Any disease process that causes derangement of the tricuspid valve apparatus (annulus, leaflets, chordae, and papillary muscles) can lead to TR. Such disease processes are categorized as either primary (organic) or secondary (functional) TR. Table 16-2 lists the etiologies of TR.

C. Laboratory examination

    1. ECG. The findings are usually non-specific. Incomplete right bundle branch block may be seen.

    2. Echocardiography. The large majority of the information needed to characterize TR can be found with echocardiography alone. The most common views used for the detection of TR are the parasternal right ventricular inflow, basal short axis, and the apical four chamber.

      a. Physiologic tricuspid regurgitation. A minor degree of TR is often observed in patients with structurally normal hearts and the prevalence increases with age. Physiologic TR is usually represented by a small jet that does not extend greater than 1 cm into the atrium. Determining whether or not TR is clinically significant is much more difficult than determining its presence. The TR jet velocity in a structurally normal heart can vary from 2 to 2.6 m/sec; this is secondary to the expected pressure differential between right atrium and right ventricle during systole, and corresponds to pressure differences of 16 to 27 mm Hg. A normal TR jet duration measured on continuous wave Doppler is less than 150 milliseconds.

      b. Two-dimensional findings. These findings are often very helpful in determining the TR etiology.

        (1) Chambers, tricuspid valve annulus, and veins. With moderate to severe TR, the M-mode and two-dimensional images reveal a **right ventricular volume overload pattern** (right ventricular enlargement, ventricular septal flattening or shift to the left in diastole, and paradoxical motion in systole). The right ventricular overload pattern, however, is nonspecific and could be due to such entities as atrial septal defect (with left to right shunting) and anomalous venous return. Other two-dimensional image abnormalities likely to be present with moderate to severe TR are right atrial enlargement (the normal right atrial area is less than 20 cm^2), dilated tricuspid valve annulus (a tricuspid valve annulus greater than or equal to 3.4 cm is severe), and dilated inferior vena cava and hepatic veins (normal hepatic vein measures 0.5 to 1.1 cm). Dilatation of the right atrium and vena cava appears to occur early in the course of the TR.

        (2) Leaflets. Thickening, myxomatous changes, retraction, and increased reflectance of the leaflets should be sought when TR is detected. The tricuspid valve leaflets in carcinoid heart disease are thickened and rigid (occasionally fixed in the open position). Frequently, **rheumatic TR** has some degree of tricuspid valve stenosis. Pertinent to the evaluation of tricuspid

Table 16-2. Etiologies of tricuspid regurgitation

Primary etiologies of TR	Abnormalities of TV apparatus
Rheumatic	
Ebstein's anomaly (downward displacement of a malformed tricuspid valve)	Most diagnostic feature: apical four-chamber view, apical displacement of septal leaflet
Other congenital abnormalities of the TV	Cleft leaflet
Tricuspid annular calcification	
Carcinoid	
Connective tissue disease	Marfan syndrome, Ehlers-Danlos syndrome
Tricuspid valve prolapse myxomatous changes	Common in Marfan syndrome, occurs in 23% of mitral valve prolapse cases
Right ventricular MI or cardiomyopathy	Papillary muscle dysfunction
Trauma (motor vehicle accidents can cause blunt trauma, right ventricular contusion, and even deceleration injury)	Penetrating and nonpenetrating trauma, radiation exposure, pacemaker wire
Tumor of TV leaflet	Myxoma, fibroelastoma
Infective endocarditis (predispositions are intravenous drug abuse, chronic indwelling catheters, alcoholism, and immune deficiency states)	*Staphylococcus aureus* is the most common infecting organism. Triad (fever, narcotic addiction, multiple lung lesions) suggests clinical diagnosis of TV endocarditis.
Myocarditis	
Bioprosthetic valve dysfunction	Thrombosis and/or degeneration
SECONDARY ETIOLOGIES OF TR	PULMONARY HYPERTENSION
Left ventricular failure results in LV and RV dilatation.	Coronary artery disease, cardiomyopathy, hypertension, mitral regurgitation, aortic stenosis and/or regurgitation
Primary pulmonary hypertension	
Obstructive causes	Pulmonary embolus or emboli, pulmonary venous obstruction
COPD and sleep apnea syndrome	
Pulmonary fibrosis and or resection	
Connective tissue diseases	Systemic sclerosis
Mitral stenosis	
Atrial/ventricular septal defect	Congenital or acquired
Patent ductus arteriosis	Congenital
DIASTOLIC TR	Reversal of normal pressure gradient during diastole
Heart block (most common cause)	When an atrial contraction is not followed by a regularly timed ventricular contraction
Mechanically effective atrial fibrillation or flutter	
Restrictive cardiomyopathy	
Severe pulmonic regurgitation	

MI, Myocardial infarction; TR, tricuspid regurgitation; TV, tricuspid valve; COPD, chronic obstructive pulmonary disease.

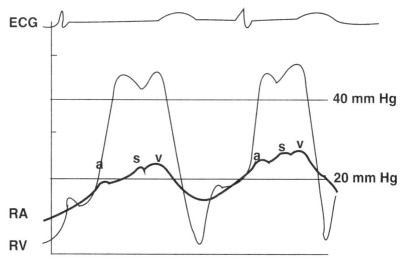

FIG. 16-2. Tracings of simultaneous right atrial (RA) and right ventricular (RV) pressure waveforms in a patient with tricuspid regurgitation.

valve dysfunction is scrutinizing **leaflet coaptation. Tricuspid valve prolapse** (one or more leaflets prolapse above the plane of the tricuspid valve annulus) should be ruled out; the four-chamber view is best for diagnosing tricuspid valve prolapse, which rarely occurs without concomitant mitral valve prolapse. Also to be ruled out are tricuspid valve annular dilatation (TR is usually central), leaflet retraction (often seen with fibrosis of the tricuspid valve leaflets), and flail cusps with ruptured chordae or papillary muscle. **Tricuspid endocarditis** is usually associated with a mass or masses on multiple valve leaflets with associated severe TR. In **Ebstein's anomaly,** a congenital deformity of the tricuspid valve, a malformed valve is displaced downward into the right ventricular cavity, although significant anatomic variability exists.

  c. **Doppler analysis. Assessment of TR involves incorporation of all of the Doppler information obtainable:** the amount of atrium containing the color jet, the presence or absence of a proximal convergence zone (on the right atrial side of the valve), the velocity profile, and even the eccentricity of the TR jet. An extremely eccentric TR jet that hugs the wall of the right atrium tends to lead to underestimation of the TR both on color flow and velocity assessment.

   (1) **Color Doppler**

      (a) **Tricuspid regurgitation direction and severity** are assessed with color flow Doppler. Severity of TR is estimated primarily by judging the size of the regurgitant jet (size of jet orifice at the valve) and the degree of the right atrium involved in the jet. The regurgitant jet area divided by the right atrial area (RJA/RAA ratio) is calculated with color Doppler.

         i. A ratio of less than 20% is consistent with mild TR.

         ii. A ratio of 20% to 40% is consistent with moderate TR.

       iii. A ratio greater than 40% is consistent with severe TR.

(b) Systolic flow reversal in the inferior vena cava or hepatic veins is consistent with severe TR (the reversed flow can sometimes be seen with color Doppler; however, the reversal of flow is best assessed by pulse wave Doppler). If the Doppler signal is weak, contrast echocardiography (injection of agitated saline) may be tried to evaluate the TR since contrast usually augments the Doppler signal.

(2) Calculating right ventricular systolic pressure

(a) The TR **jet velocity** is quantified by continuous wave Doppler sampling across the tricuspid valve in whichever view best affords a parallel orientation of the TR jet with the Doppler. The focal depth of the beam should be at the origin of the TR jet because that is where the highest velocity occurs. The value for maximal TR jet velocity is obtained by averaging 5 (sinus rhythm) to 10 (atrial fibrillation) peak velocities that are measured from beats that show the most complete envelope. The averaging is performed because of known variation in right-sided velocities with cycle length and respiration. **Not all TR velocity peak profiles can be measured;** measurable peak velocities in patients with TR range from 75% to 96%.

(b) The right ventricular systolic pressure (RVSP) needs to be calculated. First the pressure gradient (between the right atrium and right ventricle during systole) is calculated by placing the averaged TR velocity from the continuous wave Doppler sampling above into the simplified Bernoulli equation

Pressure gradient $= 4V^2$

    Adding the value for pressure gradient to the estimated right atrium pressure (RAP) gives an accurate estimation of right ventricular systolic pressure (RVSP).

RVSP $= 4V^2 +$ RAP

(c) Estimation of RAP. Many methods are used. Some simply use the value of 10 mm Hg for all patients' RAP, whereas others will estimate RAP based on an evaluation of the jugular venous pulse. Since assessment of the jugular venous pulse is not always possible, some estimate RAP based on the two-dimensional echo assessment of the inferior vena cava in the subcostal view as follows: A nondilated inferior vena cava (1.2 to 2.3 cm) that collapses at least 50% on inspiration correlates to a RAP of 0 to 5 mm Hg. A nondilated inferior vena cava that does not collapse on inspiration correlates to a RAP of 5 to 10 mm Hg. A dilated inferior vena cava that collapses at least 50% on inspiration correlates to a RAP of 10 to 15 mm Hg. A dilated inferior vena cava that does not collapse on inspiration correlates to a RAP of 15 to 20 mm Hg.

(d) The systolic pulmonary artery pressure (SPAP) is equal to the RVSP in the absence of right ventricular outflow obstruction, so long as there is no gradient across the right ventricular outflow tract or across the pulmonic valve. The severity scale for SPAP or pulmonary hypertension is as follows:

Normal: SPAP of 18 to 25 mm Hg
Mild pulmonary hypertension: SPAP of 30 to 40 mm Hg
Moderate pulmonary hypertension: SPAP of 40 to 70 mm Hg
Severe pulmonary hypertension: SPAP greater than 70 mm Hg

In the case of TR and normal pulmonary artery pressures, calculated gradients across the tricuspid valve are less than 25 mm Hg (maximal velocity of 2.5 cm/second).

3. **Cardiac catheterization**
   a. **Catheterization abnormalities** in the presence of moderate to severe TR include a dominant V wave in the right atrial pressure curve (see Fig. 16-2), a right atrial pressure curve resembling that of the right ventricle, increased right ventricular end-diastolic pressure, and low cardiac output by thermodilution and Fick techniques.
   b. **Normal or low right ventricular and pulmonary artery pressures** can be seen in some cases of isolated TR.
   c. **Angiocardiography** involves injecting contrast into the right ventricle while viewing the right anterior oblique projection. This method allows for visualization and semiquantification of the TR jet, but is rarely performed.

D. **Therapy**
   1. **Medical therapy.** If right ventricular failure develops with severe TR, **preload reduction (diuretics) and afterload reduction** should be started.
   2. **Surgical therapy.** When there is an **organic (primary) etiology** to the TR, **surgical repair or replacement** might be necessary. The appropriate prosthesis to use at the tricuspid position is controversial. Mechanical valves are more likely to thrombose (often be successfully treated with thrombolysis). Usually tricuspid repair or annuloplasty is favored over prosthetic implantation.

SUGGESTED READINGS

Key Reviews
Scully HE, Armstrong CS. Tricuspid valve replacement: fifteen years of experience with mechanical prosthesis and bioprosthesis. *J Thorac Cardiovasc Surg* 1995;109: 1035–1041.
Van Nooten GJ, Caes FL, Francois KJ, et al. The valve choice in tricuspid valve replacement: 25 years of experience. *Eur J Cardiothorac Surg* 1995;9:441–446.

Relevant Book Chapters
Braunwald E. *Heart disease: a textbook of cardiovascular medicine,* 5th ed. Philadelphia: WB Saunders; 1997:chapter 32, 1007–1076.
Feigenbaum H. *Echocardiography,* 5th ed. 1994. Baltimore: Williams & Wilkins: chapter 6, 239–349.
Reynolds T. *The echocardiographer's pocket reference.* Arizona Heart Institution Foundation, 1993:23–29.
Schiller NB, Thomas JD. Transthoracic echocardiography. In: Topol EJ, ed. *Textbook of cardiovascular medicine.* Philadelphia: Lippincott-Raven, 1998:1239–1266.
Weyman AE. *Principles and practice of echocardiography,* 2nd ed. Philadelphia: Lea & Febiger, 1994:chapter 26, 824–862.

17. PULMONARY VALVE DISEASE

Marc Penn

I. **Introduction.** The pulmonary valve is a trileaflet valve that separates the right ventricle from the pulmonary vasculature. Dysfunction of the valve can have adverse effects on the right ventricle. Although many patients have some degree of pulmonic insufficiency on echocardiogram, certain disease states can cause so much pulmonary valve stenosis or insufficiency as to alter significantly the hemodynamics in the right heart and to cause right ventricular dysfunction.

II. **Pulmonary valve stenosis**

    A. **Clinical presentation**

        1. **Signs and symptoms. Patients with pulmonary valve stenosis present in the fourth or fifth decade of life with signs and symptoms of right heart failure and dyspnea on exertion.**

        2. **Physical findings.** Pulmonary valve stenosis causes a systolic ejection murmur heard best in the third and fourth intercostal spaces. It can be heard in mild to moderate pulmonary valve stenosis. The murmur decreases with inspiration, due to a decrease in the transpulmonary valve gradient. There is also a decreased intensity of P_2. Finally, if significant right ventricular dysfunction has developed, evidence of right heart failure can be present.

    B. **Etiology**

        1. **Congenital pulmonary stenosis is the most common** pulmonary valve problem, occurring in approximately 10% of all patients with congenital heart disease (see Section VII of this book).

        2. **Rheumatic heart disease** can result in fusion of the valve cusps, resulting in pulmonary stenosis; however, the pulmonary valve is the least likely valve to be affected.

        3. Pulmonary valve stenosis can also occur in the setting of **carcinoid syndrome** secondary to local invasion of the valve.

        4. Pseudopulmonary stenosis can also occur as a result of **right ventricular outflow obstruction** from cardiac tumors or from an aneurysm of the sinus of Valsalva.

    C. **Diagnostic testing. Echocardiography** is useful in diagnosing pulmonary stenosis and for quantifying the severity of the obstruction. The best images of the pulmonary valve are from the left ventricle short-axis view at the level of the base from the parasternal short and subcostal windows. Transesophageal echocardiography is useful when the transthoracic echocardiogram images are suboptimal.

        1. **Leaflets.** In adults the leaflets can appear thickened and calcified with restricted motion. In children the leaflets are noncalcified with doming of the valve.

        2. **Right ventricle.** The right ventricle can be normal, especially in children. Right ventricle hypertrophy can be seen in adults, depending on the severity and duration of the disease.

        3. **Doppler** is used to grade the severity of pulmonary stenosis. This method of quantifying pulmonary stenosis is well correlated with direct measurement by cardiac catheterization and is now considered the **preferred methodology.** The peak gradient is measured across the pulmonary valve by using continuous wave Doppler with the Bernoulli equation:

           a. Mild disease is less than 40 mm Hg

           b. Moderate disease ranges from 40 to 80 mm Hg

           c. Severe disease is more than 80 mm Hg

D. Therapy

1. **Mild to moderate** pulmonary stenosis has a very good prognosis, and rarely is an intervention necessary.

2. **Severe pulmonary stenosis and secondary right ventricular failure** often presents in the fourth decade of life. The treatment of choice is **balloon valvuloplasty,** usually with a 75% decrement in the transvalvular gradient. Prognosis and morbidity subsequent to the procedure is based on right ventricular function at the time of the procedure.

3. Pulmonary stenosis secondary to **carcinoid syndrome** has a very poor prognosis (with a median survival of 1.6 years) and the valve often does not respond to balloon valvuloplasty. **Valve replacement** is often necessary.

III. Pulmonary valve regurgitation

A. Clinical presentation

1. **Signs and symptoms.** Patients with pulmonary regurgitation present with signs and symptoms of **right heart failure and dyspnea on exertion.**

2. **Physical findings.** The murmur of pulmonary regurgitation is a **low-pitched, diamond-shaped diastolic murmur,** heard best in the third and fourth left intercostal spaces with a widening of S_2. The murmur increases with inspiration, and P_2 is accentuated in the presence of pulmonary artery hypertension. The **Graham Steell murmur** is a high-pitched, blowing decrescendo diastolic murmur starting immediately after P_2. This characteristic murmur occurs when pulmonary artery systolic pressure exceeds 70 mm Hg in the presence of pulmonary regurgitation. Depending on the severity and duration of the regurgitant valve, signs and symptoms of right heart failure may also be present on examination.

B. Etiology

1. Unlike pulmonary valve stenosis, **pulmonary regurgitation has only rare congenital causes,** such as an absent, malformed, or fenestrated leaflet.

2. Acquired causes of pathologic pulmonary valve regurgitation are much more common. **The most common acquired cause is pulmonary artery hypertension,** followed by endocarditis. Carcinoid syndrome and rheumatic heart disease both can cause pulmonary regurgitation but are more likely to cause pulmonary stenosis. Marfan syndrome can cause pulmonary valve regurgitation secondary to dilatation of the pulmonary artery. Iatrogenic pulmonary regurgitation can be caused by placement of a pulmonary artery catheter.

C. Diagnostic testing. The pulmonary valve is **best evaluated with echocardiography,** using the left ventricle short-axis view from the parasternal and subcostal windows. In the majority of normal persons, there are minimal jets due to trivial pulmonary regurgitation. A significant jet of pulmonary regurgitation reaches 1 to 2 cm into the ventricle and occupies 75% or more of diastole. Pulsed wave Doppler should reveal regurgitant flow toward the transducer in diastole.

1. Maintenance of the regurgitant velocity during diastole suggests **pulmonary hypertension** as the cause of valve incompetence. Other evidence of pulmonary artery hypertension by echocardiogram includes loss of the a wave and a midsystolic notching in the pulmonary valve motion during M-mode. Similarly, a midsystolic notch can be observed in the pulmonary artery flow measured by Doppler. Furthermore, increasing pulmonary artery pressures correlate with decreasing acceleration times of pulmonary artery flow. Pulmonary artery pressures can be obtained using Doppler flow measurements and the following equations. Pulmonary artery diastolic pressure (PADP) is only obtainable in the setting of pulmonary regurgitation:

$$PADP = 4(V_{PR-E})^2 + RA_{PRESSURE}$$

where V_{PR-E} is the end-diastolic pulmonary regurgitation velocity.

  2. A decline of the regurgitant velocity profile during diastole suggests an **abnormality of the valve**.

D. Therapy

  1. **Primary pulmonary valve regurgitation.** The prognosis is very good; rarely is correction of the defect necessary, except in cases of intractable right heart failure.

  2. **Secondary pulmonary valve regurgitation.** The prognosis due to endocarditis, carcinoid, or pulmonary artery hypertension is tied to the prognosis and treatment of the primary disease. **Treatment options consist of valve replacement or repair of the dilated annulus.** Annulus repair is ideal in patients with coexisting left-sided valvular lesions. Fixing both often reverses pulmonary hypertension.

SUGGESTED READINGS

Relevant Book Chapters

Braunwald E. Valvular heart disease. In: Braunwald E, ed. *Heart disease: a textbook of cardiovascular medicine.* Philadelphia: WB Saunders, 1997:1059–1061.

Cheitlin MD, MacGregor JS. Acquired tricuspid and pulmonary valve disease. In: Topol EJ, ed. *Textbook of cardiovascular medicine.* Philadelphia: Lippincott-Raven Publishers, 1998:557–578.

18. PROSTHETIC HEART VALVES

Steve Lin and James Wong

I. **Indications for implantation**

A. **Types of prosthetic valves.** Prosthetic valves are classified into two major categories: mechanical and bioprosthetic. Each model differs in its durability, thrombogenicity, and hemodynamic performance. Various mechanical and bioprosthetic valves are shown in Fig. 18-1.

1. **Bioprosthetic valves.** Despite the resemblance to native valves, the hemodynamic performance of a bioprosthesis is suboptimal due to the reduction in the profile by the interposed stents and the sewing ring.

a. **Heterografts**

(1) **The Carpentier-Edwards valves** are made of either bovine pericardium (aortic position), which have a lower profile, or porcine valves attached to a cloth-covered annular ring with steel-alloy flexible stents at each of the commissures, which provide support to the leaflets.

(2) **The Hancock II porcine valve** has several new design features. Its stents are manufactured from Delrin; the sewing ring for the aortic prosthesis is supraannular to improve hemodynamic performance; and modern preservation techniques using low-pressure fixation and treatment with sodium dodecyl sulfate are expected to increase longevity.

(3) In the **stentless porcine bioprosthesis** (Medtronic Freestyles or St. Jude Medical), the leaflet commissures must be attached to the native aorta.

b. **Aortic homografts.** For the aortic position, the implantation of an aortic homograft valve is increasingly popular in selected medical centers. Homografts are harvested and cryopreserved cadavaric human aortic valves. It is typically implanted stentless with a short segment of the donor's aortic root for support and requires reimplantation of coronary arteries. The hemodynamic profile of the homograft is similar to that of the native valve. Like other human donor tissues, the availability of homografts is a limiting factor.

2. **Mechanical valves**

a. **Single-leaflet tilting disc.** The single leaflet tilting disc valve (e.g., Björk-Shiley, Medtronic-Hall, and Omniscience) consists of a metallic sewing ring attached to a disc. The tilting disc is made of pyrolytic carbon and is free to rotate about a pivot axis from the occluded position to the open position at angles between 60 and 85 degrees. The prosthesis is characterized by two orifices separated by the occluder. The major orifice is formed between the disc pivot axis as the disc swings downstream to the open position. The disc on the other side of the pivot axis swings proximally forming the minor orifice.

b. **Bileaflet tilting disc.** The St. Jude and Carbomedics valves are characterized by two semicircular pyrolytic carbon discs that rotate freely 75 to 90 degrees distally. Two large lateral orifices and a small central rectangular space are created in the open position. A built-in leakage volume is designed to reduce thrombus formation on discs.

c. **Caged ball.** The Starr-Edwards valve consists of a silicone ball within a cage attached to a metallic alloy ring. The ball is free to travel along the cage over a distance of 1 to 2 cm. Flow across the prosthesis is directed circumferentially around the ball, assuming a

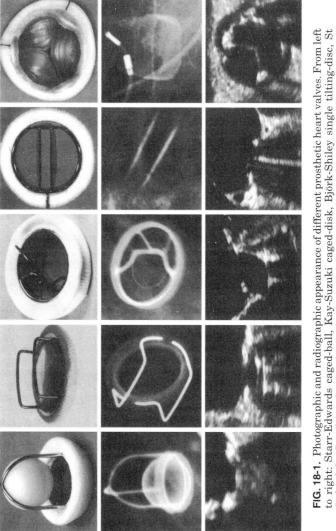

FIG. 18-1. Photographic and radiographic appearance of different prosthetic heart valves. From left to right: Starr-Edwards caged-ball, Kay-Suzuki caged-disk, Björk-Shiley single tilting-disc, St Jude's bileaflet tilting-disc mechanical valves, and Carpentier-Edwards xenograft. (From Garcia M. Principles of Imaging. In: Topol EJ. *Comprehensive Cardiovascular Medicine.* 1998, p. 610, by permission of Lippincott-Raven.)

Table 18-1. Clinical factors leading to selection of a bioprosthetic versus a
mechanical valve

Factors favoring bioprosthesis	Factors favoring homograft (aortic value)	Factors favoring mechanical prosthesis
Age >70 yr	Age <50 yr	Age <60 yr
Bleeding diathesis	Endocarditis	Combined multi-valvular placement
High risk for trauma	Composite aortic valve and conduit placement	Patients with other indications for chronic anticoagulation
Poor compliance	Female considering pregnancy (mitral valve)	Female considering pregnancy

lateral angle. The hemodynamic profile is less favorable than that
of the tilting disc prosthesis.

B. Selection of valves. Table 18-1 summarizes the clinical factors leading to
the selection of a bioprosthetic versus mechanical valve.

1. **Valve repair.** An important decision to be made before each valvular
surgery is whether repair of the native valve is feasible. **Several potential advantages of valve repair, when feasible, over replacement
include preservation of left ventricular function via conservation
of the subvalvular apparatus, lower operative mortality, higher
long-term survival rate, and freedom from anticoagulation.** The
advantages of repair and replacement are contrasted in Table 18-2.

   a. Currently, the greatest experience has been in the repair of the
   mitral valve.

   b. Bicuspid aortic valve with pure regurgitation due to prolapse, but
   without severe stenosis or calcification, can also be successfully
   repaired.

2. **Bioprosthetic valve.** The bioprosthetic valve is **indicated in patients
with contraindication for chronic anticoagulation.** It is also preferred for **patients older than 70 years,** given its adequate durability
and the freedom from chronic anticoagulation. Approximately 30% of the
heterograft bioprostheses fail within 10 to 15 years of implantation,
although the incidence of bioprosthesis failure is also age-dependent.
Table 18-3 summarizes the expected durability of bioprosthetic valves
relative to the patient's age. The complication rates for aortic bioprosthetic and mechanical valves are similar. There is a higher risk of reoperation among those who received bioprosthetic valves.

Table 18-2. Characteristics favoring valve repair versus replacement

Favoring valve replacement	Favoring valve repair
Rheumatic valve disease	Mitral valve prolapse
Endocarditis	Posterior leaflet involvement
Inexperienced surgeon	Excessive leaflet mobility
Complex mitral valve morphology	Ischemic mitral valve regurgitation
Calcified and fibrosed valve	Bicuspid aortic valve with prolapse
Restricted leaflet motion	Annular dilatation with normal Leaflets
Extensive leaflet destruction	

Table 18-3. Heterograft valve failure rate 10 years after valve replacement relative to the patient's age

Patient's age (yr)	Failure rate at 10 years (%)
<40	40
40–49	30
50–59	20
60–69	15
≥70	10

Modified from Vongpatanasin W, Hillis LD, et al. Prosthetic Heart Valves. The New England Journal of Medicine. 1996; 335:412, by permission of The Massachusetts Medical Society.

   3. **Homografts.** The homograft is the **valve of choice in aortic valve endocarditis** and has the lowest valvular gradient among the bioprosthetic valves. Although it provides durability superior to that of a heterograft, only 10% are still functioning after 20 years. Aortic homografts are appropriate for individuals under 50 years of age, women of childbearing age, those requiring composite valve-conduit grafts, patients with contraindication to anticoagulation, and especially patients with complicated endocarditis (abscess or fistula).
   4. **Mechanical valves.** Mechanical valves are **more durable than bioprosthetic valves;** some last more than 20 years. A mechanical prosthesis is generally recommended for **patients less than 60 years of age** because of its greater durability. It is also generally recommended for **patients already on permanent anticoagulation** for previous stroke or arrhythmia. The risk of stroke in a patient with a bioprosthetic valve without anticoagulation or a mechanical valve with appropriate anticoagulation management is approximately 1% per year. In **younger patients requiring combined aortic and mitral valve replacement,** mechanical valves are preferred, given the more rapid rate of prosthesis deterioration in the mitral position. **Pregnancy should be discouraged in patients with mechanical prostheses** because of the high risk to the mother and the fetus. Given its lower profile, mechanical prostheses may be preferred in **patients with small ventricles.** Once the decision to implant a mechanical prosthesis is made, the physician can select from among several types in common use. **Issues of compliance with anticoagulation and risks of trauma** should also be integrated into the selection of a mechanical valve.
      a. The St. Jude Medical and Medtronic-Hall valves are the most popular prosthetic valves because of their favorable hemodynamic performance, longevity, and low rates of complications. A major concern with the St. Jude Medical relates to the reported loss of structural integrity in a small percentage of patients, whereas the primary concern about the Medtronic-Hall valve is the potential of occluder impingement during the operation.
      b. Although the Starr-Edwards valve has the longest proven durability among all prosthetic valves, it is less popular today, given its suboptimal hemodynamic performance in comparison with the tilting disc valves.
      c. The Björk-Shiley valve has not been manufactured since 1986 after published reports of complications with strut fracture.
   C. **Follow-up post valve surgery.** There is a **wide spectrum of clinical practices** in the follow-up of the asymptomatic patient after valve surgery. A **baseline Doppler** study should be performed between 1 to 6 weeks following surgery as a baseline for future reference. For **mechanical valves, anticoagulation** should be followed permanently on a regular basis.

Table 18-4. Recommended anticoagulation therapy for patients with mechanical prosthetic valves

Level of risk	Prosthesis type	Recommended INR
Low	Single-tilting disc	3.0–4.0
	Double-tilting disc	2.5–3.0
High[a]		
	Caged disc	3.0–4.5
	Caged ball	3.0–4.5
	Multiple prostheses	3.0–4.5

[a] Patients with atrial fibrillation, left atrial thrombus, severe left ventricular dysfunction, or previous embolic events.
INR, International Normalizing Ratio.

Education regarding endocarditis prophylaxis is imperative for patients with prosthetic valves. **Annual echocardiography after the fifth postoperative year** for valve repair and replacement seems prudent.

D. Anticoagulation

1. **Immediate postoperative period**

   a. **Mechanical valves.** Table 18-4 summarizes the recommended anticoagulation therapy for patients with prosthetic heart valves. There is a **broad spectrum of practices regarding postoperative anticoagulation** for mechanical prostheses. The **embolic event rate is greater for mitral than for aortic** prostheses. Early anticoagulation increases the risk of postoperative bleeding and tamponade. Although there are many approaches, this author favors **warfarin, but not heparin, 3 to 4 days following surgery** when the pericardial wires are removed. Other centers recommend the use of **low-dose intravenous heparin,** targeted for upper normal limits of activated partial thromboplastin time within 6 to 12 hours following valve replacement, and **initiation of full-dose intravenous heparin once the chest tubes are removed. Warfarin** is initiated within 24 to 48 hours following valve replacement. **Chronic anticoagulation for mechanical valves is associated with risks** of minor hemorrhage of 2% to 4% per year, major hemorrhage of 1% to 2% per year, and death of 0.2% to 0.5% per year. The bleeding risk is 5% to 6% in patients 70 years or older. Patient-related risk factors for thromboembolism are older age, atrial fibrillation, and left ventricular dysfunction. The risk of embolization with warfarin therapy for mechanical valves is approximately 1% per year.

   b. **Bioprosthetic valves.** The **need for anticoagulation** in bioprosthetic valves is **controversial.** The risk for embolism is greatest in the early postoperative period and declines after 3 months for bioprosthetic valves. The risk for thromboembolism is greater for mitral valves (7%) than aortic valves (3%) initially. A reasonable approach is to anticoagulate patients with bioprosthetic valves at the **mitral position** for 3 months and then change to aspirin 325 mg every day. Patients with **aortic prostheses** should receive aspirin alone at 325 mg every day for 3 months unless there is another reason for anticoagulation. **Patients with prior embolic events, atrial fibrillation, or left ventricular dysfunction should be anticoagulated for the long term.**

2. **Management of anticoagulation patients with prosthetic valves undergoing noncardiac surgery.** Although the risk of thromboembolism increases when anticoagulant therapy is briefly discontinued, the decision to suspend therapy should be individualized.

    a. For **major procedures** in which substantial blood loss is expected, **warfarin should be discontinued at least 3 days prior to the procedure** to achieve an International Normalizing Ratio (INR) level of 1.6 or less. Hospital admission for **intravenous heparin administration** is often recommended for patients with **caged-ball prosthetic valves, atrial fibrillation, left atrial thrombus, severe left ventricular dysfunction, or previous embolization.**

    b. For **minor procedures** (e.g., dental extraction) where blood loss is minimal, anticoagulation can be continued.

    c. Postoperatively, intravenous heparin therapy should be **resumed when it is considered safe and continued until therapeutic anticoagulation is achieved with warfarin.**

  3. Pregnancy. Pregnant women have an increased incidence of thromboembolic complications. Given its teratogenic effects, **warfarin should be discontinued when pregnancy is considered or detected during the first trimester. Subcutaneous heparin** 15,000 U twice a day with a target activated partial thromboplastin time of 1.5 to 2.0 times the control 6 hours after injection should be administered until at least the second trimester of pregnancy, at which time warfarin may be resumed and continued until the middle third trimester. Subcutaneous heparin 5,000 U is then administered twice a day until delivery. Low-dose aspirin can be used in conjunction with anticoagulant therapy for women at higher risk for thromboembolism.

II. Clinical presentation and laboratory examination and diagnostic testing

  A. Clinical presentation. The clinical presentations of prosthetic valve dysfunction vary substantially. Discussion of the various entities occurs in Section III of this chapter.

    1. History. The history includes a thorough cardiovascular review in addition to questions pertinent to the function of the prosthesis.

      a. The **indication** for placement of valve prosthesis, **position** of implantation, **type** of prosthesis, and the **year implanted** should be elicited. The model and size of the prosthesis can be verified by the identification card provided by the manufacturer.

      b. Other important questions include **compliance with the anticoagulation** regimen, previous **endocarditis, thromboembolism, fever,** and perceived **change in the quality of the valvular click.**

    2. Physical findings

      a. The physical examination may be remarkable for a **new murmur, muffled prosthetic valve sounds, or evidence of embolic events.**

      b. Prosthetic valves are associated with **distinct auscultatory events caused by prosthesis motion or altered flow patterns.** The prosthesis sounds may mask the normal heart sounds; significant valvular dysfunction may occur without audible changes. Familiarity with the normal auscultatory findings in the prosthetic valve examination, however, can provide valuable clues on prosthesis dysfunction prior to the more definitive imaging examination. Figure 18-2 summarizes the acoustic characteristics of each valve prosthesis.

  B. Laboratory examination and diagnostic testing. The diagnosis of structural valve degeneration relies predominantly on echocardiographic findings, which can often identify degeneration prior to the onset of symptoms.

    1. Two-dimensional echocardiography. The interrogation of the prosthetic valve requires a thorough evaluation of the native structures and a systematic approach to the following: prosthetic apparatus, peak and mean gradient, and regurgitant flow. Typically, **transesophageal echocardiography** (TEE) is performed to evaluate **patients who are**

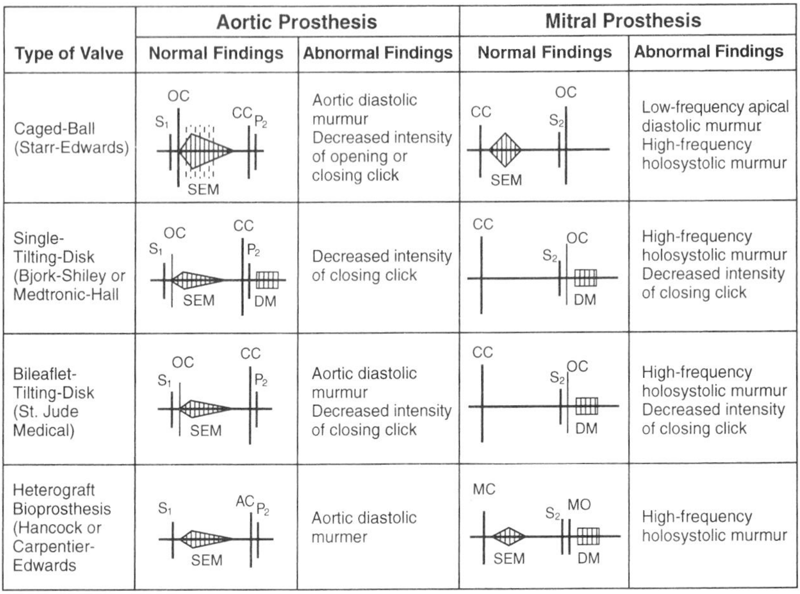

Type of Valve	Aortic Prosthesis		Mitral Prosthesis	
	Normal Findings	Abnormal Findings	Normal Findings	Abnormal Findings
Caged-Ball (Starr-Edwards)		Aortic diastolic murmur Decreased intensity of opening or closing click		Low-frequency apical diastolic murmur High-frequency holosystolic murmur
Single-Tilting-Disk (Bjork-Shiley or Medtronic-Hall)		Decreased intensity of closing click		High-frequency holosystolic murmur Decreased intensity of closing click
Bileaflet-Tilting-Disk (St. Jude Medical)		Aortic diastolic murmur Decreased intensity of closing click		High-frequency holosystolic murmur Decreased intensity of closing click
Heterograft Bioprosthesis (Hancock or Carpentier-Edwards		Aortic diastolic murmer		High-frequency holosystolic murmur

FIG. 18-2. Acoustic characteristics of various mechanical and bioprosthetic valves. (From Vongpatanasin W, Hillis LD, et al. Prosthetic Heart Valves. The New England Journal of Medicine. 1996; 335:410, by permission of The Massachusetts Medical Society.)

symptomatic or who are suspected to have endocarditis. The two-dimensional examination of prosthetic valves is similar to that of the native valve, but is limited because of reverberation artifacts and acoustic shadowing. In general, echocardiographic evaluation should assess the following:

a. Occluders and leaflets. Failure of the leaflet or occluder to open or coapt properly may be the result of pannus ingrowth (see Section III.H), thrombus formation (see Section III.E), or calcification of the bioprosthetic leaflets. Although it is important to demonstrate mobility of leaflets and occluders, their images are often suboptimal due to reverberation artifacts by transthoracic echo. Multiplane TEE provides higher temporal and spatial resolution of the prosthesis than does the transthoracic examination because TEE uses a higher frequency transducer (5 to 7 mHz) at close proximity to valvular structures (decreased depth). The cross-sectional view of an aortic bioprosthetic valve may be obtained at 40 degrees from the upper esophageal position during transesophageal examination. The area of the aortic bioprosthesis can be planimetered from this position. Increasing the array to 120 degrees provides an additional window for assessment of the aortic valve leaflet motion. Although the aortic prosthesis is less well visualized relative to the mitral prosthesis, TEE still provides a better visual inspection of the posterior aspect of the prosthesis and perivalvular structures compared to transthoracic echo. From 0 to 90 degrees in the lower esophageal position, various aspects of the mitral prosthesis can be visualized. The mitral prosthesis can be imaged in cross-sectional view from the transgastric window.

b. Sewing ring. The orientation of the prosthetic valve in the annulus can be variable; however, excessive motion ("rocking") of the

sewing ring is consistent with **dehiscence of the prosthesis.**
Adjacent echolucent structures identified in the evaluation of
endocarditis may represent abscess, fistula, or pseudoaneurysm. In
general, **flow into an adjacent echolucent space is pathologic.**
This may involve any portion of the annulus or the mitral-aortic
intervalvular fibrosa.

2. **Doppler evaluation.** Doppler evaluation complements the two-dimensional examination and provides a **reliable indirect assessment of
the prosthetic valve performance.** Color Doppler is useful in assessing regions of high-velocity, proximal flow convergence, and regurgitant
jets, whether they are valvular or perivalvular. Pulsed wave and continuous wave Doppler are used to assess transvalvular gradients, which
are then used to calculate valve areas.

   a. **Imaging planes for transthoracic echo. Prosthetic mitral and
   aortic regurgitation** can be visualized in the **parasternal long-
   and short-axis views.** Acoustic shadowing from the aortic and
   mitral prosthesis, however, can interfere with the color Doppler display in the proximal portion of the aortic and mitral regurgitant jets.
   The apical views offer the best position to assess mitral pressure gradient, but may underestimate the size of the mitral regurgitant jet
   due to acoustic shadowing. Pulmonary vein flows, which are often
   used to gauge the severity of the mitral regurgitation, may not be
   available for the same reason. **Prosthetic aortic regurgitation** can
   be characterized from the **apical window.**

   b. **Imaging planes for TEE.** At 40 degrees from the upper esophageal
   position (cross-sectional view), the origin of the aortic regurgitant
   jet (intravalvular or perivalvular) can be identified. The extent of
   the aortic regurgitant jet into the left ventricular cavity with color
   Doppler can be visualized at 120 degrees. Advancing the probe to
   the lower esophagus at 0 degrees brings forth the four-chamber
   view, which allows unimpeded visualization of the mitral regurgitant jet and measurement of transmitral gradients. Color Doppler
   interrogation of the medial and lateral aspects of the mitral prosthesis can be performed by increasing the array toward 90 degrees
   while rotating and advancing or pulling back the probe. The continuous wave Doppler is used to measure the peak velocity across
   the prosthesis.

      (1) Continuous wave Doppler evaluation of the **aortic valve** may
      be performed at the lower esophageal level using the pinch
      maneuver (simultaneous ante- and right lateral flexion of the
      probe). Inserting the probe into the stomach at 5 to 10 degrees
      with the probe anteflexed allows visualization of the origin of
      the mitral regurgitant jet. At 90 to 110 degrees, continuous
      wave Doppler evaluation of the aortic valve may be performed
      by left lateral flexion of the probe. Advancing the probe further
      to the deep transgastric view at 0 degrees with anteflexion also
      brings the aortic valve in line for Doppler interrogation.

      (2) Continuous wave Doppler can also be used to assess **mechan-
      ical prosthesis regurgitation,** especially for aortic valve
      prostheses. Continuous wave Doppler characteristics include
      low signal strength, spatial localization, and limitation to part
      of the cardiac cycle. Color Doppler is useful if a view can be
      obtained where the ultrasound beam can enter the chamber
      receiving the regurgitant flow without traversing the pros-
      thetic valve.

C. **Normal Doppler findings**

1. **Prosthetic valve clicks.** The opening and closing motion of the mechanical valve leaflet creates a brief intense Doppler signal that appears as a
narrow band on the spectral display.

Table 18-5. Normal Doppler values of prosthetic valves

Prosthetic valve	Peak velocity (m/sec)	Mean gradient (mm Hg)
AORTIC POSITION		
Starr-Edwards	3.1 ± 0.5	24 ± 4
Björk-Shiley	2.5 ± 0.6	14 ± 5
St. Jude	3.0 ± 0.8	11 ± 6
Medtronic-Hall	2.6 ± 0.3	12 ± 3
Aortic homograft	0.8 ± 0.4	7 ± 3
Hancock	2.4 ± 0.4	11 ± 2
Carpentier-Edwards	2.4 ± 0.5	14 ± 6
MITRAL POSITION		
Starr-Edwards	1.8 ± 0.4	5 ± 2
Björk-Shiley	1.6 ± 0.3	5 ± 2
St. Jude	1.6 ± 0.3	5 ± 2
Medtronic-Hall	1.7 ± 0.3	3 ± 1
Hancock	1.5 ± 0.3	4 ± 2
Carpentier-Edwards	1.8 ± 0.2	7 ± 2

Modified from Nottestad SY, Zabalgoitia M. In: Otto CM. The Practice of Clinical Echocardiography, 1997, p. 803, by permission of W.B. Saunders Company

2. **Prosthetic valve velocities/pressure gradients.** The systolic spectral Doppler contour is frequently triangular, with an early systolic peak velocity rather than semiellipsoid, resulting in a lower mean gradient for the same peak velocity. The expected normal velocities and pressure gradients for commonly used prosthetic valves are shown in Table 18-5. However, there is variation in these numbers. Therefore, a baseline study is indicated for patients with prosthetic valves.

3. **Physiologic prosthetic valve regurgitation.** Many prosthetic valves have regurgitant flow characterized by a uniform color without aliasing. For a mechanical prosthesis, the physiologic prosthetic regurgitant flow typically has a regurgitant jet area of less than 2 cm² and jet length of less than 2.5 cm in the mitral position, and a jet area of less than 1 cm² and jet length of less than 1.5 cm in the aortic position. **Most tissue valves exhibit minor regurgitant flow (closure volume) early after implantation.**

4. **Assessment of prosthetic valve dysfunction.** Loss of prosthetic valve clicks is a sensitive marker for prosthesis dysfunction.

    a. **Prosthetic valve stenosis**

        (1) **Transvalvular gradients.** Assessment of transvalvular gradients is the mainstay of the Doppler evaluation. **Each prosthetic valve is inherently stenotic with a higher peak velocity due to its small profile.** The continuous wave Doppler gradient across the prosthesis obtained within weeks following implantation serves as a control for subsequent evaluations. High gradients may be also obtained in nonobstructive situations, such as high-output states, tachycardia, anemia, severe prosthetic leaks, or the pressure recovery phenomenon. Pressure recovery occurs secondary to flow acceleration through a narrowed orifice, especially with the mechanical bileaflet prosthesis in the aortic position. With this, the highest pressure measured through the prosthesis by Doppler overestimates the true pressure gradient by approximately one third. With **prosthetic valve stenosis, pressure recovery becomes less evident.**

(2) Valve area calculations

   (a) Continuity equation. The continuity equation can be used to estimate the functional orifice area of prosthetic aortic and mitral valves. For calculation of the prosthetic valve area in the aortic position:

$$\text{Area}_{\text{aortic prosthesis}} = (\text{Diameter}_{\text{sewing ring}})^2 \times 0.785 \ \text{TVI}_{\text{LVOT}}/\text{TVI}_{\text{aortic prosthesis}}$$

   where TVI is time velocity integral and LVOT = left ventricular outflow tract.

   The LVOT diameter is replaced by the sewing ring inner diameter in the equation. The aortic prosthesis TVI is determined from continuous wave Doppler velocity through prosthesis. LVOT TVI is determined by pulsed wave Doppler. Mitral valve prosthesis TVI is determined from continuous wave Doppler. For the mitral position:

$$\text{Area} \ (\text{LVOT diameter})^2 \times 0.785 \times \text{TVI}_{\text{LVOT}}/\text{TVI mitral prosthesis}$$

(3) Pressure half time (PHT). For a mitral valve prosthesis, the PHT method is useful to assess prosthetic valvular stenosis. The empirical constant of 220 provides a reasonable approximation for mechanical prosthetic mitral valve area. The PHT method can also determine whether increased velocity is secondary to increased flow or to obstruction. If the peak velocity is increased, but the PHT is not prolonged, then the increased velocity is most likely due to increased forward flow. However, PHT may overestimate the area of the mitral prosthesis.

   Mitral prosthesis area = 220/PHT

(4) Dimensionless index. The LVOT and aortic valve prosthesis velocity ratio is helpful to evaluate prosthetic valve stenosis, particularly when the valve size is not known. The higher the index, the larger the effective orifice area, and vice versa. A value <0.23 suggests prosthesis stenosis.

   Dimensionless index = $\text{Velocity}_{\text{LVOT}}/\text{Velocity}_{\text{aortic prosthesis}}$

b. Pathologic prosthetic valve regurgitation. The pathologic flow disturbance is **larger and wider than that seen with physiologic regurgitation.** Its **severity can be reliably quantified by TEE,** which can best identify periprosthetic regurgitation. Pathologic regurgitation may be related to a scarred/calcified annulus with disrupted sutures securing the valve or a perivalvular abscess in adjacent tissue destruction. Single or multiple jets may be present.

   (1) Severe mitral prosthetic regurgitation is suggested by increased peak early diastolic velocity (more than or equal to 2.5 m/sec) and normal mitral inflow PHT (less than or equal to 150 m/sec) (see Chapter 15).

   (2) Severe aortic regurgitation is usually present when the PHT is less than or equal to 250 m/sec or when flow reversal is detected in the descending aorta (see Chapter 14).

5. Cinefluoroscopy. Cinefluoroscopy is useful for assessing **mechanical prosthetic valves.** The image intensifier is moved to a position with x-rays parallel to the valve ring plane to determine the occluder's excursions in a caged valve. Despite the radiolucency of pyrolytic carbon disc valves, the opening angle can be measured from positioning the image intensifier parallel to the plane of the open leaflets. **The mitral prosthesis is best visualized from the RAO (right anterior oblique) cranial projections. The aortic prosthesis can be viewed from RAO caudal or LAO (left anterior oblique) cranial projection.**

    a. **Diminished motion of the discs suggests valve obstruction, whereas excessive rocking of the base ring (i.e., 7 degrees for aortic prosthesis and 11 degrees for mitral prosthesis) suggests partial dehiscence of the valve.**

    b. In the setting of **suspected strut fracture in a Björk-Shiley valve,** cinefluoroscopy evaluation of the prosthesis is best performed with the tunnel view profile. Increased incidence of strut fracture has been noted in patients with an opening angle of 70 degrees or more.

6. Cardiac catheterization

    a. Invasive assessment of the left ventricle can be performed safely in patients with bioprosthetic aortic valves. Catheter-based evaluation of the mechanical aortic valve, however, must be performed with a transseptal technique in patients with a mechanical prosthesis. It may be necessary for accurate measurement of the prosthetic mitral valve gradient, as catheter-based assessment overestimates the mitral valve gradient because of a dampening of the pressure contour and intrinsic delay in the pulmonary capillary wedge tracing.

    b. **Never cross the following prosthetic valves:**

       (1) Single or bileaflet tilting-disc prosthesis

       (2) Caged-disc prosthesis

       (3) Caged-ball prosthesis

7. Magnetic resonance imaging (MRI) can be performed safely in patients with prosthetic valves. It can identify **prosthetic regurgitation, periprosthetic fistulas, and abscess if TEE is contraindicated.**

8. Computed tomography (CT) is not useful in the evaluation of prosthetic valves.

III. Valve dysfunction and complications related to prosthetic valves

  A. Atrial fibrillation. Up to 50% of patients undergoing valve surgery experience postoperative atrial fibrillation. Management of atrial fibrillation is discussed in Chapter 19.

    1. In **patients without a previous history** of atrial fibrillation, the **arrhythmia is often self-limited.**

    2. For patients with **persistent atrial fibrillation beyond 24 hours, anticoagulation, direct current cardioversion, and a short course of antiarrhythmic therapy** are warranted.

    3. Beta blockade or amiodarone prophylaxis has been found to reduce the incidence of postsurgical atrial fibrillation.

  B. Conduction disturbances. High-grade heart block requiring permanent pacemaker implantation has been described in 2% to 3% of the patients after valve replacement and 8% following repeat valve surgery. It occurs from trauma to the bundle of His or from postoperative edema of the periannular tissue. Aortic or mitral annular calcification, preoperative conduction disturbance, advanced age, infectious endocarditis, and tricuspid valve surgery have also been associated with higher rates of postoperative conduction abnormalities leading to permanent pacemaker implantation.

  C. Endocarditis. Approximately 3% to 6% of patients with prosthetic heart valves will experience prosthetic valve endocarditis. Prosthetic valve endocarditis is typically associated with large vegetations since microorganisms are sheltered from the host defense mechanisms.

    1. **Early prosthetic valve endocarditis** (60 days following prosthesis implantation) is typically caused by *Staphylococcus epidermidis.* The

clinical course is often fulminant, with high mortality rates ranging from 20% to 70%.

2. **Late prosthetic valve endocarditis** occurs most commonly in patients with multiple prostheses and bioprosthetic valves, especially in the aortic position. Its clinical course resembles that of native valve endocarditis. Streptococci are the most common infectious agents, followed by gram-negative bacteria, enterococci, and *S. epidermidis.*

3. **Transesophageal echocardiography is the imaging modality of choice** with sensitivity of 95% and specificity of 90%. It is used to establish the diagnosis; detect complications including abscess, tissue invasion, dehiscence, and fistula formation; and monitor the efficacy of medical therapy.

4. **Therapy.** The mortality of patients managed with antibiotics alone is 61% versus 38% for those having valve replacement. (See Chapter 48 for more information on diagnosis, management, and antibiotic prophylaxis for endocarditis.)

   a. **Medical therapy. Medical cure** of prosthetic valve endocarditis caused by **staphylococci, gram-negative organisms, or fungi is rare. Streptococcal** prosthetic valve endocarditis responds to medical therapy alone in **50% of the cases.**

   Patients with prosthetic valve endocarditis should **continue to receive anticoagulation.** In the absence of anticoagulation, prosthetic valve endocarditis is associated with an up to 50% incidence of stroke. Continuing anticoagulation for patients with prosthetic valve endocarditis is associated with a 10% incidence of cerebral embolization. There is no conclusive evidence for increased hemorrhage with warfarin in patients with prosthetic valve endocarditis.

   b. **Surgical therapy.** Valve replacement surgery is indicated in the setting of:

      (1) Persistent bacteremia despite intravenous antibiotics
      (2) Tissue invasion or fistula formation
      (3) Recurrent embolization
      (4) Fungal infection
      (5) Prosthesis dehiscence or obstruction
      (6) New or worsening heart blocks
      (7) Congestive heart failure

D. **Hemolysis.** Subclinical hemolysis is present in many patients with mechanical valves but **rarely results in significant anemia.**

   1. **Pathophysiology and etiology.** Clinical hemolysis occurs in 6% to 15% of patients with **caged-ball valves** but is uncommon with normal bioprosthetic or tilting-disc valves. Clinical hemolysis is also associated with **multiple prosthetic valves, small prostheses, periprosthetic leaks, and prosthetic valve endocarditis.** Mechanisms involved in the generation of hemolysis include high shear stress or turbulence across the prosthesis, interaction with foreign surfaces such as cloth, and rapid deceleration of erythrocytes following collision with adjoining structures (e.g., struts or cardiac walls).

   2. **Laboratory examination and diagnostic testing**

      a. Diagnosis is made by **elevated lactate dehydrogenase, reticulocyte count, unconjugated bilirubin, urinary haptoglobin,** and presence of **schistocytes on blood smear.**

      b. **Echocardiographic** findings consistent with mechanical hemolysis include **rocking of the prosthesis with jets of high shear stress** (e.g., eccentric or periprosthetic regurgitant jets).

   3. **Therapy**

      a. **Medical therapy.** Mild hemolytic anemia can be treated with **iron, folic acid supplement, and blood transfusion. Beta blockade and blood pressure control** may reduce the severity of hemolysis.

      b. Surgical therapy. Repair of perivalvular leaks or valve replacement is indicated in **patients with severe hemolysis requiring repeated transfusions or in those with congestive heart failure.**

E. Thrombosis. The incidence of prosthetic valve thrombosis averages 0.2% to 1.8% per year. The incidence is highest in the tricuspid position, followed by the mitral then the aortic. Thrombus is suspected in patients with **acute onset of symptoms, embolic event, or inadequate anticoagulation.**

  1. Laboratory examination and diagnostic testing. Transesophageal echocardiography is the most widely used diagnostic technique, although cinefluoroscopy can be used to document restriction in occluder mobility. No imaging modality, however, can clearly differentiate thrombus from pannus (see Section III.H). Frequently, both coexist. Echocardiographic features suggestive of thrombus include soft, irregular, or mobile mass.

  2. Therapy. The valve type or suspected duration of valve thrombosis does not influence the indications for treatment although location of prosthetic valve does.

    a. Priority of therapy

      (1) Heparin is typically initiated early in the course of evaluation.

      (2) Warfarin is continued unless surgery is planned.

      (3) Transesophageal echocardiography or cinefluoroscopy should be performed at 24 hours and, if the thrombus is still present, should be repeated serially.

    b. Medical therapy

      (1) Fibrinolytic therapy is considered the treatment of choice for **right-sided prosthetic valve thrombosis** because the consequences of distal embolization are less severe than in left-sided prosthesis. Streptokinase and urokinase are the most commonly used agents. Fibrinolytic therapy has an initial success rate of 82%, overall thromboembolism rate of 12%, and a 5% incidence of major bleeding episodes.

        (a) The recommended dosage for **streptokinase** is a 250,000-U bolus given over 30 minutes, followed by an infusion of 100,000 U/hour.

        (b) Urokinase is given as an infusion of 4,400 U/kg per hour.

        (c) Duration of thrombolytic therapy has varied **between 2 to 120 hours;** however, thrombolysis should be stopped if there is no hemodynamic improvement after 24 to 72 hours.

        (d) Following successful thrombolysis, close **follow-up of anticoagulation along with serial Doppler echocardiography** on an individual basis is recommended.

      (2) Anticoagulation with heparin and warfarin is generally recommended for **small thrombus** (less than or equal to 5 mm). The regimen consists of intravenous heparin followed by subcutaneous heparin 17,000 U twice a day and warfarin (INR 2.5 to 3.5) for up to 3 months.

    c. Surgical approach. The lowest surgical mortality reported has been approximately 5%. The risk profile of the individual patient must be balanced against the expertise and experience at each center.

      (1) Valve replacement and débridement is generally performed for **left-sided prosthetic valve thrombosis** unless the thrombus is small or the patient has a prohibitive surgical risk.

      (2) Surgery is also indicated in the case of **unsuccessful thrombolysis** 24 hours following the discontinuation of the infusion.

F. Dehiscence. Detachment of the sewing ring from the annulus might occur in the early postoperative period because of poor surgical techniques, excessive annular calcification, chronic steroid use, fragility of the annular tissue (particularly following prior valve operations), or infection. Late dehiscence occurs mainly from infectious endocarditis. **Rocking of the prosthesis** on echocardiography or cinefluoroscopy is an **indication for urgent surgery.**

G. **Patient–prosthesis mismatch.** All prosthetic valves with the exception of stentless aortic homografts have effective orifices that are smaller than that of native valves. There is an **inherent pressure gradient and relative stenosis with each prosthesis.** Occasionally, when an inappropriately small prosthesis is placed, the **ensuing low output may cause symptoms.** This mismatch occurs most frequently after valve placement for aortic stenosis.

1. In a patient with a **small annulus, a hemodynamically favorable prosthesis** like the aortic homograft or the tilting-disc valve is preferred.

2. **Aortic prostheses less than 21 mm in diameter are not recommended for a large or physically active patient.**

3. **Surgery** generally consists of replacement with a larger prosthesis and annular reconstruction.

H. **Pannus formation.** Valve obstruction occurs in up to 5% of mechanical valves per year. Valve thrombosis and pannus formation are responsible for the majority of mechanical prosthesis obstructions. **Little is known about the causes** of fibroblastic proliferation in pannus formation. Foreign body reactions to the prosthesis, inadequate anticoagulation, endocarditis, and blood flow turbulence in the mitral position have been implicated as potential causes. **Transesophageal echocardiography is generally required** to identify the etiology of prosthetic valve obstruction.

I. **Embolic stroke.** Following an embolic stroke, the risk of recurrent stroke is approximately 1% per day for the first 2 weeks.

1. **If no evidence of hemorrhage** is detected on CT scan at 24 to 48 hours, **intravenous heparin** should be administered after a small to moderate embolic stroke. **Maintaining anticoagulation** reduces this risk of recurrent stroke to one third, but **carries an increased risk of hemorrhagic transformation** of 8% to 24%, particularly during the first 48 hours.

2. In patients with **larger infarcts, anticoagulation should be withheld for 5 to 7 days.**

3. Anticoagulation is withheld for 1 to 2 weeks in the setting of **hemorrhagic transformation.**

4. **Aspirin or clopidogrel** may be necessary in the event of recurrent strokes despite adequate anticoagulation.

SUGGESTED READINGS

Landmark Articles

Acar J, Iung B, Boissel JP, et al. Multicenter randomized comparison of low-dose versus standard-dose anticoagulation in patients with mechanical prosthetic heart valves. *Circulation* 1996;94:2107–2112.

Akins CW. Results with mechanical cardiac valvular prosthesis. *Ann Thorac Surg* 1995;60:1836–1844.

Cannegieter SC, Rosendaal FR, Wintzen AR, et al. Optimal oral anticoagulant therapy in patients with mechanical heart valves. *N Engl J Med* 1995;333:11–17.

Davis EA, Greene PS, Cameron DE, et al. Bioprosthetic versus mechanical prosthesis for aortic valve replacement in the elderly. *Circulation* 1996;94:II-121–125.

Green CE, Glass-Royal M, Bream PR, et al. Cinefluoroscopic evaluation of periprosthetic cardiac valve regurgitation. *Am J Radiol* 1988;151:455–459.

Israel DH, Sharma SK, Fuster V. Anti-thrombotic therapy in prosthetic heart valve replacement. *Am Heart J* 1994;127:400–411.

Jaeger FJ, Trohman RG, Brener S, et al. Permanent pacing following repeat cardiac valve surgery. *Am J Cardiol* 1994;74:505–507.

Lengyel M, Fuster V, Keltai M, et al. Guidelines for management of left-sided prosthetic valve thrombosis: a role for thrombolytic therapy. *J Am Coll Cardiol* 1997;30:1521–1526.

Vogel W, Stoll HP, Bay W, et al. Cineradiography for determination of normal and abnormal function in mechanical heart valves. *Am J Cardiol* 1993;71:225–232.
Vongpatanasin W, Hillis LD, et al. Prosthetic heart valves. *N Engl J Med* 1996;335: 407–416.

Key Reviews
Rahimtoola SH. Prosthetic heart valve performance: long-term follow-up. *Curr Probl Cardiol* 1992:334–406.
Zabalgoitia M. Echocardiographic assessment of prosthetic heart valves. *Curr Probl Cardiol* 1992:270–325.

Relevant Book Chapters
Garcia MJ. Principles of Imaging. In: Topol EJ. *Comprehensive Cardiovascular Medicine.* Philadelphia: Lippincott-Raven, 1998:609–35.
Shaff HV. Prosthetic Valves. In: Giuliani ER, Gersh BJ, McGoon MD, et al., eds. *Mayo Clinic Practice of Cardiology,* 3rd ed. St. Louis: Mosby, 1996:1484–1495.

SECTION V. ARRHYTHMIA

Robert A. Schweikert and Gregory Kidwell

19. TACHYARRHYTHMIAS

Thomas Dresing

I. **Introduction.** The mechanisms of tachyarrhythmias have been classically divided into those of disordered impulse formation, those of disordered conduction, and combinations of both.

A. **Disorders of impulse formation.** Disorders of impulse formation include deranged automaticity as well as triggered activity.

1. Automaticity refers to the ability of a fiber of cardiac tissue to generate pacemaker activity spontaneously. **Deranged automaticity** refers to both normal and abnormal automaticity.

a. An example of accelerated **normal automaticity** would be inappropriately rapid firing rates of a normal pacemaker locus, such as the atrioventricular node or Purkinje system, due to ischemia, metabolic disturbance, or pharmacologic manipulation. A clinical example would be inappropriate **sinus tachycardia.**

b. **Abnormal automaticity** refers to discharge from a latent or ectopic locus of cells capable of generating automatic, spontaneous impulses that usurp control of the rhythm under conditions of ischemia or pharmacologic manipulation. A clinical example would be **accelerated idioventricular rhythm** (see III.A.6).

2. **Triggered activity refers to pacemaker activity that is dependent on afterdepolarizations from a prior impulse or series of impulses.** Afterdepolarizations are oscillations in the membrane potential. If these reach the threshold level for the surrounding cardiac tissue, they may trigger an action potential, thus precipitating further afterdepolarizations, perpetuating the pacemaker activity.

a. **Early afterdepolarizations (EADs)** occur before repolarization of the cardiac tissue and may be the mechanism responsible for the ventricular arrhythmias of the **long QT syndromes,** as well as **torsades de pointes** ("twisting of the points") produced by class I and class III antiarrhythmics, sympathetic discharge, and hypoxia. Antibiotics such as macrolides, certain azole antifungal agents, some psychotropic medications such as haloperidol, and several nonsedating antihistamines have been shown to produce EADs. Rapid heart rates and the administration of magnesium have been shown to suppress early afterdepolarizations.

b. **Delayed afterdepolarizations (DADs)** occur after the repolarization of the surrounding tissue is complete, and are thought to be the mechanism of triggered atrial tachycardia and the arrhythmias of **digitalis toxicity.** These have been demonstrated in various cardiac tissues, including parts of the conducting system, myocardial cells, and valve tissues. Increases in intracellular calcium are associated with delayed afterdepolarizations, such as those caused by digitalis preparations, or excessive sympathetic stimulation. Drugs that block the influx of calcium (such as calcium channel blockers and β-blockers) and drugs that decrease the sodium current (such as lidocaine and phenytoin) suppress the occurrence of delayed afterdepolarizations, whereas rapid heart rates augment DADs.

B. **Disorders of impulse conduction.** Disorders of impulse conduction include **reentry, which is the major cause of ventricular tachycardia** (VT) in the Western world. **Scar or ischemia** can produce regions anywhere in the heart that **conduct impulses inhomogeneously.** Thus, the impulse can spread into an area that has already repolarized after being previously depolarized. This can set up a circular movement of the impulse resulting in sustained tachyarrhythmias such as VT. In order for reentry to occur, **three conditions** must be met:

1. Two functionally distinct conducting pathways
2. Unidirectional conduction block in one of the pathways
3. A differential in the conduction rates in the pathways, with slow conduction via one pathway and return of conduction via the second

II. Supraventricular tachyarrhythmias

A. Sinus tachycardia

1. **Clinical presentation.** The **maximal heart rate** may be as **high as 200** beats per minute (bpm) in a young person and, **generally, 150 bpm or less in older individuals.**

2. **Etiology and pathophysiology**
   a. Sinus tachycardia generally reflects **an underlying process, metabolic state, or medication effect,** such as fever, hypovolemia, shock, congestive heart failure (CHF), anxiety, pulmonary disease including pulmonary embolism, anemia, thyrotoxicosis, caffeine, nicotine, atropine, catecholamines, or withdrawal from alcohol or drugs (both therapeutic and illicit).
   b. **Sinus tachycardia can be appropriate,** where it represents a physiologic response to maintain cardiac output, **or inappropriate,** as in defects in vagal or sympathetic tone.
   c. The **clinical consequences of sinus tachycardia vary,** based on the presence or absence of underlying heart disease. Patients with significant coronary artery disease (CAD), left ventricular dysfunction, or valve disease may not tolerate sinus tachycardia.

3. **Laboratory examination and diagnostic testing.** Electrocardiography (ECG) is used. The **heart rate is greater than 100** bpm. The **P-wave axis and morphology are normal.**

4. **Therapy** is directed generally at the elimination of the underlying etiology whenever possible.
   a. **If withdrawal from a therapeutic medication is suspected, reinstitution or slow tapering** of this medication can be attempted, if clinically appropriate.
   b. In the case of **inappropriate sinus tachycardia, β-blockers and calcium channel blockers** may be necessary to control the heart rate.
   c. In **extreme cases, sinoatrial nodal modification or atrioventricular nodal ablation** may need to be considered.

B. Atrial fibrillation (AF) is the most common sustained arrhythmia, occurring in approximately 0.4% to 1.0% of the general population. The prevalence of AF increases with age, affecting up to 10% of the population over the age of 80.

1. **Clinical presentation.** As with all arrhythmias, the clinical presentation of AF can vary widely. **Patients may be asymptomatic,** despite rapid rates of ventricular response. Common symptoms include **palpitations, fatigue, dyspnea and/or shortness of breath, dizziness, and diaphoresis.** Less commonly, patients may present with extreme manifestations of hemodynamic compromise, such as **chest pain, pulmonary edema, and syncope.** Atrial fibrillation is not infrequently noted in patients presenting with a new thromboembolic stroke, with reported rates of 10% to 40%.

2. **Differential diagnosis.** Atrial fibrillation needs to be **distinguished from multifocal atrial tachycardia** (see II.F), **frequent premature atrial contractions,** and **automatic atrial tachycardias** (see II.E.3.b).

3. **Etiology.** Atrial fibrillation is **most commonly associated with hypertension, valvular heart disease, CHF, and CAD.** It has also been associated with physiologic stress, drugs, pulmonary embolism,

chronic lung disease, hyperthyroidism, caffeine, infections, and various metabolic disturbances. Other less common cardiac associations include Wolff-Parkinson-White syndrome, pericarditis, and cardiomyopathy. Surgery, particularly **cardiac surgery, is associated with a risk of AF** that may be as high as 35% to 50%, depending on the type of cardiac-surgery. When no identifiable risk factor for AF is present, AF may be classified as lone AF.

4. **Pathophysiology**
    a. There is now a large body of evidence to support the theory of **atrial reentry as the mechanism.** According to this theory, AF is sustained by multiple reentrant wavelets that are continuously fragmented (thus spawning additional independent wavelets) by local atrial refractoriness and excitability. Other theories include disordered impulse formation, such as the theory of ectopic foci (either single or multiple), enhanced automaticity, or triggered activity. There is renewed interest in ectopic focus theory, as it has been recently shown that radiofrequency ablation (RFA) of an area in the pulmonary veins has had lasting success in eliminating AF in patients. It remains to be seen whether this technique will have broader application in the treatment of AF.
    b. Sustained or chronic AF presents a **considerable risk for thromboembolism;** even patients with lone AF are at increased risk. **The risk of stroke becomes more pronounced with increased age.** An increased risk for stroke has been shown to be associated with AF in the presence of any of the following: age greater than 65 years, history of diabetes, history of hypertension, history of CHF, history of prior stroke, or transient ischemic attacks.

5. **Laboratory examination and diagnostic testing**
    a. **ECG: P waves are absent. Atrial activity is chaotic** and fibrillatory **(F) waves are present.** The baseline of the ECG is often undulating and may occasionally have coarse, irregular activity that can resemble atrial flutter (see II.C.), but is not as stereotypic from wave to wave as atrial flutter tends to be. **Ventricular rhythm is irregularly irregular.** The **atrial rate** is generally in the **range of 400 to 700 bpm,** with a ventricular response generally in the range of 120 to 180 bpm in the absence of drug therapy.
    b. **Echocardiographic predictors of increased thromboembolic risk** include left atrial enlargement and reduced left ventricular systolic function.

6. **Therapy. It must be emphasized that the therapy of choice in any unstable patient is rapid direct current cardioversion (DCC).** The term "unstable" should include the patient who is highly symptomatic (e.g., chest pain, pulmonary edema), as well as the patient who is hemodynamically unstable. **Management of AF centers on three principles: control of the ventricular response, minimization of the thromboembolic risk, and restoration and maintenance of sinus rhythm.**
    a. **Control of the ventricular response.** The ventricular response is generally **controlled through drugs** that slow conduction through the atrioventricular node.
        (1) **β-Blockers** have a **rapid onset of action,** as well as **short half-lives in both the oral and intravenous (IV) forms.** Intravenous preparations of metoprolol, esmolol, and propranolol have their onset of action in approximately 5 minutes. Orally available β-blockers of varying durations of action can be used for rate control. These include metoprolol and propranolol, as well as atenolol, nadolol, and a number of less commonly used agents (see Appendix: Drug Index for details).

(2) **Calcium channel blockers** such as diltiazem and verapamil are available in both IV and oral forms. The IV forms are rapidly effective and have a short duration of effect. **In appropriate patients, they provide rapid control of the ventricular response.** Both diltiazem and verapamil are available in short-acting and sustained release preparations.

(3) **Digitalis** has long been used for rate control. Given its relatively long onset of action, **digoxin is ideally used in patients with decreased left ventricular function, or a contraindication** to β-blockers or calcium channel blockers (e.g., asthma, hemodynamic instability). Digoxin is usually **effective at controlling the resting heart rate;** however, it is **less effective at suppressing the ventricular response** to activity. Digoxin can be administered intravenously or orally. The **onset of action of digoxin is slow** (1 to 4 hours). Initially dosing of digoxin is 0.25 mg IV q 6 hours for a total of 1 mg every 24 hours. Then a maintenance dose is given that is based on the patient's renal function. Digoxin is **generally well tolerated, although it is associated with adverse effects,** such as gastrointestinal (GI) toxicity and neurotoxicity, and because of its long half-life (38 to 48 hours) is more likely to be associated with symptomatic bradycardia requiring intervention such as temporary pacing.

b. **Thromboembolic risk management**

(1) The **American Heart Association** recommends the following: **the patient should be anticoagulated with warfarin** (goal international normalized ratio, or INR, 2.0 to 3.0) for 3 weeks prior to undergoing cardioversion for all persons in AF for over 48 hours. **Warfarin should be continued until sinus rhythm has been maintained** for at least 4 weeks to allow for recovery of the atrial transport mechanism and for the recurrence of AF. **If cardioversion cannot be postponed for 3 weeks, patients should be systematically anticoagulated with heparin and should undergo transesophageal echocardiography (TEE)** to rule out atrial thrombus; **then warfarin** is used for 4 weeks after cardioversion.

(2) A number of major trials have attempted to compare the benefits of aspirin and warfarin in minimizing the stroke risk in patients with AF. Overall, warfarin has shown an annual average 68% reduction in relative risk for stroke, with aspirin showing a reduction anywhere from 0% to 44% (mean around 30%).

In younger patients at low risk for stroke (age less than 65, without other risk factors), aspirin may be an acceptable alternative to warfarin. **Older patients at greater risk for stroke (age 65 and older, with or without other risk factors)** should probably be anticoagulated with **warfarin with an INR of 2 to 3. Older patients who are poor candidates for warfarin** should be considered for therapy with aspirin. **Patients who have been in AF for over 48 hours are at risk** for having formed a thrombus in the atria and **should be systemically anticoagulated** whenever possible. This can be accomplished quickly with IV heparin. **Because of the increased risk of thrombus for the patient who has been in AF for over 48 hours, it is inadvisable to attempt cardioversion, either chemically or electrically, unless the patient is unstable as defined above; there is a prohibitive risk of propagation of emboli from the left atrium from DCC and the restoration of sinus rhythm.**

(3) Transesophageal echocardiography (TEE) may be able to rule out the presence of clot in the left atrium (particularly in the left atrial appendage, which is poorly seen with transthoracic echocardiography) in all patients requiring cardioversion prior to 3 weeks of supervised, therapeutic systemic anticoagulation. If the TEE is negative, cardioversion is carried out in the setting of systemic anticoagulation, which is maintained as detailed above.

(4) Cardiac output may be decreased after cardioversion in up to one-third of patients, and this can persist for as long as a week. Rarely, this leads to pulmonary edema as soon as 3 hours after cardioversion. Cardiac output should return to baseline within 4 weeks; however, the risk of thromboembolism is increased during this time period.

(5) After 4 weeks of therapy, the decision to continue anticoagulation is based on each patient's individual risks for recurrence of AF. **Patients who cannot be successfully cardioverted should be anticoagulated for the long term,** as should patients with frequent recurrences/paroxysms.

c. Restoration and maintenance of sinus rhythm. There is debate as to whether restoration to sinus rhythm is beneficial, as compared to a combined strategy of simply controlling the ventricular response and minimizing the thromboembolic risk. Some data from nonrandomized trials show an increase in mortality in patients on long-term antiarrhythmic therapy for AF.

(1) Direct Current Cardioversion (DCC). When it is determined that restoration of sinus rhythm should be attempted, this is most effectively carried out with DCC. **Direct Current Cardioversion is successful over 80% of the time,** whereas pharmacologic rates of successful cardioversion vary from 40% to 90%, depending on the clinical scenario. Whenever possible, **DCC should be carried out under sedation, with appropriate cardiac and hemodynamic monitoring, and in the presence of personnel skilled in airway control/management.** The details of DCC, including sedation and methods, are covered in detail in Chapter 53 of this book.

(2) Chemical cardioversion

(a) The success rate for chemical cardioversion is considerably lower than that for DCC. However, chemical cardioversion is often chosen by the practitioner or the patient as the first line of therapy. **Any patient who fails chemical cardioversion should be considered for DCC.** The "drugs first" approach may promote more successful DCC and/or maintenance of sinus rhythm after DCC. Similarly, it is reasonable to **attempt chemical cardioversion on any patient who fails DCC,** especially before repeated attempts at DCC.

(b) There are currently **only three IV agents available** in the United States for the chemical cardioversion of AF to sinus rhythm.

(i) Procainamide (a class IA antiarrhythmic) is often considered **the first line of therapy.** Up to one-third of patients cannot tolerate this drug due to GI, hematologic, or immunologic (lupus-like syndrome) side effects. An active metabolite of this drug, *n*-acetyl procainamide (NAPA), is cleared renally and has class III antiarrhythmic properties. Blood levels of both procainamide and NAPA need to be followed to prevent toxicity, especially in the setting of renal and/or hepatic insufficiency.

(ii) **Amiodarone** is generally **reserved for those patients who have been resistant to other agents, or in whom a contraindication** to the other available agents exists. It has been approved only for life-threatening ventricular arrhythmias. Nonetheless, it is often used for atrial or supraventricular arrhythmias. The half-life of the drug is extremely long (up to 120 days). Its long-term use is associated with many side effects, including visual disturbances, tremors and other neurologic sequelae, hepatitis, pulmonary fibrosis, photosensitivity, skin discoloration, thyroid abnormalities, and cardiac conduction disturbances. It is recommended that a **baseline eye examination, liver function tests, and thyroid function tests be obtained prior to initiation of therapy** with amiodarone. A chest x-ray is also advisable.

(iii) **Ibutilide** is the newest agent to be approved for the therapy of AF. The incidence of torsades de pointes [see III.A.6.c(1)(b)] is at least 1% to 2% with ibutilide, considerably higher than that seen with procainamide or amiodarone. **Dofetilide,** a medication similar to ibutilide, is currently being evaluated for this same purpose.

(c) A number of **oral agents** are available for the chemical cardioversion of AF. **Both amiodarone and procainamide are available in oral forms. These two agents are effective and in common use. Procainamide is less well tolerated for long-term use. Below are other agents for the use in treating AF.**

(i) **Sotalol** is a class III agent with β-blocking properties, which makes it useful as a **single-agent therapy for virtually all arrhythmias.** It has the additional advantages of being generally well tolerated, although it causes prolongation of the QT interval, thus **predisposing to torsades de pointes.** Its use is limited by side effects related to its β-blocking properties, such as exacerbation of reactive airway disease, depression, and negative inotropy. **Initiation of sotalol therapy should be in an inpatient setting with close monitoring of the QTs.**

(ii) **Flecainide** and **propafenone** are class IC agents that may be useful in AF. Flecainide was shown in the Cardiac Arrhythmia Suppression Trial (CAST) to be associated with increased mortality when used for the treatment and suppression of ventricular arrhythmias in patients after myocardial infarction (MI). This has led to **much concern over the use of this class of antiarrhythmics in patients with underlying CAD.** In general, they are well-tolerated medications in the appropriate patients, but should not be used in patients with CAD or any other structural heart disease

(iii) **Disopyramide** is a class IA antiarrhythmic similar to procainamide and quinidine. However, its **negative inotropic effects** are greater than those of other class IA drugs. It is also associated with **greater anticholinergic effects,** such as constipation and urinary retention, which may limit its use in older patients.

  (iv) **Moricizine** is a class I antiarrhythmic with properties from several of the subtypes (A, B, etc.). Its use should be **restricted to those patients without known or suspected CAD.**

  (v) **Quinidine is used with decreasing frequency, although it remains the most commonly used drug** for the conversion of AF and maintenance of sinus rhythm. It interacts with many drugs, including some commonly used for AF such as digoxin, warfarin, and verapamil. Although it is attractive because of its **low cost and less negative inotropic effects,** its **high incidence of side effects** (particularly GI intolerance, neurologic side effects, and hematologic suppressive effects), its **proarrhythmic potential, and frequent dosing** make other agents more desirable.

(3) Pacemakers

  (a) **Symptomatic refractory AF** is amenable to ablation of the atrioventricular node and implantation of a **rate-responsive permanent pacemaker. These patients still require systemic anticoagulation.** This approach is most appropriate for **patients who have frequent symptomatic recurrences related to rapid ventricular response.**

  (b) **Indications for permanent pacemaker for AF.** A permanent pacemaker may need to be considered in patients who become symptomatically bradycardic with therapy for AF. It is now possible to implant these devices with mode switching capabilities, so that the pacing mode changes from dual-chamber to single-chamber pacing at the onset of AF to avoid high heart rates due to the pacemaker responding to the atrial activity.

(4) An implantable atrial defibrillator is under investigation and is based on the success that has been proven in ventricular arrhythmias. Indeed, internal cardioversion of the atria via percutaneously directed transvenous devices has been very successful. However, implantable devices remain experimental at this time.

(5) Invasive therapy. These approaches have not gained widespread acceptance and are perhaps **best reserved for the patient who is undergoing other cardiac surgery** for another reason (valve repair, coronary artery bypass grafting, etc.). Various catheter-based therapies, such as atrioventricular nodal modification and catheter-directed maze procedures, are being investigated at present.

  (a) The **maze procedure** is the surgical approach that addresses most thoroughly the concerns about thromboembolic risk and normal hemodynamics. During the maze procedure, the atria are partitioned through a series of incisions, carefully placed to channel the atrial activity and prevent reentry. The maze procedure still carries with it a **high rate of complications, such as the need for a permanent pacemaker.**

  (b) The **corridor procedure,** developed earlier, sought to isolate both atria, as well as to create a corridor of conducting tissue from the sinoatrial node to the atrioventricular node. The thromboembolic risk does not lessen with this approach and does not restore normal hemodynamics.

(c) The **left atrial isolation procedure** was one of the first surgical approaches to AF. It involves isolating the fibrillating atrium from the rest of the heart, allowing normal hemodynamic transport in the right atrium and allowing chronotropic response during exercise. This does not eliminate the thromboembolic risk.

7. **Postoperative AF. Cardiac surgery, particularly valve surgery, is a unique risk factor for AF.** No single factor other than age has been consistently shown to predict the occurrence of postoperative AF. Mitral valve surgery increases the risk of postoperative AF more than any other type of cardiac surgery. Atrial fibrillation tends to occur during the first 2 to 3 days following surgery.

a. **Therapy.** The standard AF management is employed in the postoperative setting. **The risk of anticoagulation is greater in the postoperative period. Direct current cardioversion remains the most effective therapy,** with a success rate of 67% to 95%. Internal cardioversion (and possibly cardioversion via epicardial leads) increases the success rate to 91% to 96%. There is **no role for atrial overdrive pacing in the prevention of postoperative AF.** Many patients have asymptomatic AF and do not have sustained recurrence after DCC. Patients who are symptomatic, or those in whom AF recurs after cardioversion, should be considered for maintenance drug therapy as well as anticoagulation. This therapy should probably be continued for 3 to 6 weeks, though there is a paucity of data regarding the optimal length of drug therapy.

b. **Prevention.** Preoperative treatment with β-blockers has consistently been shown to reduce the incidence of postoperative AF. **Sotalol** has similarly been shown to be effective in a limited number of trials. **Amiodarone** has been recently shown to be effective as prophylaxis for postoperative AF.

8. **Atrial fibrillation in acute MI.** Patients with AF in the setting of an acute MI have a worse outcome at 30 days as compared to those in sinus rhythm. New-onset AF at the time of presentation with MI is associated with three-vessel disease, reduced TIMI (Thrombolysis in MI trial) flow, older age, renal insufficiency, and higher Killip class values. Patients with higher Killip class values and higher heart rates are at increased risk for developing AF after an MI. Thus, the presence of **AF in MI patients is an ominous marker for adverse events.**

9. **Atrial fibrillation and Wolff-Parkinson-White syndrome.** Patients with Wolff-Parkinson-White syndrome who develop AF are particularly vulnerable to ventricular fibrillation and sudden death. Atrial fibrillation can cause extremely rapid conduction over the accessory pathway. It is not always clear whether the AF is independent of Wolff-Parkinson-White syndrome or is due to other causes, such as the cycle length of the tachycardia or some electrophysiologic characteristic of the accessory pathway. The management of AF in patients with Wolff-Parkinson-White syndrome is discussed in further detail in III:A.6.b.(10).

C. **Atrial flutter.** Atrial flutter is the **second most common of the atrial tachyarrhythmias.** Atrial flutter is an inherently unstable rhythm, which generally is seen to revert either to sinus rhythm or to AF. Its reported incidence varies from 0.4% to 1.2% of hospital ECGs. The **clinical significance of atrial flutter is generally due to its association with AF** (with all of the attendant risks of AF) and/or its association with rapid rates of ventricular response.

1. **Clinical presentation.** The clinical presentation may vary widely, depending on the presence of underlying heart disease, the rate of

ventricular response, and the overall condition of the patient. It is **occasionally reported to persist for days** and, less commonly, for weeks or more. Careful examination of the jugular venous pulse may reveal **frequent, regular *a* waves** that correspond to the atrial flutter rate. Like AF, it is **commonly seen after open heart surgery, as well as with other conditions commonly associated with AF,** such as pulmonary disease, thyrotoxicosis, atrial enlargement due to any cause including mitral/tricuspid valve disease, and sinus node dysfunction.

2. **Pathophysiology.** Atrial flutter is the **result of reentry in the right atrium.** It is rarely the result of left atrial reentry.

   a. In **typical flutter the reentrant circuit travels in a counterclockwise rotation** down the right atrial free wall and up the interatrial septum. **It travels in a clockwise fashion around this same path in atypical flutter.**

   b. **Atrial flutter has been classified more recently** into type I and type II based on the following characteristics.

      (1) **Type I** atrial flutter can be terminated with rapid atrial pacing and typically has an atrial rate in the range of 240 to 340 bpm in the absence of drug therapy.

      (2) **Type II** atrial flutter cannot be terminated with rapid atrial pacing and typically has an atrial rate in the range of 340 to 430 bpm in the absence of drug therapy.

      (3) **Type I and II are not synonymous with typical and atypical.** Type I atrial flutter can include typical and atypical atrial flutter. Type II atrial flutter is less well characterized than type I with respect to etiology and therapy; thus **we refer to type I atrial flutter throughout this discussion.**

   c. There is **debate as to whether atrial flutter presents a significant risk for thromboembolism.**

3. **Laboratory examination**

   a. The **diagnosis can be difficult when the atrioventricular blockade is 2:1,** as the flutter waves may be superimposed on the QRS complex and/or the T waves. When the diagnosis is uncertain, one should **consider maneuvers or medications to slow the ventricular response,** thus revealing the atrial flutter complexes.

      (1) **Vagal maneuvers** include carotid sinus massage and Valsalva maneuver. **Caution must be exercised** in attempting carotid sinus massage **in patients with known or suspected carotid disease,** or vagal maneuvers in **patients with CAD who are at risk for ischemia.**

      (2) **Adenosine** can be administered, 6 mg rapid IV push, followed by 12 mg if there is no response (a second 12-mg dose can be given if there is no response). This will cause transient (lasting seconds), complete atrioventricular block. Alternative agents include the calcium channel blocking agents **verapamil and diltiazem,** and the β-blockers **esmolol and metoprolol.**

      (3) The clinician can place and record from a **transesophageal electrode** or record from a **temporary atrial epicardial pacing wire** (placed at open heart surgery). This results in an ECG with large atrial complexes and simplifies diagnosis. This strategy also allows a method of delivering rapid atrial pacing in an attempt to terminate the atrial flutter, as discussed in the section on therapy [II.C.4(2)].

   b. On the surface ECG, typical flutter shows the **classic negatively directed sawtooth waveform** in the inferior leads, II, III and aVF (Fig. 19-1). Conversely, the atrial depolarizations are positive in these leads in atypical flutter (Fig. 19-2).

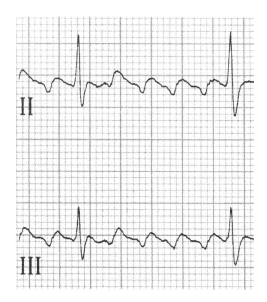

FIG. 19-1. "Typical" atrial flutter, leads II and III.

    c. In typical atrial flutter, **inverted F waves** ("sawteeth") appear in the inferior leads with constant morphology, polarity, and cycle length. No isoelectric baseline is present.

    d. The **atrial rate** in the absence of drug therapy is **240 to 340 bpm.**

    e. The **QRS complex should be the same as that seen during sinus rhythm,** although aberrant conduction may occur, and the QRS may be slightly distorted by the atrial flutter waves.

    f. The **ventricular response** can be irregularly irregular, due to varying degrees of block (2:1, 4:1, etc.), but is more **typically regular.**

4. Therapy

    a. Medical therapy differs very little from that for AF and is detailed in II.B.5.

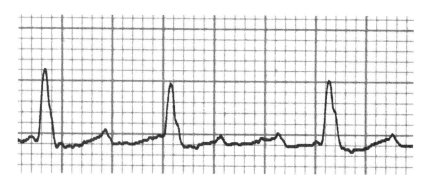

FIG. 19-2. "Atypical" flutter, lead II.

(1) **Control of the ventricular response rate with digoxin, a calcium channel blocker, or a β-blocker is critical prior to initiating therapy with agents such as the class IA or IC agents, class III agents, or moricizine.** These agents either enhance atrioventricular nodal conduction through their vagolytic effects, thus enabling 1:1 (A/V) conduction, or slow the atrial rate to a point where 1:1 conduction is possible.

(2) **The conversion from atrial flutter to AF after cardioversion is substantially lessened by the administration of class IA drugs** (quinidine, procainamide, and disopyramide) **prior to DCC, thus increasing the chance of converting to sinus.**

(3) **Anticoagulation.** At present, the decision to anticoagulate patients with atrial flutter prior to and after cardioversion **should be individualized for each patient,** based on his or her profile for thromboembolic risk.

b. **DCC**

(1) **Direct current cardioversion is the preferred and most effective therapy** for most patients. The procedure is detailed in Chapter 53. The starting energy can be as low as 25 to 50 J. Because DCC may result in conversion from atrial flutter to AF, a second shock is sometimes necessary to convert AF to sinus rhythm.

(2) **Rapid atrial pacing** should be considered as the **first line of therapy for all patients who have epicardial atrial pacing wires in place after open heart surgery.** It may be considered via a transesophageal pacing lead or via a transvenously placed pacing lead in patients who fail DCC or who are not candidates for DCC. **Before attempting to rapidly pace the atria, it must be confirmed that the ventricles are neither paced nor captured** by pacing at a safe rate while observing for such a phenomenon. Once this is confirmed, the atrium is paced at a rate of 10 to 20 bpm faster than the underlying atrial flutter rate. Once atria capture is attained, the rate is increased steadily until the hallmark negative-sawtooth waveform converts to a positive waveform. The pacing is then either halted abruptly or slowed rapidly to an acceptable atrial pacing rate. In cases that require extremely rapid rates (more than 400 bpm) of pacing or high amplitudes (more than 20 mA) of pacing stimulus strength, there is an increased tendency for the atrial flutter to convert to AF. **When pacing via a transesophageal lead, a stronger stimulus strength (up to 30 mA) might be necessary; this type of pacing can be quite painful,** so that a high enough energy to convert the atrial flutter should be used initially to minimize the number of attempts to do so.

(3) **Percutaneous therapy. Radiofrequency ablation is often curative,** with an efficacy as high as 95% for the long-term elimination of atrial flutter. It is performed by first mapping the atria during atrial flutter to identify the slow pathway in the reentrant circuit. This pathway is then ablated with radiofrequency energy. Confirmation of the absence of conduction through this pathway is then confirmed via pacing. **In patients in whom all other therapies fail, RFA of the atrioventricular node with subsequent placement of a dual-chamber permanent pacemaker** may offer the only solution.

D. **Sinus node reentry tachycardia** accounts for 5% to 10% of all supraventricular tachyarrhythmias. It is most frequently seen in patients with structural heart disease or CAD, especially in inferior MI.

1. **Clinical presentation.** The rate varies from 80 to 200 bpm.
2. **Pathophysiology.** The reentry occurs within the sinus node and then conducts via the normal conduction pathway to the rest of the heart. The morphology of the P wave is identical to the underlying sinus morphology. A block at the atrioventricular node may occur, but it does not slow the tachycardia. In fact, a Wenckebach-type block often occurs with this rhythm. The development of a bundle branch block does not affect the cycle length or the PR interval.
3. **Therapy. Vagal maneuvers or adenosine** may successfully terminate this arrhythmia. **Rapid atrial pacing** can be used to induce and terminate this tachycardia. Various agents such as β-blockers, calcium channel blockers, and digoxin may help to prevent recurrences. Sinus node ablation or modification is rarely necessary.

E. **Atrial tachycardias.** This term encompasses a number of different types of tachycardia that originate in the atria. These tachycardias account for between 10% and 15% of the tachycardias seen in older patients, usually in the setting of structural or ischemic heart disease, chronic obstructive pulmonary disease, electrolyte imbalances, or drug toxicity (particularly digitalis).

1. **Clinical presentation.** The episodes of these tachycardias are **typically paroxysmal,** but if incessant they can lead to a tachycardia-induced cardiomyopathy. These tachycardias are **infrequently seen in younger, healthy patients without underlying heart disease.**
2. **Laboratory examination and diagnostic testing**
   a. **ECG**
      (1) The **P-wave axis** or morphology is different from that of sinus rhythm.
      (2) **Atrial rhythm** is regular, except with automatic atrial tachycardia, which displays a warm-up period:(see II.E.3.b).
      (3) A **QRS complex that is generally identical to sinus rhythm** (QRS can be wide if aberrant conduction occurs) follows each P wave.
      (4) **PR interval** is within normal limits or prolonged.
      (5) **Nonspecific ST-T wave changes** may be present.
      (6) When an atrioventricular block is present, there is an **isoelectric baseline** between P waves in all leads.
   b. **Electrophysiologic study** has become critical in determining the underlying mechanism of these tachycardias, as the clinical differences are subtle and overlapping.
3. **Subclassifications.** The current subclassifications are **based on mechanisms** and include intraatrial reentry, automatic atrial tachycardia, and triggered atrial tachycardia.
   a. **Intraatrial reentry** is usually a disorder **seen in those with underlying heart disease or atrial arrhythmia history,** such as AF or atrial flutter. The mechanism is not well understood. The rate is typically 90 to 120 bpm due to the frequent occurrence of 2 : 1 atrioventricular blocks, such that hemodynamic effects are generally minimal. This rhythm can be difficult to distinguish from other supraventricular tachyarrhythmias. One clue is that despite any atrioventricular conduction block, the rhythm continues. The ability to terminate with adenosine and β-blockers is variable. **Radiofrequency ablation is the therapy of choice,** with success rates greater than 75%. **Antiarrhythmics** (the same drugs as for AF and atrial flutter) **have been disappointing in the prevention of recurrence,** though they may play a role in decreasing the frequency of recurrence.
   b. **Automatic atrial tachycardia** appears to be generated by an ectopic atrial focus, which is clustered around the crista terminalis in the right atrium and around the base of the pulmonary veins in

the left atrium. The mechanism is not well understood. Automatic atrial tachycardia is **seen more often in younger patients,** displays a **warm-up phenomenon** (the supraventricular tachyarrhythmia accelerates after its initiation), **does not respond to vagal maneuvers, and is more likely to be incessant.** Automatic atrial tachycardia can be induced with treadmill testing or with administration of isoproterenol. Atrial stimulation during electrophysiologic study has no effect on either initiating or terminating this arrhythmia. **Propranolol** has been used successfully to suppress automatic atrial tachycardia. **Catheter ablation is the preferred therapy when the tachycardia is incessant.** Although adenosine may transiently slow automatic atrial tachycardia, it is unlikely to terminate it. Likewise, verapamil has been used without success.

    c. **Triggered atrial tachycardia** is the least common of the atrial tachycardias and is virtually never incessant. It is more likely to appear in **older individuals.** It can be induced with rapid atrial pacing and is cycle length–dependent. The mechanism of triggered atrial tachycardia is thought to be due to delayed afterdepolarizations (see I.A.2) secondary to digitalis toxicity or sympathetic discharge. Catecholamines may play a role in the initiation of this arrhythmia, and thus exercise testing and isoproterenol may provoke it. Verapamil and adenosine have been shown to terminate triggered atrial tachycardia. β-blockers have been less efficacious. **RFA is preferred when the tachycardia is causing noticeable symptoms.**

F. Multifocal atrial tachycardia. This atrial arrhythmia is frequently **associated with concurrent pulmonary disease, particularly chronic obstructive pulmonary disease.** It may also be seen in CHF and can degenerate into AF. It is generally seen in adults of advanced age, though it may be seen in young patients. The atrial rate is generally 100 to 130 bpm, and the P wave is inconsistent, with three or more differing morphologies often noted. The atrioventricular interval and R-R intervals are variable. Loss of atrioventricular conduction of each P wave is infrequent, making it possible to distinguish multifocal atrial tachycardia from AF. **Therapy is directed at the underlying illness, with little role for antiarrhythmics.** Calcium channel blockers in high doses and amiodarone may be useful when antiarrhythmic therapy is deemed necessary. Maintenance of electrolyte balance, particularly potassium and magnesium, may suppress the occurrence of multifocal atrial tachycardia.

G. Atrioventricular nodal reentrant tachycardia and Atrioventricular reentrant tachycardia.

    1. **Clinical presentation.** Atrioventricular nodal reentrant tachycardia (AVNRT) is generally seen with subjects without underlying heart disease. Palpitations and anxiety are common presenting complaints. Angina, CHF, and even shock may be seen in those with a history of underlying heart disease. Syncope may occur due to rapid ventricular rates or due to the asystole or bradycardia often seen when this tachycardia terminates. It is a tachycardia with a narrow QRS complex and a ventricular rate typically in the range of 150 to 250 bpm, although faster rates are infrequently observed.

        Atrioventricular reentrant tachycardia (AVRT) is a narrow QRS tachycardia with ventricular rates similar to those of AVNRT, although it more often tends to have a ventricular rate greater than 200. The clinical features are very similar to those of AVNRT but are distinct on an electrophysiologic basis.

    2. **Pathophysiology**

      a. **Atrioventricular nodal reentrant tachycardia.** The mechanism in AVNRT appears to be a reentrant circuit composed of separate fast and slow atrial pathways into the atrioventricular node, or a slow pathway in the atrioventricular node and a fast pathway in an accessory pathway that traverses the atrioventricular groove. In 90% to 50% of patients with AVNRT, the antegrade conduction to the ventricles travels over the slow pathway and the retrograde conduction to the atria occurs over the fast pathway. The initiating event may be either an atrial premature complex (APC) or a ventricular premature complex (VPC). The APC blocks the fast pathway antegradely and conducts down the slow pathway, then back up the now repolarized fast pathway. Less commonly, a VPC conducts retrogradely to the atria via the fast pathway, then returns to the ventricles via the slow pathway. In the remaining 5% to 10% of patients, the antegrade conduction is down the fast pathway and retrograde via the slow pathway. The cycle length is thus dependent on the ability of the slow pathway to conduct, as the fast pathway generally has the ability at high rates and has a longer refractory period. Termination of the tachycardia is often the result of a block in the slow pathway. However, atrioventricular dissociation may develop during the tachycardia because the ventricles are not involved on the reentry circuit. This does not affect the rate of tachycardia, nor does the development of bundle branch block.

b. **Atrioventricular reentrant tachycardia.** The mechanism in AVRT relies on the presence of a concealed (not detectable with surface ECG) accessory pathway that conducts retrogradely to the atria from the ventricles. **(Unlike AVNRT, the circuit involves the ventricles; thus the development of bundle branch block can prolong the cycle length of the tachycardia if the block occurs in the ventricle in which the accessory pathway exists.)** Bundle branch block, particularly left bundle branch block (LBBB), occurs more commonly in AVRT than in AVNRT.

Atrioventricular reentrant tachycardia can be distinguished from AVNRT by electrophysiologic study. The presence of atrioventricular or ventricular-atrial block with continuation of the tachycardia should exclude the presence of an accessory atrioventricular pathway.

3. **Laboratory features and diagnosis**

   a. **Atrioventricular nodal reentrant tachycardia.** P waves are generally hidden within the QRS complex in a typical AVNRT, or visible as a small r' in lead V_1, as depolarization of the atria occurs simultaneously with ventricular depolarization. The RP segment is generally less than 100 milliseconds. AVNRT is often induced abruptly by a premature atrial beat and its termination, which also tends to be abrupt, is often followed by a retrograde P wave. The termination may be followed by a brief period of asystole or bradycardia before the sinus node recovers from its tachycardia-induced depression. The cycle length may vary, especially at the beginning and the end of the tachycardia. This variation reflects the variable antegrade atrioventricular nodal conduction time. Vagal maneuvers may slow or terminate this tachycardia.

   b. **Atrioventricular reentrant tachycardia.** The P waves of AVRT are frequently inscribed on the ST segment or T wave, as the atrial depolarization must occur after ventricular depolarization. The RP segment is generally greater than 100 milliseconds.

4. **Therapy**

   a. **Radiofrequency ablation** has become the mainstay of therapy for these arrhythmias, as the approach has the advantage of curing the arrhythmia and doing away with the need for long-term suppressive therapy with medications. Vagal maneuvers may slow down or terminate both AVNRT and AVRT, and there is little harm

in attempting them while awaiting the arrival of medications and other equipment.
   b. Medications that act at the atrioventricular node such as β-blockers, calcium channel blockers, digoxin, and adenosine all slow conduction in the antegrade slow pathway, whereas class Ia and Ic agents slow the conductions in the retrograde fast pathway. Adenosine may be considered as first-line drug therapy. The β-blockers or calcium channel blockers are alternatives if adenosine is unsuccessful. The onset of action of digoxin limits its usefulness in terminating these arrhythmias, though it may be useful to prevent recurrences. Recurrences may be prevented in patients with frequent sustained episodes with any of the above-named agents.
   c. Direct current cardioversion should be considered before employing further antiarrhythmias and should always be the immediate therapy for unstable or highly symptomatic patients. Low energies of 10 to 50 J are usually sufficient to terminate AVNRT.
   d. Only if DCC and the above measures fail should the class I or class III antiarrhythmics be considered. Also, if the patient is hypotensive, correction of this with pressor agents may help to terminate AVNRT.
H. Preexcitation syndromes (including the Wolff-Parkinson-White syndrome). The incidence of preexcitation on ECG is around 1.5 per 1,000, most of which occur in otherwise healthy subjects without organic heart disease. Seven to ten percent of these patients have associated Ebstein's anomaly and are thus more likely to have multiple accessory pathways. There is a higher rate of occurrence of preexcitation in males, and the prevalence decreases with age, although the frequency of paroxysmal tachycardia increases with age.
   1. **Clinical presentation.** Approximately 50% to 60% of patients with preexcitation report symptoms such as **palpitations, anxiety, dyspnea, chest pain or tightness, and syncope.** Approximately 25% will become asymptomatic over time. Those over the age of 40 who have been asymptomatic are likely to remain symptom-free. The absence of preexcitation on ECG despite the discovery of accessory pathways in asymptomatic patients likely identifies a group of patients at low risk for developing symptoms.
   2. **Etiology.** Accessory pathways are likely congenital, as relatives of subjects with preexcitation have an increased incidence of preexcitation. Preexcitation may also be acquired.
   3. **Pathophysiology.** The underlying tachycardia is an atrioventricular reentrant tachycardia 80% to 85% of the time, with 15% to 40% of patients developing AF (see II.B) and 5% atrial flutter (II.C). VT is uncommon.
      a. Wolff-Parkinson-White syndrome. The basic abnormality lies in the existence of an accessory pathway of conducting tissue, outside of the normal conducting system, which connects the atria and ventricles. This accessory pathway permits the atrial impulse to bypass the normal pathway through the atrioventricular node to the ventricles and permits the ventricular impulse to activate the atria. These accessory pathways are frequently referred to as bundles of Kent. An impulse from the atria can conduct down both the accessory pathway and the atrioventricular node, arriving at the ventricle at nearly the same time. This results in widening of the QRS complex, analogous to a fusion beat, as a portion of the ventricle is activated via the accessory pathway (giving rise to the delta wave; Fig. 19-3) and the remainder of the ventricle is activated by the normal activation pathway. If antegrade conduction occurs exclusively via the accessory pathway, the resultant QRS is maximally preexcited and wide. These accessory pathways conduct rapidly, but

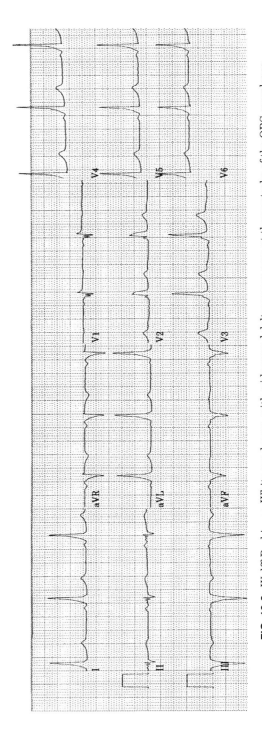

FIG. 19-3. Wolff-Parkinson-White syndrome, with widespread delta waves seen at the upstroke of the QRS complexes.

frequently have longer refractory periods than the atrioventricular node. The inciting event for AVRT is frequently an atrial premature beat that encounters a block in the accessory pathway and conducts to the ventricles via the atrioventricular node, which has recovered more rapidly. The resultant QRS complex in this instance is normal in appearance. After the QRS complex, the accessory pathway has had sufficient time to recover excitability and the impulse thus conducts retrogradely to the atria. Termed **orthodromic atrioventricular reciprocating tachycardia, this is the most common mechanism of reentry** in Wolff-Parkinson-White syndrome, accounting for approximately 97% of the reciprocating atrioventricular tachycardias. **Atrioventricular tachycardia** occurs when the antegrade circuit is the accessory pathway and the retrograde circuit is the atrioventricular node. A ventricular premature beat can also incite reentry by conducting retrogradely to the atria via the accessory pathway, followed by antegrade conduction via the atrioventricular nodal system. A small but significant percentage (5% to 10%) of patients have multiple accessory pathways.

b. **Permanent atrioventricular junctional reentrant tachycardia** is a variant form of preexcitation. It is often an incessant supraventricular tachyarrhythmia with an unusual form of accessory pathway. Here the accessory pathway behaves like the atrioventricular node in that it displays decremental conduction properties. Thus, the faster the stimulation of such an accessory pathway, the slower the conduction through the pathway. The accessory pathway is most often located in the posteroseptal region and acts as the retrograde limb of the reentrant circuit. The ventricular-atrial conduction is slowed by the decremental nature of the accessory pathway and by the long, circuitous route from the ventricle to the atrium. Due to the incessant nature of this tachycardia, a tachycardia-induced cardiomyopathy may result.

c. **Mahaim reentrant tachycardia** is another variant form of reentry. Two varieties are recognized: **atriofascicular and fasciculoventricular.** In the former, the accessory pathway is located within a few centimeters of the atrioventricular node and inserts into the right bundle branch. The reentrant tachycardia conducts antegrade via the accessory pathway, resulting in an LBBB morphology with left axis deviation. The retrograde circuit is via the atrioventricular node. In the second form of Mahaim reentry, the accessory pathway arises in the His-Purkinje fibers and allows bypass of the distal conducting system.

4. **Laboratory examination and diagnostic testing**
   a. **If an AVRT occurs in a patient with the following ECG criteria, the diagnosis of Wolff-Parkinson-White syndrome is established.**
      (1) The PR interval is short, typically less than 120 milliseconds.
      (2) The QRS complex exceeds 120 milliseconds, with some leads showing the characteristic slurred upstroke known as a delta wave (see Fig. 19-3), and a normal terminal QRS portion.
      (3) The ST-T segment is directed opposite to the major delta and QRS vectors.
   b. The most commonly seen tachycardia in Wolff-Parkinson-White syndrome is characterized by a normal QRS with a regular rate of 150 to 250 bpm. Onset and termination are abrupt.
   c. **Localization of accessory pathway.** The **surface ECG** may provide information that allows localization of the accessory pathway. The simplest classification is that of type A or B. **Type A** has a large R wave in lead V_1. It is due to a left-sided accessory pathway, which permits preexcitation to the posterobasilar segment of the left ventricle. **Type**

B has an S or QS in V_1, and is due to a right-sided accessory pathway. When present, the morphology of a retrograde P wave can be helpful in predicting the location of the accessory pathway. A positive P wave in V_1 during supraventricular tachyarrhythmia suggests a left free wall pathway, whereas a negative P wave suggests a right-sided pathway. More elaborate algorithms for localization are available. The **most precise localization method is electrophysiologic study** with ventricular pacing.

   d. **Risk stratification is necessary** for patients with preexcitation. The appearance or disappearance of preexcitation on **serial ECGs is of no predictive value.** However, **the intermittent loss or appearance of preexcitation on a beat-to-beat basis is indicative of higher risk.** Exercise testing may be helpful if the preexcitation disappears abruptly during exercise (low risk of future events) or if preexcitation persists throughout exercise (high risk). Unfortunately, these are uncommon findings during exercise testing. As the greatest danger to patients with preexcitation may be the development of AF, **the induction of AF may be most useful in risk stratification.** This can be done via transesophageal pacing. Risk stratification with medications is of no value at present.

5. **Therapy**
   a. **Emergency management of acute tachycardic episodes. A patient demonstrating hemodynamic instability or extreme symptomatology should be cardioverted rapidly.** Stable patients may be treated medically.
      (1) **If the QRS is of normal duration,** attempts to slow the atrioventricular nodal conduction are appropriate. **Vagal maneuvers are a logical first step. Adenosine** is frequently successful in terminating these tachycardias, as is **verapamil.** Amiodarone may also be considered. Atrial pacing, either transvenous or transesophageal, is also quite efficacious for terminating these types of tachycardia. DCC is rarely necessary but is frequently successful at low energies.
      (2) **If the QRS is wide, IV procainamide** is recommended (IV forms of amiodarone, flecainide, sotalol, and propafenone have all demonstrated usefulness, although only amiodarone is available in the United States). **Lidocaine, calcium channel blockers, β-blockers, and digoxin should be avoided,** as their efficacy is low and they may accelerate the ventricular response rate, precipitating VF. **If the tachycardia persists, synchronized DCC** is the treatment of choice. Energies of at least 200 J are likely to be required.
      (3) If the patient develops AF, it has been observed that **definitive therapy for the atrioventricular reentrant circuit, such as ablation of the accessory pathway, often results in termination of AF.**
   b. **Long-term management**
      (1) **Priority of therapy.** Patients who are asymptomatic when diagnosed are at low risk of sudden death. As such, it may not be justified to pursue medical or ablative therapy in these patients unless there is a family history of sudden death, or the patients are competitive athletes or are in a high-risk occupation. Patients who are symptomatic or who have a history of AF of aborted sudden death are at higher risk and warrant intervention.
      (2) **Medical therapy.** Medical therapy may be **appropriate for those with increased risk but no prior symptoms, those with accessory pathways located near the normal conduction pathway who might develop atrioventricular**

block with RFA, or those at increased risk from invasive procedures. Single-drug therapy may be attempted with **amiodarone, sotalol, flecainide, or propafenone.** These drugs work to slow conduction in both the accessory pathway and the atrioventricular node. **Combination therapy** can be accomplished with drugs that work on the atrioventricular node (calcium channel blockers, β-blockers) with drugs that work exclusively on the accessory pathway (class IA antiarrhythmics).

(3) **Percutaneous therapy.** Radiofrequency ablation is effective 90% to 98% of the time, with a recurrence rate around 5% to 8%. It should be considered for any patient at high risk, for patients with symptoms or tachycardias refractory to medical therapy, or in those who have intolerant to medical therapy.

III. **Ventricular tachyarrhythmias.** Sudden cardiac deaths are most frequently due to ventricular tachyarrhythmias. It is estimated that up to half of all cardiac deaths are sudden; thus ventricular tachyarrhythmias may be responsible for almost half of all cardiac deaths.

A. **Ventricular tachycardia (VT).** Ventricular tachycardia is defined as three or more QRS complexes of ventricular origin at a rate exceeding 100 bpm. The various types of VT and their course of disease are discussed in III.A.6.

1. **Clinical presentation.** The presentation can be quite varied and depends on the clinical setting, the heart rate, and the presence of underlying heart disease and other medical conditions. Some patients are asymptomatic or minimally symptomatic, whereas others may present with syncope or sudden death. The loss of normal atrioventricular synchrony may cause symptoms in a patient with decreased cardiac function at baseline. Heart rates less than 150 bpm are surprisingly well tolerated in the short term, even in the most compromised individuals. Exposure to these rates for more than a few hours is likely to be associated with heart failure in patients with poor ventricular function, whereas those with normal ventricular function may tolerate prolonged periods at such rates. The range of 150 to 200 bpm is tolerated variably, according to the factors noted above. Once the rate reaches and exceeds 200 bpm, there are symptoms in virtually all patients. **Nonsustained VT** (NSVT) is generally defined as less than 30 seconds in duration, though some define it as less than 1 minute or less than 10 beats. Ventricular tachycardia is **generally very regular in rate and appearance,** though it can be polymorphic in appearance, slightly irregular with respect to rate, and may have capture and/or fusion beats within it.

2. **Differential diagnosis.** Ventricular tachycardia needs to be distinguished from **supraventricular tachyarrhythmia with aberrant intraventricular conduction, bundle branch block, and morphologic changes of the QRS complex secondary to metabolic derangement or pacing.**

a. **Brugada criteria.** Distinguishing VT from **supraventricular tachyarrhythmia with aberrancy** can be very challenging. Various criteria have been proposed. The **criteria of Brugada are most helpful in making this distinction and are both sensitive** (99%) **and specific** (96.5%) in patients without a preexisting bundle branch block. As shown in Fig. 19-4, a stepwise approach is applied. In the first step, the precordial leads are examined for the presence or absence of an RS complex. If an RS is uniformly absent, VT is established. If an RS is present in at least one precordial lead, one moves to the second step, which is measuring the interval from the onset of the QRS complex to the nadir of the S wave. If this distance is greater than 100 milliseconds in at least one precordial lead, then the diagnosis of VT is made. If there is no RS interval

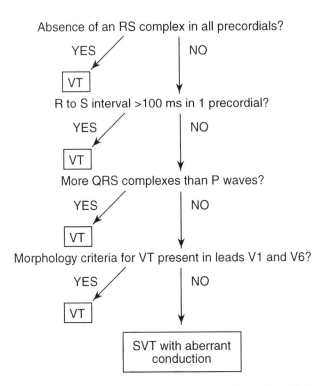

FIG. 19-4. Bruguda criteria for differentiating ventricular tachycardia from supraventricular tachycardia with aberrant intraventricular conduction.

greater than 100 milliseconds, the third step is used. In the third step, evidence for atrioventricular dissociation is looked for. If there are more QRS complexes than P waves, then the diagnosis is VT. If not, then one moves to the fourth step, which involves examining the morphology of the QRS in the precordial leads V_1 and V_6. If the morphology criteria for VT (Fig. 19-5) are present in these leads, then the diagnosis of VT is established. If not, the diagnosis is supraventricular tachyarrhythmia with aberrant intraventricular conduction.

b. The Brugada criteria have been further refined to distinguish between VT and supraventricular tachyarrhythmia with antegrade conduction over an accessory pathway. After applying the above criteria, a second stepwise algorithm is applied (Fig. 19-6). This **second algorithm has a sensitivity of 75% and a specificity of 100% to diagnose VT and exclude preexcited tachycardia.** In the first step, leads V_4 to V_6 are examined to see if the QRS is predominantly negative in these leads. If so, then VT is favored. If not, then the second step, examining leads V_2 to V_6 for the presence of a QR complex in one or more of these leads, is applied. If there is a QR complex in any of these leads, then the diagnosis is VT. The third criterion, presence of atrioventricular dissociation, is 100% specific for VT. If there is no atrioventricular dissociation, then supra-

1. QRS width > 0.14 s
2. Superior QRS axis
3. Morphology in precordial leads:

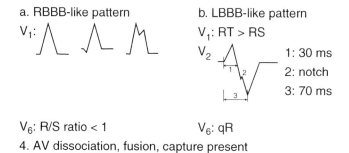

a. RBBB-like pattern

V_1:

b. LBBB-like pattern

V_1: RT > RS

V_2

1: 30 ms
2: notch
3: 70 ms

V_6: R/S ratio < 1

V_6: qR

4. AV dissociation, fusion, capture present

FIG. 19-5. Classic morphology criteria for ventricular tachycardia.

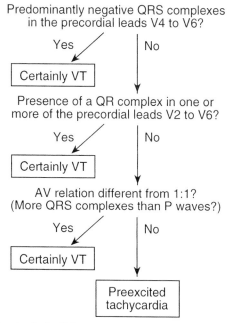

Predominantly negative QRS complexes
in the precordial leads V4 to V6?

Yes

No

Certainly VT

Presence of a QR complex in one or
more of the precordial leads V2 to V6?

Yes

No

Certainly VT

AV relation different from 1:1?
(More QRS complexes than P waves?)

Yes

No

Certainly VT

Preexcited
tachycardia

FIG. 19-6. Bruguda criteria for differentiating ventricular tachycardia from antidromic tachycardia over an accessory pathway.

ventricular tachyarrhythmia with antegrade accessory pathway conduction is favored.

3. **Therapy**

   a. **Priority of therapy.** A patient who has no hemodynamic compromise can be treated medically, at least initially. As with most types of tachyarrhythmias, **the treatment of any unstable patient with VT is rapid DCC.** Current guidelines for advanced cardiac life support (ACLS) from the American Heart Association call for early DCC, with initiation of drug therapy, followed, if necessary, by a repeated DCC for those who fail to respond to initial DCC.

   b. **Medical therapy. Intravenous lidocaine or procainamide** may be given initially. **Intravenous amiodarone** should **be considered early in the treatment of ventricular arrhythmias,** especially if the above agents are unsuccessful in terminating VT. Whenever possible, a **reversible cause for VT** should be sought. Elimination of **ischemia** is the best therapy for the VT associated with ischemia. Correction of **electrolyte abnormalities** may terminate VT. **Bradycardia** may cause frequent premature ventricular contractions or VT. Maneuvers and agents that increase heart rate should be employed for these bradycardias. **Hypotension** should be promptly corrected. Therapy for CHF should be optimized with the agents known to promote survival in this disorder. **Offending agents** should be stopped whenever possible, and **antidotes** should be administered in the case of overdosage and poisoning.

   c. **Direct current cardioversion. Rapid DCC is used on unstable patients,** with at least 100 J of electricity. The treatment of pulseless VT is unsynchronized DCC with a starting energy of 200 J. If the patient is conscious but has unstable vital signs or is extremely symptomatic, **synchronized DCC** is recommended.

4. **Prevention and prophylactic treatment.** Since the CAST trial data have become available, there has been a shift away from the use of class I agents and toward the **use of class III agents for prophylactic maintenance therapy** of VT. The development of **curative catheter-based therapies and surgical procedures** has lessened the role of antiarrhythmics in the prevention of recurrence. Foci of abnormal or enhanced automaticity, as well as reentrant circuits, should be ablated or resected when possible. The greatest impact on survival in sudden death has been made by the implantation of **automated cardiac defibrillators.**

   a. **Medical therapy**

      (1) Although drug therapy continues to have a role in the prevention of VT and sudden death, this role has become more limited. The Electrophysiologic Studies versus Electrocardiographic Monitoring (ESVEM) trial studied the efficacy of 7 antiarrhythmics (imipramine, mexilitene, pirmenol, procainamide, propafenone, quinidine, and sotalol) in preventing the recurrence of sustained VT. Sotalol was seen to be the most effective, although even with sotalol, the recurrence rate was disappointing. The European Myocardial Infarct Amiodarone Trial (EMIAT) and the Canadian Amiodarone Myocardial Infarction Arrhythmia Trial (CAMIAT) investigations were designed to study the effectiveness of empiric amiodarone for the prevention of VT after MI. Although both of these trials showed a decrease in arrhythmic deaths, no survival benefit was obtained. Thus the **role of antiarrhythmics remains uncertain,** and their use as the sole method of recurrence prevention should be questioned.

(2) **Combination therapy.** Drug therapy is becoming **an adjunct to implantable cardiac defibrillator therapy** in this high-risk population. At present, fully half of those with implantable cardiac defibrillators remain on antiarrhythmic therapy. The rationales for this combined therapy include preventing atrial tachyarrhythmias and decreasing the frequency of VT, and thus the frequency of implantable cardiac defibrillator discharge.

(3) **Calcium channel blockers** are primarily used in the treatment of supraventricular tachyarrhythmia. However, some of the idiopathic monomorphic VTs described in III.A.6 (the VTs originating in the right ventricular outflow tract [RVOT], with LBBB morphology, and VTs originating in the left ventricular apex, with right bundle branch block, or RBBB, morphology) and the VTs of digitalis toxicity are responsive to calcium channel blocking agents such as verapamil and diltiazem. Radiofrequency ablation is potentially curative for idiopathic VTs and should be considered despite effective termination with calcium channel blockers.

b. **Percutaneous therapy**

(1) **Implantable cardiac defibrillators.** Two large trials comparing implantable cardiac defibrillators with amiodarone in high-risk patients with prior infarction, the Multicenter Automatic Defibrillator Implantation Trial (MADIT) and the Antiarrhythmics versus Implantable Defibrillator (AVID) trial, have recently been completed. High risk implies either an ejection fraction of 35% or less or the presence of inducible sustained VT at electrophysiologic study. Both trials showed a **decided advantage for implantable cardiac defibrillators,** with 30% to 50% reductions in mortality with implantable cardiac defibrillators. In fact, the AVID trial found no survival benefit from amiodarone, β-blockers, or any other antiarrhythmic. Newer implantable cardiac defibrillators often have antitachycardia pacing capabilities, can recognize monomorphic ventricular rhythms with rates of less than 200 bpm, and can rapidly pace the ventricles to restore sinus rhythm, aborting the need for countershock (see Chapter 21).

(2) **Catheter-based therapy.** Radiofrequency ablation is used to eliminate the slow conducting pathway in a reentrant circuit. The success in eliminating VT has ranged from 50% to 70% to date; however, this is likely to improve with upgrades in the delivery technology. Until the technique is more reliable, it will likely serve as an adjunct to implantable cardiac defibrillators to prevent frequent firings.

5. **Types of VT and their course of disease.** The clinical presentation and course of VT can be divided into VT related to ischemia and nonischemic VT, including **torsades de pointes.**

a. **Ischemic VT**

(1) **Etiology and pathophysiology.** At the cellular level, ischemia may alter action potentials, prolong refractoriness of cells, and uncouple the cell-to-cell propagation of depolarization. The biochemical milieu in which the cells exist with respect to ion concentrations, acid–base balance, etc., can be altered. Also, the damage of infarction is inhomogeneous. Thus, scar tissue and functioning tissue are admixed in the region of the infarction. A reentrant circuit requires two functionally distinct pathways with unidirectional block in one pathway and slowed conduction down a second pathway. The changes associated with ischemia provide the anatomic substrate for reentry.

The VT of ischemia tends to be **polymorphic** in character. Ischemia has been shown to prolong the QT interval in some subjects, often with associated T-wave inversion. The **QT interval in ischemic-mediated polymorphic VT is not as prolonged** as that in torsades de pointes, another polymorphic VT. Ischemia is by far the **most common cause of polymorphic VT with normal QT interval.**

(2) **Predictors of VT.** As might be expected, **larger infarcts with greater resultant impairment of left ventricular systolic function** are more likely to be associated with VT. In fact, left ventricular systolic function is the single most important predictor of sudden death due to arrhythmia. Similarly, the presence of an **open artery appears to reduce the occurrence of VT and other arrhythmias.** Other proposed predictors include syncope, abnormal signal averaged ECG (SAECG), NSVT, absence of heart rate variability, abnormal electrophysiologic study, and possibly T-wave alternans.

(3) **Laboratory examination and diagnostic testing.** The various noninvasive tests for risk stratification (SAECG, heart rate variability, T-wave alternans, etc.) have shown poor specificity for VT and poor positive predictive value for VT, **and thus should not be used alone to guide therapy.** The decision to proceed to **electrophysiologic study** should be based on the combination of clinical grounds, results of left ventricular function testing, and noninvasive testing.

(4) **Accelerated idioventricular rhythm** (Fig. 19-7) is a form of VT seen almost exclusively in ischemic heart disease, particularly during an MI or after reperfusion of an occluded territory. It may also be seen with digitalis toxicity. The accelerated idioventricular rhythm often seen **after MI is rarely of clinical significance.**

(a) **The ECG features** include regular or slightly irregular ventricular rhythm, rate of 60 to 110 bpm, a QRS morphology resembling that of premature ventricular complexes, and, often, atrioventricular dissociation as well as fusion beats and capture beats.

(b) **Pathophysiology.** The ectopic ventricular pacing focus competes with the sinus node and usurps control of the ventricular rate when the sinus rate slows or when sinoatrial or atrioventricular block occurs. Enhanced automaticity is the likely underlying mechanism.

(c) Accelerating the sinus rhythm with atropine or atrial pacing can be useful to suppress the accelerated idioventricular rhythm. **Therapy is rarely necessary unless** the loss of atrioventricular synchrony results in hemodynamic compromise, a more rapid VT intervenes, the accelerated idioventricular rhythm falls on the T wave of the preceding beat (R on T phenomenon), the ventricular rate is rapid enough to produce symptoms, or VF occurs.

b. **Nonischemic VT.** This category includes bundle branch reentry, VT originating in the RVOT, VT originating in the left ventricular apex, congenital long QT syndrome and other genetically associated VT, idiopathic polymorphic VT, drug-induced VT, arrhythmogenic right ventricular dysplasia, Wolff-Parkinson-White syndrome, and the VTs associated with various inflammatory and infectious conditions.

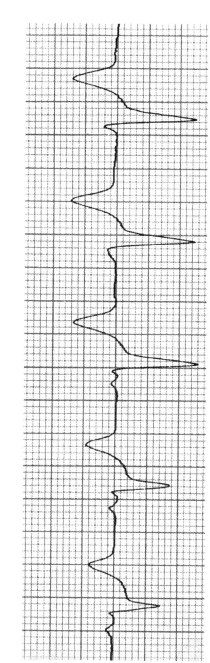

FIG. 19-7. Accelerated idioventricular rhythm (beats 3 through 5), interspersed with normal sinus rhythm (beats 1 and 2), lead IV.

(1) **Drug-induced VT. Drugs are a well-known cause of VT,** both polymorphic and monomorphic. This is particularly true in ischemic or infarcted hearts. Phenothiazines, tricyclic antidepressants, digitalis, epinephrine, cocaine, nicotine, alcohol, and glue (inhaled) are some of the wide variety of drugs that have been implicated in the development of monomorphic VT. The CAST and other trials of the late 1980s showed an increase in mortality from the use of class I antiarrhythmic agents employed to suppress asymptomatic ventricular ectopy after MI. NSVT and depressed left ventricular function remain risk factors for sudden death, and the agents studied in CAST did decrease the occurrence of ventricular ectopy; however, it is believed that these drugs (flecainide, encainide, and moricizine) generated VT, causing sudden death in recipients. These agents have in common their sodium channel blocking activities. Other drugs in this class, including procainamide, quinidine, disopyramide, lidocaine, tocainide, and mexiletine, have all been shown either experimentally or clinically to be associated with increased mortality compared with controls in the periinfarction period. The results of CAST caused a major shift away from the sodium channel blocking agents (class I antiarrhythmics) in the periinfarction period.

(2) The generation of torsades de pointes due to effects on the QT interval is discussed in III.A.2.c.

(3) **Digitalis toxicity can propagate delayed afterdepolarizations,** which generate action potentials, leading to VT. The VT of digitalis toxicity is typically monomorphic and often responds to calcium channel blockers. Rarely, digitalis toxicity manifests as a bidirectional VT, meaning that it has a regular rhythm with an axis that alternates from –60 to –90 degrees to +120 to +130 degrees, with a ventricular rate from 140 to 200 bpm. Because digitalis toxicity may have a narrow QRS complex and may respond to calcium channel blockers, it may be confused with supraventricular tachyarrhythmia. This type of VT is best treated by removing the offending agent, digoxin, with its binding antibody. The treatment for digitalis toxicity is the same in the face of bidirectional VT.

(4) **Bundle branch reentry is commonly seen in patients with dilated cardiomyopathy.** The presence of underlying His-Purkinje system disease and intraventricular conduction delay on surface ECG are universal findings in patients with bundle branch reentry. This form of VT typically has a LBBB morphology, although the less common forms may have a RBBB morphology. The mechanism in the most common form involves antegrade conduction over the right bundle and retrograde conduction via the left bundle. The VT of bundle branch reentry tends to be 200 bpm or greater. The diagnosis needs to be confirmed by electrophysiologic study, although it may be suspected clinically.

(5) **Idiopathic VT** occurs in otherwise structurally normal hearts with no significant CAD, no family history of arrhythmia or sudden death, and normal surface ECGs. It may be of LBBB morphology or RBBB morphology.

   (a) The **VT of RVOT** origin is typically a monomorphic VT with a LBBB morphology and inferior rightward axis. This is likely a VT secondary to abnormal impulse formation and may be triggered by delayed afterdepolarizations, perhaps during exercise or other periods of increased adrenergic stimulation. As such, it is often responsive to calcium channel blockers, which may lead to its being mistaken for supraventricular tachyarrhythmia. Other agents that may prove useful include β-blockers and class IA, IC, and III antiarrhythmics. **Adenosine** has often proven efficacious in terminating these VTs, which suggests that cAMP may be a mediator in the sustainment of this type of VT. This fact may also lead to misinterpretation of the VT as a supraventricular tachyarrhythmia.

- (b) **Repetitive monomorphic VT is a subtype of RVOT** and has all of the properties of RVOT already discussed. It is generally not associated with any risk of sudden death; thus **therapy is undertaken only to alleviate symptoms. Catheter ablation** is often successful in curing these forms of VT.

- (c) **Ventricular tachycardia of left ventricular apex origin** is a second type of **monomorphic VT that occurs in otherwise normal hearts.** It has a RBBB morphology with a superior axis. It is also often **responsive to calcium channel blockers.** It most likely is a reentrant VT that originates in the left-sided His-Purkinje system, resulting in a fascicular tachycardia. When incessant, this type of VT **can lead to tachycardia-induced cardiomyopathy.** It is possible to cure this type of VT with catheter-based ablation, although this represents a complex ablation procedure.

- (d) Less commonly, **monomorphic VTs occur in normal hearts** that are not typified by the characteristics of RBBB-shaped or LBBB-shaped VT. These, too, often respond to β-blockers and calcium channel blockers.

(6) **Both dilated cardiomyopathy and hypertrophic cardiomyopathy have increased risk of VT and sudden death.**

- (a) **Dilated cardiomyopathy.** It is particularly difficult to predict which patients with dilated cardiomyopathy are at increased risk for sudden death, as SAECG and electrophysiologic study are not reliable predictors in this population, and asymptomatic ventricular arrhythmias are common. The current recommendations are to place implantable cardiac defibrillators in patients with dilated cardiomyopathy who manifest life-threatening arrhythmias, although ablation may be curative if bundle branch reentry is the mechanism.

- (b) **Hypertrophic cardiomyopathy.** Supraventricular tachyarrhythmia and AF are particularly poorly tolerated by these patients, as is ischemia, and may lead to VT. Electrophysiologic study may be helpful in stratifying risk for VT and sudden death. Patients at low risk with hypertrophic cardiomyopathy include those with infrequent or brief episodes that are asymptomatic or mildly symptomatic. Patients at higher risk include those with syncope, a family history of sudden death in first-degree relatives, or the presence of NSVT on ambulatory ECG recordings. **Amiodarone** may be beneficial in this population, as may **Dual-chamber pacing,** which tends to decrease the outflow gradient.

(7) **Muscular dystrophies, particularly Duchenne's muscular dystrophy and myotonic dystrophy, have been associated with frequent defects** in the conduction system. Heart block and bundle branch block as well as sudden death due to ventricular tachyarrhythmias are well-recognized complications of these muscular disorders.

(8) **Structural abnormalities** such as **repaired tetralogy of Fallot and mitral valve prolapse** have been associated with increased risk of VT and sudden death. In tetralogy of Fallot, the VT often originates in the RVOT, at the site of a previous repair. It can be cured by catheter ablation or surgical resection. Mitral valve prolapse has been uncommonly linked to sudden death, though ventricular arrhythmias are not uncommon. **The prognosis with respect to VT is quite good in mitral valve prolapse.**

(9) **Arrhythmogenic right ventricular dysplasia** is a cardiomyopathy that begins in the right ventricle and often progresses to involve the left ventricle. It results in right ventricular dilatation with resultant poor contractile function. The right ventricular muscle becomes increasingly replaced by adipose and fibrous tissue as the disease progresses. Ventricular tachycardia arising in the right ventricle is often an early manifestation of this disorder. The **VT is a reentrant type and has an LBBB morphology;** although in sinus rhythm, there is often inversion of the T waves in the anterior leads and a slurring of the terminal portion of the QRS complex known as an epsilon wave (Fig. 19-8). These patients frequently have a positive SAECG for late potentials. The combination of the scarring and the late potentials provides the anatomic substrate for reentry. During electrophysiologic study it may be possible to elicit VT of varying morphologies, due to the prolific scarring of the myocardium. The **risk of VT correlates with the extent of myocardial involvement.** Therapy with sotalol or high-dose amiodarone may meet with some success. Ablation via catheters is often successful, but only temporizing, as the generalized involvement tends to give rise to arrhythmias at a different locus later in the disease course. Implantable cardiac defibrillators are often the only reliable therapy to prevent sudden death in this disorder.

(10) **Wolff-Parkinson-White syndrome** predisposes patients to very rapid rates of VT and ventricular fibrillation. As mentioned in II.B.8, AF can lead to rapid conduction over the accessory pathway, causing VT which can easily degenerate into ventricular fibrillation. Curative therapy via catheter-based ablation is the best approach to this disorder, with success rates in excess of 90%.

(11) **Several inflammatory or infectious conditions** have been associated with VT.

   (a) **Sarcoidosis** is frequently cited as a cause of heart block, and may also cause VT and ventricular fibrillation. **Amiodarone** and **sotalol** are the most efficacious agents in this disorder, though an implantable cardiac defibrillator may be necessary in addition to the drug therapy.

   (b) **Acute myocarditis** has been associated with both polymorphic and monomorphic VT. **Antiarrhythmic therapy and anti-inflammatory therapy** are generally combined in the treatment of these patients.

   (c) Chagas' disease, caused by the parasite *Trypanosoma cruzi,* is a well-known cause of cardiomyopathy, particularly in South and Central America. Ventricular tachycardia and other arrhythmias due to conduction system involvement are common complications. Therapy involves antiparasitic treatment, standard therapy for CHF, antiarrhythmics, and pacemakers or implantable cardiac defibrillators as appropriate.

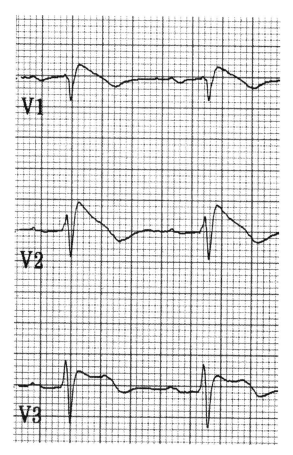

FIG. 19-8. Leads V_1–V_3, demonstrating large epsilon waves in the ST segment.

(12) **The long QT syndrome is an uncommon disorder** whose molecular basis is only now being elucidated. A full discussion of this syndrome can be found in Chapter 23.

(13) **Idiopathic polymorphic VT** has been described in patients with **structurally normal hearts and normal QT intervals.** Various characteristics have been described in these subjects. One group was noted to have persistent ST elevation despite any evidence for ischemia or CAD. Another group had reproducible arrhythmias with exercise and were responsive to β-blocker therapy. A third group had polymorphic VT triggered by an early premature ventricular beat and a high incidence of sudden death that was not prevented by β-blocker therapy, although verapamil had some benefit.

c. Torsades de pointes is a type of polymorphic VT associated with delayed myocardial repolarization, most often manifested as a prolonged QT interval. Though the duration of torsades de pointes is typically brief (less than 20 seconds), it can be sustained and can degenerate into ventricular fibrillation. It generally has an irregular ventricular rate in excess of 200 bpm and displays a polymorphic structure with an undulating appearance. The QRS complexes appear to twist around an isoelectric axis.

   (1) **Etiology.** QT prolongation can be congenital or acquired.

      (a) The **congenital** forms are seen in the long QT syndrome, discussed in Chapter 23.

      (b) The **acquired forms are most often drug-induced,** although polymorphic VT with a prolonged QT can be caused by electrolyte abnormalities, hypothyroidism, cerebrovascular events, MI or ischemia, starvation diets, organophosphate poisoning, myocarditis, severe CHF, and mitral valve prolapse.

      The **most commonly implicated drugs have** been the **class IA drugs,** although less frequent occurrences have been reported with all subclasses of class I antiarrhythmics. The class III drugs, such as sotalol and, less commonly, amiodarone, have been implicated. The incidence of torsades de pointes with sotalol is in the range of 2% to 5%. Ibutilide is a new antiarrhythmic for supraventricular tachyarrhythmias that has an incidence of torsades de pointes at least as high as sotalol. Other drugs implicated include the phenothiazines, haloperidol, and the tricyclic antidepressants. Antibiotics including erythromycin and other macrolides, as well as trimethoprim-sulfamethoxazole combinations, have been implicated. The macrolides are particularly prone to causing torsades de pointes when combined with certain antihistamines such as astemizole and terfenadine. These antihistamines have also been found to cause torsades de pointes when combined with certain azole antifungal agents such as ketoconazole.

      Bradycardia can promote torsades de pointes in patients with prolonged QT intervals, though it is not clear that bradycardia by itself predisposes to torsades de pointes.

      Ionic contrast media has been noted to cause torsades de pointes.

      Promotility agents such as cisapride have likewise been associated with torsades de pointes.

      Electrolyte disorders. Hypokalemia is the electrolyte disorder most reliably linked to torsades de pointes. **Hypomagnesemia** has been proposed as a logical cause, as its administration frequently terminates torsades de pointes. However, there is scant evidence to confirm this. Likewise, although **hypocalcemia** is associated with prolongation of the QT interval, there are only rare reports of torsades de pointes associated with hypocalcemia.

      A variety of **cerebrovascular events** have been associated with torsades de pointes, most notably subarachnoid hemorrhage. The prolongation of the QT interval sometimes seen with intracranial bleeding is usually transient, resolving within weeks.

   (2) **Therapy. Acute management** is aimed at terminating the arrhythmia.

      (a) If torsades de pointes is sustained or associated with hemodynamic compromise, prompt DCC should be carried out. Starting voltages are generally 50 to 100 J, and can be advanced to 360 J if necessary.

      (b) **Correction of hypokalemia, hypomagnesemia, and hypocalcemia** should be undertaken promptly. Magnesium can be given in bolus form at a dose of 1 to 2 g, with a total dose of 2 to 4 g given over 10 to 15 minutes. This successfully terminates torsades de pointes within 5 minutes in up to 75% of patients, and within 15 minutes in virtually all patients.

(c) **Bradycardia** can be corrected with either isoproterenol infusion or temporary transvenous pacing. Pacing may be preferable when readily available, due to the potential complications of isoproterenol therapy (worsened ischemia, hypertension). Offending agents should be discontinued. β-blockers and lidocaine may be useful, though the latter is inconsistently effective.

B. Ventricular fibrillation

1. Ventricular fibrillation is a **chaotic ventricular rhythm that reflects no organized electrical activity and hence no cardiac output** from the ventricle. It is devoid of the distinct elements that make up the usual electrical complex of ventricular activity. It is a **rapidly fatal rhythm, and if resuscitation is not begun within 5 to 7 minutes, death is virtually certain.** Ventricular fibrillation is often preceded by VT. Virtually all of the risk factors and conditions discussed for VT are applicable to ventricular fibrillation. It may arise without any inciting cardiac rhythm or event.

2. **Course of disease.** Of patients who experience an out-of-hospital cardiac arrest, 75% have ventricular fibrillation as their initial cardiac rhythm. Of those successfully resuscitated, 75% have significant CAD, and 20% to 30% have a transmural infarction. Patients without an ischemic etiology have an increased risk of further episodes of sudden death, while those who have an MI associated with sudden death have a 1-year recurrence rate of sudden death of 2%. Anterior MI complicated by ventricular fibrillation represents a subgroup at high risk for recurrence of sudden death. Predictors of sudden cardiac death include evidence of ischemia, decreased left ventricular systolic function, ten or more premature ventricular complexes per hour on telemetry, inducible or spontaneous VT, hypertension and left ventricular hypertrophy, smoking, male sex, obesity, elevated cholesterol, advanced age, and excessive alcohol use.

3. **Therapy.** As noted above, VF is a rapidly fatal rhythm, which virtually never terminates spontaneously. CPR must be initiated promptly, and rapid, unsynchronized DCC carried out. Starting energy should be at least 200J and should progress to 300 and then 360J, if unsuccessful. Successive shocks should be 360J. If after 3 shocks there has been no return of spontaneous circulation, then epinephrine, 1 mg should be rapidly administered and DCC repeated. Epinephrine may be repeated every 3–5 minutes, if necessary. Lidocaine is generally administered if there is still no response. Additional pharmacologic agents to consider are procainamide, bretylium and amiodarone. The current American Heart Association guidelines for Emergency Cardiac Care state that, "With greater experience, amiodarone may become a preferred antiarrhythmic agent for intravenous therapy of life-threatening ventricular arrhythmias in lidocaine failures."

See "Sudden Cardiac Death" (Chapter 21) for long term treatment of survivors of VF.

SUGGESTED READINGS

Key Reviews

American Heart Association. Medical/scientific statement. Management of patients with atrial fibrillation: a statement for healthcare professionals from the Subcommittee on Electrocardiography and Electrophysiology, American Heart Association, Eric N. Prystowsky MD, Chair. *Circulation* 1996;93:1262–1277.

Antiarrhythmics versus Implantable Defibrillators (AVID) Investigators. A comparison of antiarrhythmic-drug therapy with implantable defibrillators in patients resuscitated from near-fatal ventricular arrhythmias. *N Engl J Med* 1997;337: 1576–1583.

Antunes E, Brugada J, Steurer G, Andries E, Brugada P. The differential diagnosis of a regular tachycardia with a wide QRS complex on the 12-lead ECG: ventricular tachycardia, supraventricular tachycardia with aberrant intraventricular conduction, and supraventricular tachycardia with anterograde conduction over an accessory pathway. *Pacing Cardiac Electrophysiol* 1994;17:1515–1524.

Cairns JA, Connolly SJ, Roberts R, Gent M. Randomised trial of outcome after myocardial infarction in patients with frequent or repetitive ventricular premature depolarisations: CAMIAT. Canadian Amiodarone Myocardial Infarction Arrhythmia Trial Investigators. *Lancet* 1997;349(9053):675–682. [Published erratum appears in *Lancet* 1997 Jun 14;349(9067):1776.]

Cardiac Arrhythmia Suppression Trial (CAST) Investigators. Preliminary report: effect of encainide and flecainide on mortality in a randomized trial of arrhythmia suppression after myocardial infarction. *N Engl J Med* 1989;321:406–412

Cardiac Arrhythmia Suppression Trial II Investigators. Effect of the antiarrhythmic agent moricizine on survival after myocardial infarction. *N Engl J Med* 1992;327: 227–233.

Fontaine G, Fontaliran F, Lascault G, et al. In: Zipes DP, Jalife J, eds. *Cardiac electrophysiology: from cell to bedside,* 2nd ed. Philadelphia: WB Saunders, 1995: 754–768.

Julian DG, Camm AJ, Frangin G, et al. Randomised trial of effect of amiodarone on mortality in patients with left-ventricular dysfunction after recent myocardial infarction: EMIAT. European Myocardial Infarct Amiodarone Trial Investigators. *Lancet* 1997;349(9053):667–674. [Published errata appear in *Lancet* 1997 Apr 19; 349(9059):1180 and 1997 Jun 14;349(9067):1776.]

Klein AL, Grimm RA, Black IW, et al. Cardioversion guided by transesophageal echocardiography: the ACUTE pilot study. *Ann Intern Med* 1997;126:200–209.

Mason JW. A comparison of seven antiarrhythmic drugs in patients with ventricular tachyarrhythmias. Electrophysiologic Study versus Electrocardiographic Monitoring Investigators. *New Engl J Med* 1993;329:452–458.

Moss AJ, Hall WJ, Cannom DS, et al. Improved survival with an implanted defibrillator in patients with coronary disease at high risk for ventricular arrhythmia. Multicenter Automatic Defibrillator Implantation Trial Investigators. *N Engl J Med* 1996;335(26): 1933–1940.

O'Keefe JH, Hammill SC, Freed M. *The complete guide to ECGs.* Birmingham, MI: Physicians Press, 1997.

Prystowksy EN, Katz A, Waldo AL, et al. In: Topol EJ, ed. *Textbook of cardiovascular medicine.* Philadelphia: Lippincott-Raven Publishers, 1998 (Chapters 55, 60, 61, 62, 63).

Wolf PA, Abbott RD, Kannel WB. Atrial fibrillation as an independent risk factor for stroke: the Framingham study. *Stroke* 1991;22:983–988.

Zipes DP. In: Braunwald E, ed. *Heart disease: a textbook of cardiovascular medicine,* 5th ed. Philadelphia: WB Saunders, 1997 (Chapters 20–22).

20. BRADYARRHYTHMIAS, ATRIOVENTRICULAR BLOCK, ASYSTOLE, AND PULSELESS ELECTRICAL ACTIVITY

Christopher Cole

I. **Introduction. Bradyarrhythmias** and **conduction blocks** are common electrocardiographic findings. Many of these arrhythmias are asymptomatic and do not require specific therapy, whereas others can be life threatening, requiring rapid action. **Myocardial ischemia** is an important cause of acute and potentially dangerous bradyarrhythmia.

II. **Anatomy**

   A. **Sinoatrial node.** The sinus beat originates in the **sinoatrial node,** a focus of automatic cells near the junction of the superior vena cava and right atrium.

   1. The blood supply to the sinoatrial node is from the **sinus node artery,** which arises from the proximal **right coronary artery** in 55% of the population (Fig. 20-1) and from the **circumflex artery** in 35%. The sinoatrial node receives a dual supply of blood from both the right coronary artery and circumflex artery in 10% of the population.

   2. If the sinoatrial node fails to generate an impulse, other foci in the atrium, atrioventricular node, or ventricle can act as "backup" pacemaker sites. The automaticity of the sinoatrial node is affected by both the parasympathetic and sympathetic nervous systems.

   B. **Atrioventricular node.** The atrioventricular node is located in the anteromedial portion of the right atrium just anterior to the coronary sinus.

   1. The impulse generated by the sinoatrial node progresses through the atrium to the atrioventricular node. The atrioventricular node is also enervated by both the parasympathetic and sympathetic nervous systems.

   2. The atrioventricular node receives its blood supply from the atrioventricular nodal artery, which arises from the posterior descending artery in 80% of the population (see Fig. 20.1), from the circumflex artery in 10%, and from both arteries in 10%.

   3. Receipt of collateral blood supply from the left anterior descending artery makes the atrioventricular node somewhat less prone to ischemic damage than the sinoatrial node.

   C. **His bundle and bundle branches**

   1. After a delay of less than 0.2 seconds in the atrioventricular node, the electrical impulse is propagated down the His bundle to the right and left bundle branches. The **left bundle branch splits further into anterior and posterior fascicles.** The autonomic nervous system does not play a major role in conduction below the atrioventricular node.

   2. The **His bundle and right bundle branch** receive their blood supply from the atrioventricular nodal artery and from septal penetrating branches of the left anterior descending artery. The **left bundle branch** receives blood for the anterior fascicle from the septal perforating branches of the left anterior descending artery. The posterior fascicle has a dual blood supply from the septal perforating branches of the left anterior descending artery and branches of the posterior descending artery.

III. **Sinus node dysfunction.** Sinus node dysfunction encompasses any dysfunction of the sinus node and includes **inappropriate sinus bradycardia, sinoatrial exit block, sinoatrial arrest,** and **tachycardia-bradycardia syndrome.**

   A. **Clinical presentation.** There is a wide range of presentations, and some patients may be asymptomatic.

   1. **Syncope** and **presyncope** are the most dramatic presenting symptoms. **Fatigue, angina,** and **shortness of breath** are more subtle consequences of sinus node dysfunction.

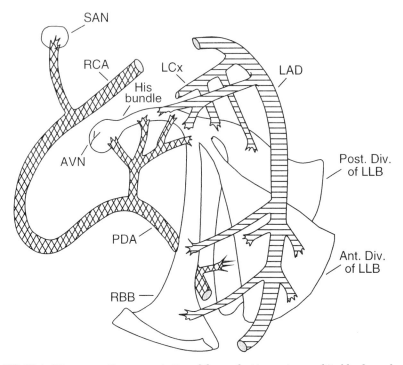

FIG. 20-1. Diagrammatic representation of the conduction system and its blood supply.

    2. In the tachycardia-bradycardia syndrome, the primary complaint may be palpitation. Documentation of the arrhythmia may be difficult because of the sporadic and fleeting nature of the problem.

B. Etiology. The intrinsic and extrinsic causes of sinus node dysfunction are listed in Table 20-1. **Idiopathic degenerative disease** is the most common cause of intrinsic sinus node dysfunction, and the incidence increases with age. **Acute coronary syndromes** are a common cause of bradyarrhythmias, occurring in 25% to 30% of patients with myocardial infarction (MI) (Table 20-2).

C. ECG findings

    1. Inappropriate sinus bradycardia is defined as a sinus rate of less than 60 that does not increase appropriately with exercise. The QRS complex is narrow and is preceded by a P wave. Inappropriate sinus bradycardia must be differentiated from a low resting heart rate, which may be normal in athletes and sleeping individuals.

    2. Sinus arrest, or sinus pause, occurs when the sinus node fails to depolarize on time. Pauses of less than 3 seconds may be seen on Holter monitoring in up to 11% of normal adults (especially athletes) and are not cause for concern. **Pauses longer than 3 seconds, however, are generally considered abnormal and are suggestive of an underlying abnormality.**

    3. Sinoatrial exit block, although similar to sinus arrest on the ECG tracing, may be distinguished by the fact that the **duration of the pause is a multiple of the sinus PP** interval. High-grade sinoatrial exit block cannot be differentiated from prolonged sinus arrest and is treated in the same manner.

Table 20-1. Etiology of sinus node dysfunction

INTRINSIC CAUSES

Idiopathic degenerative disease
Coronary artery disease
Cardiomyopathy
Hypertension
Infiltrative disorders (amyloidosis, hemochromatosis, tumors)
Collagen vascular disease (scleroderma, systemic lupus erythematosus)
Inflammatory processes (myocarditis, pericarditis)
Surgical trauma (valve surgery, transplantation)
Musculoskeletal disorders (myotonic dystrophy, Friedreich's ataxia)
Congenital heart disease (postoperative or in absence of surgical correction)

EXTRINSIC CAUSES

DRUG EFFECTS
  β-Blocking agents
  Calcium channel blocking agents
  Digoxin
  Sympatholytic antihypertensives (clonidine, methyldopa, reserpine)
  Antiarrhythmic drugs
      Type IA (quinidine, procainamide, disopyramide)
      Type IC (flecainide, propafenone)
      Type III (sotalol, amiodarone)
  Others (lithium, cimetidine, amitriptyline, phenytoin)

AUTONOMIC INFLUENCES
  Excessive vagal tone
  Carotid sinus syndrome
  Vasovagal syncope
  Well-trained athletes

ELECTROLYTE ABNORMALITIES
  Hyperkalemia
  Hypercarbia
  Endocrine disorders—hypothyroidism
  Increased intracranial pressure
  Hypothermia
  Sepsis

From Topol EJ, ed. *Textbook of cardiovascular medicine,* 1st ed. Philadelphia: Lippincott-Raven Publishers, 1998.

Table 20-2. Incidence of bradyarrhythmia in the setting of acute myocardial infarction

Rhythm	Incidence (%)
Sinus bradycardia	25
Junctional escape rhythm	20
Idioventricular escape rhythm	15
First-degree AV block	15
Second-degree, type I AV block	12
Second-degree, type II AV block	4
Third-degree AV block	15
Right bundle branch block	7
Left bundle branch block	5
Left anterior fascicular block	8
Left posterior fascicular block	0.5

AV, atrioventricular.

4. **Tachycardia-bradycardia syndrome,** also referred to as sick sinus syndrome, is characterized by episodes of sinus or junctional bradycardia interspersed with atrial tachycardia, usually paroxysmal atrial fibrillation.

D. **Diagnostic testing.** Invasive testing is used when noninvasive methods have failed to make a diagnosis but sinus node dysfunction is still strongly suspected.

1. **Noninvasive testing**

a. **ECG.** The first step when sinus node dysfunction is suspected is 12-lead ECG, followed by 24-to 48-hour ambulatory ECG monitoring, if necessary. Use of a diary during the recording period can help to correlate symptoms with the cardiac rhythm. For less frequent events, a loop recorder or event recorder may be used to assess symptoms over a 2-to 4-week period. Stress testing can be used to document the severity of chronotropic incompetence.

b. **Autonomic testing** includes physical maneuvers, such as carotid sinus massage and tilt-table testing, as well as pharmacologic interventions to test the autonomic reflexes.

(1) **Carotid sinus massage** distinguishes intrinsic sinus pause/ sinus arrest from a pause due to **carotid sinus hypersensitivity,** which is a 3-second or longer pause and/or a 50 mm Hg or greater drop in blood pressure that occurs with massage of the carotid sinus (firm pressure applied to one carotid sinus at a time for 5 seconds). **Carotid sinus massage should not normally precipitate sinus pause/sinus arrest,** although it will slow conduction in the atrioventricular node and decrease the rate of depolarization of the sinoatrial node.

(2) **Tilt-table testing** may help to differentiate between syncope caused by sinus node dysfunction and that due to autonomic dysfunction. **Bradycardic episodes precipitated by tilt table are usually due to autonomic dysfunction and not sinus node dysfunction.**

(3) **Pharmacologic testing** may be used to differentiate between sinus node dysfunction and autonomic dysfunction. Total autonomic blockade is achieved after administration of atropine 0.04 mg/kg and propranolol 0.2 mg/kg. The resulting intrinsic heart rate represents the sinus node rate devoid of autonomic influences. If the normal intrinsic heart rate (in beats per minute, bpm) is defined by the formula:

Intrinsic heart rate = $118.1 - (0.57 \times \text{age})$

then an intrinsic heart rate lower than predicted using this formula is consistent with sinus node dysfunction; an intrinsic heart rate close to the predicted rate in a patient with a clinical presentation of sinus node dysfunction is suggestive of an autonomic dysfunction as a cause of the bradyarrhythmia.

2. **Invasive testing.** The two most common tests use indirect measurements of sinoatrial node function. Direct measurement of sinoatrial node function is laborious and rarely performed.

a. **Sinus node recovery time** is the time it takes the sinoatrial node to recover following paced overdrive suppression of the node.

(1) **A delay of longer than 1,400 milliseconds is considered abnormal.** This measurement may be corrected by subtracting the intrinsic sinus cycle length (in milliseconds) from the recovery time. **A corrected sinus node recovery time of greater than 550 milliseconds is suggestive of sinus node dysfunction.**

(2) The limitations of this test are:
   (a) It is an indirect measurement of sinoatrial node function and reflects both sinoatrial node conduction time and automaticity.
   (b) It may be falsely shortened by sinoatrial node entrance block during atrial pacing (due to failure of the paced impulse to reset the sinus node) or falsely prolonged by a sinoatrial node exit block (the sinus node is normal but the impulse cannot leave the node).
   (c) The sinus node recovery time is not prolonged in all patients with sinus node dysfunction.
  b. Sinoatrial conduction time (SACT)
   (1) The steady-state atrial rate is determined (A_1–A_1 interval or the time between P waves). Then premature atrial **extra stimuli** (A_2) are introduced by pacing high in the right atrium starting in late diastole at progressively shorter intervals until atrial refractoriness is found (i. e., A_2 does not result in a P wave). The duration before the next spontaneous atrial impulse (A_3) is measured and the baseline rate is subtracted.

$$SACT = (A_2\text{–}A_3 \text{ interval}) - (A_1\text{–}A_1 \text{ interval})$$

   (2) The test assumes that sinoatrial node automaticity is not affected by pacing, that conduction time into the node is equal to conduction time out of the node, and that there is no shift in the principal pacemaker site.
 E. Therapy. Treatment for symptomatic sinus node dysfunction may be pharmacologic, pacing, or a combination of both.
  1. Indications for pacing in sinus node dysfunction are determined by symptoms (e. g., correlation with a documented arrhythmia; Table 20-3). Another common indication is when drug therapy that causes sinus node dysfunction cannot be stopped or changed.
  2. Medications that suppress sinus node automaticity should be stopped if possible. If this is not possible, it may be necessary to place a temporary or permanent pacemaker (see Table 20-3)
  3. For patients with **tachycardia-bradycardia syndrome,** a pacemaker is often placed for treatment of the bradyarrhythmia, and antiarrhythmic drugs are added for treatment of the tachycardic episodes.
  4. Acute treatment for patients with **symptomatic sinus node dysfunction** includes:
   a. Atropine (0.04 mg/kg intravenous bolus).
   b. Temporary pacing for patients who fail to respond to drug therapy.
   c. Isoproterenol (starting at 1 µg/minute intravenously), which may be used as a bridge drug to pacemaker placement. Isoproterenal is not indicated in most patients with cardiac arrest.
IV. Atrioventricular conduction disturbances. These disturbances are classified as first-, second-, or third-degree block, depending on the severity of conduction abnormality.
 A. Classification
  1. First-degree atrioventricular block is characterized by prolongation of the PR interval beyond 0.20 seconds. This finding may occur as a normal variant in 0.5% of asymptomatic young adults without overt heart disease. In older individuals, it is most often caused by idiopathic degenerative disease of the conducting system.
  2. Second-degree atrioventricular block
   a. Second-degree atrioventricular block is characterized by **a failure of one or more atrial impulses to conduct to the ventricles.** The block may be at any level of the atrioventricular conduction system.

Table 20-3. Indications for permanent pacing

Indication	Class I	Class II	Class III
SND	1. SND documented in association with symptomatic bradycardia and due to factors that are irreversible, or due to essential drug therapy. 2. Symptomatic chronotropic incompetence.	IIa. No clear association between SND with heart rate <40 bpm and symptoms can be documented. IIb. In minimally symptomatic patients, chronic heart rate <30 bpm while awake	1. SND with marked sinus bradycardia or pauses, but no associated symptoms including that due to long-term drug therapy. 2. SND in patients with symptoms suggestive of bradycardia that are clearly documented as not associated with a slow heart rate. 3. SND with symptomatic bradycardia due to nonessential drug therapy.

Acquired AV block	1. 3° AV block at any anatomic level, associated with any one of the following conditions:
	  a. Bradycardia with symptoms presumed to be due to AV block.
	  b. Arrhythmias and other medical conditions that require drugs that result in symptomatic bradycardia.
	  c. Documented periods of asystole ≥3.0 sec or any escape rate <40 bpm in awake symptom-free individuals.
	  d. After catheter ablation of the AV junction.
	  e. Postoperative AV block that is not expected to resolve.
		IIa. 1. Asymptomatic 3° AV block at any anatomic site with average awake ventricular rates ≥40 bpm.
		2. Asymptomatic type II 2° AV block.
		3. Asymptomatic type I 2° AV block at intra-His or infra-His levels found incidentally at EP study performed for other indications.
		4. 1° AV block with symptoms suggestive of pacemaker syndrome and documented alleviation of symptoms with temporary AV pacing.
			1. Aysmptomatic 1° AV block
			2. Asymptomatic type I 2° AV block at the supra-His (AV node) level or not known to be intra- or infra-Hisian.
			3. AV block expected to resolve and unlikely to recur (e.g, drug toxicity, Lyme disease).

Condition	Class	Recommendation
	I	f. Neuromuscular diseases with AV block such as myotonic muscular dystrophy, Kearns-Sayre syndrome, Erb's dystrophy (limb-girdle), and peroneal muscular dystrophy. 2. 2° AV block regardless of type or site of block, with associated symptomatic bradycardia.
	IIb	1. Marked 1° AV block (>0.30 sec) in patients with LV dysfunction and symptoms of congestive heart failure in whom shorter AV interval results in hemodynamic improvement, presumably by decreasing left atrial filling pressure.
	III	1. Transient AV block without intraventricular conduction defect. 2. Transient AV block in the presence of isolated left anterior fascicular block. 3. Acquired left anterior fascicular block in the absence of AV block. 4. Persistent first-degree AV block in the presence of bundle branch block that is old or age indeterminate.
Postmyocardial infarction	I	1. Persistent 2° AV block in the His-Purkinje system with bilateral bundle branch block or third-degree AV block within or below the His-Purkinje system after acute myocardial infarction. 2. Transient advanced (second- or third-degree) infranodal AV block and associated bundle branch block. If the site of block is uncertain, an EP study may be necessary. 3. Persistent and symptomatic second- or third-degree AV block.
	IIa	None
	IIb	1. Persistent second- or third-degree AV block at the AV node level.
Chronic bifascicular (BF) and trifascicular (TF) block	I	1. Intermittent 3° AV block. 2. Type II second-degree AV block.
	IIa	1. Syncope not proved to be due to AV block when other likely causes have been excluded, specifically ventricular tachycardia. 2. HV interval >100 msec. 3. Pacing induced block below the His that is not physiologic.
	IIb	None
	III	1. Fascicular block without AV block or symptoms. 2. Fascicular block with first-degree AV block without symptoms.

(Continued)

Table 20-3. *Continued*

Indication	Class I	Class II	Class III
Carotid sinus hypersensitivity (carotid sinus irritability) and neurally mediated syncope	1. Recurrent syncope caused by carotid sinus stimulation; minimal carotid sinus pressure induces ventricular asystole of >3 sec duration in the absence of any medication that depresses the sinus node or AV conduction.	IIa. 1. Recurrent syncope without clear, provocative events and with a hypersensitive cardioinhibitory response. 2. Syncope of unexplained origin when major abnormalities of sinus node function or AV conduction are discovered or provoked in EP studies. IIb. 1. Neurally mediated syncope with significant bradycardia reproduced by a head-up tilt with or without isoproterenol and other provocative maneuvers.	1. A hyperactive cardioinhibitory response to carotid sinus stimulation in the absence of symptoms. 2. A hyperactive cardioinhibitory response to carotid sinus stimulation in the absence of symptoms. A hyperactive cardioinhibitory response to carotid sinus stimulation in the presence of vague symptoms such as dizziness, light-headedness, or both. 3. Recurrent syncope, light-headedness, or dizziness in the absence of a hyperactive cardioinhibitory response. 4. Situational vasovagal syncope in which avoidance behavior is effective.

Class I: Conditions for which there is evidence and/or general agreement that pacing is beneficial, useful, and effective.
Class II: Conditions for which there is conflicting evidence and/or a divergence of opinion about the usefulness/efficacy of pacing.
IIa: Weight of evidence/opinion is in favor of usefulness/efficacy.
IIb: Usefulness/efficacy is less well established by evidence/opinion.
Class III: Conditions for which there is evidence and or general agreement that pacing is not useful/effective and in some cases may be harmful.
SND, Sinus node dysfunction; AV, atrioventricular; LV, left ventricular; EP, electrophysiologic; HV, half-value.
From Gregoratos G, Cheitlin MD, Conill A, et al., ACC/AHA guidelines for implantation of cardiac pacemakers and antiarrhythmia devices: a report of the American College of Cardiology/American Heart Association Task Force on Practice Guidelines (Committee on Pacemaker Implantation). *J Am Coll Cardiol* 1998;31:1175–209.

    b. When more than one atrial impulse is present for each ventricular complex, the rhythm may be described by the number of atrial impulses to the number of ventricular complexes (for three P waves preceding each QRS complex, 3:1 second-degree atrioventricular block is present).

        (1) Lesser degrees of atrioventricular block (i. e., 4:3 or 3:2) with a variable PR interval and Wenckebach periodicity are described as **Mobitz I atrioventricular block** (also known as Wenckebach block).

            (a) The conducted impulse of a **Mobitz I block** will generally be narrow, and the site of block is often in the atrioventricular node above the His bundle.

            (b) A Mobitz I block with a bundle branch block is still likely to be above the His bundle, but a His bundle ECG is needed to confirm the level of block.

        (2) High-grade atrioventricular block (3:1, 4:1, or greater) is typically described as **Mobitz II atrioventricular block.** The conducted impulse will generally have a wide QRS morphology (RBBB or LBBB pattern), and the site of block often is below the atrioventricular node. A **Mobitz II block** is usually intra-or infra- Hisian and has an increased incidence of progressing to third-degree atrioventricular block.

        (3) Pure 2:1 conduction patterns cannot be reliably classified as Mobitz I or II.

  3. Third-degree atrioventricular block, or **complete heart block,** may be acquired or congenital.

    a. Of patients with **congenital complete heart block,** 60% are female. Of children with congenital complete heart block, 30% to 50% of their mothers have connective tissue disease, usually systemic lupus erythematosus.

    b. Acquired atrioventricular block occurs most frequently in the seventh decade and more commonly affects males.

B. Clinical presentation

  1. Signs and symptoms

    a. First-degree atrioventricular block is generally not a cause of symptoms.

    b. Second-degree atrioventricular block seldom results in symptoms, although high-grade second-degree atrioventricular block may progress to third-degree atrioventricular block, which can cause symptoms.

    c. Depending on the ventricular escape rate, patients with **third-degree atrioventricular block** may experience **fatigue** or **syncope.**

  2. Physical findings. The amplitude of the arterial pulse varies, depending on the timing of atrial filling of the ventricles.

    a. Second-degree atrioventricular block is associated with a periodic change in amplitude. In patients with **third-degree atrioventricular block,** amplitude is constantly changing, e. g., periodic appearance of cannon a-waves (large-amplitude waves in the venous pulsations seen in the neck when the atria contracts against a closed tricuspid valve).

    b. Heart sounds are similarly affected by the change in filling duration of the ventricles.

        (1) S_1 **becomes softer** as the PR interval is prolonged, resulting in a soft S_1 in first-degree atrioventricular block, a progressively softening S_1 in type I second-degree atrioventricular block, and a constantly changing S_1 in third-degree atrioventricular block.

        (2) Third-degree atrioventricular block may also result in a functional systolic ejection murmur.

C. **Etiology.** The causes of atrioventricular block are listed in Table 20-4; the most common is **idiopathic fibrosis. Acute MI** results in atrioventricular block in 14% of patients with inferior infarction and 2% of those with anterior infarction, usually within the first 24 hours.

D. **Diagnostic testing**

1. **First-degree atrioventricular block.** Diagnosis is made by measuring a PR interval longer than 0.20 second in adults and 0.18 second in children who are not receiving any drugs that prolong the PR interval. AP wave precedes each QRS and both the P and QRS are morphologically normal.

2. **Second-degree atrioventricular block**

   a. The diagnosis of **Mobitz type I** is made when the following criteria are met on the ECG:

      (1) Sequential and gradual prolongation of the PR interval terminated by a nonconducted P wave
      (2) Prolongation of the RR interval occurring in progressively shorter increments
      (3) Duration of the pause following the nonconducted P wave less than the sum of any two consecutively conducted beats
      (4) Decreased PR interval following the pause when compared to the prepause PR interval
      (5) "Grouped beating," a pattern of repeated groups of QRS complexes characteristic of Wenckebach block

   b. **Mobitz type II** second-degree atrioventricular block is less common than type I.

      (1) The PR interval is constant with a sudden nonconducted P wave (Fig. 20-2), in contrast to nonconducted premature atrial contractions, which have a varying PR interval.
      (2) Each QRS complex may have multiple P waves, which are designated by the number of P waves before each conducted QRS (3:1, 4:1, etc.). The QRS complex typically is not narrow (a narrow QRS complex is suggestive of a Mobitz I block).

3. **Third-degree atrioventricular block** (Fig. 20-3)

   a. Third-degree atrioventricular block is characterized by identification of **complete dissociation of the atrial and ventricular electrical activity** (no temporal relationship exists between the P waves and the QRS complexes). Using calipers, it is possible to march out the progression of the P waves to determine the atrial rate.
   b. Third-degree atrioventricular block is only one cause of atrioventricular dissociation; **not all atrioventricular dissociation is third-degree atrioventricular block.**

E. **Therapy.** Patients with first-degree and Mobitz I atrioventricular block usually do not require therapy. Permanent pacing is indicated for Mobitz II atrioventricular block and third-degree atrioventricular block (see Table 20-3 for complete indications for pacing).

1. **Medical therapy** may be used as a bridge to pacing but has no role in long-term treatment.

   a. The principal drug used as a bridge to pacing is **atropine,** which:

      (1) Reduces heart block due to hypervagotonia but not due to atrioventricular node ischemia
      (2) Is more useful for atrioventricular block in inferior MI than anterior MI
      (3) Does not increase infranodal conduction (will not improve third-degree atrioventricular block or second-degree atrioventricular block that is below the atrioventricular node)
      (4) Is ineffective in the denervated hearts of transplant patients
      (5) Is used with caution (if at all) in Mobitz II atrioventricular block due to a possible paradoxical decrease in heart rate (as atrial rate increases, atrioventricular conduction decreases,

Table 20-4. Causes of atrioventricular block

Drug effects
    Digoxin
    Beta blockers
    Certain calcium channel blockers
    Membrane-active antiarrhythmic drugs
Ischemic heart disease
    Acute myocardial infarction
    Chronic coronary artery disease
Idiopathic fibrosis of the conduction system
    Lenegre's disease
    Lev's disease
Congenital heart disease
    Congenital complete heart block
    Ostium primum atrial septal defect
    Transposition of the great vessels
    Maternal systemic lupus erythematosis
Calcific valvular disease
Cardiomyopathy
Infiltrative disease
    Amyloidosis
    Sarcoidosis
    Hemochromatosis
Infectious/inflammatory diseases
    Endocarditis
    Myocarditis (Chagas' disease, Lyme disease, rheumatic fever, tuberculosis, measles, mumps)
Collagen vascular diseases (scleroderma, rheumatoid arthritis, Reiter's syndrome, systemic lupus erythematosis, ankylosing spondylitis, polymyositis)
Metabolic
    Hyperkalemia
    Hypermagnesemia
Endocrine—Addison's disease
Trauma
    Cardiac surgery
    Radiation
    Catheter trauma
    Catheter ablation
Tumors
    Mesothelioma
    Hodgkin's disease
    Malignant melanoma
    Rhabdomyosarcoma
Neurally mediated
    Carotid sinus syndrome
    Vasovagal syncope
Neuromyopathic disorders
    Myotonic muscular dystrophy
    Slowly progressive X-linked muscular dystrophy

From Topol EJ, ed. *Textbook of cardiovascular medicine,* 1st ed. Philadelphia: Lippincott-Raven Publishers, 1998.

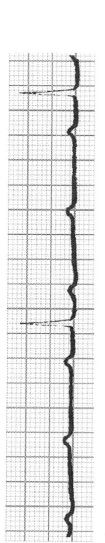

FIG. 20-2. Mobitz type II second-degree atrioventricular block with 3:1 conduction.

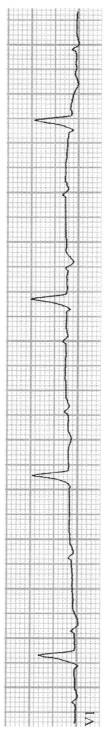

V I

FIG. 20-3. Third-degree atrioventricular block with sinus tachycardia and right bundle branch block.

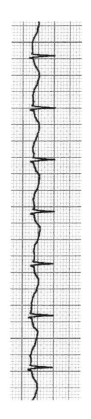

FIG. 20-4. Accelerated junctional rhythm.

and a 2:1 block with an atrial rate of 80 and a ventricular rate of 40 may be converted to a 3:1 block with an atrial rate of 90 and a ventricular rate of 30)

    b. Digoxin-specific Fab fragments may be used to treat patients with symptomatic atrioventricular blocks related to use of digitalis. The number of vials = weight (Kg) × diagoxin serum concentration (nannograms/mL) ÷ 100.

2. **Pacing**

    a. Third-degree atrioventricular block as a complication of inferior MI is usually temporary and may only require **temporary pacing.**

    b. Complete heart block as a result of anterior MI, however, often requires **permanent pacing** (see Table 20-3).

    c. Acquired third-degree atrioventricular block usually requires pacing, but patients with congenital third-degree atrioventricular block often have a fast enough escape rhythm to prevent symptoms and avoid permanent pacemaker implantation.

V. Junctional rhythms. Junctional rhythms arise from the area surrounding the atrioventricular node, including the approaches to the node, the node itself, and the bundle of His. This area has an intrinsic rate of 30 to 60 bpm and serves as an escape mechanism to prevent ventricular asystole in case of complete atrioventricular block. Junctional rhythm that is faster than the sinus rhythm is referred to as **accelerated junctional rhythm.**

  A. Clinical presentation. Patients usually do not develop symptoms directly attributable to accelerated junctional rhythm. The **physical findings of atrioventricular dissociation may be noted** and are the same as those seen in third-degree atrioventricular block.

  B. Etiology

    1. Accelerated junctional rhythm is seen in approximately **10% of patients with acute MI.** Over half of these patients have inferior MI and about one-third have anterior infarctions.

    2. **Digitalis toxicity** by itself does not seem to cause accelerated junctional rhythm, as evidenced in persons with normal hearts who take accidental overdoses of digoxin. **Concomitant heart disease** is required to develop accelerated junctional rhythm.

    3. Other causes of accelerated junctional rhythm are valve surgery, acute rheumatic fever, direct current cardioversion, cardiac catheterization, serious infection, chronic obstructive pulmonary disease, systemic amyloidosis, and uremia with hyperkalemia.

  C. ECG findings

    1. **Accelerated junctional rhythm**

      a. The P wave is normal in morphology. The QRS complex has a normal duration, unless there is concomitant bundle branch block. The distinguishing characteristic of accelerated junctional rhythm is the atrioventricular dissociation and changing PR interval (Fig. 20-4).

      b. The difference between accelerated junctional rhythm and third-degree atrioventricular block is the fact that the ventricular rate is faster than the atrial rate in accelerated junctional rhythm and slower than the atrial rate in third-degree atrioventricular block.

    2. **Junctional rhythm.** In the absence of a sinus beat, the atrioventricular node can act as a backup pacemaker. The ECG findings are an absence of P waves, a narrow QRS complex, and a rate of 30 to 60 bpm.

  D. Therapy

    1. Therapy for junctional rhythm secondary to sinoatrial node failure or atrioventricular block is as previously outlined for atrioventricular conduction disturbances.

    2. Patients with accelerated junctional rhythm do not usually require therapy for the arrhythmia, although treatment of the underlying cause is indicated.

3. Suppression of accelerated junctional rhythm may be achieved by **increasing the atrial rate with drugs** (e. g., atropine, adrenergics, etc.) or **pacing.**

4. Digitalis-induced accelerated junctional rhythm is an indication to stop digoxin but does not usually require administration of digoxin-specific Fab fragments.

VI. **Intraventricular conduction disturbances.** Conduction disturbances due to block below the atrioventricular node are classified on the basis of the intraventricular conduction system. An intraventricular conduction disturbance does not itself cause bradyarrhythmia, but may be associated with any of the other rhythms that cause bradycardia. When associated with an acute MI an intraventricular conduction disturbance predicts a worse outcome.

A. **Etiology**

1. The causes of intraventricular conduction disturbances are similar to those that cause atrioventricular block (see Table 20-4); **idiopathic degenerative conduction disease** and **acute ischemic syndromes** are the most common causes.

2. Intraventricular conduction disturbances increase with age and affect up to 2% of individuals older than age 60 years.

3. The incidence of intraventricular conduction disturbances is increased in persons with structural heart disease, especially those with coronary artery disease.

B. **ECG findings**

1. The ECG findings of intraventricular conduction disturbances are summarized in Table 20-5, and examples are presented in Figs. 20-5 to 20-8. As shown, **intraventricular conduction disturbances may be further classified by the number of fascicles they affect.**

2. **Fascicular blocks**

a. **Unifascicular blocks** affect only one of the three fascicles. Examples are right bundle branch block, left anterior fascicular block, and left posterior fascicular block.

b. **Bifascicular block** is present when conduction disturbances affect two of the fascicles, most commonly the RBBB with left anterior fascicular block. Approximately 6% of these patients progress to complete heart block. Right bundle branch block with left posterior fascicular block is less common, but the progression to complete heart block is more common.

c. **Trifascicular block** is present when there is a combination of bifascicular block and first-degree atrioventricular block (see Fig. 20-8).

C. **Therapy. Pacing** is indicated in patients with bifascicular block who have intermittent symptomatic complete heart block and in patients with bifascicular or trifascicular block with asymptomatic intermittent Mobitz II atrioventricular block (see Table 20-3).

VII. **Postsurgical bradyarrhythmias**

A. **Etiology.** Bradyarrhythmias following cardiac surgery are common.

1. **Valvular surgery and septal myectomy** can cause mechanical damage to the conduction system, leading to atrioventricular blocks and intraventricular conduction disturbances.

2. **Prolonged ischemic time during cardiac transplantation** can lead to sinus node damage.

B. **Therapy.** Because postsurgical bradyarrhythmias may be only temporary, the decision to proceed to **permanent pacing** should be made after 5 to 7 days. The same criteria listed in Table 20-3 are used to determine the need for a pacemaker. Permanent pacing is required in 2% to 3% of patients following valve surgeries and in upward of 10% of transplant patients.

VIII. **Pulseless electrical activity.** Pulseless electrical activity is defined as the absence of a pulse or blood pressure measured by usual methods with the continued presence of electrical activity of the heart.

Table 20-5. Electrocardiographic features for the fascicular and bifascicular blocks

ECG finding	LBBB	LAFB	LPFB	RBBB	RBBB & LAFB	RBBB & LPFB
QRS axis		≥−45°	+90° to +120°		−60° to −120°	≥+120°
QRS duration	≥120 ms	Normal	Normal	≥120 ms	≥ 120 ms	≥ 120 ms
Leads I and aVL	Broad monophasic R	qR	rS	qRS with wide terminal S	qR	rS
Leads II, III, aVF		rS	qR		rS	qR
Leads V1 and V2	rS or QS			rsR' or rSR'	rsR' or rSR'	rsR' or rSR'
Leads V5 and V6		S	no Q's	qRS		

LBBB, Left bundle branch block; LAFB, left anterior fascicular block; LPFB, left posterior fascicular block; RBBB, right bundle branch block.

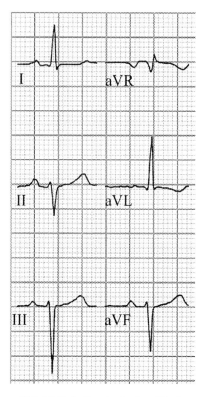

FIG. 20-5. Left anterior hemiblock.

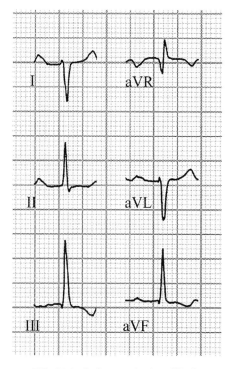

FIG. 20-6. Left posterior hemiblock.

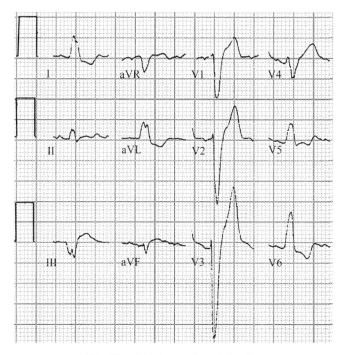

FIG. 20-7. Left bundle branch block.

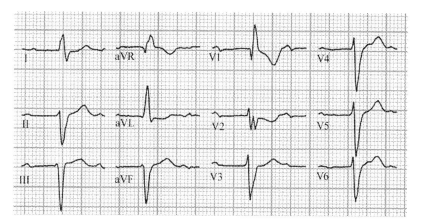

FIG. 20-8. First-degree atrioventricular block with right bundle branch block and left anterior hemiblock.

A. **Etiology**

1. Pulseless electrical activity may result from a variety of **rhythm disturbances,** such as electrical mechanical dissociation, idioventricular rhythms, and ventricular tachycardias. When the electrical activity is organized and within the physiologic range, the term **electrical mechanical dissociation** is used.

2. A variety of clinical situations are also associated with pulseless electrical activity, a potentially treatable condition if certain actions are undertaken rapidly (Table 20-6).

B. **Therapy**

1. **Specific treatment of the underlying cause** is most likely to result in a successful outcome (see Table 20-6).

2. **Emergency intervention** should be initiated at once, including:

   a. Cardiopulmonary resuscitation (CPR) and airway management with intubation to treat any possible hypoxia

   b. Epinephrine, 1 mg intravenous push every 3 to 5 minutes

   c. Atropine, 1 mg intravenously, if the rate is more than 60 bpm; may be repeated every 3 to 5 minutes to a total dose of 0.03 to 0.04 mg/kg

   d. Empiric intravenous volume infusion

IX. **Asystole**

A. **Clinical presentation.** Asystole is defined as the absence of myocardial electrical activity. It should be confirmed by switching between several leads or changing the position of the defibrillation paddles.

1. Most patients with asystole present in a code situation. Persons outside of the hospital who are found to be asystolic by the initial responding team usually have asystole resulting from **profound myocardial ischemia.** The possibility of a successful outcome in this situation is extremely small.

2. Hospital inpatients monitored by telemetry, on the other hand, may have a favorable outcome.

B. **Etiology.** Asystole may be due to profound parasympathetic suppression of both atrial and ventricular activity, stunning of the myocardium due to electrical defibrillation, complete heart block, or prolonged myocardial ischemia.

C. **Therapy.** Management consists of **CPR, intubation,** and **atropine** to unmask the possibility of profound parasympathetic suppression of both atrial and ventricular activity.

1. **Routine shocking is strongly discouraged.** Electrical shocks have not been demonstrated to have any benefit in the treatment of asystole and may in fact produce a stunned myocardium, leading to a delay in the return of a rhythm.

2. **Pacing for asystole is controversial.** If pacing is to have any effect, it must be initiated early. Asystole due to myocardial ischemia is unlikely to respond to pacing, but asystole due to other causes might respond.

X. **Carotid sinus hypersensitivity.** Carotid sinus hypersensitivity, defined as a sinus pause of 3 seconds or greater and/or a drop in blood pressure of 50 mm Hg or more with carotid sinus massage, is common, affecting up to one-third of older men with coronary artery disease. Carotid sinus hypersensitivity may be purely cardioinhibitory, purely vasodepressive, or a combination of both. **Carotid sinus syndrome** is present when carotid sinus hypersensitivity is accompanied by syncope or near-syncope.

A. **Etiology and pathophysiology**

1. The **cause of carotid sinus hypersensitivity and carotid sinus syndrome is unknown.** It is more common in older individuals, particularly those with atherosclerotic disease. Carotid sinus syndrome may be precipitated by the patient stretching his or her neck (such as with shaving or turning the head) or wearing a tight collar, but often a precipitating event cannot be found.

2. **Sites of potential lesions** causing carotid sinus hypersensitivity are the sternocleidomastoid muscle, central nervous system, and the feedback loops between the cardiovascular and central nervous systems.

Table 20-6. Conditions that cause pulseless electrical activity

Condition	Clues	Management
Hypovolemia	History, flat neck veins	Volume infusion
Hypoxia	Cyanosis, blood gases, airway problems	Ventilation
Cardiac tamponade	History (trauma, renal failure, thoracic malignancy), no pulse with CPR, vein distention; impending tamponade—tachycardia, hypotension, low pulse pressure—changing to sudden bradycardia as terminal event	Pericardiocentesis
Tension pneumothorax	History (asthma, ventilator, chronic obstructive pulmonary disease, trauma), no pulse with CPR, neck vein distention, tracheal deviation	Needle decompression
Hypothermia	History of exposure to cold, central body temperature	Warming
Massive pulmonary embolism	History, no pulse felt with CPR	Pulmonary arteriogram, surgical embolectomy, thrombolytics
Drug overdose (tricyclics, digoxin, β-blockers, calcium channel blockers)	Bradycardia, history of ingestion, empty bottles at the scene, pupils, neurologic exam	Drug screens, intubation, lavage, activated charcoal, lactulose per local protocols
Hyperkalemia	History of renal failure, diabetes, recent dialysis, dialysis fistulas, medications	Calcium chloride (immediate); then combination of insulin, glucose, sodium bicarbonate; then sodium polystyrene sulfonate/sorbitol; dialysis (long-term)
Preexisting acidosis	History of bicarbonate-responsive preexisting acidosis, renal failure	Sodium bicarbonate, hyperventilation
Acute massive MI	History, ECG, enzymes	Treat for cardiogenic shock

CPR, Cardiopulmonary resuscitation. From *Essentials of ACLS.*

3. It has been demonstrated that the **carotid sinus function is intact** and the sinus is not hypersensitive in the true sense. Some investigators have suggested that carotid sinus syndrome be renamed carotid sinus irritability to better reflect its pathophysiology.

B. **Diagnostic testing.** A patient with suspected carotid sinus hypersensitivity/carotid sinus syndrome should be tested lying down with ECG and blood pressure monitoring.

1. **Carotid sinus massage** is performed by placing firm manual pressure over the carotid sinus located at the bifurcation of the carotid artery for no more than 5 seconds. Only one sinus at a time is compressed, and the temporal artery should be lightly palpated to ensure that complete occlusion of the artery does not occur.

2. **Potential risks** of carotid sinus massage are transient ischemic attack and stroke. This test should not be performed if a carotid bruit is present. Tilting the patient to an upright position will increase the diagnostic yield of the test but may also result in false positives.

C. **Therapy**

1. Carotid sinus hypersensitivity by itself generally does not require treatment. Therapy is warranted, however, if carotid sinus hypersensitivity is demonstrated to be the cause of syncope or near-syncope.

2. For purely cardioinhibitory or the mixed type of carotid sinus syndrome, the therapy of choice is pacing (see Table 20-3).

3. Treatment of vasodepressive carotid sinus syndrome is more difficult, and pacing is generally ineffective.

SUGGESTED READINGS

Landmark Articles

American College of Cardiology/American Heart Association. Guidelines for pacemaker implantation after acute myocardial infarction. What is persistent advanced block at the atrioventricular node? *Am J Cardiol* 1997;80:770–774.

Gregoratos G, Chetlin MD, Conill A, et al. ACC/AHA guidelines for implantation of cardiac pacemakers and antiarrhythmia devices: a report of the American College of Cardiology/American Heart Association Task Force on Practice Guidelines (Committee on Pacemaker Implantation). *J Am Coll Cardiol* 1998;31:1175–1209.

Kusumoto FM. Goldschlager N. Cardiac pacing. *N Engl J Med* 1996; 334:89–97.

Maloney JD, Jaeger FJ, Rizo-Patron C, Zhu DW. The role of pacing for the management of neurally mediated syncope: carotid sinus syndrome and vasovagal syncope. *Am Heart J* 1994;127:1030–1037.

Rotman M, Wagner GS, Wallace AG. Bradyarrhythmias in acute myocardial infarction. *Circulation* 1972;45:703–722.

21. SUDDEN CARDIAC DEATH

Robert A. Schweikert

I. **Clinical presentation.** Sudden cardiac death (SCD) refers to any natural death from cardiac causes occurring within an hour of the onset of symptoms. The incidence of SCD in the United States is estimated to be approximately 200,000 to 400,000 cases annually, possibly accounting for over half of all cardiovascular deaths in this country. High-risk subgroups of patients include those with reduced left ventricular (LV) ejection fraction (EF), history of congestive heart failure (CHF), and survivors of out-of-hospital cardiac arrests. It is estimated that 80% of victims of SCD do not survive to hospital discharge, and 50% of those who do survive die within 3 years.

   Sudden cardiac death is therefore a significant public health problem, and there has been a great deal of research directed at its primary and secondary prevention.

II. **Etiology**

   A. The majority of episodes of SCD occur in those individuals with structural heart disease, most commonly coronary artery disease (CAD). Approximately 80% of episodes of SCD are primary; that is, no precipitating factor can be identified. The risk of recurrent SCD for these patients is high and may be more than 20% within the first year. A secondary episode of SCD is one in which a precipitating factor can be identified, such as acute myocardial ischemia or infarction, drug toxicity or proarrhythmia, decompensated CHF, or severe electrolyte imbalance. Evaluation and treatment of such patients is generally directed at the precipitating cause, as there is less risk of recurrent SCD in such patients.

   B. **Etiologies of SCD** (Table 21-1)

      1. Most episodes of SCD (about 65% to 85%) that are documented electrocardiographically are due to malignant arrhythmias such as ventricular fibrillation (VF). Monomorphic ventricular **tachycardia** (VT) is uncommonly documented as a cause of out-of-hospital SCD, probably due to the rapid degeneration of unstable VT to VF. The rhythm documented by medical personnel depends on the time elapsed since the arrest. If a rhythm tracing is obtained within 4 minutes of the arrest, the overwhelming majority of the rhythms will be VF.

      2. Asystole and electromechanical dissociation (EMD) are found in greater proportions as the time since arrest increases. These observations suggest that asystole and EMD are usually preceded by prolonged VF and are not commonly the primary rhythm disturbance for SCD episodes. However, it must be remembered that bradyarrhythmias are also a potential cause of SCD and may degenerate into VF prior to documentation of the arrhythmia.

III. **Diagnostic and prognostic testing**

   A. Survivors of SCD should have a detailed cardiovascular evaluation. Reversible precipitating factors must be identified and corrected. Underlying diseases must be identified and treated, and the risk of recurrent SCD must be determined.

   B. Diagnostic and prognostic testing to be considered for the survivor of SCD:

      1. **Electrocardiogram** for evidence of myocardial infarction (MI) or ischemia, intraventricular conduction delay, accessory pathway (Wolff-Parkinson-White syndrome), and prolonged QT interval.

      2. **Laboratory data** to rule out reversible causes, such as creatine kinase–MB (CK-MB), electrolytes, antiarrhythmic drug levels, and urine screening for illicit drugs such as cocaine.

Table 21-1. Etiologic basis of sudden cardiac death

Etiology	Proportion of SCD (%)
Coronary heart disease (acute ischemic events, chronic ischemic heart disease)	80
Cardiomyopathies (dilated cardiomyopathies, hypertrophic cardiomyopathies)	10–15
Valvular inflammation/infiltration	±5
Uncommon, subtle, ill-defined lesions, e.g., right ventricular dysplasia	?
Lesions of molecular structure, e.g., congenital long QT syndromes	?
Definable functional abnormalities	?
"Normal" hearts—idiopathic ventricular fibrillation	?

SCD, Sudden cardiac death.

3. **ECG monitoring** to assess frequency, duration, and symptomatology of arrhythmias.
4. **Echocardiography** for assessment of left ventricular function, valvular disease, cardiomyopathy (including hypertrophic cardiomyopathy). Nuclear or angiographic determinations of left ventricular function may be used but do not provide as much information as echocardiography.
5. **Coronary angiography** for assessment of CAD or coronary anomalies.
6. **Exercise or pharmacologic stress testing with radionuclide imaging or echocardiography** if CAD is present and myocardial ischemia and/or viability is in question.
7. **Electrophysiologic (EP) testing.** For the survivor of SCD, the need for EP testing is somewhat controversial, especially in light of the superiority of the implantable cardioverter-defibrillator (ICD) over antiarrhythmic drugs in this population. There are some electrophysiologists who advocate EP testing for the survivor of SCD prior to implantation of an ICD to identify and characterize an inducible tachyarrhythmia, particularly one that may be cured with catheter ablation techniques, or to rule out a supraventricular arrhythmia that might complicate management of an ICD. In addition, EP testing may guide the clinician in the selection of a particular ICD or identify the need for concomitant cardiac pacing.
8. **Cardiac magnetic resonance imaging (MRI).** Particularly for the patient with normal left ventricular function, cardiac MRI may be useful to evaluate for arrhythmogenic right ventricular dysplasia.

IV. **Therapy**
   A. **Acute therapy for SCD**
      1. **Cardiopulmonary resuscitation (CPR).** Early response is crucial. Studies have shown that survivors of SCD are more likely to be discharged from the hospital if they received early CPR from bystanders.
      2. **Advanced cardiac life support (ACLS).** Early defibrillation is crucial to improved survival. Approximately 40% of SCD victims are found to have VF upon arrival of paramedical personnel. There are currently at least two ongoing prospective randomized clinical trials studying the use of amiodarone in shock-refractory VF for patients with out-of-hospital SCD. Preliminary results of one trial suggest that amiodarone is an effective acute therapy for such patients.
      3. **Survival to hospital.** The two most crucial factors that determine the value of out-of-hospital resuscitation are citizen bystander CPR and rapid emergency medical response. The use of automated external defi-

brillators (AEDs) may have a significant impact in this area (discussed below). Some centers in the United States with rapid emergency medical response and early bystander CPR have reported that of the 40% of SCD victims found in VF, up to 60% to 70% survive to be admitted to the hospital, and approximately 25% are subsequently discharged from the hospital (therefore, only approximately 10% of SCD victims survive overall). As most cities in the United States do not achieve quite as rapid a response, it is clear that the primary prevention of SCD would be a more effective focus.

B. Primary prevention of SCD

1. **Identifying individuals at risk for SCD.** No single factor has been identified that accurately predicts the occurrence of SCD, although combinations of factors have been more useful. In general, the specificity and positive predictive value of these tests are poor, while the negative predictive value is much better (particularly for combinations of tests). Table 21-2 summarizes the incidence of sustained ventricular arrhythmias or SCD for patients after myocardial infarction for combinations of various tests.

2. **Pharmacologic agents and surgical/percutaneous techniques.** As the majority of episodes of SCD occur in patients with CAD, agents that reduce myocardial ischemia, prevent or limit the extent of myocardial infarction, or alter ventricular remodeling after MI should reduce the incidence of SCD. Early studies of surgical myocardial revascularization have shown a reduction in SCD for patients with triple-vessel CAD and LV dysfunction compared with those patients treated medically. Combined surgical revascularization and aneurysmectomy to remove the arrhythmogenic myocardial substrate had variable results; however, catheter-based VT mapping and ablation methods continue to be investigated and may play a role in select patient populations, particularly in those patients with incessant arrhythmias despite optimal antiarrhythmic drug and/or implantable device therapy. More recently, myocardial reperfusion and revascularization with thrombolytic agents and/or percutaneous interventions have decreased the mortality from SCD.

   Several studies have demonstrated the efficacy of β-blockers for the prevention of SCD and the reduction of total mortality in survivors of MI. The evidence for angiotensin-converting enzyme (ACE) inhibitors is less compelling, with a few studies suggesting a reduction in SCD for patients with CHF and LV dysfunction.

Table 21-2. Incidence of documented sustained ventricular arrhythmias or sudden cardiac death in patients after myocardial infarction

Test	Percent adverse outcomes	
	For normal test results	For abnormal test results
SAECG and ejection fraction <0.40	0–1	31–38
SAECG and Holter monitor	0–1	27–35
Ejection fraction <0.40 and Holter monitor	7	29
SAECG, ejection fraction <0.40, and Holter monitor	0	50
SAECG and programmed stimulation	2	27
SAECG and HRV	7	33
SAECG, HRV, and Holter monitor	4	43

HRV, Heart rate variability; SAECG, signal-averaged ECG.
Modified from Ref. 18, with permission.

More than a decade ago, ventricular ectopy in survivors of MI was recognized as a risk factor for SCD. Suppression of ventricular ectopy with antiarrhythmic drugs in such patients was therefore thought to be beneficial. However, the Cardiac Arrhythmia Suppression Trial (CAST) demonstrated that the proarrhythmic and/or adverse effects of the class IC antiarrhythmic drugs may produce greater harm than the benefit achieved through arrhythmia suppression (1, 2). Other studies have demonstrated that survivors of MI with poor LV function are particularly at risk for proarrhythmia or excess mortality from certain antiarrhythmic drugs, including the class IC agent encainide (3) and, more recently, the class III agent d-sotalol in the Survival With Oral d-Sotalol (SWORD) study (4). To date, no study has demonstrated a benefit with any of the antiarrhythmic agents other than amiodarone for the prevention of SCD, and the evidence for amiodarone has been mixed.

Amiodarone, a complex antiarrhythmic agent with a broad spectrum of electropharmacologic activity (primarily class III activity), was thought to be particularly promising given its lack of significant negative inotropy, and therefore less propensity to exacerbate CHF. While initial small trials of amiodarone therapy for survivors of MI (including a meta-analysis of these trials) demonstrated reduced mortality, the more recent larger controlled trials of amiodarone have not corroborated these findings. The European Myocardial Infarct Amiodarone Trial (EMIAT) was designed to study the efficacy of amiodarone in reducing mortality for survivors of MI with left ventricular dysfunction (EF 40%). There was no difference in all-cause or cardiac mortality, although there was a significant reduction in arrhythmic deaths (5). The Canadian Amiodarone Myocardial Infarction Arrhythmia Trial (CAMIAT) was designed to study the efficacy of amiodarone in reducing mortality for survivors of MI with frequent ventricular ectopy. There was no difference in all-cause mortality; however, similar to EMIAT, there was a significant reduction in a composite end point of resuscitated VF or arrhythmic death (6).

Amiodarone treatment for the prevention of SCD for patients with CHF has also been studied, with conflicting results. The Grupo de Estudio de la Sobrevida en la Insuficiencia Cardiaca en Argentina (GESICA) trial studied the efficacy of amiodarone for the prevention of SCD in patients with severe CHF. There was a significant reduction in all-cause mortality and SCD for the patients treated with amiodarone (7). However, this trial has been criticized for its nonblinded design and the lack of uniform follow-up strategies among the study groups. The Survival Trial of Amiodarone in Patients with Congestive Heart Failure (CHF-STAT) did not demonstrate a difference in SCD or all-cause mortality with prophylactic amiodarone therapy for patients with CHF, LV dysfunction (EF 40%), and asymptomatic ventricular ectopy. However, in a subgroup analysis those patients with nonischemic cardiomyopathy did have a trend toward reduction in SCD (8).

3. **Implantable devices.** In light of evidence for the inefficacy and hazards of antiarrhythmic drugs for the prevention of SCD, attention shifted to the ICD. Several randomized trials comparing the ICD and medical therapy for the primary prevention of SCD were initiated. In the Multicenter Automatic Defibrillator Implantation Trial (MADIT), the ICD was more effective than conventional antiarrhythmic drug therapy in the primary prevention of SCD for patients with nonsustained VT, poor LV function after MI, and inducible ventricular arrhythmia at the time of EP testing that was not suppressed with procainamide (9). However, the recently reported Coronary Artery Bypass Graft (CABG) Patch Trial demonstrated that prophylactic ICD implantation at the time of CABG for patients with LV dysfunction and an abnormal signal-averaged ECG (SAECG) did not improve survival (10).

4. Other ongoing trials of primary prevention of SCD in specific high-risk patient subgroups include the following:

   a. Multicenter Unsustained Tachycardia Trial (MUSTT) (11). This study will evaluate the effect of EP-guided antiarrhythmic drug therapy on SCD and total mortality in patients with CAD, left ventricular EF less than 0.40, asymptomatic nonsustained VT, and inducible sustained VT at EP testing. Also, the study will evaluate the ability of the SAECG to identify patients at high risk for SCD.

   b. Sudden Cardiac Death in Heart Failure Trial (SCD-HeFT). This study will evaluate the ICD, amiodarone, and placebo for the primary prevention of SCD in patients with ischemic and nonischemic heart disease and a left ventricular EF of 0.35.

   c. Second Multicenter Automatic Defibrillator Implantation Trial (MADIT II). This study will evaluate the efficacy of the ICD versus conventional therapy for reduction of total mortality in patients with CAD and a left ventricular EF of 0.30.

C. Secondary prevention

   1. Pharmacologic agents. As with primary prevention of SCD, the disappointments regarding the efficacy and safety of class I antiarrhythmic drugs also shifted attention to non–class I antiarrhythmic drugs for the secondary prevention of SCD. In the Cardiac Arrest in Seattle Conventional versus Amiodarone Drug Evaluation (CASCADE) study, amiodarone was demonstrated to be superior to conventional class I antiarrhythmic drugs in the secondary prevention of SCD (12). In addition, the Electrophysiologic Study Versus Electrocardiographic Monitoring (ESVEM) trial demonstrated that the class III antiarrhythmic drug sotalol was more efficacious than several class I agents in the reduction of total mortality, cardiac mortality, arrhythmic mortality, and VT recurrence for patients with a history of VT, VF or syncope, ventricular ectopy by Holter monitoring of more than 10 PVCs (Premature Ventricular Contractions)/hour, and reproducibly inducible ventricular arrhythmias by EP testing (13,14). These studies supplied further evidence supporting the abandonment of class I antiarrhythmic drugs as first-line therapy for malignant ventricular arrhythmias. However, emergence of the ICD led to randomized trials comparing the efficacy of best medical therapy and ICDs for the secondary prevention of SCD.

   2. Implantable devices. The Antiarrhythmics Versus Implantable Defibrillators (AVID) Trial was designed to study the efficacy of ICD therapy versus the antiarrhythmic drugs amiodarone or sotalol for the secondary prevention of SCD for patients with a history of VF or sustained VT and LV dysfunction or hemodynamically compromising VT. Less than 10% of patients randomized to antiarrhythmic drug therapy received sotalol. The AVID trial was recently terminated prematurely due to significant benefit in total mortality for the patients receiving an ICD (15).

   Two other large trials of secondary prevention of SCD have recently been completed: the Cardiac Arrest Study Hamburg (CASH) was designed to study the efficacy of the ICD versus propafenone, amiodarone, or metoprolol in the secondary prevention of SCD. The propafenone arm of the study was terminated in 1992 due to excess mortality in this group compared with the ICD group (16). Preliminary results of CASH suggest significantly lower mortality in the ICD group compared to the amiodarone and metoprolol groups. Interestingly, there was no significant difference in mortality between the amiodarone and metoprolol groups. The Canadian Implantable Defibrillator Study (CIDS) is similar to AVID in its investigation of the efficacy of ICD versus amiodarone for the secondary prevention of SCD (17). Preliminary results from this trial showed a strong trend toward improved survival in the ICD group (approximately 20% reduction in total mortality), although this did not reach statistical significance. Of note, a potentially important difference between AVID and CIDS is that the latter study included patients with undocumented syncope and either inducible sustained VT at EP study or 10 seconds of VT by monitor. A metaanalysis of the AVID, CASH, and CIDS trials is in progress.

D. Summary: Antiarrhythmic drugs versus ICDs. From the available data there is good evidence that many antiarrhythmic drugs are not efficacious and may be deleterious in the primary prevention of SCD. The ICD has been proven to be highly effective in the termination of malignant ventricular arrhythmias and is more effective than antiarrhythmic medications for the prevention of SCD for patients who fit the criteria for MADIT (nonsustained VT, poor LV systolic function post MI, inducible and nonsuppressible VT at EP Study). However, the superiority of the ICD has not yet been proven in other high-risk subgroups. Patients with LV dysfunction and an abnormal SAECG undergoing CABG did not benefit from prophylactic ICD implantation. The ongoing trials outlined above, which are designed to compare antiarrhythmic drug therapy and the ICD for primary prevention of SCD for patients with heart failure or nonsustained VT, will hopefully provide valuable information regarding these high-risk patients.

The treatment of survivors of SCD is much less controversial. The evidence from several recent randomized trials demonstrates the superiority of the ICD over antiarrhythmic drugs for this population. Perhaps more controversial for this group of patients is the type of ICD to implant, given the fact that the majority of these patients only require protection from sudden death. The choice of device and its associated technological features should be considered on an individual basis and are beyond the scope of this book.

E. Key Suggestions
1. A thorough evaluation of the SCD survivor for reversible triggers of the episode, particularly myocardial ischemia, is crucial.
2. Risk stratification for recurrent SCD is also important, especially determination of LV function and the extent and severity of CAD.
3. If CAD is present, stress testing with radionuclide or ECG imaging for determination of myocardial ischemia and/or viability may be indicated.

F. Controversies. Electrophysiologic testing for SCD survivors may be limited by the low incidence and unknown significance of inducible ventricular arrhythmias in this population.

G. Future
1. **Prevention.** Several areas of research should have an impact on the occurrence of SCD. The majority of episodes of SCD are secondary to underlying CAD. Therefore, efforts to prevent CAD and improve treatment modalities for myocardial ischemia and MI may have the greatest impact on the incidence of SCD. Advances in the understanding of the mechanisms and triggers of SCD may lead to more specific and efficacious treatments aimed at prevention, such as new medications, gene therapies, or advanced catheter ablation techniques. Technological advances will continue to improve the efficacy and safety of the ICD, and improved telemetry storage within these devices for arrhythmic events may provide valuable insight into the mechanisms of SCD. Perhaps most importantly of all, there should be continued support for large-scale, controlled randomized trials designed to investigate the therapeutic strategies for populations at risk for SCD.
2. **Dual-chamber pacemaker-defibrillators.** These devices are a promising development, particularly for patients who require a pacemaker and an ICD. Such patients would only require one implantation procedure, and the incorporation of the two devices into one virtually eliminates the potential for pacemaker–ICD interaction (see Chapter 46). Also, the combined device should increase the specificity of ventricular arrhythmia detection via information gained through the atrial and ventricular leads, which would decrease the incidence of inappropriate shocks for supraven-

tricular arrhythmias. These devices may also incorporate such technology as rate adaptation for chronotropic incompetence and automatic mode switching to avoid inappropriate tracking of atrial arrhythmias.

3. **Automated external defibrillator (AED) and public access defibrillation.** An automated external defibrillator is designed to be used by emergency personnel and perhaps even minimally trained lay rescuers, particularly for victims of out-of-hospital SCD. The device monitors the patient's electrocardiogram via self-adhesive defibrillation electrode pads applied to the chest wall and is programmed with a VF detection algorithm. When the device detects VF, an alarm is emitted, followed by delivery of a defibrillation shock or an indicator for the rescuer to press a button to deliver the shock. There is evidence that the use of these devices results in more rapid delivery of a defibrillation shock than that achieved with manual defibrillation, particularly in those areas served by personnel with less training. There has been an effort to provide AEDs at specific locations for public access defibrillation, including airplanes, airports, and shopping malls.

SUGGESTED READINGS

References

1. The Cardiac Arrhythmia Suppression Trial (CAST) Investigators. Preliminary report: effect of encainide and flecainide on mortality in a randomized trial of arrhythmia suppression after myocardial infarction. *N Engl J Med* 1989;321: 406–412.
2. The Cardiac Arrhythmia Suppression Trial II Investigators. Effect of the antiarrhythmic agent moricizine on survival after myocardial infarction. *N Engl J Med* 1992;327:227–233.
3. The Encainide-Ventricular Tachycardia Study Group. Treatment of life-threatening ventricular tachycardia with encainide hydrochloride in patients with left ventricular dysfunction. *Am J Cardiol* 1988;62:571.
4. Waldo AL, Camm AJ, deRuyter H, et al. Effect of *d*-sotalol on mortality in patients with left ventricular dysfunction after recent and remote myocardial infarction. The SWORD Investigators. Survival With Oral *d*-Sotalol. [Published erratum appears in *Lancet* 1996 Aug 10;348:416.] *Lancet* 1996;348:7–12.
5. Julian DG, Camm AJ, Frangin G, et al. Randomised trial of effect of amiodarone on mortality in patients with left ventricular dysfunction after recent myocardial infarction: EMIAT. European Myocardial Infarct Amiodarone Trial Investigators. [Published errata appear in *Lancet* 1997 Apr 19:349:1180 and 1997 Jun 14; 349:1776.] *Lancet* 1997;349:667–674.
6. Cairns JA, Connolly SJ, Roberts R, Gent M. Randomised trial of outcome after myocardial infarction in patients with frequent or repetitive ventricular premature depolarisations: CAMIAT. Canadian Amiodarone Myocardial Infarction Arrhythmia Trial Investigators. [Published erratum appears in *Lancet* 1997 Jun 14; 349:1776.] *Lancet* 1997;349:675–682.
7. Doval HC, Nul DR, Grancelli HO, Perrone SV, Bortman GR, Curiel R. Randomised trial of low-dose amiodarone in severe congestive heart failure. Grupo de Estudio de la Sobrevida en la Insuficiencia Cardiaca en Argentina (GESICA). *Lancet* 1994;344:493–498.
8. Singh SN, Fletcher RD, Fisher SG, et al. Amiodarone in patients with congestive heart failure and asymptomatic ventricular arrhythmia. Survival Trial of Antiarrhythmic Therapy in Congestive Heart Failure. *N Engl J Med* 1995;333:77–82.
9. Moss AJ, Hall WJ, Cannom DS, et al. Improved survival with an implanted defibrillator in patients with coronary disease at high risk for ventricular arrhythmia. Multicenter Automatic Defibrillator Implantation Trial Investigators. *N Engl J Med* 1996;335:1933–1940.
10. Bigger JT Jr. Prophylactic use of implanted cardiac defibrillators in patients at high risk for ventricular arrhythmias after coronary artery bypass graft surgery. Coronary Artery Bypass Graft (CABG) Patch Trial Investigators. *N Engl J Med* 1997;337:1569–1575.

11. Buxton Ae, Fisher JD, Josephson ME, et al. Prevention of sudden death in patients with coronary artery disease: the Multicenter Unsustained Tachycardia Trial (MUST). *Prog Cardiovasc Dis* 1993;36:215–226.
12. The CASCADE Investigators. Randomized antiarrhythmic drug therapy in survivors of cardiac arrest (the CASCADE study). *Am J Cardiol* 1993;72:280–287.
13. Mason JW. A comparison of seven antiarrhythmic drugs in patients with ventricular tachyarrhythmias. Electrophysiologic Study versus Electrocardiographic Monitoring Investigators. *N Engl J Med* 1993;329:452–458.
14. Mason JW. A comparison of electrophysiologic testing with Holter monitoring to predict antiarrhythmic-drug efficacy for ventricular tachyarrhythmias. Electrophysiologic Study versus Electrocardiographic Monitoring Investigators. *N Engl J Med* 1993;329:445–451.
15. The Antiarrhythmics versus Implantatable Defibrillators (AVIC) Investigators. A comparison of antiarrhythmic-drug therapy with implantable defibrillators in patients resuscitated from near-fatal ventricular arrhythmias. *N Engl J Med* 1997;337:1576–1583.
16. Siebels J, Kuck KH. Implantable cardioverter defibrillator compared with antiarrhythmic drug treatment in cardiac arrest survivors (the Cardiac Arrest Study Hamburg). *Am Heart J* 1994;127:1139–1144.
17. Connolly SJ, Gent M, Roberts RS, et al. Canadian Implantable Defibrillator Study (CIDS): study design and organization. CIDS Co-Investigators. *Am J Cardiol* 1993;72:103F–108F.
18. Cain ME, Anderson JL, Arnsdoft MF, Mason JW, Scheinman MM, Waldo AL. American College of Cardiology Expert Consensus Document: signal-averaged electrocardiography. *J Am Coll Cardiol* 1996;27:238–249.

Landmark Articles

Antiarrhythmics Versus Implantable Defibrillators (AVID) Investigators. A comparison of antiarrhythmic-drug therapy with implantable defibrillators in patients resuscitated from near-fatal ventricular arrhythmias. *N Engl J Med* 1997;337:1576–1583.

Buxton AE, Fisher JD, Josephson ME, et al. Prevention of sudden death in patients with coronary artery disease: the Multicenter Unsustained Tachycardia Trial (MUST). *Prog Cardiovasc Dis* 1993; 36:215–226.

CABG Patch Trial Investigators and Coordinators. The Coronary Artery Bypass Graft (CABG) Patch Trial. *Prog Cardiovasc Dis* 1993; 36:97–114.

Cairns JA, Connolly SJ, Roberts R, Gent M. Randomised trial of outcome after myocardial infarction in patients with frequent or repetitive ventricular premature depolarisations: CAMIAT. Canadian Amiodarone Myocardial Infarction Arrhythmia Trial Investigators. *Lancet* 1997;349:675–682.

Cardiac Arrhythmia Suppression Trial (CAST) Investigators. Preliminary report: effect of encainide and flecainide on mortality in a randomized trial of arrhythmia suppression after myocardial infarction. *N Engl J Med* 1989;321:406–412.

CASCADE Investigators. Randomized antiarrhythmic drug therapy in survivors of cardiac arrest (the CASCADE Study). *Am J Cardiol* 1993; 72:280–287.

Connolly SJ, Gent M, Roberts RS, et al. Canadian Implantable Defibrillator Study (CIDS): study design and organization. CIDS Co-Investigators. *Am J Cardiol* 1993; 72:103F–108F.

Doval HC, Nul DR, Grancelli HO, Perrone SV, Bortman GR, Curiel R. Randomised trial of low-dose amiodarone in severe congestive heart failure. Grupo de Estudio de la Sobrevida en la Insuficiencia Cardiaca en Argentina (GESICA). *Lancet* 1994;344:493–498.

Julian DG, Camm AJ, Frangin G, et al. Randomised trial of effect of amiodarone on mortality in patients with left-ventricular dysfunction after recent myocardial infarction: EMIAT. European Myocardial Infarct Amiodarone Trial Investigators. *Lancet* 1997; 349:667–674.

Mason JW. A comparison of electrophysiologic testing with Holter monitoring to predict antiarrhythmic-drug efficacy for ventricular tachyarrhythmias. Electrophysiologic Study versus Electrocardiographic Monitoring Investigators. *N Engl J Med* 1993;329:445–451.

Moss AJ, Hall WJ, Cannom DS, et al. Improved survival with an implanted defibrillator in patients with coronary disease at high risk for ventricular arrhythmia. Multicenter Automatic Defibrillator Implantation Trial Investigators. *N Engl J Med* 1996;335:1933–1940.

Siebels J, Cappato R, Ruppel R, Schneider MA, Kuck KH. Preliminary results of the Cardiac Arrest Study Hamburg (CASH). CASH Investigators. *Am J Cardiol* 1993; 72:109F–113F.

Singh SN, Fletcher RD, Fisher SG, et al. Amiodarone in patients with congestive heart failure and asymptomatic ventricular arrhythmia. Survival Trial of Antiarrhythmic Therapy in Congestive Heart Failure. *N Engl J Med* 1995;333:77–82.

Waldo AL, Camm AJ, deRuyter H, et al. Effect of *d*-sotalol on mortality in patients with left ventricular dysfunction after recent and remote myocardial infarction. The SWORD Investigators. Survival With Oral *d*-Sotalol. *Lancet* 1996;348:7–12.

Key Reviews

Domanski MJ, Zipes DP, Schron E. Treatment of sudden cardiac death. Current understandings from randomized trials and future research directions. *Circulation* 1997;95:2694–2699.

Furberg CD. Effect of antiarrhythmic drugs on mortality after myocardial infarction. *Am J Cardiol* 1983;52:32C–36C.

Myerburg RJ, Interian A Jr, Mitrani RM, Kessler KM, Castellanos A. Frequency of sudden cardiac death and profiles of risk. *Am J Cardiol* 1997;80:10F–19F.

Yusuf S, Peto R, Lewis J, Collins R, Sleight P. Beta blockade during and after myocardial infarction: an overview of the randomized trials. *Prog Cardiovasc Dis* 1985; 27:335–371.

Zipes DP, Wellens HJ. Sudden cardiac death. Circulation 1998; 98:2334–2351.

Relevant Book Chapters

Dunbar SB, Ellenbogen K, Epstein AE. *Sudden cardiac death: past, present, and future.* American Heart Association Monograph Series. Armonk, NY: Futura Publishing, 1997:417.

Myerburg RJ, Castellanos A. Cardiac arrest and sudden cardiac death. In: Braunwald E, ed. *Heart disease: a textbook of cardiovascular medicine.* Philadelphia: WB Saunders, 1997:742–779.

Poole JE, Bardy GH. Sudden cardiac death. In: Zipes DP, Jalife J, eds. *Cardiac electrophysiology: from cell to bedside.* Philadelphia: WB Saunders, 1995:812–832.

22. SYNCOPE

Vasant B. Patel

I. **Introduction**
   A. Syncope is a common medical problem that accounts for approximately 6% of medical admissions and 3% of emergency room visits. Syncope is defined as a **sudden transient loss of consciousness with associated loss of postural tone. Recovery is spontaneous, without neurologic deficit and without requiring electrical or chemical cardioversion.** Generally, a fall in systolic blood pressure below 70 mm Hg or a mean arterial pressure of 40 mm Hg results in loss of consciousness. Cerebral blood flow usually decreases with aging, making the elderly at higher risk for syncope.
   B. Syncope as a symptom can be caused by **a variety of medical diseases that produce a transient interruption of cerebral blood flow.**
      1. A genuine effort should be made to **determine a specific cause of syncope.** Identifying a specific cause can help in the selection of therapy, prevent recurrences, minimize expensive evaluations, and decrease morbidity.
      2. **Patients with cardiac syncope have higher rates of mortality and sudden death** at follow-up; thus, identifying and treating cardiac syncope can improve outcome.
II. **Clinical presentation.** Although a variety of diagnostic tests are available for evaluation of syncope, a thorough history and physical examination is crucial to determine the etiology and the best diagnostic approach. A good history and physical examination can provide a clue to a diagnosis in up to 50% of cases.
   A. **Signs and symptoms.** Accurately described symptoms can lead to specific diagnostic considerations, as illustrated in Tables 22-1A and 22-1B.
      1. Important during history taking is to **determine the symptoms prior to syncope (the prodrome),** association with any particular activity, exertion or change in position, and frequency of syncope.
      2. The initial approach to any patient with syncope should include a **search for the presence of structural heart disease such as valvular stenosis, cardiomyopathy, or myocardial infarction.** This suggests more malignant etiologies such as ventricular tachycardia.
      3. **Symptoms of vasovagal syncope.** Calkins et al. reported that a careful history could diagnose vasovagal syncope (1). They reported that **young women (younger than than 55 years) with a postsyncopal recovery period that included fatigue,** and patients with **clear precipitating factors, diaphoresis, palpitations preceding syncope, and severe fatigue following syncope** were more likely to have vasovagal syncope than ventricular tachycardia or complete heart block.
      4. **Convulsive syncope.** Occasionally, a syncopal episode is accompanied by **mild muscular jerking** as a result of cerebral anoxia. This phenomenon is not true epilepsy, and one must make every effort to distinguish between syncope and seizure.
      5. Other entities that make diagnosis difficult are **vertigo, transient ischemic events, and conversion disorder.**
      6. One should always **carefully review the medications of a patient with syncope** for their potential role directly or by interaction with other medications.
   B. **Physical findings**
      1. The **physical examination is especially important when the patient is unable to describe the event** and no witnesses are available, as certain findings on examination can direct the physician in the diagnostic evaluation.

Table 22-1a. Cardiovascular causes of syncope

Neurally mediated (vasovagal)
Situational
    Micturition
    Defecation
    Postprandial
    Swallowing
    Coughing
    Sneezing
Glossopharyngeal neuralgia
Orthostatic syncope
Carotid sinus syncope
    Cardioinhibitory
    Vasodepressor
    Mixed
Mechanical
    Aortic stenosis
    Hypertrophic cardiomyopathy
    Left atrial myxoma
    Mitral stenosis
    Pulmonic stenosis
    Pulmonary hypertension/embolism
    Right atrial myxoma
    Myocardial infarction
    Cardiac tamponade
Electrical
    Second- and third-degree atrioventricular block
    Sick sinus syndrome
    Supraventricular tachycardia
    Ventricular tachycardia
    Torsade de pointes
    Pacemaker malfunction

2. The **comprehensive evaluation** should include a fundoscopic examination of the eye for an embolic source. The evaluation should also search for the presence of carotid bruit and carotid upstroke, subtle neurologic deficits that may be due to a stroke or neuropathy, cardiac murmurs with attention given to valvular findings, extra heart sounds such as tumor plop, peripheral pulses for evidence of peripheral vascular disease and entities such as subclavian steal, and dermatologic clues that may suggest collagen vascular disease or vasculitis.

3. In examining a patient with syncope, it is important to **check blood pressure in both arms and orthostatic blood pressure. Repeated orthostatic blood pressure measurements** may be needed when there is a high clinical suspicion of orthostatic syncope (see II.C.1.c).

C. **Etiology and pathophysiology**

1. **Neurally mediated syncope.** Vasovagal or neurally mediated syncope is the **most common cause of syncope.** Many situations can lead to vasovagal faint. Examples include unpleasant smell, sudden pain, acute blood loss, and sustained upright posture. Vasovagal reactions are often preceded by increase in heart rate and blood pressure.

a. **Neurocardiogenic syncope** is thought to be the result of **autonomic overactivity followed by a fall in peripheral vascular resistance without a significant rise in cardiac output.** In susceptible individuals, the stimulation of mechanoreceptors located in the inferior and posterior wall of the left ventricle by stretch, cardiac

Table 22-1b.   Clinical features suggestive of specific causes

Symptom or finding	Diagnostic consideration
After sudden unexpected pain, unpleasant sight, sound, or smell	Vasovagal syncope
During or immediately after micturition, cough, swallow, or defecation	Situational syncope
With neuralgia (glossopharyngeal or trigeminal)	Bradycardia or vasodepressor
Upon standing	Orthostatic hypotension
Taking hypotensive medication	Drug-induced syncope
Symptoms within 1 hr after meals	Postprandial hypertension
Prolonged standing at attention	Vasovagal
Well-trained athlete after exertion	Vasovagal
Changing position (from sitting to lying, bending, turning over in bed)	Atrial myxoma, thrombus
Syncope with exertion	Aortic stenosis, pulmonary hypertension, mitral stenosis, HOCM, coronary artery disease
With head rotation, pressure on carotid sinus	Carotid sinus syncope
Associated with vertigo, dysarthria, diplopia	TIA, stroke
With arm exercise	Subclavian steal syndrome

HOCM, Hypertrophic obstructive cardiomyopathy; TIA, Transient ischemic attack.
Adapted from Kapoor WN, et al. *J Am Geriatr Soc* 1994, with permission.

distention, or rapid systolic contraction leads to increased neural discharges through unmyelinated C fibers to the vasomotor center in the medulla, resulting in enhanced parasympathetic and decreased sympathetic activity. The withdrawal of the sympathetic nervous system results in sudden bradycardia and/or hypotension. Animal studies suggest that cardiac afferents may not be required all of the time to initiate a vasodepressor response and that other potential mechanisms, such as release of endogenous opioids or nitric oxide inhibition of sympathetic nerve firing and primary central nervous system activation, may play a role in vasodepressor syncope.

b. Situational syncope. Patients often recall situational syncopal episodes. **Micturition, defecation, cough, and trumpet playing** are examples. The action causes a reflex vasodilatation (vagally mediated) that is made worse if the patient undergoes a Valsalva maneuver, which would decrease the blood return to the right heart.

c. Orthostatic syncope. Postural hypotension is reported in up to 24% of elderly people. Normally when one stands, the systolic blood pressure drops only 5 to 15 mm Hg, and the diastolic pressure rises a little. In orthostasis, the decrease in systolic blood pressure is higher than 20 mm Hg; frequently, the diastolic pressure drops by more than 10 mm Hg. This finding demands that one search for a potential cause.

   (1) Common etiologies include **volume depletion, medications, diabetes, alcohol, infection, and varicose veins.**

   (2) Dysautonomic syndromes causing orthostatic hypotension are divided into two categories: primary and secondary. Primary autonomic failure is idiopathic and includes pure autonomic failure (Bradbury-Eggleston syndrome) and multiple system atrophy (Shy-Drager syndrome). Secondary causes include amyloidosis, tabes dorsalis, multiple sclerosis, spinal tumors, and familial dysautonomia.

d. Carotid sinus syncope. Fewer than 1% of patients presenting with syncope have been given a diagnosis of carotid sinus syncope. This entity should be considered in patients with spontaneous symptoms while shaving, turning the head, or wearing a tight collar and in older patients with recurrent syncope. A cardioinhibitory response (bradycardia) occurs in about 70% and a vasodepressor response (hypotension) in 10%. The remainder have a mixed response (bradycardia with hypotension). Carotid sinus syncope is elicited by pressure on the carotid sinus and can be blocked by atropine. Clinical presentation along with findings of carotid sinus hypersensitivity in the absence of other potential causes is enough to make the diagnosis. Symptom reproduction during carotid massage is not necessary for a diagnosis. A positive carotid test is defined by a cardiac asystole of 3 seconds or longer, a drop in systolic blood pressure of greater than 50 mm Hg, or a drop of more than 30 mm Hg and symptoms.

2. Cardiac syncope

a. Mechanical

   (1) Syncope or symptoms frequently occur with exertion and usually from left ventricular outflow obstruction, as seen in aortic stenosis or hypertrophic obstructive cardiomyopathy (HOCM). With exertion, peripheral vascular resistance falls but the cardiac output is fixed, leading to hypotension.

   (2) Right ventricular outflow obstruction can also result in syncope. This condition can also trigger a vasodepressor component by mechanisms similar to neurocardiogenic syncope.

   (3) Myocardial ischemia and infarction, pulmonary embolus, and cardiac tamponade should be kept in mind. **Syncope may be the initial complaint in 7% of patients over the age of 65 presenting with myocardial infarction.**

b. Electrical. Ventricular tachycardia, sick sinus syndrome, and atrioventricular block are the most common causes of arrhythmic syncope. One must also consider supraventricular tachycardia, Wolff-Parkinson-White syndrome, and torsades de pointes. Arrhythmic syncope carries the worst prognosis and must be thoroughly evaluated.

   (1) Primary cardiac arrhythmias are the most common cause of syncope in patients with known cardiac disease, such as previous myocardial infarction, left ventricular dysfunction, or cardio-myopathy.

   (2) Medications and electrolyte abnormalities should also be considered as etiologies of arrhythmic syncope.

   (3) Patients with pacemakers should have their pacemaker inter-rogated for possible malfunction. Individuals with pacemaker or implantable defibrillators should be educated about the devices and followed regularly.

3. Noncardiovascular syncope

a. Neurologic causes include stroke, transient ischemic attacks, normal pressure hydrocephalus, and seizures.

b. Metabolic causes include arrhythmias induced by hypoglycemia, hypoxia, and hypokalemia.

c. Psychogenic causes include anxiety disorder, panic disorder, hyperventilation, somatization, depression, hysterical syncope (no change in blood pressure or pulse), and conversion disorder.

d. Drugs that can cause syncope include **nitrates, angiotensin-converting enzyme inhibitors, calcium channel blockers, β-blockers, quinidine, procainamide, disopyramide, flecai-**

nide, amiodarone, diuretics, vincristine, insulin, cocaine, and digoxin. The α-blockers (i.e., prazosin) are potent agents and commonly cause orthostatic hypotension, especially in the elderly. These agents should be initiated with careful monitoring and prescribed to be taken in the evening.

4. **Unknown/unexplained.** This is a diagnosis of exclusion and carries a very good prognosis. The studies in the past indicate that anywhere from 33% to 50% of patients with syncope had no identifiable cause, but this more often provides reassurance. Newer diagnostic tools such as tilt-table testing, loop recorders, signal-averaged electrocardiography (SAECG), and electrophysiologic study assist physicians in identifying a previously unknown cause of syncope.

III. **Laboratory examination**

A. **A single electrocardiogram offers the possible diagnosis in approximately 5% of cases;** it demonstrates sinus pause, high-degree atrioventricular block, prolonged QT interval, or Wolff-Parkinson-White syndrome.

B. **Laboratory tests** including stress testing, electroencephalogram, computed tomographic scan of head, and cerebral angiography all have a very low yield unless there is a history of trauma, stroke, or seizures.

C. **Echocardiography** has a low yield unless the physical examination reveals evidence of structural heart disease (aortic stenosis, HOCM).

IV. **Diagnostic testing.** Holter monitoring, loop recorders, SAECG, electrophysiologic testing, and tilt-table testing are major diagnostic tools. Their yield depends on presence or absence of underlying structural heart disease.

A. In evaluating a patient with syncope, **it is important to differentiate patients with and without structural heart disease.** Furthermore, the goal of evaluation should be to obtain a sufficiently strong correlation between symptoms and an abnormal finding during diagnostic testing. The key points to remember are as follows:

1. Cardiac syncope carries a high mortality rate, and thus one should **admit an individual suspected of having cardiac syncope** for evaluation.

2. The cause of **47% of syncope cases remains unexplained;** the prognosis in these cases, however, often is good.

3. **Syncope in the elderly** is frequently multifactorial (e.g., drugs, structural heart disease, anemia, volume depletion, decreased baroreceptor sensitivity)

4. The **workup should be individualized** to be cost-effective and accurate, as suggested in Fig. 22-1.

B. **Holter monitoring.** Holter or prolonged ECG monitoring is one of the most commonly utilized tests for the evaluation of syncope. However, symptomatic correlation of a cardiac arrhythmia with a syncopal spell is rare and seen only in about 4% of cases. **A completely normal or negative Holter may be just as helpful as a captured arrhythmia.** The sensitivity and specificity of ECG monitoring for arrhythmic syncope are not known because of the lack of criteria for abnormal results or a gold standard that is independent of arrhythmias diagnosed by monitoring. The difficulty is to establish a correlation between arrhythmia and a syncopal spell.

1. Gibson et al. reviewed 1,512 Holter recordings of patients referred for evaluation of syncope; a total of 255 (17%) patients reported syncope or related symptoms of which only 30 (2%) were correlated with arrhythmias (2). Ventricular tachycardia was predominant in the syncope group, whereas supraventricular and sinus tachycardia were common in the presyncope group. In addition, there was an increasing incidence with age of supraventricular and ventricular tachycardia, but the correlation with syncope remained obscure.

2. Pratt et al. studied 80 patients with structural heart disease through Holter monitors and follow-up electrophysiologic study. They concluded that the combination of a clinical presentation of syncope, presence of coro-

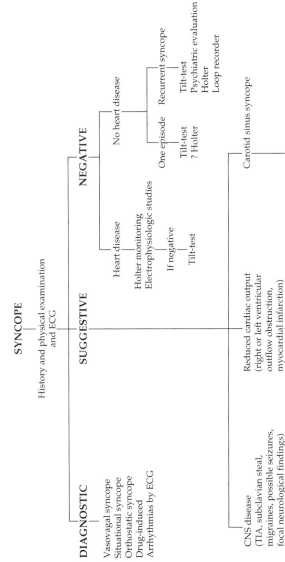

FIG. 22-1. Schematic algorithm for evaluation of patients presenting with syncope. Reproduced from Kapoor WN. *Am J Med* 1991;90:91–106, with permission.

nary artery disease, and left ventricle ejection fraction less than 30% had a better positive predictive value in terms of inducibility of sustained ventricular tachycardia than any ambulatory ECG monitoring criteria (3).

3. Studies have shown that **sinus pause longer than 2 seconds, Mobitz II or complete atrioventricular block, and runs of nonsustained ventricular tachycardia on Holter should be taken seriously.**

4. The duration of ECG monitoring is an important issue. It appears that **48 hours is optimum.**

C. **Loop recorder.** When used correctly, **loop recorders effectively couple arrhythmias and syncope.** Loop recorders are **useful in patients with recurrent frequent syncope** who benefit from prolonged monitoring for weeks to months. When activated by the patient, loop recorders permanently record the previous 4 to 5 minutes of rhythm data. The recorder can capture arrhythmias during a syncopal episode if the patient activates it after regaining consciousness. The next-generation loop recorders will be implantable devices similar to a pacemaker, and they continuously record a single-lead ECG (i.e., Medtronic-Reveal). These devices have the capability to store a 15-minute segment of cardiac rhythm when activated either during or after a syncopal episode, and the physician can later retrieve this information.

D. **Signal-averaged electrocardiography** is useful in predicting inducibility of ventricular arrhythmias by electrophysiologic testing, especially in patients with ischemic heart disease, but it does not address the presence of sinus pauses or blocks that require electrophysiologic testing.

1. Signal-averaged electrocardiography is a collection of 100 to 300 single QRS complexes, which are amplified, filtered for noise, and averaged to determine the presence of late potentials. Late potential refers to the presence of low-amplitude/high-frequency signals in the terminal segment of the amplified QRS. The **late potentials seem to identify the presence of a reentrant substrate and may indicate an independent risk factor of future life-threatening ventricular arrhythmias.**

2. When **combined with an ejection fraction of less than 40%, the presence of late potentials can be used to identify patients with an even higher risk for ventricular tachycardia.** Studies evaluating this profile of patients have demonstrated sensitivity of 90% and specificity of 95% to 100% in predicting inducible sustained ventricular tachycardia.

3. Various commercially available devices utilize different filters, lead configurations, and processing algorithms; therefore, the **criteria for abnormal SAECG may vary among various manufacturers.** Abnormal SAECG findings include total QRS duration greater than 114 milliseconds, root mean square voltage of the terminal 40 milliseconds of the complex (RMS40) less than 20 μV, or duration of low-amplitude signals in terminal QRS (LAS) greater than 38 milliseconds. The total duration of the QRS complex, including the late potential, has been shown to be independent of other measures of cardiac risk. RMS40 is probably the most sensitive and specific of all three variables.

4. **A positive SAECG suggests the need for further electrophysiologic testing,** especially in individuals with known heart disease.

5. The **absence of late potentials has a high negative predictive value** (94%). In patients with syncope and a negative SAECG, electrophysiologic study is not absolutely indicated. A normal SAECG has less than a 5% risk of inducible ventricular tachycardia by electrophysiologic testing.

6. **No satisfactory method of analysis is available at present to include patients with bundle branch block** because it would be virtually impossible to distinguish between late activation due to the conduction defect and reentrant substrate.

E. **Electrophysiologic study.** Electrophysiologic study should be considered in **patients with underlying structural heart disease or in elderly patients with recurrent syncope.** Similar to Holter monitoring, induced arrhythmias during electrophysiologic study do not usually produce syncope in the laboratory; therefore, a cause-and-effect relationship often has to be assumed. Regardless, electrophysiologic testing is useful in better delineating a cardiac etiology of syncope, especially in people with baseline bundle branch or bifascicular block.

1. **Indications** for electrophysiologic study generally include:

> Known or suspected ventricular tachyarrhythmias, especially to guide therapy
> Uncertainty about the origin of wide QRS tachycardia
> Patients with unexplained syncope and history of heart disease
> Patients with nonsustained ventricular tachycardia, impaired left ventricular function, and late potentials on SAECG, to stratify prognosis and guide therapy
> Patients with drug-refractory malignant ventricular arrhythmias who are candidates for ablative therapy
> Patients being considered for implantable cardioverter-defibrillator

2. The **electrophysiologic findings** considered important in the etiology of syncope are:

> Sustained monomorphic ventricular tachycardia
> Sinus node recovery time greater than 3 seconds
> Spontaneous or pacing-induced infranodal or infrahisian block
> Baseline HV interval greater than 100 milliseconds or significant prolongation post procainamide challenge
> Paroxysmal supraventricular tachycardia with symptomatic hypotension

3. The sensitivity and specificity of induced sustained monomorphic ventricular tachycardia is greater than 90%. However, the sensitivity of prolonged sinus node recovery time is low (69%), although the specificity is reported as high as 100% when electrophysiologic studies are compared with results of Holter monitoring.

4. Patients with no known heart disease, ejection fraction greater than 40%, normal ECG and Holter, and multiple syncopal episodes (more than five per year) often have **negative electrophysiologic studies.** A 3-year follow-up of patients with negative electrophysiologic tests revealed a 24% recurrence rate of syncope and a mortality rate of 15%; however, **a 3-year follow-up after positive electrophysiologic studies and treatment revealed a 32% recurrence rate and higher mortality (61%)** (4).

5. The **limitations and disadvantages of electrophysiologic testing** are high cost, lower specificity if a more aggressive electrical stimulation protocol is utilized, and poor prediction of bradyarrhythmias and several other arrhythmias of unknown clinical significance without symptoms.

F. **Upright tilt-table testing**

1. **Mechanism.** It is believed that a surge in catecholamines may paradoxically enhance the susceptibility to bradycardia and hypotension, resulting in syncope by activation of cardiac mechanoreceptors. Vasovagal syncope can be induced by keeping susceptible individuals upright on a tilt table with or without chemical stimulation. The mechanism is not completely understood, but it is believed to be similar to activation of Bezold-Jarisch reflex.

2. The best candidate for a tilt-table study is **a person with unexplained recurrent syncope, with underlying heart disease and a negative electrophysiologic study, or with no known structural heart disease.** In reviewing various tilt-table studies, Kapoor et al. found that 49% of patients had positive response during tilt testing, 66% had positive response using isoproterenol with tilt testing, 65% had a cardioinhibitory response, and 30% had a vasodepressor response. The **number of positive responses increased with an increasing angle of tilt and longer duration;** however, there was no correlation between posi-

Table 22-2. Medical therapy in syncope

Etiology	Treatment
Vasodepressor syncope	β-Blockers, disopyramide, fluoxetine, sertraline, dual-chamber pacing, theophylline, and scopolamine
Dysautonomic syncope	Elastic support hose, water exercise, increased sodium intake, fludrocortisone, ephedrine sulfate, midodrine, erythropoietin, and methylphenidate
Situational syncope	Stool softeners, urinating while sitting down
Carotid sinus syncope	Avoidance of tight collars, surgical removal of carotid sinus tumor, pacemaker in patients with predominantly cardioinhibitory syncope
Tachyarrhythmias	Antiarrhythmic agents, such as amiodarone or sotalol, or implantable defibrillators

tive responses and maximum dose of isoproterenol (5). Although limited information is available on the sensitivity of upright tilt-table testing, it is reported to be around 70%. The specificity has ranged from 35% to 92% with isoproterenol. Kapoor et al. reported higher false-positive rates with isoproterenol, especially at higher angle of tilt, indicating lower specificity.

3. It appears that **tilt-table testing when used in the appropriate setting is beneficial in diagnosing previously unexplained syncope,** thus preventing recurrences and reducing morbidity. A detailed discussion of head-up tilt-table testing is provided in Chapter 48.

V. Treatment. In general, the treatment of syncope is individualized and depends on the etiology of syncope.

  A. Medical therapy. Table 22-2 addresses the various etiologies of syncope and potential medical treatment. Appropriate medical therapy is associated with a low recurrence rate (10%).

    1. **Electrolyte abnormalities must be corrected** if they are suspected in the etiology of arrhythmias (e.g., prolonged QT secondary to hypomagnesemia or hypocalcemia).

    2. **Particular attention should be given to the patient's medications** as these might have drug–drug interactions or proarrhythmic potentials, and might be causing orthostatic hypotension. Unnecessary medications should be discontinued when feasible.

  B. Device therapy

    1. **Symptomatic bradyarrhythmias and atrioventricular blocks require pacemaker implantation.**

      a. Patients with an HV interval (impulse time from atrioventricular node to the ventricle) of more than 100 milliseconds are at a high risk for **progression to heart block** and may benefit from a pacemaker.

      b. Although the mode of pacing is debated, in **patients with carotid sinus syncope,** a dual-chamber pacer is desirable with rate responsiveness.

      c. VVIR pacing should be used only in the setting of **bradycardia without a vasodepressor component or chronic atrial fibrillation.**

    2. **Antiarrhythmic therapy** appears to decrease the frequency of syncope; however, it has not been shown to improve survival. In patients with malignant or life-threatening ventricular arrhythmias or inducible sustained monomorphic ventricular tachycardia, **implantable defibrillators** are the current best option based on recent studies.

  C. Surgical therapy

    1. **Patients who have exertional cardiac syncope** due to left or right heart outflow obstruction should be instructed to **avoid exertional**

activities that precipitate syncope and **should be considered for surgical repair.**

2. Surgical septal myomectomy is procedure of choice in **patients with HOCM;** however, percutaneous septal ablation is now being investigated.

3. Coronary artery bypass graft surgery or percutaneous coronary intervention should be considered in **patients with life-threatening arrhythmias (usually polymorphic ventricular tachycardias) due to ischemia.**

VI. **Follow-up.** The follow-up of patients with syncope is often dependent on the etiology and the therapy being instituted.

A. **Patients with frequent spells of syncope without an identifiable etiology** have a favorable prognosis and should be followed regularly.

B. **Patients with cardiac syncope** require very close follow-up as their mortality is significantly higher than that of patients with other causes of syncope.

C. **Elderly patients** may require closer monitoring about their home situation, their need for assistance with activity of daily living, and changes in medications.

D. A consultant who diagnoses syncope should **communicate with the patient's primary physician about etiology, therapy, and important warning signs** if devices such as pacemakers or defibrillators are implanted.

SUGGESTED READINGS

References

1. Calkins H, Shyr Y, Frumin H, et al. The value of the clinical history in the differentiation of syncope due to ventricular tachycardia, atrioventricular block, and neurocardiogenic syncope. *Am J Med* 1995;98:365–373.

2. Gibson TC, Heitzman MR. Diagnostic efficacy of 24-hour electrocardiographic monitoring for syncope. *Am J Cardiol* 1984; 53:1013–1017.

3. Pratt CM, Thornton BC, Margo SA, et al. Spontaneous arrhythmia detected on ambulatory electrocardiographic recording lacks precision in predicting inducibility of ventricular tachycardia during electrophysiology study. *J Am Coll Cardiol* 1987;10:97–104.

4. Bass EB, Elson JJ, Fogoros RN, et al. Long-term prognosis of patients undergoing electrophysiologic studies for syncope of unknown origin. *Am J Cardiol* 1988;62: 1186–1191.

5. Kapoor WN, Smith M, Miller NL. Upright tilt testing in evaluating syncope: a comprehensive literature review. *Am J Med* 1994; 97:78–88.

Landmark Articles

Kapoor WN. Diagnostic evaluation of syncope. *Am J Med* 1991;90:91–106.

Kapoor WN, Karpf M, Wieand S, et al. A prospective evaluation and follow-up of patients with syncope. *N Engl J Med* 1983;309:197–204.

Sra JS, Anderson AJ, Sheikh SH, et al. Unexplained syncope evaluated by electrophysiologic studies and head-up tilt testing. *Ann Intern Med* 1991;114:1013–1019.

Teichman SL, Felder SD, Matos JA, et al. The value of EPS in syncope of undetermined origin: report of 150 cases. *Am Heart J* 1985; 110:469–479.

Key Reviews

Benditt G, Remole S, Milstein S, et al. Syncope: causes, clinical evaluation, and current therapy. *Annu Rev Med* 1992;43: 283–300.

Kapoor WN, Smith M, Miller NL. Upright tilt testing in evaluating syncope: a comprehensive literature review. *Am J Med* 1994;97:78–88.

Klein GJ. Syncope. *Cardiol Clin North Am* 1997;15(2):165–341.

Relevant Book Chapter

Benditt DG. In: Topol E, ed. *Textbook of cardiovascular medicine.* Philadelphia: Lippincott-Raven Publishers, 1998:1807–1831.

23. LONG QT SYNDROME

Rodolfo D. Farhy

I. **Introduction.** The long QT syndrome (LQTS) is a rare congenital disorder characterized by QT interval prolongation and repetitive episodes of syncope and cardiac arrest related to rapid, polymorphic ventricular tachycardia. The acquired form of the syndrome is mainly secondary to drug administration or electrolyte imbalances that prolong the QT interval.

II. **Epidemiology**
   A. **Incidence:** Congenital LQTS has an incidence of 1:10,000 to 1:15,000 and an equal gender distribution. The average age of symptom onset is 14 years, and 60% of patients have a family history of LQTS or sudden death.
   B. Untreated patients with LQTS have a 10-year mortality rate of up to 50%. However, this risk can be decreased to less than 10% with appropriate treatment.

III. **Diagnostic testing**
   A. The diagnostic criteria for congenital LQTS are listed in Table 23-1.
   B. The most common clinical presentation in LQTS is syncope or sudden death, and may be triggered by exertion or emotional stress.
   C. Electrocardiographic findings
      1. The degree of QT interval prolongation may vary in the same patient from one time to another.
      2. A corrected QT interval (QT_c) of more than 460 milliseconds has a positive predictive value of 92% and a negative predictive value of 94%.
      3. There is no clear correlation between the degree of QT interval prolongation and the incidence of syncope or malignant arrhythmias.
   D. **QT dispersion.** Patients with LQTS have a marked heterogeneity in the repolarization of different regions of the myocardium. This heterogeneity may be reflected by measurement of QT dispersion. Treatment with β-blockers and/or left cardiac sympathetic denervation (LCSD) may normalize the QT dispersion. Recent studies have suggested that patients in whom the QT dispersion does not normalize with β-blockers therapy may be a high-risk group that should be considered for LCSD.
   E. **T-Wave alternans.** Patients with LQTS may demonstrate alternation in the T-wave polarity or amplitude. This is a marker of significant electrical instability and identifies a patient at high risk for torsades de pointes (TdP). T-Wave alternans may be transient or sporadic and may be more evident when the patient is under emotional or physical stress.
   F. **T-Wave morphology.** In addition to the abnormal duration of repolarization, patients with LQTS may have an abnormality in the morphology of the T wave. The T-wave morphology in the precordial leads may be biphasic, bifid, or notched in the terminal portion, similar to a T-U wave fusion. The morphology of the T wave may be characteristic of the underlying genotype (Fig. 23-1).
   G. **Bradycardia.** Patients with LQTS often have inappropriately slow heart rates and may have sinus pauses. The bradycardia may precipitate TdP. Patients with frequent sinus pauses prior to initiation of TdP may benefit most from implantation of a permanent pacemaker.

IV. **Molecular biology of LQTS**
   A. **Jervell and Lange-Nielsen (JLN) syndrome**
      1. Described in 1957 by Jervell and Lange-Nielsen in several families of Scandinavian origin.
      2. This form is associated with bilateral sensorineural deafness at birth and has an autosomal recessive inheritance pattern.

Table 23-1. Diagnostic criteria for LQTS

Criteria	Points
ELECTROCARDIOGRAPHIC FINDINGS[a]	
A. QTc[b]: >480 msec	3
460–470 msec	2
450 (male) msec	1
B. Torsade de pointes[c]	2
C. T-wave alternans	1
D. Notched T wave in at least 3 leads	1
E. Low heart rate for age[d]	0.5
CLINICAL HISTORY	
A. Syncope[e]: with stress	2
without stress	1
B. Congenital deafness	0.5
FAMILY HISTORY[e]	
A. Family members with definite LQTS[f]	1
B. Unexplained sudden cardiac death younger than age 30 years among immediate family members	0.5

[a] In the absence of medications or disorders known to affect these electrocardiographic features.
[b] QTc calculated by Bazett's formula where $QTc = QT/\sqrt{RR}$.
[c] Mutually exclusive.
[d] Resting heart rate below the 2nd percentile for age.
[e] The same family member cannot be counted in A and B.
[f] Definite LQTS is defined by an LQTS score >4.
Scoring: <1 point = low probability of LQTS
        2–3 points = intermediate probability of LQTS
        >4 points = high probability of LQTS
Modified from Ref. 1, with permission.

   B. Romano-Ward (RW) syndrome
      1. Described in 1963 by Romano and Ward.
      2. Autosomal dominant inheritance pattern.
   C. Previously it was thought that the JLN syndrome gene was different from the RW syndrome gene. Recently, it has been discovered that both forms are due to mutations in the same gene, KVLQT1. This gene also controls production of potassium-rich endolymph in the inner ear. When both copies of the gene are abnormal, deafness occurs. The inheritance of the JLN syndrome is complex. It is thought that the portion responsible for the prolonged QT interval is inherited by autosomal dominant transmission, whereas the portion responsible for deafness is inherited by autosomal recessive means.
   D. Molecular basis of LQTS
      1. LQT1: Mutant KVLQT1 gene on chromosome 11.
        a. Encodes a protein for the phase 3 slowly activating delayed rectifier potassium current (I_{Ks}).
        b. A homozygous mutation of KVLQT1 is thought to be responsible for the JLN syndrome.
      2. LQT2: Mutant HERG gene on chromosome 7.
        a. Encodes a protein for the phase 3 rapidly activating delayed rectifier potassium current (I_{Kr}).
      3. LQT3: Mutant SCN5A gene on chromosome 3.
        a. Encodes a protein for the phase 0 sodium channel (I_{Na}).
      4. LQT4: Mutant gene on chromosome 4 (not well characterized yet).
      5. LQT5: Mutant KCNE1 gene on chromosome 21.

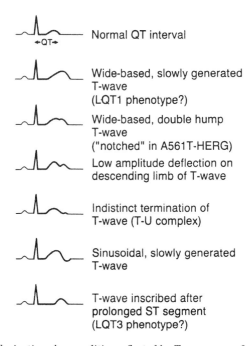

FIG. 23-1. Repolarization abnormalities reflected by T wave on surface electrocardiogram (lead II) in some patients with long QT syndrome. Possible phenotypes demonstrated here include LQT1 (second tracing), LQT2 (third and fourth tracings), and LQT3 (seventh tracing). HERG, human ether-a-go-go related gene. Modified from Ref. 2, with permission.

> **a.** Encodes proteins for potassium channel β subunits (minK) that coassemble with KVLQT1 α subunits to form I_{Ks} and complexes with HERG to regulate I_{Kr}.
> **b.** Mutation of KCNE1 reduces I_{Ks}.

V. Therapy

  A. Every symptomatic patient should receive treatment. Asymptomatic patients should at least be followed closely, and some authorities recommend treatment with β-blockers for these patients. Family members of patients with LQTS must be screened and followed closely.

  B. An increase in sympathetic activity is the most common trigger for the syncopal episodes in LQTS, primarily mediated by the left cardiac sympathetic nerves. Therefore, antiadrenergic therapy is the treatment of choice. Other treatment options include implantation of a pacemaker or defibrillator and a surgical procedure to produce LCSD.

    1. β-blockers are the preferred therapy unless specific contraindications exist; they have been shown in several studies to significantly reduce the incidence of syncope and sudden death. Propranolol in a dose of 2 to 3 mg/kg or nadolol is the commonly prescribed treatment. β-blockers are ineffective in up to 25% of cases.

    2. Cardiac pacing. Patients who develop symptomatic bradycardia with β-blocker therapy should have a pacemaker implanted with continuation of the drug. Patients with LQTS and bradycardia or pause-dependent ventricular arrhythmias should also receive a pacemaker. The benefit of cardiac pacing in the absence of concomitant β-blocker therapy or LCSD is controversial.

3. **Left sympathetic cardiac denervation.** If therapy with full-dose β-blockers is not effective, another option is LCSD. This procedure involves removal of the first four or five thoracic ganglia. The most cephalic portion of the left stellate ganglion should not be ablated so as to avoid Horner's syndrome. Left sympathetic cardiac denervation has been shown to reduce the incidence of syncope and cardiac arrest for patients with LQTS with or without concomitant β-blocker therapy. The fact that cardiac denervation is efficacious for patients already receiving β-blockers raises the issue as to whether β-blockers may be useful for those patients in whom β-blockers are ineffective.

4. **Implantable cardioverter-defibrillator (ICD).** The role of ICDs in LQTS is controversial. Some authorities recommend that they should be reserved for patients who continue to have malignant arrhythmias or syncope in spite of full-dose β-blockers and LCSD, whereas others consider the ICD to be first-line therapy in patients with marked QT_c prolongation (more than 550 milliseconds). The episodes of TdP in the LQTS are often self-terminating and may lead to frequent unnecessary ICD therapies.

5. **Tailored therapy.** Identification of specific genetic and ion channel defects of patients with various forms of LQTS has led to more specific therapies.
   a. Patients with LQT3 and consequently abnormal sodium channel inactivation may benefit from sodium channel blockers such as mexiletine.
   b. Patients with LQT1 or LQT2 may benefit from treatments targeting the potassium channel. Treatments designed to increase the extracellular potassium concentration, such as oral potassium supplements with or without potassium-sparing agents, may be effective for patients with LQT2. Potassium channel openers are under investigation.

SUGGESTED READINGS

References
1. Schwartz PJ. The long QT syndrome. *Curr Probl Cardiol* 1997;22(6)297–351.
2. Ackerman MJ. The long QT syndrome: ion channel diseases of the heart. *Mayo Clin Proc* 1998;73(3):250–69.

Landmark Articles
Kass RS, Davies MP. The roles of ion channels in an inherited heart disease: molecular genetics of the long QT syndrome. *Cardiovasc Res* 1996; 32 (3):443–54.
Jervell A, Lange-Nielsen F. Congenital deaf-mutism, heart disease with prolongation of the QT interval, and sudden death. *Am Heart J* 1957;54:59–68.
Romano C, Gemme G, Pongiglione R. Aritmie cardiache rare dell eta pediatrica. *Clin Pediatr* 1963;45:656–683.
Schwartz PJ, Moss AJ, Vincent GM, Crampton RS. Diagnostic criteria for the long QT syndrome. An update. *Circulation* 1993;88 (2):782–784.
Vincent GM. Heterogeneity in the inherited long QT syndrome. *J Cardiovasc Electrophysiol* 1995;6 (2):137–146.
Ward OC. A new familial cardiac syndrome in children. *J Irish Med Assoc* 1964;54: 103–106.

Key Reviews
Keating MT. The long QT syndrome. A review of recent molecular genetic and physiologic discoveries. *Medicine* 1996;75 (1):1–5.
Roden DM, Lazzara R, Rosen M, Schwartz PJ, Towbin J, Vincent GM. Multiple mechanisms in the long-QT syndrome. Current knowledge, gaps, and future directions. The SADS Foundation Task Force on LQTS. *Circulation* 1996;94 (8):1996–2012.

Tan HL, Hou CJ, Lauer MR, Sung RJ. Electrophysiologic mechanisms of the long QT interval syndromes and torsade de pointes. *Ann Intern Med* 1995;122 (9):701–714.

Vincent GM. Genetics and molecular biology of the inherited long QT syndrome. *Ann Med* 1994;26 (6):419–425.

Relevant Book Chapters

Keating MT, Curran ME. Molecular genetics. In: Topol E, ed. *Textbook of cardiovascular medicine.* Philadelphia: Lippincott-Raven Publishers, 1998:2371–2387.

Schwartz PJ, Locati EH, Napolitano C, Priori SG. The long QT syndrome. In: Zipes DP, Jalife J, eds. *Cardiac electrophysiology: from cell to bedside.* Philadelphia: WB Saunders, 1995:788–811.

24. ANTIARRHYTHMIC DRUGS

Wakkas Tayara and Robert A. Schweikert

I. **Introduction.** Antiarrhythmic medications have been used to control a wide variety of arrhythmias. Lessons from past trials have taught us that the risks of arrhythmia suppression in certain patient populations may exceed the benefits. The decision to use an antiarrhythmic drug must generally be made with the goal of symptom relief or mortality reduction. Furthermore, the physician must then choose the appropriate antiarrhythmic drug for the particular patient, with consideration for such issues as the type of arrhythmia, drug toxicity, proarrhythmic potential, side effect profile, and potential drug interactions. Therefore, it is crucial that the prescribing physician have a thorough knowledge of the characteristics of the available antiarrhythmic drugs.

II. **Classification of antiarrhythmic drugs.** There have been many proposed classification schemes for antiarrhythmic drugs, and controversy still exists regarding this complex issue. Classification of the antiarrhythmic drugs has been difficult, in part due to incomplete knowledge of the complex and often nonspecific actions of these medications. Therefore, the classification systems that are easier for clinicians to use are also criticized for oversimplification.

   A. **Vaughan Williams classification** (Table 24-1).

      1. This descriptive classification is the most widely accepted and is based on the physiologic effects of the drugs.

      2. The drugs are divided into four basic classes:

         a. Class I agents: Decrease phase 0 of the rapid depolarization phase of the action potential (rapid sodium channel).

         b. Class II agents: Inhibit spontaneous depolarization (phase 4).

         c. Class III agents: Block the outward potassium channels to prolong action potential duration (↑refractoriness).

         d. Class IV agents: Inhibit the inward calcium channel.

   B. **Harrison subclassification of the class I antiarrhythmic drugs** (Table 24-2). The Vaughan Williams classification was subsequently modified to produce three subdivisions of the class I antiarrhythmic drugs.

   C. **The Sicilian gambit**

      1. This is an approach to antiarrhythmic drug classification that attempts to account for the complex characteristics of antiarrhythmic drugs as well as the particular arrhythmia. The system was in part a response to the perceived oversimplification of other classification systems. The name was derived from the Queen's Gambit, an opening move in chess that provides the player with a variety of options for subsequent moves, and the fact that the meeting was held in Sicily.

      2. The system consists of four steps:

         a. Identification of the arrhythmia mechanism.

         b. Identification of the vulnerable parameter of the arrhythmia (that property of the arrhythmia most susceptible to a modification that will result in suppression or prevention).

         c. Identification of a specific target most likely to influence the vulnerable parameter.

         d. Identification of an antiarrhythmic drug that will modify the target.

III. **Future directions.** There has been significant progress in our understanding of the molecular and genetic aspects of cardiac ion channels and the mechanisms of arrhythmia. Such knowledge should lead to the development of more specific and less toxic antiarrhythmic drugs, and perhaps an improved classification system (Table 24-3).

Table 24-1. Vaughan Williams classification of antiarrhythmic drugs

Class	Action	Predominant channel effects
I	Direct membrane action	Blocks fast sodium channels (phase 0)
II	β-Adrenergic blocker	Indirect closure of calcium channels (phase IV)
III	Prolongation of repolarization	Blocks outward potassium channels (phase III)
IVA	Calcium channel blocker	Blocks slow inward (AV nodal) calcium channels (phase II)
IVB	Indirect calcium channel blocker	Opens potassium channels (hyperpolarization)

AV, atrioventricular.

Table 24-2. Harrison subclassification of class I antiarrhythmic drugs

Class	Action	ECG
IA	Intermediate inhibition of fast sodium channel (phase 0 of action potential) Prolongs repolarization via inhibition of K^+ channels ($\uparrow$ action potential duration)	Prolongs QRS and QT
IB	Less inhibition of sodium channel (more in abnormal tissue) Shortens repolarization ($\downarrow$ action potential duration)	Minimal effect on QRS and QT
IC	Marked inhibition of fast sodium channel Minimal effect on repolarization	Prolongs QRS (QT prolongs due to change in QRS)

Table 24-3. Characteristics of antiarrhythmic drugs

Drug	Loading dose	Maintenance dose	$t_{1/2}$ (hr)	Therapeutic range	Metabolism and elimination	Side effects and precautions	Drug interactions
CLASS IA							
Quinidine (Quinaglute, Quinidex)		PO: 1.2–1.6 g/day divided doses (not IV due to hypotension risk)	7–9	2.3–5 µg/mL	Hepatic: 80% Renal: 20%	GI, hematologic, hepatic, hypotension, TdP	↑ Digoxin level Potentiates warfarin Class III agents (TdP)
Procainamide (Procan SR, Procanbid)	IV: 17 mg/kg at 20–30 mg/min	IV: 2–6 mg/min	3.5	4–10 µ/mL (metabolized to NAPA)	Hepatic: 40% Renal: 60%	GI, CNS, hematologic, hypotension, lupus (limit use to 6 mo)	Class III agents (TdP)
NAPA: major metabolite		PO: 2–6 q day divided doses	6–8	9–20 µg/mL	Renal: 85%		Class III activity Tdp
Disopyramide (Norpace)	PO: 300 mg	PO: 100–200 mg q 6 hr	8	3–6 µg/mL	Hepatic: 50% Renal: 50%	Anticholinergic, negative inotropic, hypotension, Tdp	Class III agents (TdP)
CLASS IB							
Lidocaine (Xylocaine)	IV: 1–1.5 mg/kg followed by 0.5 mg/kg every 10 min up to total of 3 mg/kg	IV: 2–4 mg/min	2	1.4–5.0 µg/mL	Hepatic: 90% Renal: 10%	CNS effects at high dose; Reduce dose if low hepatic blood flow (severe CHF and shock)	↑ Levels by β-blockers (↓ hepatic blood flow) and cimetidine (↓ metabolism)

(Continued)

Table 24-3. *Continued*

Drug	Loading dose	Maintenance dose	$t_{1/2}$ (hr)	Therapeutic range	Metabolism and elimination	Side effects and precautions	Drug interactions
Mexiletine (Mexitil)	PO: 400 mg	PO: 100–400 mg q 8 hr	10–17	1–2 μg/mL	Hepatic: 90% Renal: 10%	CNS, GI, bradycardia, hypotension	↓ Levels by rifampin and phenytoin; ↑ theophylline levels
Tocainide (Tonocard)	PO: 400–800 mg	PO: 400–800 mg q 8 hr	13.5	4–10 μg/mL	Hepatic: 40% Renal: 60%	CNS, GI, hematologic	
Phenytoin (Dilantin)	IV: 10–15 mg/kg over 1 hr	PO: 400–600 mg q day	24	10–18 μg/mL	Hepatic	CNS, hypotension, anemia	↑ Levels by amiodarone, fluconazole, and cimetidine; ↓ levels by carbamazepine and rifampin
*Moricizine (Ethmozine)		PO: 200–300 q 8 hr	6–13		Hepatic: 99% Renal: 40%	CNS, GI, proarrhythmia (esp. with LV dysfunction)	
CLASS IC							
Flecainide (Tambocor)		PO: 50–200 mg q 12 hr	12–27	0.2–1.0 μg/mL	Hepatic: 65% Renal: 35%	CNS, negative inotrope, proarrhythmia. Contraindicated with structural heart disease	↑ Levels by amiodarone; highdegree AV block with β– or calcium channel blockers

Drug	Dose	Half-life	Therapeutic level	Metabolism	Side effects	Drug interactions
Propafenone (Rythmol)	PO: 150–300 mg q 8 hr	2–32	0.2–3.0 µg/mL	Hepatic: 50% Renal: 50%	GI, negative inotrope, proarrhythmia. ↑ Mortality in SCD survivors	↑ Digoxin levels; potentiates β-blocker effect
CLASS II						
Metoprolol (Lopressor)	IV: 5 mg q 5 min PO: 25–100 mg q 8–12 hr	3–4	50–100 ng/mL	Hepatic	Negative chronotrope, negative inotrope, bronchospasm, CNS, impotence	Potentiated by calcium channel blockers
Propranolol (Inderal)	IV: 5 mg q 5 min PO: 10–120 mg q 8 hr	3–4	50–100 ng/mL	Hepatic	Negative inotrope, negative chronotrope, bronchospasm, CNS, impotence	Potentiated by calcium channel blockers
Esmolol (Brevibloc)	IV: 0.5 mg/kg IV: 0.05–3 mg/kg/min	9 min	0.15–1.0 µg/mL	Blood esterases	Negative chronotrope, negative inotrope, bronchospasm	Potentiated by calcium channel blockers
CLASS III						
Amiodarone (Cordarone, Pacerone)	PO: 1.2–1.6 g/q day IV: 5 mg/kg then 10–20 mg/kg/day PO: 200–400 mg day	25–110 days	1.0–2.5 µg/mL	Hepatic	Pulmonary, ophthalmologic, thyroid and hepatic dysfunction, ↑ QT, negative chronotrope	Potentiates warfarin effects; ↑ flecainide and digoxin levels; ↑ risk of TdP with class IA agents

(Continued)

Table 24-3. *Continued*

Drug	Loading dose	Maintenance dose	$t_{1/2}$ (hr)	Therapeutic range	Metabolism and elimination	Side effects and precautions	Drug interactions
Sotalol (Betapace)	IV: 5–10 mg/ kg, repeat to maximum of 30 mg/kg	PO: 80–320 mg q 12 hr	15–17	< 3 µg/mL	Renal excretion (not metabolized)	Negative chronotrope, AV block, negative inotrope, TdP, bronchospasm	Potentiates effects of calcium channel blockers; ↑ risk of TdP with class IA or diuretics
Bretylium tosylate		IV: 1–2 mg/min	7–9	0.5–1.0 µg/mL	Hepatic: 20% Renal: 80%	Hypotension, GI	Augments hypotensive effects of diuretics and vasodilators
Ibutilide (Corvert)	IV: 0.015– 0.025 mg/ kg over 5 min		2–12		Hepatic: 90%	TdP, hypotension, headache, GI	Avoid other agents that prolong QT interval
CLASS IVA							
Verapamil	IV: 2.5– 10 mg	PO: 80–120 mg/ 8 hr	6–12		Hepatic	Negative chronotrope, negative	Potentiates negative inotropic

Drug	Dose			Adverse Effects	Interactions
				inotrope, CHF exacerbation	and chronotropic effects of other agents
Diltiazem	IV: 0.25 mg/kg	IV: 10–15 mg/hr PO: 30–120 mg q 8 hr	3–4		Hepatic	Negative chronotrope, negative inotrope, CHF exacerbation	Potentiates negative inotropic and chronotropic effects of other agents
CLASS IVB					
Adenosine (Adenocard)	IV: 6-mg bolus, if no effect then 12-mg bolus		10 sec		Flushing, dyspnea, chest pain, asystole, bronchospasm (contraindicated in asthma)	Potentiated by dipyridamole; attenuated by caffeine, theophylline
OTHER					
Digoxin	IV/PO: 0.25–0.5 mg	IV/PO: 0.1–0.75 mg q 6–8 hr up to day; 1 mg over 24 hr	36–48	0.8–2 ng/mL	Renal	CNS, GI, AV block, arrhythmias	↑ Level with quinidine, verapamil, amiodarone, propafenone

IV, Intravenous; PO, per oral; NAPA, N-acetylprocainamide; GI, gastrointestinal; CNS, central nervous system; Tdp, torsade de pointes; CHF, congestive heart failure; LV, left ventricular; SCD, sudden cardiac death; AV, atrioventricular.

SUGGESTED READINGS

Key Reviews

Kowey PR. Pharmacological effects of antiarrhythmic drugs. Review and update. *Arch Intern Med* 1998;158:325–332.

Nattel S. Antiarrhythmic drug classifications. A critical appraisal of their history, present status, and clinical relevance. *Drugs* 1991;41:672–701.

Singh BN. Antiarrhythmic drugs: a reorientation in light of recent developments in the control of disorders of rhythm. *Am J Cardiol* 1998;81:3D–13D.

Task Force of the Working Group on Arrhythmias of the European Society of Cardiology. The Sicilian gambit. A new approach to the classification of antiarrhythmic drugs based on their actions on arrhythmogenic mechanisms. *Circulation* 1991;84:1831–1851.

Relevant Book Chapters

Marcus FI, Opie LH. Antiarrhythmic agents. In: Opie LH, ed. *Drugs for the heart,* 4th ed. Philadelphia: WB Saunders, 1997:207– 247.

Rosen MR, Strauss HC, Janse MJ. The classification of antiarrhythmic drugs. In: Zipes DP, Jalife J, eds. *Cardiac electrophysiology: from cell to bedside,* 2nd ed. Philadelphia: WB Saunders, 1995:1277–1286.

Vaughan Williams EM. Classification of antiarrhythmic drugs. In: Sandoe E, Flensted-Jensen E, Olsen KH, eds. *Cardiac arrhythmias.* Sodertalje, Sweden: Astra, 1970: 449–472.

SECTION VI. DISEASES OF THE AORTA AND PERICARDIUM

Steven P. Marso and Richard A. Grimm

25. AORTIC ANEURYSM AND AORTIC DISSECTION

John P. Gassler

I. **Introduction**
  A. **Aorta.** The aorta is the **principal conductance vessel** in the body. Anatomically, the aorta is divided into the ascending, arch, descending thoracic, and abdominal components.
    1. The **ascending aorta** includes the aortic root, which contains the sinuses of Valsalva. The left and right coronary arteries arise from the left and right coronary sinuses, respectively.
    2. The **aortic arch** gives rise to the great vessels of the head and upper extremities. These usually include the brachiocephalic, the left common carotid, and the left subclavian arteries.
    3. The **descending thoracic aorta** gives off the intercostal vessels as it courses through the posterior mediastinum. The vascular supply to the anterior spinal artery is included among these vessels.
    4. The **abdominal aorta** begins just after the aorta crosses the diaphragm. It provides the splanchnic and renal arteries before bifurcating to become the common iliac arteries.
  B. **Histology.** The aorta comprises **three layers:** the intima, the media, and the adventitia.
    1. The **intima** is the lining layer of the aorta and is easily damaged.
    2. The **media** is the main structural layer of the aorta. It consists primarily of laminar layers of elastic tissue and smooth muscle in varying amounts. This structure allows for the high tensile strength and elasticity that the aorta requires to withstand the pressure changes of each heartbeat throughout the life of the individual.
    3. The **adventitia** is the thin outer layer that assists with anchoring the aorta within the body, as well as providing nourishment to the outer half of the wall through the vasa vasorum.
  C. **Physiology**
    1. The **elasticity of the aortic wall allows it to distend** under the pressure created during ventricular systole. In this way the kinetic energy that was developed during ventricular systole is stored as potential energy in the distended aortic wall. Then, during ventricular diastole, the potential energy is converted back to kinetic energy by elastic recoil of the wall. Thus, forward blood flow is maintained throughout the cardiac cycle.
    2. Another role of the aorta relates to control of **systemic vascular resistance.** Pressure receptors found in the ascending aorta as well as the aortic arch signal the vasomotor centers of the brain via the vagus nerve. When blood pressure is elevated, the reflex response is to lower heart rate and decrease systemic vascular resistance. The converse is true when blood pressure is decreased.
II. **Aortic aneurysm.** An aortic aneurysm is defined as a pathologic dilatation to more than 1.5 times the normal diameter of the aorta. The aneurysm can be either fusiform (symmetric dilatation) or saccular (asymmetric outpouching). Pseudoaneurysms, which are well-defined pockets of blood and connective tissue, must be distinguished from true aneurysms. Overall, 13% of patients with a single aneurysm have one or more additional aneurysms, and 25% of patients with a thoracic aneurysm have abdominal aneurysms as well. There are no well-defined guidelines for screening other vascular beds in patients upon diagnosis of aortic aneurysm. However, given the high incidence of multiple aneurysms, a chest and abdominal computed tomographic (CT) scan on diagnosis to rule out other sites would be reasonable.

A. **Abdominal aortic aneurysms (AAAs)** are much more common than thoracic aortic aneurysms; **up to 75% of aortic aneurysms involve the abdominal aorta. The incidence has increased** from 8.7/100,000 person-years to 36.5/100,000 in the last 30 years. The prevalence of the disease in those 50 years and older is at least 3%. Risk factors include hypertension, hyperlipidemia, tobacco abuse, diabetes mellitus, genetics, and age. The incidence increases after age 55 in males and age 70 in females. There is a **male-to-female ratio of 9:1,** and most cases (95%) involve the infrarenal aorta.

   1. **Clinical presentation. The majority of AAAs are discovered incidentally** on physical examination or during radiologic or ultrasound evaluation of the abdomen.

      a. **Signs and symptoms. The vast majority of patients are asymptomatic;** thus, it is important to consider the diagnosis of AAA in patients with an appropriate risk profile.

         (1) **The predominant symptom associated with rapid enlargement or rupture/impending rupture is severe back or flank pain.** This is often described as sudden in onset, constant, and not affected by movement or position. Occasionally, there is radiation to the legs, buttocks, or groin.

         (2) Findings consistent with shock (hypotension, pallor, diaphoresis, oliguria, and obtundation) can develop rapidly with a ruptured aneurysm.

      b. **Physical examination**

         (1) **A palpable, pulsatile mass may be felt** on examination, variably extending from the xyphoid process to below the umbilicus. This is more difficult to palpate in obese individuals. Accurate sizing is nearly impossible on physical examination. Palpation should be gentle, especially if the aneurysm is tender, as this can be an indication of impending rupture.

         (2) Often evidence of **associated vascular disease** can be found (abdominal or femoral bruits), as can decreased pulses.

         (3) Physical evidence of **thromboembolism** is sometimes found. Either atheromatous material or mural thrombus may be embolized. Patients can exhibit livedo reticularis, painful blue toes, hypertension, and renal insufficiency.

   2. **Etiology**

      a. **Atherosclerosis has long been considered the underlying etiology** for abdominal aneurysms, with interactions of multiple cofactors, including:

         (1) The relative lack of nutrient vessels (vasa vasorum) in the infrarenal aorta

         (2) The relative decrease in elastic lamellae compared to smooth muscle layers

         (3) Ongoing hypertensive states

      b. **Genetic factors may also play a role,** with family studies showing up to 28% of patients having a first-degree relative with an abdominal aneurysm. First-degree male relatives of AAA patients have a 12 times greater risk of having an aneurysm.

      c. Less common causes include infection *(Salmonella, Staphylococcus aureus)* and trauma.

   3. **Pathophysiology and clinical course**

      a. **Cellular and molecular factors** play a role.

         (1) Histologically, a decrease in quantities of elastin and collagen are found in aortic aneurysms relative to normal aortic tissue.

         (2) Increased activity of elastase and other proteolytic enzymes has been found on biochemical evaluation of samples from patients with aneurysms. Recent evidence suggests that inflammation may lead to activation of these metalloproteases.

(3) These two factors decrease the elastic and tensile strength of the aorta and increase the risk of developing an aneurysm.

b. The risk of rupture is proportional to aneurysm size.

    (1) Available data suggest that aneurysms larger than 7.0 cm have greater than 20% per year risk of rupture, whereas those between 5 and 6 cm have approximately 6% risk of rupture per year.

    (2) The majority of aneurysms enlarge at a rate of 0.4 cm/year. (Rapidly expanding ones enlarge more than 0.5 cm/year.)

    (3) The larger the aneurysm grows, the faster it will continue to expand.

c. Laplace's law defines the parameters for growth of aneurysms.

Wall tension (WT) = transmural pressure (TP) × radius *(r)*

Therefore, with luminal dilatation (increased *r*), the wall tension will increase at a given blood pressure (TP). This leads to a further increase in radius and to a self-perpetuating cycle and growth of the aneurysm.

d. Rupture usually occurs into the left retroperitoneal space (80%). This may initially be contained; ultimately, however, it will extend, causing shock and death if untreated.

e. Abdominal aortic aneurysm can also rupture into the inferior vena cava (causing aortovenous fistula formation), and the gastrointestinal tract (causing aortoenteric fistula formation). Hence, **the patient with a gastrointestinal bleed and history of aortic aneurysm or AAA repair should always be suspected of potentially having an aortoenteric fistula.**

f. Prior to the surgical era, the 3- and 5-year survival rates for AAA were 49% and 19%, respectively. Current data suggest that out-of-hospital mortality for a ruptured aneurysm approaches 60%. Typically, the **operative mortality for emergent surgery is 50%.**

4. Diagnostic testing

a. Abdominal ultrasound is the most commonly used screening tool for abdominal aneurysms. It has the capacity to acquire both longitudinal and transverse images of the aneurysm.

    (1) **Advantages.** Abdominal ultrasound has been verified to accurately measure size to within ±0.3 cm. It is also widely available, relatively low in cost, and does not involve radiation exposure. It is a reasonable choice to follow aneurysm growth serially.

    (2) **Disadvantages.** Abdominal ultrasound cannot adequately define involvement of branch vessels and therefore is insufficient for preoperative evaluation.

b. Computerized tomography

    (1) **Advantages.** Computed tomography allows for a **more accurate evaluation of the aneurysm shape** and its spatial relations to the branch vessels. The technique allows for evaluation of extravasated blood in acute or subacute rupture, as well as measurements that have been validated to within ±0.2 cm.

    (2) **Disadvantages.** Computed tomography is more expensive, involves moving the patient to a less accessible location, is less available, uses ionizing radiation, and requires intravenous (IV) contrast. It does not allow evaluation of luminal impingement of branch vessels by the aneurysm, thus limiting its usefulness in preoperative evaluation.

c. Aortography is limited to preoperative evaluation

    (1) **Advantages** include its ability to define suprarenal and iliofemoral involvement, and branch vessel impingement. Current

indications for aortography include clinical suspicion of visceral ischemia; occlusive ileofemoral vascular lesions; severe hypertension/chronic renal insufficiency, possibly due to renal artery stenosis; suspicion of a horseshoe kidney; suspicion of suprarenal/thoracoabdominal extension; and presence of femoral or popliteal aneurysms.

    (2) **Disadvantages.** Aortography tends to underestimate size, especially when mural thrombus is present. It has an invasive nature, is expensive, and uses IV contrast and ionizing radiation.

  d. **Magnetic resonance imaging/angiography (MRI/MRA)**

    (1) **Advantages.** Magnetic resonance imaging allows for **excellent definition of aneurysm size** as well as suprarenal and iliofemoral extension. Magnetic resonance angiography allows for improved visualization of compromised flow to branch vessels. The technique has an advantage over aortography in that it is noninvasive and requires no IV contrast.

    (2) **Disadvantages.** Magnetic resonance angiography lacks sensitivity to absolutely define obstruction in the renal vessels. The technique is expensive, and there is a limited availability of scanners and qualified radiologists to read the study.

  5. **Therapy**

    a. **Medical therapy. The goal is to decrease aortic dP/dt**. Medical therapy is limited in extent and effect.

      (1) **β-Blockers** have been shown to decrease the rate of enlargement and risk of rupture in animal models and early human trials. This is due both to the decrease in dP/dt (shear stress) and a yet unspecified effect on aortic wall breakdown. Table 25-1 lists drugs and doses.

        (a) These agents are for use in acute management of impending AAA rupture as the first-line agent.

        (b) Oral equivalents can be used in the stable AAA patient.

        (c) Calcium channel blockers are a reasonable alternative in patients with contraindications to β-blockers.

      (2) **Risk factor modification** with hypertension and hypercholesterolemia control are important, although studies are limited.

Table 25-1. Intravenous dosing for acute medical management

Drugs	Loading dose	Maintenance dose
FIRST-LINE AGENTS		
Propranolol	1 mg IV q 3–5 min (max. 6.15 mg/kg)	2–6 mg IV q 4–6 hr
Labetolol	10 mg IV over 2 min, then 20–80 mg q 10–15 min (max 300 mg)	2 mg/min IV drip titrate to 5–20 mg/min
Esmolol	30 mg IV bolus	3–12 mg/min drip
Metoprolol	5 mg IV q 5 min to effect	5–10 mg IV q 4–6 hr to effect
SECOND-LINE AGENTS IN PATIENTS WITH CONTRAINDICATIONS FOR β-BLOCKERS		
Enalaprilat	0.625 mg IV	0.625 mg IV q 4–6 hr
Diltiazem	0.25 mg/kg IV over 2 min 0.35 mg/kg IV after 15 min if no effect	5 mg/hr titrate by 2.5 to 5 mg/hr increments; max 15 mg/hr
Verapamil	0.075–0.1 mg/kg to 2.5-5 mg/kg over 2 min	5–15 mg/hr IV drip

IV, intravenous.

(3) **Cigarette smoking should be eliminated.**

(4) **Serial ultrasound or CT scans** are indicated in asymptomatic patients. Studies should be obtained every 3 to 6 months depending on the patient's risk of rupture.

b. **Percutaneous therapy.** Percutaneous catheter repair is a relatively new approach that involves **percutaneous placement of an intraluminal stent/graft.** The stent/graft acts as a bridge to allow circulation to the lower extremities while decreasing the transmural pressure on the aortic wall.

(1) Animal data for this procedure look promising.

(2) Early human implantation ($n = 50$) was successful in 80% of high-risk cases (deployment), but with a 10% periprocedural mortality rate. Success was defined as complete exclusion of the aneurysm with restoration of normal flow (1).

(3) Long-term data are lacking.

c. **Surgical therapy.** The technical details of repair are beyond the scope of this book. The basic premise is for a Dacron tube graft to be inserted in place of the diseased aorta. The major branches are then reimplanted to the graft.

(1) **Preoperative evaluation.** Given the strong association of coronary artery disease (CAD) and AAA, and the high operative mortality with untreated CAD, **all patients being considered for surgical repair of AAA need preoperative risk assessment.** A detailed description of the preoperative evaluation can be found in Chapter 35.

(2) **Timing**

(a) Aneurysms enlarge at varying rates, but in general:

(i) The larger the aneurysm, the faster is the ongoing expansion.

(ii) The larger the aneurysm, the higher is the risk of rupture.

(b) Perioperative mortality in elective procedures is 4% to 6% (less than 2% in low-risk patients).

(c) Based on limited available data, the consensus recommendation from the Society for Vascular Surgery and the International Society for Cardiovascular Surgery (1992) is for **elective repair of aneurysms 5.0 cm or greater in diameter, or those expanding at greater than 0.5 cm/year.**

(3) **Complications** are shown in Table 25-2.

(4) **Long-term outcomes.** Kiell and Ernst (2) reviewed approximately 2,500 patients with surgical repair. Their 1-, 5-, and 10-year data show survival rates of 93%, 63%, and 40%, respectively.

B. **Thoracic aortic aneurysms (TAAs)** are much less common than the abdominal variety discussed above (incidence 5.9/100,000 person-years). Thoracic aneurysms are defined as 1.5 times the normal aortic diameter and

Table 25-2. Complications in patients undergoing AAA repair

Complication	Incidence (%)
Death	9.6
Myocardial infarction	7.2
Cerebrovascular accident	4.8
Paralysis/paresis	6.0
Non-Q-wave myocardial infarction.	8.4
Distal emboli/thrombosis	6.0

are classified according to the segment involved. The etiology of aneurysms in these different segments is varied (see II.B.2). Extension of a descending thoracic aneurysm below the diaphragm creates a thoracoabdominal aneurysm.

1. **Clinical presentation.** Up to 40% of patients with thoracic aneurysms are asymptomatic at the time of diagnosis. They are discovered as incidental findings on chest radiograph or other radiologic studies.

   a. **Signs and symptoms.** The various presenting complaints can be collected into three groups.

      (1) Some patients present with **vascular complications of the aneurysm.** These include aortic insufficiency (AI) with left ventricle dilatation and congestive heart failure (CHF), myocardial ischemia due to coronary artery compression, sinus of Valsalva rupture into the right atrium/ventricle with left-to-right shunt and CHF, or thromboembolic phenomena.

      (2) **Compression of external structures by the aneurysm** causes the second group of symptoms. Examples of this include superior vena cava syndrome, dysphagia from esophageal compression, or hoarseness from recurrent laryngeal nerve compression. Also, compression of the trachea or main-stem bronchus can lead to wheezing, dyspnea, tracheal shift, cough, or hemoptysis. Chest or back pain from compression and bony involvement is described as constant, boring, and deep.

      (3) **Rupture presents with sudden, severe, sharp chest or back pain.** In order of decreasing frequency, TAAs rupture into the left pleural space, the pericardium (presenting as tamponade), and the esophagus (presenting as hematemesis).

   b. **Physical examination. Specific physical findings** directly referable to the TAA **are usually absent.**

      (1) **Cardiac.** The diastolic murmur of AI (classically right lower sternal border, or RLSB) and a laterally displaced point of maximal impulse are sometimes noted with chronic ascending aortic dilatation. Signs of congestive heart failure can be seen in these circumstances. Unilateral jugulovenous distention can be seen in patients with venous compression.

      (2) **Vascular.** Rarely, a pulsatile mass can be palpated in the suprasternal notch. Differential pulses in the extremities can sometimes be found. Evidence of thromboembolic events can be seen when examining the digits. If the aneurysm compresses the venous return, evidence of superior vena cava syndrome or lower extremity edema may be found.

      (3) **Pulmonary.** If the aneurysm compresses part of the bronchial tree, decreased air movement or stridor is auscultated.

   c. **Laboratory examination**

      (1) The **chest radiograph** frequently shows widening of the mediastinum, unusual aortic contours, or displacement of the trachea or bronchi in the presence of a large TAA.

      (2) In patients exhibiting some of the cardiac findings above, the **ECG** may show evidence of left ventricular hypertrophy with strain.

2. **Etiology**

   a. Table 25-3 gives the various classifications of TAAs as well as the segment involved and pathophysiology.

   b. Approximately 5% to 10% of patients undergoing surgery for AI are secondary to **annuloaortic ectasia,** which is a clinicopathologic diagnosis in which the aortic root, ascending aorta, and aortic annulus dilate, resulting in AI.

      (1) This variant is more common in men and is typically seen in the fourth, fifth, and sixth decades of life.

Table 25-3. Etiology of thoracic aortic aneurysm

Etiology	Aortic segment involved	Pathophysiology
Marfan syndrome	Ascending aorta and root, aortic arch	Defective fibrillin; secondary cystic medial degeneration
Ehlers-Danlos syndrome	Ascending aorta, predominantly aortic arch	Defective collagen; secondary cystic medial degeneration
Cystic medial degeneration	Ascending aorta, aortic arch	De novo cystic medial degeneration
Atherosclerotic	Descending aorta	Atherosclerotic plaques, weakening vessel walls
Traumatic	Aortic isthmus, proximal descending aorta	Damaged vessel wall, intramural hematoma
Inflammatory	Variable	Takayasu's arteritis, giant cell arteritis, HLA-B27-associated spondyloarthropathies
Infectious	Aortic root (syphilis), variable (mycotic)	CMD (syphilis), inflammatory changes (mycotic)
Poststenotic	Ascending (aortic stenosis), descending (coarctation)	Hemodynamic insult
Postsurgical	Aortic valve replacement, s/p aortic anastamosis	Weakening of the anastamotic walls

HLA, Human leukocyte antigen; CMD, xxx.

> (2) Histologically, all of these patients have evidence of cystic medial necrosis. This is defined by fragmentation of elastic fibers, increase in collagen content, and replacement of tissue with interstitial cysts of basophilic ground substance.
> (3) Angiographically
>> (a) Flask shape (most common)
>> (b) Diffuse symmetric dilatation
>> (c) Localized to root dilatation

3. **Pathophysiology and clinical course.** The natural history and progression of TAA is not as well defined as that of AAA.
   a. **The rate of dilatation, as well as the TAA's propensity to rupture, may be related to its underlying etiology.** Onset of symptoms usually heralds a more rapid course, as do larger dimensions at baseline.
   b. There appears to be a dichotomy in the rate of growth according to data from Dapunt et al. (3). In looking at all TAAs, aneurysms less than 5.0 cm at baseline have a mean growth rate of 0.17 cm/year, while those larger than 5.0 cm grew at a mean rate of 0.79 cm/year.
   c. According to the limited data available, 1-, 3-, and 5-year survival rates for nonrepaired thoracic aneurysms were 65%, 36%, and 20%, respectively, in one study, whereas others suggest 50% 5-year and 70% 10-year mortality rates.
   d. **Rupture is the most common cause of death in these patients** (32% to 47% of all deaths), followed by complications of co-existing atherosclerosis. Rupture has been reported in 32% to 68% of all untreated cases. Location of the aneurysm does not appear to influence mortality; however, diastolic hypertension, advanced age, size

greater than 6 cm, and associated coronary or cerebrovascular disease increase the risk of death.

 e. **Complications of TAA vary by location of the aneurysm.**
   (1) **Ascending aneurysms** may be complicated by AI with consequent CHF, coronary artery compression, rupture into the pericardial space (tamponade) or right ventricle (CHF).
   (2) Marfan syndrome or annuloaortic ectasia involvement of the **ascending aorta** is prone to dissection as well.
   (3) **Arch aneurysms** may involve the great vessels or shower distal emboli.
   (4) Descending aneurysms may progress to involve the abdominal aorta with compromise of the branch vessels, as well as being a source for distal emboli.

4. **Diagnostic testing**
  a. **Computed tomography** allows for good definition of the size and extent of aneurysmal involvement. In addition, laminated mural thrombus can be readily defined by CT images. It is useful for serial examinations in following the expansion of smaller aneurysms. Drawbacks to CT are similar to those noted for CT in AAA (see Section II.A.4). CT is the test of choice.
  b. **Magnetic resonance imaging/magnetic resonance angiography is also useful for detecting and defining the extent of aneurysmal involvement.** It allows for evaluation of the entire aorta, branch vessels, aortic valve, and pericardium. Disadvantages and other advantages are similar to those noted for AAA (see II.A.4).
  c. **Aortography allows for evaluation of the segment involved by the aneurysm as well as the branch vessels off the aorta.** Disadvantages and other advantages are similar to those noted for AAA (see II.A.4). This procedure is currently reserved for preoperation evaluation to establish branch vessel patency.
  d. **Transthoracic and transesophageal echocardiography.** Transthoracic echocardiography is of limited use in evaluating the thoracic aorta, except for the ascending portion. Transesophageal echocardiography has a well-defined role in evaluating aortic dissection, but its role in aneurysm evaluation is under evaluation. Its major limitation is difficulty in obtaining composite longitudinal images of the aorta. Additionally, it is a semiinvasive technique.

5. **Therapy**
  a. **Medical therapy.** Although long-term data on medical management for TAA are lacking, **the medical management of these patients is similar to that of those with AAA** (Table 25-1). One small prospective trial of patients with Marfan syndrome evaluated the effect of propranolol over 10 years of follow-up on several end points. The data showed a slower rate of dilatation, decreased incidence of death, dissection, AI, and decreased mortality from year 4 onward in the treated group.
  b. **Percutaneous therapy.** Recently, use of a percutaneous stent-graft has been reported from one site for descending thoracic aneurysms distal to the takeoff of the left subclavian artery. This procedure has the advantage of being less invasive and potentially decreasing the incidence of paraplegia. Larger studies and longer follow-ups must be evaluated before widespread use of this technology can be encouraged.
  c. **Surgical therapy.** The **timing of surgical repair is less clear than in AAA.**
   (1) Several factors contribute to this lack of clarity. First, **data are limited** on natural history, progression of dilatation, and short- and long-term surgical outcomes. Second, there are **significant risks and complications associated with repair,** especially if the aneurysm involves the arch or descending aorta.

(2) **Current recommendations are for surgical repair when the maximal diameter is greater than 6.0 cm** (7.0 in high-operative-risk patients).

  (a) The cutoff is lowered to 5.5 cm for Marfan syndrome, given the proclivity of TAAs to dissect and/or rupture in this population. In the presence of AI, the threshold for operating on a patient with Marfan syndrome is lower.

  (b) Smaller aneurysms can be followed with serial CT scans. The frequency of evaluation is controversial and depends on the aneurysm size. Usually every 6 to 12 months is sufficient if the patient is asymptomatic and the aneurysm is less than 5 cm in diameter. More frequent evaluation is necessary if the aneurysm is larger than 5 cm (3 to 6 months).

(3) The technical details of repair are beyond the scope of this book. The basic premise is for a Dacron tube graft to be inserted in place of the diseased aorta. The main branches are reimplanted to the graft (coronary arteries, great vessels, mesenteric, and T_8 to L_2 intercostals/lumbricals). When the aortic valve is involved with aortic root dilatation, a Bentall procedure (composite prosthetic aortic valve with Dacron graft) or aortic valve homograft is performed. The aortic valve homograft is a cryopreserved cadaveric aortic valve with a portion of the original ascending aorta intact.

(4) **Overall perioperative survival** is reported to be 90% to 95% for elective repair (ascending aorta) in most institutions. One- and five-year survival rates are improved to higher than 70% and 50% to 60%, respectively, after elective reconstruction.

(5) The **major complications** associated with TAA repair include myocardial infarction (MI) (7.2%), cardiovascular accident (CVA) (4.8%), acute renal failure (2.4%), perioperative hemorrhage (7.2%), and paraplegia (6.0%).

  (a) Paraplegia is particularly associated with repair of the descending aorta due to perioperative ischemia of the anterior spinal cord. Even with proper reimplantation of the T_8–L_2 arteries the reported rate of paraplegia is 5% to 6%.

  (b) Another late complication is the development of graft margin aneurysms.

(6) **Factors associated with increased surgical risk** include emergent surgery, greater age, prolonged cross-clamp time, diabetes, prior aortic surgery, and intraoperative hypotension.

III. **Aortic dissection**

  A. **Epidemiology.** The incidence of aortic dissection is thought to be around 2,000 cases per year in the United States. The male-to-female ratio is 2:1, with the peak incidence in the sixth and seventh decades of life. The mortality for untreated acute aortic dissection is approximately 1% per hour within the first 48 hours. Around 65% of dissections originate in the ascending aorta (just above the right or noncoronary sinus), 20% in the descending thoracic aorta, 10% in the aortic arch, and the remainder in the abdominal aorta.

  B. **Classification schemes**

    1. Currently in use are **three classification schemes** based on anatomy. These are the DeBakey, Stanford, and anatomic classifications. (See Table 25-4 and Fig. 25-1 for a description of the DeBakey and Stanford classifications; anatomic classification refers to the portion(s) of aorta involved.)

    2. **Dissections are further classified according to chronicity:** acute (less than 2 weeks from onset) or chronic (greater than 2 weeks). The mortality curve rises during the first 2 weeks and levels off at 75% to 80%, thereby providing a natural breakpoint.

Table 25-4. Aortic dissection classification systems

Classification	Pathologic description
STANFORD	
Type A	Any dissection involving the ascending aorta
Type B	Any dissections *not* involving the ascending aorta
DEBAKEY	
Type I	Entry point in the ascending aorta, extends to the aortic arch and often beyond
Type II	Confined entirely to the ascending aorta
Type III	Entry in the descending aorta (distal to left subclavian); extends distally (usually) or proximally (rarely)

3. The classification according to each type (anatomic involvement and chronicity) affects the optimal treatment approach (to be discussed later).
C. Clinical presentation
    1. Signs and symptoms
        a. Severe chest and/or back pain is the presenting symptom in 74% to 90% of acute aortic dissections. This pain is of sudden

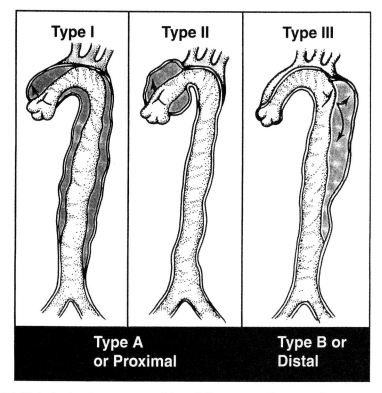

FIG. 25-1. Anatomic appearance of three different aortic dissection classifications.

onset, at its maximal level, which contrasts with the pain of MI, which is more gradual in onset. The pain is usually described as tearing, ripping, or stabbing. The location of the most severe aspect can help localize the dissection. Anterior chest discomfort is often associated with ascending aorta involvement. Intrascapular pain is often associated with DeBakey type I or III dissections.

b. **Less common presentations** include CHF (usually due to severe AI in proximal dissection), syncope (in 4% to 5% of cases, due to rupture into pericardial space with resultant tamponade), CVA, paraplegia, or cardiac arrest.

2. **Physical examination**
   a. **Cardiac**
      (1) **Hypertension is often seen with aortic dissection,** frequently as the cause and occasionally as a complication. In distal dissections, which involve the renal artery, the increase in blood pressure is a response to renal ischemia.
      (2) **Hypotension can be seen in proximal dissection** with aortic root involvement, hemopericardium, and tamponade.
      (3) **Pseudohypotension** occurs when the subclavian artery is involved with resultant compression of the vessel.
      (4) The diastolic murmur of **AI** (16% to 67%) often indicates root involvement, with disturbance of normal aortic valve coaptation. If AI is severe, CHF symptoms are usually found because the left ventricle cannot dilate sufficiently to allow the regurgitate volume to be tolerated. Approximately 1% to 2% of proximal dissections involve the coronary ostia (usually the right coronary ostia), resulting in acute MI picture.
   b. **Vascular. Pulse deficits,** which wax and wane, may be seen in up to 50% of cases.
   c. **Neurologic. Findings of cerebrovascular accident occur in 3% to 6% of proximal dissections.** Rarely, a dissection of the descending aorta involves the primary vessel to the spinal cord with resultant paraplegia.

3. **Laboratory examination**
   a. **Chest radiograph findings are suggestive of dissection** in more than 80% of cases. Findings include a widened aortic silhouette (80% to 90% of cases), widened mediastinum, or the calcium sign (displacement of intimal Ca greater than 1 cm from outer aortic soft tissue), pleural effusion, and CHF. These findings should cause one to consider the diagnosis of aortic dissection in the proper setting.
   b. **ECG. The most common finding is left ventricular hypertrophy.** Other less common findings include ST depression, T-wave changes, or ST elevation. Acute injury patterns are found if the coronary arteries are involved. It is important to consider this diagnosis in the setting of MI with an unusual pain presentation. Rarely, pericarditis changes and atrioventricular block have been reported.

D. **Etiology and pathology**
   1. **Medial degeneration, as in Marfan and Ehlers-Danlos syndromes, is felt to play a major role** in aortic dissection. Any process that weakens the aortic media can predispose the patient to dissection.
      a. **Aging and uncontrolled hypertension** (found in up to 80%) are two of the most commonly associated factors.
      b. **Other associated findings** include congenital bicuspid or unicuspid aortic valves, coarctation of the aorta, Noonan's syndrome, Turner's syndrome, and, rarely, giant cell arteritis.
   2. **Pregnancy increases the risk of dissection,** with up to 50% of events in women younger than 40 years occurring in the third trimester or postpartum period. This is especially true of women with Marfan syndrome and preexisting aortic root dilatation.

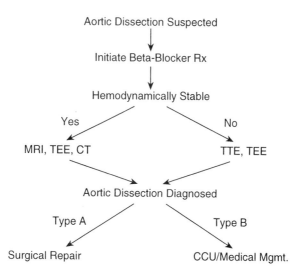

MRI–magnetic resonance imaging; TEE–transewophageal echocardiography; CT–computed tomography; TTE–transthoracic echocardiography. (See text for details)

FIG.25-2. Aortic dissection diagnostic/therapeutic algorithm.

3. **Direct trauma** is also associated with dissection. Blunt trauma causes transection or mural hematoma more commonly; it also, however, rarely causes dissection. Instrumentation with arterial catheterization or intraaortic balloon pump can cause intimal damage and dissection, as may cardiac surgery (at the site of cannulation, cross clamping, or graft insertion).

E. **Diagnostic testing**
   1. **Evaluation.** Fig. 25-2 provides an algorithm to aid in diagnosis. The following characteristics are important in defining the diagnosis of aortic dissection: ascending versus descending aortic involvement; site of the intimal tear; presence or absence of AI; presence/absence of pericardial effusion/tamponade; and coronary involvement.
   2. **Magnetic resonance imaging/magnetic resonance angiography.** Despite its disadvantages, **MRI is currently held as the gold standard for diagnosis of aortic dissection.** It allows multiple planes to be reproduced, thereby providing the most information to determine the presence of a dissection, its extent, and, often, branch vessel involvement. Magnetic resonance imaging has a 98% sensitivity and specificity in the recent series by Nienaber. In addition, it is 88% sensitive for the site of the intimal tear, 98% for the presence of mural thrombus, and 100% for pericardial effusion. When cine-MRI is incorporated, this technique is 85% sensitive for AI as well.
      a. **Advantages** of high sensitivity, specificity, noninvasive nature, and lack of contrast agent are offset by several disadvantages.
      b. **Disadvantages** include the length of the study, lack of available scanners for emergency cases in many hospitals, and limited detection of branch vessel involvement and AI. Patients with metal surgical clips, pacemakers, older heart valves, and multiple drips cannot be studied in the strong magnetic field.

3. **Transesophageal echocardiography/transthoracic echocardiography**

   a. **Transthoracic echocardiography allows a quick (within minutes), easy, noninvasive evaluation at the bedside.** This study, however, has been shown to have an overall sensitivity of 59% to 85% and a specificity of 63% to 96%. These values are dramatically different in the ascending and descending aorta. The sensitivity in the ascending aorta is 78% to 100%, but it drops off to 31% to 55% in the descending portion. Emphysema, patient ventilation, and obesity further decrease the utility of this technique.

   b. **Transesophageal echocardiography overcomes many of the problems with TTE and has the advantage over other imaging modalities of rapid acquisition** at the bedside, thus enabling immediate triage. Overall sensitivity for TEE is 98% to 99% in two large studies. The detection of an intimal tear and intramural thrombus were 73% and 68%, respectively. Detection of AI and/or pericardial effusion was 100%. The specificity (77% to 97%) in detection of dissection can be a problem; however, it is dependent on the experience of the operator and the number of criteria used to define the diagnosis. Diagnostic accuracy can be significantly improved by looking for a flow disturbance associated with an intimal flap.

4. **Computed tomography.** According to two recent prospective studies, the sensitivity of CT for dissection ranges from 83% to 94%, while the specificity is 87% to 100% (4,5). The further development of ultrafast CT and helical CT may improve the sensitivity of this diagnostic test.

   a. **Advantages** are ready availability, noninvasive nature, and detection of thrombus in the false lumen or pericardial effusion.

   b. **Disadvantages** include low sensitivity, inability to define the intimal tear or branch vessel involvement, and inability to define the presence of AI. The need for IV contrast is a minor disadvantage.

5. **Aortography.** This was the first means available to evaluate patients with suspected dissection. Visualization of the false lumen or intimal flap are considered diagnostic; in one study, these findings are present in 87% and 70% of cases, respectively. Recent studies comparing aortography to CT, MRI, and TEE show the overall sensitivity and specificity to be 88% and 95%, respectively. False negatives can occur with thrombosis of the false lumen, intramural hematoma, or equal filling of the false lumen.

   a. **Advantages** of aortography include definition of coronary anatomy, branch vessel involvement and extent of the dissection, as well as its wide availability.

   b. **Disadvantages,** beyond its low sensitivity, are risks of an invasive procedure, contrast administration, and prolonged time to diagnosis and treatment.

6. **Comparison.** The relative advantages and disadvantages of the four modalities are outlined in Table 25-5. **The technique chosen should be based on local expertise and clinical availability,** rather than the published literature. Each method has advantages and disadvantages. In doubtful or puzzling cases (e.g., inconclusive TEE) multiple modalities may be necessary. The aim in type A dissections is to get the patient to the operating room as soon as possible.

   a. Transesophageal echocardiography and CT offer the most rapid answer in most emergency situations. Transesophageal echocardiography is preferred because of its portability, rapid access, greater sensitivity, additional information provided, and relative safety. However, in centers where this is not available, CT is a reasonable alternative.

   b. Magnetic resonance imaging allows the most detail, as well as the greatest sensitivity and specificity. In the unstable setting of acute

Table 25-5. Comparison of imaging modalities in aortic dissection

Factor	Angiography	CT	MRI	TEE
Intimal tear definition	++	+	+++	++
False Lumen Thrombus +/−	+++	++	+++	+
Involvement of branch vessels	+++	+	++	+
Pericardial effusion	−	++	+++	+++
Coronary involvement	+++	−	−	++
AI presence	+++	−	+	+++
Overall sensitivity (%)	88	83–94	98	98–99
Overall specificity (%)	95	87–100	98	77–97

CT, Computed tomography; MRI, magnetic resonance imaging; TEE, transesophageal echocardiography; AI, aortic insufficiency.
Modified with permission from Jaselbacher EM, Eagle RA, DeSanctis RW, 1997.

dissection, the lack of access to the patient and length of the procedure make this a less desirable alternative. **Magnetic resonance imaging is best suited for serial evaluation of patients with chronic dissection, whether treated medically or surgically.**

c. Aortography is the most difficult to obtain rapidly in an emergent situation and may simply delay a life-saving surgical procedure. Thus, **aortography should be reserved for when a definitive diagnosis is not obtained with other studies or definition of coronary anatomy is imperative** to surgical planning.

F. **Therapy.** Death in aortic dissections results not from the intimal flap but from progression of the dissection resulting in either vascular compromise or rupture. **Proximal (type A) aortic dissection is universally felt to mandate immediate surgical treatment.** This greatly reduces the risk of poor outcomes (acute AI, CHF, tamponade, and neurologic sequelae) from progression of the dissection and halts the 1% per hour mortality rate. **Management of distal (type B) aortic dissections is controversial,** but it is generally believed that medical management is initially indicated. Surgical interventions are reserved for complications of dissection or treatment failure. Table 25-6 recommends course of treatment for various types of dissections. The 5-year survival rate for patients leaving the hospital with appropriate treatment (medical or surgical) ranges from 75% to 82%.

1. **Priority of therapy.** The initial management of patients with suspected aortic dissection is directed toward **reducing dP/dt and lowering blood pressure.** Close hemodynamic monitoring with an arterial line and sufficient venous access for volume replacement should be established simultaneously. This initial aggressive dP/dt and blood pressure management applies to all patients regardless of the type of dissection or the long-term management (medical or surgical).

2. **Caveats**

a. **Hypotension and dissection.** The most likely causes are aortic wall rupture or tamponade. In either event, **aggressive volume replacement should be initiated and the patient taken to the operating room promptly.** In a small nonrandomized series (seven patients), three of the four who underwent pericardiocentesis died

Table 25-6. Surgical versus medical therapy for aortic dissection

Medical therapy	Surgical therapy
Uncomplicated type III dissection	Acute, type I or II dissection
Stable, lone arch dissection	Acute, complicated type III dissection
	End-organ dysfunction
	Rupture/impending rupture
	Aortic insufficiency
	Associated with Marfan syndrome
	Retrograde extension into the
	ascending aorta
Stable, chronic dissection (more than 2 weeks after onset of symptoms)	

suddenly 5 to 40 minutes after the procedure. All three of the patients who went to the operating room without the procedure survived. It is possible that the hemodynamic improvement that was seen after pericardiocentesis, with its accompanying increase in dP/dT, caused rapid and fatal progression of the dissection. If pericardiocentesis becomes an absolute requirement to get the patient to the operating room, enough fluid to raise the blood pressure to an acceptable level, but no more, should be removed. **If vasopressors are required for hemodynamic stabilization, norepinephrine and phenylephrine are the drugs of choice, as neither has a demonstrable effect on dP/dT. Epinephrine and dopamine should be avoided.**

    b. **Acute MI** can be seen in association with a type A dissection. In this setting, **thrombolysis is absolutely contraindicated.** Lack of flow in the proximal coronary artery or a flap obstructing the coronary may be visible on TEE. In the acute setting, coronary angiography is a higher risk procedure with low yield. Downstream thromboembolism and mechanical progression of the dissection are possible complications. **A time delay to surgical repair with the resultant increase in preoperative mortality is a complication of angiography in the acute setting.**

3. **Medical therapy**

    a. **β-Blockers should be initiated immediately** if aortic dissection is being considered in the differential diagnosis. They should be titrated to effect (heart rate of less than 60, mean arterial pressure of 60 to 70 mm Hg). In patients intolerant of β-blockers, calcium channel blockers are acceptable alternatives (see Table 25-1 for drugs and doses).

    b. **Once the patient is adequately β-blocked, sodium nitroprusside can be initiated.** It is an effective, rapid onset, IV medication that can be titrated to the desired blood pressure. Initial infusion is at 20 µg/min, with titration to maintain a mean arterial pressure of 60 to 70 mm Hg.

4. **Surgical therapy**

    a. **Patients with proximal or type A dissection** should be taken to the operating room upon diagnosis.

    b. **Patients with type B dissection in whom pain and/or hypertension cannot be controlled medically, or who have evidence of rupture or end-organ involvement,** signifying progression of the dissection, should receive surgical repair.

    c. **Perioperative risk** is affected by age, comorbidities (especially CAD or chronic obstructive pulmonary disease), tamponade or rupture, shock, or compromise of vital organs (brain, kidneys, heart). The longer the preoperative diagnostic period, the higher is the perioperative mortality.

d. **Surgical repair.** Details are beyond the scope of this book. The general approach is to remove the intimal flap, oversew the entry and exit sites of the false lumen, and usually reinforce the aorta with a Dacron graft. In the event that the aortic valve is not able to be repaired or resuspended, a Bentall procedure is performed with a prosthetic valve sewn onto a Dacron graft and used to replace the native valve. The coronary arteries are reimplanted into the graft. In similar fashion the visceral arteries and T_8 to L_2 intercostal/lumbar arteries are reimplanted if needed.

e. **Complications** from this procedure include bleeding, infection, ischemic acute tubular necrosis, and/or mesenteric ischemia.

   (1) **Paraplegia is one of the most feared complications** in repair of descending thoracic dissections. As discussed in the section on thoracoabdominal aneurysms, paraplegia is due to the disruption of blood flow to the anterior spinal artery via the intercostal arteries.

   (2) **Late complications** include progressive AI (if the valve was not replaced at surgery), anastomotic aneurysm formation, and recurrent dissection at the previous or a secondary site.

5. **Percutaneous therapy. New techniques** are emerging in the treatment of aortic dissections. The newest of these, the percutaneous intraluminal stent-graft, has shown early success in dog models of distal dissections. Success is defined by deployment, occlusion of the proximal intimal tear, and thrombosis of the false lumen in 2 hours. Early experience in human trials is promising; however, long-term data are lacking at this time.

6. **Long-term management**

   a. **Chronic management of distal (type B) aortic dissections is an extension of the acute management.** Aggressive blood pressure control is obtained with oral agents such as atenolol, metoprolol, labetalol, or diltiazem.

      (1) **Vasodilators,** such as hydralazine or minoxidil, which increase dP/dt, **should be used only in conjunction with a negative inotrope** (β-blocker).

      (2) **In the event of treatment failure,** these patients should always be considered for surgical treatment. Failure is defined as evidence of aortic leak, progression with visceral organ involvement, recurrent pain, or AI.

   b. **Long-term therapy is the same for all patients,** regardless of whether they had surgical repair. It consists of **blood pressure and dP/dT control** as described above.

      (1) **Target systolic blood pressure** should be 130 mm Hg or below.

      (2) Late deaths are due, in about 30% of cases, to rupture of a second aneurysm or recurrence of the dissection. A majority of these secondary aneurysms will develop within 2 years of the initial treatment. **The goal of the follow-up visits is early detection of these secondary aneurysms.** Careful physical examination, blood pressure evaluation, and plain chest radiograph are important; however, serial evaluations of the aorta with TEE, CT, or MRI are vital. **Magnetic resonance imaging is the gold standard** and offers the most data for the procedure. Since the period of highest risk is the first 2 years, the visits and radiographic follow-up should occur at 3 and 6 months post discharge, and then every 6 months for 2 years, after which patients can be followed every 6 to 12 months depending on their risk.

G. Atypical variants of dissection

1. **Intramural hematoma** may represent rupture of the vasa vasorum, without tearing through the intima of the aorta. This hematoma may dissect locally in the layer between the outer media and the adventitia. **The difference between this phenomenon and a classic dissection is the lack of communication with the lumen of the aorta,** although some theories have this process converting to frank dissection via rupture through the intima. The presentation of these patients is usually the same as for classical dissection. The lack of an intimal tear as seen on TEE or MRI is what differentiates this process from a true dissection. Intramural hematomas have a similar natural history to classic dissection. Therefore, management for this entity is similar to that for a true dissection.

2. **Penetrating atherosclerotic ulcer is an atherosclerotic plaque that ulcerates into the media,** allowing formation of a local hematoma. The risk factors for this process include older age and uncontrolled hypertension. The descending aorta is the most common site. The presentation is similar to other types of dissection, with sudden onset back and/or chest pain. Complications include local dissection, pseudoaneurysm formation, true aneurysm formation, and transmural erosion with rupture. The diagnostic study of choice for this process is aortography, which defines the presence of contrast protruding into an atherosclerotic plaque. Since the natural history and outcomes of this entity are not well elucidated, treatment is individualized to the patient. In the event that a patient presents with this process with hemodynamic instability, urgent surgical repair is necessary. Otherwise, medical management with β-blockers and frequent radiologic follow-up for signs of progression should be undertaken. Follow-up studies should be performed every 6 to 12 months, or more frequently if clinically indicated.

IV. Controversies

A. **The major controversy that exists in the evaluation of AAA concerns the screening of asymptomatic patients.** At present no controlled clinical trials have addressed this issue. A metaanalysis has suggested that physical examination screening in males aged 60 to 80 years was cost-effective but offered little survival benefit. In the same population ultrasound offered greater benefit but at significantly greater cost. The current consensus for screening is for ultrasound in high-risk patients, especially those with a family history.

B. There are **two instances in which coronary anatomy plays a role in decision making at surgery.** The first is with occlusion of the coronary ostium by the dissection flap. The second instance is when patients with chronic coronary disease have a proximal aortic dissection. In many circumstances, the coronary ostia can be evaluated with TEE to define the presence or absence of obstruction from the intimal flap. Additionally, the presence or absence of a wall motion abnormality can be helpful in defining significant coronary obstruction. If this is not possible, then intraoperative (palpation, angioscopy) evaluation can be performed. In either case, the time delay in waiting for angiography to be performed has not proven valuable, in small retrospective and autopsy studies, in a disease process wherein mortality increases by the hour. Others have shown good outcomes with combined dissection repair and coronary artery bypass graft and therefore argue for coronary angiography in all stable aortic dissections. **Coronary angiography should be reserved for patients with known or strongly suspected CAD,** especially in the setting of acute aortic dissection.

C. **Management of uncomplicated type III aortic dissections remains controversial.** The general belief, as described earlier, is that medical treatment is as effective and safe as surgical repair in these patients. This is based on collected retrospective data from the University of Alabama, Duke University, Stanford University, Massachusetts General Hospital, and Crawford groups over the 1960s to 1980s. In general, these studies have shown the following:

The criteria used to determine which patients go to surgery are the very complications that increase the risk of surgery.

Over the years the perioperative mortality has declined to acceptable levels in appropriately chosen patients (6% to 12% between series).

The uncomplicated, low-surgical-risk patients become the focal point for discussion on this topic. Over time, the perioperative mortality has declined from the 30% range to under 10% in Crawford's report. The largest reported series with defined low-risk patients (no end-organ damage, cardiac or renal comorbidities, or vessel rupture) belongs to the Duke-Stanford group. Of 136 patients overall, 30 (19 medical versus 11 surgical) fell into this low-risk category. The survival curves show no significant difference over 1-, 5-, and 10-year intervals (94%, 87%, 32% medical treatment versus 90%, 80%, 50% surgical treatment); in the surgical group, however, a trend toward long-term benefit is seen. **This one subgroup of patients should be looked at in a prospective manner to determine whether surgery is truly advantageous over medical management.**

SUGGESTED READINGS

References

1. Parodi J. Endovascular repair of abdominal aortic aneurysms and other arterial lesions. *J Vasc Surg* 1995;21:549–555.
2. Kiell CS, Ernst CB. Advances in management of abdominal aortal aneurysm. *Adv Surg* 1993;26:73–98.
3. Dapunt OE, et al. The natural history of thoracic aortic aneurysms. *J Thorac Cardiovasc Surg* 1994;107:1323–1332.
4. Erbel R, et al. Echocardiography in the diagnosis of aortic dissection. *Lancet* 1998; 1 (8636):457–461.
5. Nienaber CA, et al. The diagnosis of thoracic aortic dissection by noninvasive imaging procedures. *N Engl J Med* 1993;328:1–9.

Landmark Articles

Gadowski GR, Pilcher DB, Ricci MA. Abdominal aortic aneurysm expansion rate: effect of size and blockade. *J Vasc Surg* 1994;19:727–731.
Nienaber CA, von Kodolitsch Y, Nicholas V, et al. The diagnosis of thoracic aortic dissection by noninvasive imaging procedures. *N Engl J Med* 1993;328:1–9.
Parodi JC. Endovascular repair of abdominal aortic aneurysms and other arterial lesions. *J Vasc Surg* 1995;21:549–557.
Slonim SM, Nyman U, et al. Aortic dissection: percutaneous management of ischemic complications with endovascular stents and balloon fenestration. *J Vasc Surg* 1996;23:241–253.
Williams DM, Lee DY, et al. The dissected aorta. Percutaneous treatment of ischemic complications: principles and results. *J Vasc Intervent Radiol* 1997;8:605–625.

Key Reviews

Cigarroa JE, Isselbacher EM, et al. Diagnostic imaging in the evaluation of suspected aortic dissection. *N Engl J Med* 1994;328:35–43.
Coselli JS, de Figueiredo LFP. Natural history of descending and thoracoabdominal aortic aneurysms. *J Cardiovasc Surg* 1997;12 (Suppl): 285–291.
Furthmayr H, Francke U. Ascending aortic aneurysm with or without features of Marfan syndrome and other fibrillinopathies: new insights. *Semin Thorac Cardiovasc Surg* 1997;9:191–205.
Fuster V, Halperin JL. Aortic dissection: a medical perspective. *J Cardiovasc Surg* 1994;9:713–728.
Kouchoukos NT, Dougenis D. Surgery of the thoracic aorta. *N Engl J Med* 1997;336 (26):1876–1888.

Lindsay J Jr. Diagnosis and treatment of diseases of the aorta. *Curr Probl Cardiol* 1997;22:485–548.

Miller DC. The continuing dilemma concerning medical versus surgical management of patients with acute type B dissections. *Semin Thorac Cardiovasc Surg* 1993;5:33–46.

Pitt MPI, Bonser RS. The natural history of thoracic aortic aneurysm disease: an overview. *J Cardiovasc Surg* 1997;12 (Suppl): 270–278.

Pretre R, Von Segesser LK. Aortic dissection. *Lancet* 1997;349:1461–1464.

Svensson LG. Natural history of aneurysms of the descending and thoracoabdominal aorta. *J Cardiovasc Surg* 1997;12 (Suppl): 279–284.

Relevant Book Chapters

Berstein EF. Computed tomography, ultrasound, and magnetic resonance:imaging in the management of aortic aneurysms. In: Vieth et al., eds. *Vascular surgery: principles and practice,* 2nd ed. New York: McGraw-Hill, 1994:565–575.

Coselli JS. Aneurysms of the transverse aortic arch. In: Baue AE, et al., eds. *Glenn's thoracic and cardiovascular surgery,* 6th ed. Norwalk, CT: Appleton and Lange, 1996:2239–2253.

Crawford ES, Crawford JL. Thoraco-abdominal aortic aneurysm. In: Vieth et al., eds. *Vascular surgery: principles and practice,* 2nd ed. New York: McGraw-Hill, 1994:539–549.

Ergin MA, Griepp RB. Dissections of the aorta. In: Baue AE, et al., eds. *Glenn's thoracic and cardiovascular surgery,* 6th ed. Norwalk, CT: Appleton and Lange, 1996: 2273–2298.

Fann JI, Miller DC. Descending thoracic aortic aneurysms. In: Baue AE, et al., eds. *Glenn's thoracic and cardiovascular surgery,* 6th ed. Norwalk, CT: Appleton and Lange, 1996:2255–2272.

Freischlag JA, Crawford ES, Bernstein EF, et al. Abdominal aortic aneursyms. In: Vieth, et al., eds. *Vascular surgery: principles and practice,* 2nd ed. New York: McGraw-Hill, 1994:539–549.

Isselbacher EM, Eagle KA, et al. Diseases of the aorta. In: Braunwald E, ed. *Heart disease: a textbook of cardiovascular medicine,* 5th ed. Philadelphia: WB Saunders, 1997:1546–1581.

Kouchoukos NT. Aneurysms of the ascending aorta. In: Baue AE, et al., eds. *Glenn's thoracic and cardiovascular surgery,* 6th ed. Norwalk, CT: Appleton and Lange, 1996:2225–2237.

Spittell PC. Diseases of the aorta. In: Topol EJ, ed. *Textbook of cardiovascular medicine.* Philadelphia: Lippincott-Raven Publishers, 1998:2519–2540.

Jenny Wu

I. **Introduction**
   A. Pericarditis is a **clinical syndrome resulting from inflammation of the pericardium and is associated with chest pain, a friction rub, and characteristic ECG changes.** The incidence is 2% to 6% in autopsy series although it is diagnosed clinically in only 1 in 1,000 admissions. It is more **common in men.**
   B. **Types of pericarditis and etiology.** There are a vast number of etiologies; the most common causes are idiopathic, viral, bacterial, tuberculous, uremic, post myocardial infarction (MI), neoplastic, and traumatic (Table 26-1).
II. **Idiopathic pericarditis.** Most cases of acute pericarditis are idiopathic. Frequently when the etiology is unknown or idiopathic, it is **most likely to be of viral origin** (see Section III of this chapter). For discussion of other types of pericarditis, see Sections IV (purulent pericarditis), V (tuberculous pericarditis), VI (post-MI pericarditis), VII (uremic pericarditis), and VIII (neoplastic pericarditis).
   A. **Clinical presentation**
      1. **Signs and symptoms**
         a. **Chest pain** from pericarditis is usually retrosternal, sharp, and severe, and often radiates to the neck, shoulders, and back. Classical features include worsening with lying supine, coughing, and inspiration. The pain is often alleviated by leaning forward.
         b. There may be a **prodrome of fever and myalgias.**
         c. **Dyspnea** can also occur as a result of shallow breathing from pleuropericardial chest pain.
         d. Patients are often **in distress and uncomfortable.**
      2. **Physical findings**
         a. The **pericardial friction rub is pathognomic for pericarditis.** It is characterized by a **scratchy, grating, high-pitched sound.** It is often evanescent and may change in quality. Additionally, it may be absent with subsequent examinations or may change in intensity with respiration. Classically, it has three components, corresponding to atrial systole, ventricular systole, and early ventricular diastole. Most often, only the atrial and ventricular systolic components are heard. Occasionally, only one component is heard.
         b. The best place to **auscultate the rub is at the lower left sternal border,** using the diaphragm of the stethoscope, with the patient sitting forward, and during inspiration.
   B. **Laboratory examination and diagnostic testing.** Pericarditis is a **clinical diagnosis based on history, physical examination, chest radiograph, and serial electrocardiographic (ECG) changes.** Some patients may need further testing, such as tuberculin skin testing, fungal tests, viral serologies, cold agglutinins, thyroid function tests, heterophile antibodies, antinuclear antibodies (ANAs), and rheumatoid factor.
      1. Typically, the **ECG changes** evolve through **four stages** (Table 26-2). These changes occur in most patients, although their absence does not exclude acute pericarditis. These ECG changes are typical regardless of etiology for pericarditis.
         a. The first stage usually occurs within hours of onset of chest pain and is diagnostic of acute pericarditis (Fig. 26-1). The presence of **stage 1 ECG changes is most useful in confirming the diagnosis of acute pericarditis** along with the clinical presentation, yet such changes are often **difficult to distinguish from changes**

Table 26-1. Etiologies of pericarditis

IDIOPATHIC (nonspecific)

Viral infections: coxsackievirus A, coxsackievirus B, echovirus, adenovirus, mumps virus, infectious mononucleosis, varicella, hepatitis B, acquired immunodeficiency syndrome

Bacterial infections: *pneumococcus, staphylococcus, streptococcus,* gram-negative septicemia, *Neisseria meningitidis, Neisseria gonorrhoeae,* tularemia, *Legionella pneumophila,* mycobacterium tuberculosis

Fungal infections: histoplasmosis, coccidioidomycosis, *Candida,* blastomycosis

UREMIA

Neoplasm: lung cancer, breast cancer, leukemia, Hodgkin's disease, lymphoma

RADIATION

Autoimmune diseases: acute rheumatic fever, systemic lupus erythematosus, rheumatoid arthritis, scleroderma, mixed connective tissue disease, Wegener's granulomatosis, polyarteritis nodosa

Inflammatory disease: sarcoidosis, amyloidosis, inflammatory bowel disease, Whipple's disease, temporal arteritis

DRUGS

Hydralazine, procainamide, phenytoin, isoniazid, phenylbutazone, doxorubicin, penicillin

TRAUMA

Postmyocardial-pericardial injury syndromes: postmyocardial infarction (Dressler's syndrome), postpericardiotomy syndrome

Dissecting aortic aneurysm

Adapted from Braunwal E, 1997, p. 1482, with permission.

Table 26-2. Typical ECG evolution of acute pericarditis

Stage	J-ST	T waves	PR segment
"EPICARDIAL" LEADS (I, II, AVL, AVF, V3-6)			
I	Elevated	Upright	Depressed or isoelectric
II early	Isoelectric	Upright	Isoelectric or depressed
II late	Isoelectric	Low to flat to inverted	Isoelectric or depressed
III	Isoelectric	Inverted	Isoelectric
IV	Isoelectric	Upright	Isoelectric
"ENDOCARDIAL" LEADS (AVR, OFTEN V1, SOMETIMES V2)			
I	Depressed	Inverted	Elevated or isoelectric
II early	Isoelectric	Inverted	Isoelectric or elevated
II late	Isoelectric	Shallow to flat to to upright	Isoelectric to elevated
III	Isoelectric	Upright	Isoelectric
IV	Isoelectric	Inverted	Isoelectric

Modified from Spodick DH. Electrocardiographic changes in acute pericarditis. *Am J Cardiol* 1974; 33:470 with permission.

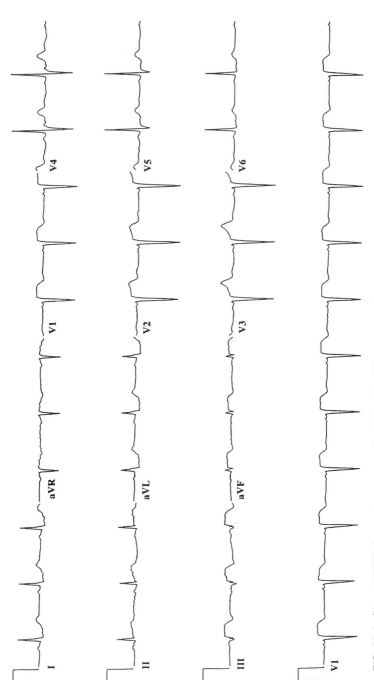

FIG. 26-1. Stage 1 ECG changes in acute pericarditis. Note PR segment elevation in lead aVR, and diffuse ST elevation and the upsloping nature of ST segments as compared to acute myocardial infarction.

associated with early repolarization and acute infarction. There is diffuse ST-segment elevation with upright T waves in all leads except aVR and V_1. PR-segment depression is seen in all leads except aVR and V_1.

- b. **Stage 2,** occurring several days later, is characterized by resolution of PR/ST segments to baseline and T-wave flattening.
- c. T-Wave inversions mark **stage 3.**
- d. **Stage 4** occurs when T waves become upright again, which may take days to weeks.

2. If an **effusion** is present, there may be **electrical alternans or low voltages on the ECG.**
3. A chest radiograph may reveal **cardiomegaly suggestive of a pericardial effusion;** otherwise, it does not help in establishing the diagnosis.
4. **Blood cultures along with sputum and gastric aspirate** for tuberculosis should be done in complex cases (over 1 week in duration) to rule out bacteremia or endocarditis.
5. **Blood tests** may reveal leukocytosis, elevated erythrocyte sedimentation rate, and creatine phosphokinase MBs. However, these are all **nonspecific indicators of inflammation.**
6. **Echocardiography. Pericarditis is not an echocardiographic diagnosis.**
    - a. Echocardiography should be done when **symptoms last longer than a week, to evaluate for hemodynamic abnormalities or thickening in routine cases.** Pericardial thickening is often difficult to assess accurately; trivial or small effusions can be seen in 8% to 15% of asymptomatic individuals.
    - b. On the other hand, **if the patient has had recent cardiac surgery, is elderly, or if there is a suspicion for pericardial effusion,** then echocardiography should be done as part of initial workup.
7. **Computed tomography, magnetic resonance imaging, or transesophageal echocardiography** can be done in select cases to investigate the pericardium.
8. **Radionuclide scans** have been used to identify pericarditis, though this has not been clinically established as an effective diagnostic tool in this setting.

C. **Differential diagnosis.** The differential should be considered in any patient with suspected pericarditis.
1. Chest pain of acute pericarditis can mimic **aortic dissection, pulmonary embolism, pneumothorax, or MI.**
2. ECG changes can also mimic **myocardial ischemia.** However, ST segments concave upward in myocardial ischemia. Echocardiography can also help in differentiating pericarditis from ischemia in unclear cases of patients with chest pain and diffuse ST elevations, by assessing for segmental wall motion abnormalities.

D. **Therapy**
1. **Priority of therapy. Most cases** of acute pericarditis are **uncomplicated and self-limited and usually respond to medical therapy.**
    - a. First-line therapy should be **nonsteroidal anti-inflammatory drugs** (NSAIDs).
    - b. Management of complications such as pericardial effusions and constrictive pericarditis are discussed in Chapters 27 and 28.
2. **Medical therapy**
    - a. **Ibuprofen,** 600 to 800 mg PO three times a day for 3 weeks, **or indomethacin** 25 to 50 mg PO three times a day for 3 weeks.
    - b. **Alternatively,** if patient does not respond to the NSAIDs or in cases of recurrent pericarditis, **prednisone,** 40 to 60 mg, is given PO every day, tapering over 3 weeks, or, if care is inpatient, intravenous

methylprednisolone. **Colchicine** may also be tried at 1 mg/day for at least a year, with gradual tapering off.

   3. **Percutaneous therapy** (for cardiac tamponade). As most cases of pericarditis are self-limited, there is no role for routine pericardiocentesis or pericardial biopsy. However, in cases of tamponade or suspected purulent effusion pericardiocentesis should be performed urgently (see Chapter 27 and Section IV of this chapter).

      a. **Pericardiocentesis.** This should only be done when there is a large pericardial effusion with evidence of hemodynamic compromises, or cardiac tamponade, or when pericardial fluid is needed for diagnosis and treatment. For technique, see Chapter 52.

      b. Percutaneous balloon pericardiotomy can be done in cases of malignant effusion.

   4. **Surgical therapy**

      a. **Subxiphoid pericardiostomy** is usually performed for neoplastic pericarditis (see VIII.C.2).

      b. **Pericardiectomy** is usually performed for severe recurrent pericarditis or constrictive pericarditis.

III. **Viral pericarditis.** The most common viruses involved are Coxsackie virus group B and echovirus. **A prodrome of upper respiratory tract symptoms preceding the onset of chest pain along with a fourfold rise in viral convalescent antibody titers** support this diagnosis. Most cases are self-limited, with infrequently occurring complications that include myocarditis, recurrent pericarditis, pericardial effusion, tamponade, and constrictive pericarditis. Diagnosis and management are discussed in Section II of this chapter.

IV. **Purulent pericarditis.** The diagnosis of purulent pericarditis early in its course is paramount as **cardiac tamponade often develops and is associated with high mortality.**

   A. **Clinical presentation. Purulent pericarditis** is characterized by **acute onset of fever, shaking chills, night sweats, and dyspnea** of a few days duration. **Chest pain or pericardial friction rub are not necessarily present.**

   B. **Etiology.** Purulent pericarditis usually occurs as a **complication of pneumonia or empyema** with staphylococci, pneumococci, or streptococci. It can occur from direct extension via subdiaphragmatic abscess, infective endocarditis, or hematogenous spread.

   C. **Diagnosis.** The clinician needs to have a high degree of suspicion. When one suspects purulent pericarditis, pericardiocentesis needs to be done, along with fluid sent for appropriate lab studies including cell counts, Gram stain, and cultures. The **fluid should be cultured** for bacteria, acid-fast bacillus (AFB), fungi, and malignancy, and sent for hematocrit, white blood cell count with differential, glucose, and protein.

   D. **Therapy. Early surgical pericardial fluid drainage and intravenous antibiotic administration can be life saving.**

V. **Tuberculous pericarditis. If the clinical suspicion is high, the patient should be hospitalized. Presumptive triple antituberculous therapy should be started and not delayed while waiting for AFB isolation.**

   A. **Clinical presentation. Any patient who has fever and a pericardial effusion, especially if immunocompromised or with human immunodeficiency virus risk factors, should be suspected of having tuberculous pericarditis.**

      1. **Clinical onset typically is slow** and chronic, with nonspecific constitutional symptoms of **dyspnea, fever, chills, and night sweats.**

      2. **Congestive heart failure symptoms** are more common than chest pain and a pericardial rub.

   B. **Etiology.** Tuberculosis usually manifests as a pericardial effusion often leading to constrictive pericarditis. Pericardial involvement occurs in 1% to 2% of cases of pulmonary tuberculosis and develops from lymphangial, direct, or hematogenous spread.

C. **Laboratory examination and diagnostic testing**
   1. **The fluid is commonly serosanguinous to grossly bloody** and is predominantly composed of polymorphonuclear leukocytes early, with lymphocytosis later.
   2. The **classic ST-segment elevations** of acute pericarditis are **usually absent.**
   3. A **chest radiograph** may reveal a **pulmonary infiltrate** suggestive of active pulmonary tuberculosis or cardiomegaly.
   4. The **diagnosis of tuberculous pericarditis** can be made either by AFB culture from the fluid or by pericardial biopsy, although a normal biopsy does not exclude the diagnosis. Laboratory tests such as a high adenosine deaminase level in pleural or pericardial fluid (more than 40 U/L) or polymerase chain reaction positive for AFB from biopsy sample support the diagnosis. Testing with purified protein derivative is not as helpful.
   5. **Echocardiography** may show a pericardial effusion with fibrinous stranding or a thickened pericardium with an echodense intrapericardial density consistent with an exudate.
D. **Therapy**
   1. **Rifampin** (600 mg/day), **isoniazid** (300 mg/day) **with pyridoxine** (50 mg/day), **and either streptomycin** (1 g/day) **or ethambutol** (15 mg/kg per day) are recommended for at least 9 months, with 6 months of treatment post culture conversion (1).
   2. **Early pericardiectomy** is recommended for recurrent tamponade or the presence of pericardial thickening consistent with development of constrictive pericarditis.
VI. **Post-MI pericarditis.** Because pericarditis is associated with extensive necrosis, these **patients are at increased risk for congestive heart failure and have higher 1-year mortality rates** than those without pericarditis. A lower incidence of pericarditis has been noted with the use of thrombolytic therapy. As infarct size has been correlated with the incidence of pericarditis, **earlier institution of thrombolytic therapy has in turn reduced the occurrence of pericarditis** (see Chapter 3).
   A. **Clinical presentation.** Pericarditis in the **postinfarction patient is diagnosed by recurrent pleuritic pain and a friction rub.** Because incidental small pericardial effusions occur post infarction, **clinical symptoms are required to make the diagnosis.**
   B. **Etiology.** Pericarditis is associated with large, usually anterior wall MIs, within the first few hours to days post infarction.
   C. **Laboratory examination. The T waves may be positive for more than 2 days** or previously inverted T waves may become positive. However, the typical ECG changes are not usually present.
   D. **Therapy**
      1. Treatment with **aspirin** is the first-line recommended therapy.
      2. **Contraindications.** Nonsteroidal antiinflammatory drugs cause coronary vasoconstriction, and prednisone is associated with myocardial rupture in postinfarction pericarditis.
   E. **Dressler's syndrome** usually **occurs weeks to several months after MI,** with an incidence of about 1%. Its etiology is unclear, although it has been proposed to be autoimmune. Patients present with **fever, pleuritis, pericardial and pleural friction rubs, malaise, and severe chest pain, which may mimic a recurrent MI.** This syndrome should be treated with **aspirin or NSAIDs and bedrest. Anticoagulation should be avoided** to prevent the possibility of hemorrhage into the pericardium. Occasionally, there is recurrence of the syndrome, which should be treated with a short course of prednisone. There is **no adverse prognosis** associated with this syndrome.

   F. Postpericardiotomy syndrome is similar to Dressler's syndrome in
   its presentation and it **occurs usually one week after cardiac surgery.**
   The incidence varies from 10% to 40% and is thought to be mediated by the
   autoimmune system. **Clinical course is self-limited,** although it is often
   prolonged. Treatment is with **aspirin, NSAIDs,** and only **corticosteroids**
   for refractory symptoms. Complications include cardiac tamponade and,
   rarely, constrictive pericarditis.
 VII. Uremic pericarditis
   A. Clinical presentation
   1. Uremic pericarditis usually develops in **patients who are just begin-
       ning dialysis; the majority present with a rub.**
   2. The presence of a **small pericardial effusion without a rub or chest
       pain does not establish the diagnosis.**
   3. It is usually **associated with large pericardial effusions.**
   B. Etiology. The etiology is currently unknown and does not seem related to
   the level of circulating uremic catabolites or toxins.
   C. Therapy
   1. **Medical therapy.** NSAIDs have limited use, although steroids may be
       of benefit.
   2. **Percutaneous therapy. Intensive dialysis, even daily, is the treat-
       ment of choice** for symptomatic uremic pericarditis. **Dialysis is not
       necessary for patients who are asymptomatic** with relatively small
       pericardial effusions. **If the pericardial effusion is large,** with ele-
       vated white blood cell count, fever, or cardiac tamponade, then **percu-
       taneous pericardiocentesis** should be considered, as it is unlikely that
       dialysis will be effective.
   3. **Surgical therapy.** Interventions such as **subxiphoid pericardiotomy
       or limited pericardiectomy should be reserved for patients with
       recurrent pericardial effusions** who have failed pericardiocente-
       sis or with loculated effusions that cannot be accessed readily percuta-
       neously.
 VIII. Neoplastic pericarditis. Tumors involving the pericardium are usually of
   metastatic origin (lung, breast, Hodgkin's disease, non-Hodgkin's lymphoma,
   and leukemia). Primary tumors of the pericardium such as mesothelioma, sar-
   coma, teratoma, or fibromas are rare.
   A. Clinical presentation
   1. Patients are **usually asymptomatic,** and neoplastic pericarditis is an
       incidental finding at autopsy.
   2. **Shortness of breath is a common symptom and may represent
       either pleural effusion or pericardial effusion with impending
       cardiac tamponade.**
   3. It is important to **suspect cardiac tamponade in patients with
       known malignancy and symptoms of relatively acute onset, such
       as fatigue, dyspnea, or edema,** since such patients have a high like-
       lihood of developing significant pericardial effusions.
   B. Laboratory examination and diagnostic testing
   1. The **typical ECG changes of acute pericarditis are not present;**
       rather, the ECG shows nonspecific ST and T-wave abnormalities. Elec-
       trical alternans may be present with pericardial effusions.
   2. **Cytologic examination** of pericardial fluid or open pericardial biopsy
       aids in the diagnosis. There is a higher chance of finding malignant cells
       on cytology with lung and breast cancer, but a lower chance with hema-
       tologic and other malignancies. Elevated levels of carcinoembryonic anti-
       gen have been associated in patients with malignant effusions.
   3. **Surgical biopsies are rarely required** for diagnosis.
   4. Serial echocardiograms should be obtained, initially to establish the loca-
       tion and size of pericardial effusion and to evaluate any hemodynamic
       compromise, and later, after pericardiocentesis, to monitor for reaccu-
       mulation of the effusion.

C. **Therapy**
   1. **Percutaneous therapy**
      a. **Pericardiocentesis with catheter drainage, preferably with echo guidance,** is recommended for symptomatic patients.
      b. **Percutaneous balloon pericardiotomy** has also been performed as an alternative but has been **associated with a higher morbidity** than with catheter-drainage pericardiocentesis.
   2. **Surgical therapy**
      a. **Subxiphoid pericardiostomy,** a common surgical procedure, can also be performed. It involves an incision into the parietal pericardium with placement of a tube initially for drainage, which results in subsequent drainage into the anterior mediastinum upon tube removal (2).
      b. **Pericardial sclerosis** also has been performed with tetracycline in normal saline. It is infused into the pericardial space and allowed to dwell for several hours. This is done about every 1 or 2 days until there is no reaccumulation of fluid. Aside from this being a **painful procedure, arrhythmias and fevers are common side effects.**
      c. Pericardiectomy, which involves stripping of the parietal pericardium with drainage into either the left or the right pleural cavity, is not recommended as first-line management of malignant pericardial effusions.

IX. **Follow-up**
   A. Most patients with idiopathic or viral pericarditis **should be followed up in approximately a month** to see if their symptoms have resolved and that constrictive pericarditis has not developed.
   B. **Patients with pericardial effusions** should have serial echocardiograms in follow-up to ensure there has not been recurrence or increase in the size of the effusion.

X. **Complications**
   A. **Recurrent pericarditis** can occur after an episode of acute idiopathic pericarditis, open heart surgeries, cardiac trauma, or Dressler's syndrome. Natural history studies suggest that recurrent pericarditis occurs in 20% to 30% of patients.
      1. **Clinical presentation is similar to that of acute pericarditis,** with **variable onset** from months to years after the initial episode.
      2. **Therapy. Nonsteroidal antiinflammatory drugs or indomethacin** should be given initially for treatment with slow tapering over months. **If patients fail to respond, then prednisone,** 40 to 60 mg/day, can be prescribed over 1 to 3 weeks, or intravenous methylprednisolone can be given, depending on the severity of symptoms. Most patients respond within a few days. **Surgical pericardiectomy is reserved for those patients who have persistent recurrent pericarditis accompanied by severe chest pain despite aggressive medical therapy.**
      3. **Prevention.** Data over the past decade have shown that **colchicine seems to be safe and effective for prevention of recurrent pericarditis,** although large, controlled, prospective studies are still needed. The recommended dose of colchicine is 1 mg/day for at least a year with slow tapering off. It may also have a sparing effect on steroids, which cause severe systemic side effects in the long term. On the other hand, colchicine is usually well tolerated with only minor side effects (3).
   B. **Cardiac tamponade** will occur in about 15% of patients (see Chapter 27).
   C. **Constrictive pericarditis.** Approximately 9% of patients develop mild constrictive physiology, but this usually resolves after 3 months (see Chapter 28).

SUGGESTED READINGS
References
1. Fowler NO. Tuberculous pericarditis. *JAMA* 1991;266:99–103.
2. Kirkland LL, Taylor RW. Pericardiocentesis. *Crit Care Clin* 1992;8:669–711.

3. Adler Y, Finkelstein Y, Guindo J, et al. Colchicine treatment for recurrent pericarditis: a decade of experience. *Circulation* 1998;97:2183–2185.

Key Reviews
Shabetai R, ed. Diseases of the pericardium. *Cardiology Clin* 1990;8(4):579–716.
Spodick DH. Pericarditis, pericardial effusion, cardiac tamponade, and constriction.
Crit Care Clin 1989;5:455–475.

Relevant Book Chapters
Braunwald E, ed. *Heart disease:a textbook of cardiovascular medicine,* 5th ed. Philadel-
phia: WB Saunders, 1997.
Topol EJ, ed. *Textbook of cardiovascular medicine.* Philadelphia: Lippincott-Raven
Publishers, 1998.
Alexander RW, Schlant R, Fuster V. *Hurst's the heart,* 9th ed. New York: McGraw-
Hill, 1998.

27. PERICARDIAL EFFUSION

Stanley Chetcuti

I. **Introduction.** Pericardial effusions are a common clinical entity and are routinely diagnosed by echocardiography. They may be asymptomatic or present as life-threatening tamponade. The presenting syndrome depends on the volume, rate of accumulation, and characteristics of the fluid. Large effusions may be found unexpectedly and be asymptomatic, whereas rapidly accumulating small effusions may result in tamponade.

II. **Pericardial effusions without tamponade.** The pericardial space contains 15 to 30 cc of fluid. An unstretched pericardium accommodates only 80 to 200 cc of rapidly accumulating fluid, without a significant change in hemodynamics. **In patients with pericarditis,** increased central venous pressure with decreased venous return, and lymphatic drainage, this fluid may increase significantly. The pericardial space may slowly accumulate up to 2 L of fluid without any hemodynamic or clinical sequelae. **Compressive physiology** may occur with rapid accumulation of smaller amounts of fluid if the pericardium is stiff from fibrosis or infiltration by a tumor.

   A. **Clinical presentation**
   1. **Signs and symptoms**
      a. **Slowly developing pericardial effusions,** with no elevation of intrapericardial pressures, are **usually asymptomatic.**
      b. Occasionally, patients may complain of a **constant dull ache or pressure in the chest.**
      c. There may also be a variety of symptoms from the space-occupying effects of the pericardial fluid on other organs in the chest. These include **dysphagia** from esophageal compression, **dyspnea** from lung compression and atelectasis, **hiccups** from compression of the phrenic nerve, and **nausea and abdominal fullness** from pressure on adjacent abdominal organs.
   2. **Physical findings**
      a. If the **effusion is small, there is a lack of findings** on clinical examination.
      b. **Large-volume effusions** may be associated with muffled heart sounds, Ewart's sign (dullness to percussion, bronchial breath sounds, and egophony below the angle of the left scapula), and rales in the lung field secondary to compression.

   B. **Etiology.** Any cause of acute or chronic pericarditis (see Chapter 26) may lead to the development of a pericardial effusion. Common causes of large chronic effusions include idiopathic pericarditis, uremia, pericarditis from malignancy or myxedema, congestive heart failure, nephrotic syndrome, cirrhosis, hypothyroidism, pregnancy, postcardiac surgery, and drugs. There are numerous other causes (Table 27-1).

   C. **Laboratory examination and diagnostic testing**
   1. **Electrocardiogram (ECG).** The classic ECG finding consists of a **low-voltage tracing. Electrical alternans** is a marker of a massive pericardial effusion.
   2. **Chest x-ray.** The parietal pericardium is normally within 1 to 2 mm of epicardial fat. A **pericardial line of greater than 2 mm from the lower heart border is** diagnostic of pericardial effusion. This is best seen on the lateral projection. Cardiomegaly may occur if more than 250 cc of fluid have accumulated. Cardiomegaly with a large prominent superior vena cava, azygous vein, and decreased pulmonary vascularity should lead one to consider the diagnosis of pericardial effusion.

Table 27-1. Etiology of pericardial effusion

Idiopathic
Acute myocadial infarction
Delayed postmyocardial-pericardial injury syndromes:
    Postmyocardial infarction (Dressler's) syndrome
    Postpericardiotomy syndrome.
Metabolic
    Uremia
    Myxedema
    Hypoalbuminemia
Radiation
Dissecting thoracic aneurysm
Trauma
    Pericardiotomy
    Indirect trauma to the chest
    Percutaneous cardiac interventions
    Perforation of the heart by indwelling catheters
Viral infections
    Coxsackie A, B5, B6
    Echovirus
    Adenovirus
    Mumps virus
    Hepatitis B
    Infectious mononucleosis
    Influenza
    Lymphogranuloma venereum
    Varicella
    Human immunodeficiency virus
Bacterial infections
    Staphylococcus
    Streptococcus
    Pneumococcus
    Hemophilus influenzae
    Neisseria gonorrhoeae
    Neisseria meningitidis
    Legionella hemophilia
    Tuberculosis
    Salmonella
    Psittacosis
    Tularemia
    Bacterial endocarditis
Fungal infections
    Histoplasmosis
    Aspergillosis
    Blastomycosis
    Coccidioidomycosis
    Fungal endocarditis
Other infections
    Amebiasis
    Echinococcus
    Lyme disease
    Mycoplasma pneumonia
    Rickettsia

Table 27-1. *Continued*

Tumors
    Primary
        Mesothelioma
        Teratoma
        Fibroma
        Leiomyofibroma and sarcoma
        Lipoma angioma.
    Metastatic
        Breast carcinoma
        Bronchogenic carcinoma
        Lymphoma
        Leukemia melanoma
        Others
Immunologic/inflammatory disorders
    Rheumatic fever
    Systemic lupus erythematosus
    Ankylosing spondylitis
    Rheumatoid arthritis
    Vasculitis
    Wegener's granulomatosis
    Polyarteritis nodosa
    Scleroderma
    Dermatomyositis
    Sarcoidosis
    Inflammatory bowel disease
    Whipple's disease
    Behçet's syndrome
    Reiter's syndrome
    Temporal arteritis
    Amyloidosis
    Familial Mediterranean fever
Drugs
    Procainamide
    Hydralazine
    Heparin
    Warfarin
    Phenytoin
    Phenylbutazone
    Cromolyn sodium
    Dantrolene
    Methysergide
    Doxorubicin
    Penicillin
    Minoxidil
    Colony-stimulating factor
    Interleukin-2

     3. **Transthoracic echocardiography (TTE)** is the **modality of choice** for diagnosing and following pericardial effusions. It allows for accurate diagnosis, ensures the adequacy of drainage procedures, and enables a qualitative assessment in following pericardial effusions. Echocardiography is not useful in differentiating among the different etiologies.
       a. **Two-dimensional echocardiographic** findings are as follows:
         (1) An **echo-free space** is found between the visceral and parietal pericardium.

          (2) The **motion of the parietal pericardium is decreased.**

          (3) When the effusion is large, the **entire heart swings in the pericardium.** This swinging or rocking may occur along both the anteroposterior and the mediolateral axis of the heart, and is thought to be the mechanism for electrical alternans seen on the ECG.

     b. The size of a pericardial effusion may be determined by the degree of separation of the pericardial surfaces and the pattern of distribution of the effusion.

          (1) Small effusions (less than 100 mL) tend to localize at the posterior wall distal to the atrioventricular ring. These tend to be less than 1 cm in width.

          (2) Moderate effusions (100 to 500 mL). A moderate effusion could also be classified as one that surrounds the heart but is 1 cm or less at its greatest width.

          (3) Large effusions (more than 500 mL). Here, although the posterior accumulation continues, the heart seems to settle posteriorly with a greater expansion of the pericardial space laterally, apically, and anteriorly. The effusion is greater than 1 cm at its widest.

     c. The following may mimic a pericardial effusion on two-dimensional echocardiography.

          (1) Pericardial fat tends to be localized anteriorly. Unless loculated, a pericardial effusion localized to the anterior wall is very rare.

          (2) Seventy percent of **pericardial cysts** are found adjacent to the right cardiophrenic junction and adjacent to but separate from the right atrium in the apical four-chamber view.

          (3) A pleural effusion can be differentiated from a pericardial effusion by virtue of the position of the descending thoracic aorta in the parasternal long-axis view. If the fluid is based in the pericardium, the aorta is displaced posteriorly to the effusion away from the posterior wall of the left atrium. If the fluid is pleural-based, the aorta retains its position immediately below the left atrium. Lung parenchyma may be seen within the pleural fluid.

          (4) Other mimics of pericardial effusions are pericardial fibrous bands and pericardial calcification, anterior mediastinal tumors, peritoneal fluid, and a giant left atrium.

4. Magnetic resonance imaging (MRI). Although not usually required, MRI detects pericardial effusions with a high sensitivity. It outlines the distribution and provides an estimate of the pericardial fluid volume that correlates well with echocardiography. It is very effective in detecting loculated pericardial effusions and pericardial thickening. Due to its high tissue contrast, MRI allows the visualization of the pericardium in multiple planes. It can also differentiate simple from complex effusions, and pericardial fat from pathologic thickening.

5. Electron beam computed tomography (EBCT). Using 1.5- to 3.0-mm, high-resolution axial images, EBCT provides excellent detail of the pericardium. The size of the pericardial effusion and its manner of distribution are easily obtained by this technique. Moreover, differentiation among blood, exudate, chyle, and serous fluid may be achieved due to the different attenuation coefficients for these substances.

6. Diagnostic pericardiocentesis and pericardial fluid examination. A diagnostic pericardiocentesis should be considered in patients with large effusions and without clear etiology. Aspirated pericardial fluid should be carefully inspected and immediately placed in sterile tubes for biochemical, microbiologic, and cytologic examination.

     a. Inspection. The initial inspection may indicate the etiology of the effusion. Hemorrhagic pericardial effusions suggest recent bleeding into the pericardial space. However, sanguinous and serosanguinous effusions are seen in a variety of infections and inflammatory disorders. **If the fluid is grossly hemorrhagic,** a small sample is placed on a gauze sponge; if it is thick and clots easily, its origin is most likely a vascular compartment. Confirmation may be obtained by sending samples of pericardial fluid and blood for a complete blood count. **Frank pus** is indicative of an infectious etiology, most likely bacterial. **Chylous fluid** implies injury or obstruction of the thoracic duct.

    b. Culture. Consideration should be given to all possible infectious etiologies, including fungal and viral causes. The etiology of a viral pericardial effusion may also be isolated by in situ hybridization, viral isolation, and microneutralization.

D. Therapy. The management of pericardial effusions depends on the underlying etiology, volume, and hemodynamic significance.

    1. Pericardiocentesis. Although the etiology is important, it can often be determined without pericardiocentesis by virtue of the clinical, systemic, and laboratory features of the presenting condition.

        a. Pericardiocentesis is indicated if malignancy, bacterial, mycobacterial, or fungal pericardial effusion is suspected.

        b. With large effusions of recent onset, close clinical and echocardiographic follow-up is warranted. Pericardiocentesis **may be warranted in large asymptomatic pericardial effusions.**

        c. Pericardiocentesis may **not be indicated** because its yield for incidental pericardial effusions is small.

    2. Anticoagulation is best avoided until resolution of a pericardial effusion.

II. Pericardial effusion with cardiac compression or cardiac tamponade. When an increase in pericardial fluid results in an increase in the intrapericardial pressure with the impairment of cardiac diastolic filling, cardiac tamponade may ensue. Tamponade is characterized by **elevated intracardiac pressure, progressive limitation of ventricular diastolic filling, and reduction of cardiac output.**

A. Clinical presentation

    1. Signs and symptoms. These are all reflective of a low cardiac output: **restlessness, agitation, drowsiness, and stupor; decreased urine output; dyspnea; chest discomfort;** and **weakness, anorexia, and weight loss with a chronic effusion.**

    2. Physical findings. Raised central venous pressure, with prominent x descent and attenuated or absent y descent; **tachypnea; tachycardia; pericardial rub; diminished heart sounds;** sign of **right heart failure** with pleural effusions and hepatomegaly; **hypotension,** which may initially be absent due to the increased adrenergic tone; and **pulsus paradoxus,** which is defined as an inspiratory decline in systolic blood pressure greater than 10 mm Hg. Its mechanism appears to be related to an increased venous return during inspiration. Because there is increased pressure surrounding the heart, the septum of the right ventricle bows into the left ventricle, resulting (due to the negative intrathoracic pressure in inspiration) in decreased left ventricular filling. This phenomenon, combined with the decreased pulmonary venous return to the left ventricle, results in a decreased blood pressure with inspiration. Pulsus paradoxus is **not specific for cardiac tamponade** and may also be seen in severe obstructive pulmonary disease, RV infarction, pulmonary embolism, or asthma. There may be **no pulsus paradoxus when the pericardial tamponade is associated with severe left ventricular dysfunction and elevated diastolic pressures, atrial septal defects, aortic insufficiency, or regional tamponade.**

B. Pathophysiology

    1. There appears to be an **inverse relationship between the volume of the pericardial effusion and cardiac output beyond a critical volume.** Beyond this, small increments in pericardial volume result in large increases in pressure. This volume depends on the compliance of the pericardium, the rate of fluid accumulation, and the status of the pericardial lining (infiltrations, calcification, or fibrosis).

2. The raised intrapericardial pressure results in a **decreased transmural distending pressure that results in decreased diastolic filling.**

3. The **cardiac output is initially maintained** by a heightened adrenergic tone resulting in a resting tachycardia and peripheral vasoconstriction.

4. **In severe tamponade, the compensatory mechanisms fail,** resulting in a decreased cardiac output. Reduced coronary perfusion may cause subendocardial hypoperfusion, further compromising the stroke volume and cardiac output. The finite space around the heart chambers also results in the equalization of filling pressures and the pericardium.

C. **Laboratory examination and diagnostic testing**

1. **Transthoracic echocardiography** should always be performed when the diagnosis of cardiac tamponade is suspected. Echocardiographs readily identify patients with large pericardial effusions.

a. **The differential for patients with elevated central venous pressure and hypotension includes tamponade, right ventricular infarction, and constrictive pericarditis.**

b. The raised pericardial pressures in tamponade and its hemodynamic consequences on the heart, especially the lower pressured right ventricle and atrium, give rise to a number of easily discernible echocardiographic signs of cardiac tamponade. Signs of cardiac tamponade include the following:

(1) **Pericardial effusion.**

(2) **Right atrial diastolic collapse** typically begins in late diastole and continues into ventricular systole. It is best seen in the parasternal short-axis view, the subcostal view, and the apical four-chamber view. It is a very sensitive sign, but its specificity drops to 82%, with a positive predictive value of 50%.

(3) **Right ventricular early diastolic collapse** (or right ventricular diastolic inversion). Although very sensitive in medical patients, it is less so in surgical patients due to the loculated nature of these effusions and the presence of adhesions. When present, the collapse is described as a persistent posterior or inward movement of the right ventricular free wall in diastole. It is seen most commonly in the anterior right ventricular free wall and infundibulum with patients in the supine position. The parasternal long- and short-axis views of the heart are the best for evaluating this sign; M-mode recording through the area best seen helps to outline the timing and duration of the event. Isolated right ventricular diastolic collapse appears to occur before the onset of clinical tamponade. Conditions that raise right ventricular intracavity volume and right ventricular pressure (pulmonary hypertension, right ventricular hypertrophy, right ventricular infarction) delay the occurrence of right ventricular diastolic collapse to higher intrapericardial pressures.

(4) **Left atrial diastolic collapse.**

(5) Abnormal inspiratory increase of **right ventricular dimensions** with abnormal inspiratory decrease of left ventricular dimensions.

(6) **Inspiratory decrease of mitral valve DE excursion** (anterior leaflet opening) and EF slope (initial anterior leaflet closing).

(7) **A respiratory variation in atrioventricular valve flow pattern, with an abnormal inspiratory increase in tricuspid valve flow and abnormal inspiratory decrease of mitral valve flow** (Fig. 27-1). Doppler echocardiography com-

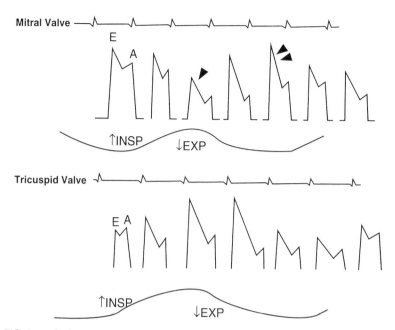

FIG. 27-1. Pulsed wave Doppler for the mitral and tricuspid valves in a patient with cardiac tamponade. Note the marked respiratory variation of the inflow pattern, which is typical tamponade physiology.

bined with the use of a nasal thermistor allows direct quantitation of transmitral, transtricuspid, and systemic venous flow patterns and their variation with respiration. Normally inspiration causes a decrease in mitral valve flow of up to 10% and an increase in tricuspid valve flow of up to 7%. A decrease on inspiration of the transmitral E wave of more than 25% is highly suggestive of significant tamponade. A reduction of the tricuspid E wave of more than 40%, together with prominent hepatic venous flow reversal in expiration, also suggests tamponade.

(8) **Inferior vena cava plethora.** Failure to decrease the proximal diameter by at least 50% on sniff or deep inspiration has a 97% sensitivity but only a 40% specificity.

(9) **Left ventricular pseudohypertrophy.**

Key Suggestions: Performing Transthoracic Echocardiography

When performing TTE it is important to increase the visualization of an echo-free space and decrease background reverberations by decreasing the receiver gain or damping the output signal to a point where the epicardial and pericardial signals are clearly visible.

When a large pericardial effusion is present, an echocardiographic diagnosis of the following entities should be deferred until the effusion has resolved: mitral valve prolapse, tricuspid valve prolapse, aortic valve prolapse, pulmonic valve prolapse, systolic anterior motion of the mitral valve, and middiastolic notching of the pulmonary and aortic valve.

Pleural effusions can be differentiated from a pericardial effusion by virtue of the position of the descending thoracic aorta in the parasternal long-axis view. If the fluid is based in the pericardium, the aorta is displaced posteriorly to the effusion away from the posterior wall of the left atrium. If the fluid is pleural-based, the aorta retains its position immediately below the left atrium.

2. **Right heart catheterization** is important both from a diagnostic and a therapeutic standpoint. It allows confirmation of the diagnosis of tamponade, quantitation of the hemodynamic compromise and cardiac output, and following of the hemodynamic improvement and adequacy of drainage with pericardiocentesis.

   a. The **hemodynamic findings** include equalization (within 4 mm Hg) of the right arterial pressure, pulmonary capillary wedge pressure (PCWP), pulmonary artery diastolic pressure, and right ventricle mid-diastolic pressure, which are raised usually between 10 to 30 mm Hg; the RAP tracing of the right arterial pressure reveals a preserved x descent with an absent or attenuated y descent; during expiration, the PCWP is slightly greater than the intrapericardial pressure that promotes filling of the left heart. With inspiration, the PCWP decreases (transiently), rendering a low or negative pressure gradient between the pulmonary venous circulation and the left heart.

   b. **With pericardiocentesis,** the initial finding is a decrease in all pressures (right atrium, right ventricle diastolic, intrapericardial, PCWP, and left ventricular end-diastolic). As the intrapericardial pressures continue to fall below the right atrium pressure, the y-descent recovers to baseline. This may take as little as 50 cm³ of fluid aspiration, due to the steep ratio of the pressure volume curve of the pericardium. These changes are accompanied by an increase in the carbon monoxide level, blood pressure, and abolition of the pulsus paradoxus. Only with adequate hemodynamic monitoring, including arterial line and right heart catheterization, can these changes be followed.

D. **Therapy**

   1. **Priority of therapy.** Once the diagnosis of tamponade is made, one needs to consider **drainage.** The timing and method of drainage ultimately depend on the etiology of the effusion, the patient's level of acuity, and the availability of trained physicians. The options include needle pericardiocentesis, surgical drainage (subxiphoid pericardiectomy, pericardial window, and subtotal pericardiectomy), or percutaneous balloon pericardiotomy. **Patients in the immediate postoperative period following cardiac surgery** have a high incidence of loculated effusions; for this reason, surgical drainage tends to be the preferred treatment. Unless the situation is immediately life threatening, pericardiocentesis should be performed by staff experienced with the procedure in a controlled setting equipped with hemodynamic monitoring and after an echocardiogram has been performed. Fluoroscopic capabilities are also helpful in minimizing possible complications. During the preparation for the procedure the patient should be supported hemodynamically.

   2. **Medical therapy.** Optimal medical management is important and includes volume expansion, inotropic support such as norepinephrine and dobutamine if the patient is hypotensive, and avoidance of vasodilators such as nitroprusside and nitroglycerin.

   3. **Percutaneous therapy**

      a. **Pericardiocentesis.** The technique for pericardiocentesis is described in detail in Chapter 52. Pericardiocentesis allows the rapid drainage of pericardial tamponade. **It can be done quickly, is less** invasive than other methods, and requires minimal prepara-tion. Complications include laceration of the heart, coronary arter-ies, and lung. There is also the possibility of recurrence or incomplete drainage. It should be avoided if less than 1 cm effusion is present, or in the presence of loculation, adhesion, or fibrinous strands.

b. **Percutaneous balloon pericardiotomy.** With more experience, this **may become the treatment of choice** for medical pericar-dial effusion, especially malignant effusions. It avoids major sur-gical procedures; complications in experienced hands are limited; and recurrences are uncommon. After performing subxiphoid peri-cardiocentesis in the usual manner, 20 cm^3 of 50% radiographic contrast media is injected into the pericardial space through the drainage catheter. A 0.038-in. J-tipped stiff guide wire is looped in the pericardial space and the catheter is removed, taking care to leave the wire in the pericardial space. A 10-Fr dilator is used to widen the track, followed by an 18- to 25- by 30-mm Mansfield or Inoue balloon until it lies at the border of the pericardium where it is inflated to create a window. The balloon is removed and the catheter readvanced over the wire. A repeated injection of 10 cm^3 of diluted contrast media should reveal easy egress from the pericar-dial space. The catheter may then be left in place until drainage ceases completely.

4. **Surgical therapy. Surgical drainage allows for more complete drainage and is preferred if there is a high likelihood of recur-rence.** It allows the examination of the pericardium, access to the peri-cardial tissue for histopathologic and microbiologic diagnosis, and the capability to drain loculated effusions. It is also associated with none of the blind injuries seen with needle pericardiocentesis. It is, however, more painful, with a longer recovery period due to the morbidity associ-ated with the surgical procedure, which also makes it more expensive. There are three frequently employed surgical techniques.

a. **Subxiphoid pericardectomy.** This may be done under local anes-thesia by an experienced surgeon. It is ideal for patients who do not require extensive pericardial incision. It involves the resection of a small portion of the pericardium under direct visualization and the insertion of a tube into the pericardium for extrathoracic drainage. However, unless a ring is used to maintain patency, these incisions tend to close, giving rise to the possibility of recurrences.

b. **Pericardial window.** This allows a connection between the peri-cardial space and the left pleural cavity. The immediate result is to alleviate the pressure in the pericardium, but by virtue of the larger surface of exposure, it also promotes easier absorption of the fluid. This procedure requires a left thoracotomy, and not all available pericardial tissue is excised.

c. **Total and subtotal pericardiectomy.** In the total version, the pericardium is resected from the right phrenic nerve to the left pul-monary veins, sparing the left phrenic nerve, and from the great vessels to the middiaphragm, whereas the subtotal version is lim-ited to the great vessels. This requires greater surgical technique than the other two procedures. It is the procedure of choice in the presence of loculated effusions or effusoconstrictive pericarditis.

SUGGESTED READINGS

Landmark Articles

Appleton PA, Hatle LK, Popp RL. Cardiac tamponade and pericardial effusion: respi-ratory variation and transvalvular flow velocities studied by Doppler echocardiogra-phy. *J Am Coll Cardiol* 1988;11:1020.

Burstow DJ, Oh JK, Baileys KR, et al. Cardiac tamponade: characteristic Doppler observations. *Mayo Clin Proc* 1989;64:312.

Guberman BA, Fowler NO, Engel PJ, et al. Cardiac tamponade in medical patients. *Circulation* 1981;64:633.

Reddy PS, Curtiss EI, O'Toole JD, Shaver JA. Cardiac tamponade: hemodynamic considerations in man. *Circulation* 1978;58:265.

Singh S, Wenn LS, Schuchard GH, et al. Right ventricular and right atrial collapse in patients with cardiac tamponade: a combined echocardiographic and hemodynamic study. *Circulation* 1984;70:960.

Key Reviews
Pericardial heart disease. *Curr Probl Cardiol* 1988 (Aug);22.

Relevant Book Chapters
Feigenbaum H. Pericardial disease. In:Feigenbaum H, ed. *Echocardiography,* 5th ed. Baltimore: Williams & Wilkins, 1994:511–555.

Klein A, Scalia G. The pericardium, restrictive cardiomyopathy, and diastolic function. In: Topol EJ, ed. *Textbook of cardiovascular medicine.* Philadelphia: Lippincott-Raven Publishers, 1998:639–707.

Lorell BH. Pericardial diseases. In: Braunwald E, ed. *Heart disease: a textbook of cardiovascular medicine.* 5th ed. Philadelphia: WB Saunders, 1997:1478–1534.

Lorell BH, Grossman W. Profiles in constrictive pericarditis, restrictive cardiomyopathy and cardiac tamponade in cardiac catheterization. In: Baim DS, Grossman W, eds. *Angiography and intervention,* 5th ed. Baltimore: Williams & Wilkins, 1996:801–822.

SanFillpo AJ, Weyman AE. Pericardial disease. In: Weyman AE, ed. *Principles and practice of echocardiography,* 2nd ed. Philadelphia: Lea & Febiger, 1994:1102–1134.

28. CONSTRICTIVE PERICARDITIS

Joel P. Reginelli and Tom A. Grady

I. **Introduction.** Constrictive pericarditis results from a fibrous thickening of the pericardium, secondary to chronic inflammation from a variety of injuries. Essentially, the heart is encased by the rigid pericardium, leading to a decrease in diastolic filling, an increase in intracardiac pressures, and a dissociation of intracardiac pressure from intrathoracic pressure. The elevated cardiac pressures and diminished diastolic filling lead to increased venous pressure, both pulmonary and systemic, and thus to progressive signs and symptoms of right and left heart failure. Although constrictive pericarditis is a relatively uncommon cause of heart failure, recognition of this entity is important, as its **prevalence appears to be increasing and the diagnosis is often missed.**

II. **Clinical presentation**

A. **Signs and symptoms**

1. The **early symptoms** of constrictive pericarditis are often insidious in nature, and the patient may have nonspecific complaints such as **malaise, fatigue, and decreased exercise tolerance.**

2. As the disease progresses, symptoms consistent with left-sided heart failure such as **exertional dyspnea, orthopnea, and paroxysmal nocturnal dyspnea** may predominate.

3. Additionally, with **advanced disease,** there are often features of right-sided heart failure such as **peripheral edema, abdominal distention, and ascites.**

B. **Physical findings**

1. **Examination of jugular veins.** Nearly all patients have **jugular venous distention,** which simply reflects the elevated right-sided pressures. Many patients demonstrate an inspiratory increase in venous distention known as **Kussmaul's sign.** This finding is sensitive but lacks specificity as other conditions such as right ventricular hypertrophy and right ventricular infarction also produce this sign. Observation of the jugular venous pulsations reveals a **prominent y descent that is produced by the rapid ventricular filling in early diastole.**

2. **Cardiac examination.** Cardiac auscultation may reveal **muffled heart sounds** due to decreased transmission through the thickened pericardium. Given that the mitral and tricuspid valves are nearly closed by end diastole, there may be a **soft S_1. Occasionally, one may observe a pericardial knock** in early diastole (60 to 120 milliseconds after S_2). This represents the abrupt cessation of diastolic filling that occurs when further ventricular relaxation is impeded by the rigid pericardium. The pericardial knock **must be differentiated from other early diastolic sounds** such as an opening snap, S_3, and tumor plop. In general, the pericardial knock is of a higher frequency and occurs slightly earlier than an S_3. An opening snap may be similar in frequency and timing, but is nearly always followed by a diastolic rumble.

3. **Pulmonary examination.** Auscultation of the lung fields may reveal **decreased breath sounds at the bases,** attributed to pleural effusions. Although **rales due to pulmonary edema** have been reported, it is a **relatively rare** finding.

4. **Abdominal examination.** The abdominal exam may reveal evidence of right-sided heart failure, with **hepatomegaly and splenomegaly** frequently noted. In **severe cases, there may be "cardiac cirrhosis"** as evidenced by liver dysfunction and the presence of **ascites.**

5. **Examination of the extremities.** Elevated central venous pressures due to right ventricular impairment and sodium retention due to

Table 28-1. Common etiologies of constrictive pericarditis

Idiopathy
Infectious disease
    Tuberculosis
    Bacterial
    Viral (e.g., Coxsackie B, echovirus)
    Fungal
    Parasitic
Trauma (including cardiac surgery)
Radiation
Inflammatory/immunologic disorder
    Rheumatoid arthritis
    Systemic lupus erythematosus
    Scleroderma
    Sarcoidosis
Neoplastic disease
    Breast cancer
    Lung cancer
    Lymphoma
    Mesothelioma
    Melanoma
End-stage renal disease

---

left ventricular impairment contribute to the development of **peripheral edema.**

III. **Etiology.** The etiologies of constrictive pericarditis are numerous; however, they share a common pathophysiologic pathway that leads to chronic inflammation and pericardial fibrosis. Neoplastic disease is an exception because tumor infiltration of the pericardium is often responsible for constriction. Table 28-1 lists common etiologic factors. The causes of constrictive pericarditis in decreasing order of frequency are idiopathic, radiation therapy, post-surgical therapy, and infectious disease. This represents a significant change from the early part of this century when infectious disease, namely tuberculosis, predominated.

  A. Since the advent of effective antitubercular medications, the **number of cases due to tuberculosis has dropped precipitously in the United States.** However, tuberculosis does remain the primary cause of constrictive pericarditis in most developing regions of the world.

  B. Similarly, **bacterial infections of the chest** continue to represent a large number of cases on a global scale but **have largely disappeared in the United States** following the introduction of antibiotics and improved drainage procedures. **Most idiopathic cases are likely infectious in nature,** due to viral infections such as Coxsackie virus and echovirus; however, a clear etiologic link cannot be established in most cases. Less common infectious etiologies include fungal and parasitic infections.

  C. Constrictive pericarditis is a **late complication of radiation therapy,** generally occurring many years after the administration of radiation. Risk factors for developing constrictive pericarditis include duration of therapy, total amount of radiation administered, and volume of the heart in the radiation field. In contrast to other etiologies of constrictive pericarditis, where the myocardium is typically normal in structure and function, there may be **associated radiation damage to the myocardium as well.**

  D. Constrictive pericarditis is a well-documented **late complication of cardiac procedures involving the pericardium.** It is most **frequently observed following extensive procedures** such as coronary artery bypass grafting or valvular surgery. **Risk factors** for developing postoperative constrictive pericarditis include **intraoperative hemorrhage into the pericardium, postoperative pericarditis,** and the occurrence of **postpericardiotomy syndrome.**

E. **End-stage renal disease, neoplastic disease (primarily breast, lung, and lymphoma), and connective tissue disease are less common etiologies** but need to be considered in the initial differential.

IV. **Pathophysiology**

A. The pericardium is composed of an inner monocellular visceral layer adherent to the myocardium and an outer thicker parietal layer, which is joined to adjacent intrathoracic structures by means of ligaments. Interspersed between the two layers is a small amount of pericardial fluid, generally less than 60 mL. The normal pericardium is quite distensible and permits unimpeded expansion of the ventricles during diastole. Normally, changes in intrathoracic pressure are easily transmitted to the heart, resulting in increased venous return to the right side of the heart with inspiration and increased pulmonary venous return to the left side of the heart with expiration.

B. In constrictive pericarditis there is **thickening and fibrosis of the pericardium,** often with superimposed calcification, resulting in decreased ventricular compliance.

Ventricular compliance = Δend-diastolic volume/Δend-diastolic pressure

As the pericardium thickens and limits ventricular compliance, there is an increased end-diastolic pressure for any given end-diastolic volume. This increase in pressure affects both ventricles equally, and effectively decreases diastolic filling and thus end-diastolic volume of both ventricles. The increased pressure is transmitted backward and results in elevated pulmonary venous and systemic venous pressures.

1. The myocardium is generally normal in structure and function; therefore, **systole is unimpaired.**

2. **Diastolic function,** on the other hand, **is markedly altered** by the constrictive process. In early diastole, the ventricles expand normally, and there is rapid filling secondary to the elevated pulmonary and systemic pressures. Once the ventricles reach the confines of the rigid pericardium, there is an immediate increase in ventricular pressure, and diastolic filling comes to an abrupt halt.

3. The result is that **nearly all ventricular filling occurs in the second phase of diastole (early filling)** with little contribution from the third phase (diastasis) and the fourth phase (atrial systole).

V. **Laboratory examination**

A. **Electrocardiography. Low voltage** is frequently seen with **generalized flattening of the T waves.** There may be **left atrial enlargement. Atrial fibrillation** is a common finding.

B. **Chest x-ray**

1. **Pericardial calcification** is relatively common in advanced disease. The calcification is usually best appreciated with a lateral film and frequently involves the right ventricle and atrioventricular groove.

2. **Pleural effusions** occur frequently, and there may be evidence of both **left and right atrial enlargement.**

3. **Pulmonary edema** is an uncommon finding.

VI. **Diagnostic testing.** Confirming the diagnosis of constrictive pericarditis often presents a challenge as there exists no diagnostic gold standard. **The clinician must rely on a collection of findings from multiple diagnostic modalities to detect both anatomic and pathophysiologic abnormalities.** Perhaps the greatest challenge lies in differentiating constrictive pericarditis from restrictive cardiomyopathy. This is discussed more fully in Chapter 9.

A. **Echocardiography.** M-Mode, two-dimensional, and Doppler echocardiography all provide valuable clues in determining the diagnosis of constrictive pericarditis. While many of the signs are not highly sensitive or specific, a combination of findings often suggests the diagnosis and assists in differentiating it from other diagnoses, such as restrictive cardiomyopathy and pericardial tamponade.

1. **M-mode echocardiography**
   a. **Flattening of the left ventricular free wall.** Early diastolic motion is normal; however, there is flattening of the free wall once the limit of the pericardial case is reached.
   b. **Thickened pericardium.** Thickening may be represented by a single thick line or multiple lines in parallel. Precise measurement of pericardial thickening is difficult with M-mode; computed tomography, magnetic resonance imaging, and transesophageal echocardiography are better suited for precise measurement of the pericardium.
   c. **Premature opening of the pulmonary valve.** The elevated end-diastolic pressure in the right ventricle exceeds the pulmonary artery pressure; therefore, the pulmonic valve opens prior to the onset of systole.
   d. **Septal motion during atrial systole.** Diastolic relaxation is limited by the rigid pericardium; therefore, the additional volume provided by atrial systole results in bowing of the interventricular septum toward the right ventricle. On M-mode, this is manifested as an anterior motion of the septum following the P wave. Just prior to this anterior movement, there is a brief posterior displacement of the septum occurring in the middle of the P wave. This to-and-fro motion of the septum can also be seen on two-dimensional echocardiography.
2. **Two-dimensional echocardiography**
   a. **Septal bounce.** This is the two-dimensional correlate to M-mode findings of septal motion during diastole. On apical four-chamber images, the motion appears as a bounce.
   b. **Inferior vena cava plethora**
   c. **Decreased angle between left atrium and left ventricle.** Pericardial constriction impedes ventricular motion to a greater degree than it impedes atrial motion. The result is a normally expanding atrium juxtaposed with a restricted ventricle and thus a more acute angle at the junction of the two.
3. **Doppler echocardiography.** Although M-mode and two-dimensional findings may suggest pericardial constriction, most of the findings described above are relatively low in sensitivity and specificity. Doppler echocardiography has emerged as an **excellent tool in evaluating diastolic function.** Doppler assessment of diastolic flow patterns and the respiratory changes in these patterns can provide **compelling evidence for the presence of pericardial constriction** and assist in **excluding competing diagnoses** such as restrictive cardiomyopathy and cardiac tamponade.
   a. **Respiratory variation in mitral and tricuspid flow.** In constrictive pericarditis, the thickened pericardium isolates the cardiac chambers from respiratory changes in intrathoracic pressures.
      (1) During **inspiration,** the drop in intrathoracic pressure is transmitted to the pulmonary veins, but not to the left ventricle. This reduces the driving pressure gradient required for diastolic filling of the left ventricle; therefore, a **decrease in mitral flow is observed during inspiration.** Conversely, there is an **increased tricuspid flow during inspiration.**
         (a) **Mitral valve inflow.** Peak E velocity decreased by 33% and isometric volume time increased by 50% (Fig. 28-1).
         (b) **Tricuspid valve inflow.** Peak E velocity increased by 44% and Peak A velocity increased by 38% (Fig. 28-2).
      (2) Opposite changes can be seen with **expiration.** Increased intrathoracic pressure is transmitted to the pulmonary veins and thus increases the driving pressure for left ventricular filling. There is a **decreased tricuspid flow. The wide respiratory variation in peak E velocities helps to differentiate constrictive pericarditis from restrictive**

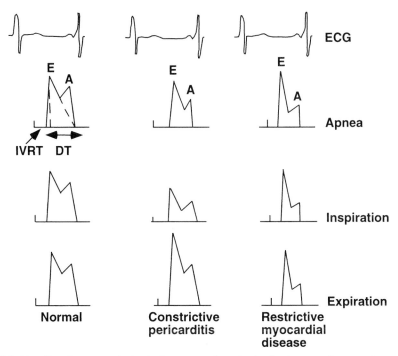

FIG. 28-1. Respiratory variation in flow across the mitral valve in normals, constrictive pericarditis, and restrictive cardiomyopathy. The peak early diastolic filling velocity is denoted as E and the peak late diastolic filling velocity (from atrial contraction) is denoted as A. The isovolumetric time (IVRT) is the period between aortic valve closure and mitral valve opening. The deceleration time (DT) is the time it takes to go from peak E velocity to cessation of flow. In constrictive pericarditis, expiration results in a decreased IVRT and a marked increase in peak E and peak A velocities across the mitral valve. Similar changes are not observed in normals and those with restrictive disease. Patients with restriction have an increased E/A and shortened DT; however, there is no significant respiratory variation. Adapted from Klein AL, et al., 1993, with permission.

cardiomyopathy where minimal respiratory variation occurs (see Figs. 28-1 and 28-2).

(3) The variations in respiratory flow across the atrioventricular valves are further compounded by the **ventricular interdependence** observed in constrictive pericarditis. As one ventricle experiences enhanced filling, depending on the phase of respiration, the septum bows toward the opposite ventricle to accommodate the increased volume. This septal bowing increases the pressure and decreases the volume of the opposite ventricle and thus further impairs its ability to fill. These respiratory variations in filling, seen on Doppler echocardiography (see Figs. 28-1 and 28-2), can assist in making the diagnosis of constriction. Normal values for left and right ventricular filling are listed in Tables 28-2 and 28-3.

b. **Pulmonary vein flow.** In a normal individual, pulmonary vein flow consists of a peak velocity during ventricular systole (S wave) and a smaller peak velocity during ventricular diastole (D wave); there is normally little respiratory variation in these velocities. In

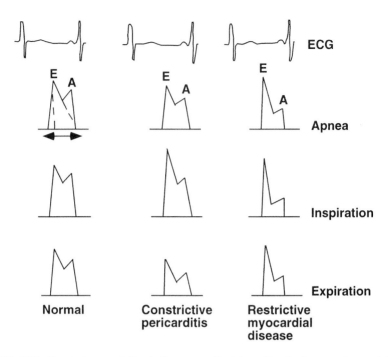

FIG. 28-2. Respiratory variation in flow across the tricuspid valve in normals, constrictive pericarditis, and restrictive cardiomyopathy. Constrictive pericarditis results in changes in flow across the tricuspid valve that are opposite to those described for the mitral valve in Fig. 28–1. In constrictive pericarditis, inspiration results in increased peak E and peak A velocities across the tricuspid valve. Similar changes are not observed in normals and those with restrictive cardiomyopathy. Patients with restriction have an increased E/A and shortened DT; however, there is no significant respiratory variation. Adapted from Klein AL, et al., 1993, with permission.

constrictive pericarditis, there is an increase in early diastolic flow manifested as a larger D wave; therefore, the **pulmonary systolic/ diastolic (S/D) flow ratio is decreased.** Additionally, **both systolic and diastolic pulmonary vein flow are markedly increased during expiration.** This increase in expiratory pulmonary venous flow assists in differentiating constrictive pericarditis from restrictive cardiomyopathy (Fig. 28-3).

c. **Respiratory variation in hepatic vein flow.** Hepatic venous flow reflects right-sided filling in much the same manner that pulmonary venous flow reflects left-sided filling. It is represented similarly as both an S wave and a D wave as well as a reversal in flow during atrial systole (AR wave) and a reversal in flow due to late ventricular systole (VR wave). Both normal individuals and those with constrictive pericarditis have a more prominent systolic flow than a diastolic flow; however, the normal individual has little respiratory variation in these flow velocities. **In constrictive pericarditis there is a marked increase in the D wave during inspiration and a significant blunting during expiration. Expiration also results in a more prominent AR and VR.** In restrictive disease there is a reversal in systolic-to-diastolic flow ratios, and no respiratory variation exists in these flow velocities (Fig. 28-4).

Table 28-2. Normal left ventricular filling dynamics

	Patients <50 yr	Patients >50 yr
LEFT VENTRICULAR INFLOW		
Peak E (cm/sec)	72 ± 14	62 ± 14
Peak A (cm/sec)	40 ± 10	59 ± 14
E/A	1.9 ± 0.6	1.1 ± 0.3
DT (msec)	179 ± 20	210 ± 36
IVRT (msec)	76 ± 11	90 ± 17
PULMONARY VEIN		
Peak S (cm/sec)	48 ± 9	71 ± 9
Peak D (cm/sec)	50 ± 10	38 ± 9
Peak AR (cm/sec)	19 ± 4	23 ± 14

Peak E =   ;peak A =   ;E/A =   ;DT =   ;IVRT =   ;peak S =   ;peak D =   ;peak AR =
DT, Deceleration time; IVRT, isovolumic relocation time.
Adapted from Klein AL, et al. Differentiation of constrictive pericarditis from restrictive cardio-myopathy by Doppler transesophageal echocardiographic measurements of respiratory variations in pulmonary venous flows. *J Am Coll Cardiol* 1993; 22:1935–1943.

B. Cardiac catheterization. The hemodynamics obtained in the catheteriza-tion laboratory assist in both diagnosing constrictive pericarditis and differ-entiating it from restrictive cardiomyopathy. In general, both right and left heart catheterizations are performed to obtain simultaneous ventricular pres-sure readings.

    1. Atrial pressures. The right atrial pressure waveform has been de-scribed as having a **W-shaped configuration.** This morphology is pro-duced by a prominent "a" wave as the atria contracts against an elevated ventricular pressure, an exaggerated x descent, and a steep y descent, due to rapid ventricular filling in early diastole (Fig. 28-5).

    2. Ventricular pressures

        a. Ventricular pressure waveforms demonstrate the classic dip-and-plateau physiology, commonly referred to as the square root sign (Fig. 28-6). The initial downward deflection reflects the drop in pres-sure during the isovolumetric relaxation period. The subsequent

Table 28-3. Normal right ventricular filling dynamics

	Patients <50 yr	Patients >50 yr
RIGHT VENTRICULAR INFLOW		
Peak E (cm/sec)	51 ± 7	41 ± 8
Peak A (cm/sec)	27 ± 8	33 ± 8
E/A	2.0 ± 0.5	1.34 ± 0.4
DT (cm/sec)	188 ± 22	198 ± 23
SUPERIOR VENA CAVA		
Peak S (cm/sec)	41 ± 9	42 ± 12
Peak D (cm/sec)	22 ± 5	22 ± 5
Peak AR (cm/sec)	13 ± 3	16 ± 3

Peak E =   ;peak A=   ;E/A =   ;DT =   ;peak S =   ;peak D =   ;peak AR =
DT, Deceleration Time.
Adapted from Klein AL, et al. Differentiation of constrictive pericarditis from restrictive cardio-myopathy by Doppler transesophageal echocardiographic measurements of respiratory variations in pulmonary venous flows. *J Am Coll Cardiol* 1993;22:1935–1943.

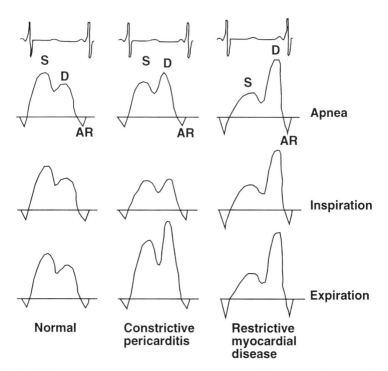

FIG. 28-3. Respiratory variation in pulmonary venous flow in normals, constrictive pericarditis, and restrictive cardiomyopathy. The peak pulmonary venous velocities during systole are denoted as the S wave and peak diastolic velocities are denoted as the D wave. The AR wave represents the small reversal in flow noted with atrial contraction. In constrictive pericarditis, there is a slight decrease in the S/D ratio and a marked increase in both velocities during expiration as compared to inspiration. This respiratory variation in pulmonary venous flows is not observed in normals or those with restrictive disease. Adapted from Klein AL, et al., 1993, with permission.

upward deflection reflects early diastolic filling. The terminal plateau represents the cessation of flow that occurs once the limit of the rigid pericardium has been reached.

   b. The end-diastolic pressures of both ventricles are not only elevated but also equal, with a less than 5 mm Hg difference between the two. The right ventricular systolic pressure is generally less than 55 mm Hg, with a right ventricular end-diastolic pressure that is greater than one-third the right ventricular systolic pressure. These findings assist in differentiating constrictive pericarditis from restrictive cardiomyopathy.

VII. Therapy. Pericardiectomy is preferred in most cases, although there are certain patient populations in whom medical therapy would be appropriate.

   A. Medical therapy

   1. Patients who have functional class I symptoms may initially be managed with diuretics and a low-sodium diet; however, the vast majority of these patients ultimately require pericardiectomy.

   2. Medical therapy is also appropriate in **patients with severe comorbid illnesses** that limit life expectancy and/or place them at an unacceptably high risk for operative mortality.

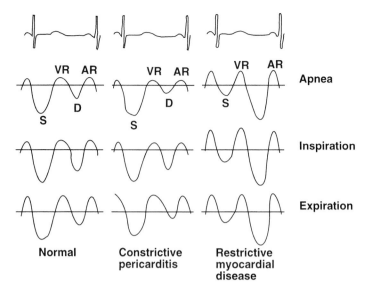

FIG. 28-4. Respiratory variation in hepatic vein flow in normals, constrictive pericarditis, and restrictive cardiomyopathy. Similar to pulmonary vein flow, the S wave represents peak systolic flow velocity and the D wave represents peak diastolic flow velocity. VR denotes reversal in flow noted in late systole, and AR is the reversal in flow due to atrial contraction. In both normal subjects and those with constrictive pericarditis, there is an increase in both S and D waves with inspiration. In expiration, there is little change in normal subjects; however, those with constrictive pericarditis will have a marked drop in both S and D waves and an increase in both VR and AR. Adapted from Klein AL, et al., 1993, with permission.

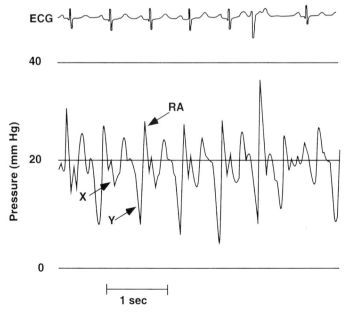

FIG. 28-5. Right atrial pressure waveform in constrictive pericarditis. The preserved x descent and the prominent y descent contribute to the classic W-shaped atrial waveform. Adapted from Baim DS, Grossman W, 1996, with permission.

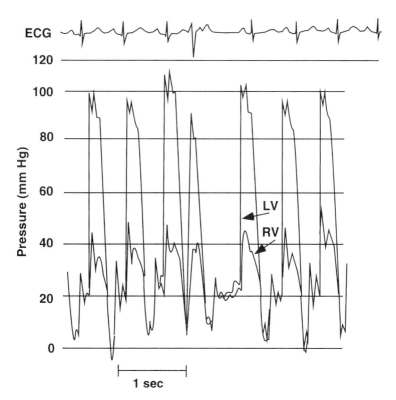

FIG. 28-6. Right and left ventricular waveforms in constrictive pericarditis. Note the equalization of left ventricular and right ventricular end-diastolic pressures, generally within 5 mm Hg of one another. The rapid early diastolic filling and subsequent abrupt cessation of flow due to the rigid pericardium produces a dip-and-plateau waveform (square root sign) appreciated best in this waveform following the premature ventricular contraction (PVC). Adapted from Baim DS, Grossman W, eds., 1996, with permission.

B. Surgical therapy
1. **The treatment of choice is pericardiectomy.** Over 90% of patients will report symptomatic improvement following the procedure.
2. Pericardiectomy carries an **operative mortality** reported to range from **5% to 20%.** Those patients with a poor preoperative functional class are at highest risk for perioperative death; therefore, most physicians advocate **early surgical intervention.**

SUGGESTED READINGS

Landmark Articles

Hansen AT, et al. Pressure curves from the right auricle and the right ventricle in chronic constrictive pericarditis. *Circulation* 1961;3:881–888.

Hatle LK, et al. Differentiation of constrictive pericarditis and restrictive cardiomyopathy by Doppler echocardiography. *Circulation* 1989;79:357–370.

McCaughan BC, et al. Early and late results of pericardiectomy for constrictive pericarditis. *J Thorac Cardiovasc Surg* 1985;89:340–350.

von Bibra H, et al. Diagnosis of constrictive pericarditis by pulsed Doppler echocardiography of the hepatic vein. *Am J Cardiol* 1989;63:483–488.

White PD. Chronic constrictive pericarditis (Pick's disease), treated by pericardial resection. *Lancet* 1935;2:539–548, 597–603.

Key Reviews
Brockington GM, Zebede J, Pandian NG. Constrictive pericarditis. In: Shabetai R, ed. Diseases of the pericardium. *Cardiol Clin* 1990;8(4):645–661.
Cameron J, et al. The etiologic spectrum of constrictive pericarditis. *Am Heart J* 1987;113:354–360.
Fowler N. Constrictive pericarditis: its history and current status. *Clin Cardiol* 1995;18:341–350.
Klein AL, et al. Differentiation of constrictive pericarditis from restrictive cardiomyopathy by Doppler transesophageal echocardiographic measurements of respiratory variations in pulmonary venous flows. *J Am Coll Cardiol* 1993;22:1935–1943.
Klein AL, Cohen GI. Doppler echocardiographic assessment of constrictive pericarditis, cardiac amyloidosis, and cardiac tamponade. *Cleveland Clin J Med* 1992;59:278–290.
Oh J, et al. Diagnostic role of Doppler echocardiography in constrictive pericarditis. *J Am Coll Cardiol* 1994;23:154–162.

Relevant Book Chapters
Braunwald E, Lorell BH. Pericardial diseases. In: Braunwald E, ed. *Heart disease: a textbook of cardiovascular medicine,* 5th ed. Philadelphia: WB Saunders, 1997:1496–1505.
Feigenbaum H. Pericardial disease—constrictive pericarditis. In: Feigenbaum H, ed. *Echocardiography.* Baltimore: Williams & Wilkins, 1994:577–583.
Grossman W, Lorell BH. Profiles in constrictive pericarditis, restrictive cardiomyopathy, and cardiac tamponade. In: Baim DS, Grossman W, eds. *Cardiac catheterization, angiography, and intervention.* Baltimore: Williams & Wilkins, 1996:801–821.
Topol EJ, Klein AL, Scalia GM. Diseases of the pericardium, restrictive cardiomyopathy, and diastolic dysfunction. In: Topol EJ, ed. *Comprehensive cardiovascular medicine.* Philadelphia: Lippincott-Raven Publishers, 1998:669–733.

SECTION VII. ADULT CONGENITAL HEART DISEASE

J. Donald Moore and Douglas S. Moodie

29. ATRIAL SEPTAL DEFECT

J. Donald Moore and Douglas S. Moodie

I. **Introduction**
   A. Atrial septal defects (ASDs) constitute approximately 5% to 10% of congenital heart defects. With the exception of bicuspid aortic valve and mitral valve prolapse, ASDs are the most common form of congenital heart disease found among adults.
   B. Most infants and children with ASD are asymptomatic and physical findings may be unimpressive, making survival into adulthood common.
   C. Life expectancy overall is decreased in patients with unrepaired ASD. Although most patients have few symptoms, long-term exposure to chronic right heart volume loading can have deleterious effects such as atrial arrhythmias (increasing risk with age), irreversible pulmonary vascular disease (5% to 10%, increased in females), and, eventually, congestive heart failure. The presence of an atrial communication is also a potential source of paradoxical embolus

II. **Anatomy**
   A. **Embryology.** The primitive atrium is first partitioned by growth of the **septum primum.** An atrial communication initially persists as the **foramen primum** near the endocardial cushions. Before closure of the foramen primum, fenestrations develop in the septum primum which will coalesce to form the **foramen secundum.** As the foramen primum then fuses with the endocardial cushions, an atrial communication is maintained that is important for right-to-left shunting in the fetal circulation. The **septum secundum** then develops to the right of the septum primum, developing toward the endocardial cushions. The **foramen ovale** (fossa ovalis) constitutes the opening through the septum secundum on the right atrial side with a flap valve on the left atrial side composed of remaining septum primum tissue. At birth, when left atrial pressure increases, the septum primum flap closes and eventually fuses to anatomically close the atrial septum. Probe patency can remain in 25% to 30% of adults (patent foramen ovale) but does not represent a congenital ASD. When deficiencies in septal development or resorption occur, atrial septal defects result.
   B. Types of atrial septal defects (Fig. 29-1).
      1. **Ostium secundum** (fossa ovalis) defects constitute the most common type of ASD, accounting for 60% to 70% of all forms of ASD. This defect is located in the middle portion of the atrial septum within or including the fossa ovalis. Defects result from either deficient septum primum or an abnormally large foramen secundum. Isolated secundum ASD has been associated with mitral valve prolapse. This defect is more common in female patients (2:1).
      2. **Ostium primum defects** account for 15% to 20% of atrial septal defects. These defects occur in the inferoanterior portion of the atrial septum, frequently in association with a cleft in the anterior leaflet of the mitral valve.
      3. **Sinus venosus defects** compose the remaining 5% to 10% of septal defects. The location of these defects typically is superior and posterior in relation to the fossa ovalis or, less frequently, located inferiorly to the fossa ovalis. These defects require a high index of suspicion as they are typically difficult to visualize by standard transthoracic echocardiography. The superior sinus venosus defects are almost always associated with partial anomalous pulmonary venous return of the right pulmonary veins to either the superior vena cava (SVC) or the high right atrium.

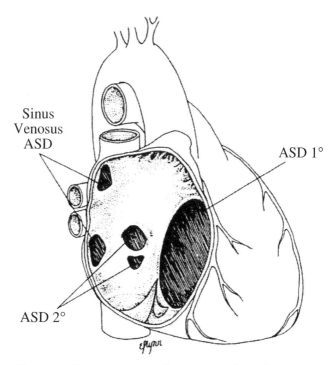

FIG. 29-1. Diagrammatic representation of common atrial septal defects. ASD, atrial septal defect; 1°, primum; 2°, secundum. From Fyler DC, ed. *Nadas pediatric cardiology.* Philadelphia: Hanley & Belfus, 1992, with permission.

    4. A less common type of atrial septal defect is the **coronary sinus type,** which is located inferior and slightly anterior to the fossa ovalis. These defects are commonly associated with other forms of congenital heart disease such as complete atrioventricular septal defect. These defects may occur with an absent coronary sinus and a left SVC that drains to the left atrium.

III. Clinical presentation. The signs and symptoms of an ASD result from the effects of long-term left-to-right shunting and subsequent volume loading of the right heart.

  A. Signs and symptoms if present at all typically include fatigue and dyspnea in the younger patient. Late findings include supraventricular dysrhythmias such as atrial fibrillation or flutter, severe irreversible pulmonary vascular disease, and, eventually, congestive heart failure.

  B. Physical findings may include a hyperdynamic cardiac impulse, characteristic widely and fixed split second heart sound, and a soft systolic murmur at the second left intercostal space secondary to increased flow to the pulmonary arteries.

  C. The differential diagnosis includes systemic arteriovenous malformation and total or partial pulmonary venous return.

IV. Laboratory exam

  A. The **ECG** can reveal several typical findings.

    1. Secundum ASD:

      a. RSR or rSR in lead V_1

      b. QRS less than 0.11 second

      c. Right axis deviation
      d. Right ventricular hypertrophy
      e. First-degree atrioventricular block (20%)
      f. Right atrial enlargement (about 50%)
    2. Primum ASD:
      a. RSR in lead V_1
      b. Left axis deviation
      c. First-degree atrioventricular block
      d. Possibly biventricular hypertrophy
 B. The **chest x-ray** may reveal cardiomegaly due to right heart enlargement. With large left-to-right shunts, the pulmonary arteries and vascular markings may appear prominent. In the setting of later pulmonary vascular disease, however, the pulmonary arteries may appear large but with oligemic peripheral lung fields.

V. Diagnostic testing
 A. Echocardiography is the primary means by which an ASD is diagnosed. In the younger patient, the diagnosis can usually be made by transthoracic imaging alone. In the adult, transesophageal studies are often required.
    1. Typical transthoracic views for imaging an ASD include the parasternal short-axis view, apical four-chamber view, and the subcostal coronal and sagittal views. Findings include right atrial and right ventricular enlargement. An estimate of right ventricular pressure should be deduced in the presence of tricuspid insufficiency. Evidence of left-to-right (or right-to-left) shunting across the defect should be demonstrated using color Doppler techniques. Sinus venosus defects are often missed by transthoracic imaging alone and should prompt further investigation by transesophageal echocardiography or contrast study.
    2. **Transesophageal echocardiography** is usually required in the adult patient. Particular attention must be paid to unusual atrial defects such as the sinus venosus type which can be associated with partial anomalous pulmonary venous return of the right pulmonary veins. Contrast studies are sometimes helpful in confirming the presence of atrial shunting. The four-chamber view is preferred with injection of agitated saline through an upper extremity vein. Injection into the left arm may be particularly helpful to establish the presence of a persistent left SVC that drains to the coronary sinus or directly to the left atrium.
 B. Cardiac catheterization is typically not required for diagnostic purposes except to assess pulmonary pressures and resistance, to assess for coronary artery disease prior to planned surgical closure in the adult patient, or as part of transcatheter device closure. Catheterization can be performed in most cases using a standard multipurpose end-hole catheter. The lateral camera is helpful in directing the catheter posterior prior to advancing across the ASD. This catheter or a balloon-directed catheter can be used to complete the remainder of the study, which includes complete right heart oximetry and hemodynamic assessment.
    1. Saturations during catheterization demonstrate a step-up within the right atrium due to shunting across the defect. Careful interrogation of innominate vein saturation and SVC saturation is also important to exclude a step-up in the SVC that would support the diagnosis of associated partial anomalous pulmonary venous return. Anomalous pulmonary veins should be selectively entered if present. Desaturation in the left atrium and systemically confirms right-to-left shunting and should prompt further investigation of right ventricular and pulmonary artery pressures. Pulmonary vein saturations should be measured in this case to exclude pulmonary venous desaturation. Other diagnoses producing a similar picture include large VSD with tricuspid regurgitation, partial or complete atrioventricular canal, or systemic arteriovenosus fistulae.
    2. Hemodynamic assessment may reveal modest elevations in right ventricular and pulmonary artery pressures. An important assessment is

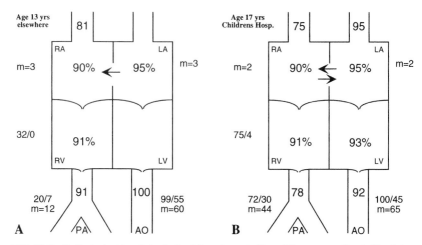

FIG. 29-2. Catheterization data derived from two studies of the same patient. The data obtained at age 13 **(A)** were interpreted as compatible with a small atrial septal defect of insufficient size to require closure. Some years later she had developed pulmonary vascular obstructive disease **(B)** and was no longer shunting enough to recommend surgery. Death occurred 5 years later. RA, right atrium; LA, left atrium; RV, right ventricle; LV, left ventricle; PA, pulmonary artery; AO, aorta; numeric values within schematic, oxygen % saturation; numeric values outside schematic, pressure in mm Hg. Adapted from Fyler DC, ed. *Nadas pediatric cardiology.* Philadelphia: Hanley & Belfus, 1992, with permission.

comparison of right ventricular pressure to systemic pressure and measurement of pulmonary vascular resistance. If elevated pulmonary pressures are detected, the response to oxygen should be assessed. Examples of the usual catheterization findings with and without pulmonary vascular disease are illustrated in Fig. 29-2.

    3. Angiography is typically not necessary for diagnostic purposes. Some transcatheter closure device protocols include angiography, typically performed in the right pulmonary vein or levophase from a right pulmonary artery injection in the left anterior oblique/cranial projection. This may be more important if partial anomalous pulmonary venous return is suspected.

VI. Therapy. Medical intervention is typically not required preoperatively as many patients will be asymptomatic. Congestive symptoms may be improved with standard diuretic therapy. Rhythm disturbances such as atrial fibrillation obviously require attention with respect to rate control and anticoagulation. Antibiotic prophylaxis is not required in the setting of an isolated atrial septal defect prior to surgery. The mainstay of therapy is closure of the defect either by surgical or transcatheter means. Due to the reduced life expectancy associated with ASDs, closure is recommended in most adults. Indications for closure generally include symptomatology, a significant left-to-right shunt (more than 2:1), or history of a cerebrovascular event. In the setting of pulmonary hypertension (pressure greater than 2/3 systemic, resistance greater than 2/3 systemic), pulmonary reactivity to vasodilators must be documented and a net left-to-right shunt shown at catheterization (greater than 1.5:1).

    A. Primary surgical closure has been the standard approach for many years. Depending on the defect size and location, the ASD can be closed by primary suture or, if needed, by autologous pericardial patch.

1. Important preoperative risk factors include older age at operation, presence of atrial fibrillation, and elevated pulmonary pressures and resistance.
2. Postoperatively patients are at risk for postpericardiotomy syndrome, more so than following other surgery for congenital defects. Atrial arrhythmias may persist in short- and long-term follow-up as the right atrial and ventricular sizes may take time to return to normal. In some centers, prophylactic β-adrenergic blockade is advocated empirically for 3 to 6 months following surgery. Antibiotic prophylaxis is continued for 6 months following uncomplicated surgical closure.

B. Transcatheter closure of secundum atrial septal defects has recently become an attractive alternative to surgical closure despite advances in minimally invasive surgical techniques. Any patient with an isolated secundum ASD may be suitable for transcatheter closure. Depending on the device, defects of up to 15 to 20 mm may be considered. The defect must be located centrally with adequate room for the device to be positioned without interference of other intracardiac structures such as the AV valves, coronary sinus, or right pulmonary veins. It is for this reason that only secundum-type defects can be approached with a transcatheter technique. Although promising with regard to closure results, complication rates, patient convalescence, and cost, all current ASD closure devices remain investigational and under Food and Drug Administration clinical trials in the United States.

SUGGESTED READINGS
Key Reviews

Connelly MS, Webb GD, Sommerville J, et al. Canadian Consensus Conference on Adult Congenital Heart Disease 1996. *Can J Cardiol* 1998;14:395–452.

Gatzoulis MA, Redington AN, Somerville J, Shore DF. Should atrial septal defects in adults be closed? *Ann Thorac Surg* 1996;61:657–659.

Latson LA. Per-Catheter ASD Closure. *Pediatr Cardiol* 1998;19:86–93.

Mahoney LT. Acyanotic congenital heart disease: atrial and ventricular septal defects, atrioventricular canal, patent ductus arteriosus, pulmonic stenosis. *Cardiol Clin* 1993;11:603–616.

Mandelik J, Moodie DS, Sterba R, et al. Long-term follow-up of children after repair of atrial septal defects. *Cleveland Clin J Med* 1994;61:29–33.

Relevant Book Chapters

Brecker SJD. Atrial septal defect. In: Redington A, Shore D, Oldershaw P, eds. *Congenital heart disease in adults: a practical guide.* London: WB Saunders, 1994:103–110.

Perloff JK. Survival patterns without cardiac surgery or interventional catheterization: a narrowing base. In: Perloff JK, Child JS, eds. *Congenital heart disease in Adults,* 2nd ed. Philadelphia: WB Saunders, 1998:15–53.

Snider AR, Serwer GA, Ritter SB. Defects in cardiac septation. In: Snider AR, Serwer GA, Ritter SB, eds. *Echocardiography in pediatric heart disease,* 2nd ed. St. Louis: Mosby, 1997:235–246.

Vick GW. Defects of the atrial septum including atrioventricular septal defects. In: Garson A, Bricker JT, Fisher DJ, Neish SR, eds. *The science and practice of pediatric cardiology,* 2nd ed. Baltimore: Williams & Wilkins, 1998:1141–1179.

30. VENTRICULAR SEPTAL DEFECT

J. Donald Moore and Douglas S. Moodie

I. **Introduction**
   A. Excluding the bicuspid aortic valve, a ventricular septal defect (VSD) is the most common congenital defect in children, accounting for 25% of all congenital heart defects in childhood.
   B. In contrast, an isolated VSD is found in approximately 10% of adult patients with congenital heart disease, which reflects the natural tendency for spontaneous closure as well as improved diagnosis in childhood with subsequent surgical closure.
   C. **Natural history** varies according to the defect size, location, and associated findings.
      1. Of small VSDs, 75% to 80% close spontaneously by late childhood. Of those that do persist, their restrictive nature protects the patient from pulmonary vascular injury. Of large VSDs, 10% to 15% will still close spontaneously. Life expectancy is thought to be essentially normal for patients with small defects that persist into adulthood.
      2. Endocarditis remains a risk in the unoperated patient due to the presence of a high-velocity, turbulent jet into the right ventricle.
      3. A large VSD during childhood may be associated with significant left-to-right shunt. This may eventually lead to pulmonary vascular disease and Eisenmenger physiology if left untreated. As pulmonary vascular resistance increases, the patient gradually begins to shunt right to left instead of left to right. Once this physiology has ensued, these patients rarely survive beyond their 40s. Complications in these patients include pulmonary hemorrhage, endocarditis, cerebral abscess, ventricular arrhythmias, and the complications associated with erythrocytosis. Poor prognostic factors in this population include syncope, congestive failure, and hemoptysis.
      4. Risk factors for decreased survival in the unoperated patient include cardiomegaly on chest x-ray (CXR), elevated pulmonary artery systolic pressure (more than 50 mm Hg), or cardiovascular symptoms.
      5. Associated aortic insufficiency in some defects may lead to left ventricular (LV) dysfunction if left untreated and thus will complicate the clinical outcome.
II. **Anatomy**
   A. **Embryology.** Partitioning of the ventricular mass begins as a muscular ridge in the floor of the ventricle near the apex. This ridge later undergoes active growth which forms the muscular ventricular septum. Concomitantly, the endocardial cushions fuse and the two regions meet, completing closure of the interventricular foramen.
   B. Types of Ventricular Septal Defects
      1. **Perimembranous defects** are the most common type, accounting for approximately 70% to 80%. They are less likely to be associated with additional intracardiac defects and have the highest rate of spontaneous closure.
      2. **Muscular or apical defects** (5% to 20%) also typically occur in isolation and have a high spontaneous closure rate unless multiple defects are present.
      3. **Inlet or atrioventricular (AV) canal–type defects** (5% to 8%) rarely close spontaneously, are usually large, and are associated with abnormalities of the AV valves. These abnormalities range from cleft mitral and/or tricuspid valves to the common AV valve as seen in complete AV canal. This type of defect, in association with complete AV canal, is commonly seen in Down's syndrome.

4. **Supracristal or subaortic VSDs** are less common (about 5% to 7%). They vary in size but are often small. However, due to their position beneath the aortic valve, they can lead to development of aortic insufficiency, which often prompts their closure despite small size.

C. **Associated lesions.** Of patients who present with a VSD, 5% to 10% will develop aortic regurgitation. In addition, there is a small percentage (less than 10%) who will develop subvalvar pulmonary stenosis or an obstructive muscle bundle referred to as a double-chamber right ventricle.

III. **Clinical presentation**

A. **Signs and symptoms.** The most common symptoms in adult patients with VSD are dyspnea on exertion, exercise intolerance, and shortness of breath. The symptoms are related to the degree and chronicity of left-to-right shunt and the resultant increase in pulmonary pressure and resistance.

B. **Physical findings.** The auscultatory findings classically include a holosystolic murmur of varying intensity. Smaller muscular defects may produce a high-frequency early systolic murmur that ends before S_2 due to its closure from muscular contraction of the septum. Another important feature is intensity of the second heart sound, which if increased suggests increased pulmonary pressures. A diastolic flow rumble at the apex may be heard in large left-to-right shunts due to increased flow across an otherwise normal mitral valve. Depending on associated lesions, other findings may also be present such as the diastolic murmur of aortic insufficiency that may occur with subaortic defects. A prominent systolic ejection murmur at the left upper sternal border suggests subvalvar pulmonic stenosis or double-chamber right ventricle.

C. The **differential diagnosis** on exam includes tricuspid regurgitation, acyanotic tetralogy of Fallot, isolated subvalvar pulmonic stenosis, and hypertrophic cardiomyopathy.

IV. **Laboratory exam**

A. The **electrocardiogram (ECG)** may be unremarkable or reveal left atrial and LV enlargement in the larger defect. An inlet or AV canal defect can be diagnosed from the ECG based on the presence of marked left axis deviation. Right axis deviation suggests elevated right ventricular (RV) and pulmonary artery pressure. Following surgical repair, right bundle branch block is not uncommon.

B. **CXR** is often helpful in determining degree of left-to-right shunt. A small or normal-sized heart with normal pulmonary vascular markings on CXR supports a hemodynamically insignificant lesion whereas cardiomegaly and left atrial and LV enlargement will be seen with large left-to-right shunts. A large defect associated with a small heart and oligemic lung fields should raise the suspicion of pulmonary vascular disease.

V. **Diagnostic testing**

A. **Echocardiography** is the diagnostic modality of choice for VSDs and associated lesions. Transthoracic imaging is almost always sufficient in the child and younger adult, but transesophageal imaging may be required in the older adult. Defect size and location should be defined using both two-dimensional and color Doppler techniques. Complete scans of the ventricular septum should be made to rule out additional defects. Optimal images are usually obtained from the parasternal long- and short-axis views and the apical four-chamber view. In the younger patient, subcostal coronal and sagittal views may also be helpful. Quantification of shunt velocity provides an estimate of the restrictive nature across the defect. The higher the velocity, the more restrictive the defect and the less likely the patient has experienced pulmonary vascular insult. Systemic blood pressure should be noted when the velocity across the VSD is measured. Assuming no LV outflow obstruction, RV pressure can then be estimated based on the gradient across the VSD. This pressure can also be estimated if tricuspid insufficiency is present. A complete evaluation is always indicated to exclude other associated findings such as atrial septal defect, patent ductus arteriosus, aortic insufficiency, and RV or left heart outflow tract obstruction.

B. Catheterization is seldom needed in the current management of isolated VSD in the infant or child. Surgical correction, when indicated, proceeds in most cases based on echocardiographic evaluation. In the adult, catheterization should be considered if anatomic questions remain despite transthoracic and transesophageal echocardiography, or if pulmonary hypertension is suspected based on these studies. Hemodynamic assessment should include quantification of cardiac index and careful oximetric definition of the shunt level and quantity. An elevated pulmonary artery saturation confirms persistent left-to-right shunt across the defect and should correlate with acceptable pulmonary artery pressures and resistance. Evidence of low pulmonary artery saturations is expected with elevations of pulmonary resistance. Simultaneous comparison of RV pressure to systemic pressure is mandatory in these cases with documentation of changes in response to oxygen or nitric oxide administration. Left ventriculography performed with **left anterior oblique and cranial angulation** demonstrates the defect in most cases. If an inlet type of defect is present, the hepatoclavicular view (about 40 degrees left anterior oblique and 40 degrees cranial) is usually adequate. Right ventriculography will not opacify the left ventricle unless there is suprasystemic RV pressure. Coronary angiography should be performed during the case in patients felt to be at risk for coronary artery disease.

VI. Therapy. Factors supporting intervention include cardiomegaly on CXR, significant left-to-right shunt (pulmonary to systemic flow ratios greater than 1.5:1), elevated but responsive pulmonary vascular resistance, symptoms of congestive failure or associated lesions such as aortic insufficiency, RV or LV outflow tract obstruction, or recurrent endocarditis. Management of the VSD following myocardial infarction is discussed separately in Chapter 51.

A. Medical management in symptomatic cases without Eisenmenger's physiology involves anticongestive measures such as the use of diuretics, digoxin, and afterload reduction. Efforts should then be focused on addressing suitability for surgical closure. Endocarditis is a recognized complication of VSD. In the patient with culture-proven endocarditis, 4 to 6 weeks of antibiotics should be administered parenterally prior to consideration of intervention. This must be tailored to the individual patient's clinical status and the infective organism's identification and sensitivity.

B. Transcatheter device closure of selected VSDs is being performed on an investigational or compassionate use basis in select pediatric centers. Small apical or muscular defects, either congenital or postinfarction, can technically be closed by device, often performed if the surgical risk is exceedingly high. The long-term outcome of this approach has yet to be determined. Active investigation and device development for this purpose continue.

C. Surgical closure is the primary means of repair. Current surgical practice proceeds with earlier closure in the symptomatic infant or child. Outcome following VSD closure is good in children with low mortality rates of 2% to 3%. Thus, the adult is more likely to present following surgical repair or with a small defect that is hemodynamically insignificant. Surgical closure in the symptomatic adult appears to also be well tolerated with acceptable mortality and improved functional status. Irreversible pulmonary vascular disease with Eisenmenger's physiology, however, is a contraindication for surgical closure as right heart failure will almost certainly develop thereafter. Depending on the defect size and location, many defects are closed via a transatrial approach or across the pulmonary valve. Direct suture is used for the smaller defect and either Dacron or autologous pericardial patch material for the larger defect. Postoperative sequelae include residual patch leaks, as well as supraventricular and ventricular arrhythmias.

D. Antibiotic prophylaxis is recommended for 6 months following surgical closure of VSDs. A prior history of endocarditis or residual lesions following repair warrants continued antibiotic prophylaxis postoperatively.

E. The Eisenmenger syndrome is usually referred to in the context of irreversible pulmonary hypertension from long-standing exposure of the pulmonary vasculature to left-to-right shunting across a VSD. However, this physiology can occur as a result of any left-to-right shunting lesion including patent ductus arteriosus and, less commonly, isolated atrial septal defect. As a result of the elevated pulmonary pressures, the direction of shunting is reversed across the defect, producing systemic cyanosis and its associated complications.

SUGGESTED READINGS

Key Reviews
Bridges ND, Perry SB, Keane JF, et al. Preoperative transcatheter closure of congenital muscular ventricular septal defects. *N Engl J Med* 1991;324:1312–1317.
Connelly MS, Webb GD, Sommerville J, et al. Canadian Consensus Conference on Adult Congenital Heart Disease 1996. *Can J Cardiol* 1998;14:395–452.
Ellis JH, Moodie DS, Sterba R, Gill CC. Ventricular septal defect in the adult: natural and unnatural history. *Am Heart J* 1987;114:115–120.
Folkert M, Szatmari A, Utens E, et al. Long-term follow-up after surgical closure of ventricular septal defect in infancy and childhood. *J Am Coll Cardiol* 1994;24: 1358–1364.
Lock JE, Block PC, McKay RG, et al. Transcatheter closure of ventricular septal defects. *Circulation* 1988;78:361–368.
Mahoney LT. Acyanotic congenital heart disease: atrial and ventricular septal defects, atrioventricular canal, patent ductus arteriosus, pulmonic stenosis. *Cardiol Clin* 1993;11:603–616.
O'Fallon MW, Weidman WH, eds. Long-term follow-up of congenital aortic stenosis, pulmonary stenosis, and ventricular septal defect. Report from the Second Joint Study on the Natural History of Congenital Heart Defects (NHS-2). *Circulation* 1993;87[Suppl II]:II-1–II-126.
O'Laughlin MP, Mullins CE. Transcatheter closure of ventricular septal defect. *Catheter Cardiovasc Diagn* 1989;17:175–179.
Somerville J. How to manage the Eisenmenger syndrome. *Int J Cardiol* 1998;63:1–8.

Relevant Book Chapters
Brecker SJD. Ventricular septal defect. In: Redington A, Shore D, Oldershaw P, eds. *Congenital heart disease in adults: a practical guide.* London: WB Saunders, 1994:111–117.
Gumbiner CH, Takao A. Ventricular septal defect. In: Garson A, Bricker JT, Fisher DJ, Neish SR, eds. *The science and practice of pediatric cardiology,* 2nd ed. Baltimore: Williams & Wilkins, 1998:1119–1140.
Perloff JK. Survival patterns without cardiac surgery or interventional catheterization: a narrowing base. In: Perloff JK, Child JS, eds. *Congenital heart disease in adults,* 2nd ed. Philadelphia: WB Saunders, 1998:15–53.
Snider AR, Serwer GA, Ritter SB. Defects in cardiac septation. In: Snider AR, Serwer GA, Ritter SB, eds. *Echocardiography in pediatric heart disease,* 2nd ed. St. Louis: Mosby, 1997:246–265.

31. PATENT DUCTUS ARTERIOSUS

J. Donald Moore and Douglas S. Moodie

I. **Introduction. Patent ductus arteriosus (PDA)** has been reported to occur in approximately 1 in 2,000 to 5,000 live births but is relatively uncommon among the adult population. The natural history depends on the size of the ductus arteriosus and resultant left to right shunt. If **PDA is left untreated, congestive heart failure** can occur because of chronic left heart volume overload. The adult with this condition may seek evaluation because of atrial flutter or fibrillation. Pulmonary vascular disease is a rare complication of isolated PDA among adults. **Endocarditis** is an extremely rare complication but the possibility necessitates lifelong antibiotic prophylaxis. Spontaneously occurring aneurysms of the ductus arteriosus have been reported but typically among very young or very old persons or in association with endocarditis.

II. **Anatomy**
  A. **Embryology.** The ductus arteriosus is a **normal and essential component** of cardiovascular development. In normal fetal development, the ductus arteriosus originates from the distal sixth left aortic arch. The communication persists in fetal circulation between the descending aorta usually just distal to the left subclavian artery and the main pulmonary artery near the bifurcation. Variations in the side on which the arch is situated or branch vessels originate can cause abnormally positioned or bilateral ductus arteriosus. The presence of the ductus arteriosus in the fetal circulation is essential to allow preferential **shunting of nutrient rich, oxygenated blood from the placenta to the fetal systemic circulation bypassing the pulmonary circuit.**
  B. Several important **changes occur at birth** to initiate normal functional **closure of the ductus arteriosus within the first 15 to 18 hours of life.** At birth, blood oxygen tension increases with the onset of spontaneous respirations. This is coupled with a decrease in circulating prostaglandins in part because of increased metabolism within the pulmonary circulation and removal of the primary source of production, the placenta. These factors allow normal functional closure of the ductus arteriosus followed by eventual fibrosis and anatomic closure by the 15th to 21st day of life. The **fibrotic remnant** of this structure persists in the adult as the **ligamentum arteriosum.** Failure of this process by 3 months of age results in persistent patency of this normal fetal structure.

III. **Clinical presentation**
  A. **Signs and symptoms.** As with other acyanotic congenital lesions, **nonspecific symptoms** are the most common presentation. These include exercise intolerance, dyspnea, and shortness of breath.
  B. **Physical findings** classically include a **harsh continuous murmur** auscultated at the left infraclavicular area or left upper sternal border. With a large left to right shunt, pulse pressure is widened because of ductal runoff with sometimes bounding peripheral pulses. A diastolic rumble may be audible at the apex from increased flow across the mitral valve. An increased left ventricular (LV) impulse may be present. In the setting of long-standing left to right shunting, however, pulmonary hypertension may occur, reduce the left to right shunt, and mask the auscultatory findings. In this setting other findings may be evident, including increased right ventricular impulse and an increased intensity of the S_2, which reflects increased pulmonary pressures. The variability or lack of clinical findings underscores the importance of a high index of suspicion in the evaluations of adult patients.
  C. The **differential diagnosis** of PDA based on the clinical findings includes arteriovenous malformations such as pulmonary arteriovenous fistula, coronary artery fistula, systemic arteriovenous fistula, ruptured sinus of Valsalva,

ventricular septal defect with aortic insufficiency, the presence of systemic aortopulmonary collateral vessels with pulmonary atresia and ventricular septal defect, and innocent venous hum.

IV. **Laboratory examination**

   A. An **electrocardiogram (ECG)** usually is nonspecific. The findings range from normal to evidence of left atrial enlargement with LV hypertrophy. Right ventricular hypertrophy may become apparent late in the setting of pulmonary hypertension.

   B. **Chest radiography** may reveal cardiomegaly and increased pulmonary vascular markings in the presence of a large left to right shunt in a young patient. Similar findings may occur among older patients after years of chronic left atrial and LV volume overload. The double density that appears with left atrial enlargement may be apparent. Normal chest radiographic findings support the presence of a hemodynamically insignificant lesion.

V. **Diagnostic testing.** Standard transthoracic echocardiographic images reliably confirm the diagnosis of PDA in most instances. Cardiac catheterization is typically spared for interventional purposes.

   A. **Transthoracic echocardiography** often demonstrates the aortic origin of the PDA, typically with suprasternal notch views. The complete course of a PDA may be difficult to find in some patients because of its tortuosity. Color Doppler imaging often can reveal the complete course to insertion into the pulmonary artery. It is imperative to demonstrate color Doppler flow within the pulmonary artery, typically on a parasternal short-axis view. Quantitative assessment of shunt velocity is valuable to estimate degree of restriction across the PDA. This measurement becomes important in planning transcatheter intervention. Associated left atrial and LV enlargement suggests a hemodynamically significant lesion.

   B. **Cardiac catheterization** is **rarely needed** for diagnostic purposes. The typical course of the catheter must be recognized, but in unexpected cases PDA is not diagnosed by means of physical examination or noninvasive testing.

      1. A PDA can be readily crossed antegrade from the main pulmonary artery or can be crossed in a retrograde direction from the descending aorta best guided on the lateral projection. Oximetric sampling typically demonstrates an increase in saturation within the main pulmonary artery with variable increases in the branch pulmonary arteries. Pressures within the pulmonary arteries and right ventricle are near normal or slightly elevated but typically remain below systemic levels. The presence of systemic pulmonary pressures alerts one to the presence of pulmonary vascular disease or left heart obstructive lesions such as pulmonary venous stenosis or mitral stenosis.

      2. A PDA is best demonstrated by means of angiography in the lateral projection of a **descending aortogram** performed with a standard angiographic catheter positioned just below the ductal ampulla. If biplanar imaging is used, the right anterior oblique–cranial projection is sometimes helpful.

   C. **Magnetic resonance imaging (MRI)** can be of assistance in unusual situations, such as PDA aneurysm or endocarditis. For the most part, MRI is seldom needed.

VI. **Therapy.** Because of the natural history of persistent PDA, **closure is recommended.** Indications for closure include symptoms, history of endocarditis, and acceptable pulmonary vascular pressures and resistance. Closure of a small, silent PDA found incidentally in a patient who does not have symptoms remains debatable.

   A. **Surgical closure** traditionally has been the standard therapy for PDA. This usually is performed by means of double ligation and division through a left thoracotomy. High closure rates with low complications are expected. The procedure can be painful for adults and necessitates inpatient recovery. Investigational thorascopic techniques are being developed but are not yet widely available. Caution is exercised in the care of older patients because they may have ductal calcification. Extensive patch reconstruction of the ductal ampulla and pulmonary artery may be needed to manage short but wide PDA. Some centers advocate surgical ligation under cardiopulmonary bypass in these cases.

B. **Transcatheter techniques** have become the standard **first-line therapy** for most instances of PDA from infancy to adulthood. Many centers use single or multiple stainless steel coils to achieve complete closure. Numerous devices have been adapted or are under clinical investigation to allow transcatheter closure of larger defects. These procedures can often be performed on an outpatient basis and appear to have long-term closure rates comparable with those of surgical ligation. Mortality is typically less than 1% at experienced centers. Success has been reported even in instances in which ductal calcification has been apparent, but large clinical series are lacking. This procedure is performed by an interventional cardiologist experienced with transcatheter occlusion techniques on adults.

C. **Antibiotic prophylaxis** is typically continued for 6 months after complete occlusion with surgical or transcatheter techniques.

SUGGESTED READINGS

Key Reviews

Burke RP, Wernovsky G, van der Velde M, et al. Video-assisted thoracoscopy surgery for congenital heart disease. *J Thorac Cardiovasc Surg* 1995;109:499–508.

Connelly MS, Webb GD, Sommerville J, et al. Canadian Consensus Conference on Adult Congenital Heart Disease 1996. *Can J Cardiol* 1998;14:395–452.

Fisher RG, Moodie DS, Sterba R, Gill CC. Patent ductus arteriosus in adults: long-term follow-up—nonsurgical versus surgical management. *J Am Coll Cardiol* 1986; 8:280–284.

Harrison DA, Benson LN, Lazzam C, et al. Percutaneous catheter closure of the persistently patent ductus arteriosus in the adult. *Am J Cardiol* 1996;77:1084–1097.

Ing FF, Mullins CE, Rose M, et al. Transcatheter closure of the patent ductus arteriosus in adults using the Gianturco coil. *Clin Cardiol* 1996;19:875–879.

Mahoney LT. Acyanotic congenital heart disease: atrial and ventricular septal defects, atrioventricular canal, patent ductus arteriosus, pulmonic stenosis. *Cardiol Clin* 1993;11:603–616.

Schenk MH, O Laughlin MP, Rokey R, et al. Transcatheter occlusion of patent ductus arteriosus in adult patients. *Am J Cardiol* 1993;72:591–595.

Relevant Book Chapters

Mullins CE, Pagotto L. Patent ductus arteriosus. In: Garson A, Bricker JT, Fisher DJ, Neish SR, eds. *The science and practice of pediatric cardiology,* 2nd ed. Baltimore: Williams & Wilkins, 1998:1181–1197.

Perloff JK. Survival patterns without cardiac surgery or interventional catheterization: a narrowing base. In: Perloff JK, Child JS, eds. *Congenital heart disease in adults,* 2nd ed. Philadelphia: WB Saunders, 1998:15–53.

32. COARCTATION OF THE AORTA

J. Donald Moore and Douglas S. Moodie

I. **Introduction.** Coarctation of the aorta has been estimated to occur with a frequency of 7% to 9%. It is usually diagnosed in infancy or early childhood but can go undetected to become apparent well into adulthood. The natural history suggests that isolated coarctation may represent one aspect of more diffuse arteriopathy. Late **complications** can include aneurysm formation and dissection of the ascending aorta rather than the region of prior repair or intervention. Cerebrovascular events from rupture of berry aneurysms may occur before or after surgical repair of coarctation. Persistent hypertension has been reported despite apparently complete repair. Life expectancy beyond the sixth decade is unusual if the coarctation is not repaired. The mean survival time is approximately 35 years.

II. **Anatomy**

   A. **Embryology.** No single explanation has emerged to explain the cause of coarctation of the aorta. Multiple contributing factors have been proposed, including altered fetal blood flow across the aortic arch, excessive posterior tissue development that produces a discreet shelf, and the presence of ductal tissue in this area.

   B. The coarctation typically lies **just beyond the origin of the left subclavian artery across from the ampulla of the ductus arteriosus.** Medial thickening at the site coarctation has been a relatively consistent histologic finding. Extension of ductal tissue may occur among neonates and contribute to the obstruction as ductal closure ensues. Additional intimal thickening has been found in older patients. Medial elastic fiber disarray comparable with cystic medial necrosis of the aorta associated with Marfan syndrome has been described in some but not all surgical specimens.

   C. **Collateral circulation** often is present in older patients. The collateral vessels bypass the coarctation and provide blood flow to the lower extremities. The most common origins of these vessels are from the subclavian arteries through the internal thoracic arteries and the thyrocervical and costocervical branches. These vessels communicate with the intercostal arteries, which then perfuse the descending aorta distal to the coarctation. This can produce diminished but palpable lower extremity pulses and mask substantial coarctation.

III. **Clinical presentation**

   A. **Signs and symptoms.** Coarctation must be excluded in any adult with hypertension. Infants may have congestive heart failure, whereas adults may have headaches, epistaxis or claudication.

   B. **Physical examination**

      1. **Blood pressure** in the upper extremities is elevated with variable gradients detected between the upper and lower extremities. Because the left subclavian artery can be partially involved in the coarctation, four extremity blood pressures are obtained.

      2. The femoral **pulses** are diminished or absent and delayed in comparison with easily palpable upper extremity pulses. A diminished left brachial or radial pulse suggests involvement of the left subclavian artery in the coarctation. A diminished pulse in the right arm suggests anomalous origin of the right subclavian artery, which can sometimes originate below the coarctation.

      3. A systolic ejection **murmur** may be heard over the back with continuous murmurs audible throughout the precordium from multiple collateral vessels. A murmur of aortic insufficiency may be audible because of involvement of the bicuspid aortic valve. This association may produce a systolic ejection sound.

C. The most common **associated cardiovascular malformation** is bicuspid aortic valve. Other associated lesions include valvular aortic stenosis, ventricular septal defects, aneurysm of the circle of Willis, or a more complex congenital cardiovascular abnormality. Coarctation of the aorta is a common cardiovascular abnormality in Turner's syndrome.

IV. **Laboratory examination**

   A. An **electrocardiogram (ECG)** might be normal but commonly reveals left ventricular (LV) hypertrophy.

   B. A **chest radiograph** may appear normal. Subtle findings include rib notching caused by erosion from the development of large collateral vessels. A classic "3" shape of the aorta may be visualized in the posteroanterior projection at the site of the coarctation. LV enlargement is variably present.

   C. **Stress exercise testing** of adults typically demonstrates marked systolic hypertension with elevated systolic pressures.

V. **Diagnostic testing**

   A. **Echocardiography** is the primary diagnostic tool for the diagnosis of coarctation in infants and children. Clear images and accurate Doppler velocities may be difficult to obtain for adult patients.

      1. The finding of a **bicuspid aortic valve** prompts careful interrogation of the aortic arch to rule out associated coarctation.

      2. Careful investigation of the **left heart** is necessary to rule out associated left heart defects such as mitral stenosis, LV outflow tract obstruction, or ventricular septal defect.

      3. Attention is paid to the **aortic arch and the head and neck vessels.** Doppler interrogation may be inaccurate in the presence of patent ductus arteriosus or multiple collateral vessels because the gradient may be artificially lowered in these circumstances.

      4. Attention also is focused on the **abdominal aorta** with respect to size and pulsatility.

   B. **Magnetic resonance imaging (MRI)** is particularly helpful in the evaluation of coarctation among adult patients. In many instances, transthoracic or transesophageal echocardiography may provide only limited visualization of the descending aorta, even in younger patients. MRI can provide noninvasive, detailed anatomic information concerning the location of the coarctation, the anatomic features of the rest of the aortic arch, and presence or absence of collateral vessels. Cine MRI can provide hemodynamic information, which may help further define the type and timing of intervention.

   C. **Cardiac catheterization**

      1. Direct hemodynamic assessment of the gradient, associated lesions, and LV pressure and function can be helpful in deciding whether or when to proceed with intervention.

      2. For adult patients with **recurrence of coarctation** following surgical repair in childhood, catheterization is coordinated to include the option of transcatheter intervention if indicated.

      3. **Oximetric values** are normal in isolated coarctation. Cardiac index is measured before intervention. Careful hemodynamic assessment across the coarctation is essential to find a peak systolic gradient. Intervention typically is indicated when the peak gradient is greater than 20 to 30 mm Hg, but other clinical factors must also be considered (congestive heart failure, LV hypertrophy, abnormal stress test result, uncontrolled upper extremity hypertension). This gradient may be artificially decreased in the presence of collateral vessels.

      4. If MRI is performed first, much of the baseline anatomic and general hemodynamic information can be obtained so that adequate preparation can be made for intervention.

VI. **Therapy**

   A. **Neonatal coarctation** generally is repaired by means of **surgical resection** and end-to-end anastomosis. Few pediatric centers strongly advocate primary balloon angioplasty for native coarctation in neonates because of a high incidence of recurrence of coarctation and an increased prevalence of femoral artery complications.

B. Native coarctation **beyond infancy** may be approached by means of **balloon angioplasty** but again at the expense of possible recurrence of coarctation and aneurysm formation at the angioplasty site. For selected older patients, stent placement may be considered as primary intervention. Whether to perform stent placement must be considered in light of the need for growth of the aorta and risk for aneurysm formation. The long-term outcome is yet to be established. This procedure is approached with caution in the care of patients with native coarctation.

C. Recurrence of coarctation after surgical repair is a known complication. Some centers advocate reoperation for recurrent coarctation. Many centers, however, recommend balloon angioplasty alone or stent placement in adolescents and young adults. Early studies reveal promising short-term outcomes with a low complication rate. However, the long-term outcome into late adulthood after stent placement has yet to be determined, and investigation continues.

SUGGESTED READINGS

Key Reviews

Connelly MS, Webb GD, Sommerville J, et al. Canadian Consensus Conference on Adult Congenital Heart Disease 1996. *Can J Cardiol* 1998;14:395–452.

Ebeid MR, Prieto LR, Latson LA. Use of balloon expandable stents for coarctation of the aorta: initial results and intermediate-term follow-up. *J Am Coll Cardiol* 1997; 30:1847–1852.

Kaplan S. Natural history and postoperative history across age groups. *Cardiol Clin* 1993;11:543–556.

Mathew P, Moodie D, Blechman G, Gill CC. Long-term follow-up of aortic coarctation in infants, children and adults. *Cardiol Young* 1993;3:20–26.

Mendelsohn AM. Balloon angioplasty for native coarctation of the aorta. *J Intervent Cardiol* 1995;8:487–508.

Ovaert C, Benson LN, Nykanen, Freedom RM. Transcatheter treatment of coarctation of the aorta: a review. *Pediatr Cardiol* 1998;19:27–44.

Relevant Book Chapters:

Brecker SJD. Coarctation of the aorta. In: Redington A, Shore D, Oldershaw P, eds. *Congenital heart disease in adults: a practical guide.* London: WB Saunders, 1994:119–125.

Morriss MJH, McNamara DG. Coarctation of the aorta and interrupted aortic arch. In: Garson A, Bricker JT, Fisher DJ, Neish SR, eds. *The science and practice of pediatric cardiology,* 2nd ed. Baltimore: Williams & Wilkins, 1998:1317–1346.

33. TETRALOGY OF FALLOT

J. Donald Moore and Douglas S. Moodie

I. **Introduction.** Tetralogy of Fallot occurs among about 6% of infants with congenital heart disease and is the most common form of cyanotic heart disease among adults. Current surgical practice warrants early repair, usually within the first year of life. Without surgical intervention, only about 10% of patients survive beyond the age of 20 years. Adults with tetralogy of Fallot usually have undergone surgical repair or palliation.

II. **Anatomy**

   A. **Embryology.** The embryonic abnormalities produce the **four classic defining features** of tetralogy of Fallot. Varying degrees of supravalvular or branch pulmonary artery stenosis with pulmonary artery hypoplasia also may be present. The four defining features are as follows:

   1. Severe infundibular or valvular pulmonic stenosis
   2. Large malalignment ventricular septal defect (VSD)
   3. Aortic override
   4. Right ventricular hypertrophy (RVH)

   B. Two **theories** have been advanced in attempts to explain the embryologic basis of this congenital cardiac defect. The first is related to an **abnormality of truncal septation** that causes relative hypoplasia of one outflow (the future right ventricular [RV] outflow) and leaves relative enlargement of the other (the future aorta). Because of diminished RV outflow, stenosis develops, and malalignment of the ventricular septum causes a VSD with override of the aorta. The second theory explains the findings in tetralogy of Fallot as a result of **infundibular hypoplasia.** This leads to malalignment of the infundibular septum and ventricular septum producing a VSD with aortic override. In both situations RVH is a secondary result of the anatomic findings. The resultant decrease in blood flow to the distal pulmonary arteries leads to variable degrees of hypoplasia.

   C. Tetralogy of Fallot is associated with several **other abnormalities.** Anomalous origin of the left anterior descending coronary artery from the right coronary artery or a prominent conal branch from the right coronary artery can occur. These vessels cross the RV outflow tract. This anatomic feature is important to surgeons because infundibular resection or future conduit placement may be needed in this location. Right aortic arch occurs in 25% of cases. A secundum atrial septal defect occurs in 15% of cases. Among adult patients, aortic insufficiency can occur naturally from long-term dilatation of the aortic root, after endocarditis, or as a postoperative sequela.

III. **Clinical presentation**

   A. **Patients who have not undergone surgical repair**

   1. These patients may have central cyanosis, the degree of which varies with the degree of RV outflow tract obstruction. Clubbing of the fingers and toes may be apparent, as may erythrocytosis.
   2. The examination is remarkable for a prominent systolic ejection **murmur** at the left upper sternal border, possibly with a thrill. The shorter the murmur the more severe is the infundibular pulmonic stenosis. A prominent RV impulse may be appreciated because of equalization of RV and left ventricular pressures. The murmur of aortic insufficiency may be audible. Continuous murmurs may be audible because of the presence of aortopulmonary collateral vessels. These vessels are more likely in the setting of pulmonary atresia but can be acquired should progressive RV outflow tract stenosis develop.

   B. **Patients who have undergone palliative treatment** have variable clinical findings depending on the type of palliation performed.

1. Most palliative treatments consist of a **systemic to pulmonary artery shunt** initially performed to supplement the deficiency of antegrade pulmonary blood flow. The modified Blalock-Taussig shunt is most commonly used but serves only as a bridge to complete repair in the first year of life. Adults who have undergone palliative treatment may have classic Blalock-Taussig shunts (subclavian artery to pulmonary artery), Potts shunts (descending aorta to left pulmonary artery), or Waterson shunts (ascending aorta to right pulmonary artery).

2. With time the shunts may remain patent and produce characteristic continuous **murmurs or may be silent** if they have occluded. Continuous murmurs from collateral formation may be audible. Branch pulmonary artery stenosis at prior shunt insertion sites can produce unilateral systolic or continuous murmurs. Prior resection of the RV outflow with or without a conduit may produce variable degrees of pulmonary insufficiency. Depending on the degree of antegrade flow across the outflow tract, systolic ejection murmurs may be audible, as they are in a patient who has not undergone surgical repair.

C. Patients who have undergone surgical repair

1. These patients typically first have undergone palliation with a shunt. Complete repair consists of patch closure of the VSD, variable degrees of RV outflow tract resection, and reconstruction, pulmonary valvotomy, or placement of an RV to pulmonary artery conduit, either bioprosthetic or homograft. Distal branch pulmonary arterial stenosis may have been repaired, or residual lesions may be present. Examination focuses on the detection of residual lesions.

2. Some degree of turbulence almost always remains across the RV outflow tract. This produces a variable systolic ejection **murmur** at the left upper sternal border with radiation to the back and peripheral lung fields. Of importance is the presence of associated pulmonary insufficiency, which also is audible in this location, sometimes producing a to-and-fro murmur. In this setting, chronic volume loading of the right ventricle occurs and can lead to diminished exercise tolerance, dysrhythmias, and right heart failure. A higher-frequency systolic murmur at the left lower sternal border suggests the presence of a residual VSD commonly caused by a small VSD patch leak. The diastolic murmur of aortic insufficiency must also be actively considered.

IV. Laboratory Examination

A. **Chest radiographic** findings vary depending on the surgical history. The presence of a right aortic arch is determined. A concave deficiency of the left heart border reflects variable degrees of pulmonary arterial hypoplasia. Upturning of the apex from RVH causes the classic finding of a boot-shaped heart. Differences in pulmonary vascular markings are sought because they might reflect discrete pulmonary arterial branch stenosis and differential pulmonary blood flow. The size of the heart is important because cardiomegaly can occur among adults. Calcification or aneurysmal dilatation of surgical conduits or RV outflow tract repair may be visible on plain radiographs.

B. An **electrocardiogram** typically demonstrates sinus rhythm with RVH. A patient who has undergone surgical repair typically has right bundle branch block, which reflects prior surgical intervention. Both atrial and ventricular late rhythm disturbances can be present. Marked ventricular hypertrophy in patients who have undergone surgical repair suggests hemodynamically significant residual lesions that must be investigated.

V. Diagnostic testing

A. Echocardiography

1. For a child or young adult, transthoracic echocardiography may be the only modality necessary. For adults or patients who have undergone surgical intervention, more information may be needed. The primary objectives are to **determine which residual lesions are present and their locations.**

    a. Adequate **views** are obtained of the right heart, RV outflow tract, and proximal pulmonary arteries. Helpful views include the parasternal long-axis, parasternal short-axis, and apical four-chamber views. Further definition of residual lesions in the branch pulmonary arteries may be possible with a high parasternal short-axis view. Residual VSDs and the presence of aortic insufficiency are sought on these views.

    b. Palliative shunts are often best visualized in the suprasternal notch view where the subclavian arteries course distally.

    c. Continuous flow is typically demonstrated with **color Doppler** techniques. Less common shunts may be difficult to image in adult patients. Aortopulmonary collateral vessels are difficult to visualize but may be seen in suprasternal notch views of the descending aorta.

  2. Transesophageal echocardiography may allow improved imaging of the intracardiac anatomic structures in adults but limitations often remain with regard to the distal pulmonary arteries, and additional testing frequently is necessary.

B. Quantitative pulmonary flow scans are useful to determine discrepancies in pulmonary flow that may be caused by branch pulmonary arterial stenosis. These scans also provide an objective baseline for scans obtained after surgical or transcatheter intervention.

C. Magnetic resonance imaging often is better for demonstrating the distal pulmonary arterial anatomic features. It also provides hemodynamic information about residual lesions. Previously placed shunts and possibly aortopulmonary collateral vessels can be identified. The anatomic information may be sufficient to proceed with surgical treatment or to guide the interventional cardiologist in planning a transcatheter procedure.

D. Cardiac catheterization can be used for diagnostic and potentially for interventional purposes.

  1. Residual shunts are actively sought at the atrial, ventricular, and pulmonary arterial levels.

    a. RV pressure is systemic in a patient who has not undergone surgical repair.

    b. After surgical repair, elevated RV pressure supports the presence of residual obstructive lesions, the levels of which are documented.

    c. Careful pullback recordings are performed from the branch pulmonary arteries to the right ventricle because stenosis at each level is possible.

    d. The presence of stenosis at a prior shunt site is expected. RV end diastolic pressures may be elevated in the setting of pulmonary insufficiency.

  2. Left heart catheterization is performed if noninvasive studies suggest residual VSDs.

    a. **Angiography** includes a cranialized right ventriculography and possibly selective pulmonary arterial injections if hemodynamic findings suggest stenosis.

    b. **Left ventriculography** better demonstrates residual VSDs in the presence of subsystemic RV pressures.

    c. **Aortic root injection** demonstrates the presence of aortic insufficiency, confirms the presence of grossly abnormal coronary artery origins or branching patterns, and reveals prior surgical shunts or aortopulmonary collateral vessels. If present, shunts and collateral vessels are best visualized in the posteroanterior and lateral projections after selective injection by hand.

    d. **Selective coronary arteriography** is recommended in the care of adult patients to exclude coronary artery disease before surgical intervention.

VI. Therapy and follow-up care
A. Medical treatment
1. The medical treatment of an **infant** with cyanosis and tetralogy of Fallot primarily entails expectant observation for worsening cyanosis or hypercyanotic episodes. β-Blockade may be considered for patients with episodic hypercyanosis. Consideration also may be given to proceeding with systemic to pulmonary arterial shunt placement or complete surgical repair.
2. If an **adult** has not been surgically treated or has undergone palliative treatment, a relatively well-balanced situation must exist. However, the following problems are to be expected:
   a. Long-term effects of RV outflow obstruction
   b. Progressive infundibular pulmonary stenosis
   c. Exposure of the pulmonary circulation to systemic shunt flow
   d. Development of distal pulmonary arterial stenosis, typically at shunt sites
   e. Erythrocytosis
   f. Chronic hypoxemia
   g. Increased risk for aortic insufficiency over time
   h. Endocarditis
3. Because more children are undergoing earlier repair, follow-up care will increasingly involve **patients who have undergone surgical repair** and management of residual postoperative lesions.
   a. Rhythm disturbances are common among postoperative patients. The rate of sudden death is reported to be approximately 3%, the deaths are presumed to be caused by arrhythmia. Regular **Holter monitoring** is warranted for this reason.
   b. There have been no reports that prophylactic antiarrhythmic therapy lowers risk for sudden death among this patient population.
   c. An increased incidence of ventricular rhythm abnormalities has been associated with RV volume overload and QRS prolongation from pulmonary insufficiency.
B. Although the mainstay of therapy has been surgical, **transcatheter techniques** are being used to treat patients who have not undergone surgical repair and those who have.
1. Investigation has begun to explore the efficacy of **early pulmonary balloon valvuloplasty** in the care of **infants** to provide increased pulmonary blood flow before consideration for systemic to pulmonary arterial shunting. Increased size of the pulmonary valve annulus and pulmonary arterial growth have been reported. This approach is not yet widely accepted.
2. For the most part, transcatheter therapies in the care of **adult patients** with tetralogy of Fallot are limited to patients who have undergone surgical treatment with attention to residual obstructive lesions in the main pulmonary artery, RV to PA conduit, or distal pulmonary arteries. Prior shunt sites may become stenotic with time and necessitate **balloon angioplasty** and possibly stent placement. Success has been achieved in these situations, but most residual lesions necessitate surgical reintervention.
C. The primary therapeutic consideration for patients with tetralogy of Fallot is **surgical intervention.** The objective is to relieve the outflow obstruction while maintaining competency of a preferably native pulmonary valve with closure of the VSD.
1. Some **younger patients** need extensive reconstruction of the RV outflow tract with early placement of a bioprosthetic valved conduit or homograft. These will usually become restrictive to flow and insufficient with time. The result is progressive right heart hypertrophy, fibrosis, and failure if revision is not performed.

2. Replacement or revision of conduits or homografts is indicated for **adult patients** because risk is acceptably low and outcome is favorable in most series.
3. Factors that weigh in favor of reintervention include residual VSD with reasonable (approximately 1.5:1) shunt, RV pressures greater than two-thirds systemic pressures because of residual obstructive lesions and RV enlargement in the setting of pulmonary insufficiency and tricuspid insufficiency. Reduced exercise tolerance, rhythm disturbances often related to hemodynamic abnormalities, and symptomatic or progressive aortic insufficiency also may be grounds for advocating further intervention.

SUGGESTED READINGS

Key Reviews

Connelly MS, Webb GD, Somerville J, et al. Canadian Consensus Conference on Adult Congenital Heart Disease 1996. *Can J Cardiol* 1998;14:395–452.

Cullen S, Celermajer DS, Franklin RCG, et al. Prognostic significance of ventricular arrhythmia after repair of tetralogy of Fallot: a 12-year prospective study. *J Am Coll Cardiol* 1994;23:1151–1155.

Harrison DA, Harris L, Siu SC, et al. Sustained ventricular tachycardia in adult patients late after repair of tetralogy of Fallot. *J Am Coll Cardiol* 1997;30:1368–1373.

Kreindel MS, Moodie DS, Sterba R, Gill CC. Total repair of tetralogy of Fallot in the adult: the Cleveland Clinic experience 1951–1981. *Cleve Clin Q* 1985;52:375–381.

Murphy JG, Gersh BJ, Mair DD, et al. Long-term outcome in patients undergoing surgical repair of tetralogy of Fallot. *N Engl J Med* 1993;329:593–599.

Nollert G, Fischlein T, Bouterwek S, et al. Long-term survival in patients with repair of tetralogy of Fallot: 36-year follow-up of 490 survivors of the first year after surgical repair. *J Am Coll Cardiol* 1997;30:1374–1383.

Warnes CA. Tetralogy of Fallot and pulmonary atresia/ventricular septal defect. *Cardiol Clin* 1993;11:643–650.

Yemets IM, Williams WG, Webb GD, et al. Pulmonary valve replacement late after repair of tetralogy of Fallot. *Ann Thorac Surg* 1997;64:526–530.

Relevant Book Chapters

Neches WH, Park S, Ettedgui JA. Tetralogy of Fallot and Tetralogy of Fallot with pulmonary atresia. In: Garson A, Bricker JT, Fisher DJ, Neish SR, eds. *The science and practice of pediatric cardiology,* 2nd ed. Baltimore: Williams & Wilkins, 1998: 1383–1411.

Perloff JK. Survival patterns without cardiac surgery or interventional catheterization: a narrowing base. In: Perloff JK, Child JS, eds. *Congenital heart disease in adults,* 2nd ed. Philadelphia: WB Saunders, 1998:15–53.

Redington A, Shore D, Oldershaw P. In: Tetralogy of Fallot. Redington A, Shore D, Oldershaw P, eds. Congenital heart disease in adults: a practical guide. London: WB Saunders, 1994:57–67.

Snider AR, Serwer GA, Ritter SB. Defects in cardiac septation. In: Snider AR, Serwer GA, Ritter SB, eds. *Echocardiography in pediatric heart disease,* 2nd ed. St. Louis: Mosby, 1997:235–246.

34. MISCELLANEOUS DEFECTS

J. Donald Moore and Douglas S. Moodie

I. **Congenitally corrected transposition of the great arteries (ccTGA).**
Ventricular inversion or ccTGA is a rare congenital anomaly that occurs among less than 1% of children with congenital cardiovascular defects. Among these patients, it is equally rare to have no other associated structural abnormalities. The natural history of ccTGA is gradual congestive failure caused by systemic atrioventricular AV valve insufficiency and systemic ventricular dysfunction even in the absence of other associated malformations. The presence of associated defects and conduction abnormalities contributes to a further decrease in life expectancy without intervention. Life expectancy is good but does not reach normal.

A. **Anatomy**

1. The **defining feature** of this congenital abnormality of cardiac looping is AV and ventriculoarterial discordance. Blood flows from the right atrium across a mitral valve into a right-sided, morphologic left ventricle that is related to the pulmonary artery, which typically is more posterior and rightward than usual. Pulmonary venous return is normal to the left atrium but then flows across an anatomic tricuspid valve into a left-sided, morphologic right ventricle, which is related to an anterior and leftward aorta.

2. The anatomic coronary arteries, like the AV valves, follow their respective ventricles. The left-sided coronary artery resembles the anatomic right coronary artery as it courses in the AV groove and gives rise to infundibular and marginal branches. The right-sided coronary artery resembles the morphologic left coronary artery, which branches into the anterior descending and circumflex arteries (Fig. 34-1).

3. The conduction system likewise follows the respective ventricle as the right-sided, morphologic left ventricle depolarizes first. Accessory AV nodal tissue is located anteriorly with respect to normal and His's bundle must traverse anterior to the pulmonary artery and along the superior margin of a ventricular septal defect (VSD) if present. As a result of this abnormal course, approximately 30% of adolescents and adults will have complete heart block, the rate of which increases at 2% per year without surgical intervention.

4. Isolated ccTGA is the exception. **Associated lesions** are common and are considered in the diagnostic evaluation. These include VSD, pulmonary outflow obstruction, or abnormalities of the left-sided, systemic tricuspid valve. There is increased risk for acquired complete heart block in this lesion because of the abnormally placed AV node and its extended course. Accessory pathways have been described and are typically left sided in the presence of an Ebstein's anomaly–like malformation of the left-sided (tricuspid) AV valve.

B. **Clinical presentation**

1. Because physiologic blood flow is preserved, patients may have no symptoms through adulthood in the absence of other structural lesions or associated complications. This scenario is rare, however, because the commonly occurring associated lesions dictate the clinical features.

2. Without associated structural abnormalities, **failure of the systemic, morphologic right ventricle** with varying degrees of systemic AV valve (tricuspid) insufficiency is the norm. In this setting the patient has nonspecific descriptions of fatigue, shortness of breath, and exercise intolerance or congestive failure. Patients may have syncope or presyncope caused by conduction abnormalities or complete heart block.

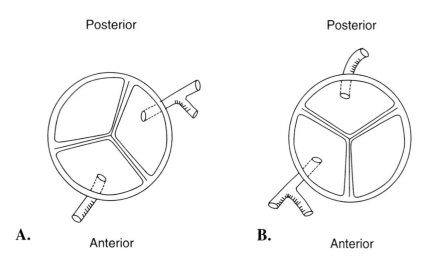

FIG. 34-1. Schematic representation of coronary artery origins and branching in the normal heart (**A**) and in congenitally corrected transposition (**B**).

C. Laboratory examination
    1. In the usual anatomic configuration of ccTGA, the aorta is anterior and to the left, which produces a **chest radiograph** with a straight left heart border. The left pulmonary artery is not well defined. The chest radiograph may appear normal or reflect the presence of associated lesions, such as increased pulmonary flow from a VSD or decreased pulmonary flow in the setting of pulmonary stenosis.
    2. The typical **electrocardiographic (ECG)** findings include left axis deviation. Among pediatric patients there is loss of the usual Q waves in the precordial leads with deep Q waves in leads II and aVF. A variety of AV node conduction abnormalities may become manifest with time and progress to complete heart block.
D. Diagnostic evaluation
    1. In the most instances the diagnosis can be made with **echocardiography.** The essential findings of AV and ventriculoarterial discordance must be demonstrated. Close attention must be paid to the morphologic detail of each chamber.
        a. The **right ventricle** is identified through the presence of trabeculations, an inferiorly placed AV valve with respect to the mitral valve, and discontinuity between the AV and the semilunar valve.
        b. The **left ventricle** is identified on the basis of its smooth wall, more superiorly positioned AV valve, and continuity between the AV and semilunar valves. In the case of ccTGA these relations are preserved though reversed.
        c. Continuity is lacking between the **left-sided (tricuspid) AV valve and aorta** but is present between the **right-sided (anatomic mitral) valve and pulmonary artery.** The left-sided AV valve is displaced inferiorly relative to the right-sided (mitral) valve and may appear malformed or have the characteristics of Ebstein's anomaly.
        d. Apical four-chamber and subcostal images are particularly helpful. Comparable transesophageal images may be needed for adult patients.
        e. The **aortic arch** typically lies to the left of midline in the sagittal plane and can often be visualized from the high left parasternal

position. Because variations in great vessel position occur, the spatial orientation must be clarified.

    f. Associated defects with ccTGA must be excluded or defined (systemic AV valve insufficiency, VSD, outflow tract obstruction).

  2. Catheterization is **not necessary** for diagnosis of ccTGA but may be helpful in preoperative planning with regard to the hemodynamic significance of associated lesions. In rare instances ccTGA is diagnosed in the catheterization that was not recognized at routine echocardiography. An unusual arterial catheter course is caused by the anterior and leftward position of the aorta in most instances. The left-sided coronary artery typically arises from the posterior sinus and assumes a right coronary branching distribution, whereas the right-sided coronary artery arises from the anterior and rightward sinus and assumes a typical left coronary branching distribution (see Fig. 34-1). The ventricular septum often lies in the sagittal plane, so ventriculography is usually best performed in the straight posteroanterior and lateral projections.

E. Therapy

  1. Medical management is dictated primarily by the associated malformations. In the rare case of isolated ccTGA, the risk for development of conduction abnormalities is cumulative over time. Permanent pacemaker placement often is needed. The systemic AV valve and ventricle also show signs of failure that necessitate initiation of anticongestive measures in the form of diuretics and afterload reduction. Associated lesions such as pulmonary stenosis or atresia, severe systemic AV valve regurgitation, or VSD may likewise contribute to the medical treatment of these patients but often also necessitate surgical intervention. Periodic Holter monitoring is warranted because of the increased risk for acquired conduction abnormalities.

  2. Surgical treatment

    a. Infants and children who are brought to medical attention early often need surgical intervention in the form of relief of pulmonary outflow tract obstruction or placement of palliative shunts, depending on the associated lesions.

    b. For selected **children,** a double switch procedure may be performed but may necessitate a period of retraining of the left ventricle by means of pulmonary artery banding. The double switch procedure consists of baffling atrial blood to the appropriate ventricle (oxygenated blood diverted from the left atrium rightward to the right-sided left ventricle and vice versa). Arterial switch is performed in the same operation to restore physiologic AV and anatomic ventriculoarterial concordance. The long-term results of this procedure have yet to be determined.

    c. Adult patients with symptoms of progressive systemic AV valvular insufficiency may need valve repair or replacement. Most centers that have reported results with this procedure have found improved functional status after surgical treatment and acceptable risks. The timing of surgical intervention among patients with less severe symptoms is a topic of debate.

II. Ebstein's anomaly. This anomaly of the tricuspid valve represents less than 1% of congenital heart defects. The natural history of this lesion varies from early death to adult survival depending on the degree of tricuspid valve involvement and the presence and type of arrhythmias. An increased risk for sudden death irrespective of functional class, presumably caused by arrhythmia, has been observed. Predictors of poor outcome include earlier age at presentation, cardiomegaly, severe right ventricular (RV) outflow abnormalities, and disproportionate dilatation of the right atrium relative to the other chambers. There is an association with maternal lithium administration.

A. Anatomy
1. The **tricuspid valve** is morphologically and functionally abnormal. The basic features include adherence of the posterior and septal leaflets to the myocardium, which lowers the functional annulus toward the RV apex. This results in a classic atrialization of the right ventricle (Fig. 34-2). The anterior leaflet usually is not displaced.
2. **Associated structural anomalies** include a patent foramen ovale or atrial septal defect and pulmonary stenosis.

B. Clinical presentation
1. **Signs and symptoms**
   a. The presence of a severely insufficient valve can be apparent **at birth** because of cyanosis caused by right to left shunting at the atrial level. In subtle cases, the anomaly may not come to attention until **adulthood** and then causes nonspecific descriptions of fatigue, shortness of breath, palpitations, near syncope, or syncope. Because the spectrum of involvement varies greatly, a high index of suspicion must be maintained.
   b. Ebstein's anomaly is **associated** with the presence of accessory pathways and clinical Wolff-Parkinson-White syndrome in 10% to 25% of patients. Arrhythmias are not uncommon; they include supraventricular tachycardia mediated by an accessory pathway or caused by atrial arrhythmias from progressive atrial dilatation. The combination of atrial fibrillation or flutter conducted rapidly across an accessory pathway is poorly tolerated.
2. **Physical examination**
   a. **General inspection** usually reveals normal jugular venous pulsations despite severe tricuspid regurgitation, which is masked by a large, compliant atrium. Cyanosis may be present as a result of right to left shunting at the atrial level.
   b. The most common **auscultatory findings** are the regurgitant murmur of tricuspid insufficiency, gallop rhythms, multiple systolic ejection sounds, and a widely split S_2.

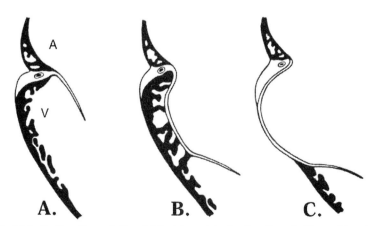

FIG. 34-2. Section through the right atrioventricular junction. **A:** Normal heart. *A*, Right atrium; *V*, right ventricle. **B:** Mild degree of Ebstein's anomaly. **C:** Severe Ebstein's anomaly. In **B** and **C** apparent displacement of the tricuspid valve is present. (From Adams FH, Emmanouilides GC, Riemenschneider TA, eds. *Moss' Heart Disease in Infants, Children, and Adolescents*, 4th ed. Baltimore: Williams & Wilkins, 1989, with permission.)

C. Laboratory examination
   1. **Chest radiography** may reveal cardiomegaly caused by right atrial enlargement from the tricuspid insufficiency.
   2. **ECG** can demonstrate PR prolongation, right atrial enlargement, and superior axis with or without right bundle branch block (Fig. 34-3). The preexcitation pattern if present is almost always type B (left bundle branch pattern).

D. Diagnostic evaluation
   1. The diagnosis can be confirmed with transthoracic or transesophageal **echocardiography** with the tricuspid valve readily visualized in the parasternal short axis, apical four-chamber, and subcostal views. Left lateral decubitus positioning may be helpful in examinations of older patients.
      a. Echocardiographic assessment of the **tricuspid valve** describes the degree of displacement of the posterior and septal leaflets and the degree of dysplasia. In less obvious cases, only tethering of the septal leaflet may be apparent with careful and directed inspection. An imperforate valve may rarely occur and should be interrogated for Doppler evidence of antegrade flow.
      b. The **anterior leaflet** may produce functional obstruction of the pulmonary outflow tract. The leaflet in this circumstance often is called *sail-like*. The pulmonary outflow is carefully studied to discern functional obstruction from such a leaflet as opposed to true anatomic atresia of pulmonary outflow.
      c. Views of the **atrial septum** are included in all studies to assess the size of the atrial septal defect and degree of shunting if present.
      d. The size of the **right ventricle** and true tricuspid annulus are assessed because size guides the feasibility of surgical intervention.
      e. The size and function of the **left ventricle** are assessed. The shape of the left ventricle may be unusual because of extreme leftward bowing of the ventricular septum. Left ventricular function can thus be affected; abnormalities may affect long-term outcome.
      f. **Associated lesions** must be excluded, such as atrial septal defect, RV outflow tract obstruction, patent ductus arteriosus, and in rare instances mitral valve abnormalities with associated insufficiency.
   2. **Cardiac catheterization** is **not necessary** for diagnostic evaluation of Ebstein's anomaly except to exclude coronary artery disease among adult patients with risk factors for whom surgical intervention is planned. Increased risk for cardiac arrest during catheterization has been reported. Diagnostic study may be indicated in the presence of associated hemodynamic abnormalities as part of preoperative planning.

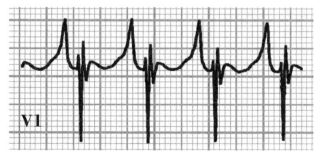

FIG. 34-3. Lead V1 of an electrocardiogram from a newborn infant with Ebstein's anomaly demonstrates marked right atrial enlargement and an rSR′ pattern.

   3. Formal **electrophysiologic study** may be considered for patients with arrhythmias or who are to being considered for surgical treatment. Radiofrequency ablation of accessory pathways is performed.
E. **Treatment**
   1. A large number of adult patients may undergo **medical treatment.** Particular attention must be focused on the management of atrial dysrhythmias, which become more common with age.
   2. **Surgical correction** usually is recommended for patients with symptomatic atrial enlargement and rhythm disturbances. The tricuspid valve may be repaired primarily, or complete replacement may be necessary. Patients with symptomatic cardiomegaly, cyanosis, or arrhythmias are considered for surgical intervention. Favorable results have been achieved at experienced centers in the care of adult patients, and functional class has improved after therapy.
III. **Marfan syndrome**
A. **Introduction.** Marfan syndrome is estimated to affect one in 10,000 persons. The genetic basis for this multisystem connective tissue disorder is now known to be mutations in the fibrillin (*FBN1*) gene on chromosome 15. An increasing number of different mutations of the gene have been found, which explains the heterogeneity of this autosomal dominant disorder within and between affected families. The family history is positive among 65% to 75% of patients, the others representing sporadic cases. A median age at death 30 to 35 years has been reported among untreated patients. Life expectancy is markedly reduced because of the risk for aortic root dilatation and subsequent regurgitation, dissection, or rupture. Prompt diagnosis, careful follow-up examinations, and earlier surgical intervention have improved outcome drastically.
B. **Clinical features**
   1. **Signs and symptoms.** Patients with Marfan syndrome usually come to attention because of **phenotypic features** rather than symptoms. Most symptoms when present are caused by **associated cardiovascular abnormalities.** Congestive symptoms may be caused by aortic insufficiency. Classic descriptions of tearing chest pain may be inapparent. Thus the index of suspicion remains high for **any patient with even vague chest or abdominal discomfort.** This is especially true for patients with a family history of aortic dissection or rupture.
   2. **Physical examination** of the cardiovascular system may reveal systolic clicks or murmurs of mitral causation or the diastolic murmur of aortic insufficiency. A diastolic murmur at presentation has been associated with a poor prognosis. Among children mitral valve regurgitation can predominate and be followed by aortic root dilatation and insufficiency.
   3. The diagnosis of Marfan syndrome is made when specific criteria are met. The **diagnostic criteria** have been revised in an attempt to avoid overdiagnosis or misdiagnosis. These more stringent major and minor criteria are summarized in Table 34-1.
   4. The **differential diagnosis** can be extensive (Table 34-2.)
C. **Laboratory examination**
   1. **Chest radiography** may reveal cardiomegaly, which has been associated with a poor long-term prognosis. In rare instances a dilated aortic arch is apparent on plain radiographs.
   2. **ECG** typically reveals sinus rhythm. Left ventricular hypertrophy and left atrial enlargement also may be seen.
D. **Diagnostic evaluation**
   1. **Echocardiography** remains the primary means by which cardiovascular involvement is diagnosed. Aortic root measurements are made from the parasternal long-axis view at the level of the annulus, sinus of Valsalva, supraaortic ridge, and transverse aorta. Published nomograms are available for comparison. Values above the 95th percentile for body surface area are to be considered abnormal. Equally critical in the evaluation are serial examinations to document **rates of progression** if any.

Table 34-1. Diagnostic criteria for Marfan syndrome

Major criteria	Minor criteria
SKELETAL[a]	
Pectus carinatum	Pectus excavatum
Pectus excavatum necessitating surgical treatment	Joint hypermobility
	High arched palate
Reduced upper-to-lower segment ratio *or* arms span–to–height ratio >1.05	Facial
	Dolichocephaly
Wrist and thumb signs	Malar hypoplasia
Scoliosis >20 degress *or* spondylos- listhesis	Enophthalmos
	Retrognathia
Reduced extension at the elbows (<170 degrees)	Down-slanting palpebral fissures
Medial displacement of the medial malleolus causing pes planus	*Involvement: 2 major criteria or 1 major and 2 minor*
Protrusio acetabulli of any degree (ascertained on ragiographs)	
OCULAR	
Ectopia lentis	Flat cornea
	Increased axial length of the globe (<23.5 mm)
	Hypoplastic iris *or*
	Hypoplastic ciliary muscle causing decreased miosis
	Involvement: 2 minor criteria
CARDIOVASCULAR	
Dilatation of the ascending aorta with or without aortic regurgitation and involving at least the sinuses of Valsalva	Mitral valve prolapse with or without regurgitation
Dissection of the ascending aorta	Dilatation of the main pulmonary artery in the absence of valvular or periph- eral pulmonic stenosis before 40 years of age
	Dilatation or dissection of the descend- ing thoracic or abdominal aorta before 50 years of age
	Involvement: 1 minor criterion
PULMONARY	
—	Spontaneous pneumothorax
	Apical blebs
	Involvement: 1 minor criterion
SKIN AND INTEGUMENT	
—	Striae atrophica
	Recurrent incisional hernia
	Involvement: 1 minor criterion
DURA	
Lumbosacral dural ectasia at computed tomography or magnetic resonance imaging	—

(Continued)

Table 34-1. *(continued)*

Major criteria	Minor criteria
FAMILY AND GENETIC HISTORY	
First-degree relative who independently meets the diagnostic criterion: presence of mutation in *FBN1*	—
Presence of haplotype around *FBN1* inherited by descent and unequivocally associated with diagnosed Marfan syndrome in the family	

Diagnostic criteria for index case: major criteria in two different organ systems and involvement of a third system or in the presence of a known Marfan mutation, one major criterion in an organ system, and involvement of a second organ system. For a relative of an index case; one major criterion in family history with presence of one major criterion in a single organ system and involvement of a second organ system.
a Presence of at least four major criteria.
Adapted from Milewicz DM, 1998, with permission.

Associated echocardiographic findings include mitral valve prolapse, mitral regurgitation, and aortic regurgitation.
2. **Magnetic resonance imaging** is commonly used at many centers to provide a reliable means of tracking changes in the entire aorta, which is often poorly visualized in adults. Aortic dissection localized to the descending or abdominal aorta is better visualized with this modality.
E. **Therapy**
1. **Medical management**
   a. **Genetic counseling** is provided to patients and their families. Women with Marfan syndrome are counseled with regard to the high risk for maternal aortic complications with childbearing and the 50% chance of passing on this autosomal dominant disorder.
   b. **β-Adrenergic blockade** has been used to slow the rate of aortic dilatation and reduce the risk for aortic complications.
   c. Patients with Marfan syndrome are **advised against contact sports** because of ophthalmologic, cardiac, and skeletal risks. Strenuous isometric exercises should be avoided.
   d. Preoperative **antibiotic prophylaxis** is advised for patients with valvular involvement associated with insufficiency. It also is administered after surgical repair.

Table 34-2. Differential diagnosis of Marfan syndrome

Congenital contractural arachnodactyly
Ehlers-Danlos syndrome
Familial aortic dissection
Familial ectopia lentis
Familial Marfan-like habitus
Homocystinuria
Klinefelter's syndrome
MASS phenotype (myopia, mitral valve prolapse, mild aortic dilatation, skin and skeletal involvement)
Multiple endocrine neoplasia type II (MEN II)
Osteogenesis imperfecta
Shprintzen-Goldberg syndrome
Sotos' syndrome
Stickler syndrome

2. **Surgical therapy** in the form of aortic root replacement is generally recommended when the aortic root exceeds 50 to 55 mm in adults, preferably before the onset of aortic insufficiency. The exact dimension remains a matter of debate because other factors are considered. A rapid rate of dilatation, regardless of the absolute measurement, prompts earlier consideration for surgical intervention. This is particularly true among families with a history of aortic dissection or rupture. Some patients may need mitral valve repair or replacement separately or in the same operation. Current postoperative outcome at experienced centers has improved with early mortality rates approaching 1% to 2%. Results have been much lower, however, in the setting of aortic dissection.

F. **Pregnancy and Marfan syndrome**
   1. There is a 50% risk for transmission of this autosomal dominant disorder to offspring. Of importance is the wide variability of clinical expression such that offspring may be more or less affected.
   2. The risk for **maternal death during pregnancy** is increased but varies with respect to cardiovascular findings.
      a. Women in whom the **aortic root measures less than 40 mm** before or early in pregnancy are thought to be at acceptable risk. Aortic dissection, however, remains a potential complication and prompts continued serial follow-up examinations throughout gestation.
      b. Pregnancy is **discouraged** among patients with cardiovascular findings such as aortic dilatation (generally greater than 40 mm or with a previously documented rapid rate of increase), aortic insufficiency, or marked mitral regurgitation. Family history of aortic dissection also is a risk factor.
      c. Patients are closely observed in a multidisciplinary setting. Serial transthoracic or transesophageal echocardiography at 6- to 10-week intervals has been advocated, but the schedule is tailored to the individual patient.
      d. The use of β-**blockers** during pregnancy is generally accepted but is weighed against the reported adverse side effects to the fetus such as intrauterine growth retardation, fetal bradycardia, hyperbilirubinemia, hypoglycemia, and apnea after delivery.

IV. **Index of postoperative anatomy among adult patients with congenital heart disease**
   A. **Postoperative states for single-ventricle physiologic mechanisms.** A patient with a functional single ventricle typically proceeds with palliation, including the Norwood, Glenn, and ultimately Fontan procedures. Examples of congenital defects that may necessitate such palliation include hypoplastic left heart, tricuspid atresia, pulmonary atresia with intact ventricular septum, or unbalanced complete AV canal.
      1. The **Norwood** operation or its modification is usually the first of three stages toward palliation of a single-ventricle physiologic status. The procedure establishes a single outlet for the single ventricle by incorporating native aorta and pulmonary artery (one of which may be hypoplastic or atretic) to produce a "neoaorta." The main pulmonary artery is transected from the heart. Pulmonary flow is maintained with placement of a Blalock-Taussig shunt from the subclavian artery or innominate artery to the right or left pulmonary artery. Atrial septectomy is typically performed in this setting to allow complete mixing at the atrial level. Infants soon outgrow the Blalock-Taussig shunt and need a Glenn or larger shunt.
      2. The bidirectional **Glenn** procedure involves anastomosis of the superior vena cava to the pulmonary artery, usually with takedown of a previously placed systemic to pulmonary artery shunt and repair of pulmonary arterial branch stenosis if necessary. The pulmonary arteries usually remain in continuity; thus the term *bidirectional* is used in descriptions of this procedure. This operation usually is performed when the patient is 4 to

6 months of age if pulmonary arterial anatomy, pressures, and resistance are adequate.

3. The **Fontan** procedure represents the final palliative procedure for single-ventricle physiologic status. This procedure completes the direction of the remaining systemic venous blood from the inferior vena cava and hepatic veins to the pulmonary arteries. This is accomplished in most cases by means of an intraatrial lateral tunnel, which courses from the lateral and inferior aspect of the right atrium. The atrial appendage or superior vena caval stump transected during the Glenn procedure is directed to the pulmonary artery, effectively "septating" the circulation. Pulmonary blood flow is achieved passively without the assistance of a ventricular pumping chamber. For this reason it is imperative to have low pulmonary pressures and vascular resistance.

B. Repair or palliation of **d-transposition of the great arteries** (dTGA). In this lesion, there is ventriculoarterial discordance such that the aorta is anterior and related to the right ventricle, whereas the pulmonary artery is committed to the left ventricle and is positioned posterior and leftward.

1. **Arterial switch (Jantene procedure)** is the preferred surgical procedure for neonates with uncomplicated TGA and is performed on an increasing number of patients who need follow-up therapy as young adults. The arterial switch restores ventriculoarterial concordance. The great arteries are transected and reanastomosed to the appropriate ventricle. The coronary arteries are removed with a button of surrounding tissue and reimplanted to the appropriate sinuses.

2. A **Mustard or Senning** operation is a palliative procedure that essentially redirects blood at the atrial level in patients with dTGA. Either baffle material (Mustard) or native atrial tissue (Senning) is used to baffle pulmonary venous blood to the right ventricle, which is connected to the aorta. Systemic venous blood is baffled at the atrial level leftward to the left ventricle, which is committed to the pulmonary artery. Normal saturations are established in the absence of baffle leaks.

3. The **Rastelli procedure** allows complete anatomic repair of dTGA, VSD, and pulmonary stenosis. The VSD is closed with a patch in such a manner that left ventricular blood is routed across the VSD to the aorta. RV outflow is established by means of placement of a conduit from the right ventricle to the pulmonary artery.

C. Systemic to pulmonary artery **shunts** are commonly used to produce or supplement pulmonary arterial flow. They are typically needed when deficiencies of the RV outflow tract are present, such as pulmonary atresia or tetralogy of Fallot with hypoplastic pulmonary arteries.

1. A **classic Blalock-Taussig** shunt simply directs the native subclavian artery to the right or left pulmonary artery.

2. A **Waterson** shunt is an anastomosis between the ascending aorta and right pulmonary artery.

3. A **Potts** shunt is an anastomosis between the descending aorta and left pulmonary artery.

4. A **modified Blalock-Taussig** shunt is a communication between the subclavian artery or innominate artery and the pulmonary artery and is usually of expanded polytetrafluoroethylene (Gore-Tex) material of variable diameter.

SUGGESTED READINGS

Landmark Articles

Connelly MS, Liu PP, Williams WG, et al. Congenitally corrected transposition of the great arteries in the adult: functional status and complications. *J Am Coll Cardiol* 1996;27:1238–1243.

De Paepe A, Devereux RB, Dietz HC, et al. Revised diagnostic criteria for the Marfan syndrome. *Am J Med Genet* 1996;62:417–426.

Dietz HC, Cutting GR, Pyeritz RE, et al. Marfan syndrome caused by a recurrent de novo missense mutation in the fibrillin gene. *Nature* 1991;352:337–339.

Dimas AP, Moodie DS, Sterba R, Gill CC. Long-term function of the morphologic right ventricle in adult patients with corrected transposition of the great arteries. *Am Heart J* 1989;118:526–530.

Elkayam U, Ostrzega I, Shotan A, Mehra A. Cardiovascular problems in pregnant women with the Marfan syndrome. *Ann Intern Med* 1995;123:117–122.

Gillinov AM, Zehr KJ, Redmond JM, et al. Cardiac operations in children with Marfan's syndrome: indications and results. *Ann Thorac Surg* 1997;64:1140–1145.

Gray JR, Davies SJ. Marfan syndrome. *J Med Genet* 1996;33:403–408.

Kainulainen K, Pulkkinen L, Savollainen A, et al. Location on chromosome 15 of the gene defect causing Marfan syndrome. *N Engl J Med* 1990;323:935–939.

Karl TR, Weintraub RG, Brizard CP, et al. Senning plus arterial switch operation for discordant (congenitally corrected) transposition. *Ann Thorac Surg* 1997;64:495–502.

Lundstrom U, Bull C, Wyse RKH, Somerville J. The natural and unnatural history of congenitally corrected transposition. *Am J Cardiol* 1990;65:1222–1229.

Marsalese DL, Moodie DS, Vacante M, et al. Marfan's syndrome: natural history and long-term follow-up of cardiovascular involvement. *J Am Coll Cardiol* 1989;14:422–428.

Penny DJ, Somerville J, Redington AN. Echocardiographic demonstration of important abnormalities of the mitral valve in congenitally corrected transposition. *Br Heart J* 1992;68:498–500.

Presbitero P, Somerville J, Rabajoli F, et al. Corrected transposition of the great arteries without associated defects in adult patients: clinical profile and follow up. *Br Heart J* 1995;74:57–59.

Pyeritz RE, McKusick VA. The Marfan syndrome: diagnosis and management. *N Engl J Med* 1979;300:772–777.

Roman MJ, Devereux RB, Kramer-Fox R, O'Loughlin J. Two-dimensional echocardiographic aortic root dimensions in normal children and adults. *Am J Cardiol* 1989;64:507–512.

Shores J, Berger KR, Murphy EA, et al. Progression of aortic dilatation and the benefit of long-term B-adrenergic blockade in Marfan's syndrome. *N Engl J Med* 1994;330:1335–1341.

Smith JA, Fann JI, Miller DC, et al. Surgical management of aortic dissection in patients with the Marfan syndrome. *Circulation* 1994;90 [Part II]:II-235–II-242.

Van Son, JAM, Danielson GK, Huhta JC, et al. Late results of systemic atrioventricular valve replacement in corrected transposition. *J Thorac Cardiovasc Surg* 1995;109:642–653.

Key Reviews

Connelly MS, Webb GD, Sommerville J, et al. Canadian Consensus Conference on Adult Congenital Heart Disease 1996. *Can J Cardiol* 1998;14:395–452.

Edwards W. Embryology and pathologic features of Ebstein's anomaly. *Progress in Pediatric Cardiology* 1993;2:5–15.

Liao P, Feldt RH. Clinical profile of Ebstein's anomaly. *Progress in Pediatric Cardiology* 1993;2:16–21.

Milewicz DM. Molecular genetics of Marfan syndrome and Ehlers-Danlos type IV. *Curr Opin Cardiol* 1998;13:198–204.

Olson TM, Porter CJ. Electrocardiographic and electrophysiologic findings in Ebstein's anomaly. *Prog Pediatr Cardiol* 1993;2:38–50.

Simpson LL, Athanassious AM, D'Alton ME. Marfan syndrome in pregnancy. *Curr Opin Obstet Gynecol* 1997;9:337–341.

Tuzcu EM, Moodie DS, Ghazi F, et al. Ebstein's anomaly: natural and unnatural history. *Cleve Clin J Med* 1989;56:614–618.

Relevant Chapters

Perloff JK. Survival patterns without cardiac surgery or interventional catheterization: a narrowing base. In: Perloff JK, Child JS, eds. *Congenital heart disease in adults,* 2nd ed. Philadelphia: WB Saunders, 1998:15–53.

Bishop A. Corrected transposition of the great arteries. In: Redington A, Shore D, Oldershaw P, eds. *Congenital heart disease in adults: a practical guide.* London: WB Saunders, 1994:145–153.

Snider AR, Serwer GA, Ritter SB. Abnormalities of ventriculoarterial connection. In: Snider AR, Serwer GA, Ritter SB, eds. *Echocardiography in pediatric heart disease,* 2nd ed. St. Louis: Mosby, 1997:317–323.

MacLellan-Tobert SG, Porter CJ. Ebstein's anomaly of the tricuspid valve. In: Garson A, Bricker JT, Fisher DJ, Neish SR, eds. *The science and practice of pediatric cardiology,* 2nd ed. Baltimore: Williams & Wilkins, 1998:1303–1315.

SECTION VIII. COMMON CARDIOLOGY CONSULTS

Harpreet Bhalla and Brian P. Griffin

35. ASSESSING AND MANAGING CARDIAC RISK IN NONCARDIAC SURGICAL PROCEDURES

Vasant B. Patel

I. Introduction

A. Background. The number of people older than 65 years and the prevalence of cardiovascular disease in the United States are increasing. The number of noncardiac surgical procedures performed on older persons may increase from 6 million to nearly 12 million per year over the next three decades. Major abdominal, thoracic, vascular, and orthopedic procedures carry high risk for perioperative cardiovascular morbidity and mortality, making preoperative risk assessment an important evaluation to reduce perioperative morbidity and mortality. In 1977, Goldman et al. (1) developed a multifactorial index of risk for cardiac morbidity and mortality. Since then, extensive work has been done in various areas of cardiac evaluation—clinical factors and noninvasive testing. The variety of strategies and practices used has led to high costs associated with preoperative risk assessment. The American Heart Association and American College of Cardiology (AHA/ACC) task force committee has developed practice guidelines aimed at providing a more efficient approach to preoperative evaluation.

B. Objective. The purpose of preoperative evaluation is not to clear patients for an operation. The purpose is to **assess current medical status, assess cardiac risks posed by the planned operation,** and **recommend strategies to decrease risk.** The stepwise approach recommended by the AHA/ACC task force in Fig. 35-1 is used to screen patients at substantial risk for cardiac complications during noncardiac operations.

1. Although the preoperative assessment is a complex process, a few **basic questions and observations** by a physician with regard to patient's general health, functional capacity, cardiac risk factors, comorbid medical illnesses, and type of anticipated operation can assist in evaluating cardiac risk.

2. It is not prudent to order noninvasive tests for every patient. The physician tries to obtain as much information as possible by means of **history and physical examination.** Noninvasive tests are requested only if the results are likely to influence treatment.

3. Coronary intervention usually is not necessary to lower the risk of a surgical procedure.

4. Communication is vital between primary physicians, consulting physicians, anesthesiologists, and surgeons for long-term care of patients recognized to be at increased cardiac risk that necessitates long-term management.

II. Clinical presentation

A. Signs and symptoms

1. The clinician needs to **identify cardiac conditions that place a patient at increased risk,** such as recent myocardial infarction (MI), decompensated congestive heart failure (CHF), unstable angina, substantial arrhythmias, and valvular heart disease.

2. Attention is directed at serious **comorbid diseases,** such as diabetes mellitus, peripheral vascular disease, history of stroke, renal disease, and pulmonary disease.

3. **Functional capacity** is determined on the basis of the patient's ability to perform certain daily tasks (Table 35-1).

B. Physical findings. A thorough examination is crucial, and specific findings are addressed.

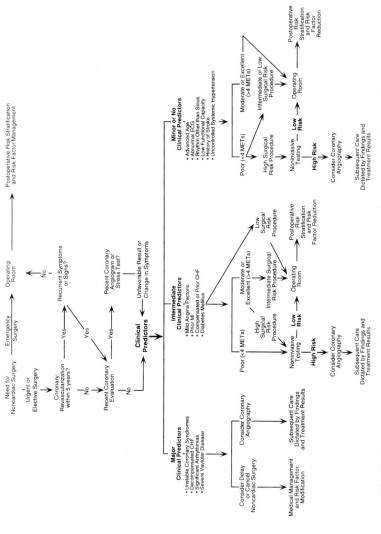

FIG. 35-1. A stepwise approach to preoperative cardiac evaluation of a patient undergoing a non-cardiac operation. (Adapted from Eagle KA, 1996, with permission.)

Table 35-1. Estimated energy requirements for various activities

1 MET

Eat, dress, or use the toilet
Walk indoors around the house
Walk on level ground at 2 mph (3.2 km/hr)
Do light housework such as washing dishes

4 METs

Climb a flight of stairs
Walk on level ground at 4 mph (6.4 km/hr)
Run a short distance
Heavy work such as vacuuming or lifting heavy furniture
Play games such as golf or doubles tennis

>10 METs

Participate in strenous activities such as swimming, singles tennis, basketball, or
    skiing

MET, metabolic equivalent.

1. The **physical examination** includes blood pressure in both arms (supine and standing) and evaluation of carotid arterial pulse (character, volume, and upstroke), jugular venous pulsation, cardiac rhythm, heart sounds (murmurs, gallops, or rub), and extremity pulses.
2. **Lung fields** are auscultated and the **abdomen palpated** for a possible aneurysm.
3. **High surgical risk** is suggested by findings of severe aortic stenosis murmur, elevated jugular venous pressure, pulmonary edema, or S_3 gallop.

C. **Clinical markers and functional assessment.** In general, it is important to evaluate clinical markers (Table 35-2) that identify high risk in the context of the person's functional capacity (see Table 35-1). For example, a sedentary person without history of coronary artery disease who has clinical markers that suggest increased surgical risk may benefit from a more thorough evaluation, whereas a person with known coronary artery disease (CAD) who has excellent functional capacity and no symptoms may need no further evaluation.

III. **Type of operation.** In addition to clinical markers and functional capacity, the proposed operation is an important factor. The consultant uses all the information available to estimate cardiac risk and provide recommendations to minimize perioperative risk.

A. **High-risk operations** are emergency major procedures, especially on the elderly, aortic or peripheral vascular operations, or extensive operations with large volume shifts.

B. **Intermediate-risk operations** are orthopedic, urologic, thoracic, and abdominal procedures, carotid endarterectomy, or head and neck procedures.

C. **Low-risk operations** include cataract or breast operations, endoscopic procedures, or superficial biopsy.

IV. **Laboratory examination**

A. **Routine laboratory tests** such as creatinine, hemoglobin, platelets, potassium, liver profile, and oxygen saturation are important to ascertain whether a patient needs special attention. Patients who do are those with bleeding risk, renal failure, or liver disease.

B. Patients with **pulmonary disease** (chronic obstructive pulmonary disease or pulmonary fibrosis) undergo a preoperative **arterial blood gas evaluation.**

C. An **electrocardiogram (ECG)** may provide additional clues to assist a consultant in determining whether additional preoperative testing and therapy are needed. ECG **findings of relevance** are rhythm other than sinus, more

Table 35-2. Clinical predictors of increased perioperative cardiovascular risk
(myocardial infarction, congestive heart failure, death)

MAJOR PREDICTORS

Unstable coronary syndromes
   Recent myocardial infarction[a] with evidence of important ischemic risk on the
   basis of clinical symptoms or results of noninvasive studies
   Unstable or severe[b] angina (Canadian class 3 or 4)[c]
Decompensated congestive heart failure
Marked arrhythmias
   High-grade atrioventricular block
   Symptomatic ventricular arrhythmias in the presence of underlying heart disease
   Supraventricular arrhythmias with uncontrolled ventricular rate
Severe valvular disease

INTERMEDIATE PREDICTORS

Mild angina pectoris (Canadian class 1 or 2)
Prior myocardial infarction on the basis of history or pathologic Q waves
Compensated or prior congestive heart failure
Diabetes mellitus

MINOR PREDICTORS

Advanced age
Abnormal ECG findings (left ventricular hypertrophy, left bundle branch block,
   ST-T abnormalities)
Rhythm other than sinus (e.g., atrial fibrillation)
Low functional capacity (e.g., inability to climb one flight of stairs with a bag of
   groceries)
History of stroke
Uncontrolled systemic hypertension

---

[a] The American College of Cardiology National Database Library defines recent myocardial infarction as having occurred 7 to 30 days before coming to medical attention.
[b] May include stable angina among patients who are unusually sedentary.
[c] Campeau L. Grading of angina pectoris. *Circulation* 1976;54:522–523.
ECG, electrocardiogram.
From Eagle KA, et al., 1996, with permission.

than five premature ventricular contractions per minute, heart block (especially Mobitz type II or complete heart block), sinus pauses, symptomatic ventricular arrhythmias (ventricular tachycardia, torsades de pointes), supraventricular tachycardia with rapid ventricular rate (atrial fibrillation, flutter, or atrial tachycardia), left ventricular (LV) hypertrophy, prior MI, and bundle branch block.

V. **Criteria for estimating risk.** Cardiac risk is a function of patient characteristics and the proposed operation.

   A. **Goldman criteria.** Goldman et al. (1) developed the Goldman Multifactorial Cardiac Risk Index (Table 35-3) based on their experience with 1,001 consecutive general surgical procedures (1). Goldman et al. identified nine independent variables that predicted perioperative cardiac events and assigned them a point value. Because the Goldman index often underestimated perioperative cardiac risk, Detsky et al. (2) developed a modified multifactorial index to address the severity of CAD and heart failure (Table 35-4). Although the original and modified cardiac risk indices help one ascertain whether a patient is at high surgical risk, these indices do not include important variables such as diabetes mellitus, hypertension, stable angina, or history of stroke.

   B. **Eagle criteria.** Eagle et al. (3) used additional clinical markers and perfusion imaging (see **VI.B** and **VI.C**) for risk stratification. The Eagle criteria,

Table 35-3. Original Goldman multifactorial cardiac risk index

Criteria	Points
History	
Age older than 70 yrs	5
MI in previous 6 months	10
Physical examination	
S_3 gallop or JVD	11
Important valvular AS	3
Electrocardiogram	
Rhythm other than sinus or PACs on last peroperative ECG	7
>5 PVCs/min documented at any time preoperatively	7
General status	
PO_2 <60 or PCO_2 > 50 mm Hg, K <3.0 or HCO3 <20 mEq/L, BUN >50 or Cr >3.0 mg/dL, abnormal AST, signs of chronic liver disease, or patient bedridden from noncardiac causes	3
Operation	
Intraperitoneal, intrathoracic, or aortic operation	3
Emergency operation	4
Total	53

Class	Points	Cardiac deaths (%)
I	0–5	0.2
II	6–12	2.0
III	13–25	2.0
IV	≥26	56.0

MI, Myocardial infarction; *JVD,* jugular venous distention; *AS,* aortic stenosis; *PAC,* premature atrial contractions; *PVC,* premature ventricular contractions; *BUN,* blood urea nitrogen; *Cr,* creatinine; *AST,* aspartate aminotransferase.
Adapted from ref. 1, with permission.

which include age greater than 70 years, Q waves on an ECG, diabetes mellitus, a history of ventricular arrhythmias necessitating treatment, and history of angina or CHF, were found to be independent correlates of postsurgical cardiac events.

1. Patients **at high risk** (50% rate of postsurgical cardiac complications, even in the absence of thallium redistribution) were those with three or more clinical markers.
2. Patients **at intermediate risk** with normal results of thallium imaging studies had a 3.2% rate of postsurgical events, whereas patients at intermediate risk with abnormal results of thallium studies had a 30% likelihood of postsurgical cardiac events.
3. Patients **at low risk** (3.1% postsurgical cardiac complication rate) were those with no clinical markers. Eagle et al. (3) recommended a perfusion imaging study only for patients at intermediate risk undergoing vascular operations.

C. The **ACC/AHA** task force developed a more comprehensive (although less user friendly) set of guidelines for preoperative cardiac evaluation for noncardiac operation (see Fig. 35-1). These guidelines help physicians systematically identify clinical predictors and determine appropriate noninvasive and, when indicated, invasive tests to prepare a patient for an operation.

VI. **Diagnostic testing.** The medical history, physical examination, basic laboratory tests, and ECG help determine whether the surgical risk for a patient is low,

Table 35-4. Modified multifactorial index

Variables	Points
Coronary	
MI within 6 months	10
MI more than 6 months in past	5
Canadian class of angina	
Class 3	10
Class 4	20
Unstable angina within 3 months	10
Alveolar pulmonary edema	
Within 1 week	10
Ever	5
Valvular disease	
Suspected critical aortic stenosis	20
Arrhythmias	
Sinus plus atrial premature beats or rhythm other than sinus on last preoperative electrocardiogram	5
>5 ventricular premature beats at any time before operation	5
Poor general medical status[a]	5
Age older than 70 years	5
Emergency operation	10
Total	120

[a] $P_{O_2} < 60$ mmHg, $P_{CO_2} >50$ mm Hg, $K^+ <3.0$ or $HCO_3 < 20$ mEq/L, BUN ≥ 18 mmol/L, serum Cr >260 mmol/L, abnormal AST, signs of chronic liver disease, or patient bed-ridden because of noncardiac causes.
MI, Myocardial infarction; *BUN,* blood urea nitrogen; *Cr,* createnine; *AST,* aspartate aminotransferase.
Adapted from Detsky AS, 1986, with permission.

moderate, or high. In general, a patient who is at low risk needs no further evaluation. Those who are at high risk usually undergo coronary angiography. Patients who are at intermediate risk usually need additional testing. The following are functional studies for assessing myocardium at risk and functional capacity.

A. Exercise ECG testing is the **modality of choice** when a noninvasive test is necessary to assess functional capacity and the patient can walk.

  1. Cutler et al. (4) reported that patients who can achieve greater than 75% of maximum predicted heart rate without ischemic ECG changes are at the lowest risk for postoperative cardiac complications. Those with an abnormal ECG response at greater than 75% of maximum predicted heart rate are at intermediate risk. Those with an abnormal ECG response at less than 75% of maximum predicted heart rate have the highest rate of complications.

  2. The **advantages** of this modality are that it provides an estimate of functional capacity, helps detect myocardial ischemia, and provides information about hemodynamic response during stress.

  3. The **limitations** are abnormal baseline ECGs because of LV hypertrophy, digitalis effect, and bundle branch block.

  4. The mean **sensitivity and specificity** of exercise testing for obstructive coronary disease are 68% and 77%, respectively. The sensitivity and specificity for multivessel disease are 81% and 66% and for three-vessel or left main coronary disease, 86% and 53%.

B. Stress myocardial perfusion imaging

  1. For patients with known CAD, abnormal baseline ECG, LV hypertrophy, or bundle branch blocks, perfusion imaging with thallium 201, technetium Tc 99m sestamibi, or technetium Tc 99m teboroxime is performed to assess myocardial regions at risk for ischemia.

2. For patients with two or more Eagle criteria or those undergoing high-risk operations, stress myocardial perfusion imaging is preferred over routine exercise stress testing.

3. Perfusion imaging improves the overall sensitivity and specificity of regular exercise treadmill testing to 90% and 95%, respectively. The positive predictive value is only 15% to 30% for postoperative events.

C. **Pharmacologic myocardial perfusion imaging** is an alternative modality to exercise testing and is used most in the care of patients who are undergoing orthopedic, neurosurgical, or vascular surgical procedures and are unable to exercise. Dipyridamole myocardial perfusion imaging and dobutamine echocardiography are commonly used tests. These imaging modalities help ascertain whether a patient is at surgical risk for perioperative cardiac complications, and the results have long-term prognostic value.

1. **Dipyridamole perfusion imaging.** Qualitative and quantitative assessment of thallium redistribution helps ascertain whether a patient is at high surgical risk.

   a. **Important findings** at dipyridamole imaging are as follows:

      (1) More than four myocardial segments demonstrating redistribution, which indicates greater risk for perioperative events than redistribution in three or fewer segments (16% versus 4%).

      (2) Redistribution in three coronary artery territories, which indicates higher risk for events than redistribution in two coronary artery territories (43% versus 17%).

      (3) Reversible LV cavity dilatation, which indicates that a cardiac event is likely.

   b. Stratmann et al. (5) evaluated late cardiac events among 172 medically treated patients undergoing peripheral vascular operations after preoperative technetium Tc 99m dipyridamole sestamibi scans. Late cardiac events occurred among 15% of the patients. Those who had abnormal sestamibi scan results had a significantly greater event rate than those with normal sestamibi scan results (26% versus 4%). The rate of late cardiac events was 33% among patients with a reversible defect and 23% in those with a fixed defect (Fig. 35-2). The study points to the fact that **although patients survive the operation, they retain preoperative cardiac risk.**

   c. **Dipyridamole imaging is avoided** in the evaluation of patients taking long-term theophylline therapy and patients with severe pulmonary obstructive disease or critical carotid stenosis.

2. **Dobutamine stress echocardiography (DSE)** is an excellent tool in assessing risk among patients with significant CAD, especially if there is a question of valvular disease. Although the criteria for positive and negative test results differed in the studies reported thus far, the study protocols were similar.

   a. **Important findings** include new wall motion abnormalities, the degree of wall motion abnormality, and the presence of wall motion abnormalities at low infusion rates. Poldermans et al. (6) studied late cardiac events among patients with clinical risk factors who underwent dobutamine echocardiography before vascular operations. **Extensive ischemia** (three or more segments) or **limited ischemia** (one or two segments) at DSE and **previous MI** at clinical evaluation were independent predictors of late cardiac events.

   b. Kontos et al. (7) found **DSE to be comparable with dipyridamole thallium testing** as a preoperative evaluation tool in predicting major cardiac complications of noncardiac operations.

   c. DSE is **especially useful** in evaluations of **women.**

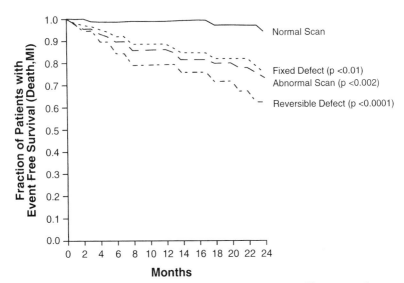

FIG. 35-2. Late cardiac events after vascular operations assessed by means of preoperative technetium 99m Tc dipyridamole sestamibi myocardial tomography. Patients with normal scan findings had higher event-free survival rates than patients with abnormal scan findings. Patients with reversible defects had lower event-free survival rates than those with fixed defects. (Adapted from ref. 5, with permission.)

       d. Dobutamine is avoided in evaluations of patients with severe hypertension, hemodynamically significant ventricular arrhythmias, or poor echocardiographic images.

  D. Ambulatory ECG monitoring. Although several studies have reported the favorable utility of ECG monitoring in preoperative evaluation, there are several **limitations,** including abnormal baseline ECGs and an inability to quantify myocardium at risk. However, this modality may be used for **monitoring in the postoperative period** for ischemic ECG changes.

  E. The indications for **coronary angiography** before noncardiac operation are the same as the indications for angiography in general. It is most helpful in the following situations:

    1. Evaluation of patients with **angina pectoris** unresponsive to medical therapy or with unstable angina pectoris

    2. Evaluation of patients whose results at noninvasive testing placed them in the high-risk category

    3. Nondiagnostic, noninvasive testing for patients at high risk undergoing a high-risk procedure

    4. An urgent noncardiac operation on a patient recovering from acute MI

VII. Therapy

  A. Preoperative management of specific cardiac conditions

    1. Valvular heart disease. It is important to recognize and manage critical valvular lesions before an operation.

      a. Critical **aortic stenosis** must be recognized promptly and if symptomatic managed with valve replacement, or for selected patients valvuloplasty, before a noncardiac operation.

      b. Mitral stenosis when mild and asymptomatic is managed medically with heart rate control. When mitral stenosis is severe or symptomatic, mitral valvuloplasty or valve replacement is considered before a high-risk operation is performed.

   c. For patients with **aortic or mitral regurgitation** the medical regimen is optimized with diuretics and afterload reduction as needed. Appropriate prophylaxis for bacterial endocarditis is administered.

   d. Patients with **prosthetic valves** who need oral anticoagulation can safely undergo minimally invasive procedures such as dental work or skin biopsy if the international normalized ratio is briefly reduced to a low or subtherapeutic range. Full anticoagulation is resumed after the procedure. For patients undergoing extensive surgical procedures with prosthetic valves, heparin therapy is initiated. Oral anticoagulants are resumed after the procedure. Appropriate antibiotic prophylaxis for bacterial endocarditis is administered.

2. **Arrhythmias and conduction disease.** For patients with arrhythmias, the metabolic profile and medications are reviewed and any underlying derangement managed.

   a. Most **supraventricular tachycardias** necessitate rate control until the underlying cause is managed. In the setting of hemodynamic compromise or ongoing myocardial ischemia, electrical cardioversion is the therapy of choice.

   b. **Ventricular arrhythmias** for the most part do not require special attention except in the care of patients with sustained or symptomatic ventricular tachycardia. These patients are treated with preoperative suppressive therapy with lidocaine or procainamide.

   c. Symptomatic **bradyarrhythmias are** managed with temporary pacing and a permanent pacemaker implanted when indicated.

   d. **Permanent pacemakers** are checked. In operations on patients who are totally pacemaker dependent, electrocautery is used only briefly and with caution. Bipolar pacing minimizes the risk of electrocautery. After the operation, all pacemakers are interrogated to ensure that the settings are optimal and that no changes occurred during the operation or electrocautery. Implanted defibrillators are programmed to *off* and then reprogrammed to *on* after the procedure.

3. **Hypertension.** In general, patients with hypertension **are monitored closely during an operation** because they have a tendency toward intraoperative hypotension.

   a. Patients with **mild to moderate** hypertension may undergo elective operations with continued medical therapy.

   b. **Severe** hypertension (diastolic pressure greater than 110 mm Hg) is controlled before the operation. If possible, the operation is delayed until the pressure is consistently controlled. If urgent surgical intervention is needed, rapid-acting agents are used. β-Blockers are preferred, especially because they act as antiischemic agents.

   c. Withdrawal of β-blockers and clonidine from patients undergoing long-term therapy with these agents **must be avoided** to prevent a rebound phenomenon.

4. **Cardiomyopathy.** The treatment of patients with cardiomyopathy **depends on the cause** and overall clinical status.

   a. Patients with **severe LV dysfunction** may benefit from placement of pulmonary arterial catheters to optimize hemodynamic status before and during an operation.

   b. Patients **with hypertrophic cardiomyopathy** need close monitoring of volume status, heart rate, and systemic vascular resistance to avoid intraoperative hypotension or heart failure.

5. **Coronary artery disease.** In evaluations of patients with known coronary atherosclerosis, the **important issues** to clarify are the amount of myocardium at risk, the threshold of stress at which ischemia occurs, and whether the patient is a candidate for revascularization.

   a. Presurgical revascularization

     (1) Patients who are candidates for revascularization undergo noninvasive testing to assess ischemic threshold and undergo revascularization if indicated before the noncardiac operation. Patients who are not candidates for coronary revascularization may need no further testing.

   (2) **Coronary artery bypass grafting (CABG)**

      (a) There are no results of randomized controlled trials to assess the benefit of **coronary artery bypass grafting (CABG)** before noncardiac operations. Results of several retrospective studies, however, have indicated that patients with severe CAD who underwent CABG before the other operation had a low perioperative mortality with the noncardiac operation.

      (b) When the **appropriate subset** of patients undergoes revascularization before a noncardiac operation, **the outcome is favorable,** as reported in the European Coronary Surgery Study Group, data from the Cleveland Clinic in 1984 and the Coronary Artery Surgery Study (CASS) registry. Eagle et al. for the CASS investigators reported results for 3,368 patients who underwent noncardiac operations (8). The mean follow-up period was 4.1 years. The patients who underwent CABG before an abdominal, vascular, thoracic, or head and neck operation had a significantly lower rate of postoperative death and MI than patients who underwent preoperative medical treatment.

      (c) In contrast, patients undergoing urologic, orthopedic, breast, and skin operations had a similar mortality regardless of prior coronary revascularization. The indications for CABG are similar to those recommended by the ACC/AHA task force.

   (3) **Coronary angioplasty** may be a reasonable alternative for certain patients. Allen et al. (9) in a retrospective study reported favorable outcomes of angioplasty among patients with symptomatic CAD; however, the sample size was rather small. Because there are limited data at present, **no definite criteria exist for prophylactic angioplasty,** although it has a role in the care of selected patients with severe CAD. It is generally recommended to wait several days after angioplasty before proceeding with the noncardiac operation. An acceptable waiting period is 2 to 6 weeks to allow acute complications to resolve and allow performance of the noncardiac operation before restenosis occurs.

 b. Whether or not prophylactic revascularization is performed, the **perioperative use of β-blockers** has been shown to be beneficial in a few randomized trials. In general, perioperative β-blocker therapy is recommended in the care of patients who have **hypertension or symptomatic arrhythmias** and patients who need long-term β-blocker therapy for **angina.**

 c. **Nitroglycerin** is recommended for patients at high risk who were taking it before the operation and have active signs of myocardial ischemia without hypotension.

 d. The role of **calcium antagonists** is not well defined.

6. Carotid artery disease. Over the past 30 years, morbidity, mortality, and patient comfort have improved considerably among patients undergoing carotid endarterectomy.

 a. Cardiac events have been reported among patients undergoing carotid endarterectomy. Urbinati et al. (10) evaluated early and late cardiac events among 106 patients undergoing carotid endarterectomy with neither history nor symptoms of CAD who underwent exercise thallium imaging. Overall, there were no cardiac events within 30 days of the operation. The event-free survival rate at 7 years was

51% among patients with redistribution on stress thallium images and 98% among patients with normal scan results preoperatively.

   b. The **treatment strategy** for patients with significant carotid artery disease and CAD **remains somewhat controversial.**

      (1) Several studies have reported on the combined approach (carotid endarterectomy and CABG) versus a staged approach (carotid endarterectomy followed by CABG) to surgical revascularization. The studies, however, vary widely in stroke and mortality rates because of wide variability in patient selection criteria.

      (2) There are no compelling data to prove the superiority of one approach over the other. The staged approach is associated with a lower stroke rate (5.3%) but a higher rate of MI (11.5%) and death (9.4%). In contrast, the combined approach has yielded lower MI (4.7%) and mortality rates (5.6%) and a slightly higher stroke rate (6.2%).

      (3) In general, the **strategy is individualized.** Combined carotid and coronary revascularization is reserved for patients with severe neurologic symptoms and unstable angina. There is inadequate evidence to recommend carotid endarterectomy to manage asymptomatic disease in combination with CABG.

B. Perioperative management. Postoperative MIs are rare (less than 1%); however, the mortality rate may be as high as 50%. MIs that occur usually do so by postoperative day 3, most within 24 hours. Postoperative MIs are more often non-Q-wave and often are asymptomatic, given the lingering effects of anesthesia and postoperative analgesia.

   1. Presentation. Nonspecific findings, such as CHF, hypotension, nausea, or ST-segment depression, may be the only clues to postoperative ischemia.

   2. Anesthetic agents and techniques. Several studies have evaluated the effect of anesthetic agents and techniques on cardiac morbidity. It appears that there is **no one best myocardial protective agent or technique.** All inhalational agents cause depression of myocardial contractility and afterload reduction, which can lead to hypotension. More important is the role of perioperative pain management because it reduces postoperative catecholamine response and thus cardiac stress.

   3. Perioperative monitoring

      a. For patients with known CAD, a baseline ECG is obtained immediately after the operation and daily on the first two postoperative days.

      b. For **patients without known CAD,** no further testing is necessary unless there is intraoperative hemodynamic dysfunction or cardiac complications.

      c. In general, **cardiac enzymes** are measured for patients at high risk or those with intraoperative hemodynamic dysfunction.

   4. Although use of **transesophageal echocardiography** is increasing to monitor myocardial ischemia through wall motion abnormalities, there is insufficient information to make firm recommendations.

   5. Several studies have reported **ST-segment changes** of ischemia during an operation as an independent predictor of perioperative cardiac events. Postoperative ST-segment changes are predictive of worse long-term survival among patients at high risk. Therefore, computerized ST-segment monitoring is recommended in the care of patients at high risk.

   6. Hemodynamic monitoring. Studies on the intraoperative use of pulmonary arterial catheters as opposed to central venous catheters suggest no significant change in cardiac mortality among selected patients. Those with pulmonary arterial catheters, however, had fewer intraoperative hemodynamic complications. Therefore **pulmonary arterial catheters** are used in the care of **carefully selected patients at high risk for cardiac events,** especially those with poor LV function at risk for CHF.

C. **Postoperative management.** In most cases, the results of the preoperative determine whether a patient is at substantial cardiac risk. For these patients, postoperative care is dictated by the findings before the operation. In a few urgent cases or for patients who did not undergo preoperative evaluation, postoperative evaluation and care are individualized.

1. Once a patient has successfully undergone a procedure, the physician **assesses and manages risk factors** for coronary and peripheral atherosclerosis.

2. Management of risk factors, including smoking cessation, control of labile hypertension, aggressive management of hyperlipidemia, and glycemic control for patients with diabetes are of paramount importance.

3. Particular attention is given to **patients who sustain perioperative MI or demonstrate perioperative ischemia** because these patients are at risk for MI or cardiac death in the subsequent years. These patients are aggressively treated. Revascularization is performed if indicated after noninvasive testing.

SUGGESTED READINGS

References

1. Goldman L, Caldera DL, Nussbaum SR, et al. Multifactorial index of cardiac risk in noncardiac surgical procedures. *N Engl J Med* 1977;297:845–850.

2. Detsky AS, Abrams HB, McLaughlin JR, et al. Predicting cardiac complications in patients undergoing noncardiac surgery. *J Gen Intern Med* 1986;1:211–219.

3. Eagle KA, Coley CM, Newell JB, et al. Combining clinical and thallium data optimizes preoperative assessment of cardiac risk before major vascular surgery. *Ann Intern Med* 1989;110:859–866.

4. Cutler BS, Wheeler HB, Parakos JA, et al. Applicability and interpretation of electrocardiographic stress testing in patients with peripheral vascular disease. *Am J Surg* 1981;141:501–506.

5. Stratmann HG, Younis LT, Wittry MD, et al. Dipyridamole technetium-99m sestamibi myocardial tomography in patients evaluated for elective vascular surgery: prognostic value for perioperative and late cardiac events. *Am Heart J* 1996; 131:923–929.

6. Poldermans D, Arnese M, Fioretti PM. Sustained prognostic value of dobutamine stress echocardiography for late cardiac events after major noncardiac vascular surgery. *Circulation* 1997;95:53–58.

7. Kontos MC, Akosah KO, Brath LK. et al. Cardiac complications in noncardiac surgery: value of dobutamine stress echocardiography versus dipyridamole thallium imaging. *J Cardiothoracic Vasc Anesth* 1996;10:329–335.

8. Eagle KA, Rikal CS, Mickel MC, et al. Cardiac risk of noncardiac surgery: influence of coronary disease and type of surgery in 3368 operations. *Circulation* 1997;96:1882–1887.

9. Allen JR, Helling TS, Hartzler GO. Operative procedures not involving the heart after percutaneous transluminal coronary angioplasty. *Surg Gynecol Obstet* 1991; 173:285–288.

10. Urbinatis S, Pasquale G, Andreoli A, et al. Frequency and prognostic significance of silent coronary artery disease in patients with cerebral ischemia undergoing carotid endarterectomy. *Am J Cardiol* 1992;69:1166–1170.

Landmark Articles

Eagle KA, Coley CM, Newell JB, et al. Combining clinical and thallium data optimizes preoperative assessment of cardiac risk before major vascular surgery. *Ann Intern Med* 1989;110:859–866.

Eagle KA, Rihal CS, Mickel MC, et al. Cardiac risk of noncardiac surgery: influence of coronary disease and type of surgery in 3368 operations. *Circulation* 1997;96: 1882–1887.

Goldman L, Caldera DL, Nussbaum SR, et al. Multifactorial index of cardiac risk in noncardiac surgical procedures. *N Engl J Med* 1977;297:845–850.

Hertzer NR, Beven EG, Young JR, et al. Coronary artery disease in peripheral vascular patients: a classification of 1000 coronary angiograms and results of surgical management. *Ann Surg* 1984;199:223–233.

Mackey WC. Carotid and coronary disease: staged or simultaneous management? *Semin Vasc Surg* 1998;11:36–40.

Stratmann HG, Younis LT, Wittry MD, et al. Dipyridamole technetium-99m sestamibi myocardial tomography in patients evaluated for elective vascular surgery: prognostic value for perioperative and late cardiac events. *Am Heart J* 1996;131: 923–929.

Key Reviews

Eagle KA, Brundage BH, Chaitman BR, et al. Guidelines for perioperative cardiovascular evaluation for noncardiac surgery: report of the American College of Cardiology/American Heart Association Task Force on Practice Guidelines (Committee on Perioperative Cardiovascular Evaluation for Noncardiac Surgery). *J Am Coll Cardiol* 1996;27:910–948.

Wong T, Detsky AS. Preoperative cardiac risk assessment for patients having peripheral vascular surgery. *Ann Intern Med* 1992;116:743–753.

Relevant Book Chapter

Cohen MC, Eagle KA. The role of the cardiology consultant. In: Topol EJ, ed. *Textbook of cardiovascular medicine.* Philadelphia: Lippincott–Raven, 1998:1007–1031.

36. HYPERTENSIVE CRISIS

Harpreet Bhalla

I. **Introduction**
   A. **Systemic hypertension.** It is estimated that 60 million persons in the United States have systemic hypertension, many of whom are inadequately treated. Among the 60 million, 1% to 2% have primary hypertension that progresses to a crisis phase, accounting for more than 50% of all cases of hypertensive crisis. Uncontrolled or undercontrolled hypertension causes a high mortality from premature cardiac, vascular, and renal disease. In most instances end-organ damage occurs after decades of elevated blood pressure.
   B. **Hypertensive crisis.** In rare instances, hypertension may become acutely life threatening. This emergency situation, hypertensive crisis, occurs when an **abrupt, marked increase in blood pressure** (relative to the patient's baseline) **causes acute or rapidly progressing end-organ damage.** Unless promptly recognized and treated, hypertensive crisis can lead to cardiovascular, renal, and central nervous system complications and death. Effective and prompt antihypertensive treatment improves the prognosis.
   1. Hypertensive crisis can present de novo, but most patients have a **history of chronically elevated blood pressure that has been poorly controlled or untreated.**
      a. Public health campaigns aimed at educating and treating patients with hypertension have markedly decreased the incidence of hypertensive crisis. Nevertheless, it continues to represent a large portion of **emergency department visits.**
      b. Because the cardiovascular system is imminently threatened, cardiologists are called on to provide expert management of these emergencies. In addition, patients with severe elevations in blood pressure often go to a cardiologist for initial care. The cardiologist must be able to **differentiate an emergency** from urgency and a pseudoemergency; understand the underlying pathophysiologic mechanisms, potential complications, and treatment options; and guide the evaluation.
      c. Overzealous treatment can cause severe morbidity and even death. Therefore, a working knowledge of the **pharmacologic characteristics and side effects** of the various therapeutic agents is essential.
   2. **Classification.** Hypertensive crisis traditionally has been classified as emergency or urgency depending on the presence of acute or progressive end-organ damage. This distinction, although not absolute, aids in formulating an effective and safe treatment plan.
      a. **Hypertensive emergencies** include conditions characterized by **rapid decompensation of vital organ function** caused by inappropriate elevations in blood pressure. Treatment requires immediate reduction in blood pressure and parenteral medication, usually in an intensive care unit (ICU). Delay may cause irreversible organ damage and death.
         (1) A number of different clinical syndromes can present hypertensive emergencies (Table 36-1).
         (2) Accelerated or malignant hypertension and hypertensive encephalopathy are the prototypical hypertensive emergencies.
            (a) **Accelerated or malignant hypertension** is a systemic disease characterized by an extreme elevation in blood pressure (mean arterial blood pressure [MAP] greater than 120 mm Hg), bilateral retinal hemorrhage, and exudates

Table 36-1. Hypertensive emergencies

In general, diastolic blood pressure exceeds 120 mm Hg
Malignant hypertension with papilledema
Hypertensive encephalopathy
Severe hypertension in the setting of stroke, subarachnoid hemorrhage, head trauma
Acute aortic dissection[a]
Hypertension and left ventricular failure[a]
Hypertension and myocardial ischemia and infarction[a]
Hypertension after coronary artery bypass operation
Pheochromocytoma crisis[b]
Food or drug interactions with monoamine oxidase inhibitors[b]
Cocaine abuse[b]
Rebound hypertension after sudden drug withdrawal (clonidine)[b]
Idiosyncratic drug reactions (e.g., atropine)[b]
Eclampsia

[a] Exceptions include cardiovascular dysfunction in which low blood pressure may represent an emergency.
[b] Considered emergencies when associated with end-organ damage; otherwise treated as urgencies.

(accelerated) or papilledema (malignant). This hypertensive emergency demands emergency treatment and close follow-up care.

   (b) Hypertensive encephalopathy causes headache, irritability, and an altered state of consciousness from a sudden marked increase in blood pressure. Hypertensive encephalopathy occurs when cerebral edema is induced by markedly elevated blood pressures that overwhelm the autoregulatory capabilities of the brain. This condition tends to affect a person with previously normal blood pressure who has a rapid rise in blood pressure (see **IV.C**). Persons with chronic hypertension are relatively resistant to encephalopathy because their autoregulatory systems have adapted to the chronically elevated blood pressure. When persons with chronic hypertension do have encephalopathy, it is usually in the setting of markedly elevated blood pressure (diastolic blood pressures higher than 150 mm Hg). Mental status reverts to normal with the lowering of blood pressure.

   b. Hypertensive urgencies (Table 36-2) present as **marked elevations in blood pressure** (diastolic blood pressure higher than

Table 36-2. Hypertensive urgencies

Diastolic blood pressure exceeds 120 mm Hg, but patients have no symptoms and there are no signs of tissue damage
Severe hypertension, accelerated hypertension
Pheochromocytoma crisis
Food or drug interactions with monoamine oxidose inhibitors
Rebound hypertension after sudden drug withdrawal
Idiosyncratic drug reactions
Preoperative hypertension
Postoperative hypertension

120 mm Hg) **without evidence of acute or progressive target organ damage** and minimal, if any, symptoms. The risk for tissue damage is not immediate. Blood pressure can be lowered over a period of hours to days. Patients usually can be treated with oral medication, often as outpatients.

    c. **Pseudoemergencies** must be differentiated from true hypertensive emergencies because the treatments differ markedly. The increase in blood pressure in a pseudoemergency is caused by massive sympathetic outflow as the result of pain, hypoxia, hypercarbia, hypoglycemia, anxiety, or the postictal state. Treatment is directed at the underlying cause.

II. Clinical presentation. If an **emergency** is suspected, appropriate arrangements for ICU admission and parenteral treatment are made without waiting for the results of further tests. Chest pain, shortness of breath, headache, blurred vision and signs of altered mental status, focal neurologic signs, grade III-IV retinopathy, rales, S_3, and pulse deficits all point toward an emergency. Severe hypertension in the presence of chronic organ damage without associated symptoms does not constitute an emergency. Pseudo-emergencies must be ruled out.

    A. Signs and symptoms. The following **history** is elicited from patients with increased blood pressure.

        1. Presence of constitutional symptoms, such as nausea, vomiting, weight loss, or anorexia. Symptoms also can include shortness of breath, chest pain, headache, blurred vision, and abdominal pain. Patients with accelerated or malignant hypertension often have oliguria.

        2. Chronology of symptoms. Among patients with hypertensive encephalopathy, the symptoms typically have progressed over a period of several days.

        3. History of hypertension. Most patients with accelerated or malignant hypertension have an underlying history of chronic essential hypertension, although a high percentage of patients have secondary forms of hypertension. A search for correctable causes is indicated.

        4. Concurrent medications—cardiac medications, antihypertensive agents, oral contraceptives, diuretics, psychotropic agents, monoamine oxidase inhibitors.

        5. Use of **recreational drugs** (cocaine, amphetamines).

        6. Smoking history. Smokers are at increased risk for progression to malignant hypertension.

    B. Physical findings

        1. Vital signs. Blood pressure is measured in both upper and lower extremities. Severe hypertension is confirmed with two blood pressure measurements separated by 15 to 30 minutes. No absolute level of blood pressure differentiates emergency from an urgency; the distinction is based on a thorough clinical evaluation.

        2. Optic fundi—signs of retinopathy, including exudates, hemorrhages, and papilledema.

        3. Central nervous system—mental status, focal neurologic signs. Patients with hypertensive encephalopathy may manifest focal neurologic signs, confusion, or seizure activity.

        4. Heart and lungs—edema, S_3, or S_4.

        5. Vascular system—pulses and bruits.

III. Etiology. Table 36-3 lists the underlying clinical conditions that can precipitate a hypertensive crisis. Patients with chronic hypertension usually progress to an accelerated or malignant phase or have severe blood pressure elevations and progressive end-organ damage (e g., aortic dissection). A thorough search for secondary causes and precipitants is indicated in the evaluation of all patients with hypertensive crisis. Twenty percent to 56% of patients have an identifiable underlying cause, compared with less than 5% of those with uncomplicated hypertension.

Table 36-3. Conditions that may precipitate a hypertensive crisis

Essential hypertension (most common)
Renovascular hypertension
Parenchymal renal diseases
Drug-induced causes (interactions, idiosyncratic reactions, exaggerated effects, abrupt withdrawal)
Head injuries, central nervous system events (stroke, hemorrhage)
Vasculitis
Collagen vascular disease

A. A common situation is that a patient has been **inadequately treated** or has been noncompliant with a medical regimen.

B. **Risk factors** for progression to hypertensive crisis include male sex, African-American race, cigarette smoking or tobacco abuse, oral contraceptive use, and low socioeconomic status. Unlike essential hypertension, the incidence of which increases with age, the peak incidence of hypertensive crisis occurs among persons 40 to 50 years of age.

C. **Underlying diseases** that can precipitate hypertensive crisis include renal parenchymal disease, renovascular hypertension, collagen vascular disease, pheochromocytoma, vasculitis, preeclampsia, burns, and head trauma.

D. A number of **medications and illicit drugs** can cause marked elevations in systemic blood pressure. The most common offenders are oral contraceptives, sympathomimetic agents (diet pills, amphetamines), nonsteroidal antiinflammatory drugs (NSAIDs), cocaine, tricyclic antidepressants, and monoamine oxidase inhibitors.

E. In rare instances a hypertensive crisis is the first manifestation of disease. These patients tend to have secondary forms of hypertension, most commonly renovascular or renal parenchymal disease or a reaction to medications or illicit drugs.

F. **Left ventricular failure or pulmonary edema.** Elevated blood pressure poses an enormous workload on a failing heart. Even patients with normal systolic function can have pulmonary edema in the setting of markedly elevated blood pressures (afterload mismatch).

G. **Myocardial ischemia.** Blood pressure, heart rate, and preload determine myocardial oxygen demand. Elevated blood pressure can induce ischemia or complicate myocardial infarction (MI).

H. Hypertensive crisis associated with **hypercatecholaminemia.** A hypercatecholamine state can cause severe elevations in blood pressure that threaten tissue function and necessitate parenteral treatment. Hypercatecholamine states most commonly are induced by the exaggerated effects of medications, recreational drugs, or food-drug interactions. The common culprits include clonidine withdrawal; abuse of cocaine, amphetamines, LSD, and diet pills; and drug and food interactions with monoamine oxidase inhibitors. In rare instances pheochromocytoma can cause marked blood pressure elevations.

I. **Postoperative hypertension.** Severe hypertension can complicate the postoperative course after coronary and peripheral vascular procedures. The elevated pressure threatens suture lines and promotes excessive bleeding.

IV. **Pathophysiology**

A. Although the exact pathophysiologic mechanism is unknown, it is believed that hypertensive emergencies are triggered by an **abrupt increase in systemic vascular resistance (SVR) caused by increases in circulating vasoconstrictors** (e.g., norepinephrine, angiotensin II). The resulting increase in blood pressure leads to **arteriolar fibrinoid necrosis** characterized by endothelial damage, platelet and fibrin deposition, and loss of autoregulatory function. Ensuing **ischemia and dysfunction** in the target organ cause further release of vasoactive substances, producing a cycle of increasing SVR, elevated systemic blood pressure, decreased cardiac output, vascular injury, and tissue damage.

B. **An alternative explanation is that elevated blood pressure complicates a primary disease process and accelerates tissue injury.** The specific organ system affected defines the hypertensive crisis (e.g., aortic dissection, acute left ventricular failure, stroke).

C. **Autoregulation**

1. The kidney, brain, and heart all possess autoregulatory **mechanisms that maintain blood flow at near constant levels despite fluctuations in blood pressure.** Because the brain is encased in a finite space and because it maximally extracts oxygen at baseline, it is most vulnerable when its autoregulatory systems fail. Excess blood flow results in cerebral edema, elevated intracranial pressure, and ischemia.

2. Cerebral blood flow normally is maintained at a near constant level despite variations in cerebral perfusion pressure. The relation between cerebral blood flow, cerebral perfusion pressure, MAP, and intracranial pressure (ICP) is described with the following equations:

CBF varies with CPP

$$CPP = MAP - ICP$$

$$MAP = DBP - \tfrac{1}{3}PP$$

where DBP is diastolic blood pressure, PP is pulse pressure, CBF is cerebral blood flow, and CPP is cerebral perfusion pressure.

3. An **elevated MAP causes an increase in cerebral perfusion pressure,** whereas a decreasing MAP causes decreased cerebral perfusion pressure. Despite changes in cerebral perfusion pressure, cerebral autoregulatory mechanisms maintain cerebral blood flow; as MAP rises, vasoconstriction occurs, and as MAP decreases, vasodilatation occurs. This system has upper and lower limits beyond which cerebral blood flow can no longer be controlled.

   a. When **cerebral perfusion pressure decreases below the lower limits of autoregulation,** brain hypoxia ensues and symptoms of hypoperfusion manifest themselves: headache, nausea, dizziness, altered sensorium, lethargy. If uncorrected or extreme, this may ultimately cause infarction.

   b. When **MAP exceeds autoregulatory capabilities,** hyperperfusion occurs, leading to an increase in ICP, cerebral edema, and progressive organ dysfunction.

4. Most persons with normal blood pressure maintain autoregulation of MAP between 50 and 150 mm Hg, although this is highly variable. These values generally increase among patients with chronic hypertension. These patients consequently may have cerebral hypoperfusion at an MAP that is considered normal. In addition, elderly persons and patients who have had cerebrovascular accidents, subarachnoid hemorrhage, hypertensive encephalopathy, or accelerated or malignant hypertension have altered autoregulation.

5. Treatment must be tempered by the fact that **overzealous blood pressure reduction can lead to permanent neurologic damage.** Cerebrovascular accidents, blindness, paralysis, coma, MI, and death have been reported as consequences of overaggressive blood pressure reduction.

D. **Prognosis**

1. The prognosis of a patient who has undergone hypertensive crisis and not been treated is poor. Before the introduction of effective antihypertensive agents, more than 90% of patients with accelerated malignant hypertension died within 1 year of diagnosis.

2. Modern pharmacotherapy and the availability of dialysis have substantially increased survival rates, with recent studies reporting greater than 70% survival rates at five-year follow-up.

V. **Laboratory examination and diagnostic testing.** The diagnostic evaluation must be brief because **time to treatment is crucial.** Diagnostic imaging if clinically indicated can be performed after treatment has been instituted.

   A. **Complete blood count and blood smear.** Azotemia and hemolysis indicate an emergency.

   B. **Blood chemistries** to rule out uremia.

   C. **Urinalysis** to look for proteinuria, hematuria, and casts. **Hematuria** and moderate to severe **proteinuria** indicate an emergency.

   D. **Finger-stick glucose** to rule out hyperglycemia as a cause of changes in mental status.

   E. **Electrocardiography (ECG). Ischemic changes** on the ECG indicate an emergency.

   F. **Chest radiography. Pulmonary edema** on a chest radiography indicates an emergency.

   G. **Computed tomography (CT)** may be needed in the setting of a possible cerebrovascular accident.

VI. **Therapy.** The presence of **acute or rapidly progressive end-organ damage not the absolute blood pressure reading determines whether the situation is an emergency or urgency.** This determination dictates the type of treatment (oral versus parenteral) and the setting (ICU, hospital ward, outpatient) in which it is implemented. For example, a blood pressure of 120/80 mm Hg may represent a hypertensive emergency for a patient with aortic dissection, whereas a blood pressure of 200/120 mm Hg for a person with asymptomatic chronic hypertension usually does not necessitate emergency therapy. The appropriate diagnostic evaluation and therapeutic plan also are dictated by the specific disease. For example, the specific pharmacologic regimen for a pregnant woman with preeclampsia differs from that for an elderly man who has had a stroke. Regardless of drug regimen, the **goal of treatment** is to break the cycle of increasing SVR and blood pressure, preserve cardiac output and renal blood flow, and limit end-organ damage.

   A. **Neurologic emergencies.** Patients with neurologic findings and severe hypertension present a particular challenge. Neurologic emergencies can result from hypertensive emergencies or may cause markedly elevated blood pressures, which may exacerbate neurologic damage. The key differentiating point is that **neurologic alterations caused by elevated blood pressure are reversed when blood pressure is controlled** whereas primary diseases are not. The insidious progression of symptoms in hypertensive encephalopathy aids in differentiating hypertensive encephalopathy from cerebrovascular accidents, which usually present abruptly. Nevertheless, the diagnosis is one of exclusion because other hypertensive emergencies, such as cerebrovascular accident, subarachnoid hemorrhage, intraparenchymal bleeding, and primary seizure disorder, share many symptoms and signs. Evaluation often **necessitates further diagnostic imaging, such as CT, and consultation with a neurologist.**

   B. **Hypertensive emergencies**

   1. **Priority of therapy.** The goal of therapy is **immediate, controlled reduction in blood pressure.** The pharmacologic characteristics and potential toxic side effects of antihypertensive agents must be understood and anticipated.

      a. Patients are **treated in an ICU,** where clinical status and vital signs can be constantly monitored with the aid of an arterial line.

      b. Attention is focused on the **ABCs** (airway, breathing, and circulation). Ancillary measures such as intubation and dialysis are instituted if necessary.

      c. **Blood pressure is reduced in a controlled, predictable manner.** The lower limit of autoregulation among both persons with normal blood pressure and those with hypertension is approximately 25% of MAP. Therefore it is recommended that **blood pressure initially be reduced by no more than 25% of MAP over minutes to hours** and that further reductions occur over a prolonged period of time (days to weeks) for the autoregulatory mechanisms to reset. Exceptions include aortic dissection, left ventricular failure, and pulmonary edema, which demand more aggressive blood pressure reduction to limit tissue damage.

d. Specific antihypertensive therapy is tailored to the underlying disease (e.g., aortic dissection, angina).

e. Diagnosis and treatment are reassessed if the clinical condition, especially neurologic status, deteriorates with reduction of blood pressure.

2. Medical therapy. A number of parenteral antihypertensive medications are available to manage hypertensive emergencies. The specific clinical scenario dictates the agents used. Characteristics of an ideal agent include rapid onset and cessation of action, a predictable dose-response curve, and few side effects.

a. Patients with **hypertensive emergencies** have excessive elevations in SVR, decreased cardiac output and renal blood flow, and volume depletion. Therefore the most useful agents are **vasodilating agents** such as nitroprusside. Diuretics and β-blockers are avoided unless the patient has aortic dissection, MI, or pulmonary edema.

b. For hypertensive encephalopathy, cerebrovascular accidents, or other **conditions in which mental status must be monitored,** agents that have prominent CNS side effects (e.g., sedation) are **avoided.**

c. For conditions associated with **elevated ICP,** such as cerebrovascular accident, subarachnoid hemorrhage, or hypertensive encephalopathy, agents that directly increase cerebral blood flow are **avoided.**

d. The agent selected has the most favorable hemodynamic and side-effect profile on the basis of the specific hypertensive emergency.

e. Table 36-4 lists parenteral antihypertensive agents, dosages, side-effect profiles, and specific indications. The drug of choice for most hypertensive crises is sodium nitroprusside. Effective alternatives include labetalol; in certain circumstances, nitroglycerin or hydralazine may be preferred.

(1) Sodium nitroprusside (SNP) is the **drug of choice** for most hypertensive emergencies. The favorable hemodynamic profile, rapid onset, and cessation of action of SNP make it the preferred parenteral agent for most emergencies. A potent direct vascular smooth-muscle relaxant, SNP decreases afterload and preload by means of dilating arterioles and increasing venous capacitance. Hemodynamic effects include a decrease in MAP, afterload, and preload, an increase or no change in cardiac output, and increased renal blood flow and glomerular filtration rate. Although the direct action of SNP on the cerebral vasculature may cause increased cerebral perfusion, this is counteracted by a potent effect on MAP. Most patients with neurologic crisis who need blood pressure control tolerate SNP without a worsening of neurologic status. However, the possibility of an increase in ICP and further clinical deterioration despite a decrease in MAP must be kept in mind as a potential side effect among patients with severely increased ICP.

(a) Administration. SNP must be administered by means of constant intravenous infusion in an intensive care setting with constant monitoring of arterial blood pressure. It has a rapid onset of action, and its effect ceases within 1 to 5 minutes of cessation of infusion.

Table 36-4. Parenteral medications used to manage hypertensive emergencies

Drug	Dosage	Onset/duration	Indications	Side effects
Nitroprusside sodium (Nipride, Nitropress)	Infusion: 0.25–10 µg/kg per min	Immediate/3–5 min	Most emergencies	Nausea, vomiting, sweating, thiocyanate and cyanide poisoning
Glyceryl trinitrate (Nitro-Bid)	Infusion: 5–200 µg/min	Immediate/3–5 min	Myocardial ischemia, myocardial infarction, LV failure	Headache, methemeaglobinemia, tolerance with prolonged infusion
Labetolol (Normodyne, Trandate)	Bolus: 20 mg/5 min until desired effect (max 80 mg) Infusion: 1–2 mg/min	5–10 min/1–8 hr	Most emergencies except those complicated by LV failure	Heart block, orthostatic hypotension Avoid if patient has asthma, heart failure, heart block greater than first degree
Nicardipine (Cardene)	Infusion: 5–15 mg/hr	5–10 minutes/1–4 hr	Most emergencies except those complicated by LV failure	Reflex tachycardia, headache, nausea, flushing Avoid in heart failure
Enalapril (Vasotec)	1.25–5 mg every 6 hr	15 min/6 hr	LV failure, scleroderma crisis	Marked decreases in blood pressure in high-renin states, renal failure hyperkalemia
Phentolamine (Regitine)	Bolus: 5–15 mg IV Infusion: 0.2–5.0 mg/min	1–2 min/3–10 min	Pheochromocytoma crisis Catecholamine crisis	Tachycardia, headache, flushing
Hydralazine (Apresoline)	Bolus: 10–20 mg IV every 30 min until desired effect achieved or side effects occur	10–20 min/3–8 hr	Eclampsia	Marked hypotension, tachycardia, flushing Contraindicated in myocardial ischemia and aortic dissection

LV, Left ventricular.

(b) **Side effects.** Red blood cells and muscle cells metabolize SNP to cyanide, which is converted to thiocyanate in the liver and excreted in the urine. **Thiocyanate levels rise in patients with renal insufficiency; cyanide accumulates in patients with hepatic disease.** Signs of thiocyanate toxicity include nausea, vomiting, headache, fatigue, delirium, muscle spasms, tinnitus, and seizures. Monitoring for signs and symptoms of toxicity and maintaining thiocyanate levels less than 12 mg/dL allow safe use of SNP.

(2) **Labetalol** is useful in most hypertensive crises. The main disadvantage is its relatively long duration of action. Labetalol is an α- and nonselective β-blocker with partial β_2 agonist activity. When given through continuous intravenous infusion, the relative β to α blocking effects of labetalol are 7 : 1.

   (a) The **hemodynamic effects** of labetalol include a decrease in SVR, MAP, and heart rate, and a decrease or no change in cardiac output. Cardiac output often is spared because of the decrease in afterload. Labetalol has little direct effect on cerebral vasculature, does not increase ICP, and is **considered by some to be the drug of choice in situations characterized by markedly elevated ICP.** Labetalol begins to lower blood pressure within 5 minutes, and its effects can last 1 to 3 hours after cessation of the infusion.

   (b) **Contraindications.** Labetalol is contraindicated in congestive heart failure, bradycardia, heart block (more than first degree), and reactive airway disease.

(3) **Nitroglycerin** is considered the drug of choice for managing hypertension in the setting of myocardial ischemia, acute MI, and pulmonary edema and after coronary artery bypass grafting. The role of intravenous nitroglycerin therapy is limited to hypertension complicating myocardial ischemia, MI, and congestive heart failure. Nitroglycerin is primarily a venodilator and has modest effects on afterload at high doses. The decrease in preload and afterload decreases myocardial oxygen demand. Nitroglycerin also dilates the epicardial coronary arteries, inhibits vasospasm, and favorably redistributes blood flow to the endocardium. Nitroglycerin directly increases cerebral blood flow and is **not used in situations characterized by high ICP.**

(4) **Hydralazine.** The role of intravenous hydralazine is limited to the treatment of pregnant women with preeclampsia. Hydralazine is a direct arterial vasodilator with no effect on venous capacitance. It crosses the uteroplacental barrier but has minimal effects on the fetus. It is usually administered in boluses of 10 to 20 mg and has a long duration of action. Hydralazine decreases SVR, induces compensatory tachycardia, and increases ICP. It can exacerbate angina and is **contraindicated in the care of patients with ongoing coronary ischemia, aortic dissection, or increased ICP.**

3. **Management of specific emergencies**

  a. **Accelerated or malignant hypertension**

    (1) In the **acute phase** the pharmacologic agent of choice is **SNP.** Labetalol is an effective alternative.

    (2) **Contraindications.** Because patients usually have marked elevations of SVR and volume depletion, β-blockers and diuretics are contraindicated.

  b. **Hypertensive encephalopathy**

    (1) The treatment of choice is **SNP or labetalol.** Agents that depress the sensorium or increase ICP are avoided.

(2) Management of markedly elevated blood pressure in the setting of hypertensive encephalopathy is tempered by **concerns about further reducing blood flow to underperfused areas of the brain.**

(3) Most patients with hypertensive encephalopathy improve within hours of blood pressure reduction; neurologic deficits persist in the other conditions. **If there is no improvement despite a decrease in blood pressure, the diagnosis must be reconsidered.**

c. **Neurologic complications,** including cerebrovascular accident, embolic stroke, intraparenchymal hemorrhage, and subarachnoid hemorrhage.

(1) **Extreme caution** must be exercised when **lowering even markedly elevated blood pressures in the setting of a cerebrovascular accident.** Elevated ICP caused by cerebral edema or intraparenchymal hemorrhage increases the MAP needed to adequately perfuse the brain (cerebral perfusion pressure = MAP – ICP). Subarachnoid hemorrhage is characterized by intense vasospasm at and adjacent to the site of rupture. Reduction of blood pressure in these circumstances may cause global or in the case of subarachnoid hemorrhage focal hypoperfusion.

(2) **Markedly elevated blood pressures, however, may increase risk for rebleeding** in subarachnoid hemorrhage or extend a hemorrhagic infarct.

(3) Lesions that are potentially **surgically correctable** such as subarachnoid hemorrhage and neoplasms must be identified.

(4) Management of markedly elevated blood pressure in the setting of cerebrovascular accident or subarachnoid hemorrhage is tempered by **concerns about further reducing blood flow to underperfused areas of the brain.**

(5) The following **guidelines** are suggested:

(a) When blood pressure is less than 180/105 mm Hg, no treatment is recommended.

(b) When blood pressure is 180/105 to 230/120 mm Hg for longer than 60 minutes, treatment is started.

(c) When blood pressure is higher than 230/120 mm Hg for longer than 20 minutes, treatment is started.

(6) When treatment is indicated it must be **closely monitored,** often with direct ICP monitor.

(7) Target blood pressures are 160/100 to 175/110 mm Hg systolic for patients who had normal blood pressure and 180/110 to 185/120 mm Hg among persons with chronic hypertension.

(8) The drug of choice is **labetalol or SNP.**

(9) **Nimodipine,** a calcium channel blocker with modest antihypertensive effect, has been shown to be beneficial in the management of subarachnoid hemorrhage. If despite use of nimodipine blood pressure remains higher than desired, use of **SNP or labetalol** may be considered.

(10) Agents that directly increase cerebral perfusion pressure and thus ICP are avoided.

d. **Aortic dissection is an emergency.** Blood pressure must be lowered immediately. Patients with **type A dissection** have a mortality rate of 1% per hour unless medical therapy is instituted and the patient is referred for **emergency surgical intervention. Antihypertensive therapy** is the treatment of choice in **type B dissection.** SVR and shear force must be decreased. This is accomplished by means of decreasing the inotropic state of the heart and the ratio of change in ventricular pressure to change in time (dP/dT). **Labetalol** or SNP with a β-blocker is the treatment of choice. **Aggressive blood pressure reduction** is indicated even for patients with normal blood pressure because shear force and afterload must be reduced to limit tissue damage. A reasonable goal is an MAP of approximately 70 mm Hg. **Drugs that decrease afterload and induce compensatory tachycardia are contraindicated** (see Chapter 25).

  e. **Left ventricular failure or pulmonary edema.** Treatment is best accomplished with **SNP and small doses of diuretics. Nitroglycerin** is an effective alternative, especially if ischemia is present. SNP and nitroglycerin often are used concomitantly. β-Blockers and calcium channel blockers must be avoided in the decompensated state.

  f. **Myocardial ischemia.** Blood pressure reduction with nitrates and β-blockers is the treatment of choice. **SNP** is added if further blood pressure reduction is required. **Reperfusion and antithrombotic therapy** are the mainstays of management of acute MI and unstable angina.

  g. **Hypertensive crisis associated with hypercatecholaminemia.** The pharmacologic agents of choice include **SNP, labetalol, or calcium channel blockers. Phentolamine** can be useful in cases of pheochromocytoma. β-Blockers must be avoided, because they can cause a paradoxic increase in blood pressure because of the effects of unopposed α-receptor stimulation.

  h. **Postoperative hypertension.** Parenteral treatment with **SNP or labetalol** is preferred. **After coronary bypass grafting, nitroglycerin** is considered the initial drug of choice.

C. **Hypertensive urgencies.** Most patients diagnosed with hypertensive urgency actually have severe hypertension and **are not in any immediate danger of progressing to hypertensive emergency.** They are often persons with chronic hypertension who are undertreated or noncompliant.

 1. **Priority of therapy**

  a. Hypertensive urgencies usually can be managed with **oral medication without admission to the hospital.** End-organ damage is not imminent, and blood pressure can be modestly lowered over a period of hours as long as adequate follow-up care is ensured. **The great danger lies in overtreating these patients and inciting a hypotensive crisis.**

  b. Sometimes simply placing the patient in a **quiet, calm environment** can decrease blood pressure to a less alarming level. If the blood pressure is still markedly elevated, **reinstitution or enhancement of prior therapy often is effective.** MAP is not decreased more than 15% to 20%.

  c. Lower initial doses of antihypertensive medications are used to treat patients with **cerebrovascular disease or coronary artery disease, taking antihypertensive drugs, or who are volume depleted.** These patients tend to have exceptional responses to drug therapy, some of which cause hypotension. They also are especially vulnerable to **hypotension.** Lower doses of medications must be used. Monitoring for 4 to 6 hours is necessary to judge treatment effect and look for complications. Urgent follow-up care is mandatory within 24 hours. Evaluation for secondary causes of hypertension is indicated.

 2. **Drug therapy.** Oral agents used to manage hypertensive urgencies are listed in Table 36-5 The drugs of choice include captopril, clonidine, and oral labetalol.

  a. **Captopril.** Considered by some to be the drug of choice, captopril is the **fastest-acting oral angiotensin-converting enzyme inhibitor.** At small doses it rarely causes marked hypotension, although this potential exists among patients who are markedly volume-depleted or who have renal artery stenosis. Captopril begins to work

Table 36-5. Oral agents used to manage hypertensive urgencies

Drug	Dosage	Onset/duration	Indications	Side effects
Captopril	6.25–25 mg by mouth every 6 hr	15–30 min/ 4 hr	Well-tolerated in most instances	Can precipitate hypotension in high renin states, cough, renal failure
Clonidine (Catapres)	0.1–0.2 mg every hr as needed to a maximum of 0.8 mg hr	30–60 min/ 6–12 hr	Severe uncomplicated hypertension	Sedation, bradycardia, dry mouth
Labetolol	100–200 mg by month every 2–3 hr	30–120 min/ 2–8 hr	Well-tolerated in most instances	Heart failure, heart block, bronchospasm

within 15 to 30 minutes of ingestion and has a 4- to 6-hour duration of activity. Caution is advised in the treatment of patients with marked renal insufficiency and the volume depleted.

b. Clonidine acts through central α-agonist activity. It has been administered in repeated hourly doses and safely lowers blood pressure over a period of hours. Untoward effects include sedation and a proclivity for rebound hypertension. Clonidine is not administered to anyone with altered sensorium or who may not comply with treatment.

c. Labetalol. A combined α- and β-blocker, labetalol taken orally has a relative β to α blocking effect of approximately 3 : 1. Begin at 100 mg po bid and titrate to desired response. The onset of action is 30 minutes to 2 hours after administration; the duration of action is 8 to 12 hours.

d. Nifedipine. According to a number of reports, the use of sublingual nifedipine has caused hypotension, syncope, transient ischemic attacks, cerebrovascular accidents, myocardial ischemia, and infarction. Given this and the fact that the U.S. Food and Drug Administration has recommended that the drug not be approved to manage hypertensive crisis, there is **no role for sublingual nifedipine in the treatment of patients with hypertension.**

SUGGESTED READINGS

Key Reviews

Kaplan NM. Management of hypertensive emergencies. *Lancet* 1994;344:133–135.

McKindley DS, Boucher BA. Advances in pharmacotherapy: treatment of hypertensive crisis. *J Clin Pharm Ther* 1994;19:163–180.

Prisant LM, Carr A, Hawkins DW. Treating hypertensive emergencies: controlled reduction of blood pressure and protection of target organs. *Postgrad Med* 1993;93: 92–96,101–104,108–110.

Ram CV. Immediate management of severe hypertension. *Cardiol Clin* 1995;13: 579–591.

Relevant Book Chapter

Kaplan NM. Systemic hypertension: mechanism and diagnosis. In: Braunwald E, ed. *Heart disease: a textbook of cardiovascular medicine,* 5th ed. Philadelphia: WB Saunders, 1997:807–839.

37. EVALUATION OF CHEST PAIN IN THE EMERGENCY DEPARTMENT

Jason B. Wischmeyer and Samir R. Kapadia

I. **Introduction.** Chest pain is one of the most common problems evaluated in an emergency department (ED).

   A. **Rapid evaluation** of chest pain to identify life-threatening illnesses is important. **Triage** is essential for optimal utilization of resources. For patients with **myocardial infarction (MI), emergency treatment is initiated in the ED** to minimize permanent myocardial damage. Short-term observation with specific investigations can help to identify the source of chest discomfort. This approach has been implemented in many EDs for efficient and cost-effective treatment of selected patients with chest pain.

   B. Each year approximately 4 million patients who arrive at an ED with chest pain are admitted to the hospital, mainly to an intensive care unit; 1.5 million of these patients have acute MI. However, **3% to 10% of persons who arrive with chest discomfort and acute MI are inappropriately discharged** to home. This inefficiency in diagnosing MI is dangerous and is not cost effective. Not only the diagnosis but also **early recognition and treatment** are important. Time to treatment is important in the management of acute ST-elevation MI and probably is important in the management of unstable angina and non-Q-wave MI.

   C. **Assessment** of chest pain in the ED involves a careful, directed patient **history, physical examination,** and **12-lead electrocardiogram (ECG).** Biochemical and functional tests can supply additional data, but these data are not immediately available, so triage decisions are made without these data. With clinical history, physical examination, and initial ECG, 92% to 98% of acute MIs and approximately 90% of cases of unstable angina can be identified.

II. **Clinical presentation**

   A. **History**

   1. **Chest pain.** The initial history accurately characterizes the patient's discomfort, the duration of the discomfort, associated symptoms, and aggravating and alleviating factors (Table 37-1). Most patients with ischemic chest pain describe it as substernal pressure, squeezing, or a sensation of suffocation. Some patients describe aching, burning, or tightness. The pain may radiate to the shoulder, neck, jaw, left or right arm, and the fingertips. Pain below the belt or above the jaw probably is not caused by acute coronary syndrome (ACS).

   2. **Risk factors.** Although a number of clinical factors have been associated with an increased risk for cardiovascular disease, only the **age** of patient, **history of coronary artery disease,** and **male** sex are consistently predictive of ACS among patients with chest pain. In some studies diabetes and family history have been associated with ACS, but the overall power of these risk factors in predicting an ischemic event is low. The **absence of risk factors cannot be used to exclude cardiac ischemia.**

   B. **Physical examination**

   1. The physical examination helps to identify **signs of left ventricular dysfunction and occult valvular heart disease.** Presence of S_3, rales, sinus tachycardia, hypotension, and increased jugular venous distention are associated with worse outcome. The presence of these signs and symptoms indicates cardiac origin of the chest pain. A thorough physical examination also helps identify the cause of nonischemic chest pain (Table 37-2). Chest wall tenderness, skin lesions, and pleural or pericardial rub can be useful in this regard.

Table 37-1. Differentiating cardiac from noncardiac chest pain

Favoring ischemic origin	Against ischemic origin
CHARACTER OF PAIN	
Constricting	Sharp, knife-like
Squeezing	Stabbing
Burning	Jabs aggravated by respiration
Heaviness	
LOCATION OF PAIN	
Substernal	Left submammary area
Across midthorax	Left hemithorax
Radiation to both arms, shoulders, neck, cheeks, teeth, forearms, interscapular region	Discomfort localized with one finger
Associated with nausea, vomiting, diaphoresis	
FACTORS PROVOKING PAIN	
Exercise	Pain after completion of exercise
Excitement	Provoked by a specific body motion
Stress	
Cold weather	
Eating	
DURATION OF CHEST PAIN	
Minutes	Seconds
	Hours without evidence of myocardial damage

From Selzer A. *Principles and practice of clinical cardiology,* 2nd ed. Philadelphia: WB Saunders, 1983:17, with permission.

    2. Response to treatment is not reliable in unraveling the cause of chest pain. Pain relief after administration of nitroglycerin does not point to MI or unstable angina, and antacids do not always alleviate esophageal pain.

III. Diagnostic testing

    A. ECG is integral to the evaluation of chest pain and has important diagnostic and prognostic value. It is even more important in evaluations of persons with diabetes and elderly persons, who tend to have atypical symptoms.

        1. Only 50% to 60% of patients with acute MI undergo an initial diagnostic ECG. **Sensitivity** depends on a number of factors, including the time from symptom onset, coronary distribution of ischemia, baseline ECG abnormalities, patient characteristics, and the specific criteria used to define abnormal ECG findings. ECG findings normalize rapidly after resolution of chest pain. Therefore the ECG findings of a patient who does not have active chest pain are difficult to interpret. Circumflex distribution ischemia is notoriously silent on an ECG; the lateral wall is underrepresented on a conventional 12-lead ECG.

        2. Among patients with the ischemic type of chest discomfort, ST-segment elevation on an ECG has a specificity of approximately 90% and a sensitivity of approximately 50% in the diagnosis of acute MI. Sensitivity decreases to 82% and specificity increases to 69% when ST-segment elevation or depression, Q waves, or left bundle branch block (LBBB) is used to define abnormal ECG findings.

        3. The ECG can be used to identify a population of patients at low risk for MI. A normal ECG indicates less than 3% risk for MI and less than 6%

Table 37-2. Causes of chest pain

CARDIAC

Acute coronary syndromes (AMI, USA, non-Q MI)
Chest pain with normal coronaries (syndrome X)
Pericarditis
Mitral valve prolapse
Aortic stenosis
Hypertrophic cardiomyopathy

AORTIC

Aortic dissection
Penetrating ulcer of aorta

PULMONARY

Embolism

GASTROINTESTINAL

Esophageal spasm, reflux or esophagitis
Gastritis, gastric ulcer
Cholecystitis

COSTOCHONDRITIS

Tietze's syndrome

NEUROLOGIC

Cervical spondylosis and other compression neuropathy
Herpes

PSYCHOLOGIC

Panic disorder
Anxiety
Depression
Hysteria

---

for death in the following year. However, approximately one-third of the patients with unstable angina may have a normal or equivocal ECG. Therefore **ECG cannot be used alone to exclude ACS.**

4. Preexisting abnormalities, including left ventricular hypertrophy, LBBB, Q waves, preexcitation, and pacing, make ECG interpretation difficult. Comparison of the initial ECG with a prior tracing often is helpful in this setting. Whether new or old, the presence of **LBBB is an adverse prognostic finding.** New LBBB suggests left anterior descending coronary artery ischemia. Preexisting LBBB alone defines a group of patients at high risk for cardiac morbidity and mortality. Although LBBB complicates the ECG diagnosis of acute MI, criteria have been proposed for ascertaining whether a patient has acute MI and LBBB. The criteria were derived from the Global Utilization of Streptokinase and Tissue Plasminogen Activator for Occluded Coronary Arteries (GUSTO I) database (1) (see Chapter 1).

B. **Biochemical markers** of myocardial necrosis are used in conjunction with the clinical history and ECG to confirm the diagnosis of MI. Markers historically were enzymes released into the serum after myocardial cell death. Newer markers include myocardial proteins such as the cardiac **troponins and myoglobin.** These markers appear to be sensitive and specific for myocardial injury and can provide important prognostic information.

1. **Serial blood samples** are collected over a 24-hour period to measure a temporal rise and fall or change in ratio for the diagnosis of MI. All

biochemical markers follow a predictable pattern of release after the onset of myocardial injury (Fig. 37-1).

2. An **ideal serum marker** is specific to myocardium, highly sensitive, and quantitative; that is, serum concentration is proportional to the amount of myocardial tissue injured. Levels are increased rapidly to allow early diagnosis. None of the currently available markers is optimal for the diagnosis of ACS. In most cases, the combination of serial measurement of markers and interpretation of clinical data helps in the diagnosis of ACS.

3. Enzymes such as aspartate aminotransferase (AST), lactate dehydrogenase (LDH), and creatine kinase (CK) are released from dying myocytes but are relatively nonspecific for cardiac tissue. Added sensitivity and specificity are obtained when **cardiac isoenzymes** such as CK MB and LDH_1 are measured.

   a. **Creatine kinase** is a cytosolic enzyme commonly found in skeletal muscle, brain, kidney, smooth muscle, and cardiac muscles. It is a dimer composed of two subunit types, M and B, with three isoenzymes, MM, MB, and BB. The **MB subunit** is present in cardiac myocytes and intestinal muscle, uterus, and in small amounts in skeletal muscle. In athletes, however, CK MB can replace the normal MM isoform in skeletal muscle. CK isoform MM is the predominant isoform in the skeletal muscle; BB is present mainly in the brain and kidney.

      (1) **CK MB is released in the circulation after myocardial cell death.** There is some evidence in animal models that CK MB can be released with reversible myocardial injury. However, this has never been shown in humans. The M subunit of the MB isoenzyme when released in the circulation is modified through cleavage of the C-terminal lysine residue, resulting in two electrophoretically distinct isoforms, MB1 (serum) and MB2 (tissue). The change in proportion of CK MB1 to CK MB2 occurs faster than the absolute elevation of CK MB with myocardial damage. There is some evidence that this ratio can help to quickly ascertain in the ED whether a patient has ongoing chest pain, resulting in better utilization of resources. However, this test is still not widely available (2).

      (2) CK_{Total} can be measured through enzymatic activity; electrophoresis then is used to measure CK isoforms. Most studies

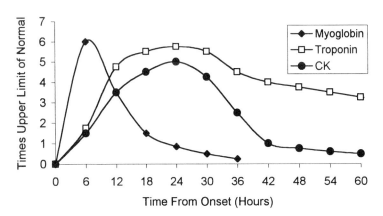

FIG. 37-1. Time of release of important biochemical markers.

have confirmed that serial measurement of CK MB for the diagnosis of acute MI has a sensitivity of approximately 92% with a specificity of 98%. The initial level of CK MB, however, does not carry equal statistical weight and does not have sufficient negative predictive value to exclude MI when used in isolation. CK MB level can be increased with normal or minimally elevated CK_{Total} levels. This sign has been associated with increased risk for cardiac events in some studies but the significance of this finding is debatable.

   (3) Immunologic methods allow rapid, accurate measurement of CK MB mass. A relative index can then be derived from the ratio of CK MB_{mass} (ng/mL) to total CK (IU). This relative index appears to be more sensitive than the CK MB/CK_{Total} percentage measured with electrophoresis.

b. **Myoglobin** is a small heme protein that is not specific to cardiac tissue. Therefore, the use of myoglobin as a marker of myocardial necrosis does not carry the specificity of CK MB measurement. The advantage of myoglobin as a marker lies in its **release kinetics.** Myoglobin is released rapidly after myocardial injury, and serum levels are detectable within 1 to 2 hours of the onset of symptoms. Peak serum levels are reached within 4 to 5 hours after MI. Within 1 to 3 hours of MI, serum myoglobin determination has a sensitivity of 62% to 100% in the detection of myocardial damage. Because of its short half-life, measurement of myoglobin may not help confirm the diagnosis for patients who seek treatment late after symptom onset. The specificity is low when there is a substantial release of skeletal muscle myoglobin and in the setting of renal failure.

c. **Troponins**

   (1) Cardiac troponin T, troponin I, and troponin C are **proteins that regulate the calcium-dependent interactions between actin and myosin.** This interaction results in myocyte contraction and relaxation. **Troponin C** is common to both skeletal and cardiac muscles; the skeletal and cardiac forms of troponin T and troponin I differ immunologically. **Troponin T** is a myofibrillary protein and as a subunit of the troponin complex is a constituent of the contractile apparatus of skeletal and cardiac muscle. In cardiac cells, 6% of troponin T is dissolved in the cytosol and 94% is structurally bound. This distribution is responsible for the unique release kinetics. Cardiac troponins, like CK MB, can be found in the serum soon after injury but remain elevated for as long as 2 weeks. Both cardiac troponin T and troponin I are useful in the diagnosis of ACS and have been shown to be very sensitive and specific markers of myocardial cell injury.

   (2) A large prospective analysis from the Global Use of Strategies to Open Occluded Coronary Arteries (GUSTO IIa) trial has provided important data on the **value of cardiac troponins for diagnosis and risk assessment** (3).

   (a) Among patients who come to medical attention within 12 hours of the onset of myocardial ischemia, elevated levels of **troponin T** (more than 0.1 mg/mL) were associated with significantly higher mortality within 30 days. This was true for all ECG subgroups examined, including those with ST depression, ST elevation, T-wave inversion, LBBB, and paced rhythms. A quantitative relation also has been demonstrated between levels of cardiac troponin T and long-term clinical outcome.

   (b) Troponin I also was shown to have prognostic value. Among patients with unstable angina and non-Q-wave MI, elevated cardiac troponin I levels (more than 0.4 ng/mL) were associated with significantly higher mortality (4). Troponin T and I show similar prognostic significance for acute MI or death among patients with unstable angina (5).

(3) **Bedside tests** for cardiac-specific troponins are **highly sensitive** for the early detection of myocardial cell injury in ACS. Qualitative and quantitative point-of-care tests for both troponin T and troponin I are fast (a few minutes), reliable, and accurate. **Negative test results have been associated with low risk** and allow rapid and safe discharge from the ED of patients with an episode of acute chest pain (6).

C. **Imaging studies.** Although clinical history, initial ECG findings, and biochemical markers have been combined to diagnose ACS with high sensitivity and specificity, atypical presentations and equivocal ECG findings can make diagnosis challenging. Investigations aimed at overcoming these problems have focused on myocardial perfusion and functional imaging.

1. **Echocardiography.** Two-dimensional echocardiography provides valuable diagnostic data on ventricular function and regional wall motion abnormalities.

   a. Myocardial ischemia can cause abnormal segmental function of the myocardium manifested as impaired relaxation, hypokinesis, akinesis, or even dyskinesia.

   b. Although echocardiography alone has moderate sensitivity in the diagnosis of acute MI, it may be a useful adjunctive test. For patients with equivocal ECG findings, two-dimensional echocardiography has been demonstrated to have a sensitivity of approximately 88% and a specificity of 78% in the detection of MI.

   c. Two-dimensional echocardiography can be used to detect regional wall motion abnormalities, but a single examination cannot help differentiate acute MI, ischemia, and old infarction.

   d. Normal findings at echocardiography cannot always be used reliably to rule out myocardial ischemia. However, echocardiography can be helpful in the evaluation of complications of MI and unexplained cardiogenic shock.

2. **Radionuclide perfusion imaging** is useful to quantify myocardium at risk. It is rarely used for the diagnosis of ACS.

   a. Thallium 201 scintigraphy has been used to detect areas of reduced or absent perfusion in acute MI. Areas of myocardium with a negative scintigraphic image, indicating decreased myocardial uptake, can be demonstrated in ischemic or infarcted myocardium within 6 hours of symptom onset. The diagnostic utility of such imaging is limited by the moment-in-time problem; perfusion defects may represent acutely ischemic myocardium or preexisting areas of scar tissue.

   b. **Technetium 99m sestamibi tomographic imaging** has the advantage that sestamibi does not redistribute after initial injection. Therefore this type of imaging allows definition of an initial ischemic zone that can be studied even after reperfusion. Perfusion imaging with sestamibi appears to have a sensitivity equivalent to that of thallium 201 imaging in defining myocardium at risk.

IV. **Differential diagnosis.** Differentiating ischemic from nonischemic causes of chest pain can be difficult. It has been estimated that more than 50% of patients initially admitted to the hospital with a diagnosis of unstable angina are later discharged with a noncardiac diagnosis. Given that there is symptom overlap among a number of clinical entities, in most diagnostic strategies it is assumed that **chest pain is cardiac in origin until proved otherwise.** It is important to understand the clinical characteristics that represent the leading noncardiac causes of chest pain (see Table 37-1). Life-threatening causes of chest pain that can be confused with ACS include aortic dissection, pericarditis, and pulmonary embolus.

A. Pericarditis (see Chapter 26) often is accompanied by substernal chest pain, but the **pain** is more likely to be pleuritic in character and aggravated by recumbency, deep inspiration, and swallowing. **Physical examination** may reveal a three-component pericardial friction rub. The **ECG** often reveals ST elevation in multiple leads without reciprocal changes and PR-segment depression in lead aVR. It is important to recognize that **pericarditis may be a late presentation of MI.**

B. Aortic dissection (see Chapter 25) requires **urgent** diagnosis because early medical and surgical intervention reduces the high short-term mortality. The **chest pain** of aortic dissection is typically described as sudden, severe, tearing pain that radiates to the back and interscapular areas. **Examination** may reveal a difference in right and left arm blood pressures, pulse deficits, and focal neurologic deficits. Aortic dissection also may involve the aortic valve or coronary ostia. The latter may be associated with myocardial ischemia and ST-segment elevation on an **ECG.**

C. Pulmonary embolism is potentially life threatening and can be associated with chest pain. The **chest pain** of pulmonary embolism is typically pleuritic in character and is associated with dyspnea and tachypnea. There is often a **history** of recent surgical intervention, malignant disease, or immobility. The cardinal **clinical findings** include hypoxia and tachycardia. An **ECG** may demonstrate an S_1–Q_3 T_3 pattern, right bundle branch block, and right axis deviation.

SUGGESTED READINGS

References
1. Sgarbossa EB, Pinski SL, Barbagelata A, et al. Electrocardiographic diagnosis of evolving acute myocardial infarction in the presence of left bundle-branch block: GUSTO-1 (Global Utilization of Streptokinase and Tissue Plasminogen Activator for Occluded Coronary Arteries) Investigators [published correction appears in *N Engl J Med* 1996;334:931]. *N Engl J Med* 1996;334:481–487.
2. Puleo PR, Meyer D, Wathen C, et al. Use of a rapid assay of subforms of creatine kinase-MB to diagnose or rule out acute myocardial infarction. *N Engl J Med* 1994;331:561–566.
3. Ohman EM, Armstrong PW, Christenson RH, et al. Cardiac troponin T levels for risk stratification in acute myocardial ischemia: GUSTO IIA investigators. *N Engl J Med* 1996;335:1333–1341.
4. Antman EM, Tanasijevic MJ, Thompson B, et al. Cardiac-specific troponin I levels to predict the risk of mortality in patients with acute coronary syndromes. *N Engl J Med* 1996;335:1342–1349.
5. Olatidoye AG, Wu AH, Feng YJ, Waters D. Prognostic role of troponin T versus troponin I in unstable angina pectoris for cardiac events with meta-analysis comparing published studies. *Am J Cardiol* 1998;81:1405–1410.
6. Hamm CW, Goldmann BU, Heeschen C, Kreymann G, Berger J, Meinertz T. Emergency room triage of patients with acute chest pain by means of rapid testing for cardiac troponin T or troponin I. *N Engl J Med* 1997;337:1648–1653.

Key Review
Jesse RL, Kontos MC. Evaluation of chest pain in the emergency department. *Curr Probl Cardiol* 1997;22:149–236.

Relevant Book Chapter
Gibler WB. Diagnosis of acute coronary syndromes in the emergency department. In: Topol EJ, ed. *Acute coronary syndromes.* New York: Marcel Dekker, 1998:193–232.

SECTION IX. PREVENTIVE CARDIOLOGY

JoAnne Micale Foody and Dennis Sprecher

38. CARDIOVASCULAR RISK FACTORS

Joanne Micale Foody

I. **Introduction.** Coronary artery disease (CAD) is the **leading cause of morbidity and mortality in the industrialized world.** According to projections, it will become the leading cause of disease globally in the twenty-first century.
   A. **Mortality. CAD is the number one killer** in the United States. One-fourth of a million people each year die within 1 hour of the onset of symptoms. Approximately 50% had no previous symptoms. CAD causes nearly 500,000 deaths in the United States per year. This represents one-half of the overall 1 million deaths caused by cardiovascular disease, which includes high blood pressure, stroke, rheumatic heart disease, and CAD. One of every five deaths in the United States is caused by CAD. More than 1.9 million people will have a myocardial infarction (MI) this year, and one-third of the MIs will be fatal. The rate of death from CAD increases with age; among persons older than 75 years the death rate is twice that among persons older than 65 years (1).
   B. **Morbidity.** There are 13.5 million Americans with a history of MI or angina pectoris (1). Seven million people have angina pectoris, which is two times more common among women than men. Clearly many more persons have CAD than is apparent on the basis of previous MI or angina. Another 13.6 million people are likely to have asymptomatic CAD. More than 50% of total MIs occur among persons older than 65 years. Although 20% more MIs are experienced by men before the age of 65 years, three times more than that are experienced by women after the age of 65 years. Congestive heart failure (CHF), the leading reason for hospitalization among persons older than 65 years, is primarily associated with previous hypertension and known CAD.
   C. **Economic consequences of cardiovascular disease.** An estimated $259.1 billion was allocated in 1997 to manage cardiovascular illness. Most cardiovascular disease costs are related to CAD (1).
   D. **Prevention of CAD.** Table 38-1 shows important targets for CAD prevention. The consequences of modest population-wide risk reduction (e.g., reduction in fat intake [currently 33% of total calories] and cholesterol levels) and life-saving technologies (e.g., surgery, angioplasty, coronary care units) have resulted in a reduction in death rate but an increase in morbidity and in the prevalence of CHF. National guidelines from the American Heart Association (AHA) and American College of Cardiology have emphasized the importance of preventive strategies in the care of patients at risk for or with CAD (2).

II. **Hyperlipidemia.** Except for age, dyslipidemia is the most **important predictive factor for CAD.** There is a strong, independent, continuous, and graded relation between total cholesterol (TC) or low-density lipoprotein cholesterol (LDL-C) level and risk for CAD events. This relation has been clearly demonstrated among men and women and in all age groups. More than one-half of U.S. adults (96 million) have TC levels greater than 200 mg/dL; one-third (38 million) have values greater than 240 mg/dL. In general a 1% increase in LDL-C level leads to a 2% to 3% increase in risk for CAD.
   A. **Physiology**
      1. **Lipoproteins** are large molecular compounds that are essential to the transport of cholesterol and triglycerides (TG) within the blood. They contain a lipid core composed of TG and cholesterol esters surrounded by phospholipids and specialized proteins known as **apolipoproteins.** The **five major families of lipoproteins** are **chylomicrons,** very-low-density lipoproteins (**VLDL**), intermediate-density lipoproteins (**IDL**), low-density lipoproteins (**LDL**), and high-density lipoproteins

Table 38-1. Important targets for prevention of coronary artery disease

Estimated LDL = TC – HDL – (TG/5)
LDL cholesterol <130 mg/dL, <100 mg/dL (CAD)
TG <150 mg/dL, <100 (CAD)
TC/HDL ratio <4. <3 (CAD)
Blood sugar <100 mg/dL
Blood pressure <130/85 mm Hg, <120/80 (CAD)
Homocysteine < 10 ng/mg
Lipoprotein(a) <30 mg/dL
20 min aerobic exercise 3 times per week
No smoking
Waist to hip ratio <0.8
Hemoglobin A, C <6.5 g/L

LDL, Low-density lipoprotein; *TC,* total cholesterol; *HDL,* high-density lipoprotein; *TG,* triglycerides; *CAD,* coronary artery disease; *Lp(a),* lipoprotein(a).

   (**HDL**). Chylomicrons are the largest, least dense lipoproteins and contain the least amount of lipid.

   2. **Apolipoproteins** are necessary for the the structure and enzymatic processes of lipids. Apolipoprotein A1 (**apo A1**) is a major component of **HDL,** and apolipoprotein B (**apo B**) is the main apolipoprotein for the remaining **non-HDL** lipoproteins.

   3. **Lipid-modifying enzymes** and **lipid transport proteins** have an important role in lipoprotein metabolism and possibly in **atherosclerosis.** Lipoprotein lipase hydrolyzes TG in chylomicrons and VLDL, binds to the surface of capillary endothelial cells, and binds to the chylomicron and VLDL. Hepatic lipase is present predominantly in the hepatic sinusoids and hydrolyzes both chylomicrons and phospholipids. Lecithin-cholesterol acyltransferase converts free cholesterol to cholesterol ester on lipoproteins by means of transferring fatty acids from phospholipid to cholesterol. The cholesterol ester transfer protein transfers cholesterol esters among lipoproteins. These enzymes act together to modulate lipoprotein transport and metabolism and have important implications for the development of atherosclerosis.

B. Lipid-lowering trials. Aggressive lipid-lowering drug treatment of persons at high risk reduces CAD morbidity and mortality rates and increases overall survival rate (3–7).

   1. **Regression trials.** A number of smaller trials evaluated the effect of aggressive lipid-lowering therapy on actual vessel blockage. These so-called regression trials assessed the degree of atherosclerotic progression and regression by means of either ultrasonography of the carotid arteries or more often coronary angiography.

      a. Although lesion regression was uncommon, the rate of lesion progression often was slowed appreciably with lipid-lowering therapy.

      b. The modest degree of change in vascular end points was disproportionate to the substantial reduction in clinical events observed in some regression trials. The small changes in luminal narrowing observed with lowering TC level are unlikely to be the principal mechanism by which lipid-lowering measures achieve a reduction in clinical events and revascularization rates.

      c. Several factors may mediate risk for plaque rupture, including the functional state of the vascular endothelium and the morphologic and biochemical composition of the atherosclerotic plaque.

      d. Endothelium-dependent vasomotor function and the cellular characteristics of plaques that seem to be intimately related to rupture and thrombosis are factors that might explain clinical success in correcting dyslipidemia.

2. **Primary prevention trials.** The **strongest evidence** that lipoproteins are causally related to the development of CAD is derived from randomized clinical primary prevention trials (Table 38-2).

   a. The West of Scotland Coronary Prevention Study (**WOSCOPS**) (5) demonstrated that treatment of men at relatively high risk with profoundly elevated cholesterol levels significantly reduced risk for heart attack and death from heart disease.

   b. The Air Force/Texas Coronary Atherosclerosis Prevention Study (**AFCAPS/TexCAPS**) (7) demonstrated benefit among patients with more typical risk profiles, including lower cholesterol values, than those in WOSCOPS. AFCAPS/TexCAPS capitalized on the increased risk among healthy persons with low HDL levels (mean of 36 mg/dL) and high TC levels (mean of 221 mg/dL). Therapy with the cholesterol-lowering drug lovastatin reduced by 36% the risk for first acute major coronary events among healthy adults with average to mildly elevated cholesterol levels and low HDL levels. By including patients with only mildly elevated TC and low HDL levels, AFCAPS/TexCAPS expanded by more than 8 million the number of persons in the United States who are possible candidates for cholesterol-lowering drug therapy.

3. **Secondary prevention trials** are shown in Table 38-2.

   a. The Scandinavian Simvastatin Survival Study (**4S**) (3) was the first secondary trial to demonstrate clearly a reduction in total mortality. Simvastatin reduced total mortality among patients with CAD by 30% because of a 42% reduction in deaths from CAD. The 4S treated 4,444 men and women with CAD and TC levels of 212 to 309 mg/dL. The mean LDL at baseline was 188 mg/dL with a range of 130 to 266 mg/dL.

   b. The Cholesterol and Recurrent Events Trial (**CARE**) (4), a randomized, controlled trial, was designed to evaluate the effects of treatment with pravastatin on 4,000 persons who had experienced acute MI 3

Table 38-2. Statin trials

Study	Intervention	End point	Risk reduction (%)
PRIMARY PREVENTION TRIALS			
WOSCOPS (5) (men only)	Pravastatin	Fatal CAD, nonfatal MI	31 MI
		Total mortality	22 total mortality
AFCAPS/TEXCAPS (7)	Lovastatin (Mevacor)	Fatal CAD, nonfatal MI	36
SECONDARY PREVENTION TRIALS USING STATINS			
4S (3)	Simvastatin	Total mortality	30
		Fatal CAD, nonfatal MI	44
CARE (4)	Pravastatin	Fatal CAD, nonfatal MI	24
LIPID (6)	Pravastatin	CAD mortality	34

WOSCOPS, West of Scotland Coronary Prevention Study; CAD, coronary artery disease; MI, myocardial infarction; AFCAPS/TexasCAPS, Air Force/Texas Coronary Atherosclerosis Prevention Study; 4S, Scandinavian Simvastatin Survival Study; CARE, Cholesterol and Recurrent Events; LIPID, Long-Term Intervention with Pravastatin in Ischemic Disease.

to 20 months before randomization and had moderately elevated TC levels (mean 209 mg/dL). The benefits of pravastatin therapy in preventing recurrent coronary events were similar in the subset analysis of age, sex, ejection fraction, hypertension, diabetes mellitus, and smoking. The results of this secondary prevention trial suggested that **risk reduction in a large portion of the population with only moderately elevated TC could have positive public-health implications.** It remains to be determined whether treatment for lower levels of LDL is beneficial.

 c. The Long-Term Intervention with Pravastatin in Ischemic Disease Study (**LIPID**) (6) was the first to examine the use of a 3-hydroxy-3-methylglutaryl coenzyme A (HMG-CoA) reductase inhibitor by patients with a history of unstable angina. The LIPID study provided new data on noncoronary mortality (stroke) and on other groups such as women and patients with diabetes, who previously had been underrepresented in clinical trials. LIPID demonstrated improved CAD outcomes among all patients, including those with unstable angina.

 4. Clinical studies of vasoregulation. Clinical and experimental evidence is available to support the hypothesis that **hypercholesterolemic states also affect the endothelium.** Hypercholesterolemic endothelial vasomotor dysfunction is responsive to cholesterol-lowering regimens. Improvement in endothelium-dependent flow reserve may represent a new mechanism by which lipid-lowering therapy may exert its beneficial effects. Small but persuasive studies have indicated that both brachial and coronary artery flow reserve increase after LDL reduction and that oxidation may be particularly influential.

C. Management of lipids. Despite national guidelines emphasizing the importance of lipid-lowering therapy, **more than two-thirds of patients treated for hyperlipidemia by primary care physicians do not reach National Cholesterol Education Program (NCEP) Adult Treatment Panel II targets.** More striking is the fact that 80% of patients with established CAD do not reach nationally proposed targets. This problem is partially caused by inconsistent strategies for the treatment of patients at risk for the development and progression of CAD.

 1. Guidelines for primary prevention of CAD events based on the NCEP Adult Treatment Panel II (8)

  a. TC and HDL-C levels. All adults 20 years of age or older, **without a history of CAD or other atherosclerotic disease,** should have TC and HDL-C measured at least once every 5 years. These values may be determined with nonfasting blood samples. Other nonlipid risk factors also should be assessed. For persons without CAD, the following classifications and follow-up care are recommended.

   (1) TC less than 200 mg/dL is classified as **desirable.** If HDL-C is greater than 35 mg/dL, follow-up care includes general education about dietary modification, physical activity, and other risk-reduction activities. Repeating TC and HDL-C measurements in 5 years is recommended. If HDL-C is less than 35 mg/dL, fasting lipoprotein analysis, including LDL-C and TG, is performed because of the increased likelihood of abnormalities of these lipid components among persons with low HDL.

   (2) TC from 200 to 239 mg/dL is classified as **borderline high.** If HDL-C is more than 35 mg/dL and no or only one other CAD risk factor is present, instruction on dietary modification, physical activity, and other risk-reduction activities is provided. TC and HDL-C measurements are repeated in 1 to 2 years. If HDL-C is less than 35 mg/dL or if two or more other risk factors are present, a fasting lipoprotein analysis is performed.

   (3) TC more than 240 mg/dL is classified as **high.** A fasting lipoprotein analysis is performed.

b. **LDL-C levels of persons without CAD or other atherosclerotic disease.** NCEP provides LDL-C cut points for initiating dietary therapy and considering drug therapy (Table 38-3). NCEP also provides a target for LDL-C concentration after therapy. Lifestyle intervention, including dietary therapy, generally is attempted for 3 to 6 months before initiation of drug treatment. Need for intervention is based on estimation of overall risk. For persons **without CAD, treatment and target cut points vary according to the presence of other risk factors for CAD.** Among young persons with no other risk factors for CAD, drug therapy may be indicated only if LDL-C exceeds 190 mg/dL. On the other hand, physicians may chose to initiate drug therapy as primary prevention at 130 mg/dL if overall risk is high on the basis of multiple risk factors.

(1) **LDL-C concentration less than 130 mg/dL** is classified as **desirable.** Persons with desirable LDL-C levels do not need further evaluation at this time. They are instructed about dietary modification, physical activity, and other risk-reduction activities. Information about dietary modification, physical activity, and other risk-reduction activities is provided. TC and HDL-C are measured in 5 years.

(2) **LDL-C concentration from 130 mg/dL to 159 mg/dL** is classified as **borderline high** in primary prevention. If no or only one other risk factor is present, information about dietary modification, physical activity, and other risk-reduction activities is provided. Lipoprotein analysis is repeated annually.

(3) Persons classified as having **borderline-high LDL-C** and who have two or more other risk factors or as having **high LDL-C** (greater than 160 mg/dL) undergo a full clinical evaluation and begin active cholesterol-lowering dietary therapy.

2. **Guidelines for secondary prevention of coronary events.** Optimal LDL-C concentration for a patient with CAD is **less than 100 mg/dL.**

   a. **Patients who have achieved this level** receive individual instruction on the AHA step II diet and physical activity. Lipoprotein analysis is conducted annually.

   b. **Patients with higher than optimal LDL-C** undergo a full clinical examination and evaluation for secondary causes of dyslipidemia and familial disorders. The physician considers the influences of

Table 38-3. Treatment cut points and targets for therapy based on low-density cholesterol level: primary and Secondary Prevention

Patient category	Initiation level (mg/dL)		Low-density cholesterol target (mg/dL)
	Diet	Drug	
No CAD, <2 other risk factors[a]	>160	>190	<160
No CAD, >2 other risk factors[a]	>130	>160	<130
With CAD or other atherosclerotic disease	>100	>130	<100

CAD, Coronary artery disease

[a] Risk factors are age less than 45 yr for men less than 55 yr for women; family (MI or sudden death of first-degree relative before 55 yr for male or 65 yr for female relative), smoking, hypertension, diabetes mellitus.

age, sex, and other CAD risk factors. Once the evaluation is complete, therapy is cholesterol-lowering therapy initiated on the basis of recommended cut points. If LDL-C remains at **100 to 130 mg/dL** in secondary prevention despite lifestyle changes, the physician uses clinical judgment about overall risk to determine whether drug therapy should be initiated.

c. For secondary prevention in adults with **evidence of CAD or other atherosclerotic disease,** lipoprotein analysis is performed after 12 hours of fasting. Definitive lipoprotein analysis is performed when the patient is not in the recovery phase from an acute event, which can lower the usual LDL-C concentration. Physicians may want to begin lipid-lowering therapy before a patient is discharged from the hospital in view of the patient's risk factors.

d. Decisions should be based on the **average of two LDL-C determinations 1 to 8 weeks apart.** If the first two LDL-C determinations differ by more than 30 mg/dL, a third test result is obtained within 1 to 8 weeks, and the average value of the tests is used.

3. **Types of therapy**

a. **Diet.** The NCEP and the AHA promote a diet in which **fat composes only 30% or less of the total calories for the day.** The first step in dietary therapy, usually the AHA step I diet, parallels NCEP recommendations. The AHA committee on nutrition uses recommendations from the World Health Organization to suggest that fat calories constitute no less than 15% of total calories. The AHA step I and II diets (Table 38-4) involve reducing the intake of saturated fat and cholesterol to lower LDL-C. A change from the average U.S. diet to the step I diet of less than 10% saturated fatty acids and less than 300 mg/day cholesterol reduces serum cholesterol levels approximately 7%. In the step II diet, further restriction to less than 7% saturated fatty acids and less than 200 mg/day cholesterol should reduce cholesterol levels an additional 3% to 7%.

b. **Pharmacotherapy.** Guidelines from the AHA and American College of Cardiology (see **I.D**) for modifying the cholesterol levels of **persons without CAD** indicate that the **goal of therapy is an LDL-C less than 130 mg/dL.** For persons **with documented CAD** the goal is to lower LDL-C levels to **less than 100 mg/dL.** The guidelines also recommend that a **statin** (HMG-CoA reductase inhibitor) be the **initial therapy in the care of patients with TG levels less than 400 mg/dL.** The high efficacy of statins in lowering LDL-C and their few side effects make them an attractive choice for patients with established CAD. Given the early benefits of cholesterol-lowering therapy among patients with CAD and substantial risk for recurrent, often fatal events, **it is inappropriate to wait several months before beginning drug therapy.** If at a patient's 4- to 6-week follow-up evaluation after MI, LDL-C levels are greater than

Table 38-4. Step I and step II diet recommendations (% of total calories)

Measure	Step I diet	Step II diet
Total fat	<30%	<30%
Saturated fat	8–10%	<7%
Polyunsaturated fat	Up to 10%	Up to 10%
Monounsaturated fat	Up to 15%	Up to 15%
Carbohydrates	50–60%	50–60%
Protein	15%	15%
Cholesterol	<300 mg/dL	<200 mg/dL

100 mg/dL, the patient should be considered a candidate for drug intervention.

(1) The second report of the NCEP Adult Treatment Panel (8) included **HMG-CoA reductase inhibitors** among the first-line alternatives in the management of hypercholesterolemia. The category includes six drugs: lovastatin, simvastatin, pravastatin, fluvastatin, atorvastatin, and cerivastatin (see Drug Index for dosages).

    (a) **Effectiveness.** When dietary measures are inadequate HMG-CoA reductase inhibitors effectively **lower TC and LDL-C among patients with mixed hyperlipidemias** (elevated cholesterol and TG). HMG-CoA reductase inhibitors are **extremely effective in reducing LDL-C among most patients with primary hypercholesterolemia.** HMG-CoA reductase inhibitors decrease TC 15% to 60% and LDL-C 20% to 60% and increase HDL-C 5% to 15%. Declines in apo B commensurate with reductions in LDL have been demonstrated. TG levels have been reduced 10% to 25%. The lowering of TG parallels the lowering of LDL in that higher doses of more potent agents produce TG reductions of more than 40%. The HMG-CoA reductase inhibitors appear to have minimal effects on apo AI, apo AII, and lipoprotein(a) [Lp(a)]. **Lovastatin, simvastatin, pravastatin, and fluvastatin are well-tolerated, efficacious,** and approximately equivalent with respect to safety profiles during monotherapy within trials. The **safety and efficacy of cerivastatin and atorvastatin have not been determined** in large clinical trials. Given their similar drug class, there is no reason to believe these agents will not perform as effectively and safely as the other statins.

    (b) **Inadequate response**

        (i) Before atorvastatin and cerivastatin became available most patients with CAD needed two or three agents to maintain LDL values less than 100 mg/dL. This may be somewhat easier with more potent agents. Combination therapy may be required in only the most extreme cases [see **II.C.3.b.(1)(c)**].

        (ii) The infrequent occurrence of a **negligible response** may be caused by poor absorption of the medication or rapid catabolism and clearance. Multiple daily dosing may be helpful in these cases. More frequently, combination therapy is needed [see **II.C. 3.b.(1)(c)**].

    (c) **Averse effects.** Fewer than 5% of patients in controlled clinical trials reported side effects with HMG-CoA reductase inhibitors.

        (i) **Minor side effects.** The most common side effects are mild gastrointestinal disturbances (nausea, abdominal pain, diarrhea, constipation, flatulence), which rarely warrant discontinuation of therapy. Headache, fatigue, pruritus, and myalgia are other minor side effects that seldom prompt termination of treatment.

        (ii) **Liver function test abnormalities.** Mild transient elevations in liver enzymes have been reported with all HMG-CoA reductase inhibitors. Elevations in serum amino transferase levels to three times the upper limit of normal occurred among less than 2% of patients in controlled clinical trials. At the usual midrange dosing, the frequency of abnormalities is less than 1%. In general, for each doubling of a statin dose, there is an 0.6% increase in risk for elevation of transaminase levels. Therapy should be discontinued when greater than threefold elevation occurs. Enzyme levels typically return to normal within 2 weeks. Either lower doses of the same medication can be reinstituted or a different HMG-CoA reductase inhibitor can be used. **Monitoring of hepatic aminotransferase levels is recommended for those taking HMG-CoA reductase inhibitors.** Levels should be measured 6 weeks and 3 months after initiation of therapy and every 6 months thereafter. Because of the excellent safety profiles of **pravastatin and simvastatin,** the U.S. Food and Drug Administration (FDA) recommends discontinuing hepatic enzyme monitoring after 3 months for pravastatin and after 6 months of continuous same-dose therapy for simvastatin.

- (iii) **Myopathy,** a rare but potentially serious side effect of HMG-CoA reductase inhibitors, occurs with muscle symptoms and elevations in serum creatine kinase (CK) level to more than 10 times the upper limit of normal. CK measurements are not needed unless symptoms occur.

- (iv) **Drug interactions.** When statins are used in combination with some pharmaceutical agents, such as erythromycin, gemfibrozil, azole antifungals, cimetidine, methotrexate, or cyclosporine, risk for CK elevation and myositis increases. These drug combinations should be either avoided or used judiciously with interval measurements of CK levels and liver function. Pravastatin and fluvastatin in combination with other drugs are considered relatively safe because these two drugs do not use the cytochrome P450 3A4 microsomal pathways.

- (d) **Combination therapy.** One-third of patients with hypercholesterolemia do not respond adequately to one-drug therapy. The target level of 100 mg/dL or less may be difficult to attain. Combination therapy, which reduces LDL 30% to 55%, often is needed.

  - (i) The combination of a **statin with a bile-acid sequestrant** is ideal. At one time therapy combining high doses of both statins and resins was administered. More recent reviews favor the addition of low-dose resins over doubling of ongoing statin agents. Addition of 4 to 8 grams of a resin to an ongoing statin regimen usually results in greater LDL lowering than doubling the statin dose. The marginal value of adding resin to a statin will likely diminish as the potency of statin agents increases. The sequestrant provides little added toxicity, and the LDL-C lowering needed may not necessitate a full sequestrant dosage. In isolated forms of LDL elevation, HMG-CoA reductase inhibitors and bile acid resins exhibit highly complementary mechanisms of action in combination therapy.

        (ii) **Combining a statin with niacin** may increase risk for drug-induced myopathy. Because risk for myopathy may be as high as 3% among patients taking this drug combination, all patients are instructed to report any muscle pain and to discontinue drug use until a medical evaluation is conducted and CK levels are determined.

       (iii) When a **statin is used with gemfibrozil,** the report of myopathy may be as high as 5%.

       (iv) **Triple-drug therapy (statin, niacin, and resin)** occasionally is necessary to lower LDL-C levels to less than 100 mg/dL. Patients need careful monitoring for liver and muscular toxicity (Table 38-5).

    (2) **Statins and stroke**

      (a) The link between elevated cholesterol level and stroke until recently has not been clear.

      (b) 4S, WOSCOPS, CARE, and LIPID provide a **clear basis for statin therapy in decreasing the incidence of fatal and nonfatal stroke.** Use of statins substantially reduces the likelihood of ischemic stroke among patients with a history of CAD both with or without elevated cholesterol level.

III. Hypertension. Hypertension contributes to MI, cerebrovascular accidents, CHF, peripheral vascular disease (PVD), and increased mortality among men and women of all ages and ethnic groups with or without signs or symptoms of CAD. Hypertension is defined as systolic blood pressure 140 mm Hg or greater, diastolic blood pressure 90 mm Hg or greater, or need for antihypertensive medication; high blood pressure, as defined, occurs among 25% of the adult population.

    A. Etiology. Hypertension is a complex disease modified by both environmental and genetic determinants. Blood pressure levels are correlated among family members.

      1. **High blood pressure does not follow the classic mendelian rules of inheritance** attributable to a single gene locus. The currently documented exceptions are a few rare forms of hypertension, such as those

Table 38-5. Clinically encountered lipid phenotypes and therapies

	Isolated LDL-C phenotype	Combined phenotype	High TG/low HDL-C phenotype
Clinical markers	**LDL-C** >100 mg/dL (CAD) >130 mg/dL (2 CAD risk factors) **HDL-C** >40 (men) >50 (women) **TG** <250 mg/dL	**LDL-C** >100 mg/dL (CAD) >130 mg/dL (2 CAD RF) **HDL-C** <40 (men) <50 women **TG** >250 mg/dL	**HDL-C** <40 mg/dL (men) <50 mg/dL (women) **TG** >250 mg/dL
Therapy	**Statin, statin/resin,** resin	**Statin** with or **without niacin, statin gemfibrozil,** niacin, gemfibrozil, fenofibrate	**Fibrate, niacin,** lifestyle intervention

Bold, Preferred therapy.

LDL-C, Low-density lipoprotein cholesterol; *TG,* triglycerides; HDL-C, high-density lipoprotein cholesterol; *CAD,* coronary artery disease.

related to a single mutation involving a chimeric 11-β-hydroxylase–aldosterone synthase gene, Liddle syndrome, and variants in the angiotensinogen locus, which cause primary hypertension among white persons. Other potential candidate genes suggested by recent experimental data include those that affect various components of the renin-angiotensin-aldosterone system, the kallikrein-kinin system, and the sympathetic nervous system. Increased left ventricular (LV) mass and thickness and altered vascular capacity and responsiveness occur more frequently among patients with a family history of hypertension.

2. Potential contributors to hypertension include variations in sodium intake, renin-angiotensin system, renal function and natriuresis, sympathetic nervous system, vascular function, cell membrane alterations, hyperinsulinemia and insulin resistance, atrial natriuretic factor, and prostaglandins.

B. Pathophysiology

1. The **positive relation between systolic and diastolic blood pressure and cardiovascular risk** has long been recognized. This relation is strong, continuous, graded, consistent, independent, predictive, and etiologically significant for those with and without CAD.

   a. The Multiple Risk Factor Intervention Trial (**MRFIT**) (9), a prospective study (11.6 years average follow-up period) with more than 361,000 subjects, has provided the most data regarding the relation between blood pressure and CAD. Baseline blood pressure was shown to be strongly and independently related to increased risk for CAD. The relation was shown to be stronger for systolic than diastolic blood pressure, the **risk for CAD progressively increasing for an increase in systolic blood pressure.** The death rate among men with systolic blood pressures of 140 to 149 mm Hg (2.4 per 1,000) and 150 to 159 mm Hg (3.1 per 1,000) was 40% higher than the death rate among men with a baseline systolic blood pressure less than 120 mm Hg.

   b. Data analysis has shown that the death rate in the follow-up period can be lowered 36% by means of primary prevention of hypertension in the general population. A reduction in rates of stroke and CAD with antihypertensive therapy has been demonstrated even in the presence of isolated systolic hypertension.

   c. Subjects with blood pressure less than 120/80 mm Hg have the fewest cardiovascular events (9). Current guidelines recommend 140/90 as the treatment cut point.

   d. The rise in blood pressure and increased prevalence of **hypertension among the elderly** are not benign occurrences and are not to be viewed as a normal consequence of aging. In some epidemiologic studies involving elderly persons, the relation between blood pressure and mortality appeared to be a U-shaped curve. After adjustment for confounding variables and exclusion of deaths within the first 3 years of the follow-up period, however, a linear relation between blood pressure and mortality from cardiovascular disease and all-cause mortality was demonstrated. Persons with isolated systolic hypertension, the prevalence of which increases as the population ages, are at increased risk for morbidity and mortality related to cardiovascular disease.

      (1) Data from the Systolic Hypertension in the Elderly Program (**SHEP**) (10) show that 8% of persons 60 to 69 years of age had isolated systolic hypertension, defined as systolic blood pressure greater than 160 mm Hg and diastolic blood pressure less than 90 mm Hg, as did 11% of those 70 to 79 years of age and 22% of those older than 80 years.

    (2) The relation of systolic blood pressure and diastolic blood pressure to cardiovascular events is more pronounced among persons 65 years and older. The association is stronger and more consistent for systolic blood pressure than for diastolic blood pressure and is evident at levels considerably less than 140 mm Hg.

2. Careful alteration in both diastolic and systolic values has not translated into the expected reductions in cardiac events. Metaanalyses suggest that a 7 to 10 mm Hg reduction in diastolic pressures reduces CAD by about 17%. The relative reduction in stroke, in contrast, is totally consistent with expectations, providing over 30% lessening in stroke rates. Generally, the yearly percent risk (risk of event by end of study, divided by duration of study) is between 0.5% and 2.5% at age 40 years or higher.

3. Over the last few years, **greater emphasis has been placed on systolic pressure in characterizing cardiovascular risk.** The age-adjusted 10-year mortality in the MRFIT trial (9) revealed systolic blood pressure to be a stronger predictor of events from CAD than did diastolic blood pressure. High systolic blood pressure conferred CAD risk regardless of diastolic blood pressure. A systolic blood pressure of 140 to 149 mm Hg confers greater CAD mortality risk than a diastolic blood pressure of 90 to 94 mm Hg. A systolic blood pressure of 150 to 159 mm Hg carries greater risk than a diastolic blood pressure of 95 to 100 mm Hg. According to the SHEP study (10), isolated systolic hypertension, which accounts for 60% of cases of hypertension among the elderly, is highly correlated with cardiovascular disease and is important to control.

C. **Clinical presentation.** Detection of hypertension begins with proper **blood pressure measurements,** which should be obtained at each health care encounter.

1. Data for evaluation are acquired through the medical history, physical examination, laboratory tests, and other diagnostic procedures. Evaluation of patients with documented hypertension has the following three **objectives:**

    a. To identify known causes of high blood pressure

    b. To assess the presence or absence of end-organ damage and cardiovascular disease, the extent of the disease, and response to therapy

    c. To identify other cardiovascular risk factors or concomitant disorders that may define prognosis and guide treatment.

2. A **medical history** should focus on identifying important risk factors or symptoms of hypertension.

3. Repeated **blood pressure measurements** determine whether initial elevations persist and necessitate prompt attention or whether blood pressure has returned to normal and the patient needs only periodic surveillance. Ambulatory blood pressure monitoring is most clinically helpful and is most commonly used to evaluate patients with suspected white-coat hypertension. It is also helpful in the care of patients with apparent drug resistance, hypotensive symptoms with antihypertensive medications, episodic hypertension, and autonomic dysfunction.

    a. **Office visits.** Clinicians should explain to patients the meaning of their blood pressure readings and advise them of the **need for periodic remeasurement.** Blood pressure is measured in a standardized manner with equipment that meets certification criteria.

        (1) Patients sit in a chair with their backs supported and their arms bared and supported at heart level.

        (2) Patients should refrain from smoking or ingesting caffeine during the 30 minutes preceding the measurement.

        (3) Measurement should begin after at least 5 minutes of rest.

(4) The appropriate cuff size must be used to ensure accurate measurement. The bladder within the cuff should encircle at least 80% of the arm. Many adults need a large adult cuff.

(5) Measurements are taken preferably with a mercury sphygmomanometer; otherwise, a recently calibrated aneroid manometer or a validated electronic device can be used.

(6) Both systolic blood pressure and diastolic blood pressure are recorded. The first appearance of sound (phase 1) is used to define systolic blood pressure. The disappearance of sound (phase V) is used to define diastolic blood pressure.

(7) Two or more readings separated by 2 minutes should be averaged. If the first two readings differ by more than 5 mm Hg, additional readings should be obtained and averaged.

b. Ambulatory blood pressure monitoring. A variety of commercially available monitors that are reliable, convenient, easy to use, and accurate are available. These monitors typically are programmed to take readings every 15 to 30 minutes throughout the day and night while patients go about their normal daily activities. The readings can be downloaded for computer analysis.

(1) **Normal** ambulatory blood pressure values are **lower than clinical readings while patients are awake** (less than 135/85 mm Hg) and are **even lower while patients are asleep** (less than 120/75 mm Hg). The blood pressure of most persons falls by 10% to 20% during the night. This change is more closely related to patterns of sleep and wakefulness than to time of day, as illustrated by the blood pressure rhythm that follows the inverted cycle of activity of night-shift workers.

(2) **Patients with hypertension.** An extensive and consistent body of evidence indicates that **ambulatory blood pressure correlates more closely than clinical blood pressure with a variety of measures of end-organ damage,** such as left ventricular hypertrophy (LVH). Prospective data relating ambulatory blood pressure to prognosis are limited to two published studies, which suggest that among patients for whom an elevated clinic pressure is the only abnormality, ambulatory monitoring may help identify a group at relatively low risk for morbidity.

4. Physical examination should include the following components:

a. Fundoscopic examination for hypertensive retinopathy (arteriolar narrowing, focal arteriolar constrictions, arteriovenous crossing changes, hemorrhages and exudates, disc edema).

b. Examination of the **neck** for carotid bruits, distended veins, or an enlarged thyroid gland.

c. Examination of the **heart** for abnormalities in rate and rhythm, increased size, precordial heave, clicks, murmurs, and S_3 and S_4.

d. Examination of the **lungs** for rales and evidence for bronchospasm.

e. Examination of the **abdomen** for bruits, enlarged kidneys, masses, and abnormal aortic pulsation. Abdominal bruits, particularly those that lateralize to the renal area or have a diastolic component, suggest renovascular disease. Abdominal or flank masses may be polycystic kidneys.

f. Examination of the **extremities** for diminished or absent peripheral arterial pulsations, bruits, and edema. Delayed or absent femoral arterial pulses and decreased blood pressure in the lower extremities may indicate aortic coarctation.

g. Neurologic assessment

h. Other assessments. Labile hypertension or paroxysms of hypertension accompanied by headache, palpitations, pallor, and perspiration suggest pheochromocytoma. Truncal obesity with purple striae suggests Cushing's syndrome.

D. Laboratory evaluation

1. It is recommended that the clinician request routine laboratory tests before initiating therapy to determine the presence of end-organ damage and other risk factors. These routine tests include **urinalysis, complete blood cell count, blood chemistry, and 12-lead electrocardiogram (ECG).**

2. Additional diagnostic procedures may be indicated to seek causes of hypertension, particularly for patients whose age, history, physical examination findings, severity of hypertension, or initial laboratory findings suggest such causes; those whose blood pressures are responding poorly to drug therapy; those with well-controlled hypertension whose blood pressures begin to increase; those with stage 3 hypertension; and those with sudden onset of hypertension. **Optional tests** include creatinine clearance, microalbuminuria, 24-hour urinary protein, blood calcium, uric acid, fasting TG levels, LDL-C, glycosylated hemoglobin, thyroid-stimulating hormone, and limited echocardiography (to determine the presence of LVH).

    a. Examples of **clues from laboratory tests** include unprovoked hypokalemia (primary aldosteronism), hypercalcemia (hyperparathyroidism), and elevated creatinine or abnormal urinalysis (renal parenchymal disease).

    b. The **presence of LVH** as determined by means of ECG or echocardiography has been known to be an important risk factor for adverse cardiovascular events and an independent predictor of high risk for CAD, cardiovascular disease, and all-cause mortality. LVH, the consequence of chronic pressure or volume overload and obesity, seems to be a stronger predictor of MI and CAD death than the degree of hypertension. LV mass, as assessed with echocardiography, is a powerful predictor of cardiovascular events, cardiovascular mortality, and all-cause mortality.

3. **More complete assessment** of cardiac anatomy and function by means of conventional echocardiography, examination of structural alterations in arteries by means of ultrasonography, measurement of ankle/arm index, and plasma renin activity and urinary sodium determination may be useful in assessing **cardiovascular status** in selected patients.

E. Risk stratification

1. Although classification of adult blood pressure is somewhat arbitrary, it is useful to clinicians who must make treatment decisions on the basis of a constellation of factors. A classification of blood pressure is shown in Table 38-6. The criteria are limited to persons who are not taking antihypertensive medication and have no acute illness. **Classification is based on the average of two or more blood pressure readings** taken. When systolic blood pressure and diastolic blood pressure fall

Table 38-6. Classification of blood pressure for adults 18 years and older

Category	Systolic/diastolic blood pressure (mm Hg)
Optimal	<120/<80
Normal	<130/<85
High-normal	130–139/85–89
Hypertension	
Stage 1	140–159/90–99
Stage 2	160–179/100–109
Stage 3	≥180/≥110

into different categories, **the higher category should be selected** to classify the patient's blood pressure.

2. Risk for cardiovascular disease among patients with hypertension is determined not only by the **level of blood pressure** but also by the **presence or absence of end-organ damage or other risk factors** such as smoking, dyslipidemia, and diabetes. These factors independently modify risk for subsequent cardiovascular disease. The presence or absence of these factors is determined during the routine evaluation of patients with hypertension (history, physical examination, laboratory tests). This empiric classification stratifies patients with hypertension into risk groups for therapeutic decisions. The World Health Organization Expert Committee on Hypertension Control recommends a similar approach. Obesity and physical inactivity are also predictors of cardiovascular risk and interact with other risk factors, but they are of less importance in the selection of antihypertensive drugs.

   a. **Risk group A** includes patients with high-normal blood pressure or hypertension at stage 1, 2, or 3 (see Table 38-6) who do not have clinical cardiovascular disease, end-organ damage, or other risk factors. Persons with stage 1 hypertension in risk group A are candidates for a longer trial (up to 1 year) of vigorous lifestyle modification with vigilant blood pressure monitoring. If the desired blood pressure is not achieved, pharmacologic therapy is added. For those with stage 2 or stage 3 hypertension, drug therapy is warranted.

   b. **Risk group B** includes patients with hypertension who do not have clinical cardiovascular disease or end-organ damage but have one or more of the risk factors but not diabetes mellitus. This group contains most patients with high blood pressure. If multiple risk factors are present, clinicians consider antihypertensive drugs as initial therapy. Lifestyle modification and management of reversible risk factors are strongly recommended.

   c. **Risk group C** includes patients with hypertension and clinically manifested cardiovascular disease or end-organ damage. According to Joint National Committee (JNC-VI) criteria (11,12), some patients who have high-normal blood pressure and renal insufficiency, heart failure, or diabetes mellitus should be considered for prompt pharmacologic therapy. Appropriate lifestyle modifications always are recommended as adjunct treatment.

F. **Therapy.** Antihypertensive treatment has proved **beneficial in the prevention and reduction of the progression of hypertension, cerebrovascular accidents, CHF, renal insufficiency, and renal failure.** Among patients with mild to moderate hypertension, antihypertensive therapy has not favorably influenced angina, MI, and other atherosclerotic diseases (such as PVD and aortic atherosclerosis). Among some subsets of patients with mild hypertension, therapy has adversely affected these CADs. The lower than expected reduction in CAD risk in most trials of antihypertensive agents has been attributed to the choice of agents, such as thiazide diuretics and β-blockers, that might negatively influence risk for CAD and to the short duration of the trials. Overall, antihypertensive treatment markedly reduces the prevalence of CAD events, CAD mortality (by 16%), and the rate of fatal stroke (by 40%) with similar numbers of deaths prevented.

1. **Nonpharmacologic therapy**

   a. **Weight reduction** reduces both systolic and diastolic blood pressure. Most clinical trials have demonstrated that weight reduction is directly related to blood pressure reduction. A weight loss of approximately 10 lb (4.5 kg) may reduce both systolic and diastolic blood pressure 2 to 3 mm Hg. Among patients with high-normal blood pressure, the need for medical therapy may be averted for one-half of these patients through weight reduction by means of physical activity and calorie restriction.

   b. Exercise reduces blood pressure by means of decreasing cardiac output and peripheral vascular resistance and modifying serum norepinephrine and insulin levels. After an increase in physical activity, both systolic and diastolic blood pressure have been demonstrated to fall 7 mm Hg with or without weight reduction. Moderate-intensity exercise is as effective as high-intensity exercise for reducing blood pressure.

   c. Diet. A modest, independent benefit of **salt reduction** has been demonstrated. Hypertension is rare in societies that consume low-salt, high-potassium diets. Although the theory that excessive salt intake produces hypertension has been difficult to prove in large clinical trials, most data support the role of dietary salt excess for some persons. In general, low-salt diets are recommended to most patients with hypertension. Pooled estimates have suggested that **salt restriction is most important for older persons, those with higher baseline levels of blood pressure, and particularly those who are salt-sensitive.** Salt restriction reduces the need for combination antihypertensive medications.

   d. Both alcohol and tobacco increase blood pressure. **Cessation of smoking and alcohol use** markedly reduces blood pressure and further reduces cardiovascular risk.

2. Medical therapy. Pharmacologic therapy should be initiated in the presence of severe blood pressure elevation, end-organ damage, clinical cardiovascular disease, or other risk factors.

   a. Priority of therapy

     (1) Therapy for most patients with **uncomplicated hypertension** at stage 1 and 2 (see Table 38-6) should **begin with the lowest dose** to prevent adverse effects. If blood pressure remains uncontrolled after 1 to 2 months, the next dosage level may be prescribed. It may take months to adequately control hypertension. Most antihypertensive agents may be taken once a day. To improve patient compliance this regimen is used whenever possible.

     (2) For patients at **higher risk** (stage 3; see Table 38-6), those in risk group 3 (see **III.E.2.c**), or those at particularly high risk for CAD or cerebrovascular accident event, drug therapy to **achieve maximum beneficial reductions** in blood pressure should **proceed without delay.**

     (3) There is **no debate regarding the need for aggressive blood pressure reduction** among patients with **diastolic pressures greater than 115 mm Hg and systolic pressures greater than 160 mm Hg.** JNC-VI aggressively targets the 135/85 mm Hg cut point and incorporates hypertensive therapy into an algorithm of overall risk.

     (4) In the setting of **symptomatic end-organ organ damage,** patients with a systolic blood pressure greater than **200 mm Hg** or a diastolic blood pressure greater than 120 mm Hg may need **hospitalization** for therapy: (see Chapter 37).

     (5) Although some patients may respond to single therapy, **two or more drugs often are required.** The intervals between changes in regimen should not be prolonged, and the maximum dosage of some drugs may be increased.

   b. Selecting the medication. Special considerations include concomitant disease, demographic characteristics, quality of life, cost, and use of other drugs that may cause drug interactions.

     (1) Concomitant diseases. Antihypertensive medications may worsen some diseases and improve others. Table 38-7 provides information on concomitant diseases and possible therapies. In selecting an agent, the physician considers coexisting disease

Table 38-7. Management of hypertension in specific clinical syndromes

Condition	Treatment
Acute coronary syndromes	β-Blockers or nitrates; CCB
Hypertension among African-Americans	Diuretic, CCB, or α-blocker
Arrhythmia	
Sinus bradycardia, SSS, or AV block	Diuretic, ACE inhibitor, or α-blocker
Afibrillation or flutter, SVT	β-Blocker, diltiazem, verapamil, or clonidine
Benign prostatic hypertrophy	α-Blocker
COPD with bronchospasm or asthma	CCB or ACE inhibitor
Diabetes	ACE inhibitor, CCB, or α-blocker
Advanced age (>65 yr)	Diuretic, CCB, ACE inhibitor, or α-blocker at lower doses to avoid postural hypotension
Gout	Any *except* diuretics
Congestive heart failure	
Systolic	ACE inhibitor, diuretic, or α-blocker
Diastolic	CCB or β-blockers
HCOM	β-blockers or verapamil
Hyperlipidemia	α-Blocker, ACE inhibitor, or CCB
Liver dysfunction	Any *except* methyldopa and labetalol
Left ventricular function	ACE inhibitor, CCB, β-blocker, or α-blocker
Post–myocardial infarction	ACE inhibitor, β-blocker, or both
Osteoporosis	Thiazide diuretics
PVD	Vasodilator, ACE inhibitor, CCB or α-blocker
Renal insufficiency (creatinine >2mg/dL)	Loop diuretics, ACE inhibitor, CCB, α-blocker, labetolol, or a combination of these
Diabetic nephropathy	ACE inhibitor
Smokers	α-blockers, ACE inhibitors, or CCB
Isolated systolic hypertension in the elderly	CCB, ACE inhibitor, diuretics

CCB, calcium channel blocker; *SSS,* sick sinus syndrome; *AV,* atrioventricular; *ACE,* angiotensin-converting enzyme inhibitor; *SVT,* supraventricular tachycardia; *COPD,* chronic obstructive pulmonary disease; *HCOM,* hypertrophic obstructive cardiomyopathy; *PVD,* peripheral vascular disease.

in an attempt to increase overall patient benefit, simplify regimens, and reduce cost.

(a) When choosing a certain drug for its favorable effect on comorbidity, clinicians must be aware that reduction of long-term cardiovascular morbidity and mortality has not been demonstrated.

(b) Regression of **LVH** has been associated with a reduction in risk for cardiovascular events. All commonly used antihypertensive agents, except direct vasodilators and weight loss, induce regression of LVH. An unanswered question is whether treatment aimed at reducing LVH will produce substantial prognostic benefit. No large trial has evaluated the prognostic relevance of regression of LVH.

(2) **Dosage.** For most patients, a **low dose of the initial drug** choice is initiated and then titrated to the desired effect. The

optimal formulation provides 24-hour efficacy with a once-daily dose, at least a 50% of the peak effect remaining at the end of 24 hours. Long-acting formulations increase adherence, incur lower cost for some patients, provide consistent blood pressure control, and protect against early-morning sudden death.

 (3) **Special populations.** Neither sex nor age usually affects responsiveness to various agents. In general, hypertension among **African-Americans** is more responsive to monotherapy with diuretics and calcium-channel blockers than with β-blockers or angiotensin-converting enzyme inhibitors. However, if a β-blocker is needed for other therapeutic benefits, differences in efficacy usually can be overcome with reduction of salt intake, higher doses of the drug, or addition of a diuretic.

 (4) **Drug interactions.** Some drug interactions may be beneficial. For example, diuretics acting on different sites in the nephron may increase natriuresis and diuresis, and diltiazem may reduce the amount of cyclosporine needed. Other interactions may be harmful: nonsteroidal anti-inflammatory drugs (NSAIDs) may blunt the action of diuretics, and β-blockers, and angiotensin-converting enzyme inhibitors.

 c. **Treatment of the elderly.** The benefit of blood-pressure lowering is evident in the elderly, with a marked **reduction in both all-cause mortality and CAD mortality,** as shown in multiple trials and studies. SHEP (10) was the first study to show that antihypertensive treatment of the elderly can reduce these events. It is not clear, however, that all agents are equally effective in reducing the rate of cardiovascular events among the elderly.

IV. Diabetes mellitus. Both insulin-dependent diabetes mellitus (IDDM) and non-insulin-dependent diabetes mellitus (NIDDM) are powerful, independent predictors of CAD. CAD, the leading cause of premature death among patients with either IDDM or NIDDM, accounts for nearly 80% of all deaths (13) and hospital admission among persons with diabetes. Nearly 8 million persons in the United States have diabetes mellitus, a disease closely associated with body mass. More than 10% of the U.S. population older than 65 years has NIDDM that has been diagnosed.

 A. **Etiology and pathophysiology**

  1. **Diabetes accelerates the natural process of atherosclerosis.** Accelerated atherosclerosis in a person with diabetes may be attributed to coexistent hypertension, hyperlipidemia, obesity, and insulin resistance.

   a. At autopsy most persons with diabetes are found to have a **greater number of affected coronary vessels, more diffuse distribution of atherosclerosis,** and **greater narrowing of the left main coronary artery** than persons without diabetes. Autopsy studies consistently demonstrate that atherosclerosis is more extensive and accelerated among persons with diabetes than among persons without diabetes. In a study in which over 7,000 sets of coronary arteries autopsy specimens were examined, diabetes was associated with an increase in the extent of lesions in the arteries whether the prevalence of CAD in the country was low or high (14).

   b. Younger persons with IDDM are not spared. Severe and extensive luminal narrowing of large coronary arteries has been found among persons who had an onset of IDDM before 15 years of age and died before the age of 40 years.

   c. Large angiographic trials have consistently demonstrated that patients with diabetes undergoing cardiac catheterization for MI, percutaneous transluminal coronary angioplasty, or planned coronary artery bypass grafting have significantly more severe CAD. Although there is an increased plaque burden, persons with diabetes have decreased coronary collateral circulation. **Diabetes is a** predictor for progression and occlusion of atherosclerotic lesions.

2. Diabetes carries a greater burden of **additional cardiovascular risk.** Persons with diabetes in the Framingham study were nearly four times more likely to have additional cardiovascular risk factors than persons without diabetes. Men in the MRFIT study were three times more likely to die of CAD if they had three risk factors in addition to baseline diabetes alone.

3. **Tight glycemia control** of IDDM **decreases microvascular complications,** such as retinopathy, nephropathy, and neuropathy; there now are similar data for patients with NIDDM. The increased incidence of hypoglycemia that frequently accompanies tight glucose control and the increase in body weight with insulin therapy must be viewed in the overall context of cardiovascular outcomes.

4. **Acute coronary syndrome** is the cause of death among a large percentage of patients with diabetes.

   a. Thirty percent of patients with acute coronary syndrome are persons with diabetes. Despite encouraging results from thrombolytic trials, the **in-hospital mortality rate among persons with diabetes with MI remains twice that of persons without diabetes.** Patients with diabetes who have survived MI have a higher late mortality than persons without diabetes.

   b. Survival and recurrent cardiovascular events among patients with diabetes after MI are closely related to post-MI ejection fraction, the presence of multivessel CAD, the prothrombotic state associated with diabetes, and increased risk for sudden death.

   c. **CHF and cardiogenic shock** are more common and more severe among patients with diabetes than among other patients. The high in-hospital mortality among persons with diabetes is related to the high incidence of CHF among this population and, to a lesser degree, to an increase in reinfarction rate and extension of the infarct.

B. **Risk factors.** In general the prevalence of known major risk factors for CAD is amplified among persons with diabetes. The major risk factors for CAD of particular importance here include alterations in lipoprotein concentration and composition (dyslipidemia), hypertension, hyperinsulinemia, and central obesity, some of which have a genetic determination.

   1. **Dyslipidemia.** One of the most profound risk factors among persons with diabetes is hyperlipidemia. Diabetes is associated with metabolic abnormalities in the transport, composition, and metabolism of lipoproteins. These abnormalities are associated with the type of diabetes, glycemia control, obesity, insulin resistance, presence of diabetic nephropathy, and genetic factors. The dyslipidemia associated with diabetes includes hypertriglyceridemia, low levels of HDL, alterations in the composition of LDL, and an increase in apo B and apo E. CAD among persons with diabetes is strongly associated with the dyslipidemia of diabetes—high TG level, small, dense LDL particles, and low HDL level.

   2. **Hypertriglyceridemia.** Elevated fasting plasma TG level is a hallmark of **insulin resistance syndrome,** a metabolic disorder characterized by hyperinsulinemia, glucose intolerance, decreased HDL-C level, and possibly central obesity and increased production of atherogenic, small, dense LDL particles. Clinicians must consider hypertriglyceridemia a severe metabolic derangement that affects lipoprotein metabolism and coagulation. The defective lipoprotein metabolism involved in hypertriglyceridemia may produce a vascular environment predisposed to atherogenesis.

   3. **Hypertension.** Hypertension is more **prevalent among persons with IDDM or NIDDM** than among persons without diabetes. The role of hypertension as a risk factor for atherosclerosis is at least as strong among persons with diabetes as for persons without diabetes. Hyper-

tension can be the result of diabetic nephropathy, although the frequency of hypertension also appears to be higher among persons with diabetes without renal complications than among the general population. In NIDDM, hypertension occurs as part of a syndrome in which it can coexist with central obesity, insulin resistance, and dyslipidemia (see Chapter 6).

4. **Tobacco.** There is strong evidence that smoking markedly increases risk for both MI and complications of PVD among those with diabetes, especially women. Smoking is believed to be associated with adverse changes in plasma lipids and lipoproteins, especially with low levels of HDL-C.

5. **Hyperinsulinemia.** Hyperinsulinemia is a clinically underrecognized risk factor. There is growing evidence that **patients who do not have frank diabetes but have marked hyperinsulinemia are at increased risk for CAD.** The identification of such a profile of a patient (**syndrome X** or **insulin resistance syndrome**) has important implications for health promotion and disease prevention programs (see Chapter 6).

   a. Persons with a prediabetic condition might have an atherogenic pattern of risk factors before the onset of clinical diabetes. Cardiovascular risk factor status was documented for study subjects who initially did not have diabetes and later participated in a population-based study of diabetes and cardiovascular disease. Later evaluation of baseline values revealed that subjects with a prediabetic condition, compared with persons without diabetes, had higher levels of TC, LDL-C, TG, fasting glucose and insulin, and 2-hour glucose; higher blood pressure and body mass index; and lower levels of HDL-C. The study results demonstrated that subjects with a **prediabetic condition have an atherogenic pattern of risk factors that may be caused by obesity, hyperglycemia, and hyperinsulinemia.** These factors may be present for a long time and may contribute to risk for CAD and clinical diabetes.

   b. Findings from the Paris Prospective Study support the hypothesis that a constellation of metabolic abnormalities, such as elevated TG level, insulin resistance, and obesity may play a deleterious role in CAD risk (15). In this long-term study of CAD risk factors in a sample of 7,028 men with a mean follow-up time of 11 years, the leading independent predictors of CAD death were blood pressure, smoking, cholesterol level, and fasting and 2-hour postload plasma insulin levels. The strongest independent predictor of subsequent CAD death in this quintile was plasma TG concentration, adding to the evidence that hyperinsulinemia and hypertriglyceridemia are related.

C. **Therapies and risk interventions.** Although our knowledge of the epidemiologic and pathophysiologic mechanisms of atherosclerosis associated with diabetes is incomplete, strategies aimed at prevention can be developed. The combination of hypertension, hyperlipidemia, and tobacco use with diabetes greatly accelerates the development of both CAD and diabetic complications. Therefore, **efforts to target all CAD risk factors among persons with diabetes must be undertaken.** With the exception of lipid-lowering therapies, strategies in the prevention of cardiovascular complications among persons with diabetes have not been extensively studied.

   1. **Control of glucose levels.** Tight control of IDDM is indicated for prevention of both microvascular and possibly macrovascular events. Whether tight control of glucose among persons with NIDDM retards progression of CAD is not known.

   2. **Lipid-lowering therapy** is considered critical in the management of NIDDM. In 4S there was 55% reduction in CAD among persons with diabetes (3) and in CARE 25% reduction (4). Although the strategy is controversial, persons with diabetes without heart disease should main-

tain an **LDL of 100 mg/dL or less** in primary prevention, rather than 130 mg/dL.

- a. The 20-year follow-up results of the Seven Countries Study (16) indicate that **decreased intake of saturated fatty acids** and **high vegetable consumption** are associated with a lower incidence of glucose intolerance and a decrease in lipid levels.
- b. The American Dietary Association recommends **mild or moderate weight loss** (10 to 20 lb [4.5 to 9 kg]), which improves diabetes control even if ideal body weight is not achieved.
- c. **Lipid-lowering pharmacologic agents** that can be used by patients with diabetes include fibric acid derivatives and HMG-CoA reductase inhibitors.
  - **(1) Nicotinic acid** has been demonstrated to increase insulin resistance and adversely effect blood glucose levels.
  - **(2) Bile acid–binding resins** may cause gastrointestinal autonomic neuropathy, increase constipation, and increase TG levels, a characteristic among most patients NIDDM. They are used with **caution.**
  - **(3)** The use of β-blockers, diuretics, estrogens, or glucocorticoids increases TG levels and is closely monitored.

3. **Management of hyperinsulinemia**
   - a. Patients are monitored closely for metabolic and physiologic derangements associated with hyperinsulinemia. Although it is not feasible in most instances to check insulin levels, a **hemoglobin A_{1c} level greater than 6.5% is a useful clinical marker** for glucose intolerance and is managed aggressively for all patients at risk.
   - b. Therapy focused at **reducing insulin levels** whether through diet or drug is considered in the care of patients at high risk.

V. **Obesity.** Obesity is established as a leading predictor of CAD and is associated with several cardiovascular risk factors—cholesterol, hypertension, and glucose intolerance, which may increase all-cause mortality and cardiovascular mortality. More than 25% of persons in the United States 18 years or older are more than 20% heavier than their desirable weight. This has come to be a critical problem for African-American women, among whom the prevalence of obesity is 50%.

A. **Pathophysiology**
   1. A positive association between body mass index (BMI), TC and TG levels, and a reduction in HDL-C has been documented in various age groups.
   2. **Distribution of fat appears to be a more important predictor than total amount of fat** because android fat patterns are more metabolically active and highly associated with dyslipidemia. Although both BMI and waist-to-hip ratios have indicated a linear association between obesity and CAD, the **waist-to-hip ratio,** which accounts for abdominal adiposity, is viewed as a more **accurate predictor of CAD.** Among obese persons, those with central adiposity are at particularly high risk. In a cohort of 1,500 women observed for 20 years, the waist-to-hip ratio but not BMI was highly predictive of the occurrence of fatal MI.
   3. The **National Center for Health Statistics still uses BMI,** defined as **weight (kg)/height (m)^2, as the recognized measurement of obesity.** Their guidelines define obesity as a BMI of 27.8 or more for men and 27.3 or more for women. Morbid obesity has been defined as a BMI of 31.1 for men and 32.3 for women. The Nurses Health Study showed that women with a BMI of 25 to 29 had an age-adjusted relative risk for CAD of 1.8 compared with the leanest women. Women with morbid obesity (BMI greater than 29) had a relative risk for CAD of 3.3.
   4. Obesity among adults is associated with **increased LV mass,** a powerful independent predictor of mortality and morbidity from cardiovascular disease. LV mass among persons with obesity but without diabetes prob-

ably depends, at least in part, on the degree of insulin resistance and hyperinsulinemia and not BMI and blood pressure.

5. Central obesity is part of the **insulin resistance syndrome, or syndrome X,** which appears to be associated with increased risk for CAD in both sexes. This condition is characterized by elevated plasma TG and low plasma HDL-C levels.

   a. An essential feature is the presence of **dense, atherogenic LDL.**

   b. Other features are hypertension, impaired glucose intolerance with hyperinsulinemia, and decreased sensitivity to the action of insulin on peripheral tissues.

   c. Hyperinsulinemia is associated with **lipid derangements, increased production of plasminogen activator inhibitor, and enhanced proliferation of cells composing atherosclerotic plaque.** Among patients with hyperinsulinemia, an increased prevalence of CAD and a relation between abnormal insulin, glucose metabolism, and severity of CAD have been reported. The physiologic response to insulin resistance is increased secretion of insulin, which may lead to glucose intolerance or frank diabetes mellitus.

B. Therapy

1. **Calorie restriction, behavior modification, and exercise** are the main treatment modalities for weight loss. The greatest weight losses have occurred with a combined regimen of diet and exercise rather than diet or exercise alone.

2. Several **medications** can be used for temporary management of obesity. Although pharmacologic agents temporarily aid in the struggle against obesity, the National Task Force on Obesity **cautions against the use of these agents for long-term maintenance because of the potential for unknown side effects.**

   a. **Noradrenergic drugs** influence weight loss through stimulation of the hypothalamus.

   b. **Orlistat,** a pancreatic lipase inhibitor, reduces weight through inhibition of fat absorption.

   c. A new class of **serotonin reuptake inhibitors,** including sibutramine, fluoxetine, and sertraline, promote weight loss with varying degrees of side effects.

   d. Use of dexfenfluramine and fenfluramine, already of concern because of rare instances of pulmonary hypertension, has been discontinued because of an increase in valvular heart defects.

3. In the most extreme cases, **surgical therapy** can be provided. Among morbidly obese patients (BMI greater than 40) and obese patients (BMI between 35 and 40) with coexisting conditions, jejunoileal shunts and gastroplasty often aid in the maintenance of weight loss. About 10 years after surgical intervention, 80% of patients maintain a weight 10% less than preoperative weight.

4. **Risk of weight loss.** Even if weight is lost, weight loss maintenance fails in most instances. Health risks that accompany weight cycling are increases in cardiovascular morbidity and mortality, abdominal fat, blood pressure, and insulin resistance.

VI. **Tobacco.** Smoking, the single most preventable cause of death in the United States, is a leading risk factor for CAD, cerebrovascular accident, and PVD. Secondhand smoke has been shown to increase risk for CAD. The causal role of smoking in cardiovascular disease has been derived from more than 20 million person-years of follow-up study (NHLBI, 1996). Twenty-eight percent of white men and 25% of white women smoke, as do 34% of African-American men, 22% of African-American women, 24% of Hispanic men and 15% of Hispanic women. It is estimated that 37% of the population is exposed to secondhand smoke. Exposure to secondhand smoke increases 30% one's risk for death of CAD. More than 90% of current smokers began their habit before they were 21 years of age.

A. Pathophysiology. Cigarette use activates platelets, increases circulating fibrinogen, increases heart rate, and elevates blood pressure. It appears to promote plaque disruption. A strong dose-response relation exists between smoking and CAD. Duration of smoking and the daily amount markedly influence risk for CAD. The number of cigarettes smoked per day is directly proportional to risk for MI. The adverse effect of smoking is present among both men and women (but may be stronger among women) of all ages and ethnic groups with or without prior CAD. Data suggest that risk for cardiac death is two to four times greater among current smokers than nonsmokers.

B. Risk reduction and therapy. Risk for cardiovascular disease begins to decline soon after smoking cessation, irrespective of age and sex. There is a 50% reduction in cardiovascular events within the first 2 to 4 years of cigarette cessation; however, increased cardiovascular risk still exists 10 years after cessation. It is thought to take as long as 20 years to regain baseline risk.

    1. Behavioral and psychosocial treatment. Several techniques have been developed to help patients stop smoking and maintain cessation.

    2. Pharmacotherapy

        a. Nicotine replacement therapy (NRT). Approximately 50% to 70% of patients discontinue cigarette use after a major cardiac event, such as MI or coronary artery bypass grafting. Cessation for another 10% to 20% can be accomplished with cigarette cessation programs, which often incorporate nicotine patches or the somewhat less efficacious nicotine gum. Programs that incorporate a nurse clinician increase cessation beyond 30%. Eight-week treatment appears to be as effective as longer periods of use.

            (1) The patch. Clinical practice guidelines support the use of the transdermal nicotine patch as the **primary pharmacologic agent for all patients who smoke.** The risk of use of the patch among patients with CAD is now considered to have been overstated. Use of the patch is contraindicated for persons who continue to smoke because it leads to nausea. **Side effects** of NRT include itching and skin rash among as many as 50% of patients. NRT approximately doubles cessation rate. One-year follow-up evaluations of patch cessation therapy indicated cessation rates of 20% to 25% versus 5% to 10% for a placebo.

                (a) Standard dosages (Nicoderm, Prostep, Nicotrol) include the maximum for 4 weeks and lesser doses for another 4 weeks.

                (b) Because baseline nicotine levels, that is, the number of cigarettes smoked per day, are inversely associated with cessation rates, **patients who smoke less than 1 pack per day** may be adequately treated with **submaximal nicotine doses.**

            (2) Nicotine gum. Use of gum for NRT appears to delay postcessation weight gain, a typical deterrent to cigarette cessation. Multipack users should use 4 mg gum, whereas patients who smoke less than 1 pack per day may need only 2 mg.

            (3) Nicotine nasal spray has been approved as a smoking cessation treatment. Nasal spray provides a more rapid rise in nicotine level than either gum or patch, peak levels occurring in less than 10 minutes. Nicotine nasal spray has markedly more severe **side effects** and appears to be best suited for patients who have not had success with other forms of NRT.

        b. Other pharmacologic agents. For selected patients supplementation with agents other than NRT may be useful, even though NRT is currently the only strategy recommended in standard smoking cessation guidelines.

            (1) Buproprion, recently approved for smoking cessation, has both dopaminergic and noradrenergic properties. Clinical trials have demonstrated the efficacy of buproprion SR (sustained release) with or without transdermal nicotine for smoking cessation. The recommended dose of buproprion is 150 mg two times per day. In clinical trials the medication was typically started 1 to 2 weeks before cessation and was continued for 7 to 12 weeks after cessation. Buproprion must be **avoided by patients with a seizure disorder or who are at risk for seizures** (e.g., patients with head injury, who abuse alcohol, or who have alcohol dependence) because the medication lowers seizure threshold. Common **side effects** of buproprion include headache, nausea, and restlessness. Buproprion has no serious adverse effects on the cardiovascular system.

(2) **Clonidine,** an α_2 agonist, **dampens the sympathetic activity associated with withdrawal.** Dosages used for smoking cessation typically range from 0.1 to 0.4 mg/day for 2 to 6 weeks in either the oral or the transdermal preparation. The most common **side effects** are dry mouth, constipation, postural hypotension, and sedation. Clonidine is **recommended for patients who prefer not to take nicotine or who have not had success with NRT.** Nasal spray clonidine has been effective among nicotine-dependent women intolerant of the patch.

VII. Sedentary lifestyle

A. Pathophysiology. A sedentary lifestyle is associated with increased risk for CAD. Sedentary persons have nearly double the risk for CAD death of active persons. In five prospective exercise studies, persons at the lowest levels of exercise conditioning had an age-adjusted CAD mortality risk 2 to 10 times that of the best-conditioned participants. Metaanalyses of epidemiologic studies suggest a nearly twofold increase in risk among sedentary persons for development of CAD and for CAD death. A sedentary lifestyle also is associated with obesity, hypertension, NIDDM, and hypercholesterolemia, which point to the need for changes in exercise patterns. More than 50% of the U.S. population does not exercise at least 20 minutes three times a week, and 40% of adults are classified as sedentary. Only 22% of U.S. adults partake in 30 or more minutes of exercise five times a week; 25% report no leisure-time physical activity.

B. Risk reduction. Even moderate physical activity provides a reduction of risk. Regular physical activity prevents obesity, may reduce weight, and promotes positive effects on blood pressure, LDL-C, HDL-C, and TG. Independent of other risk factors, physical fitness has a direct protective effect from CAD events. Among patients who have had MI, controlled cardiac rehabilitation programs significantly reduce cardiovascular mortality (20% to 25% reduction). The AHA recommends that every U.S. adult accumulate 30 minutes or more of moderate-intensity physical activity on most, preferably all days of the week.

1. Mechanism

a. Exercise **improves glucose tolerance and insulin sensitivity, increases fibrinolysis, increases HDL, improves oxygen uptake** in the heart, and **increases coronary artery diameter.** Exercise reduces the sensitivity of the myocardium to the effects of catecholamines and thus reduces risk for ventricular arrhythmias, important factors in sudden cardiovascular death. Exercise is commonly believed to increase HDL-C and lower LDL-C and as such reduce cardiac events. Exercise can alter the progression of coronary atherosclerosis. Among patients with angiographically documented CAD, exercise training may increase regression and reduce the progression of coronary lesions.

b. Studies on the effect of exercise have been difficult to conduct and suffer from difficulties in quantification of exercise. Reviews on the effects of cardiac rehabilitation on morbidity and mortality demonstrated reductions in all-cause mortality of 20% to 24% and in CAD mortality of 23% to 25%. The data support a reduction in anginal episodes and mortality, although the reduction in mortality is no better than 15%. A direct relation has been shown between exercise intensity and angiographic modifications: 1,533 kcal/week is necessary to stabilize coronary lesions, and 2,200 kcal/week is needed to induce coronary regression.

2. **Fitness** (measured in metabolic equivalents [MET] achieved) and **physical activity** (measured in caloric expenditure per time period) appear to be closely linked, although it remains unclear which of the two is the better predictor of cardiovascular morbidity and mortality.

   a. Several studies have shown that **higher degrees of physical activity** are associated with decreased risk for death of CAD. These studies suggest that **changes in fitness from low to high levels and level of current activity are the best predictors of reduction in risk for CAD.**

   b. **Death rate decreased 50% among men** 60 years or older who changed from unfit to fit status over an 18-year follow-up period. The age-adjusted cardiovascular disease mortality rate decreased 52%.

   c. An important measurement of fitness among **older postmenopausal women** is leisure-time physical activity; it can halve risk for MI.

3. **Problems with compliance.** Only 50% of persons who begin an exercise program adhere to it for more than 6 months.

   a. Physicians may need to help **tailor exercise programs for individual patients** to participate in activity that is sustained in the long term.

   b. As for healthy persons, **precautions** must be taken to **prevent injury.** The current guidelines may be **slightly modified for elderly exercisers** to emphasize a longer warm-up period to enable musculoskeletal and cardiorespiratory readiness for exercise and an adequate cool-down period to help dissipate heat.

VIII. **New risk factors.** Screening studies have shown that hypertension, hyperlipidemia, tobacco use, family history, and diabetes are predictive of less than half of all future cardiovascular events. Among patients with premature atherosclerosis, the predictive value of these traditional cardiovascular risk factors is limited. Many patients with few traditional risk factors experience life-threatening acute coronary syndromes without prior symptoms of disease. Several new potential risk factors have been identified that may enhance risk for CAD. These are levels of lipoprotein(a) [Lp(a)], homocysteine, and fibrinogen.

A. **Lp(a)** is to LDL except for the addition of apolipoprotein A (apo A), a highly glycosylated protein. Although it is a lipid, Lp(a) often is considered a **marker of thrombosis.**

   1. **Pathophysiology**

      a. There is a striking amino-acid sequence homology between apo A and plasminogen, suggesting that Lp (a) may have an important role in the connection between atherosclerosis and thrombosis. **Lp(a) may be atherogenic;** it accumulates in atherosclerotic lesions, binds to apo B–containing lipoproteins and proteoglycans, and can be taken up by foam cell precursors. It also may promote thrombosis when it binds to fibrin and blocks the fibrinolytic action of plasmin.

      b. Lp(a) may be more predictive of CAD among younger men, women, and in persons with hyperlipidemia.

      c. **Studies have had mixed results.**

         (1) Cross-sectional and retrospective case-control studies have in general supported the role of Lp(a) in CAD.

         (2) Several prospective studies have found little if any association between Lp(a) and CAD risk.

      (3) Several prospective studies have correlated baseline Lp(a) levels with vascular disease in general.

   d. Few studies have been conducted on the role of Lp(a) in **women.** Cardiovascular risk tends to increase with an Lp(a) value greater than 30 mg/dL.

  2. Therapy. The atherogenicity of Lp(a) may be modified through **substantial reductions in LDL-C level.** Evidence seems to suggest that niacin and postmenopausal estrogen replacement therapy may lower Lp(a) level. Lp(a) at present acts as a marker among patients at particular risk for poor outcome in terms of severity and progression of cardiovascular disease.

B. Homocysteine is a product of folate metabolism.

  1. Etiology and pathophysiology

   a. The mechanism by which homocysteine appears to promote vascular disease is **unclear.** Elevated homocysteine levels play a causative role in the production of arterial lesions, but deficiencies of other factors, such as vitamin B_{12} and folic acid, also may be involved, especially among the elderly.

   b. Possible mechanisms of increased risk are that hyperhomocystinemia may impair release of nitric oxide from endothelial cells, stimulate proliferation of atherogenic smooth-muscle cells, and contribute to thrombogenesis through activation of protein C.

   c. Homocysteine is derived from the sulfur-containing amino acid **methionine** and is metabolized through pathways associated with folic acid, vitamin B_6, and vitamin B_{12} as cofactors.

      (1) Deficiencies in the cofactors lead to elevated serum concentrations of homocysteine, although profound deficiencies are rare among persons with high-homocysteine CAD.

      (2) Defects in the genes for 5, 10-methylene tetrahydrofolate reductase (rare), cystathione B-synthase (0.5% prevalence), methylene tetrahydrofolate homocysteine methyltransferase (rare), and methionine synthases (rare) can lead to increases in homocysteine.

   d. Elevated plasma homocysteine levels (greater than 15 µ/L) confer an **independent risk for vascular disease,** according to cross-sectional and prospective case-control studies. The risk was first identified because of thromboembolic events, including MI and stroke, associated with homocystinuria, a rare disorder that involves homocysteine levels greater than 100 µmol/L and is related to cystathione B-synthase deficiency.

   e. Elevated homocysteine levels are found among more than 20% of patients with atherosclerotic disease, including PVD. In PVD there may be direct endothelial toxicity, smooth muscle cell proliferation, enhanced LDL oxidation, abnormalities in platelet function, or increased thrombotic risk because of abnormal clotting factors (e.g., factor V, factor VII), or altered secretion of von Willebrand's factor.

   f. The **relative risk for stroke and MI is approximately 2.0 for homocysteine levels greater than 15 µmol/L** compared with those less than 10 µmol/L. Relative risk for PVD is much greater than 3.0. Risk enhancement is continuous over the spectrum of homocysteine values.

   g. Secondary causes of increased homocysteine levels include age, male sex, menopause, renal function, and some medications (e.g., niacin, oral contraceptives with estrogen, phenytoin, methotrexate, and theophylline). Thyroid function also is relevant.

  2. Laboratory examination. For patients with abnormal homocysteine values, further evaluation includes thyroid-stimulating hormone, B_{12}, B_6, folate, and creatinine.

3. **Risk reduction and therapy.** No data are available to establish the vascular benefits of reducing homocysteine values. Treatment suggestions include 400 µg (typical amount in multivitamins) to 2 mg folate daily. Second-line therapy includes 10 to 25 mg pyridoxine (vitamin B_6) daily with or without 400 µg vitamin B_{12} for patients with vitamin B_{12} deficiency. Use of folate in the setting of vitamin B_{12} deficiency can lead to **megaloblastic anemia crisis.** This suggests that vitamin B_{12} levels, albeit of low yield, should be measure for persons with high homocysteine values before initiation of folate therapy.

C. **Fibrinogen,** a large glycoprotein made mostly in the liver, is a clotting factor that activates thrombin, aggregates platelets (through the glucoprotein IIb/IIIa receptor), and stimulates smooth muscle proliferation.

1. **Etiology and pathophysiology.** There is increasing evidence that **fibrinogen is important in the development of premature atherosclerosis.** The link is likely and plausible.

   a. Several prospective studies including the Framingham study have shown an **impressive relation between plasma fibrinogen level and the occurrence of CAD and stroke.** Plasma fibrinogen levels higher than 350 mg/dL are powerful independent risk factors for stroke and MI. High fibrinogen level is an independent risk factor for CAD with a two- to threefold increase in risk and markedly enhances risk for hypercholesterolemia.

   b. Clinical findings suggest that **high fibrinogen level also may be a risk factor for the sequelae of CAD.** In the Northwick Park Heart Study, a fibrinogen level in the upper third for the population was associated with risk for cardiovascular disease three times higher than that among patients with a plasma level in the lower third. In the Goteburg study, baseline fibrinogen level was significantly related to the incidence of MI and ischemic stroke.

2. **Cofactors.** Determinants of high fibrinogen levels include age, female sex, menopause, African-American race, smoking, obesity, stress, use of oral contraceptives, pregnancy, and a consumption of large amounts of dietary fat.

3. **Risk reduction and therapy**

   a. Factors associated with a decrease in fibrinogen level include smoking cessation, physical activity, moderate alcohol intake, normalization of body weight, and postmenopausal hormone replacement.

   b. Although no clinical trial has identified a drug that reduces fibrinogen level safely and selectively, the following medications have been shown to decreased fibrinogen level in various clinical settings: fibrates, pentoxifylline, ticlopidine, n-3 polyunsaturated fatty acids, and anabolic steroids.

SUGGESTED READINGS

References

1. 1997 Heart and Stroke Statistical Update. Dallas: American Heart Association, 1996.
2. Grundy SM, Balady GJ, Criqui MH, et al. Guide to primary prevention of cardiovascular disease: a statement for healthcare professionals from the Task Force on Risk Reduction—American Heart Association Science Advisory and Coordinating Committee. *Circulation* 1997;95:2329–2331.
3. Randomised trial of Cholesterol lowering in 4444 patients with coronary heart disease: the Scandinavian Simvastatin Survival Study (4S). *Lancet* 1994;344:1383–1389.
4. Pfeffer M, Sacks F, Lemuel A, et al. cholesterol and recurrent events: a secondary prevention trial for normolipidemic patients. *Am J Cardiol* 1995;76:98C–106C.
5. West of Scotland Coronary Prevention Group. Influence of pravastatin and plasma lipids on clinical events in the West of Scotland Coronary Prevention Study (WOSCOPS). *Circulation* 1998;97:1440–1445.

6. Prevention of cardiovascular events and death with pravastatin in patients with coronary heart disease and a broad range of initial cholesterol levels: the Long-Term Intervention with Pravastatin in Ischaemic Disease (LIPID) Study Group. *N Engl J Med* 1998;339:1349–1357.
7. Downs JR, Beere PA, Whitney E, et al. Design and rationale of the Air Force/Texas Coronary Atherosclerosis Prevention Study (AFCAPS/TexasCAPS). *Am J Cardiol* 1997;80:287–293.
8. Expert Panel on Detection, Evaluation, and Treatment of High Blood Cholesterol in Adults. Summary of the Second Report of the National Cholesterol Education Program (NCEP) Expert Panel on Detection, Evaluation, and Treatment of High Blood Cholesterol in Adults (Adult Treatment Panel-II). *JAMA* 1993;269:3015–3023.
9. Multiple risk factor intervention trial: multiple risk factor changes and mortality results—Multiple Risk Factor Intervention Trial Research Group. *JAMA* 1982;248:1465–1477.
10. Kostis JB, Davis BR, Cutler J, et al. Prevention of heart failure by antihypertensive drug treatment in older persons with isolated systolic hypertension: SHEP Cooperative Research Group. *JAMA* 1997;278:212–216.
11. Opie LH. JNC-VI guidelines. *Lancet* 1998;351:289–290.
12. Gifford RW Jr. New hypertension guidelines set aggressive goals based on risk factors: Joint National Committee on Prevention, Detection, Evaluation, and Treatment of High Blood Pressure. *Cleve Clin J Med* 1998;65:18–24.
13. Kannel WB. Lipids, diabetes, and coronary heart disease: insights from the Framingham Study. *Am Heart J* 1985;110:1100–1107.
14. Burchfiel CM, Reed DM, Marcus EB, et al. Association of diabetes mellitus with coronary atherosclerosis and myocardial lesions: an autopsy study from the Honolulu Heart Program. *Am J Epidemiol* (US) 1993;137:1328–1340.
15. Charles MA, Fontbonne A, Thebult N, et al. Risk factors for NIDDM in white population. *Diabetes* 1991;40:796–799.
16. Farchin G, Fidenza F, et al. Is diet an independent risk factor for mortality: 20 year mortality in the Italian rural cohorts of the 7 county study. *Eur J Clin Nutri* 1994;48:19–29.

39. CORONARY ARTERY DISEASE AND WOMEN

JoAnne Micale Foody

I. **Introduction.** Cardiovascular disease is the leading cause of morbidity and mortality among women. Most deaths occur in the postmenopausal years. Most of our knowledge of cardiovascular disease comes from studies involving middle-aged men. New emphasis on women's health in general and in cardiovascular health in particular has led to increasing evidence that sex differences do exist in the incidence of coronary artery disease (CAD), in risk factors, and in the modification of cardiovascular risk among women. Health care providers must coordinate their efforts to effectively manage and prevent cardiovascular disease among women to take into account the unique biologic, physiologic, and epidemiologic characteristics of cardiovascular disease among women. There is increasing evidence of the roles of traditional and nontraditional risk factors in the development of cardiovascular disease among women. New strategies must be developed to incorporate this evidence into programs of prevention.

A. Cardiovascular disease is the leading cause of mortality among women in the United States. CAD is more age dependent among women than it is among men. Women are usually 10 years older than men when coronary manifestations first appear, and myocardial infarction (MI) may occur as much as 20 years later. One in eight women 45 to 64 years of age has clinical evidence of CAD; this figure increases to nearly one in three women older than 65 years.

B. With the aging of the U.S. population, **more women than men die each year of CAD** (1); 500,000 women each year die of CAD. The number of deaths of cardiovascular disease among women is almost twice that of deaths of cancer. Approximately one of every two women in the United States will die of a cardiovascular event, most likely MI, hypertensive heart disease, or stroke. The effect of **cardiovascular disease is even greater for black women,** among whom the overall annual mortality rate due to cardiovascular disease is approximately 67% higher than among white women (2.25/1,000 versus 1.35/1,000).

C. Risk factors for CAD are similar for men and women (Table 39-1), but the **effect of individual coronary risk factors and the results of intervention differ dramatically by sex.**

D. Special emphasis must be placed on **uniquely female attributes** that modify coronary risk, specifically use of oral contraceptives, pregnancy, menopausal status, and use of postmenopausal hormone therapy.

E. Coronary **risk factors are highly prevalent among women in the United States.** Among women 20 to 74 years of age, 33% have hypertension, more than 25% have hypercholesterolemia, more than 25% are cigarette smokers, more than 25% are overweight, and more than 25% report sedentary lifestyles. Although these risk factors are more prevalent among men than women, as women age their risk-factor profiles approach and in some instances surpass those of their male counterparts.

II. **Clinical presentation of CAD among women**

A. **Angina pectoris** is the main initial and subsequent presenting symptom of CAD among women; MI and sudden cardiac death are the more common presentations among men. Women with angina pectoris are more likely to be older than men and to have hypertension, diabetes mellitus, and congestive heart failure. They also are less likely than men to have a history of either MI or percutaneous coronary intervention.

B. **MI is more ominous among women than among men,** and hospital mortality is higher for women with MI than for men. Women who survive MI have earlier and more frequent recurrence, and their 1-year mortality is

Table 39-1. Risk factors for cardiovascular disease among women

MODIFIABLE RISK FACTORS
Dyslipidemia
Hypertension
Diabetes mellitus
Cigarette smoking
Obesity
Physical inactivity
Genetics (?)

UNMODIFIABLE RISK FACTORS
Increasing age
Sex
Genetics
Race
Menopause (?)

greater. Although **sex differences lessen when older age and comorbidity among women are considered,** these differences do not completely disappear. Women with MI have higher Killip classes, more tachyarrhythmias, more atrioventricular blocks, congestive heart failure, shock, recurrent angina, and rupture of the aorta.

1. Although the presentations of MI are identical, women are less likely than men to be treated aggressively; they are half as likely to be considered for acute catheterization, angioplasty, thrombolysis, or coronary artery bypass grafting.

2. The survival benefit from thrombolysis after acute MI is similar among women and men, even though women tend to have more bleeding complications. Nonetheless, the mortality difference between sexes persists.

3. Primary **percutaneous transluminal coronary angioplasty provides an alternative to thrombolysis** among women. Women appear to have equally good outcomes after this procedure compared with men.

III. **Cardiovascular risk factors among women**

A. **Cholesterol and dyslipidemia**

1. **The higher the level of serum cholesterol, the higher is the risk for CAD** (1). Multiple studies have borne out this hypothesis.

   a. Elevated levels of high-density lipoprotein cholesterol (HDL-C) are cardioprotective among men and women.

   b. HDL-C level is a key predictor of mortality from CAD among women.

   c. Outside other biologic characteristics, menopausal women have HDL-C levels significantly lower than those of premenopausal women. This may place postmenopausal women at higher risk for CAD.

2. Lipid and lipoprotein **concentrations vary according to a woman's ovarian function.** Women who have undergone natural menopause or oophorectomy have significantly higher concentrations of total cholesterol (TC) than menstruating women or those who have undergone hysterectomy with preservation of ovarian function. Similar findings have been observed for changes in low-density lipoprotein cholesterol (LDL-C) levels.

3. There is virtually no risk for CAD among women with a desirable level of TC (less than 205 mg/dL), whereas **even a slight elevation in cholesterol** (up to a borderline high level of 220 to 250 mg/dL) results in an approximate **doubling of risk.**

      4. The incidence of CAD continues to rise steeply as cholesterol concentrations reach a high level (more than 280 mg/dL).

B. Age. Risk for **CAD correlates strongly with increasing age and serum TC** level among women. The annual incidence of CAD among women rises sharply in relation to age, plateaus at the age of 65 to 74 years, and begins to decline. Fewer than 10 of 1,000 women younger than 55 years (presumed to be pre- or perimenopausal) have CAD, whereas the incidence of CAD jumps to almost 25 of 1,000 among women between the ages of 55 and 64 years (presumed to be postmenopausal) and to more than 30 of 1000 among women between the ages of 65 and 74 years.

C. Elevated levels of **HDL-C have** a key role in protecting both men and women against the development of CAD. The Lipid Research Clinic's follow-up study (2) showed that HDL-C was the major lipid predictor of CAD mortality among women. Recent data suggest that HDL-C levels decline in association with natural menopause, placing postmenopausal women at greater risk for CAD than their male counterparts. The ratio of TC to HDL-C should be 4.0 or less. The Framingham study (3) illustrated that the ratio rises steadily with age among women (Table 39-2).

D. LDL-C. As women age and as they progress through menopause, the percentage of smaller, denser LDL-C molecules rises. The Framingham study found LDL-C level to be a significant positive predictor of CAD among women, although less a powerful predictor than HDL-C level. In contrast, The Lipid Research Clinic's study (2) did not find LDL-C level to be a significant independent predictor of cardiovascular disease among women.

      1. **Premenopausal** women are relatively protected by estrogen and a high level of HDL-C.

      2. For **postmenopausal** women, LDL-C level may be a stronger and perhaps more independent risk factor. Postmenopausal women with high levels of LDL-C are not protected by estrogen or by the generally higher level of HDL-C. The higher levels of LDL-C are most likely associated with a greater percentage of small, dense LDL-C particles.

E. Triglycerides

      1. The role of triglycerides in the development of CAD is still the subject of considerable debate. For the most part, triglycerides have not been shown to be a statistically independent predictor of CAD risk when HDL-C and LDL-C are considered in multivariate analysis. Several large studies, however, have demonstrated that **triglyceride level is a strong and independent risk factor for women.** Some experts believe triglycerides should be conscientiously addressed.

      2. **Effect of menopause.** Elevated triglyceride levels are likely to be prevalent among older postmenopausal women. The levels may be a marker for the presence of other atherogenic lipoproteins. The **presence of small, dense LDL-C molecules in older women has been**

Table 39-2. Ratio of total to high-density lipoprotein Cholesterol among women by age: The Framingham Study

Age (yr)	Mean ratio	Standard deviation
15–24	3.4	0.9
25–34	3.4	1.1
35–44	3.6	1.2
45–54	4.0	1.5
55–64	4.5	1.5
65–74	4.6	1.5
75–79	4.7	1.4

associated with hypertriglyceridemia. Small, dense LDL-C molecules may be more susceptible to oxidation and thus more atherogenic. The association between LDL-C triglycerides may explain the predictive power of triglyceride level among older postmenopausal women.

F. **Diabetes mellitus and blood glucose.** Diabetes mellitus is the single most powerful risk factor for CAD among women. Its effect is greater among women than among men.

1. Women with diabetes have a fivefold higher prevalence of cardiovascular disease than women without diabetes. Follow-up data from the Framingham study have shown that the prevalence of diabetes among women rises sharply with age (Table 39-3).

2. **High levels of blood glucose** are a strong predictor of CAD risk whether or not the person has clinical diabetes. The annual incidence of CAD increases with blood glucose level and increasing age. There is, for example, little risk for CAD among women with blood glucose levels less than 60 mg/dL (low). At levels higher than about 130 mg/dL, however, risk for CAD escalates sharply, doubling and even tripling over that associated with lower glucose glucose levels.

3. Women with **diabetes have been found to have twice the risk for MI** as women of the same age without diabetes. Among women with diabetes, the incidence of CAD is almost three times that of women without diabetes, compared with an incidence twofold higher among men with diabetes than among men without diabetes.

4. There is also some indication that diabetes predisposes women to more lethal coronary events, almost doubling case fatality rates.

5. The presence of diabetes tends to attenuate any sex-related differences in cardiovascular morbidity and mortality. The **risk for MI** among women with diabetes equals that of men of the same age without diabetes. The **risk for CAD** among women with diabetes is higher than that among both men with diabetes and women without diabetes, even after adjustment has been made for age and other CAD risk factors. The higher risk among women with diabetes may be explained in part by the clustering of multiple risk factors among persons with diabetes, such as hypertension, smoking, and obesity. As shown in Table 38-3, women with diabetes have significantly higher levels of four other risk factors for CAD, as follows:

   a. HDL cholesterol
   b. Triglycerides
   c. Systolic blood pressure
   d. Relative body weight

Table 39-3. Risk factors for coronary artery disease among women with and women without diabetes: The Framingham Study

Risk Factor	Women with diabetes	Women without diabetes
Serum cholesterol (mg/dL)	259	250
High-density lipoprotein cholesterol (mg/dL)	54[a]	58
Low-density lipoprotein cholesterol (mg/dL)	157	155
Triglycerides (mg/dL)	141[b]	133
Systolic blood pressure (mm Hg)	150[b]	139
Relative weight (% of ideal)	129[b]	121
Cigarettes/day	6	5

G. Hypertension and stroke are two other leading causes of cardiovascular mortality and morbidity among women.

1. Stroke is the **second leading cause of cardiovascular mortality among women,** accounting for nearly 100,000 deaths among women in the United States. This figure is substantially higher than the number of men who die of strokes.

2. The incidence of both fatal and nonfatal stroke rises steadily with age among both sexes. Among women 30 to 44 years of age, the estimated incidence of stroke is only 8,000 annually. This figure rises sharply to 50,000 among women between the ages of 45 and 65 years and more than triples to 179,000 among women older than 65 years. Thus **post-menopausal women are at markedly higher risk for stroke than are premenopausal women.**

3. Although the incidence of stroke is higher for men of all ages compared with women of all ages, the **mortality rate is higher among women,** mainly because of an 80% higher death rate from stoke among black women than among white women.

H. Obesity

1. The Nurses' Health Study (4), a large, prospective, cohort study, showed that women with a body mass index (BMI; weight [kg]/height [m]^2) of 25 to 29 had an age-adjusted relative risk for CAD of 1.8 compared with the leanest women. Morbidly obese women (BMI greater than 29) had a relative risk for CAD of 3.3. In 115,886 American women 30 to 55 years of age, the Nurses' Health Study found that **40% of coronary events were attributable to excess body weight.** Twenty-five percent of U.S. women 35 to 64 years of age have a BMI of 29 or higher; this category of women has a relative risk of 3.2 for nonfatal MI and 3.5 for fatal CAD.

2. Obesity has been shown to be an **independent risk factor for the development of CAD among women.** In 26 years of follow-up evaluation of participants in the Framingham heart study, relative weight among women was positively and independently associated with the presence of coronary disease and with death of coronary and cardiovascular disease. The study also showed that weight gain after the young adult years conveys increased risk for cardiovascular disease (among men and women) that cannot be attributed either to the initial weight or levels of risk factors that may have resulted from weight gain.

3. On the basis of results of other epidemiologic studies, **30% of CAD occurring among obese women can be attributed to excess weight alone,** and even mildly to moderately excess weight increases risk for CAD among middle-aged women.

4. Truncal, android, central, or male-pattern obesity, manifested as a rise in waist-to-hip ratio, correlates with higher LDL-C and lower HDL-C levels among both women and men and accounts for the increased risk for CAD associated with central obesity. **Truncal obesity is associated with high blood pressure and hyperinsulinemia,** which lead to increases in atherogenic lipoproteins and decreases in HDL-C. The mechanism is unclear. It has been hypothesized that it may somehow be related to an increase in peripheral insulin resistance. The portal venous drainage of abdominal fat may induce hepatic insulin resistance, elevated circulating insulin levels and triglyceride levels, and decreased HDL-C levels.

I. Smoking. Although diabetes is the most biologically sex-differentiated risk factor for CAD among women, **cigarette smoking may be the most psychologically and sociologically differentiating risk behavior** for men and women. Smoking is deadly, claiming nearly 200,000 lives in the United States in 1994, or nearly one fifth of all heart disease deaths. Cigarette smoking among women is an especially serious risk.

1. Cigarette smoking carries an **especially increased hazard** for women who use **oral contraceptives,** a combination that promotes thrombogenesis.

2. The sex gap in smoking prevalence has narrowed considerably. Although the prevalence of cigarette smoking among adults in the United States has declined markedly since its peak in 1965, when 40% smoked, smoking prevalence has declined more rapidly among men than women. The sex gap is likely to continue to narrow, because female adolescents are starting to smoke at the same rate as male adolescents. This is likely to contribute to a substantially greater female burden of cardiovascular disease.

3. **Risk for cardiac disease.** Although it has been clear that smoking is associated with elevated risk for CAD among men, it was believed that cigarette smoking was not associated with CAD among women. However, **positive correlations have been observed in both case-control and prospective cohort studies of nonfatal MI and fatal CAD.**

   a. The Nurses' Health Study (5) examined the incidence of CAD in relation to cigarette smoking among a cohort of 119,404 female nurses from 30 to 55 years of age. The number of cigarettes smoked per day correlated positively with risk for CAD (relative risk 5.5 for more than 25 cigarettes per day), nonfatal MI (relative risk 5.8), and angina pectoris (relative risk 2.6). Overall, cigarette smoking accounted for approximately half of these events. This attributable risk was highest among women who were already at increased risk because of older age, family history of MI, obesity, hypertension, hypercholesterolemia, or diabetes. These data emphasize the **importance of cigarette smoking as a determinant of CAD among women** and the markedly increased hazards associated with this habit in combination with other risk factors for this disease.

   b. New evidence points to the significant role of **passive smoking** in the development of CAD. Women are seriously threatened by this risk for CAD. Passive smoke reduces the ability of the blood to deliver oxygen to the myocardium and impairs the ability of the heart to utilize oxygen. After inhaling only two cigarettes, nonsmokers have platelet activity matching that of a habitual smoker. **Secondhand smoke increases intimal wall damage, accelerates atherosclerotic lesions, and increases intimal wall damage after ischemia or MI.**

J. **Physical activity.** Increasing evidence shows that **inactivity and a sedentary lifestyle may be independent risk factors for the development of CAD** among both men and women.

   1. Few studies have specifically addressed the effects of increased physical activity on CAD risk factors other than lipid levels. It appears, however, that in addition to improvement in lipid profiles, even moderately fit women have better blood sugar levels, blood pressure, and anthropometric indices than unfit or inactive women.

   2. Few studies have addressed the relation between physical fitness or habitual activity level and cardiovascular disease among women. Studies have, however, examined the link between activity and lipid levels. Cross-sectional studies with active and sedentary women showed a positive association between exercise and HDL-C level among both premenopausal and postmenopausal women. Significant differences between groups remained for HDL-C values when results were adapted for differences in percentage of body fat. Two studies examined plasma lipid level in relation to menopausal status among female runners. They showed no differences in HDL-C level between premenopausal and postmenopausal women who exercised. When inactive and exercising women were compared, however, it appeared

that younger premenopausal women responded with lipoprotein changes less strongly than did older postmenopausal women. **Exercise appeared to attenuate the age-related increase in LDL-C and decrease in HDL-C.** Otherwise, in these cross-sectional studies, women taking hormone replacement therapy (HRT) who reported exercising had higher HDL-C levels than sedentary women not taking HRT.

K. Psychosocial aspects. A large body of evidence has accumulated regarding the relation between cardiovascular disease and socioeconomic status, employment, type A behavior, hostility, depression, and social support.

   1. Socioeconomic factors, including educational attainment, are an important contributing factor to risk for CAD. Women with a low educational level have a significantly increased age-specific incidence of angina pectoris. There is no significant correlation between marital status or number of children and incidence of ischemic heart disease or overall mortality. Multivariate analyses have shown that the association between low educational level and incidence of angina pectoris is independent of socioeconomic group itself, cigarette smoking, systolic blood pressure, indices of obesity, and serum triglyceride and serum cholesterol levels.

   2. Employment. As women have assumed different roles in the workplace, the effect of these roles on cardiovascular health and women's health in general has come into question. According to several health indicators, women who work in positions beyond keeping their own homes appear to be healthier than women who work solely as homemakers and women who are unemployed. Women in the first category have fewer risk factors: they smoke fewer cigarettes, have lower fasting glucose levels, drink less alcohol, and exercise more than women in the other two categories. Mean HDL-C level is significantly higher among women in the first category than among those in the second.

L. Level of estrogen. Although women are generally viewed as being relatively protected from CAD, after menopause they rapidly develop risk equivalent to that of their male counterparts. Epidemiologic, clinical, and experimental studies suggest that **estrogen confers protection against cardiovascular disease** among premenopausal women and that in the absence of estrogen, women no longer have this advantage.

IV. Risk factor modification among women

A. Primary prevention

   1. Primary prevention of cardiovascular disease among women is problematic and faces obstacles to implementation for several reasons. The benefits of recommendations are difficult to recognize. The issue often is raised that there are insufficient data from clinical trials to justify cholesterol-lowering interventions among women because most studies have been performed with male subjects. The recommendations of the National Cholesterol Education Project (NCEP) (6) may not be appropriate for women. Some women who are screened may have TC levels in the desirable range but LDL-C or HDL-C levels that put them at risk.

   2. Clinical studies have shown that women may benefit more from risk intervention than their male counterparts.

   3. NCEP guidelines

   a. Patients are categorized according to age, sex, hormonal status, number of risk factors, and fasting LDL-C level. Patients with two or more risk factors are considered to be at high risk. Patients at low risk have one risk factor. Little consideration of sex is present in the NCEP guideline as originally published. Normal values for lipoproteins are considered to be the same for men and women.

   (1) Evaluation beyond TC and HDL-C measurement is recommended for persons with screening TC levels greater than 240 mg/dL or with TC levels of 200 to 239 mg/dL associated with other risk factors or established CAD. HDL-C level higher than 60 mg/dL allows credit of one risk factor.

(2) Persons with low levels of HDL-C (less than 35 mg/dL) are considered to have an additional risk factor, and lipoprotein analysis is recommended.

(3) Neither TC nor HDL-C is actually targeted for intervention; only LDL-C is specifically targeted.

b. Recommendations for risk modification

(1) **Dietary modification** is recommended for patients at low risk with LDL-C levels greater than 160 mg/dL and patients at high risk (two or more risk factors) with LDL-C levels less than 160 mg/dL.

(2) **Drug therapy** is recommended for patients at low risk whose LDL-C levels reach 190 mg/dL or patients at high risk whose LDL-C levels reach 160 mg/dL. Drug therapy is not recommended for men younger than 35 years or for premenopausal women unless LDL-C levels are greater than 220 mg/dL. The guidelines set higher LDL-C thresholds for drug intervention among premenopausal women (LDL-C greater than 220 mg/dL) than postmenopausal women (LDL-C greater than 190 mg/dL).

(3) **HRT** is recommended by NCEP as an option for postmenopausal women with hypercholesterolemia.

(4) **Nonpharmacologic therapy** (weight reduction, alcohol restriction, increased physical activity) is recommended for all patients with elevated triglyceride levels.

c. Difficulties of NCEP guidelines in the care of women

(1) Treatment is based on **LDL-C** levels, which are probably less important among women than levels of other lipoproteins.

(2) A cutoff of 35 mg/dL is used for **HDL-C** rather than the more relevant level of 45 or 50 mg/dL among women; 50 mg/dL is an average HDL-C value for women.

(3) **Triglyceride** levels and **diabetes** are not considered to be independent risk factors, although they have been demonstrated to be risks for some groups of women. Drugs are started to lower triglyceride level only if other lipoprotein abnormalities are present, if triglyceride levels are very high (greater than 1,000 mg/dL) to prevent acute pancreatitis, or if there is a personal or family history of CAD or other manifestations of atherosclerosis.

B. Secondary prevention. Treatment is needed to reduce risk.

1. Evaluation. All patients need lipoprotein analysis, but classification is based on LDL-C level. For these patients, **optimal LDL-C level is 100 mg/dL or less.**

2. Treatment

a. For patients with LDL-C levels greater than 100 mg/dL, **cholesterol-lowering therapy** must be initiated. A nonpharmacologic approach is used between 100 and 130 mg/dL. Drug therapy is instituted when LDL-C is 130 mg/dL or higher despite a trial of dietary therapy and physical activity. Lowering LDL-C to less than 100 mg/dL results in a 25% reduction in risk for recurrent MI and a 9% reduction in CAD mortality. Drugs to lower triglyceride levels are recommended for all patients with elevated triglycerides (greater than 200 mg/dL) in the context of tertiary prevention.

b. HRT has a position between diet and lipid-lowering drugs and is of greater benefit in secondary prevention than in primary prevention of CAD. There is a 73% reduction in CAD mortality among users of postmenopausal estrogen who have CAD at baseline, compared with a 55% reduction among all women regardless of baseline CAD status.

C. Specific measures

1. Diet

   a. The NCEP dietary intervention occurs in two steps. Step I involves an intake of saturated fat of 8% to 10% of total calories; 30% or less of total calories from fat; and less than 300 mg of cholesterol per day. If this diet proves inadequate to achieve the goals, the patient proceeds to the step II diet. Step II calls for further reductions in saturated fat intake to less than 7% of calories and in cholesterol to less than 200 mg/d. The polyunsaturated to saturated fat ratio thus is increased.

   b. All reduced-fat diets have a beneficial effect on LDL-C level but consistently also reduce levels of HDL-C, which is disadvantageous for women. There are specific sex differences for diet responsiveness. The decrease in HDL-C is more severe among women and even more extreme in postmenopausal women.

   c. Menopausal status may affect dietary responsiveness. Postmenopausal women following a low-fat diet have a lesser decline in LDL-C and triglyceride levels and a greater decline in HDL-C levels than do men of the same age.

   d. The most **important problem with dietary therapy** among women appears to be the accompanying **decrease in HDL-C level.** Given that the risk for cardiac events associated with a decrease in HDL-C level may be more important for women than the adverse risk imparted by an increase in LDL-C level, the conclusion is that **diet may have opposite the desired effect.** For women with a very high LDL-C and who are at risk for CAD, all available techniques must be used to lower LDL-C level. For women at low risk, the benefits of a low-fat diet are far from clear unless the woman has a weight problem.

2. Weight management. Efforts to prevent or manage obesity have had limited success. Striking excesses in morbidity and mortality from CAD attributable to obesity among middle-aged women have stimulated efforts to understand and treat the problem.

   a. Studies indicate that serum lipid responses to weight loss among women are different from those among men. A 10% reduction in body weight causes HDL-C level to rise in men, but to fall slightly in women. LDL-C levels decline in both men and women but to a greater extent in men. Wood (7) reported a decrease in HDL-C among women who exercised but not among men. HDL-C levels remained about the same among women who exercised and dieted and were higher than among women who only dieted but not higher than among control subjects.

   b. **Adipose tissue in postmenopausal women** can serve as a source of **estrogen synthesis.** Thus the benefits of weight reduction among older women may be offset by the loss of estrogen-producing adipose tissue.

   c. **Developments** that advanced understanding of obesity are the 1994 discovery of **ob,** the obesity gene, which produces the food-intake regulating enzyme, **leptin;** the development of **behavioral programs** that modify unhealthful eating behavior; and the use of **pharmacologic agents** such as noradrenergic and serotonin reuptake inhibitors.

   d. Several medications are available for the temporary management of obesity. These medications are categorized according to their effects on energy intake, storage, and output.

      (1) Drugs that affect the brain include **serotonergic and noradrenergic** medications. Noradrenergic drugs influence weight loss through stimulation of the hypothalamus.

      (2) **Orlistat,** a pancreatic lipase inhibitor, reduces weight through inhibition of fat absorption.

      (3) A new class of **serotonin reuptake inhibitors,** including sibutramine, fluoxetine, and sertraline, promote weight loss with varying degrees of side effects.

      (4) **Combination therapy** provides two serotonergic agents to promote weight loss while counteracting opposing side effects.

      (5) The use of dexfenfluramine and fenfluramine has been discontinued because of an increase in valvular heart defects and pulmonary hypertension.

  e. Exercise figures as one of the most important methods of weight loss for obese patients. The greatest weight losses have been reported in a combined regimen of diet and exercise rather than diet alone or exercise alone.

  f. Two issues important to the effectiveness of weight loss are **degree of loss** and **duration of loss.**

      (1) Even if weight is lost, studies indicate that **weight-loss maintenance fails** in most instances because of the many physiologic factors that contribute to obesity. Approximately two-thirds of persons who lose weight regain it within 1 year, and almost all who lose weight regain it within 5 years.

      (2) **Short-term weight loss is ineffective in modifying coronary risk factors. Additional health risks** that accompany weight cycling are increased cardiovascular morbidity and mortality, increased abdominal fat, high blood pressure, and insulin resistance.

3. Exercise is generally accepted as a mechanism for men to increase HDL-C and to lower LDL-C levels. Exercise improves lipid profile, probably less strongly for women than for men. The studies that have been performed with women have not considered potential confounding factors such as hormonal status and body composition.

  a. Postmenopausal women seem to have a response to exercise, even if some results of training studies are controversial. Exercise at least seems to attenuate the age-related modifications in **lipid profile.**

  b. The physiologic reasons for differences between men and women and their lipoprotein responses to diet, weight-loss, and exercise are not well defined. The **role of circulating estrogen** might be involved. Larosa (8) proposed that further investigation should include studies of different responses to these therapeutic modalities among postmenopausal women with and without exogenous hormone replacement.

  c. Reviews on the effects of **cardiac rehabilitation programs** on morbidity and mortality have demonstrated mortality reductions of 20% to 24% from all causes and of 23% to 25% from CAD. Only 3 of 22 studies reviewed included women, and in these three studies, women made up only 3% (143 of 4,554 patients) of the entire sample. No separate analyses have related the effect of participation in cardiac rehabilitation programs to clinical outcomes among women. Inadequate data exist for determining whether formal cardiac rehabilitation provides women with reductions in cardiovascular disease similar to those provided to men.

  d. Intervention studies in general suggest that exercise training programs in the absence of other interventions attenuate the age-related increase in TC levels but do not cause HDL-C levels to rise appreciably among **older women.** Two longitudinal investigations did not compare pre- and postmenopausal women but focused on postmenopausal women. In one study the exercise intensity was low.

  e. Among **younger women,** high volumes of exercise accompanied by decreases in body fat may increase HDL-C level.

4. Cholesterol-altering drugs. Although few studies include women, and very few analyze results for women in a separate group, recent data suggest that **aggressive lowering of cholesterol levels among women significantly decreases coronary morbidity and mortality.** That premenopausal women are at lower risk for heart disease than men of the same age has been misinterpreted by many to mean that risk factors are less important in the treatment of women than the treatment of men. Women should be treated for high cholesterol levels, and they may benefit more from the treatment than do men.

  a. Drug therapy appears to be as effective or even more effective in altering lipid levels among women than among men in both primary and secondary prevention. A consistent, albeit limited, set of data exists for women.

  b. The Scandinavian Simvastatin Survival Study (**4S**) (9) involved 4,444 patients, 18% of whom were women. Use of simvastatin decreased TC 25% and LDL-C 35% and increased HDL-C 8%. The probability that a woman avoided a major coronary event was 77.5% in the placebo group and 85.1% in the treatment group. Total mortality and risk for a major coronary event were similar for both sexes. Other benefits of treatment included a 37% reduction ($p < .00001$) in the risk for needing myocardial revascularization procedures.

  c. The Cholesterol and Recurrent Events Study (**CARE**) (10) was designed to address the question whether LDL-C lowering with pravastatin among patients with CAD and normal or only mildly elevated LDL-C conentrations provided clinical benefit. **A greater reduction in CAD death and nonfatal MI was observed in the subset of women** in this study compared with that of men. These data corroborate findings from other trials that the benefits of lipid-lowering therapy start to appear relatively soon after the initiation of therapy. Women may have a greater benefit from cholesterol reduction interventions.

  d. Postmenopausal women with a history of CAD may need more aggressive treatment for elevated cholesterol levels. The Heart and Estrogen/progestin Replacement Study (**HERS**) (11) involved 2,763 women with a known history of CAD.

   (1) Although 47% of the HERS participants were taking some form of cholesterol-lowering medication at the time of the study, 63% had LDL-C levels that exceeded NCEP guidelines. Therefore many of the women who were eligible to receive cholesterol-lowering drug therapy because of their elevated cholesterol levels either were not receiving drug treatment or were not treated aggressively enough.

   (2) Fully 91% of the study's participants had LDL-C levels that exceeded the 1993 NCEP Adult Treatment Protocol goal of less than 100 mg/dL. Most of the women were white (88.7% white, 7.9% African-American, 2% Hispanic), and most were inactive and overweight. Many were exsmokers (49%) and more than 13% still smoked. More than half (59.5%) had high blood pressure, and 23% had diabetes.

   (3) The HERS researchers found that women with one or more of the following characteristics were less likely to be taking a cholesterol-lowering agent: African-American, Hispanic, or other ethnic identity, high BMI, sedentary activity level, consumer of alcohol or tobacco, and a diagnosis of CAD before 1985. Women with lower LDL-C levels tended to have postgraduate education, participated in an exercise program, and had never married.

5. **Antioxidant therapy.** Antioxidants may suppress the formation of oxidized LDL-C and thereby influence the formation of atherosclerotic plaque. Both epidemiologic and laboratory studies suggest that antioxidants can provide a protective effect on the coronary arteries.

  a. The Nurses' Health Study (12) assessed the relative risk for a major CAD event among 87,245 female nurses followed for up to 8 years. The relative risk for major coronary disease of those in the lowest quintile of vitamin E intake was compared with risk among the highest quintile (relative risk 0.66 after adjustment for age and smoking). Adjustment for a variety of other coronary risk factors and nutrients, including other antioxidants, had little effect on the results. Although these prospective data do not prove a cause-and-effect relation, they suggest that **among middle-aged women the use of vitamin E supplements is associated with reduced risk** for coronary heart disease.
  b. No large randomized clinical trials of antioxidants have yet been reported, albeit two such trials, the Women's Health Initiative and an ancillary trial of antioxidant therapy, are in progress.
6. **Smoking cessation**
  a. In the Nurses Health Study, **risk for CAD decreased 30% within only 2 years of smoking cessation.** These benefits extended to the population with diagnosed CAD. Most studies indicate a 30% to 50% reduction in CAD mortality in the first 2 years and a more gradual decline in the next 10 to 20 years before the smoker mirrors the CAD mortality risk of someone who never smoked.
  b. In general, **women are less likely to contemplate smoking cessation** than are men and are more likely to smoke to reduce tension and control weight.
    (1) Although women stop smoking at the same rate as men, they are **less likely to maintain cessation over the long term.** Data from the Lung Health Study (13) indicate that long-term relapse rates may be higher among women than in men. The study, sponsored by the National Heart, Lung, and Blood Institute, evaluated the efficacy of early smoking cessation intervention for patients with chronic obstructive pulmonary disease. Men had significantly higher cessation rates than women, but other factors were seen to be important predictors of successful cessation. Participants who were better educated, married, and older were more likely to stay away from tobacco. Those with larger body mass were more likely to be unsuccessful, as were those who had made cessation attempts in the past without the help of nicotine gum. **Women tended to fit into the categories of participants less likely to remain abstinent.**
    (2) The Lung Health Study offered evidence for **sex differences in the subjective effects of nicotine withdrawal.** Women reported a greater dependence on cigarettes and used more nicotine gum during the study. Biochemically **nicotine clearance is more rapid among men** than among women, even after correction for body weight.
    (3) **Women's anxiety about weight gain** after smoking cessation is an impediment to attempts to stop smoking. Smoking cessation has been suggested as a possible contributing factor to the increase in prevalence of overweight in the United States. Postcessation weight gain, an average of 10 pounds over a 10-year period, appears to be caused by both increased eating and the metabolic changes produced by nicotine withdrawal. Nicotine gum has been shown to partially reduce or delay gain.
  c. The clinical implications are that smoking cessation programs may have to **emphasize strategies to help women develop confidence to stop smoking, make a commitment to stopping, maintain cessation** for extended periods of time. Smoking cessa-

tion programs for women should emphasize techniques for reducing tension and controlling weight.

7. **Aspirin therapy.** Aspirin in doses of 325 mg or less per day appears to be beneficial in preventing the incidence of MI among men and women without clinically apparent CAD. This benefit is magnified among patients older than 50 years and those with risk factors for CAD. Use of aspirin does not appear to reduce overall mortality and may be associated with increased risk for hemorrhagic stroke, particularly in larger doses.

   a. Results of the Nurses' Health Study (14) suggest that **aspirin is beneficial in the primary prevention** of cardiovascular disease among the population involved in the study. In the study 87,000 women without clinically apparent CAD were observed 6 years. Those who took one to six aspirin tablets per week had a 32% reduction in incidence of first MI compared with those who took no aspirin ($p = .005$). The benefit was limited to women older than 50 years and was greatest among smokers and those with hypertension or hypercholesterolemia. The women who took more than 15 aspirin tablets a week had a statistically significant increase in incidence of hemorrhagic stroke.

   b. Data support the use of aspirin by survivors of MI to reduce the incidence of reinfarction and death. **Aspirin may provide the best opportunity for secondary prevention** after acute MI because of its effectiveness, low cost, safety profile, and lack of strong contraindications. More than 18,000 patients have been enrolled in randomized trials to assess the role of antiplatelet therapy for secondary prevention of MI. The guidelines for treatment of acute MI published by the American Heart Association and American College of Cardiology in 1990 strongly recommend the use of aspirin for all survivors of acute MI.

8. **Estrogen** appears to be protective against many forms of cardiovascular disease, including heart attack, stroke, and blockage of the coronary blood vessels. After menopause, women often have an increase in weight, higher levels of LDL-C, and lower levels of HDL-C. Estrogen is purported to relax the blood vessels, decrease fibrinogen, decrease LDL, increase HDL, and reduce oxidation. Hormonal status must be carefully considered because of the important effects of estrogen not only on lipids, but also on endothelial function and other risk factors.

   a. **Research findings**

      (1) The results of more than 20 epidemiologic studies suggest a **reduction of cardiovascular events with the use of estrogen.** Metaanalysis suggests a 50% reduction in risk. Cohort studies of the use of unopposed estrogen generally indicate better than a 50% reduction rate of CAD. In the Nurses' Health Study (15), risk reduction was 40% for estrogen alone (ERT) and 60% for estrogen combined with progestin (HRT).

      (2) Estrogen has been shown to slow the progression of atherosclerosis in experimental studies. Observations have led researchers to hypothesize that estrogen may directly or indirectly retard the development of plaques, favorably affect the vulnerability of existing plaques, or reduce risk for coronary occlusion through prevention of the formation of an occlusive thrombus, a consequence of plaque rupture. Estrogen also may alter endothelial function and attenuate vasomotor dysfunction, possible triggers of plaque rupture.

      (3) Estrogen may protect women through modification of the lipid profile. Premenopausal women have low LDL-C and high HDL-C levels compared with men. After menopause, women

have a more atherogenic lipid profile: LDL-C levels increase, HDL-C levels fall, and lipoprotein (a) levels increase. **Estrogen reverses these adverse changes in lipoprotein profile and diminishes cardiovascular risk.**

(4) Multiple regression analyses of large-scale clinical trials indicate that the **beneficial changes in lipoprotein levels resulting from ERT account for only 25% to 50% of the observed risk reduction.** This suggests that additional factors are involved. Cardioprotective mechanisms unrelated to lipid lowering are evident among women with heterozygous familial hypercholesterolemia. Despite higher levels of TC and LDL-C, these women have a reduced incidence and a markedly delayed onset of the clinical manifestations of CAD compared with their male counterparts.

(5) In **large epidemiologic studies,** postmenopausal women taking ERT experience 50% fewer coronary events with particular benefit to women with CAD (Table 39-4). No less than 15 prospective cohort studies on postmenopausal ERT have demonstrated a **significant relative risk reduction of death or nonfatal MI.** Estrogen use appears to be protective among women with and without risk factors for heart disease. For example, among smokers and nonsmokers, women who use estrogen have a lower occurrence of CAD than do nonusers.

(6) Observational studies of ERT and HRT and CAD are numerous. Most of them, including outcomes studies, have shown a lower risk for reinfarction, CAD-related death, and coronary artery restenosis among users of HRT and ERT. Observational studies have found lower rates of CAD among postmenopausal women, this potential benefit has not been confirmed in clinical trials.

(7) **Former users of estrogen** are at higher risk for heart disease than are current users, but the risk is lower than that among women who have never taken estrogen.

(8) The HERS investigators (11) found no significant difference between HRT-treated and placebo-treated groups in primary outcome of MI or CAD death or in any of the secondary outcomes. Treatment did increase the rate of thromboembolic events and gallbladder disease, however. Because of the findings of no overall cardiovascular benefit and a pattern of early increase in risk for CAD events, **HRT and ERT cannot be recommended for secondary prevention.** However, it might be **appropriate for women already taking estrogen to continue.**

(9) Although prospective cohort data suggest one, **no clinical trials have shown that estrogen use is beneficial in primary prevention.**

(10) The **benefits for postmenopausal women at increased risk for CAD are considerable.** The Post-menopausal Estrogen/Progestin Intervention study (PEPI) (16) was designed to show the benefits of HRT in a 3-year study involving 875 postmenopausal women 45 to 64 years of age. Baseline triglyceride values were less than 500 mg/dL. Five treatment arms compared use of estrogen alone (ERT) with use of estrogen and different regimens of progestin (HRT). The various treatment regimens lowered LDL-C to levels about 15 mg/dL less than those among women who took a placebo. All regimens raised triglycerides.

(11) Several randomized clinical trials are examining the effects of HRT on CAD—the Women's Health Initiative (WHI), the

Table 39-4. Risk for cardiovascular disease and postmenopausal hormone use

Group	Person-yr	Major coronary disease			Fatal cardiovascular disease			Total stroke		
		No. of cases	RR	(95% CI)	No. of cases	RR	(95% CI)	No. of cases	RR	(95% CI)
Nonusers	179,194	250	2.50	—	129	1.0	—	123	1.0	—
Current users	73,532	45	0.51	(0.37–0.70)	21	0.48	(0.31–0.74)	39	0.96	(0.67–1.37)
Former users	85,128	110	0.91	(0.73–1.14)	55	0.84	(0.61–1.15)	62	1.00	(0.74–1.36)

RR, Relative risk; *CI*, = Confidence interval.
From Stampfer MJ, Colditz GA, Willett WC, et al. Postmenopausal estrogen therapy and cardiovascular disease: ten-year follow-up from the nurses' health study. *N Engl J Med* 1991;325:756–762, with permission.

Women's Angiographic Vitamin and Estrogen (WAVE) trial, the Women's Estrogen/Progestin and Lipid Lowering Hormone Atherosclerosis Regression trial (WELL-HART), and the Estrogen Replacement and Atherosclerosis (ERA) trial. These studies will assist in ascertaining which women will experience a cardioprotective effect of HRT and which women may be susceptible to its potential thrombogenic effects.

b. Institution of therapy

   (1) For women starting postmenopausal hormone therapy, it seems reasonable to check levels of cholesterol, triglycerides, LDL-C, and HDL-C. If triglyceride level is greater than 300 mg/dL, attention should be given to nonpharmacologic interventions, such as regular exercise and a weight-reducing diet low in simple sugars. A search for secondary causes and family screening for familial lipid disease also is reasonable. Although only a small group of women who take postmenopausal estrogen have severe hypertriglyceridemia or pancreatitis, the number might be reduced if more women were screened for lipid abnormalities.

   (2) Unopposed estrogen for **patients with a uterus** incurs an eightfold increase in risk for the development of endometrial cancer over 10 to 20 years. These patients should be treated with **combination therapy (estrogen and progesterone),** which does not appear to pose any risk to the endometrium. The **risk for breast cancer** increases 25% over 10 to 20 years with estrogen therapy. Recent evidence suggests that the incidence of breast cancer with HRT increases to as high as 43% with long-term use and compromises the benefit accrued in overall mortality the longer estrogen is administered. Breast cancer risk with combination treatment is thought to be greater than for patients not taking any form of estrogen therapy, but the degree of enhanced risk remains unclear.

   (3) HRT or ERT may be considered for the direct purpose of **vascular protection in late menopause** rather than early in the postmenopausal period. With increasing numbers of risk factors, both risk for early-onset CAD and the benefits of HRT or ERT increase. Earlier HRT or ERT must be weighed against risk factor management, such as cholesterol lowering and blood pressure control. For postmenopausal patients with CAD, HRT or ERT should be seriously considered regardless of age, particularly when the patient has no contraindications and has proper medical follow-up care.

   (4) **Dosage.** The American College of Physicians recommends the following:

   (a) For women **without a uterus:** 0.625 mg conjugated equine estrogen alone for 10 to 14 days per month

   (b) For women **with a uterus:** 0.625 mg conjugated equine estrogen in combination with either cyclic progestin, 5 to 10 mg medroxyprogesterone acetate (MPA) for 10 to 14 days per month, or continuous progestin, 2.5 mg MPA daily.

   (c) Careful maintenance supervised by a physician and other health care personnel to include **routine Papanicolaou smears and mammograms**

   (5) **Contraindications and side effects.** The presence of uterine cancer, breast cancer, and thrombotic tendencies are considered contraindications to the use of estrogen. Blood pressure is typically unaffected, if not reduced; however, blood pressure initially increases among a small percentage of patients. Risk for chole-

cystitis increases twofold with estrogen use. Increased risk for breast or uterine cancer, e.g., a family history, must temper the use of early postmenopausal estrogen therapy.

SUGGESTED READINGS

References

1. 1997 Heart and Stroke Statistical Update. Dallas: American Heart Association, 1996.
2. Bush TL, Barrett-Connor E, Cowan LD, et al. Cardiovascular mortality and non-contraceptive use of estrogen in women: results from the Lipid Research Clinics Program follow-Up. *Circulation* 1987;75:1102–1109.
3. Report of the National Cholesterol Education Program Expert Panel on detection, evaluation and treatment of high blood cholesterol in adults. *Arch Intern Med* 1988;148:36–69.
4. Manson JE, Colditz GA, Stampfer MJ, et al. A prospective study of obesity and risk of coronary heart disease in women. *N Engl J Med* 1990;322:882–889.
5. Willett W, Green A, Stampfer M, et al. Relative and absolute excess risks of coronary heart disease among women who smoke cigarettes. *N Engl J Med* 1987; 317:1303–1309.
6. Expert Panel on Detection, Evaluation, and Treatment of High Blood Cholesterol in Adults. Summary of the second report of the National Cholesterol Education Program (NCEP) (Adult Treatment Panel-II). *JAMA* 1993;269:3015–3023.
7. Wood PD. Physical activity, diet, and health: independent and interactive effects. *Med Sci Sports Exerc* 1994;26:838–843.
8. LaRosa JC. Lipids and cardiovascular disease: do the findings and therapy apply equally to men and women? *Womens Health Issues* 1992;2:102–111.
9. Scandinavian Simvastatin Survival Study Group. Randomised trial of cholesterol lowering in 4444 patients with coronary heart disease: The Scandinavian Simvastatin Survival Study (4S). *Lancet* 1994;344:1383–1389.
10. Pfeffer M, Sacks F, Lemuel A, et al. Cholesterol and Recurrent Events: a secondary prevention trial for normolipidemic patients. *Am J Cardiol* 1995;76:98C–106C.
11. Hulley S, Grady D, Bush T, et al. Randomized trial of estrogen plus progestin for secondary prevention of coronary heart disease in postmenopausal women: Heart and Estrogen/progestin Replacement Study (HERS) Research Group. *JAMA* 1998;280:605–613.
12. Stampfer M, Hennekens C, Manson J, Colditz G, Rosner B, Willett W. Vitamin E consumption and the risk of coronary disease in women. *N Engl J Med* 1993;328: 1444–1449.
13. Kanner RE, Connett JE, Williams DE, Buist AS. Effects of randomized assignment to a smoking cessation intervention and changes in smoking habits on respiratory symptoms in smokers with early chronic obstructive pulmonary disease. the Lung Health Study. Am J Med 1999;106:410–416.
14. Manson JE, Stampfer MJ, Colditz GA, et al. A prospective study of aspirin use and primary prevention in women. *JAMA* 1991;266:521–527.
15. Grodstein F, Stampfer MJ, Manson JE, et al. Postmenopausal estrogen and progestin use and the risk of cardiovascular disease [published corrections appears in *N Engl J Med* 1996;336:1406]. *N Engl J Med* 1996;335:456–461.
16. The Writing Group for the PEPI Trial. Effects of estrogen or estrogen/progestin regimens on heart disease risk factors in postmenopausal women: the Postmenopausal Estrogen/Progestin Interventions (PEPI) trial. *JAMA* 1995;273:199–208.

Landmark Articles

Ayanian J, Epstein A. Differences in the use of procedures between women and men hospitalized for coronary heart disease. *N Engl J Med* 1991;325:221–225.
Buring J, Hennekens C. The Women's Health Study: a randomized trial of aspirin, beta-carotene and vitamin E. *Myocardial Ischemia* 1992.
Colditz G, Stampfer M, Willett W, Rosner B, Speizer F, Hennekens D. A prospective study of parental history of myocardial infarction and coronary heart disease in women. *Am J Epidemiol* 1986;123:48–58.

Downs JR, Beere PA, Whitney E, et al. Design and rationale of the Air Force/Texas Coronary Atherosclerosis Prevention Study (AFCAPS/TexCAPS). *Am J Cardiol* 1997;80:287–293.

Grady D, Rubin S, Petitti D, et al. Hormone therapy to prevent disease and prolong life in postmenopausal women. *Ann Intern Med* 1992;117:1016–1037.

Wenger NK, Speroff L, Packard B. Cardiovascular health and disease in women. *N Engl J Med* 1998;329:247–256.

Willett W, Stampfer M, Colditz G. Intake of transfatty acids and risk of coronary heart disease among women. *Lancet* 1993;341:581–585.

The Writing Group for the PEPI Trial. Effects of estrogen or estrogen/progestin regimens on heart disease risk factors in postmenopausal women: the Postmenopausal Estrogen/Progestin Interventions (PEPI) trial. *JAMA* 1995;273:199–208.

Relevant Book Chapter

Barrett-Connor E, Bush TL. In:Douglas PS, ed. *Heart disease in women.* Philadelphia: FA Davis, 1989:159–172.

SECTION X. NONINVASIVE ASSESSMENT

Steven P. Marso and Thomas H. Marwick

40. EXERCISE ELECTROCARDIOGRAPHIC TESTING

Christopher Cole

I. **Introduction**
   A. The concept of exercise electrocardiographic (ECG) testing arose from observations of ST-segment depression caused by exercise-induced ischemia. Exercise ECG testing now is used alone and as a gateway to other imaging modalities such as nuclear or echocardiographic assessment.
   1. The **advantages** of exercise ECG testing are its ability to test functional capacity, which is a powerful predictor of mortality, widespread availability, safety, ease of administration, and relatively low cost. Exercise ECG is ideal for older patients with an intermediate likelihood of having coronary artery disease (CAD).
   2. **Disadvantages.** As a screening test for CAD in persons without symptoms, exercise ECG is not helpful. It has a **low sensitivity and specificity,** which can be improved with careful selection of the patient population undergoing testing.
   B. **Submaximal exercise ECG testing** (testing at submaximal heart rate; see later) is a useful assessment before hospital discharge for **patients who have had myocardial infarction** (MI). The advantages are as follows:
   1. It assists in setting **safe levels** of exercise (exercise prescription) and reassuring patients and families.
   2. It is beneficial in **optimizing medical therapy,** in triage for intensity of follow-up and care, and in recognition of exercise-induced ischemia and arrhythmias.
   3. For patients with uncomplicated MI who have received reperfusion therapy, submaximal exercise testing may be safely **performed as early as 3 days after MI** with maximal exercise testing 3 to 6 weeks later.
   C. **Exercise ECG testing of women.** The results of exercise ECG testing of women are different than those for men. Cardiovascular disease among women is addressed in Chapter 38.
II. **Indications.** The indications for exercise ECG testing are divided into three classes on the basis of degree of likelihood of disease or severity of diagnosed disease (Table 40-1).
III. **Contraindications.** Contraindications to exercise testing are divided into absolute and relative categories (Table 40-2).
IV. **Limitations of exercise ECG.** Before ordering an exercise ECG test, the physician should have an understanding of Bayes' theorem and the limitations of the test.
   A. **Bayes' theorem** is that the probability of a positive test result is affected by the likelihood (conditional probability) of a positive test result among the population that has undergone the test (pretest probability). The higher the probability that a disease is present in a given individual before a test is ordered, the higher the probability that a positive test result is a true-positive test result. Pretest probability is determined on the basis of symptoms, age, sex, and risk factors and can be divided into very low, low, intermediate, and high (Table 40-3).
   B. **Sensitivity and specificity.** The likelihood that an abnormal ECG finding indicates CAD is much higher for an older person with multiple risk factors than a young person with no risk factors. Sensitivity and specificity vary with the population being tested.
   1. Exercise ECG is **best used** in the evaluation of a patient at intermediate risk with an atypical history or a patient at low risk with a typical history.

Table 40-1. Guidelines for exercise testing

EXERCISE TESTING IN DIAGNOSIS OF OBSTRUCTIVE CORONARY ARTERY DISEASE (CAD)

Class 1
  Adult patients (including those with complete right bundle branch block or less
    than 1 mm of resting ST depression) with an intermediate pretest probability of
    CAD on the basis of sex, age, and symptoms

Class 2a
  Patients with vasospastic angina

Class 2b
  Patients with a high pretest probability of CAD on the basis of age, symptoms,
    and sex
  Patients with a low pretest probability of CAD on the basis of age, symptoms,
    and sex
  Patients with less than 1 mm of baseline ST depression and taking digoxin
  Patients with electrocardiographic (ECG) criteria of left ventricular hypertrophy
    and less than 1 mm of baseline ST depression

Class 3
  Patients with baseline ECG abnormalities[a]
  Patients with a documented myocardial infarction or prior coronary angiographic
    findings of disease and an established diagnosis of CAD (ischemia and risk can
    be determined with testing)

RISK ASSESSMENT AND PROGNOSIS AMONG PATIENTS WITH SYMPTOMS OR A HISTORY OF
CORONARY ARTERY DISEASE

Class 1
  Patients undergoing initial evaluation with suspected or known CAD (exceptions
    in Class 2b)
  Patients with suspected or known CAD previously evaluated with marked change
    in clinical status

Class 2b
  Patients with baseline ECG abnormalities[a]
  Patients with a stable clinical course who undergo periodic monitoring to guide
    treatment

Class 3
  Patients with severe comorbidity likely to limit life expectancy or are candidates
    for revascularization

AFTER MYOCARDIAL INFARCTION

Class 1
  Before discharge for prognostic assessment, activity prescription, or evaluation of
    medical therapy (submaximal at about 4–7 d)
  Early after discharge for prognostic assessment and cardiac rehabilitation if the
    predischarge exercise test was not performed (symptom-limited, about 14 to
    21 d)
  Late after discharge for prognostic assessment, activity prescription, evaluation
    of medical therapy, and cardiac rehabilitation if the early exercise test was sub-
    maximal (symptom-limited, about 3 to 6 wk)

Class 2a
  After discharge for activity counseling or exercise training as part of cardiac
    rehabilitation of patients who have undergone coronary revascularization

Class 2b
  Before discharge of patients who have undergone cardiac catheterization to iden-
    tify ischemia in the distribution of a coronary lesion of borderline severity
  Patients with the ECG abnormalities[a]
  Periodic monitoring for patients who continue to participate in exercise training
    or cardiac rehabilitation

Table 40-1. *Continued*

Class 3
  Severe comorbidity likely to limit life expectancy or candidacy for revascularization

EXERCISE TESTING FOR PERSONS WITHOUT SYMPTOMS OR KNOWN CORONARY ARTERY DISEASE

Class 1
  None
Class 2b
  Persons with multiple risk factors
  Men older than 40 years and women older than 50 years without symptoms
    Who plan to start vigorous exercise (especially if sedentary)
    Who are involved in occupations in which impairment might affect public safety
    Who are at high risk for CAD because of other diseases
Class 3
  Routine screening of men or women without symptoms

Class 1, Conditions for which there is evidence or agreement that a given procedure or treatment is useful and effective; *Class 2,* conditions for which there is conflicting evidence or a divergence of opinion about the usefulness or efficacy of a procedure or treatment; *class 2a,* weight of evidence or opinion is in favor of usefulness and efficacy; *class 2b,* usefulness or efficacy is less well established on the basis of evidence and opinion; *class 3,* conditions for which there is evidence or general agreement that the procedure or treatment is not useful or effective and in some cases may be harmful.
[a] Electrocardiographic findings include preexcitation (Wolff-Parkinson-White) syndrome, electronically paced ventricular rhythm, more than 1 mm of resting ST depression, or complete left bundle branch block.
From Gibbons RJ, et al., 1997, with permission.

  2. For the general population, the sensitivity is 68% and the specificity is 70%. Values are lower among persons at low risk.
  3. Exercise ECG has a higher sensitivity and specificity among **persons at high risk.** For most of these patients, however, invasive testing is preferred for a more definitive diagnosis and possible intervention. Excluding patients with left ventricular hypertrophy or resting ST depression and those taking digoxin also improves sensitivity and specificity.
  C. **Positive predictive value (PPV).** Once pretest probability and the sensitivity and specificity are known, PPV can be calculated. PPV is a measure of the likelihood that an abnormal test finding represents a true-positive result. It is highly dependent on pretest probability (prevalence of disease) in the population being tested. For example, in a population at low risk, the PPV of ECG exercise testing is only 21% but in a population at high risk, PPV rises to 83%.
V. **Patient preparation**
  A. **Instructions.** Table 40-4 provides a list of directions to give to patients before testing.
  B. **Medications**
    1. Before diagnostic testing, **cardiovascular drugs are withheld** at the discretion of and under the guidance of the supervising physician. This greatly increases the sensitivity of the test.
      a. **β-Blockers** pose a special problem. Patients taking β-blockers often do not have an adequate increase in heart rate to achieve the level of stress needed for the test. Abrupt withdrawal of β-blockers is to be discouraged because of reflex tachycardia. The best possible solution is to withdraw the β-blocker over several days before an exercise test. This is not always possible, however, because of

Table 40-2. Contraindications to exercise testing

ABSOLUTE CONTRAINDICATIONS

Recent (within 3–5 d) marked change in the resting electrocargiogram, suggesting infarction or other acute cardiac event

Recent complicated myocardial infarction (unless patient's condition is stable and pain free)

Unstable angina

Uncontrolled ventricular arrhythmia

Uncontrolled atrial arrhythmia that compromises cardiac function

Third-degree atrioventricular heart block without pacemaker

Acute congestive heart failure

Severe aortic stenosis

Suspected or known dissecting aneurysm

Active or suspected myocarditis, pericarditis, or endocarditis

Thrombosis of lower extremity or intracardiac thrombi

Recent systemic or pulmonary embolus

Acute infection

Acute noncardiac disorder that may affect exercise performance or be aggravated by exercise (e.g., infection, renal failure, or thyrotoxicosis)

Considerable emotional distress (psychosis)

RELATIVE CONTRAINDICATIONS

Resting diastolic blood pressure >115 mm Hg or resting systolic blood pressure >200 mm Hg

Moderate valvular heart disease

Known electrolyte abnormalities (e.g., hypokalemia, hypomagnesemia)

Fixed-rate pacemaker

Frequent or complex ventricular ectopy

Ventricular aneurysm

Uncontrolled metabolic disease (e.g., diabetes, thryotoxicosis, or myxedema)

Chronic infectious disease (e.g., mononucleosis, hepatitis, acquired immuno-deficiency syndrome)

Neuromuscular, musculoskeletal, or rheumatoid disorders exacerbated by exercise

Advanced or complicated pregnancy

Left main coronary arterial stenosis or its equivalent

Hypertrophic cardiomyopathy

Mental impairment leading to inability to cooperate

Modified from Kenney WL, 1995, and Fletcher GF, et al. Exercise Standards: a statement for healthcare professionals from the American Heart Association. *Circulation* 1995; 91:580–615, with permission.

time constraints or the necessity of drug therapy. In these cases, the clinician records that β-blockers were in use at the time of the test.

    b. Digoxin may cause problems in test interpretation. To avoid a reading that cannot be used to confirm a diagnosis, digoxin should be withheld for 2 weeks before testing.

  2. Patients undergoing diagnostic testing take their **other usual medications** on the day of the test to reproduce more closely the conditions outside the exercise laboratory.

VI. Exercise protocols. There are advantages and disadvantages to each exercise protocol (Table 40-5). Selection depends on patient characteristics, the equipment available, and the familiarity and comfort of the testing personnel with the protocol.

  A. An **optimal protocol** achieves peak workload and maximizes the sensitivity and specificity of the test.

Table 40-3. Pretest probability of coronary artery disease according to age, sex, and symptoms

Age (yr)	Sex	Typical or definite angina pectoris	Atypical or probable angina pectoris	Nonanginal chest pain	Asymptomatic
30–39	Men	Intermediate	Intermediate	Low	Very low
	Women	Intermediate	Very low	Very low	Very low
40–49	Men	High	Intermediate	Intermediate	Low
	Women	Intermediate	Low	Very low	Very low
50–59	Men	High	Intermediate	Intermediate	Low
	Women	Intermediate	Intermediate	Low	Very low
60–69	Men	High	Intermediate	Intermediate	Low
	Women	High	Intermediate	Intermediate	Low

From Gibbons RJ, et al., 1997, with permission.

1. **Workload.** An optimal protocol incorporates a **gradual increase** in the level of work so that the patient's true peak workload can be determined. If there are large increases in workload, maximum oxygen consumption ($\dot{V}O_2$ max) may fall between two levels. The test also is more comfortable for the patient if the increases in workload are not large.
2. **Duration.** The optimal duration for an exercise test is **8 to 12 minutes.** Periods longer than this measure muscular endurance rather than cardiovascular fitness. Periods shorter than this do not allow adequate time for the patient to warm up and achieve maximum workloads.
3. **Stage length.** Steady-state oxygen consumption is reached after about 2 minutes of exercise at a given workload. Thus the optimal protocol would have stage lengths of **2 to 3 minutes.**

Table 40-4. Patient preparation

Patients should refrain from ingesting food, alcohol, or caffeine or using tobacco products within 3 hours of testing.

Patients should be rested for the assessment, avoiding significant exertion or exercise on the day of the assessment.

Patients should wear clothing that allows freedom of movement, including walking or running shoes, and a loose-fitting shirt with short sleeves that buttons down the front. They should not wear restrictive undergarments during the test.

Outpatients should be warned that the evaluation may be fatiguing and that they may wish to have someone available to drive them home afterward.

If the test is for diagnostic purposes, it may be helpful for patients to discontinue prescribed cardiovascular medication after discussion with their physician. Antianginal agents alter the hemodynamic response to exercise and significantly reduce the sensitivity of ECG changes for ischemia. Patients taking intermediate or high-dose beta-blockers should taper their medication over a 2-to-4 day period to minimize hyperadrenergic withdrawal responses.

If the test is for functional purposes, patients should continue their medication regimen on their usual schedule, so that the exercise responses will be consistent with responses expected during exercise training.

Patients should bring a list of their medications with them to the assessment.

From *ACSM's Guidelines for Exercise Testing and Prescription.* Edited by Kenny WL, et al., 1995, with permission.

Table 40-5. Common exercise protocols

The five right-hand protocol columns fall under the spanning heading **Treadmill protocol**.

Functional Class	O_2 cost ml/kg per min	MET	Bruce 3-min stages mph/grade	Cornell 2-min stages mph/grade	Balke 2-min stages mph/grade	Naughton 2-min stages mph/grade	Jogger 2-min stages mph/grade
World–class athlete	70.0	20	—	—	—	—	—
	66.5	19	6.0/22	—	—	—	6.0/20.0
	63.0	18	5.5/20	—	—	—	6.0/17.5
	59.5	17	—	5.0/18	—	—	6.0/15.0
Athlete	56.0	16	5.0/18	—	4.0/20	—	6.0/12.5
	52.5	15	—	4.6/17	—	—	6.0/10.0
	49.0	14	—	4.2/16	3.5/20	—	6.0/7.5
Fit	45.5	13	4.2/16	—	—	—	6.0/5.0
	42.0	12	—	3.8/15	—	—	5.5/2.5
	38.5	11	—	3.4/14	3.0/20.0	—	5.0/2.5
Normal and 1	35.0	10	3.4/14	—	3.0/17.5	—	—
	31.5	9	—	3.0/13	3.0/15.0	—	—
	28.0	8	2.5/12	2.5/12	3.0/12.5	2.0/21.0	—
	24.5	7	—	2.1/11	3.0/10.0	2.0/17.5	—
2	21.0	6	1.7/10	1.7/10	3.0/7.5	2.0/14.0	—
	17.5	5	—	—	3.0/5.0	2.0/10.5	—
	14.0	4	1.7/5	1.7/5	3.0/2.5	2.0/7.0	—
3	10.5	3	1.7/0	1.7/0	3.0/0	2.0/3.5	—
	7.0	2	—	—	—	2.0/0	—
4	3.5	1	—	—	—	1.0/0	—

mph, Miles per hour; *MET*, metabolic equivalents.

4. **Exercise method.** Although **bicycle riding** is a better method for testing, **treadmill testing** is more common in the United States.

    a. The primary physiologic **advantage of bicycle** riding is the ability to take **direct measurements** of workload in watts, which has direct linear relation to $\dot{V}O_2$. With a **treadmill** one can only **estimate workload** because workload depends on the efficiency of walking, the weight of the patient, and the change in energy expenditure between walking and running. Other advantages of a bicycle are the stable platform that it provides for ECG and blood pressure recordings, the smaller amount of space it occupies, quieter use, and a lower initial cost of equipment.

    b. Treadmill testing is used more commonly in the United States because most Americans do not regularly ride bicycles and therefore have less training and thus a subsequent (falsely) lower peak workload than that achieved on a treadmill.

B. **Protocol options**

  1. **Bruce protocol**

    a. **Advantages.** The Bruce protocol has been widely used in the past and often is the basis of older studies; therefore **comparisons are easier.** Because the Bruce protocol has a final stage that cannot be completed, it is a good protocol for a highly fit person.

    b. **Disadvantages**

      (1) The main disadvantage of the Bruce protocol is the **large increments of change in workload between stages.** These large increases mean that for many persons peak workload falls somewhere between stages. This is a problem in evaluating functional capacity and may result in a lower sensitivity for the test.

      (2) The fourth stage of the Bruce protocol is an awkward stage that can be run or walked, resulting in divergent oxygen costs and workloads.

  2. **Modified Bruce protocol.** Developed for less fit persons, the modified Bruce protocol adds additional stages 0 and 1/2. These stages, at 1.7 mph (2.7 km/hr) with, respectively, 0% and 5% grades, provide a **lower workload for persons with poor cardiovascular fitness.** However, even these workloads may be too great for some debilitated patients and may result in premature fatigue.

  3. **Other protocols.** Protocols superior to the Bruce protocol have been developed. These protocols have more gradual increases in workload and can be modified to suit the individual.

    a. The **Naughton protocol** is good for older or debilitated persons and allows for a gradual increase in workload.

    b. The **Balke protocol** is good for younger, fit persons. It maintains a speed of 3, 3.5, or 4 mph (4.8, 5.6, or 6.4 km/hr) and increases the grade every 2 minutes.

    c. The **Cornell protocol** is good for a wider range of fitness levels depending on starting grade. It allows for a gradual increase in grade and speed and may be started at 0%, 5%, or 10% grade depending on fitness level.

    d. **Ramp protocols** are computer-driven protocols that continuously increase workload until maximum exertion is reached. This is the ultimate in continuous advancement; however, steady state may not be reached at any given workload.

VII. **Potential complications.** Complications of exercise ECG testing are rare but they do occur (Table 40-6). Exercise testing of healthy persons without CAD rarely if ever results in cardiac complications, which are most likely to occur among persons with underlying CAD. Several researchers have looked at large numbers of unselected persons involved in various activities to determine risk.

Table 40-6. Potential medical complications of exercise electrocardiographic testing

CARDIOVASCULAR COMPLICATIONS

Cardiac arrest
Ischemia
   Angina
   Myocardial infarction
Arrhythmias
   Superventricular tachycardia
   Atrial fibrillation
   Ventricular tachycardia
   Ventricular fibrillation
Bradyarrhythmias
   Bundle branch blocks
   Atrioventricular nodal blocks
Congestive heart failure
Hypertension
Hypotension
Aneurysm rupture

UNDERLYING MEDICAL CONDITIONS PREDISPOSING TO INCREASED COMPLICATIONS

Hypertrophic cardiomyopathy
Coronary artery anomalies
Idiopathic left ventricular hypertrophy
Marfan syndrome
Aortic stenosis
Right ventricular dysplasia
Congenital heart defects
Myocarditis
Pericarditis
Amyloidosis
Sarcoidosis
Long QT syndrome
Sickle-cell trait
Sudden death

PULMONARY COMPLICATIONS

Exercise-induced asthma
Bronchospasm
Pneumothorax
Exercise-induced anaphylaxis
Exacerbation of underlying pulmonary disease

GASTROINTESTINAL COMPLICATIONS

Vomiting
Cramps
Diarrhea

NEUROLOGIC COMPLICATIONS

Dizziness
Syncope (fainting)
Cerebrovascular accident (stroke)

MUSCULOSKELETAL COMPLICATIONS

Mechanical injuries
Back injuries
Joint pain or injury
Muscle cramps or spasms
Exacerbation of musculoskeletal disease

A. **Cardiac arrest**
   1. For the **general population** there is approximately 1 cardiac arrest per 565,000 person-hours of exercise.
   2. Among **persons with known CAD,** there is an estimated 1 arrest per 59,000 person-hours of vigorous activity. Acute coronary symptoms may be precipitated by exercise testing. Acute MI has been reported in approximately 1.4 in 10,000 exercise tests.
   3. Among **persons at low risk** for CAD, however, the risk for cardiac arrest during exercise testing is much lower. In one study no complications occurred in 380,000 exercise tests of young persons with presumably no heart disease.
B. **Arrhythmic complications** are a potential hazard of exercise testing (Table 40-7). Arrhythmias are more likely among persons with a history of arrhythmia. In this population they occur in 9% of tests compared with an overall incidence of 0.1%.
   1. **Atrial fibrillation** is the most common arrhythmia that occurs during testing, occurring in 9.5 per 10,000 tests.
   2. **Ventricular tachycardia** is less common, occurring in 5.8 per 10,000 tests.
   3. **Ventricular fibrillation** is even less common, occurring 0.67 times per 10,000 tests.

Table 40-7. Absolute and relative indications for termination of an exercise test

ABSOLUTE INDICATIONS

Acute myocardial infarction or suspicion of myocardial infarction
Onset of moderate to severe angina or increasing anginal pain
Drop in systolic blood pressure with increasing workload accompanied by signs or symptoms or drop below resting pressure
Serious arrhythmias (e.g., second- or third-degree atrioventricular block, sustained ventricular tachycardia or increasing premature ventricular contractions, atrial fibrillation with fast ventricular response)
Signs of poor perfusion, including pallor, cyanosis, or cold and clammy skin
Unusual or severe shortness of breath
Central nervous system symptoms, including ataxia, vertigo, visual or gait problems, or confusion
Technical inability to monitor the electrocardiogram
Patient's request

RELATIVE INDICATIONS

Pronounced electrocardiographic changes from baseline >2mm of horizontal or downsloping ST-segment depression, or >2 mm of ST-segment elevation except in aVR
Any chest pain that is increasing
Physical or oral manifestations of severe fatigue or shortness of breath
Wheezing
Leg cramps or intermittent claudication (grade 3 on 4-point scale)
Hypertensive response (systolic blood pressure >260 mm Hg, diastolic blood pressure >115 mm Hg)
Less serious arrhythmias such as supraventricular tachycardia
Exercise-induced bundle branch block that cannot be differentiated from ventricular tachycardia
General appearance

Modified from Kenney WL, et al., 1995, and Fletcher GF, et al. American Heart Association Exercise Standards. *Circulation* 1992; 86:340–344, with permission.

C. Deaths during exercise testing are exceedingly rare among well-monitored patients but may occur in 1 of 25,000 tests. If death occurs, it is usually caused by sudden cardiac death or MI.

VIII. **Data**

A. **ECG data.** Although not the only data that should be examined, ECG changes garner the most attention (Table 40-8; see Table 40-7). The **portion of the ECG most sensitive to ischemia** is the ST segment. The pathophysiologic mechanism of the ST change is net depression caused by a current of ischemia from the affected myocardial cells. The TP segment may be useful at rest and should be used when possible; however, it shortens or disappears with exercise. Baseline ECG abnormalities that can obscure the correct diagnosis of ST changes are listed in Table 40-9.

1. **ST-segment changes**

a. **Measurement of the ST segment.** There is no clear consensus as to where to measure the ST segment. Traditionally it is measured 80 msec past the J point, but some authors suggest measuring at the J point or at the midpoint of the ST segment (using either the end of the T wave or the peak of the T wave to determine the end of the segment) (Fig. 40-1A).

b. **ST-segment changes** are measured from the isoelectric baseline, which can be determined from the PR interval. If the ST segment is elevated at rest, any depression that occurs with exercise still is measured from the isoelectric line; early repolarization of the ST segment at rest is normal. If, however, the ST segment is depressed at rest, any further depression should be measured from the baseline ST segment (Fig. 40-1B)

c. **Normal response.** During exercise, there is depression of the J junction that is maximal at peak exercise and returns to baseline during recovery. This normal depression is upsloping and typically less than 1 mm below the isoelectric line 80 msec after the J point.

d. **ST depression** does not localize the area of ischemia.

Table 40-8. Newer principles of interpretation of exercise test results

Ischemic ST depression normally occurs in the lateral leads (I, V4–V6).
In the presence of Q waves, changes may be isolated (II, V2).
Change in both inferior and lateral leads suggests severe ischemia.
Isolated inferior or anterior changes often are false-positive findings.
ST depression does not localize ischemia to an area of myocardium.
ST depression without angina suggests milder coronary artery disease and lower risk.
ST depression not interpretable in left bundle branch block, previous coronary artery bypass graft, Q-wave myocardial infarction, left ventricular hypertrophy, use of digitalis, Wolff-Parkinson-White Syndrome, or use of ventricular pacemaker.
ST elevation over Q-wave areas indicates myocardial damage or aneurysm.
ST elevation over non-Q-Wave areas indicates local transmural myocardial ischemia.
Markers of poor prognosis are as follows:
  Exertional hypotension—a drop in systolic blood pressure below preexercise value
  Angina that limits exercise
  Poor exercise capacity (<5 MET)
  Downsloping ST depression especially in recovery
  ST depression starting at a low double product (<15,000)
  ST depression that persists into late recovery

From Marwick TH, 1996, with permission.

Table 40-9. Baseline abnormalities that may obscure electrocardiographic changes during exercise

Left bundle branch block
Left ventricular hypertrophy with repolarization abnormality
Digitalis therapy
Ventricular paced rhythm
Wolff-Parkinson-White syndrome
ST abnormality associated with supraventricular tachycardia or atrial fibrillation
ST abnormalities with mitral valve prolapse and severe anemia

    (1) ST depression of at least 1 mm that is horizontal or down-sloping is abnormal, as is upsloping ST depression of at least 2.0 mm.

    (2) Baseline ST abnormalities are less likely to represent exercise-induced myocardial ischemia, and the baseline ST depression should be subtracted from the peak ST depression.

    (3) Criteria that increase the probability of ischemia are the **number of leads** involved (more leads increase the probability of ischemia), the **workload** at which the ST depression occurs (lower workload increases probability), the **angle of the slope** (a downsloping angle has a higher probability than a horizontal one), **amount of time in recovery** before normalization of the ST segment (longer recovery increases the probability), and possibly the **magnitude of the depression.** Changes in the lateral leads, particularly V5, are more specific than in any of the other leads. Changes in the inferior leads alone are likely to be a false-positive result.

  e. The **meaning of ST elevation** depends on the presence or absence of Q waves of prior MI.

    (1) ST-segment elevation **with Q waves of prior MI** is a common finding among patients who have had MI. It occurs among as many as 50% of patients with anterior MI and 15% of patients with previous inferior MI and is not caused by ischemia. The mechanism is thought to be caused by dyskinetic myocardium or ventricular aneurysms. There may even be reciprocal ST-segment depression. Patients with more extensive Q waves have more pronounced ST elevation. These patients typically have a lower ejection fraction than those without elevated ST segment with a Q wave. These changes do not imply ischemia (although they may imply viability) and should be interpreted as normal.

    (2) ST-segment elevation **without Q waves of prior MI** represents marked transmural myocardial ischemia. ST elevation also may indicate the location of the ischemia. This finding should be interpreted as abnormal.

  f. ST normalization, or the lack of ST changes during exercise, **may be a sign of ischemia.** This phenomenon occurs when ischemic ST depression and ST elevation cancel one another. This effect is rare but should be considered in tests of patients with no ECG changes but with a high likelihood of CAD.

2. R waves may change in amplitude during exercise. There is no diagnostic value in these changes.

3. T-wave and U-wave changes

  a. The **T wave** normally decreases gradually in early exercise and begins to increase in amplitude at maximal exercise. One minute into recovery, the T wave should be back to baseline. T-wave

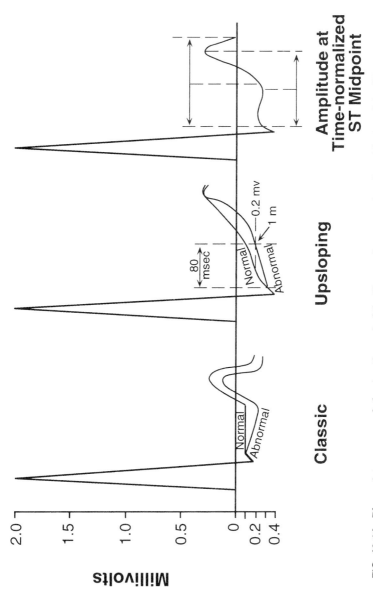

FIG. 40-1A. Blomqvist recommended using the end of the T wave for measuring the midpoint of the ST segement, but Simons used the peak of the T wave. This change was made to have a more stable end point, since the end of the T wave is much more difficult to find than the peak of the T wave.

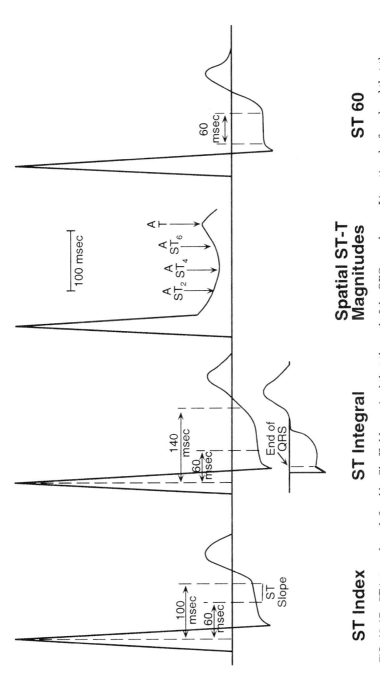

ST Index   **ST Integral**   **Spatial ST-T Magnitudes**   **ST 60**

FIG. 40-1B. ST integral, as defined by Sheffield, required that the end of the QRS complex, or J junction, be found and that the area measurement stop as soon as the ST segment crossed the isoelectric line or as the T wave began. The St integral used by most commercial systems initiates the area at a fixed period after the R wave and then ends 80 msec thereafter.

515

   inversion is not a specific marker of ischemia and may occur
   normally.
   b. If the U wave is upright at baseline, **U-wave inversion** may be
      associated with ischemia, left ventricular hypertrophy, and valvular
      disease.
   4. **Arrhythmias.** Table 40-7 lists abnormal arrhythmias that may occur
      during exercise. Ectopic atrial and ventricular beats are not predictive
      of outcome. but exercise-induced left bundle branch block is predictive of
      a worse outcome. Sustained ventricular tachycardia and ventricular fib-
      rillation are abnormal but rarely occur.
   5. **Time to resolution of changes.** The longer into recovery that it takes
      for ECG changes to resolve, the higher is the probability that they are
      important. Rapid recovery (less than 1 minute) indicates less likelihood
      of disease and that disease if present is less severe.
B. **Age-predicted maximum heart rate (APMHR).** Many formulas have
   been developed to predict maximum heart rate (MHR). These formulas are
   generated by measuring MHR in a sample population and plotting a regression line against various factors that may affect heart rate. There is a great
   deal of scatter on either side on the regression line, and the fit of the line seldom reaches an r value greater than 0.9. It is well known that MHR decreases
   with age; thus most equations incorporate age. The two most common formulas are as follows:

   APMHR = 220 − age

   APMHR = 200 − ½ age

   The APMHR may be much lower or much higher than a person's actual
   measured maximal heart rate. Therefore **heart rate should not be used
   as an indicator of maximal exertion or in the decision to terminate
   testing except in a submaximal test.** If maximal heart rate does not
   exceed 85% of APMHR during testing and there are no substantial ECG
   changes, the test is usually read as nondiagnostic. If there are substantial
   ECG changes, the test is read as abnormal, regardless of the heart rate
   achieved.

C. **Rating of perceived exertion (RPE)** is a better marker of maximal level
   of exertion.
   1. A useful indicator of percentage of maximum workload achieved is the
      RPE scale. This is a subjective scale used to rate how hard the subject
      feels they are working during an exercise test. The subject should be
      advised to rate how he or she feels overall and not an individual element
      such as leg fatigue. Although subjective, the scale has been shown to be
      reproducible, and maximum ratings correspond well with maximum
      exertion.
      a. The **Borg scale** is used most often. The original scale ranges from
         6 to 20, which is meant to correspond to a heart rate increase from
         60 to 200 beats/min during exercise.
      b. The **modified Borg scale** is 0 to 10. The scale includes word
         anchors, which are important for accurate assessment of work level.
         The scales are not linear, and at higher workloads the changes in
         RPE are closer together.
   2. A maximal level of exertion is marked by a score greater than 18 (Borg
      scale) or 9 (modified Borg scale), respiratory quotient (RQ) greater than
      1.1 (if carbon dioxide exchange is monitored), and overall patient
      appearance.
D. In addition to ECG monitoring, **blood pressure monitoring** is an important aspect of the exercise test both for safety and for diagnosis of CAD. It

Table 40-10. Work capacity (in METs) classifications, age, and sex

Age (yr)	Low	Fair	Average	Good	High
WOMEN					
20–29	<7.5	8–10.3	10.3–12.5	12.5–16	>16
30–39	<7	7–9	9–11	11–15	>15
40–49	<6	6–8	8–10	10–14	>14
50–59	<5	5–7	7–9	9–13	>13
60–69	<4.5	4.5–6	6–8	8–11.5	>11.5
MEN					
20–29	<8	8–11	11–14	14–17	>17
30–39	<7.5	7.5–10	10–12.5	12.5–16	>16
40–49	<7	7–8.5	8.5–11.5	11.5–15	>15
50–59	<6	6–8	8–11	11–14	>14
60–69	<5.5	5.5–7	7–9.5	9.5–13	>13

should be checked in each walking stage. It may not be practical to check blood pressure while the subject is running.

1. **Systolic blood pressure** (SBP) normally rises during exercise. A **failure of SBP to rise** with increasing workload or a drop in SBP usually indicates the presence of CAD and is an indication to **terminate testing.**

2. **Diastolic blood pressure** decreases with exercise and may be audible down to zero during vigorous activity. Unlike SBP, diastolic blood pressure is not useful in diagnosis or safety monitoring.

E. **Symptoms.** The presence or absence of symptoms and their change over time are included in the final report.

F. **Functional capacity.** Functional testing is a powerful marker for prognosis. Persons who achieve more than 6 metabolic equivalents (MET) workload have a significantly lower mortality rate than those who do not achieve this workload regardless of ECG changes. On the basis of age and workload achieved, functional capacity can be divided into five classifications (Table 40-10). Among 3,400 patients with no history of diagnosed CAD undergoing exercise testing at the Cleveland Clinic, those with average or better classifications had a 2.5-year mortality of less than 2% compared with 6% and 14% among those who were in the fair and poor groups. The adjusted relative risk for fair or poor functional capacity in this population was almost 4.

IX. **Termination of exercise testing.** The American Heart Association and American College of Sports Medicine have developed very similar indications for exercise termination (see Table 40-7). The decision when to terminate a test ultimately relies on the expertise and judgment of those performing the test.

Table 40-11. Information to include in exercise electrocardiography report

Exercise protocol used
Duration of exercise
Peak treadmill speed and grade
Peak workload in MET or $\dot{V}O_2$max
Functional capacity
Maximum heart rate and percentage of age-predicted maximum heart rate achieved
Resting and peak blood pressure
Symptoms
Arrhythmias
Electrocardiographic changes

Table 40–12. Guidelines for interpretation of results of exercise electrocardiography

Variable	Normal	Normal except for	Abnormal
Symptoms	Neuromuscular chest pain Fatigue, shortness of breath, leg or joint pain	Angina as an isolated finding Atypical angina Chest discomfort of questionable causation Claudication Dizziness, lightheadedness Other noteworthy symptoms	Syncope Angina when associated with ST- or T-wave changes, including borderline Angina when associated with exercise hypotension
Blood pressure response (mm Hg)	SBP increases >10 but is <230 at peak DBP increases ≤10 but is <120 at peak DBP stays the same or decreases DBP increases ≥ 12 from rest but peak is <100	SBP ≥230 at peak exercise DBP ≥120 at peak exercise DBP ≥12 increase from rest if peak is ≥ to 100	Any drop in SBP as exercise intensity increases
arrhythmias	Occasional PVCs PACs Frequent PACs or PVCs at rest that abate during exercise	Paroxysmal SVT Increased frequency of PVCs or couplets during exercise Isolated run of nonsustained VT	Sustained SVTs, AFIB, atrial flutter, or junctional rhythm Nonsustained VT Second or third degree AV block

	Chronic AFIB, atrial flutter	Ventricular couplets Paroxysmal escape rhythms	AV dissociation Exercise induced before excitation Idioventricular rhythm *Very abnormal* Sustained VT (≥ 30 sec) VF/cardiac arrest Asystole
ST segments	< 1.0 mm ST depression or elevation	Borderline ST changes (0.5–0.9 mm ST depression) ST elevation in leads in area of prior MI T-wave inversion Pseudonormalization of resting T-wave abnormalities	≥ 1.0 mm H or D ST depression ≥ 1.5 mm upsloping ST depression ≥ 1.0 mm U ST depression if associated with anginal symptoms ≥ 1.0 mm ST elevation in leads without q waves or not over a prior MI *Very abnormal* ≥ 2.0 mm H or D ST depression ≥ 2.5 mm upsloping ST depression ≥ 2.0 mm ST elevation in leads without Q waves or not over a prior MI
Functional capacity	Normal or mildly impaired exercise tolerance	Low exercise tolerance	Inability to achieve 3 MET workload

SBP, Systolic blood pressure; *DBP,* diastolic blood pressure; *PVC,* premature ventricular contractions; *PAC,* premature atrial contractions; *AFIB,* atrial fibrillation; *SVT,* supraventricular tachycardia; *VT,* ventricular tachycardia; *AV,* atrioventricular; *VF,* ventricular fibrillation; *MI,* myocardial infarction; *H,* horizontal; *D,* downsloping; *U,* Upsloping.

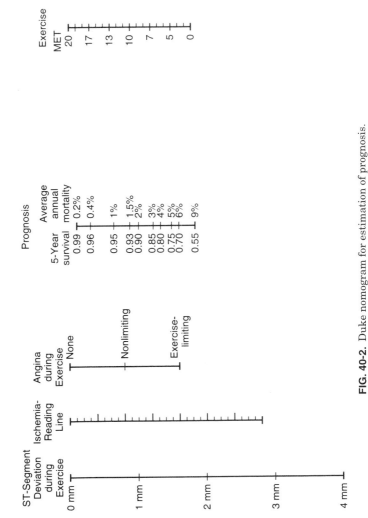

FIG. 40-2. Duke nomogram for estimation of prognosis.

A. **Absolute indications** are all serious findings. A drop in SBP with increasing workload is a particularly ominous sign and usually but not always indicates the presence of severe CAD.

B. **Relative indications** to terminate testing are findings that should increase the level of concern and vigilance among those administering the test and possibly cause cessation of testing. Relative indications for termination rely heavily on the judgment of the personnel performing the test, and the decision to continue the test should not be made lightly (see Table 40-7).

C. **Indications for termination of submaximal exercise testing** include any one of the following end points:

1. Signs or symptoms of ischemia
2. Achievement of 6 MET workload
3. Eighty-five percent of the APMHR
4. Heart rate of 110 beats/min for a patient taking β-blockers.
5. A score on the Borg RPE of 17 or modified Borg RPE of 7

D. **Postexercise recovery**

1. In **all routine exercise tests a cool-down period** adds safety to the test. The length of cool-down may vary from 30 seconds to several minutes, depending on the person. A general rule is to allow enough time for the heart rate to drop to less than 110 beats/min. A shorter cool-down period increases the sensitivity of exercise ECG because of increased venous return; resuming the supine position leads to increased wall stress. This same mechanism also increases the risk of testing.

2. The exception to observing a cool-down period may be made in exercise echocardiography, in which it is important to image the subject when he or she is as close as possible to maximum heart rate.

X. **Interpretation of data.** An exercise ECG test must be interpreted by an experienced clinician. Although the terms *positive* and *negative* often are used, these terms do not accurately describe the results of an exercise ECG test and are to be avoided. The information to include in an exercise ECG report is listed in Table 40-11.

A. Exercise ECG test results can be normal, abnormal, normal except for, or nondiagnostic (Table 40-12). Nondiagnostic tests are those in which the subject does not achieve 85% of APMHR and has no abnormal ECG changes or in which baseline ECG changes are present that obscure ST changes (see Table 40-9).

B. **Prognosis.** The Duke nomogram (Fig. 40-2). is a simple chart that factors in ST-segment deviation, amount of angina during exercise, and exercise capacity to give an estimate of 5-year survival and average annual mortality. This nomogram was derived by means of regression analysis and can be a useful tool in determining prognosis and the degree of aggressiveness needed in treating a patient.

SUGGESTED READINGS

Landmark Articles

Dubach P, Froelicher VF, Klein J, et al. Exercise-induced hypotension in a male population. *Circulation* 1988;78:1380–1387.

Gibbons L, Blair SN, Kohl HW, et al. The safety of maximal exercise testing. *Circulation* 1989;80:846–852.

Topol EJ, Burek K, O'Neill WW, et al. A randomized controlled trial of hospital discharge three days after myocardial infarction in the era of reperfusion. *N Engl J Med* 1988;318:1083–1088.

Young DZ, Lampert S, Graboys TB, et al. Safety of maximal exercise testing in patients at high risk for ventricular arrhythmias. *Circulation* 1984; 70:184–191.

Key Reviews

Gibbons RJ, Balady GJ, Beasley JW, et al. ACC/AHA guidelines for exercise testing: a report of the American College of Cardiology/American Heart Association Task

Force on Practice Guideline (Committee on Exercise Testing). *J Am Coll Cardiol* 1997;30:260–315.

Pina IL, Balady GJ, Hanson P, Labovitz AJ, Madonna DW, Myers J. Guidelines for clinical exercise testing laboratories: a statement for healthcare professionals from the Committee on Exercise and Cardiac Rehabilitation, American Heart Association. *Circulation* 1995;91:912–921.

Relevant Book Chapters

In: Chou T, Knilans TK, eds. *Electrocardiography in clinical practice.* Philadelphia: WB Saunders, 4th ed, 1996:214–239.

Kenney WL, Humphrey RH, Bryant CX, eds. *ACSM's Guidelines for Exercise Testing and Prescription.* Baltimore: Williams & Wilkins, 1995.

Marwick TH, ed. *Cardiac stress testing and imaging.* New York: Churchill Livingstone, 1996.

Wasserman K, Hansen JE, Sue DY, Whipp BJ, eds. *Principles of exercise testing.* Philadelphia: Lea & Febiger, 1987

41. NUCLEAR IMAGING

Jeffrey A. Skiles

I. **Introduction.** Nuclear cardiology has an integral role in the noninvasive detection of coronary artery disease (CAD), assessment of myocardial viability, and stratification of risk. It imparts improved sensitivity and specificity over standard exercise stress testing. The average sensitivity of single photon emission computed tomography (SPECT) with technetium 99m is reported to be 90% and the average specificity 74%. Nuclear imaging can provide functional-physiologic and prognostic information, is quantifiable and reproducible, and is readily obtainable in diverse patient populations.

II. **Indications**
   A. **Diagnosis of CAD.** Nuclear perfusion studies are performed to establish noninvasively the diagnosis of CAD in the following situations: history of **stable angina; chest pain of unclear causation; unstable angina,** after stabilization; **abnormal exercise test result** without symptoms; **screening** for risk factors; scheduled standard exercise testing in the setting of an **abnormal electrocardiogram (ECG);** and previously **nondiagnostic graded exercise test.**
   B. **Assessment of the physiologic importance of known CAD.** Perfusion imaging is indicated in the care of patients with borderline coronary stenosis (40% to 70%) and small-vessel stenosis in a distal branch. It is also useful to evaluate a specific coronary lesion before percutaneous intervention.
   C. **Assessment after therapeutic intervention.** Perfusion imaging can be performed as a routine follow-up procedure after percutaneous intervention, coronary artery bypass grafting, or medical therapy and for evaluation of recurrent symptoms.
   D. **Risk stratification.** With nuclear imaging, it is possible to stratify risk among patients with stable angina or unstable angina, those who have had myocardial infarction (MI), and those about to undergo noncardiac operations.
   E. **Identification of MI** among patients with angiographically normal coronary arteries is afforded by nuclear imaging.

III. **Contraindications.** In addition to standard contraindications to exercise stress testing, specific considerations apply uniquely to nuclear imaging in general and the subgroup of dipyridamole stress perfusion studies.
   A. **General contraindications to nuclear studies.** Nuclear imaging is contraindicated for patients who have had **iodine 131 therapy** within 12 weeks; **technetium 99m studies** within 48 hours, including bone, lung, multigated acquisition (MUGA), liver, tagged red blood cell (to evaluate gastrointestinal bleeding), and renal scans; **indium 111 scans** within 30 days; **gallium 67 scans** within 30 days; **oral intake** within 4 hours (except for water); and **caffeine** consumption within 4 hours.
   B. **Contraindications to dipyridamole** administration include allergy to dipyridamole; allergy to aminophylline; ongoing theophylline therapy (must be discontinued for 36 hours); history of asthma or reactive airway disease; caffeine consumption within 12 to 24 hours.

IV. **Equipment.** The most basic tool in nuclear imaging is the **gamma** or **scintillation camera,** which is used to detect gamma rays (also known as x-ray photons) produced by the chosen radionuclide. Three types of gamma camera exist.
   A. **A single-crystal camera** consists of one large sodium iodide crystal. Other essential elements of this camera include the **collimator** (a lead device that screens out background or scattered photons) and the **photomultiplier** (an electronic processor that translates photon interactions with the crystal into electric energy).

1. Electric signals from the photomultiplier are processed by the **pulse height analyzer** before reaching a final form. Only signals in a specified energy range are incorporated into the interpreted images. The range recognized by the pulse height analyzer is established on the basis of the radiopharmaceutical used.

2. **Digitalization** of the single-crystal camera has greatly enhanced its performance (up to 400,000 counts/sec).

B. A **multicrystal camera** works with an array of crystals with increased count-detection capability. Because of the availability of an individual crystal to detect scintillation at any given time, this type of camera can be used to detect many more counts than a single-crystal camera can (up to 600,000 counts/sec compared with 200,000 to 400,000 counts/sec for a single-crystal camera).

C. A **positron camera** is a gamma camera used to detect the photon products of positron annihilation. Interaction between a positron and an electron causes annihilation with the generation of two high-energy photons (511 keV).

1. An array of multiple concentric rings of crystals constitute a positron camera. Each crystal is linked optically to multiple photomultipliers. The crystals are oriented in pairs in such a way that each crystal must be struck simultaneously by an annihilation photon to record activity. Thus background interference and stray photon energy are automatically accounted for, and artifact is limited.

2. Most positron cameras contain **bismuth germanite** for annihilation photon detection. The clinical utility and radiopharmaceuticals for positron emission tomography (PET) are discussed in **XI**.

V. **Mechanics and techniques**

A. **Image acquisition.** Basic perfusion imaging can be performed by means of **planar** and **tomographic** techniques.

1. **Planar images** are acquired in three views: **anterior, left anterior oblique** (LAO), and **steep LAO** or **left lateral orientation** (LLAT) (Fig. 41-1). The patient is supine for anterior and LAO views but is placed in the lateral decubitus position for LLAT image acquisition. Although it allows scrutinization of specific myocardial segments, planar imaging superimposes vascular distributions and therefore can compromise the ability to implicate a specific vascular supply when a defect is present. For example, normally perfused myocardial segments may overlap perfusion defects in a separate distribution.

2. In SPECT a series of planar images usually are obtained over a 180-degree arc to reconstruct a three-dimensional representation of the heart. The arc extends from the 45-degree right anterior oblique plane to the 45-degree left posterior oblique plane with the patient in the supine position.

   a. Three orientations are analyzed in the final representation: **short axis, vertical long axis,** and **horizontal long axis.** A computer-generated display, the **polar map,** also is analyzed as a quantifiable representation of count density.

   b. Unlike planar imaging, **SPECT** can be used to **separate vascular territories** and thus improve interpretation of image. SPECT, however, also **increases the time needed** for image acquisition and requires close attention to quality-control issues.

B. **Radiopharmaceuticals** available for nuclear imaging include thallium 201, technetium 99m, and several positron imaging agents. Each possesses specific energy characteristics, kinetic profiles, and biodistribution (Tables 41-1, 41-2).

1. **Thallium 201**

   a. **General characteristics.** Thallium 201 (thallous chloride) is a metallic element in group IIIA of the periodic table; it is produced in a cyclotron. Thallium emits mercury x-rays at an energy range of 69 to 83 keV and has a **half-life of 73 hours.** The biologic activity of

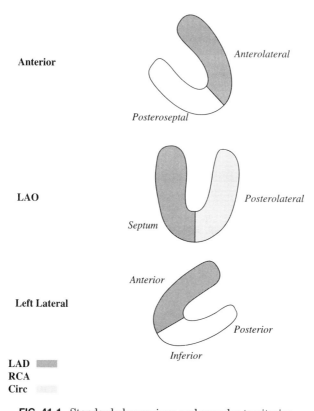

FIG. 41-1. Standard planar views and vascular territories.

Table 41-1. Characteristics of common perfusion agents

Attribute	Thallium 201	Technetium 99m sestamibi	Technetium 99m teboroxime
Energy (keV)	69–83	140	140
Dose (mCi)	2.5–3.5	20–30	20–30
Half-life (hr)	74	6	6
Cyclotron required	Yes	No	No
Perfusion imaging	Yes	Yes	Yes
Viability evaluation	Yes	Yes	No
Redistribution	Yes	Yes (minimal)	No
Gating (electrocardiogram)	No	Yes	No

Table 41-2. Radiopharmaceuticals useful in single-photon emission computed tomography

Myocardial perfusion
    Thallium 201
    [^{99m}Tc]isonitriles (sestamibi)
    [^{99m}Tc]boronic acid adduct of technetium oxime (BATO) complexes
    Thallium 201 (reinjection)
Myocardial metabolism
    [^{123}I]hexadecanoic acid
    [^{123}I]heptadecanoic acid
    [^{123}I]iodophenylpentadecanoic acid
Myocardial infarction
    [^{99m}Tc]pyrophosphate
    [^{99m}Tc]tetracycline
    [^{99m}Tc]glucoheptonate
    ^{111}In-labeled antimyosin antibody
    ^{131}I-labeled antimyosin antibody
Myocardial innervation and receptor
    [123I]metaiodobenzylguanidine (MIBG)
    [123I]3-quinuclidinyl-4-iodobenzylate (QNB)
Coronary thrombosis
    ^{111}In-labeled antifibrin antibody
    ^{111}In-labeled antiplatelet antibody
    ^{131}I-labeled antiplatelet antibody
    ^{111}In-labeled tissue plasminogen activator

Adapted from Saha GB, et al., 1992, with permission.

this element is very similar to that of potassium (the ionic radii of the two elements are virtually identical). Thus thallium is actively transported into cells by the sodium-potassium–adenosine triphosphatase (Na-K-ATPase) pump.

  b. Kinetics. Approximately 5% of the administered dose of thallium 201 is distributed to the myocardium (proportionate to the blood flow delivered to the coronary circulation). Nearly 85% of the thallium 201 is extracted by myocytes in the first pass.

    (1) The **initial uptake** of thallium 201 by myocardium is directly related to regional blood flow. The myocardial extraction of thallium 201, however, increases at low flow rates (less than 10% of basal) and decreases at high flow rates (more than twice basal rate).

    (2) Washout. After initial uptake into myocytes, a state of continuous exchange across the cell membrane occurs. The distribution of this radiotracer changes after administration, and thallium 201 washes out from the myocytes, a process called **redistribution.** Thallium 201 washout generally approaches 30% from 2 to 2.5 hours after injection.

    (3) Ischemic myocardium. Uptake of thallium 201 in ischemic myocardium is lower than uptake in nonischemic segments. Washout time from ischemic zones is slower than that from nonischemic zones.

    (4) Over time, counts become equal in the ischemic and nonischemic regions (or thallium 201 concentration may actually increase in ischemic regions) so that thallium 201 concentrations in these disparate areas approach one another.

2. Technetium 99m–labeled agents

    a. General characteristics. Technetium 99m is a radiopharmaceutical that can be produced on site in molybdenum 99–technetium 99m generators and possesses a number of ideal imaging characteristics.

        (1) Technetium 99m has a **half-life of 6 hours** and emits gamma rays with a single photopeak of 140 keV.

        (2) Technetium 99m–labeled **perfusion agents** include ⁹⁹ᵐ**Tc-sestamibi** and ⁹⁹ᵐ**Tc-teboroxime.** The former agent has been used clinically most often.

    b. Kinetics. After administration of ⁹⁹ᵐTc-sestamibi, approximately 40% to 60% of the agent is extracted by the myocardium. Initial uptake of the agent is proportional to regional myocardial blood flow and it is bound to the inner mitochondrial membrane.

        (1) Myocardial washout of ⁹⁹ᵐTc-sestamibi is very slow, and little redistribution is seen. The absence of redistribution requires two separate injections of the agent, at **rest** and at **peak exercise,** or with pharmacologic stress.

        (2) The **utility of technetium 99m** in the evaluation of viability remains **controversial.** Although redistribution is minimal, increased uptake of technetium 99m over time after rest injection is observed and suggests the presence of viable myocardium. In addition, areas that have diminished counts but retain at least 60% of the highest count density exhibit improved wall motion after revascularization.

VI. Imaging protocols

A. Thallium 201

    1. General features. Stress imaging with thallium 201 involves **injection at peak exercise** (or with pharmacologic stress) and **immediate imaging,** followed by **redistribution images** 3 to 4 hours after injection.

        a. Because of the long half-life of thallium 201 (73 hours), limited amounts are administered. Although a single injection typically is used because of the redistribution phenomenon, a second injection may be given to enhance filling-in of reversible defects.

        b. The low energy range of thallium 201 is marginal for imaging with the gamma camera because of scatter and diminished spatial resolution.

    2. Variations from standard protocol. Exact imaging techniques vary among institutions. Initial thallium 201 doses range from 2 to 3.5 mCi, acquisition times vary from 20 to 40 seconds per image, and the number of images varies from 32 to 64 depending on whether 180-degree or 360-degree image acquisition is used.

        a. The use of **360-degree versus 180-degree imaging** has been the subject of debate. Contrast is better, there is less artifact, and imaging times are shorter with 180-degree tomography. Slight variations also exist depending on the use of exercise stress testing or pharmacologic stress protocols.

        b. When **exercise thallium 201 scintigraphy** is performed, the radionuclide (2 to 3.5 mCi) usually is injected approximately 1 minute before peak exercise to allow time for distribution. Initial images are obtained within 5 to 10 minutes of injection. Redistribution images are obtained 2.5 to 4 hours after the initial images.

        c. Not infrequently, **persistent defects** that would ordinarily be interpreted as myocardial scar actually represent viable myocardium.

            (1) For this reason, some clinicians advocate **delayed (late redistribution) imaging** 18 to 24 hours after injection. Some studies indicate that as many as 40% of persistent defects exhibit radiotracer uptake after revascularization. Delayed imaging has resulted in further redistribution in as many as 45% of patients.

    (2) Alternative approaches in **differentiating viable tissue from scar** include **rest reinjection** of thallium 201, in effect to boost fill-in of perfusion defects. As many as 50% of persistent defects have been shown to exhibit improved thallium 201 uptake after rest injection of 1 mCi of thallium 201, suggesting viability.

  d. Minor changes in imaging protocol may be observed with **pharmacologic stress testing** with adenosine, dipyridamole, or dobutamine.

B. Technetium 99m. The relative lack of redistribution requires **two injections** of technetium 99m to obtain rest and stress images.

  1. Basic protocols

    a. Same-day protocol. At peak exercise, 25 to 30 mCi of technetium 99m is injected. Rest images are obtained first and stress imaging follows to minimize residual scintigraphic activity caused by the higher-dose stress injection.

      (1) Rest images are obtained with injection of 7 to 10 mCi of technetium 99m and image acquisition 1 to 1.5 hours later (imaging is delayed because of slower liver clearance with rest injection).

      (2) Stress images are obtained approximately 45 to 60 minutes after injection. Hepatic uptake of technetium 99m occurs within 15 to 30 minutes of injection, and the tracer is excreted into the gastrointestinal tract through the biliary system. Appearance of the tracer in the gastrointestinal tract can interfere with imaging of the inferior wall of the left ventricle.

    b. The **separate-day protocol** allows time for decay of activity. Larger doses of technetium 99m can be administered for rest and stress images, and there is minimal interference between the images.

      (1) From 22 to 30 mCi of technetium 99m is injected for both stress and rest imaging, separated in time by 1 to 2 days.

      (2) The higher doses possible with the 2-day protocol produce increased count density and better image quality at the cost of inconvenience.

  2. Factors that affect image quality. Consumption of a **fatty meal** can enhance biliary excretion of technetium 99m and improve image quality. Because of possible interference from noncardiac uptake, image processing with technetium 99m relies on normalization to the brightest cardiac pixel.

C. Dual isotope imaging. Use of both thallium 201 and technetium 99m substantially reduces the time required to obtain stress and rest images.

  1. The patient receives thallium 201 at rest (3.5 mCi) and immediately after rest imaging undergoes stress. At peak stress, the patient is given an injection of 25 mCi technetium 99m. Stress images are obtained 15 minutes later.

  2. This technique makes use of the dissimilar energy levels of the two radionuclides to shorten the protocol while still allowing acquisition of ECG-gated images (because of the use of technetium 99m).

  3. The sensitivity and specificity of this combination protocol (91% and 75%, respectively) have been shown to be comparable with that of conventional technetium 99m SPECT.

VII. Stress protocols

  A. Exercise stress testing. Standard exercise testing (see Chapter 40) is frequently complemented with nuclear imaging. The radioisotope is injected at peak exercise, and time is allowed for circulation of the agents (usually at least 1 minute before termination of exercise).

  B. For patients who are unable to exercise, **pharmacologic testing** is used in concert with nuclear imaging. Dipyridamole is an indirect vasodilator that is useful in noninvasive testing because of differences in coronary flow reserve. In the presence of marked coronary stenosis, the distal vessel is maximally dilated and therefore possesses little flow reserve. Dipyridamole substantially enhances coronary flow in normal beds (normal flow reserve) but much less so in distributions supplied by a stenotic artery. The resultant disproportionate flow is the basis for heterogenous radiotracer uptake.

1. **Administration.** Dipyridamole is infused over a 4-minute period (0.142 mg/kg per minute). Maximum vasodilatory effect is achieved 4 minutes after completion of the infusion, and the radiotracer is injected at this point. A slight increase in heart rate (10 beats/min) and decrease in blood pressure (10 mm Hg) frequently are observed.

2. **Side effects.** Headache, nausea, chest pain, hypotension, dizziness, and flushing have been reported. Severe side effects may necessitate reversal of the dipyridamole effect with aminophylline, given as a 50 to 100 mg intravenous bolus.

C. **Adenosine** is the vasoactive end product of dipyridamole infusion and thus acts similarly although with a substantially shorter half-life.

1. **Administration.** Adenosine is infused at 140 μg/kg per minute for 6 minutes. The radiotracer is injected after 3 minutes of infusion.

2. **Side effects** include chest pain, headache, nausea, flushing, dyspnea, and atrioventricular block.

D. **Dobutamine**

1. **Administration.** Infusion is begun at 5 μg/kg per minute and increased every 3 minutes to a maximum dose of 40 μg/kg per minute. The radiotracer is injected at maximum dose (or at 85% of age-predicted maximum heart rate), and the infusion is continued for 2 to 3 minutes.

2. **Side effects** associated with dobutamine include ectopy, headache, flushing, dyspnea, paresthesias, and hypotension.

VIII. **Image interpretation**

A. Standard view of normal anatomy. Uptake of radiotracer is homogeneous in persons with normal myocardial perfusion. The predominance of tracer is distributed to the left ventricle; the right ventricle usually appears as a faint, thin structure. Understanding and interpreting these images, however, requires an understanding of standard planar and SPECT views of left ventricular (LV) anatomic features.

1. **Planar images** are represented as LAO, anterior, and LLAT views.

2. Standard **SPECT views** include the short axis, vertical long axis, and horizontal long axis. The short-axis view is further divided into apical, midventricular, and basal views.

   a. As with planar views, SPECT images in various projections **correspond with specific myocardial segments** (Fig. 41-2).

   b. In addition to the standard SPECT sections, short-axis sections can be compiled into a so-called **bull's eye display** (also known as a **polar map**). This computer-generated bull's eye image arranges short-axis tomographic images such that the center portion represents apical slices and the periphery consists of the basal segments.

B. **Reviewing sequence.** Review of nuclear images follows an organized sequence, as follows:

1. **Examine unprocessed images** for artifact and evidence of increased lung uptake.

2. **Compare rest and stress images** for enlargement of the LV cavity.

3. **Examine rest images.** Document fixed defects and the number of segments involved.

4. **Examine stress images.** Document defects and segments.

5. **Evaluate the polar map** in comparison with pooled normal images (derived from a database of patients with low probability of having CAD).

6. **Incorporate the gated SPECT images** to establish overall ventricular function and evaluate wall function in areas of questionable artifact (segmental defects that demonstrate normal motion on gated SPECT images likely represent artifact).

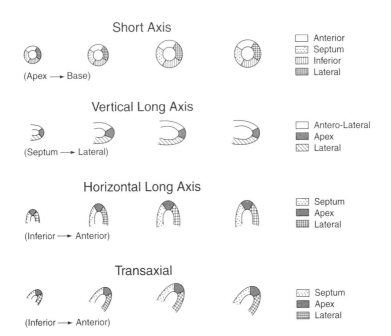

FIG. 42-2. Standard tomographic projections and myocardial segments.

C. **Characterization of defects.** Given that initial perfusion images represent regional myocardial blood flow, defects in these images represent an area of myocardium with relatively less uptake and thus diminished regional blood flow. Defects can be characterized as **fixed, reversible,** or **partially reversible** or as displaying **reverse redistribution.** (Note: The term *redistribution* is not appropriately used in context with technetium 99m imaging.)

1. **Fixed defects.** Nonreversible or fixed defects are areas of absent tracer uptake that appear unchanged on both rest and stress images. Fixed defects can **represent scar or viable myocardium.** With thallium 201 imaging, nonreversibility suggests similar rates of clearance from the two regions.

   a. **Differentiating scar from viable myocardium** in the setting of a nonreversible defect can be accomplished through the use of **metabolic radiopharmaceuticals and PET, delayed imaging, or rest reinjection** with thallium 201. The level of tracer activity reflects viability. Severe deficits (less than 50% normal counts) are less predictive of viability than are milder count deficits.

   b. Differentiating viable myocardium from scar is paramount because there is clinical and experimental evidence of improved LV function after revascularization of such hibernating regions. As methods of revascularizaton become increasingly applicable in an arena of increasingly complex patient problems, fully defining the so-called fixed defect through metabolic imaging assumes greater importance (see Chapter 43).

2. **Reversible defects** are present on initial stress images but resolve on rest or delayed images. This pattern is consistent with the presence of **ischemic myocardium** in the region of reversibility.

    a. In the setting of **thallium 201 imaging,** resolution of the defect is a function of variable tracer concentrations in ischemic and nonischemic segments, which approach one another as redistribution (and continuous exchange of myocyte and blood pool thallium 201) occurs.

    b. Technetium 99m imaging, which lacks redistribution, demonstrates reversibility on the basis of differential uptake during stress compared with rest.

    c. Fill-in of reversible defects on thallium 201 images can be enhanced by means of delayed imaging or rest reinjection.

  3. Partially reversible defects are present on stress images and partially resolve on rest images but do not fill in completely. This type of defect is thought to reflect a **mixture of scar and ischemic myocardium.** Nonetheless, reversibility may be incomplete even in the absence of nonviable tissue and represent purely ischemic myocardium.

  4. A pattern of **reverse redistribution** occurs when a defect appears larger on rest images, or is absent on stress images but present on rest images.

    a. Such a pattern is seen in the presence of **acute MI** when the infarct artery has been rendered patent through thrombolysis, primary angioplasty, autolysis, or another form of revascularization.

    b. The pattern is thought to reflect post-MI hyperemia with excess radiotracer uptake in a region of reperfused myocardium followed by accelerated myocardial washout of radiotracer in the defect region.

    c. The regions in question may demonstrate viability at PET imaging and are not indicative of ischemia.

  5. Artifacts. Apparent perfusion defects can be attributed to soft-tissue attenuation, a problem that occurs more often with thallium 201 imaging than when a higher-energy agent (technetium 99m) is used.

    a. Common causes of the presence of artifacts include **breast attenuation** (affecting the anterolateral, septal, anteroseptal, and posterolateral walls of the ventricle) and **diaphragmatic attenuation** (predominantly altering the inferior and posterior walls).

    b. Planar images with perfusion defects seen in only a single view are suspect, and the presence of artifact must be considered.

    c. SPECT artifacts may be more elusive because of processing and reconstruction of tomographic images; however, with good technique most are avoidable.

  6. High-risk perfusion scan. Specific patterns of perfusion imaging that suggest high-risk coronary anatomic features include **perfusion defects in more than one vascular distribution, increased lung thallium uptake,** and **transient LV dilatation.**

D. Quantitative analysis. The principles of image analysis rely on visual inspection, which is fraught with observer variability.

  1. Computer-aided analysis of planar data involves comparison of regional radionuclide activity on stress and rest images; count discordance coincides with reversibility. **SPECT** data are quantitatively analyzed by means of comparing count densities on short-axis images (displayed as a polar map) with normal count profiles. Although they improve sensitivity, these methods are **used in concert with visual analysis.**

  2. PET imaging, although evaluated in large part in a visual manner, also possesses great clinical utility with the application of **quantitative analysis** (similar in principle to that used with SPECT) **of coronary flow reserve.** On the basis of comparison of baseline blood flow and hyperemia induced by pharmacologic agents, this analysis may have great clinical utility in ascertaining whether a patient needs revascularization and in evaluating the success of revascularization. The administration of adenosine or dipyridamole has demonstrated at least a two- to threefold increase in coronary blood flow over baseline. Quantitative analysis of coronary flow reserve may prove useful in overcoming the Achilles heel of the angiographically present but clinically enigmatic coronary lesion.

IX. Clinical applications
A. Perfusion analysis
1. Detection of CAD
a. **Sensitivity and specificity.** Since the introduction of thallium 201 imaging in 1975, the utility of perfusion agents in the diagnosis of CAD has been well established. Quantitative planar imaging and SPECT demonstrate 90% or greater sensitivity.

(1) **Sensitivity** is affected by the number of vessels involved. Single-vessel disease is the most likely to produce a false-negative finding. Multivessel CAD rarely produces a normal perfusion scan result. The **specificity** of planar imaging has been reported to be 83% and that of SPECT 60% to 70%.

(2) In general radionuclide imaging is best used to evaluate a population at intermediate risk for CAD. The choice of radionuclide seemingly has little effect on the accuracy of these techniques.

(3) The introduction of **PET,** however, has brought with it **advanced diagnostic accuracy,** approximately 10% to 15% improvement over SPECT. The ability to detect CAD in a noninvasive manner offers numerous additional applications in risk stratification, prognosis, and imaging of acute infarction.

b. Causes of **false-positive** perfusion study results include attenuation defect, technical inadequacies, coronary vasospasm, anomalous coronary circulation, cardiomyopathy, conduction defects such as left bundle branch block, and recanalization of a thrombosed coronary artery.

c. Causes of **false-negative** perfusion study results include a submaximal exercise stress test, antiischemic medical therapy, presence of nonobstructive CAD, collateral or overlap circulation, inaccurate interpretation of perfusion images or angiograms, acquisition of suboptimal images, presence of balanced coronary stenoses, and delay in stress imaging.

2. Risk stratification.
In addition to indicators of higher risk taken from perfusion images, such as increased lung uptake, determinants in the assessment of risk are as follows:

a. **Presence of reversible as opposed to fixed defects** is associated with greater likelihood of cardiac events at follow-up evaluation. This relation has clinical utility in a number of settings, including risk stratification after MI or in the preoperative setting. In one study involving patients who had had MI without complications, patients with single, fixed defects on thallium 201 images had a 6% cardiac event rate compared with a rate of 51% among those with thallium 201 scans that indicated high risk.

b. Radionuclide **imaging abnormalities** have been identified as **independent predictors of subsequent infarction or death.** In general the number of abnormal segments identified on nuclear images can be seen as inversely proportional to survival rate. Normal findings on a nuclear perfusion study, however, suggest an excellent prognosis with a yearly mortality rate less than 1%. The application of such prognostic information to the care of patients preparing for noncardiac operations reflects significantly on the patient's surgical risk and has an established role in preoperative evaluation and clearance. For this population, evidence of ischemia on perfusion images portends higher risk for a perioperative cardiac event.

3. Myocardial perfusion imaging
may aid in diagnosis and risk stratification for patients with **acute coronary syndromes.**

a. Patients with **chest pain of ill-defined origin** can be given an injection at rest of thallium 201 or technetium 99m. In the presence of true ischemia (without infarction), **reversible defects** are documented, and insight into **regional distribution of ischemia** and extent of myocardium involved is gained. The **absence of any perfusion defect with ongoing chest pain makes a diagnosis of angina unlikely.**

b. Injection of thallium 201 or technetium 99m within 6 hours of the onset of **chest pain in acute infarction** allows imaging of both non-Q-wave and Q-wave events. As the time from onset of pain to injection increases, perfusion defects tend to normalize, probably as a result of autolysis or administration of thrombolytic therapy.

c. In the setting of **thrombolysis,** imaging with technetium 99m can provide important information about reperfusion or lack thereof. Injection of technetium 99m before initiation of thrombolysis captures a picture of hypoperfusion, which can, because of the extensive half-life, be imaged at a later time. Subsequent injections reveal the status of perfusion as the postthrombolysis period proceeds (a persistent, large defect that represents failed reperfusion). Such applications in the setting of thrombolysis and in acute coronary syndromes have limited clinical utility because of the logistics of staffing and availability of radiopharmaceuticals.

d. A further application that affects the arena of revascularization and management of ischemic syndromes involves **assessment of myocardial viability** (see Chapter 43).

B. **Assessment of ventricular function.** In addition to its use in perfusion analysis, radionuclide imaging can serve to establish cardiac performance. Radionuclide-based assessment of ventricular function includes first pass radionuclide angiocardiography and gated blood pool imaging.

1. **First-pass radionuclide angiocardiography** involves injection of a radionuclide and analysis as the agent passes through the central circulation.

   a. Technetium 99m–labeled agents typically are administered in bolus form, and scintigraphic data are recorded for 15 to 30 seconds after injection. Multicrystal cameras oriented in a straight anterior projection are used for detection of high count rates.

   b. This method of ventricular function analysis is more useful in evaluating **right ventricular function** than is gated blood imaging. In patients with **severe LV dysfunction,** the radiotracer may be dispersed, and proximal venous access and rapid administration may be necessary.

2. **Gated blood-pool imaging,** or MUGA (Multigated Acquisition), relies on ECG gating to correlate multiple individual images of the cardiac blood pool to specific phases of the cardiac cycle.

   a. The blood pool is labeled by means of removing a 2 to 3 mL sample of the patient's blood (after the intravenous administration of stannous pyrophosphate), which is labeled with technetium 99m.

   b. A single-crystal gamma camera is used in the LAO, anterior, LLAT, and left posterior oblique projections to obtain serial static images of the cardiac blood pool gated to the R-R interval.

   c. Because multiple cardiac cycles are averaged to obtain the final images, this technique is not optimal for evaluating regional wall motion.

3. **ECG-gated perfusion imaging.** Perfusion imaging with technetium 99m–labeled tracers produces sufficient count densities on individual images to allow ECG gating. The standard injection of 20 to 30 mCi of technetium 99m allows evaluation of **perfusion and function in a single study.** Comparison of this method with two-dimensional echocardiography in the evaluation of regional wall motion has shown

good correlation between the two. This correlation is not applicable to stress echocardiography, however, because of the time lag from the period of stress to the acquisition of nuclear images. The greatest utility of ECG-gated perfusion imaging may be in elucidating perceived artifacts on perfusion images.

X. PET in the evaluation of CAD allows blood flow imaging and evaluation of metabolic activity. Positron imaging agents can be considered blood flow tracers and metabolic radiopharmaceuticals.

 A. Blood flow tracers. A number of radiopharmaceuticals exist for the assessment of myocardial blood flow, both cyclotron produced and generator produced.

  1. **Rubidium 82,** the most readily used blood-flow tracer, can be generated on site without the use of a cyclotron. Much like thallium 201, rubidium 82 is a potassium analogue that is actively transported into myocytes through the the Na-K pump. **Uptake into myocardium** is proportionate to regional blood flow. Approximately 65% of the radiotracer is extracted at first pass. Because of a short half-life (76 seconds), rubidium 82–based imaging protocols can be used to assess myocardial blood flow rapidly (within 1 hour).

  2. **Copper 62 pyruvaldehyde *bis* (*N*-methylthiosemicarbazone) copper (II) ([^{62} Cu] PTSM)** is a blood-flow tracer produced by cyclotron. Image quality is comparable to that with rubidium 82, but gastrointestinal activity may interfere with evaluation of specific distributions (inferior wall in particular).

  3. Other cyclotron-produced perfusion agents include **nitrogen 13 ammonia** and **oxygen 15 water.** Image quality with **oxygen 15 water** is poor and requires extensive processing to subtract the blood pool. **Nitrogen 13 ammonia** image quality is excellent, although the impracticality of cyclotron production is a limiting factor for both agents.

 B. Metabolic radiopharmaceuticals. Metabolic imaging with PET depends on the use of radiolabeled substrates of cardiac metabolism, largely in the form of [^{18}F] fluoro-2-deoxyglucose (FDG), carbon-11 palmitate, and carbon-11 acetate.

  1. **FDG** is a glucose analogue used by ischemic myocardium because of a transition to alternative fuel sources in the hypoxic state. Ischemic myocardium diminishes the oxidation of long-chain fatty acids and incorporates glucose as a secondary fuel source. FDG is phosphorylated to FDG-6-phosphate after transport across the cell membrane. FDG imaging therefore reflects myocardial utilization of exogenous glucose, and FDG is a widely used metabolic radiopharmaceutical.

  2. [^{11}C] Palmitate is taken up by myocytes, converted to acyl-CoA, and either relegated to triglyceride stores or β-oxidized to produce [^{11}C] carbon dioxide. The release of this product of β-oxidation is reflective of long-chain fatty acid oxidation in myocardium.

  3. [^{11}C] Acetate is metabolized to [^{11}C] carbon dioxide after entering the tricarboxylic acid cycle. Measuring the production of [11C] carbon dioxide in this setting correlates with myocardial oxygen consumption.

 C. Metabolic imaging with SPECT. Metabolic imaging with SPECT cameras allows application of higher-energy photons even when PET is unavailable.

  1. FDG has been imaged with SPECT when outfitted with a high-energy collimator. Various fatty-acid radiopharmaceuticals now are available that are SPECT compatible.

  2. These techniques allow **perfusion, ischemia,** and **viability assessment** with standard SPECT equipment.

 D. Protocols. Image acquisition with PET is similar to that with SPECT in that tomographic images are obtained in short-axis, horizontal long-axis (sagittal), and vertical long-axis (coronal) views. A positron camera consists of an array of crystals arranged in a circle. Unlike in SPECT, the camera remains stationary in PET.

1. The heart is localized with the patient's arms extended above the head. An **attenuation scan** is performed that allows the density of the surrounding thorax to be subtracted to leave only cardiac count activity. This ability to make **allowance for noncardiac interference** adds a great deal to the accuracy of PET.
2. After the attenuation scan, the positron **radiopharmaceutical is injected,** and **images are obtained** 2 to 5 minutes later. As many as 21 tomographic images can be obtained concomitantly.
3. Metabolic imaging can be undertaken after flow imaging with the administration of 5 to 10 mCi of FDG. Tomographic images are typically obtained 30 to 50 minutes after FDG injection.

E. **Patterns of perfusion and metabolic imaging.** Specific patterns of perfusion and metabolic imaging are identifiable. For example, **normal flow–normal FDG (match)** indicates normal perfusion and normal metabolic activity. **Reduced flow–normal or increased FDG (mismatch)** demonstrates viability (hibernating myocardium). **Reduced flow–reduced FDG** identifies scar tissue.

F. **Clinical applications**
   1. **Diagnosis of CAD.** Flow imaging with PET is highly sensitive and highly specific for the detection of coronary stenosis, approaching 93% for both.
      a. Certain perfusion agents allow for quantitative analysis of coronary flow reserve (oxygen 15 water) and thus aid greatly in assessment of the functional significance of a stenotic lesion.
      b. Higher energy photons (511 keV), higher count densities, shorter half-life, and the ability to correct for attenuation place PET substantially ahead of SPECT in the accurate detection of CAD.
   2. **Assessment of myocardial viability.** The use of **PET with metabolic radiotracers is the standard for identifying viable myocardium.** The presence of a flow-metabolism mismatch, which indicates underperfusion in the presence of metabolically active myocytes, is reflective of hibernating myocardium. Revascularization of these zones as identified with PET has been shown to result in improvement in wall motion. This utility of nuclear imaging finds increasing application as the ever-growing population of patients with heart failure and increasingly complex CAD experience demands better methods of viability assessment.

SUGGESTED READINGS

Landmark Articles

Beller GA, Watson DD, Ackell P, Pohost GM. Time course of thallium-201 redistribution after transient myocardial ischemia. *Circulation* 1980;61:791–797.

Marshall RC, Tillisch JH, Phelps ME, et al. Identification and differentiation of resting myocardial blood flow in man with positron emission tomography, 18F-labeled fluorodeoxyglucose and N-13 ammonia. *Circulation* 1983;67:766–778.

Strauss HW, Harrison K, Langan JK, Lebowitz E, Pitt B. Thallium-201 for myocardial imaging: relation of thallium-201 to regional myocardial perfusion. *Circulation* 1975;51:641.

Wackers FJ, Berman DS, Maddahi J, et al. Technetium-99m hexakis 2-methoxyisobutyl isonitrile: human biodistribution, dosimetry, safety, and preliminary comparison to thallium-201 for myocardial perfusion imaging. *J Nucl Med* 1989:30:301–311.

Key Reviews

Alexander C, Oberhausen E. Myocardial scintigraphy. *Semin Nucl Med* 1995;25: 195–201.

Beller GA. Current status of nuclear cardiology techniques. *Curr Probl Cardiol* 1991; 16:451–535.

Berman D, Hachamovitch R, Lewin H, et al. Risk stratification in coronary artery disease: implications for stabilization and prevention. *Am J Cardiol* 1997;79:10–16.

Cerqueira MD, Harp GD, Ritchie JL. Evaluation of myocardial perfusion and function by single photon emission computed tomography. *Semin Nucl Med* 1987;17: 200–213.

Gould KL. Positron emission tomography perfusion imaging and nuclear cardiology. *J Nucl Med* 1991;32:579–606.

Hor G. What is the current status of quantification and nuclear medicine in cardiology? *Eur J Nucl Med* 1996;23:815–851.

Iskandrian AS, Heo J, Askenase A, et al. Thallium imaging with single photon emission computed tomography. *Am Heart J* 1987;114:852–865.

Maddahi J, Rodriquez E, Berman DS, et al. State of the art myocardial perfusion imaging. *Cardiol Clin* 1994;12:199–222.

Saha GB, Go RT, MacIntyre WJ. Radiopharmaceuticals for cardiovascular imaging. *Nucl Med Biol* 1992;19:1–20.

Schelbert HR, Buxton D. Insight into coronary artery disease gained from metabolic imaging. *Circulation* 1988;78:496–505.

Schwaiger M, Hutchins GD. Evaluation of coronary artery disease with positron emission tomography. *Semin Nucl Med* 1992;22:210–223.

Zaret BL, Wackers FJ. Nuclear cardiology. *N Engl J Med* 1993;329:775–783.

Wackers FJ. Radionuclide evaluation of coronary artery disease in the 1990s: choosing the best stress, best tracer, best technique. *Cardiol Clin* 1994;12:385–389.

Relevant Book Chapters

Iskandrian AE, Verani MS. Nuclear imaging techniques. In: Topol EJ, ed. *Textbook of cardiovascular medicine.* Philadelphia: Lippincott–Raven, 1998:1367–1393.

Johnson LL, Pohost GM. *Nuclear Cardiology.* In: Schlant RC, Alexander RW, eds. *Hurst's the heart,* 8th ed. New York: McGraw-Hill, 1994:2281–2323.

Schelbert HR. Positron emission tomography. In: Schlant RC, Alexander RW, eds. *Hurst's the heart,* 8th ed. New York: McGraw-Hill, 1994:2281–2323.

Wackers FJ, Soufer R, Zaret BL. Nuclear cardiology. In: Braunwald E, ed. *Heart disease: a textbook of cardiovascular medicine,* 5th ed. Philadelphia: WB Saunders, 1997:273–316.

42. STRESS ECHOCARDIOGRAPHY

Matthew Deedy

I. **Introduction.** Echocardiography combined with exercise stress, pacing, or pharmacologic stress is an effective method of **screening for the presence of coronary artery disease** (CAD) and for the **localization of coronary artery lesions.**

II. **Technology.** Advances in computer software and ultrasound technology have made it possible to acquire good-quality stress echocardiographic images. Echocardiographic images are digitally acquired. This allows cine loop recording and side-by-side comparison of rest and stress images (Fig. 42-1). **A single cardiac cycle in each view** is all that is necessary for digital acquisition. Therefore, peak- and post-exercise imaging is completed rapidly, and this improves sensitivity.

  A. **Imaging modalities**

   1. **Two-dimensional echocardiography.** Stress echocardiographic data can be obtained with transthoracic or transesophageal imaging. Harmonic imaging and myocardial contrast agents improve endocardial border definition, particularly among patients who are difficult to image. This may result in improved sensitivity and specificity in these patients.

   2. **Doppler echocardiography.** In certain circumstances, Doppler data obtained during stress provide additional useful information. Doppler assessment of a left ventricular (LV) outflow tract gradient at rest and with stress is important in the care of patients with **suspected hypertrophic cardiomyopathy** or patients with **systolic anterior motion of the mitral valve leaflet with stress.** Doppler echocardiography also is useful in the care of patients with **aortic stenosis** to establish pressure gradients across the aortic valve and aortic valve area at rest and with stress.

   3. **Doppler tissue imaging** is being studied as a method to provide **objective support to the more subjective visual assessment of myocardial response** to exercise. Tissue imaging by means of pulsed wave Doppler and color Doppler ultrasound is undergoing evaluation.

  B. **Image processing and presentation.** Rest, submaximal, peak, and post-peak stress images are digitized on line and recorded on videotape. Once all the digitized images are obtained, they are displayed for review in a continuous-loop at the same speed as one another.

   1. For **exercise echocardiography,** the images usually are arranged in a side by side manner with a rest image on the left and a stress image on the right. The low-level exercise images are helpful in determining the time of onset of wall motion abnormalities (WMA), which can be helpful in establishing the severity of disease.

   2. For **nonexercise stress echocardiography,** the images are routinely displayed in a four-screen format with the rest images top left, low-dose images top right, submaximal images bottom left, and peak images bottom right. Each view is displayed on a separate screen.

III. **Physiology**

  A. **Exercise stress.** Stress echocardiography is based on ability to detect a new or worsening WMA with stress.

   1. **Response to stress**

    a. A **normal** heart responds to exercise with a global increase in contractility, development of hyperdynamic wall motion, and a gradual rise in heart rate. These changes produce an increase in LV ejection fraction (LVEF) and a decrease in the LV end-systolic volume.

    b. An **abnormal** response to exercise may be detected as a **decrease or lack of increase in LVEF or deterioration or lack of improvement in segmental myocardial function.** Numerous conditions

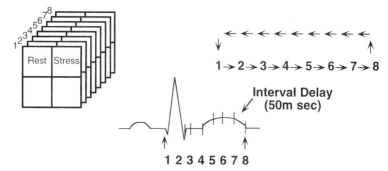

FIG. 42-1. Schematic representation of digital cine loop recording and presentation in stress echocardiography. Eight equally spaced echocradiographic images are captured and digitized. Capture of the first image is triggered by the R wave and each subsequent image is captured at a preset interval (50 msec in this example). Rest and stress images are displayed side by side on the screeen in a continuous loop format.

attenuate the normal hyperdynamic response, including but not limited to use of medications (β-blockers), poor exercise capacity, cardiomyopathy, valvular heart disease, and ischemia.

2. Supine v. upright exercise
   a. During **supine exercise, end-diastolic volume is near maximal at rest.** Therefore, the change in cardiac output with exercise is predominantly mediated by an increase in heart rate.
   b. With **upright exercise, end-diastolic volume is lower at rest** than it is in the supine position. End-diastolic volume increases more significantly with upright stress, resulting in a more dramatic increase in LVEF.

3. The sequence of events that result in the echocardiographic determination of ischemia is termed the **ischemic cascade.** Myocardial ischemia causes regional diastolic and systolic dysfunction, ST-segment depression on an electrocardiogram (ECG), and ultimately with anginal symptoms. **Regional myocardial dysfunction,** manifested by decreases in endocardial excursion and wall thickening, is **specific for myocardial ischemia.**

B. Three basic categories of nonexercise stress are cardiac pacing, vasodilator stress, and use of positive inotropic medications or exercise-simulating agents.
   1. **Exercise-simulating agents.** The greatest experience in the United States is with dobutamine and its isomer arbutamine. These agents produce stress through an **increase in myocardial oxygen demand.**
      a. Low-dose **dobutamine** has positive inotropic effects mediated through cardiac α_1 and β_1 receptors. At higher doses, dobutamine has positive chronotropic effects mediated through β_2 receptors. The plasma half-life is 2 to 3 minutes. The normal response to dobutamine involves an increase in heart rate and hyperdynamic wall motion with only minimal effect on end-diastolic LV volume.
         (1) The most common **side effect** is arrhythmia, followed by hypotension and, rarely, nausea.
         (2) When **combined with atropine** as needed for the patient to reach 85% of age-predicted maximum heart rate (APMHR), **dobutamine echocardiography** is a good alternative to exercise echocardiography for **patients who are unable to exercise adequately.**
      b. **Arbutamine** is approved for use in the United States to detect CAD when combined with ECG, echocardiography, or scintigraphy.

Arbutamine has inotropic and chronotropic effects similar to those of dobutamine; however, it has less α_1 activity and a slightly longer half-life (7 to 12 minutes). The inotropic effect is slightly less than that of dobutamine.

2. A **vasodilator stress** test is performed with either **dipyridamole** or **adenosine** infusion. These agents cause perfusion abnormalities when blood is preferentially shunted away from myocardial segments supplied by stenotic coronary arteries. Because both of these agents are potent vasodilators, the most common **side effects** include hypotension, flushing, headache, and nausea. Adenosine may produce atrioventricular (AV) block. Adenosine has fewer side effects because it has a shorter half-life; however, because of the shorter duration of action, the **echocardiographic findings tend to be less pronounced and of shorter duration, resulting in a lower sensitivity** than that of dipyridamole testing.

3. **Atrial pacing** with either a transvenous or transesophageal approach has been used to achieve stress. Transesophageal atrial pacing combined with transesophageal echocardiography and transthoracic echocardiography often is limited by patient discomfort, inability to consistently capture the atria, and by AV block at high heart rates. AV block may be avoided with the use of atropine. There is little change in blood pressure; therefore the peak rate pressure product achieved often is less than that achieved by means of exercise stress or inotropic stress. **This method is the most invasive and is not used unless necessary.**

IV. **Indications and contraindications.**

A. The **indications and contraindications** for echocardiographic stress testing are the same as for ECG stress testing (see Chapter 40). In certain circumstances, it is helpful to combine ECG stress testing with an imaging modality. Patients who would benefit include those who have an abnormal resting ECG that precludes interpretation with stress and patients who are more likely to have a nondiagnostic stress ECG, such as women. It may be preferable to perform stress echocardiography rather than nuclear stress testing in situations in which resting echocardiography may provide helpful information that a nuclear study cannot, as when a patient has valvular heart disease and symptoms that suggest angina.

B. **Exercise stress is preferred** over nonexercise stress because it more closely reproduces daily activity, and is more sensitive if the patient is able to achieve an adequate level of stress. No single exercise modality has been shown to have superior sensitivity. Therefore patient factors such as preference, stability in walking, and the presence of comorbid conditions are considered when deciding on which exercise modality to use.

C. If exercise is not an option, then **nonexercise techniques** are available. Inotropic agent produce ischemia by increasing myocardial oxygen demand. This mimics exercise more closely than does use of vasodilators. For this reason, inotropic agents are more commonly used in echocardiography than are vasodilators. A few studies have shown better sensitivity with dobutamine than vasodilator echocardiography.

1. As many as up to 30% of patients referred for exercise echocardiography may **not be able to achieve an adequate level of exercise stress** because of peripheral vascular disease, chronic obstructive pulmonary disease, or musculoskeletal problems. **Nonexercise echocardiography is indicated** for these patients.

2. Patients with **LV dysfunction and severe aortic stenosis** may be evaluated with dobutamine echocardiography to determine whether the measured aortic valve area represents true aortic stenosis or pseudostenosis. Aortic valve area is calculated at rest and stress. Patients with pseudostenosis, or a small calculated aortic valve area caused by low cardiac output, have an increase in aortic valve area at a higher cardiac output. Patients with true aortic stenosis generally do not have an increase in aortic valve area with stress (see Chapter 14).

V. Technique
 A. Patient preparation
  1. Patients fast 4 hours before the test.
  2. The primary physician instructs the patient about **medications to take or discontinue before the study.** Consideration is given to the importance of attaining at least 85% of APMHR in an effort to maximize the sensitivity of the test. Extreme hypertensive responses to stress also may lower the specificity of the study.
  3. The **standard connections for a 12-lead ECG** may be used with minor modifications to allow imaging in the parasternal and apical windows without affecting the accuracy of the exercise ECG results.
  4. Patients undergoing **nonexercise stress echocardiography** need an **intravenous (IV) line** for administration of medication.
 B. Equipment needed. All stress echocardiographic studies are conducted with **exercise ECG and standard hemodynamic monitoring equipment.** Most **cardiac ultrasound machines** can be linked with a digital processor to allow on-line digitization of echocardiographic images.
 C. Performing the test
  1. Exercise echocardiography. Regardless of the exercise modality, a quick, complete **baseline** echocardiographic scan is obtained for all patients. Rest images are digitized on line in the parasternal long- and short-axis and apical two- and four-chamber views.
   a. Treadmill exercise is performed with standard protocols according to the functional status of the patient. Exercise is **continued until a predetermined end point** is reached, usually perceived maximal exertion (see Chapter 40). **Postpeak, or stress, images** are obtained in the left lateral decubitus position after the patient transfers from the treadmill to the imaging table at the end of exercise. Stress images in the same views as the baseline study are digitized on line and recorded on videotape. All postpeak images are **obtained within 90 seconds of completing exercise** to maximize sensitivity.
   b. During **upright bicycle echocardiography, baseline images** are obtained in the standard left lateral position and are repeated with the patient in the upright position on the cycle ergometer. Adequate parasternal images may be recorded by having the patient lean forward on the cycle ergometer. These images are recorded and digitized to allow comparable windows for the rest and peak-stress images. Cycle ergometry is started at a workload of 25 W and increased by 25 to 50 W every 2 to 3 minutes until the patient reaches perceived maximal effort. During upright bicycle echocardiography, **images are obtained and digitized at rest, prepeak, peak, and postexercise. After-stress images** are obtained in the standard left lateral decubitus position.
   c. With **supine bicycle exercise,** the entire study is performed in the left lateral decubitus position and images are obtained and digitized at **rest, prepeak, peak, and postexercise.**
  2. Pharmacologic stress echocardiography
   a. Dobutamine
    (1) Dobutamine **infusion** is started at 5 µg/kg per minute and increased every 3 minutes to 10, 20, 30 and 40 µg/kg per minute. If the patient has not reached 85% of APMHR by the end of the 40 µg/kg per minute dose, a 3-minute dosage of 50 µg/kg per minute may be used. Images are digitized at rest, low-dose (5 to 10 µg/kg per minute), prepeak (30 µg/kg per minute), and peak doses.
    (2) Atropine is used as needed to reach 85% of APMHR if dobutamine alone is not effective. Atropine is given 0.25 to 0.5 mg IV every minute starting at the 40 µg/kg per minute dosage until an end point is reached or a total dose of 1.0 mg is given.

    (3) End points include 85% APMHR, angina, substantial ST-segment changes, hypertension, hypotension, marked arrhythmia, or development of a large WMA. **If angina develops,** the effects of dobutamine may be reversed more rapidly with IV β-blockade. This can be done with 0.5 mg/kg IV esmolol given over 1 minute, or 0.5 to 1.0 mg IV propranolol. Like dobutamine, esmolol has a very short half-life and therefore may be preferable.

b. Arbutamine is delivered with a computerized closed-loop delivery system. The system follows the patient's heart rate response and adjusts the dose delivered to maintain a steady preset rate of increase in heart rate, usually 8 beats/min.

    (1) The **imaging setup** is the same as for dobutamine echocardiography.

    (2) End points include 85% APMHR, a maximal infusion rate of 0.8 µg/kg per minute, a maximal dose of 10 µg/kg, heart rate plateau, ischemia, substantial ST-segment changes, hypertension, hypotension, marked arrhythmia, and development of a large WMA. **Angina** is managed the same way as during dobutamine echocardiography.

    (3) Atropine is not used during arbutamine testing.

c. Dipyridamole echocardiography

    (1) If the purpose of the study is to **rule out CAD, antianginal medication is stopped** before the test.

    (2) Patients with hypotension, substantial AV block, or a history of severe bronchospasm **should not undergo** testing with this method.

    (3) Different **protocols** of dipyridamole infusion have been studied. **A high-dose** regimen of 0.84 mg/kg given over 10 minutes has been developed to improve the sensitivity of the test in comparison with low-dose protocols. Several approaches have been tried in combination with the high-dose protocol to improve sensitivity, but they have not been standardized. These approaches include isometric handgrip, atropine infusion, and dobutamine infusion. If a high-dose dipyridamole test result is negative, either atropine or dobutamine can be given.

    (4) End points include substantial ST-segment depression, third-degree AV block, severe hypotension, and intolerable side effects. In the event of an ischemic end point or severe hypotension, aminophylline may be given to counteract the effects of dipyridamole. Aminophylline is given 25 to 50 mg IV over 1 to 2 minutes. Symptoms should begin to resolve within 60 seconds.

d. Adenosine echocardiography

    (1) If the purpose of the study is to **rule out CAD, then antianginal medications are stopped** before the test.

    (2) Patients with a history of bronchospasm, second- or third-degree heart block, hypotension, or severe heart failure **should not undergo** testing with this method.

    (3) Adenosine is given as a **continuous infusion** because of its very short half-life. A typical protocol starts at low dosage of 80 µg/kg per minute and is increased every 3 minutes by 30 µg/kg per minute to a peak dose of 170 to 200 µg/kg per minute. Isometric handgrip may be performed at the peak infusion rate to improve the sensitivity of the test.

    (4) Imaging is performed throughout the infusion. Peak images are digitized for review in a four-screen format.

    (5) Any **symptoms resolve promptly** because of the very short half-life of adenosine.

(6) **End points** include substantial ST-segment depression, third-degree AV block, hypotension unresponsive to a decrease in the rate of infusion, and intolerable side effects.

3. **Atrial pacing** may be combined with either transthoracic or transesophageal imaging.

a. Although this technique is feasible and has been shown to have reasonable diagnostic accuracy, it is **poorly tolerated** by nonsedated patients. Induction of atrial fibrillation also is possible.

b. **Images are obtained** at rest and at incrementally higher pacing rates until peak heart rate is achieved or intolerable side effects occur.

c. Atropine 0.2 to 0.5 mg IV may be used **if AV block** occurs. The most common AV block is Mobitz type 1.

VI. Interpretation

A. **Interpretation of stress echocardiographic findings is subjective** compared with that of nuclear testing. The person who interprets the images must be well trained to maintain an acceptable level of accuracy. Experienced readers have better interpretive accuracy than those without experience. However, after instruction and 100 studies of experience, the difference in accuracy between experts and less experienced readers is not significant (1). There has been concern regarding the reproducibility of stress echocardiographic interpretation between readers and between centers. Concordance within centers generally is good; however, concordance between different centers may be less than 80%, particularly with technically difficult studies and studies of patients with mild CAD (2).

B. **Prognostic value.** Stress echocardiography is emerging as a valuable tool for assessing future risk for cardiac events for a patient and for predicting recovery in myocardial function after myocardial infarction (MI). Most of the prognostic information is based on the test result, that is, the amount of ischemia and LVEF, and on the pretest probability of the existence of CAD, which is determined on the basis of patient demographic factors, comorbidity, and the presence of symptoms. For example, normal treadmill echocardiographic findings for a young, female patient with atypical chest pain and mitral valve prolapse is more predictive of a good prognosis than are normal treadmill echocardiographic findings for a patient with a history of percutaneous transluminal coronary angioplasty (PTCA) and recurrent chest pain.

1. In general patients with **normal stress echocardiographic findings** are at low risk for future cardiac events. In patients at medium risk for CAD with normal stress echocardiographic findings, the 1-year cardiac event rate (MI, PTCA, coronary artery bypass grafting, or death) has been reported to be from 5% to 10% (3–5). Patients at medium risk for CAD, normal exercise echocardiographic findings, and good functional capacity (more than 6-minute Bruce protocol; see Chapter 40), have very low event rates of less than 5% per year (6, 7).

2. **Ischemia.** Regardless of symptomatic status, abnormal findings at stress echocardiography indicate high risk for future cardiac events. Patients at medium risk for CAD who have abnormal stress echocardiographic findings have been reported to have a 1-year cardiac event rate (MI, PTCA, coronary artery bypass grafting, or death) of 26% to 50%.

3. **Viability.** In general the mass of viable myocardium correlates with the degree of improvement in LVEF after revascularization. Patients with evidence of large areas of viability at dobutamine echocardiography are likely to show improvement in LV function after revascularization. Patients with large areas of viability who do not undergo revascularization are at high risk for future events. Dobutamine and dipyridamole echocardiography has been used with about 80% accuracy to predict recovery of function among patients who have had MI.

4. **Scar.** Patients with scar only at dobutamine echocardiography are unlikely to have improved ventricular function after revascularization. Compared with patients with the same pretest probability of disease,

these patients have higher rates of cardiac events than patients with normal stress echocardiographic findings but fewer events than patients with evidence of ischemia at stress echocardiography. Heart failure is a more common end point among these patients.

C. Exercise echocardiography

1. A **normal response** to exercise stress involves a global increase in contractility, development of hyperdynamic wall motion, and a gradual rise in heart rate. This is manifested by increased wall thickness and increased endocardial excursion with stress. Although both measurements are analyzed, reduced wall thickening is a more specific marker of ischemia than of wall motion.

2. Regional wall motion is assessed with the 16-segment model outlined by the American Society of Echocardiography; the model is shown in Fig. 42-2. Results are generally reported as outlined in Fig. 42-3. In general, **the number of coronary arteries with marked stenosis is directly related to the number of myocardial segments found to be ischemic.** Wall motion is subjectively graded as normal, mildly hypokinetic, severely hypokinetic, akinetic, or dyskinetic. Each myocardial segment in the rest and stress images is graded in this manner. Possible myocardial responses to stress and their interpretations are outlined in Table 42-1.

D. Nonexercise echocardiography. With only a few exceptions, the principles of interpretation of dobutamine and arbutamine echocardiographic findings are the same as those for exercise echocardiography.

1. The **typical ischemic response** is characterized by normal resting wall motion and an initial hyperdynamic response with low-dose dobutamine followed by a decline in function at higher doses. Ischemia also may be identified on the basis of deterioration of normal wall motion without any transient hyperdynamic response.

2. A useful feature of dobutamine echocardiography is its ability **to depict viable myocardium,** either stunned or hibernating.

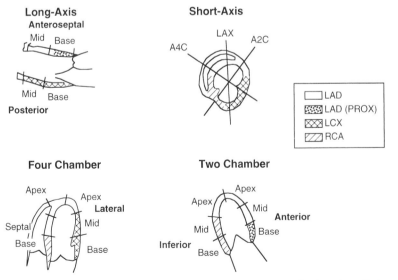

FIG. 42-2. The relation between the 16 myocardial segments in the American Society of Echocardiography ASE classification system and their coronary artery supply. The four standard views are used to delineate the relation between coronary artery distribution and the segments.

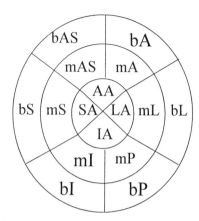

FIG. 42-3. Typical bull's-eye representation used for reporting the 16 myocardial segments model. *b*, Basal; *m*, mid; *A*, anterior; *L*, lateral; *P*, posterior; *I*, inferior; *S*, septal; *AS*, anteroseptum; *AA*, anteroapex; *LA*, lateral apex; *IA*, inferoapex; *SA*, septal apex.

a. Myocardial stunning after MI is common. **Improvement of a resting WMA** with low-dose dobutamine is predictive of **improvement in function** in this setting.

b. Patients with **chronic ischemia** may experience **myocardial hibernation.** This may be identified with a biphasic response to dobutamine in which there is improvement of a resting all motion abnormality with a low dosage of dobutamine (5 to 10 µg/kg per minute) with subsequent deterioration in function at high doses because of the development of ischemia.

Table 42-1. Interpretation of wall motion responses during exercise and pharmacologic stress echocardiography

Interpretation	Baseline	Low-dose	Peak and poststress function
Normal	Normal	Normal or hyperdynamic response	Hyperdynamic response
Ischemia	Normal	Normal or deteriorates if severe CAD	Deterioration
? Ischemia versus normal	Normal	No change	No change
Viable, nonischemic	Rest WMA	Improvement	Sustained improvement
Viable, ischemic	Rest WMA	Improvement	Deterioration
Scar	Rest WMA	No change	No change

CAD, Coronary artery disease; *WMA,* wall motion abnormalities (severe hypokinesis, akinesis, or dyskinesis).
From Topol EJ, ed. *Comprehensive Cardiovascular Medicine.* Lippincott-Raven Publishers, 1998, with permission

    c. Interpretation of results obtained with vasodilators requires detection of a new or worsening regional wall WMA during the infusion. There is only a mild increase in cardiac contractility during vasodilator stress.

E. Causes of false-negative results

1. **Single-vessel CAD.** Stress echocardiography is less sensitive for the detection of single-vessel CAD than for multivessel CAD, probably because of the presence of rapidly resolving or subtle WMA with single-vessel or well-collateralized CAD. Image acquisition must be completed within 60 to 90 seconds in stress protocols that include poststress imaging. Protocols that allow imaging while the patient continues to exercise at a peak level are more sensitive than postexercise imaging protocols.

2. **Mild CAD.** Moderate coronary stenosis, less than 60% luminal narrowing, may not be severe enough to cause a WMA or anginal symptoms. However, if CAD is defined as more than 50% luminal narrowing, the test is interpreted as a false-negative result for research purposes even if the patient has no symptoms.

3. **Inadequate level of stress.** An inadequate level of stress, less than 85% APMHR, may result in the termination of exercise before the development of a WMA. Likewise, mild ischemia with a rapidly resolving WMA may be missed if stress imaging is performed after the peak. Patients who continue antianginal therapy through the stress test may not attain an adequate level of stress to produce ischemia.

4. **LV cavity obliteration.** High-dose dobutamine, or peak exercise may result in a significant reduction in LV volume, with cavity obliteration making segmental wall motion analysis difficult.

5. **Image quality.** Poor image quality may cause incorrect interpretation. Technical advances may make this less of a concern in the future.

F. Causes of false-positive results

1. **Abnormal septal motion.** Patients with abnormal septal motion caused by left bundle branch block or postoperative status may have difficult-to-interpret studies. In this situation, particular emphasis is placed on **septal thickening rather than septal motion;** however, with vasodilators, the amount of myocardial thickening may be small. Patients who have recently undergone an operation may have substantial translational motion of the heart during systole. Particular emphasis again is placed on wall thickening rather than motion. Computer programs are available that allow correction of translational motion.

2. **Nonischemic cardiomyopathy.** Patients with nonischemic cardiomyopathy may develop WMA with stress that are not caused by coronary stenosis. Several theories exist as to why this may occur, including regional differences in myocardial fibrosis; the exact mechanism is not clear.

3. **Hypertensive response to exercise.** Patients who have a hypertensive response to exercise, systolic blood pressure greater than 230 mm Hg or diastolic blood pressure greater than 120 mm Hg, may have WMA with stress because of excessive afterload. Careful attention is paid to hemodynamic measurements with exercise before making a final interpretation.

4. **Image quality.** Poor image quality may result in incorrect interpretation of a study.

5. **Overinterpretation.** Interpreter bias may result in a lower threshold for calling a study result positive. It is **helpful for interpreters to be blinded about the patient's history** during interpretation of a study to minimize bias.

G. Controversies

1. Controversy exists about **interpretation of normal wall motion at rest that fails to augment with exercise.** This may be evidence of ischemia. In this situation, special attention is paid to the exercise measurements, hemodynamic and ECG responses to exercise, and

the timing of the stress images to help determine the most appropriate interpretation.

2. A myocardial segment may thicken and contract normally but later than other segments, a condition called **tardokinesis.** This may be normal or may represent mild ischemia.

3. Some controversy exists over the utility of stress echocardiography as a tool to determine cardiac reserve among patients with **valvular heart disease,** including mitral regurgitation, aortic regurgitation, and aortic stenosis. Some studies suggest that a decline in LVEF with exercise among patients with valvular heart disease represents occult myocardial dysfunction and indicates that the patient may benefit from surgical intervention (see Chapters 14 and 15).

4. **Treadmill versus bicycle exercise echocardiography.** It is believed that the higher level of stress with treadmill exercise offsets its drop in sensitivity with postpeak imaging, making treadmill and bicycle exercise comparable. Only a few small studies have been done comparing treadmill echocardiography with bicycle echocardiography, and these showed **no significant difference between the modalities.**

   a. **Treadmill** exercise is the most commonly used method and is the most widely accepted means of achieving a maximal level of stress. Imaging, however, must be performed after the peak, which may result in more false-negative results.

   b. **Bicycle** exercise in both the upright and supine positions allows imaging to be performed while the patient continues to exercise at a peak level, which potentially improves sensitivity. However, it is more difficult to reach maximal levels of stress during bicycle exercise, possibly due to early leg fatigue and the smaller muscle mass utilized during bicycle exercise when compared to treadmill exercise. An issue unique to stress echocardiography is **body position during exercise.** Although exercise echocardiography in upright and supine positions on a bicycle has been validated individually, the results of testing when the same patient uses the two positions have not been compared.

H. **Key suggestions**

1. Any WMA is **confirmed in a second view.** If digitized images are not adequate for confirmation, the videotape is used.

2. Care is taken to **avoid overestimating the presence of abnormalities at the cardiac base,** particularly in the inferior wall, where there may be less vigorous contractility among healthy persons, and in the posterior wall, where there may be dropout caused by the presence of the posterolateral papillary muscle.

3. **Endocardial border definition may be poor** in the lateral wall because of lateral endocardial dropout. In this situation, the **parasternal short-axis view and the videotape are used** to confirm suspected WMA. Myocardial contrast agents may prove to be most helpful in this setting.

4. In the four-screen display, the **rest and stress images are compared** to ensure that alignment is the same. If one of the images in a particular view is foreshortened, that view is not to be used alone to call an abnormal study.

5. The **timing of images is checked** to ensure that they represent systole. Image acquisition is triggered to start with the R wave so that the mitral valve is closed during most of the frames.

6. **Wall motion** of individual segments is **compared from rest to stress** in the four-screen display to define ischemia and infarction.

7. **Myocardial segments** are compared in the **stress images.** Differences in contraction and the development of "hinge points" are helpful for defining an abnormal segment.

8. Both the **digital and videotape images are reviewed** before a final decision on a study is made.

VII. Comparison of stress echocardiography with other modalities
  A. Exercise echocardiography
    1. **Cardiac catheterization.** Exercise echocardiography compared with cardiac catheterization as the standard has had a sensitivity of 80% to 85% and a specificity of 85% to 90%; however, all calculations of sensitivity and specificity depend on the definition of CAD.
    2. **Nuclear stress testing.** Studies comparing stress echocardiography with perfusion imaging have generally shown comparable sensitivities and slightly superior specificity for stress echocardiography.
      a. Compared with stress nuclear perfusion testing, **stress echocardiography** provides **more information on cardiac structure and function** and is **more convenient.** The test is performed within 30 to 45 minutes, and the results can be interpreted immediately with rapid feedback to the patient and referring physician. Stress echocardiography also **avoids exposure to radioactive tracers** and is substantially **less expensive.** Despite its lower sensitivity compared with perfusion scintigraphy, echocardiography provides useful information about ventricular size and function, valvular function, and the presence of LV hypertrophy.
      b. **Nuclear stress testing allows more objective interpretation** with quantitation of perfusion abnormalities. There is more support in the literature for the prognostic value of nuclear stress testing because this modality has been established for many years. Perfusion scintigraphy depicts differential flow in the myocardium, whereas stress echocardiography depicts WMA. Because WMA is farther down the ischemic cascade, and not all perfusion defects result in WMA, **perfusion scintigraphy is more sensitive than vasodilator echocardiography.** Perfusion scintigraphy theoretically offers an advantage over stress echocardiography with regard to sensitivity, albeit at the price of decreased specificity.
      c. Comparison of **exercise thallium scintigraphy** with exercise stress echocardiography has shown the two techniques to have comparable sensitivity. Exercise echocardiography has slightly higher specificity.
      d. Comparison of **radionuclide angiography** with exercise stress echocardiography has shown superior sensitivity and specificity with exercise echocardiography because of better resolution of regional wall motion with echocardiography.
    2. Exercise echocardiography has been shown to be more sensitive and specific than **exercise ECG.** This is most apparent in situations in which exercise ECG is nondiagnostic or has a high false-positive rate. This occurs most often among patients with left bundle branch block, digitalis effect, or LV hypertrophy and among female patients.
  B. Nonexercise echocardiography
    1. **Cardiac catheterization**
      a. Dobutamine echocardiography has been found to have a sensitivity ranging from 68% to 96% and a specificity of 80% to 85%. Arbutamine echocardiography has been reported to have a similar sensitivity range.
      b. **Adenosine echocardiography** has a sensitivity ranging from 40% to 91% and a specificity ranging from 87% to 100%.
      c. **Dipyridamole echocardiography** has been found to have a sensitivity ranging from 52% to 92% and a specificity of 80% to 100%. In general, the specificity of vasodilator stress echocardiography is superior to that of other echocardiographic stress techniques.
    2. **Perfusion scintigraphy.** Compared with dipyridamole thallium scintigraphy, dipyridamole echocardiography is believed to be less sensitive but more specific; however, there are few data comparing the two tests in the same patients. **Conclusive comparative data** from com-

parisons between adenosine echocardiography and adenosine scintigraphy are **not available.**

SUGGESTED READINGS

References

1. Picano E, Lattanzi F, Orlandini A, et al. Stress echocardiography and the human factor: the importance of being expert. *J Am Coll Cardiol* 1991;17:666–669.
2. Hoffman R, Lethen H, Marwick T, et al. Analysis of interinstitutional agreement in interpretation of dobutamine stress echocardiography. *J Am Coll Cardiol* 1996;27:330–336.
3. Krivokapich J, Child JS, Gerber RS, et al. Prognostic usefulness of positive or negative exercise stress echocardiography for predicting coronary events in ensuing twelve months. *Am J Cardiol* 1993;71:646–651.
4. Afridi I, Quinones Ma, Zoghbi WA, et al. Dobutamine stress echocardiography: sensitivity, specificity, and predictive value for future cardiac events. *Am Heart J* 1994; 127:1510–1515.
5. Poldermans D, Fioretti PM, Boersma E, et al. Dobutamine-atropine stress echocardiography and clinical data for predicting late cardiac events in patients with suspected coronary artery disease. *Am J Med* 1994;97:119–125.
6. Krivokapich J, Child JS, Gerber RS, et al. Prognostic usefulness of positive or negative exercise stress echocardiography for predicting coronary events in ensuing twelve months. *Am J Cardiol* 1993;71:646–651.
7. Sawada SG, Ryan T, Conley MJ, et al. Prognostic value of a normal exercise echocardiogram. *Am Heart J* 1990;120:49–55.

Landmark Articles

Feigenbaum H. Exercise echocardiography. *J Am Soc Echocardiogr* 1988;1:161–166.
Hecht HS, DeBord L, Shaw R, et al. Digital supine bicycle stress echocardiography: a new technique for evaluating coronary artery disease. *J Am Coll Cardiol* 1993; 21:950–956.
Ryan T, Segar DS, Sawada SG, et al. Detection of coronary artery disease with upright bicycle exercise echocardiography. *J Am Soc Echocardiogr* 1993;6:186–197.
Marwick TH, Nemec JJ, Pashkow FJ. Accuracy and limitations of exercise echocardiography in a routine clinical setting. *J Am Coll Cardiol* 1992;19:74–81.
Iliceto S, Galiuto L, Marangelli V, Rizzon P. Clinical use of stress echocardiography: factors affecting diagnostic accuracy. *Eur Heart J* 1994;15:672–680.
Marwick TH, Brunken R, Meland N, et al. Accuracy and feasibility of contrast echocardiography for detection of perfusion defects in routine practice: comparison with wall motion and technetium-99m sestamibi single-photon emission computed tomography. *J Am Coll Cardiol* 1998;32:1260–1269.

Key Reviews

Armstrong WF. Emerging technology in stress echocardiography. *Eur Heart J* 1995; 16[Suppl J]:5–9.
Beckman S, Schartl M, Bocksch W, Fleck E. Diagnosis of coronary artery disease and viable myocardium by stress echocardiography: diagnostic accuracy of different stress modalities. *Eur Heart J* 1995;16[Suppl J]:10–18.
Marwick TH. Recent advances in stress echocardiography. *Curr Opin Cardiol* 1995; 10:619–625.

Relevant Book Chapters

Geleijnse ML, Fioretti PM. Selection of myocardial perfusion or function for the diagnosis of CAD. In: Marwick TH, ed. *Cardiac stress testing and imaging.* New York: Churchill Livingstone. 1996:97–112.
Marwick TH. Pharmacologic stress testing. In: Marwick TH, ed. *Cardiac stress testing and imaging.* New York: Churchill Livingstone, 1996:233–260.
Marwick TH. Stress echocardiography. In: Topol EJ, ed. *Comprehensive cardiovascular medicine.* Philadelphia: Lippincott–Raven, 1998:1407–1440.
Ryan T. Left ventricular functional response to stress for the diagnosis of CAD. In: Marwick TH, ed. *Cardiac stress testing and imaging.* New York: Churchill Livingstone, 1996:67–96.

43. MYOCARDIAL VIABILITY

C. Patrick Green

I. **Introduction.** The identification of viable myocardium is an important clinical issue among patients who have coronary artery disease (CAD) and left ventricular (LV) systolic dysfunction.

   A. **Revascularization procedures** such as coronary artery bypass grafting may improve severe regional or global LV dysfunction caused by CAD and improve functional capacity, symptoms of heart failure, and long-term survival compared with medical therapy or cardiac transplantation. However, these patients are at **higher surgical risk** than those with normal resting LV function (1).

   B. The **goal** is to identify and offer revascularization procedures only to patients who are more likely to achieve an improved quality of life or prolonged survival.

      1. Such **benefits** can be achieved by **patients with dysfunctional yet viable myocardium** caused by ischemia, stunning, or hibernation, even in the absence of symptoms.

      2. The LV systolic function of patients with LV dysfunction caused by **myocardial necrosis and scarring** (nonviable myocardium) **does not recover** after revascularization procedures. These patients have higher perioperative mortality and morbidity rates and no benefit in terms of long-term survival from revascularization compared with similar patients with viable myocardium.

   C. **Clinical information** gained from coronary angiography, resting two-dimensional echocardiography, and electrocardiography (ECG) **is not reliable in prediction of recovery of LV function.**

      1. When the anatomic features of the coronary arteries allow revascularization, techniques that predict recovery of LV function after revascularization **must allow differentiation of viable from nonviable myocardium.**

      2. Improvement after myocardial revascularization represents a complex interaction between patient selection, anatomic features of the coronary arteries, and surgical outcome. **Even though myocardial viability may be present, some patients may not have improvement of regional or global LV function.**

      3. Recovery of LV function after coronary revascularization is the standard for determining the accuracy of any technique designed to assess myocardial viability. However, the ultimate **outcomes** of interest are improved mortality, patient functioning, and quality of life.

II. **Clinical presentation.** Ischemia, stunning, hibernation, scarring, and normal myocardium may coexist in the same patient or even in the same segment of myocardium.

   A. Physiologic requirements for cellular **viability** include adequate blood flow to deliver substrates and wash out metabolites, metabolic processes to generate high-energy phosphates, and intact sarcolemmal function to maintain electrochemical gradients across the cell membrane. Dysfunctional yet viable myocardium has the potential for recovery of contractile function after revascularization.

   B. Myocardial necrosis causes formation of **scar and nonviable myocardium.** Nonviable myocardium can be defined as dysfunctional myocardium that does not improve after revascularization.

   C. **Stunning** refers to myocardium that is **viable and has the potential for recovery of function.** It is a transient myocardial dysfunction that occurs after an acute episode of ischemia and may occur despite the return of normal myocardial blood flow. Myocardial dysfunction caused by stunning may last for several days or weeks before resolving. Recovery of contractile function may occur with or without revascularization, as after thrombolysis or primary angioplasty.

    1. Etiology. Common clinical scenarios that may cause myocardial stunning include acute coronary occlusion and reperfusion after administration of thrombolytic agents in the management of acute myocardial infarction or ischemia caused by critical coronary stenosis that occurs with exertion. Either an increase in demand or a reduction in supply can cause the ischemic episode.

    2. Pathophysiology. Proposed mechanisms for the stunning phenomenon include impairment of myocardial energy production (2), calcium overload (3), detrimental effects of oxygen-free radicals released during reperfusion and causing membrane lipid peroxidation (4), and ischemic damage to the extracellular matrix (5).

D. Hibernation also describes viable myocardium with the potential for the recovery of function. The presence of hibernating myocardium implies the presence of segments of persistently dysfunctional myocardium. Recovery of function is unlikely without revascularization and may progress to necrosis unless perfusion is restored.

    1. Etiology. Hibernation is caused by repetitive ischemic injury or chronic reduction in myocardial blood flow.

    2. Pathophysiology. The chronic low-flow state and repeated injury cause structural and metabolic changes that reduce metabolic demand with resultant contractile dysfunction. The overall effect minimizes myocardial energy expenditure and possibly enhances myocyte survival.

III. Assessment of myocardial viability. Assessment for the presence and extent of myocardial viability is **indicated** for patients who have chronic CAD and LV dysfunction or LV dysfunction after acute infarction and are suitable candidates for revascularization (percutaneous techniques or coronary artery bypass grafting). Chronic heart failure is caused by CAD in approximately 70% or more of patients. Because heart failure caused by CAD carries a less favorable long-term prognosis than nonischemic cardiomyopathy, CAD should be excluded as the cause of cardiomyopathy. Among patients with CAD and LV dysfunction treated medically, the presence of viable myocardium is associated with poor prognosis (6). Therefore evaluation for the presence and extent of CAD and viability should be part of the diagnostic evaluation of all patients with marked LV systolic dysfunction (ejection fraction less than 30%).

A. Positron emission tomography (PET) is a noninvasive nuclear imaging technique currently considered to be the **standard for assessment of myocardial viability.** Positron-emitting isotopes of carbon, hydrogen, nitrogen, and oxygen can be readily incorporated into biologically active molecules that depict naturally occurring cellular processes. This allows imaging and quantification of metabolic processes and blood flow by means of PET. In the most commonly used technique nitrogen 13–labeled ammonia is used as a perfusion tracer and fluorine 18–labeled fluorodeoxyglucose ([18F] FDG) is used as a metabolic marker of glucose utilization.

    1. Assessment of myocardial metabolism. The myocardium metabolizes free fatty acids, glucose, ketone bodies, lactate, pyruvate, acetate, and amino acids. Utilization of these various substrates depends on regional blood flow, arterial substrate concentration, oxidative capacity of the myocardium, and the neurohormonal milieu.

        a. Physiology

            (1) In the fasting state, oxidation of free fatty acids is preferred and accounts for most myocardial oxygen consumption, and myocardial glucose utilization is suppressed.

            (2) After ingestion of carbohydrates, plasma levels of insulin rise, and glucose is more readily transported into the myocyte and is metabolized through glycolysis.

   (3) Ischemia impairs mitochondrial oxidative metabolism and is associated with enhanced glycogenolysis and anaerobic glycolysis. Therefore glucose consumption (both anaerobic and aerobic) is enhanced after episodes of ischemia and may persist beyond the acute episode of ischemia itself.

   (4) Oxygen extraction is enhanced under conditions of reduced myocardial blood flow, allowing oxygen consumption to remain normal or near normal despite an almost 50% reduction in blood flow. Reduced flow beyond this point, however, causes sharp declines in oxygen consumption and glucose utilization.

  b. Metabolic tracers. Primarily three positron-emitting tracers of myocardial metabolism are currently used clinically, although a variety of tracers has been synthesized and studied.

   (1) [^{18}F] FDG is the metabolic tracer most commonly used in clinical PET. FDG, a glucose analog, is transported across the cell membrane and becomes a marker for regional rates of glucose uptake and utilization. Dysfunctional yet viable myocardium can be identified by means of metabolic PET with [^{18}F] FDG as a marker of glucose utilization with near-simultaneous assessment of regional myocardial blood flow with another PET agent.

    (a) FDG is attractive for the assessment of viable myocardium because of the effects of ischemia on myocardial tissue. When the myocardium is ischemic, mitochondrial oxidative metabolism is impaired, leading to enhanced glycogenolysis and anaerobic glycolysis. The ultimate effect is enhanced glucose consumption.

    (b) **In the fasting state, interpretation is difficult** because there is relatively little uptake of FDG with heterogeneity among myocardial regions even in normal myocardium.

    (c) Studies are **typically performed after a loading dose of oral glucose** to enhance myocardial accumulation of [^{18}F] FDG and to study specificity. The standard oral glucose load is 50 to 100 mL of a dextrose-containing solution given 1 to 2 hours before the injection of FDG. Clinical PET with FDG usually is performed 30 to 40 minutes after the intravenous bolus of 5 to 10 mCi of [^{18}F] FDG. Images are then recorded for 20 to 30 minutes.

    (d) It may be helpful to **monitor blood glucose levels** during the study.

    (e) **Patients with diabetes** may need insulin supplementation to increase glucose utilization and improve FDG image quality.

   (2) Carbon 11 palmitate and carbon 11 acetate are two other positron-emitting tracers of myocardial metabolism, but they are rarely used. Carbon 11 palmitate was one of the first tracers used in conjunction with PET to assess myocardial metabolism.

2. Assessment of myocardial blood flow

  a. Positron-emitting tracers of myocardial perfusion or blood flow most commonly used for clinical imaging are rubidium 82, nitrogen 13 ammonium, and oxygen 15 water. All three perfusion agents provide comparable diagnostic information about regional myocardial perfusion.

   (1) Rubidium 82 and nitrogen 13 ammonium are transiently trapped in the myocardium in proportion to regional distribution of blood flow. The distribution of nitrogen 13 ammonium is heterogeneous with a modest reduction of relative tracer activity in the posterolateral wall of the left ventricle. For most patients, this does not affect the clinical interpretation of the PET perfusion images.

    (2) Oxygen 15 water is a freely diffusible tracer that accumulates in and clears from the myocardium as a function of blood flow.

  b. The **water-perfusable index** is another perfusion imaging method to assess myocardial viability. The water-perfusable index is based on the principle that viable myocardium exchanges oxygen 15 water rapidly, as scar or nonviable myocardium do not.

3. Quantitative perfusion measurements. PET perfusion images depict proportionate tissue tracer concentrations that represent only relative myocardial perfusion. The severity of the perfusion defect is expressed as the reduction in regional activity relative to peak myocardial activity (as in conventional planar or single-photon emission computed tomography [SPECT]). It is assumed that the highest tissue counts reflect normal myocardium.

  a. Dynamic PET images allow one to determine the absolute rate of myocardial perfusion in milliliters of blood flow per minute per gram of tissue. The myocardium is unlikely to harbor considerable viability if resting blood flows are less than 0.25 mL/min per gram, although flows greater than 0.25 mL/min per gram do not guarantee the presence of clinically significant viability.

  b. Most imaging facilities rely on static images for the assessment of myocardial viability. This allows the patient to leave the scanner during myocardial uptake of the tracer and allows more patients to be imaged at one time.

  c. Dysfunctional myocardial segments with areas of pronounced perfusion defects (less than 40% to 50% of normal tracer activity) are less likely to improve after revascularization (7). Segments that have 40% to 60% of normal tracer activity improve approximately one-half of the time (8). Because of its low predictive power, the relative severity of perfusion defects is not used to identify viable myocardium alone, especially for patients with moderately severe perfusion defects.

4. Testing procedures

  a. The patient is carefully positioned in the scanner and is made as comfortable as possible.

  b. After localization of the heart, a 10- to 20-minute transmission scan is obtained to correct all subsequent emission images for attenuation of activity by the thorax.

  c. **It is important that the patient not move** between acquisition of the transmission and acquisition of the emission images to prevent introduction of artifacts into the emission images.

  d. **Emission images** are obtained after administration of the radioactive tracer to the patient.

  e. **Static image acquisition** refers to images acquired at the time of peak myocardial uptake of the tracer relative to background.

  f. An **alternative is sequential acquisition** of a series of images (dynamic image acquisition), which depicts changes in myocardial tracer concentration as a function of time. This allows quantification of absolute rates of blood flow and metabolic processes.

  g. Images may be **gated** to the patient's electrocardiogram for measurement of segmental wall motion and thickening, ventricular volumes, and ejection fractions. Images are obtained in a tomographic manner with reconstruction along cardiac planes similar to that of SPECT studies for semiquantitative analysis.

5. Findings. FDG metabolic PET is combined with myocardial perfusion imaging to accurately identify viable myocardium that is likely to improve after revascularization procedures. Three patterns are observed on the basis of regional blood flow (perfusion) and metabolic activity (Table 43–1). Patterns of [^{18}F] FDG uptake and normal perfusion.

  a. Normal blood flow and normal glucose uptake indicate **normal, viable myocardium.**

Table 43-1. Patterns of [¹⁸F]FDG uptake and regional perfusion

Technique	Normal myocardium	Viable myocardium	Nonviable myocardium
⁸²Rb (perfusion tracer)	Normal	Decreased	Decreased
[¹⁸F]FDG (marker of metabolism)	Normal	Normal/mildly increased	Decreased

[¹⁸F]FDG, [¹⁸F] Fluorodeoxyglucose; *⁸²Rb,* rubidium 82.

b. Decreased blood flow with normal or mildly increased glucose utilization relative to normal myocardium indicates a **viable myocardium–mismatch pattern.**

c. **Decreased blood flow and decreased glucose uptake** relative to normal myocardium is consistent with myocardial scar or irreversible damage–match pattern.

d. Several studies have shown that the blood flow–metabolism mismatch (reduced or normal myocardial perfusion with increased glucose uptake) pattern on PET is representative of viable myocardium and is **likely to improve after revascularization.** In a pooled analysis of 12 studies, the sensitivity of [¹⁸F] FDG PET to predict **segmental functional recovery** among patients undergoing revascularization ranged from 71% to 100% (mean 88%) with a specificity from 38% to 91% (mean 73%).

e. Patients with two or more viable dysfunctional segments are more likely to have improvement in **global LV function,** whereas patients with one viable dysfunctional segment or no viable segments at [¹⁸F]FDG PET cannot expect improvement in global LV function after myocardial revascularization (9).

B. Single-photon imaging techniques. Single-photon imaging techniques have achieved a prominent role in the detection of myocardial viability because of their ability to assess myocardial perfusion, cell membrane integrity, and metabolic activity. For a tracer to be useful for the detection of viable myocardium, it should depend on active cellular metabolism for cellular accumulation so that it will be retained in viable cells but not necrotic ones. Cellular accumulation should not be limited by low flow. Thallium 201 and technetium 99m sestamibi are myocardial flow tracers that satisfy these requirements.

1. Thallium 201 is produced in a cyclotron and emits mercury x-rays at 69 to 83 keV (88%) and gamma rays at 135, 165, and 167 keV (12%). Thallium 201 has a relatively long half-life (physical half-life 74 hours, biologic half-life 58 hours), so a relatively small amount can be administered. For SPECT, 3.5 to 4.0 mCi is administered. The estimated absorbed radiation dose to the whole body is 0.21 rad/mCi and to the kidney is 0.24 rad/mCi.

a. Physiology

(1) The first-pass myocardial extraction of thallium 201 is 85%. Initial accumulation is proportional to regional myocardial blood flow.

(2) Entry of thallium 201 into the myocyte depends on the Na-K-ATPase pump, which allows continuous exchange across the cellular membrane. **Irreversibly injured (necrotic) myocardium cannot concentrate thallium 201.**

(3) After the initial distribution of thallium within the myocardium, a continuous exchange of the tracer over the sarcolemmal membrane takes place. This process accounts for reaccumulation of thallium 201 (redistribution) and thus its usefulness in the assessment of myocardial viability.

(4) Simply put, **redistribution is a continuous exchange of myocardial thallium and thallium in the blood pool.** Continued accumulation of thallium into ischemic segments depends on blood levels of the tracer. Ischemic **segments may retain the tracer longer if coronary stenosis is severe or if perfusion pressure is low. Redistribution can only occur in viable myocardium.** If myocardial necrosis is present, there is no uptake or delayed redistribution of thallium in these segments.

(5) Redistribution implies resolution of initial defects at repeated imaging. With computer-assisted techniques, the ratio of ischemic-zone to normal-zone thallium activity can be quantified and used to determine the amount of redistribution.

b. **Rest-redistribution thallium imaging** might be used to assess myocardial viability. However, many clinical situations dictate simultaneous assessment of both myocardial viability and stress-induced ischemia.

c. **Stress-redistribution imaging.**   In this traditional method of assessment of regional myocardial blood flow, thallium 201 is injected at peak exercise with immediate imaging; delayed or redistribution imaging is performed 2.5 to 4 hours later. This conventional protocol with 2.5 to 4 hour delayed imaging typically underestimates the presence of viable myocardium. Detection of viable myocardium is improved if a third set of images is obtained 18 to 72 hours after the stress injection of thallium. Late redistribution, when present, is an accurate indicator of viable myocardium. However, image quality and sensitivity for myocardial viability can be further improved by means of thallium reinjection (see **III.B.1.d.**).

d. **Stress-redistribution-reinjection protocol.** Reinjection of a new dose of thallium 201 (1 mCi) at rest immediately after the 2.5 to 4 hour delayed images or injection of thallium 201 at rest on the day after can be done to assess regional blood flow at rest relative to that with stress. Fifty percent of the dose injected during exercise is readministered. Because late 24-hour imaging after reinjection does not appear to enhance detection of viable myocardium (10), many laboratories acquire reinjection images immediately after reinjection of thallium. Elimination of the 2.5 to 4 hour images though (redistribution images) and the performance of only reinjection of thallium at 4 hours and reimaging (reinjection images) convert segments that would have shown redistribution at 4 hours into irreversible defects at delayed imaging. Therefore the redistribution images should not be eliminated with this protocol.

e. **Rest-redistribution imaging** may be the **procedure of choice for** patients whose clinical question pertains to the **presence of viable myocardium only and not inducible ischemia.** Images are taken 15 minutes after a resting injection of thallium 201 (early images) and again 4 hours later (delayed resting images). Stress-redistribution-reinjection and rest-redistribution protocols have roughly the same predictive accuracy for the detection of viable myocardium (11).

f. **Rest imaging after acute MI.** Resting thallium 201 scintigraphy may be used to **assess the extent of reflow and myocardial salvage** after acute MI managed with thrombolytic therapy. This is most useful 24 hours or more after the acute event. The degree of regional thallium uptake is proportional to the mass of viable myocardium. Improvement in regional LV systolic function can be predicted if there is preserved thallium uptake in the territory of the infarction-related vessel before angioplasty.

g. **Thallium quantitation.** Quantitation of myocardial thallium activity may be predictive of the presence of viable myocardium (12). **The presence of normal tracer uptake and the presence of completely or partially reversible defects indicate the presence of viable myocardium.** Mild to moderately severe fixed defects (defined as greater than 50% of normal thallium uptake) have been confirmed to be viable at PET in more than 95% of cases, even in the absence of redistribution. Severe defects with **less than 50% of normal thallium uptake** most often reflect **nonviable myocardium or scar** (12). The use of nitrates with reinjection has been shown to improve thallium uptake and detection of viability in ischemic myocardium (13).

h. **Criteria for determining viability from thallium scans**
  (1) Normal thallium uptake on early scan
  (2) Complete thallium redistribution on delayed images
  (3) Defect fill-in after reinjection of thallium
  (4) Partial redistribution of an initial defect on delayed images if defect counts are greater than 50% of peak counts
  (5) Mild fixed defect, with defect counts greater than 50% of peak counts

i. **Diagnostic accuracy**
  (1) **Regional functional improvement.** The diagnostic accuracy of thallium 201 stress-redistribution-reinjection imaging for prediction of regional functional improvement after revascularization was analyzed in seven studies (9). The sensitivity of predicting improvement was 80% to 100% (mean 86%) with a relatively low specificity of 38% to 80% (mean 47%). These results suggest an overestimation of the potential for recovery at stress-redistribution-reinjection imaging.
  (2) **Global improvement.** The sensitivity and specificity for predicting global improvement in LV function (at least 5% improvement in ejection fraction) have been reported to be 72% and 73%, respectively.
  (3) **Comparison with other methods.** Analysis of studies involving rest-redistribution imaging protocols for the prediction of regional and global improvement in LV function was similar. The presence or absence of viable myocardium was shown to be 88% concordant between thallium 201 stress-redistribution-reinjection and [18F] FDG PET (9).

j. **Limitations.** The limitations of imaging with thallium 201 are related primarily to its low-energy photons, which are readily scattered and attenuated, and to dosimetric considerations.

2. **Technetium 99m sestamibi.** The limitations of thallium 201 have led to interest in the use of technetium 99m–based myocardial perfusion agents, which in recent years have undergone clinical testing for their efficacy in detecting viable myocardium. Of these agents, the most useful is technetium 99m methoxyisobutylisonitrile (^{99m}Tc-sestamibi), which is a lipophilic monovalent cation that emits gamma rays at 140 keV and has a physical half-life of 6 hours. Mitochondrial function and sarcolemmal integrity are required for the uptake and retention of ^{99m}Tc-sestamibi. This allows its use as a marker of viability. Necrotic myocardium does not retain sestamibi.

  a. Quantitation of ^{99m}Tc-sestamibi activity increases the ability to detect viable myocardium. The presence of segments with greater than 50% of normal sestamibi uptake correlates well with regional thallium activity, and PET allows **successful prediction** of which myocardial segments may improve after revascularization. Severe defects (less than 50% of normal activity) most commonly reflect nonviable myocardium but have been shown to be viable up to 38% of the time. The high photon flux of ^{99m}Tc-sestamibi allows acquisition of ECG-gated images. Thus assessment of regional wall thickening and wall motion improves the ability to detect viable myocardium. Administration of the tracer after nitrate administration has been shown to further improve the detection of viable myocardium.

   b. Comparison of ^{99m}Tc-sestamibi with other imaging modalities including thallium 201 stress-redistribution-reinjection, thallium 201 rest-redistribution, thallium 201 rest protocols, and [^{18}F] FDG PET consistently have shown **^{99m}Tc-sestamibi to be less accurate in the detection of myocardial viability.**

   c. The **sensitivity** of ^{99m}Tc-sestamibi in predicting segmental functional improvement ranges from 73% to 100% (mean 81%), with a specificity of 35% to 86% (mean 60%) (9). Administration of nitrates before ^{99m}Tc-sestamibi imaging may improve the specificity of the study. There currently are no available data regarding the prediction of global improvement of LV function with ^{99m}Tc-sestamibi.

C. Two-dimensional echocardiography

   1. Resting echocardiography can help quantify the extent of LV dysfunction in patients with chronic CAD or those who have had an acute MI. Regional wall motion analysis typically is performed with a 16-segment model standardized by the American Society of Echocardiography.

   a. Wall thickening is highly predictive of viable myocardium, whereas systolic wall thinning or dyskinesis is predictive of nonviable myocardium. Akinetic or dyskinetic wall segments with preserved diastolic wall thickness may represent a mixture of viable and nonviable myocardium.

   b. Although wall thickness may correlate with the extent of myocardial viability in patients with chronic CAD (especially wall thinning or scar), wall thickness is not useful after acute MI because thinning of the wall does not occur until several weeks after the event.

   c. Because resting echocardiography does not always allow accurate prediction of myocardial viability, further evaluation is necessary.

   2. Dobutamine echocardiography

   a. Findings

      (1) Improvement of regional wall motion and thickening in myocardial wall segments (that are abnormal at rest) during infusion of dobutamine at incremental doses up to 5 to 20 µg/kg per minute suggests the presence of viable myocardium in both acute and chronic ischemic myocardial dysfunction. This is known as **contractile reserve.**

      (2) Failure of a segment to improve suggests that it is nonviable.

      (3) Dobutamine echocardiography has been shown to be predictive of reversible dysfunction soon after acute MI and in patients with LV ischemic dysfunction caused by chronic CAD.

   b. Dosage. The detection of inducible ischemia generally involves infusion of **dobutamine at doses up to 40 µg/kg per minute. Low-dose dobutamine** infusion used for assessment of viability usually involves **doses of 5 to 10 µg/kg per minute.**

   c. Regional contractile response to inotropic stimulation with dobutamine. There are four basic patterns, as follows:

      (1) Biphasic—initial improvement at low dose followed by worsening at higher doses

      (2) Sustained improvement

      (3) Sustained worsening

      (4) No change

d. The biphasic response of improved contractile function during low-dose dobutamine infusion was the best predictor of recovery of segmental wall motion after revascularization in one study (14).

e. Comparison

(1) The sensitivity of low-dose dobutamine echocardiography for the prediction of regional improvement of LV function after revascularization is 71% to 97% (mean 84%) with a specificity of 63% to 96% (81%) (9).

(2) Global improvement in LV function is linearly related to the number of segments that are viable.

(3) Overall, compared with other imaging modalities, **dobutamine echocardiography may have a higher positive predictive value for the determination of myocardial viability** (14). The negative predictive value for predicting the lack of functional improvement after revascularization is either comparable with or better than that of thallium 201 imaging. The differences in predictive values are explained by a higher sensitivity but lower specificity of thallium 201 viability criteria compared with dobutamine echocardiography viability criteria.

f. Limitations

(1) Changes in regional wall motion and thickening during low-dose dobutamine infusion can be **very subtle**. Highly expert interpretation and sophisticated digital processing techniques are needed. **Interobserver variation** among experts in the field of stress echocardiography can be as high as 10%. More objective measurement of changes in regional systolic function is needed to reduce the subjectivity of dobutamine stress echocardiography. As the method comes to be used by less experienced observers, the accuracy will likely decline.

(2) The **number of patients for whom appropriate diagnostic information cannot be obtained** is high and also varies with operator experience. Patients with severe multivessel CAD and hibernating myocardium may manifest ischemia even at very low doses of dobutamine (less than 5 μg/kg), thus limiting its usefulness in this setting.

g. Future directions. Ongoing research is evaluating the ability of contrast echocardiography to reflect the status of microvascular perfusion and thus the presence of myocardial viability. Currently, this method is limited to the cardiac catheterization laboratory, where microbubbles are injected into the coronary circulation directly. Newer contrast agents that can cross the pulmonary capillary bed and allow peripheral intravenous injection may be available for wider clinical applicability in the future.

IV. Choice of imaging technique. The key to appropriate treatment of a patient with CAD and LV dysfunction is accurately ascertaining whether a patient has viable myocardium that may potentially benefit from revascularization. There is no doubt that patients with angina are candidates for revascularization. Patients with asymptomatic substantial LV dysfunction also may benefit from coronary revascularization if they harbor viable myocardium. Patients with a large amount of hibernating myocardium have better survival rates when treated with revascularization compared with patients treated medically. How much viability is enough? Which test modality, criteria, protocol, and tracers should be chosen? To a large extent, the answer to the last question is determined by the experience and expertise of the local physicians and by available resources.

A. Most patients with CAD and LV dysfunction initially undergo **evaluation for both ischemia and viability** with either stress SPECT or dobutamine echocardiography.

1. After a review and quantification of the stress-redistribution images (4 hours), a decision can be made regarding the need for reinjection and reimaging.

2. No other viability test is needed if after these images are obtained, there is evidence of induced ischemia and a large amount of tracer uptake in the dysfunctional area.
3. If tracer uptake is low in the dysfunctional area (less than 50%) with only a small area of ischemia, or no ischemia (that is, a fixed defect), PET, if available, can be performed. Flow-metabolism mismatch and relative FDG uptake are believed to be the two best-documented criteria for determining the presence of viability.

B. If the clinical question pertains only to the **presence or absence of myocardial viability** and not to the detection of inducible ischemia, rest-redistribution thallium 201 imaging or low-dose dobutamine echocardiography may be the procedure of choice.

V. **Therapy. Therapeutic options** currently available to most patients with heart failure caused by CAD are **medical treatment alone, myocardial revascularization,** or **cardiac transplantation.** Marked improvement in survival, heart failure symptoms, and functional capacity has been demonstrated among patients treated with revascularization compared with medical therapy, especially if angina or other objective evidence of reversible ischemia exists. Although cardiac transplantation can extend survival and improve quality of life, this should be reserved as a last resort because of the limited number of donor hearts available and the high cost of treatment.

A. Identification of viable myocardium is only one factor in the total equation for considering revascularization for a patient with CAD and LV dysfunction. The decision also is based on patient preference of treatment modality, clinical presentation, suitability of coronary anatomy for bypass, and presence of comorbid conditions.

B. Improvement after revascularization represents a complex interaction between compensatory mechanisms, coronary anatomy, surgical outcome, and patient selection. **Factors that may affect improvement in LV function after coronary revascularization** include presence and degree of viable myocardium, completeness of revascularization, presence of perioperative myocardial injury or necrosis, graft patency, and the presence of concomitant primary cardiomyopathy.

C. Although recovery of LV function after coronary revascularization is the standard for determining the accuracy of any technique designed to assess myocardial viability, this may or may not be the most important clinical benefit of revascularization of viable but dysfunctional myocardium. **Other important benefits** include the attenuation of LV dilatation and remodeling, improved exercise capacity and quality of life, stabilization of the electrical milieu with a reduction of ventricular arrhythmias, and a reduction in risk for future ischemic events. These considerations have to be tested in future clinical trials.

D. Improvement in LV function may not be apparent or complete immediately after revascularization or at the time of hospital discharge.
1. Most **follow-up assessment of LV function** is performed 3 months after revascularization. Full recovery, however, may not occur for as long as 6 to 12 months (15).
2. Deterioration of LV function immediately after revascularization is not uncommon and is caused by several mechanisms, including myocardial stunning from perioperative injury. **Late improvement** may be detected 2 to 3 months later.

E. **Viability assessment after acute MI**
1. Patients who have had acute MI with resultant severe regional dysfunction and marked residual stenosis in the infarct related artery may benefit from revascularization if viable myocardium is present.
2. Myocardial stunning after acute MI may complicate interpretation of diagnostic studies.
3. Most studies of reversible LV dysfunction have involved patients with chronic CAD. Extrapolation of data from these studies to patients who have had acute MI should be done with caution.

SUGGESTED READINGS
References
1. Mickleborough LL, Maruyama H, Takagi Y, et al. Results of revascularization in patients with severe left ventricular dysfunction. *Circulation* 1995;92 [Suppl II] : II-73–II-79.
2. Swain JL, Sabina RL, McHale PA, Greenfield JC Jr, Holmes EW. Prolonged myocardial nucleotide depletion after brief ischemia in open-chest dogs. *Am J Physiol* 1982;242:H818–H826.
3. Grinwald PM, Brosnahan C. Sodium imbalance as a cause of calcium overload in post-hypoxic reoxygenation injury. *J Mol Cell Cardiol* 1987;19:487–495.
4. Bolli R. Oxygen-derived free radicals and postischemic myocardial dysfunction ("stunned myocardium"). *J Am Coll Cardiol* 1988;12:239–249.
5. Zhao MJ, Zhang H, Robinson TF, Factor SM, Sonnenblick EH, Eng C. Profound structural alterations of the extracellular collagen matrix in postischemic dysfunctional ("stunned myocardium") but viable myocardium. *J Am Coll Cardiol* 1987;10:1322–1334.
6. Cuocolo A, Petretta M, Nicolai E, et al. Coronary revascularization improves survival and functional outcome in patients with previous myocardial infarction and evidence of viable myocardium at thallium-201 imaging. *Eur J Nucl Med* 1998;25:60–68.
7. Tamki N, Kawamoto M, Tadamura E, et al. Prediction of reversible ischemia after revascularization. *Circulation* 1995;91:1697–1705.
8. Duvernoy CS, vom Dahl J, Laubenbacher C, Schwaiger M. The role of nitrogen-13 ammonia positron emission tomography in predicting functional outcome after coronary revascularization. *J Nucl Cardiol* 1995;2:499.
9. Bax JJ, Wijns W, Cornel JH, Visser FC, Boersma E, Fioretti PM. Accuracy of currently available techniques for prediction of functional recovery after revascularization in patients with left ventricular dysfunction due to chronic CAD: comparison of pooled data. *J Am Coll Cardiol* 1997;30:1451–1460.
10. Dilsizian V, Smeltzer WR, Freedman NM, Dextras R, Bonow RO. Thallium reinjection after stress-redistribution imaging: does 24–hour delayed imaging after reinjection enhance detection of viable myocardium? *Circulation* 1991;83: 1247–1255.
11. Dilsizian V, et al. Concordance and discordance between stress-redistribution-reinjection and rest-redistribution thallium imaging for assessing viable myocardium: comparison with metabolic activity by positron emission tomography. *Circulation* 1993;88:941.
12. Gibson RS, Watson DD, Taylor GJ, et al. Prospective assessment of regional myocardial perfusion before and after coronary revascularization surgery by quantitative thallium-201 scintigraphy. *J Am Coll Cardiol* 1983;1:804–815.
13. He ZX, Darcourt J, Guignier A, et al. Nitrates improve detection of ischemic but viable myocardium by thallium–201 reinjection SPECT. *J Nucl Med* 1993;34:1472.
14. Afridi I, Kleinman NS, Raizner AE, Zoghbi WA. Dobutamine echocardiography in myocardial hibernation. optimal dose and accuracy in predicting recovery of left ventricular function after coronary angioplasty. *Circulation* 1995;91:663–670.
15. Vanoverschelde JL, Melin JA, Depre C, Borgers M, Dion R, Wijins W. Time-course of functional recovery of hibernating myocardium after coronary revascularization [Abstract]. *Circulation* 1996;90 [Suppl I]:I-378.

Landmark Articles
Bonow RO, Dilsizian V, Cuocolo A, Bacharach SL. Identification of viable myocardium in patients with chronic coronary artery disease and left ventricular dysfunction: comparison of thallium scintigraphy with reinjection and PET imaging with 18F-fluorodeoxyglucose. *Circulation* 1991;86:1125–1137.
Di Carli MF, Davidson M, Little R, et al. Value of metabolic imaging with positron emission tomography for evaluating prognosis in patients with coronary artery disease and left ventricular dysfunction. *Am J Cardiol* 1994;73:527–533.

Dilsizian V, Freedman NM, Bacharach SL, Perrone-Filardi P, Bonow RO. Regional Tl uptake in irreversible defects. Magnitude of change in Tl activity after reinjection distinguishes viable from nonviable myocardium. *Circulation* 1992;85: 627–634.

Gibson RS, Watson DD, Taylor GJ, et al. Prospective assessment of regional myocardial perfusion before and after coronary revascularization surgery by quantitative thallium-201 scintigraphy. *J Am Coll Cardiol* 1983;1:804–815.

Marwick TH, MacIntyre WJ, Lafont A, Nemec JJ, Salcedo EE. Metabolic responses of hibernating and infarcted myocardium to revascularization: a follow-up study of regional perfusion, function and metabolism. *Circulation* 1992;85:1347–1353.

Marwick TH, Nemec JJ, Lafont A, Salcedo EE, MacIntyre WJ. Prediction by post exercise fluoro-18-deoxyglucose positron emission tomography of improvement in exercise capacity after revascularization. *Am J Cardiol* 1992;69:854–859.

Tamaki N, Yonekura Y, Yamashita K, et al. Positron emission tomography using F-18 deoxyglucose in evaluation of coronary artery disease. *Am J Cardiol* 1989;64:860.

Tillisch J, Brunken R, Marshall R, et al. Reversibility of cardiac wall motion abnormalities predicted by positron tomography. *N Engl J Med* 1986;314:884–888.

Relevant Book Chapters
In: Marwick TH, ed. *Cardiac stress testing and imaging.* New York: Churchill Livingstone, 1996 (Chapters 20-23).

Beller GA. *Assessment of myocardial viability.* In: *Clinical nuclear cardiology.* Saunders WB, Chapter 9:293–336.

SECTION XI. ELECTROPHYSIOLOGY

Robert A. Schweikert and Patrick Tchou

44. ELECTROPHYSIOLOGIC STUDIES

Ayman S. Al-Khadra

I. **Introduction.** Electrophysiologic studies (EPS) are a specialized form of cardiac catheterization that helps identify, characterize, and manage cardiac arrhythmias. Over the past 25 to 30 years, EPS have advanced our knowledge of mechanisms of cardiac arrhythmias and revolutionized the way these arrhythmias are managed. The studies should be performed by adequately trained clinicians with the help of skilled nurses in adequately equipped laboratories. A joint task force of the American College of Cardiology and the American Heart Association in collaboration with the North American Society of Pacing and Electrophysiology has published guidelines outlining the accepted indications and the required training for personnel performing EPS (1, 2).

II. **Indications** for EPS can be divided into three broad categories—bradyarrhythmias, tachyarrhythmias, and syncope.

    A. **Bradyarrhythmias** can be caused by sinus node dysfunction, atrioventricular (AV) nodal disease, or infranodal conduction system disease. Among patients with underlying bradyarrhythmias, EPS are rarely necessary because the decision to implant a pacemaker depends primarily on correlation between symptoms and documented bradycardia or demonstration of severe bradycardia or prolonged pauses. EPS should complement clinical evaluation, including comprehensive history and physical examination, conventional 12-lead electrocardiogram (ECG), and Holter monitoring. EPS can be of value in identifying disorders associated with adverse outcome, such as severe infranodal conduction system disease.

    B. More often, EPS may suggest bradycardia as the underlying disorder among patients with **syncope** of unknown causation.

    C. EPS are of tremendous value in the evaluation of **tachyarrhythmias.** They are generally more successful in reproducing reentrant cardiac rhythms than those caused by triggered activity or enhanced automaticity. Among patients with reentrant tachyarrhythmias, EPS are useful in documenting the presence of the anatomic or physiologic substrate responsible for the arrhythmia, defining electric properties of and hemodynamic response to the arrhythmia, and guiding therapy. Response to various drugs or maneuvers also is helpful in further defining the underlying substrate and prognosis.

III. **Equipment and setting**

    A. The most important element in the performance of safe EPS is the presence of **well-trained personnel.** The presence of at least one physician, a nurse, and an engineer to repair equipment is necessary. Personnel involved should be familiar with basic electrophysiologic and electropharmacologic principles, the indications for EPS, and the various diagnostic and therapeutic modalities that can be used in the laboratory.

    B. It is important that the laboratory is equipped with appropriate high-quality **radiographic equipment.**

    C. Appropriate selection of **tools** is a very important aspect of the performance of safe and cost-effective EPS. The minimum instrumentation required for a complete study is a stimulator, an amplifier, display monitors, and reliable recording devices.

        1. The **stimulator** must have capability for burst pacing, delivery of at least three or four extra stimuli, and synchronization of the stimulator to appropriate electric events during intrinsic or paced rhythms and an adjustable output. An appropriate unit should have a constant current source and minimal current leakage. It also must be relatively easy to manipulate.

2. The **junction box** connects electrode catheters to the recording apparatus and to the stimulator.

3. **Recording** is best achieved on solid media, for example, CD or other optical media.

4. The presence of at least two functioning **external defibrillators** is extremely important, particularly during studies in which the ventricular arrhythmias may be induced.

5. The presence of a cardiac surgical team in the same institution is not mandatory for routine EPS or radiofrequency (RF) ablation procedures.

D. **Intracardiac signals** are recorded using various **electrode catheters.**

1. The most common catheters used are **quadripolar woven Dacron polyester** or **polyurethane.** The distal poles of these catheters can be used for pacing.

2. For general-purpose sensing and pacing in the atrium or ventricle, a **nondeflectable catheter** usually is sufficient. Deflectable catheters facilitate mapping and ablation by allowing precise movement.

3. Some catheters have a lumen through which a guidewire can be inserted and dye can be injected.

4. Interelectrode distance varies from 2 to 10 mm. Smaller interelectrode distance is useful for precise mapping and timing.

5. For most EPS, **bipolar recording** is used, but in some situations, especially during mapping of tachyarrhythmias, unipolar recording can be of value in localizing the earliest sites of activity.

IV. Techniques and procedures

A. **Preprocedure preparation**

1. Before the patient is taken to the EPS laboratory, detailed **discussion** of the indications and proposed procedure is conducted with the patient, and informed consent is obtained.

2. For most indications, EPS is an **elective** procedure. The patient's condition should be clinically **stable** at the time of the study. EPS on patients whose condition is unstable, including those with active, recent, or untreated coronary disease or in those with clinical heart failure, carry much higher risk for complications.

3. **Electrolytes, serum digoxin level, and bleeding measurements** are checked and verified as within the normal range.

4. A mild **sedative** is administered (e.g., a benzodiazepine).

5. The patient is attached to continuous ECG and blood pressure **monitoring** devices.

B. **Access and catheter placement**

1. The usual approach to the insertion of electrode catheters is through the **femoral veins under local anesthesia** unless there is a clear contraindication to this approach, such as the presence of deep venous thrombosis or an inferior vena caval filter. In the latter situations or when a coronary sinus catheter is difficult to insert, a superior vein approach is used.

2. Up to three **introducers** are placed in each femoral vein depending on the planned procedure. For patients with **left-sided bypass tracks or left ventricular (LV) tachycardia,** access to the left side of the heart is necessary. This can be achieved through the retrograde transaortic approach, or transseptal puncture. Systemic heparin is used for all left-sided procedures.

3. For complete EPS, **three catheters** are needed.

a. One catheter is placed in the **high right atrium,** preferably in the appendage or against the high lateral wall. Another is placed in the **right ventricular (RV) apex,** and the third is placed across the **tricuspid valve** to obtain a His electrogram.

b. To obtain a **His electrogram,** the electrode catheter is advanced into the right ventricle across the anterior septal portion of the tricuspid valve. Under gentle clockwise torque, the catheter is then slowly withdrawn. A high-frequency sharp deflection occurs at about the same time that a small atrial signal appears. This represents a **distal His** or **proximal right bundle potential.** If the catheter is drawn farther, this sharp signal occurs slightly earlier. A satisfactory position of the His catheter is achieved when a large atrial signal is recorded simultaneously with the early sharp signal. A catheter with 1 cm interelectrode spacing is preferable for this purpose.

3. In **supraventricular tachycardia (SVT)** studies when a left-sided accessory pathway or left atrial origin is suspected, a quadripolar or octapolar catheter may be placed in the coronary sinus rather than in the high right atrium. This more stable catheter position allows mapping of the left AV groove. Although the coronary sinus is easily entered from the superior venous approach, successful catheterization is expected in most attempts through the femoral approach. The catheter is placed with the proximal electrode just beyond the ostium.

C. **Baseline assessment**
1. When all the catheters are in place, a baseline ECG (generally leads I, aVF, V_1, and V_6) and intracardiac electrogram are recorded (Fig. 44-1).
2. In general, **cycle lengths** rather than rates per minute are measured. The following measurements are made at baseline: sinus cycle length and PR, QRS, QT, AH, and HV intervals.
   a. The **AH interval** is measured from the onset of local A deflection to the H deflection on the His electrogram.
   b. The **HV interval** is measured from the H deflection on the His electrogram to the earliest ventricular activity in any lead.
3. When measurements are made during pacing, it is important to **measure from the resulting deflection** rather than from the pacing artifact to avoid errors caused by latency (delay between the pacing artifact and capture).
4. All measurements are recorded in **milliseconds.** Interpretation of baseline intervals is discussed in **IX.**

D. **Programmed stimulation**
1. After baseline measurements are made, programmed stimulation is performed. The protocol used depends on the indication for the study and varies among institutions. During programmed stimulation, the **hemodynamic response** of the patient to pacing and induced tachycardia is closely monitored.
2. **Pacing stimuli** are delivered for 1 or 2 msec and are twice diastolic pacing thresholds. This is important during ventricular stimulation, because pacing at higher outputs increases the risk for inducing nonclinical rhythms. There are two main types of programmed stimulation—burst pacing and the extra stimulus technique.
   a. **Burst pacing** involves continuous pacing at rates faster than the patient's intrinsic rate.
   b. In the **extra stimulus technique,** premature beats are introduced either during intrinsic rhythm (sensed extra stimuli) or after paced drive train (paced extra stimuli). Extra stimulus techniques are useful in evaluating refractory periods of AV node, atrial tissue, ventricular tissue, and accessory pathways. It is possible to evaluate infranodal conduction system refractory periods with atrial or ventricular stimulation. Extra stimulus techniques also are useful in inducing, terminating, and identifying reentrant arrhythmias.
      (1) In the **sensed extra stimulus** technique, a single extra stimulus is introduced initially with a coupling just below the intrinsic rate (sinus or other mechanism). The coupling interval is reduced progressively by 10 to 20 msec until the premature stimulus no longer captures. A pause of 2 to 5 seconds is allowed between stimulation sequences. A second extra stimulus (S_3) can be added if necessary and the sequence repeated.

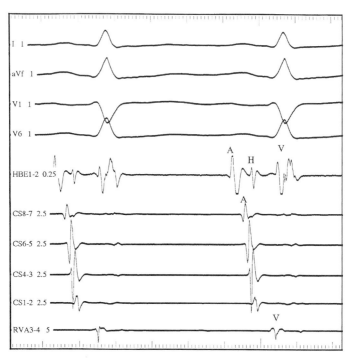

FIG. 44-1. Normal baseline intervals. Typically, up to 4 surface electrocardiograms (I, aVF, V1, and V6) are displayed along with atrial (CS), His (HBE), and ventricular (RVA) electrograms. CS 7–8 refers to the bipolar distal CS electrogram. Fast sweep speeds are used, ranging from 100 to 400 mm/sec. On the time scale, each large division is 100 msec, and each minor division is 10 msec. In addition to intervals, pattern of atrial and ventricular activation should be evaluated. If the CS catheter is placed correctly (see text), the earliest A in sinus rhythm is seen on the HRA electrogram (not shown), then on the His electrogram, and progressively later along the CS electrograms. In the absence of bundle branch block or left sided accessory pathway, the earliest ventricular activity is seen on right sided electrograms (His and RV electrograms).

(2) In the **paced extra stimulus** technique, a drive train of 8 to 10 beats at a fixed cycle length is followed by the premature beat. The drive train cycle length (S_1S_1) ranges from 350 to 800 msec (most frequently 400 to 600 msec) depending on resting heart rate. When this technique is used, testing at two drive-train cycle lengths is recommended. The premature stimulus (S_2) is introduced with a coupling interval just below S_1S_1 cycle length. The coupling interval of the premature stimulus is decreased progressively by 10 to 20 msec until it no longer captures. The longest coupling interval (S_1S_2) that does not capture is the refractory period. S_3 and S_4 are added in ventricular studies if necessary. This protocol can be varied depending on the indication and operator preference.

3. **Continuous monitoring** and recording of external and intracardiac electrograms is maintained throughout programmed stimulation. When a particular event occurs, stimulation is stopped and the event is evaluated.

One should be ready to react depending on the stage of the study. For example, during ventricular stimulation the operator should be ready for overdrive pacing or cardioversion if ventricular tachycardia is induced and for evaluation of atrial activation and ventricular pacing if SVT is induced.

V. Atrial stimulation

A. An atrial study is an integral part of EPS. The only time an atrial study is not performed is in the presence of persistent atrial fibrillation.

  1. **Burst pacing** stresses the AV node and can induce tachycardia, including AV node reentry tachycardia, AV reentrant tachycardia, atrial flutter, atrial fibrillation, atrial tachycardia, and certain forms of idiopathic ventricular tachycardia.

  2. Burst pacing is performed by means of **continuous pacing** (20 to 30 stimuli) at a fixed cycle length starting 100 msec below the sinus cycle length. Repeat burst pacing is performed at progressively shorter cycle lengths until 1:1 conduction through the AV node is no longer maintained. The shortest cycle length consistent with 1:1 conduction in the AV node is recorded.

  3. If a patient is believed to have **atrial flutter or atrial tachycardia,** repeat burst pacing at even shorter cycle lengths is performed until 1:1 atrial capture is no longer maintained.

B. After burst pacing is performed, **paced extra stimulus** sequences are initiated.

  1. The **effect of atrial premature beats** on the AH interval is assessed. Normal response of the AH interval is to progressively prolong with shorter A_1A_2 coupling. This is a direct demonstration of the normal decremental conduction properties of the AV node.

  2. At a critical A_1A_2, the AV node fails to conduct, and on the His electrogram an atrial signal is seen without a His or ventricular deflection. This indicates that **block has occurred in the AV node.** It is important to continue stimulation until the atrial refractory period is reached, because a gap phenomenon may occasionally exist if there are dual AV nodal pathways.

  3. The **gap phenomenon** is demonstrated by apparent achievement of the AV nodal refractory period and resumption of conduction. It reflects functional differences in conduction or refractoriness in several regions or areas of the AV node.

  4. If **narrow, complex tachycardia** is induced, it is evaluated with regard to type, mechanism, response to maneuvers, and method of termination (see **IX.B.3**).

C. **Sinus node evaluation.** For patients who may have underlying sinus node dysfunction, sinus node tests are sometimes performed.

  1. **Sinus node recovery time (SNRT)** is evaluated by means of burst pacing at various cycle lengths in the atrium for 30 to 60 seconds and then abrupt termination of pacing. SNRT is the escape interval between the last paced atrial beat and the first atrial recovery beat. A **corrected SNRT** (CSNRT) is calculated by means of subtracting baseline sinus cycle length from SNRT. A normal value for CSNRT is less than 550 msec. SNRT is used to evaluate the automaticity mechanism of the sinus node.

  2. **Sinoatrial conduction time (SACT)** is a combined measure of conduction in the atrial tissue that includes the area of the sinus node and sinus node automaticity. It is measured with one of two methods.

     a. In the **Strauss method,** a sensed premature atrial beat is used to reset the sinus node, and the return cycle length after the premature beat is measured. Basic cycle length is subtracted from return cycle length, leaving the time necessary to penetrate and leave the sinus nodal tissue. SACT is half this interval.

     b. In the **method proposed by Narula,** the same measurements are obtained after pacing for eight beats at a rate slightly faster than sinus rate.

VI. Ventricular stimulation

A. Ventricular stimulation is performed in evaluations of suspected SVT or ventricular tachyarrhythmia. Supraventricular arrhythmias, particularly those with a concealed bypass tract, may be more easily induced with ventricular stimulation. To characterize SVT the response to premature ventricular beats has to be assessed.

1. When ventricular stimulation is performed in the evaluation of ventricular or wide complex tachyarrhythmias, **pacing at two sites** is necessary. These sites typically are the RV apex and the RV outflow tract.

2. Before programmed stimulation is begun, pacing thresholds are determined, and the output of the pacing stimulus is set to twice the diastolic capture threshold. Higher outputs or coupling intervals shorter then 200 msec may cause induction of nonclinical arrhythmias.

B. Burst pacing in the right ventricle is the initial technique used when ventricular stimulation is performed in the evaluation of SVT.

1. The presence of **retrograde atrial activation** is documented, and a sequence or pattern of atrial activation is evaluated.

2. The **earliest atrial activity** typically is recorded on the His electrogram (Fig. 44-2) This indicates that retrograde conduction has proceeded through the AV node fast pathway. **Absence of ventriculoatrial (VA) conduction,** with one exception, excludes the presence of a bypass track (the exception is the Mahaim type of accessory pathway). The **presence of eccentric atrial activation** (late atrial activation on the His electrogram; Fig. 44-3) suggests the presence of a retrograde conducting bypass track.

3. For some patients with no evidence of retrograde VA conduction, infusion of low doses of **isoproterenol** restores this property to the AV node.

4. The **shortest paced cycle length** capable of conducting 1:1 to the atrium is documented.

   a. If **retrograde conduction** is present, the refractory periods of the conducting pathways are determined with the extra stimulus technique.

   b. In patients with **retrograde VA conduction through the AV node,** block frequently occurs in the His-Purkinje system rather than in the AV node. His-Purkinje conduction block is more likely to occur at long drive trains. Such drive trains therefore are more likely to induce AV reentry tachycardia (along a bypass track) through facilitating His-Purkinje block and allowing a retrograde conducted beat to propagate antegrade through the AV node.

C. In patients being evaluated for **ventricular arrhythmias,** programmed stimulation with extra stimuli is the initial technique used. Pacing at two drive-train cycle lengths (for example, 600 and 400 msec) is performed with single, double, and triple extra stimuli. Simultaneous atrial pacing at the same drive-cycle length sometimes is necessary to avoid competition from the intrinsic atrial pacemaker.

D. Like the A_1A_2 technique described earlier, V_2 **is introduced at progressively shorter coupling intervals** (V_1V_2) until V_2 no longer captures (ventricular refractory period). V_3 **is then introduced** at progressively shorter coupling intervals until it no longer captures. The use of **triple extra stimuli** (V_3V_4) is usually reserved for patients being evaluated for ventricular arrhythmias.

1. A pause of 4 to 5 seconds is allowed after each cycle to assess response and for the patient to recover after ventricular pacing. The increase in a number of extra stimuli increases sensitivity of the study at the cost of lower specificity.

2. There is higher risk for inducing nonclinical arrhythmias, including ventricular fibrillation, with this technique. Stimulation with more than three extra stimuli is not recommended.

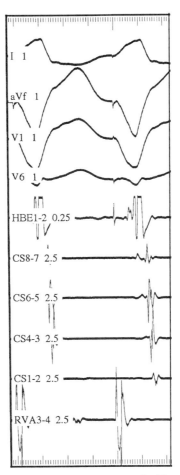

FIG. 44-2. Programmed ventricular stimulation using double extrastimuli in a patient with AV node reentry tachycardia. Note that the earliest retrograde atrial activity is seen on the His electrogram.

3. If programmed stimulation with ventricular extra stimuli does not induce ventricular tachycardia in a patient at very high risk, other techniques may be used. One is **burst pacing in the ventricle.**
   a. A series of 10 paced ventricular beats are introduced at a constant cycle length.
   b. Paced cycle length is decreased by 50 to 100 msec until reaching within 50 msec of the predicted refractory period of the right ventricle, when the decrements proceed at 10-msec intervals until 1:1 capture is no longer maintained.
4. Burst pacing in the atrium can induce idiopathic LV tachycardia in susceptible persons.
E. Some patients, particularly those with underlying dilated cardiomyopathy, may experience **bundle branch reentry (BBR) tachycardia** (Fig. 44-4)

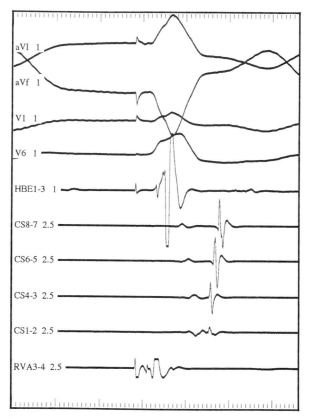

FIG. 44-3. This is an example from a 17-year-old patient with left lateral manifest pathway. Ventricular stimulation results in retrograde atrial activation with the earliest A seen in CS1-2 (eccentric atrial activation).

1. This type of tachycardia involves the right bundle branch as an antegrade limb and the left bundle branch as a retrograde limb to cause rapid and hemodynamically intolerable tachycardia.
2. Because His bundle refractoriness increases after a pause, a short-long-short sequence is used to cause block in the right bundle so that paced stimulus can conduct retrograde up the left bundle branch and possibly initiate tachycardia if the right bundle branch is not refractory.
3. The sequence most commonly used consists of a six-beat drive train at 400 msec followed by V_2 coupled at 600 to 700 msec. V_3 is then introduced at a coupling interval 100 msec longer than the refractory period of the ventricle. V_2V_3 is progressively decreased until V_3 no longer captures. V_4 can be introduced if necessary.

VII. **Induction of ventricular fibrillation.** Under certain circumstances, the operator may decide that induction of ventricular fibrillation is necessary. This is of value when testing implant defibrillators for detection of arrhythmias and during assessment of defibrillation thresholds. Ventricular fibrillation can be induced by means of direct application of alternating current or rapid ventricular pacing at high output. The current can be delivered through the catheter electrode or through the implantable cardioverter refibrillator (ICD).

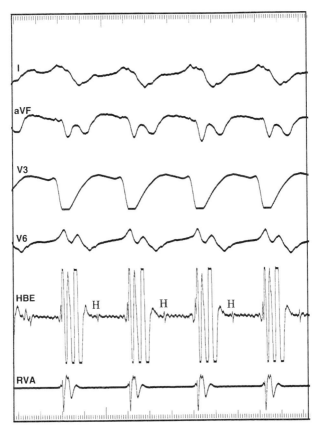

FIG. 44-4. Bundle branch reentry tachycardia. This example is from a 52-year-old man with dilated cardiomyopathy who presented with syncope. This ventricular tachycardia exhibits left bundle branch block morphology, and there is an H deflection preceding every V on the His electrogram. To be absolutely certain of this diagnosis (as opposed to myocardial VT with retrograde His), one has to look for cycle length variation and document that changes in the H-H interval precede changes in the V-V interval.

VIII. **Use of cardioactive drugs during EPS.** Cardioactive drugs can be used during EPS as diagnostic or therapeutic agents. The drugs most commonly used are isoproterenol, procainamide, atropine, and adenosine.

   A. **Isoproterenol** in doses ranging from 0.5 to 5 µg per kg per minute is used during EPS to facilitate induction of SVT and ventricular tachyarrhythmia.

   1. For patients with SVTs that are AV node dependent, isoproterenol facilitates conduction through the AV node by means of shortening its refractoriness.

   2. It is not absolutely certain how isoproterenol facilitates induction of ventricular tachycardia, but possible mechanisms include enhanced conduction, altered refractoriness, and enhanced automaticity related to delayed afterdepolarization.

   3. Isoproterenol is particularly useful in examinations of patients with exercise-induced ventricular tachycardia and patients with the special

type of RV outflow tract tachycardia. Isoproterenol is contraindicated in EPS of patients with critical coronary artery disease.

B. Procainamide is used less frequently during EPS. Among patients believed to have advanced underlying conduction disease, the response of the infranodal conduction system to procainamide infusion (10 to 15 mg/kg) is assessed during sinus rhythm and with atrial pacing.

    1. Considerable prolongation of the HV interval or induction of infranodal block with atrial pacing at cycle lengths longer than 400 msec is considered by many experts to be evidence of His-Purkinje disease. Procainamide can facilitate the induction of atrial and ventricular arrhythmias by means of slowing conduction.

    2. Procainamide often is used in examinations of patients with recurrent atrial fibrillation when programmed atrial stimulation is necessary. An example would be a patient with atrial flutter who is being evaluated for ablation and is easily induced into atrial fibrillation during programmed stimulation.

    3. Procainamide was widely used in the past for risk assessment among patients with inducible ventricular tachycardia. Studies have shown that patients with suppressible ventricular tachycardia have better long-term prognosis (lower rate of clinical recurrence and lower mortality) than those with nonsuppressible ventricular tachycardia. With the wide use of ICDs, however, and evidence of their superiority even among persons with suppressible ventricular tachycardia, this application of procainamide will be of historical interest.

C. Adenosine (6 to 18 mg) is used frequently in EPS of patients with supraventricular arrhythmias to define the mechanism of the tachycardia, establish AV node dependence, or document the presence or absence of accessory pathway conduction before and after RF ablation.

IX. Interpretation of findings in EPS

A. Bradyarrhythmia evaluation. EPS are not indicated when symptomatic bradycardia is documented. Among patients who have a clear indication for implantation of a permanent pacemaker, findings of EPS are unlikely to alter that decision. EPS, however, are more helpful to patients believed to have underlying **sinus node or conduction system disease and symptoms** but for whom noninvasive monitoring has failed to document a correlation between bradycardia and symptoms. EPS also are helpful to patients who continue to have symptoms after permanent pacemaker implantation.

    1. Baseline evaluation. Sinus bradycardia, sinus arrest with junctional or ventricular escape, various degrees of heart block, and intraventricular conduction delay, isolated or in various combinations, may occur among patients with bradycardia and can be evaluated by means of examination of the surface ECG.

        a. Conduction velocities are measured and evaluated. Disease in the AV node often produces prolongation in the AH interval, whereas disease in the infranodal conduction system produces prolongation in the HV interval.

        b. A long HV interval is suggestive but not diagnostic of an underlying bradyarrhythmia. It is commonly associated with wide QRS on surface ECG. A long HV interval at rest can be considered an indication for prophylactic pacemaker implantation (class IIa) if it exceeds 100 msec.

        c. Documented intermittent spontaneous infranodal block or infranodal block in response to atrial pacing (Fig. 44-5) or administration of procainamide also is an argument for implanting a permanent pacemaker.

    2. Programmed stimulation

        a. After baseline intervals are measured, **SNRT and SACT** are determined. SNRT is used to evaluate automaticity of the sinoatrial node.

        b. Rapid pacing causes overdrive suppression. Among patients with sinus node dysfunction, recovery time after cessation of pacing is

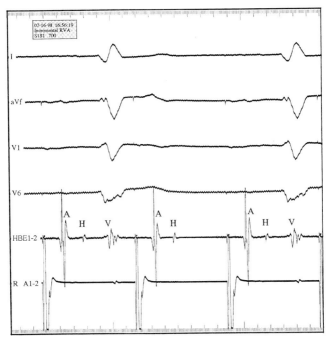

FIG. 44-5. Infrahisian block in response to slow atrial pacing. This tracing is from a 70-year-old man who presented with syncope. Baseline H-V was 110 msec. As shown in this tracing, burst pacing in the right atrium at cycle length of 700 msec resulted in intermittent infrahisian block (H deflections not followed by V). This patient had a dual chamber pacemaker implanted.

prolonged. The situation is similar to sudden termination of atrial fibrillation, which can be followed by a prolonged pause.

c. After cessation of pacing, the **longest SNRT at a particular pacing cycle length and secondary pauses** are documented. Secondary pauses are those that occur after the first escape beat. CSNRT, which is calculated by means of subtracting baseline cycle length from SNRT, is considered abnormal if it exceeds 550 msec.

d. **SACT** is used to evaluate conduction velocities in the atrium and in tissues surrounding the sinoatrial node. SACT is performed with the methods described earlier. A normal SACT is between 50 and 125 msec. When CSNRT and SACT both are normal, symptoms are uncommon. The sensitivities of CSNRT (54%) and SACT (51%) combined are higher (64%), and the specificity is approximately 88%. The low sensitivity of these tests limits their value in predicting future symptoms in a patient without symptoms.

e. **AV node and infranodal conduction system integrity** is tested with atrial stimulation techniques. Attention is paid to the AH and HV intervals during atrial pacing.

(1) The refractory period of the AV node is determined at two cycle lengths. The shortest 1:1 burst pacing cycle length also is determined.

(2) The normal AV nodal response to burst pacing at short cycle lengths is second-degree Mobitz I AV block. HV interval prolongation or infrahisian block is not typically observed. If

it occurs at cycle lengths longer than 400 msec, HV interval prolongation suggests significant underlying His-Purkinje disease.

    (3) Prolongation of the AV nodal refractory period is most frequently caused by high vagal tone or concomitant use of medications. It has no predictive or diagnostic value in evaluations of patients believed to have bradycardia. However, a long AV nodal refractory period may mask underlying abnormal His-Purkinje refractoriness, and enhancement of AV nodal conduction with atropine or isoproterenol may be necessary.

  3. Carotid sinus massage is performed on all patients undergoing evaluation of bradycardia or syncope.

    a. Firm pressure is applied over the carotid artery pulsation, behind the angle of the mandible.

    b. A **positive cardioinhibitory response** is present if pauses of 3 seconds or more occur. A vasodepressor response is present if blood pressure decreases more than 50 mm Hg in the absence of marked bradycardia.

    c. At least 70% of patients with a positive response have a cardioinhibitory response; 15% have a vasodepressor response. The others have a mixed response.

B. SVT evaluation. One of the most important elements in the evaluation of tachyarrhythmias is careful analysis of the surface ECG during clinical tachycardia. This can give several clues to the underlying diagnosis and make EPS more focused. Most SVTs that occur in the EPS laboratory are reentrant. They include AV nodal reentry tachycardia, orthodromic AV reentry tachycardia, atrial flutter, and reentrant atrial tachycardia. Automatic tachyarrhythmias are relatively uncommon except in acutely ill patients. They characteristically exhibit a warm-up phenomenon, are difficult to induce with extra stimulus techniques, and may be induced or accelerated with drugs such as isoproterenol.

  1. Baseline evaluation

    a. Resting ECG and intracardiac recordings can provide important information about a possible cause even before any tachycardia is induced. The presence of a short PR interval on the ECG and wide QRS complex suggests preexcitation.

    b. Absence of preexcitation at rest does not rule out the presence of an accessory pathway. For the diagnosis of SVT an atrial and a ventricular study have to be performed.

    c. If tachycardia is not induced at the baseline study, programmed stimulation in the atrium and ventricle are repeated with isoproterenol.

    d. Some SVTs, particularly those with a concealed bypass track, are more easily induced with ventricular stimulation, whereas atrial flutter and to a lesser extent atrial tachycardia rarely are induced by means of ventricular stimulation.

  2. Programmed stimulation begins with burst pacing in the ventricle to document and characterize VA conduction. Absence of VA conduction practically excludes a concealed bypass track, and ventricular extra stimulus technique is not performed unless ventricular tachycardia is suspected.

    a. Earliest retrograde atrial activity usually is seen on the His electrogram. Early retrograde atrial activity on the distal coronary sinus electrogram, if the position of the coronary sinus catheter position is correct, suggests the presence of a left-sided accessory pathway (see Fig. 44-4). Early atrial activity in the proximal coronary sinus electrodes suggests a posteroseptal pathway or AV node slow-pathway conduction.

      (1) Evidence of eccentric atrial activation may not be clear during burst pacing when there is fusion of retrograde impulses, arriving through the AV node and the accessory pathway.

(2) The retrograde 1:1 cycle length should be documented.

(3) Programmed ventricular stimulation is performed with single premature beats at two drive-train cycle lengths (eg., 600 and 400 msec). During programmed stimulation the following are recorded:

  (a) Retrograde refractory periods

  (b) The pattern and any change in the pattern of retrograde atrial activation

  (c) The site of retrograde VA block

  (d) The presence of dual retrograde AV node function

(4) If an accessory pathway is found, its retrograde 1:1 conduction cycle length and its refractory period are documented. With premature ventricular stimulation, retrograde VA block commonly occurs in the His-Purkinje system and not in the AV node. It is more likely to occur with longer drive-train cycle lengths.

b. During atrial stimulation particular attention is paid to the **AH and the HV intervals.**

(1) Sudden prolongation of A_2H_2 of more than 50 msec in response to a decrement of 10 msec in A_1A_2 is called a **jump** (Fig. 44-6). This is a sign of dual AV nodal function. This is not clinically equivalent to induction of AV nodal reentrant tachycardia.

(2) Induction of tachycardia generally depends on the occurrence of **critical block and conduction delay.** In the case of AV nodal reentry, antegrade block in the fast pathway combined with critical delay in the slow pathway allows the impulse to conduct retrograde on the fast pathway and excite the atrium. This first retrograde-conducted atrial depolarization is called an **echo beat** (See Fig. 44-6) If this echo beat succeeds in conducting antegrade down the slow pathway again and retrograde up the fast pathway, sustained AV nodal reentry occurs.

(3) **Induction of AV node reentry** is facilitated by use of shorter drive-train cycle lengths, if necessary by use of more than one extra stimulus, or by use of rapid burst atrial pacing.

(4) In the presence of an accessory pathway, the site of critical delay also is the AV node. However, to induce orthodromic AV reentry tachycardia, antegrade block has to occur in the accessory pathway (by means of pacing or concealment of the pathway) so that it is excitable by the time the impulse arrives to conduct back to the atrium (Fig. 44-7)

3. Evaluation of induced tachycardia

a. If a tachycardia is induced, the first reaction is to evaluate its **hemodynamic consequences.** Hemodynamically unstable tachycardia is immediately terminated. Only if the tachycardia is hemodynamically stable can further EPS be conducted.

(1) Whether the QRS is narrow or wide, the relation between atrial rate and ventricular rate is discerned, and AV association or dissociation is evaluated.

(2) Lack of a 1:1 AV relation excludes AV reentry tachycardia, and for practical purposes AV nodal reentry. In rare instances AV node reentry tachycardia can exhibit 2:1 AV block.

(3) If the atrial rate is faster than the ventricular rate with 2:1 or greater relation, the diagnosis is **atrial tachycardia or atrial flutter,** depending on the rate and pattern of atrial activation.

(4) If the ventricular rate is faster than the atrial rate the diagnosis is ventricular tachycardia.

b. When a **1:1 AV relation** exists, **further evaluation** is necessary. The following observations and techniques are helpful in arriving at the most likely mechanism:

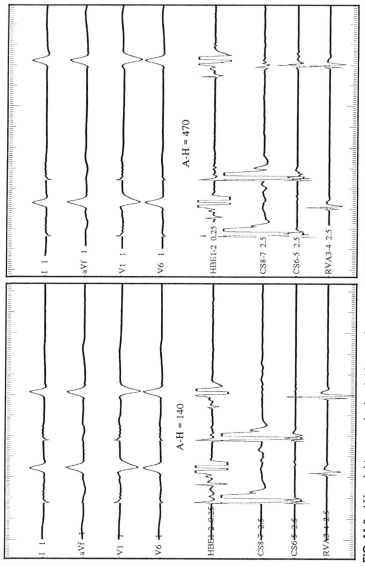

FIG. 44-6. AV nodal jump and echo. A 10 msec decrement in S1S2 resulted in marked prolongation of A2H2 by more than 300 msec. In addition, an echo beat with a short H-A is seen on the CS electrogram, a definite evidence of dual AV node physiology. The atrial premature beat blocked in the fast pathway with sufficient delay to encounter a non-refractory retrograde fast pathway.

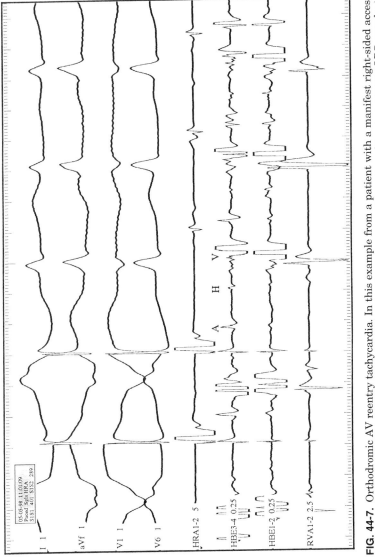

FIG. 44-7. Orthodromic AV reentry tachycardia. In this example from a patient with a manifest right-sided accessory pathway, premature atrial stimulation (S) blocks in the accessory pathway (resulting in a narrow QRS complex), conducts with a longer A-V, and re-excites the atrium. The tachycardia is narrow complex, with an H-A interval of 180 msec. The earliest A is seen on the HRA catheter.

577

(1) **Atrial activation.** The sequence of atrial activation during tachycardia is important in the differential diagnosis of SVT. Accurate placement of catheters is extremely important; catheter misplacement can lead to inappropriate conclusions or interventions. The **earliest A** in the distal coronary sinus electrogram suggests left atrial tachycardia or AV reentry with a left-sided concealed accessory pathway. If the accessory pathway is located in the posterior septum, the earliest A is seen in the proximal coronary sinus electrogram. This also is true if the atria are being activated through the slow pathway of the AV node.

(2) The presence of **cycle length variation** during tachycardia helps in prediction of activation sequence. For example, a change in AA coupling interval before an equal change in HH or VV interval (with changing VA) suggests a diagnosis of atrial tachycardia.

   (a) In cases of wide complex tachycardia in which there appears to be a 1:1 relation between H and V, HH interval change preceding VV interval change suggests supraventricular or BBR tachycardia.

   (b) Cycle length variation may also be helpful when there is **slowing of tachycardia with the development of bundle branch block and acceleration with resolution of the block.** This finding is diagnostic of AV reentry with an ipsilateral accessory pathway as the retrograde limb. This diagnosis can be made even on the surface ECG. On the intracardiac electrograms, this change in tachycardia cycle length is caused by prolongation of the VA interval. The activation wavefront must travel down the contralateral bundle and cross the intraventricular septum before it reaches the pathway. The change in cycle length is more pronounced with lateral than with septal pathways.

(3) **HA and VA intervals.** A constant HA or V relation despite cycle length variation (occurring in the absence of bundle branch block) is highly suggestive of **AV node reentry or accessory pathway mediated tachycardia.** The change in tachycardia cycle length is caused by changing conduction time through the AV node. The VA time can be used to differentiate AV nodal reentry from AV reentry. A VA interval less than 70 msec is rarely seen with AV reentry and strongly suggests the diagnosis of AV nodal reentry (Fig. 44-8) VA times in excess of 70 msec are seen with AV reentry and atypical AV nodal reentry (so-called fast-slow AV nodal reentry).

(4) **Introduction of premature beats during tachycardia.** Premature ventricular beats typically are introduced during tachycardia at a time when the His bundle is refractory. Because the normal retrograde path (His-AV node) is refractory, preexciting the atrium with a premature ventricular beat is diagnostic of the presence of an accessory pathway capable of retrograde conduction. Consistent termination of tachycardia with such premature beats without retrograde conduction to the atrium is diagnostic of AV reentry. An important clue to the presence of a second accessory pathway is a change in the retrograde atrial activation sequence with a premature ventricular beat when the His bundle is refractory. The introduction of a premature atrial beat is not as helpful.

(5) **Initiation and termination.** To understand the mechanism of tachycardia, it is important to know the mechanism of initi-

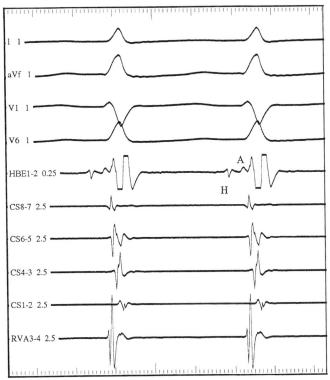

FIG. 44-8. AV node reentry tachycardia. Tachycardia is narrow complex, and is characterized by very short V-A interval and H-A interval less than 70 msec.

ation. For reentry to occur, block in one limb and slow conduction in the other limb must take place. It is important to review the stimulation sequences that did not induce tachycardia and compare them with those that induced tachycardia. A sudden jump in the AH interval suggests AV nodal reentry. Orthodromic AV reentry tachycardia develops during atrial stimulation after antegrade block in the accessory pathway takes place in combination with a critical delay in the AV node. With ventricular stimulation, AV reentry tachycardia develops when block in the distal AV node or His-Purkinje system occurs. Termination of the tachycardia in the AV node (A and no H or V on the His-bundle electrogram) suggests AV node dependence and is helpful in excluding AV node-independent tachycardia (atrial tachycardia and flutter).

4. **Significance of induced tachycardia.** With the exception of atrial fibrillation, induced reentrant supraventricular tachyarrhythmia signifies the presence of an established anatomic circuit. Comparison with the clinical arrhythmia is important, and unless significant differences exist, it can safely be assumed that the induced tachycardia is clinically significant. If a wide complex tachycardia with a supraventricular mechanism is induced, the recording is compared with a clinical recording. If the QRS structure is different between induced and clinical arrhythmias, a search for ventricular arrhythmia may be warranted.

   5. Atrial flutter, a special type of atrial tachycardia that involves a well-defined anatomic circuit, has become amenable to curative catheter ablation techniques.

   a. In the typical variety of atrial flutter, the waveform travels counterclockwise around the tricuspid annulus. The circuit is bounded anteriorly by the tricuspid annulus and posteriorly by the crista terminalis and its inferior medial continuation the eustachian ridge. The site of functional block appears to be in the isthmus region, which is the narrow corridor between the inferior tricuspid annulus and the eustachian ridge.

   b. To induce counterclockwise atrial flutter, progressively rapid (approximately 200 msec) burst pacing appears to be most successful and is performed anywhere medial to the isthmus. The impulses block in the isthmus and conduct counterclockwise around the tricuspid ring with sufficient delay to sustain atrial flutter. If burst pacing is used lateral to the isthmus, clockwise atrial flutter may be induced. Successful ablation of typical atrial flutter necessitates interruption of the flutter circuit by a lesion that spans from the posterior barrier to the anterior barrier.

C. Evaluation of accessory pathways

   1. The **most common locations** for accessory pathways in descending order of frequency are left free wall, posterior region, posteroseptal region, right free wall, and anteroseptal region. Concealed (no evidence of antegrade conduction) are more common than manifest pathways.

   a. Right-sided accessory pathways are more likely than left-sided accessory pathways to be associated with **congenital heart disease.**

   b. Multiple accessory pathways are more frequently encountered on the right side and in survivors of sudden death. In these patients the most frequent combination is posteroseptal and right free wall pathways. Rare types include atriofascicular accessory pathways, which originate in the right atrium, traverse the right anterior region of the tricuspid valve annulus, and insert in the region of the right bundle. These accessory pathways have unidirectional (antegrade) decremental conduction properties and cause the Mahaim type of preexcitation.

   c. Antidromic and orthodromic AV reentrant tachycardia both require participation of the accessory pathway. In rare instances tachycardia involves one accessory pathway antegrade and another retrograde.

   2. Evidence of preexcitation is supported by the presence of **short HV interval** (less than 35 msec) **at rest** or with atrial pacing, and the appearance of or increasing preexcitation with atrial pacing, administration of drugs, and autonomic maneuvers. The Electrophysiologic properties of the accessory pathway are examined, including its antegrade and retrograde conduction and refractory periods. If during atrial or ventricular stimulation tachycardia is induced, its mechanism is defined according to the techniques discussed earlier. This depends on whether the tachycardia is narrow or wide complex.

   3. Orthodromic AV reentry tachycardia is commonly initiated by a ventricular premature stimulus that blocks in the His-Purkinje system or AV node but conducts in a retrograde direction over the accessory pathway. It also can be induced by an atrial premature stimulus (echo beat) that blocks the accessory pathway and conducts slowly over the AV conducting system. Induction is facilitated by the presence of a relatively long accessory pathway antegrade refractory period, or a long His–Purkinje system–AV node retrograde refractory period.

   4. Antidromic AV reentry tachycardia (Fig. 44-9) can be initiated with burst pacing in the atrium or with a premature atrial stimulus that blocks in the AV node and conducts with delay over the accessory pathway. Less

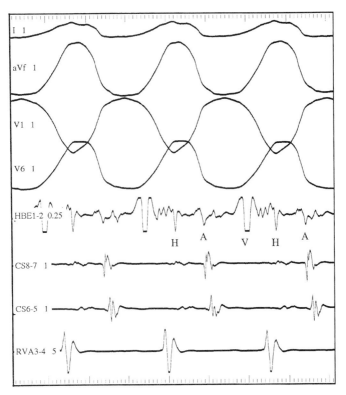

FIG. 44-9. Antidromic AV reentry tachycardia. This tachycardia was induced with atrial burst pacing in a young patient with two right-sided manifest accessory pathways. The tachycardia is rapid, wide-complex, with the earliest retrograde A seen in HBEI-2, consistent with retrograde activation through the AV node. AV node reentry with antegrade activation using the accessory pathway (bystanding accessory pathway) was excluded by lack of evidence of dual AV node physiology.

often it can be induced with a premature ventricular stimulus that blocks the accessory pathway in a retrograde manner and conducts over the AV node. Induction of antidromic tachycardia necessitates excellent retrograde conduction over the His–Purkinje system–AV node, almost always involves the free wall accessory pathway as the antegrade limb, and is frequently associated with the presence of multiple accessory pathways.

5. **Localizing accessory pathways**
   a. **Surface ECG localization**
      (1) **Delta wave vectors**
          (a) Left lateral –I and aVL, +II, III, aVF, +V_1–V_6
          (b) Left posterior wall +I and aVL, –II, III, aVF, +V_1–V_3/4
          (c) Posteroseptal +I and aVL, –II, III, aVF, R/S <1 in V_1
          (d) Right free wall +I and aVL, +II, –III, biphasic V_1 and V_2
          (e) Anteroseptal +I and aVL, +II > III, –V_1–V_6
      (2) **P-wave morphology during orthodromic tachycardia**
          (a) Left lateral –I and aVL, +III > aVF > II, –V5 and V_6
          (b) Posteroseptal +aVR > aVL, –II, III, aVF
          (c) Right free wall +I and aVL, +II, –III, biphasic V_1 and V_2

     b. Localization during EPS
- **(1)** Pacing from multiple atrial sites: shortest A-delta occurs with pacing close to the atrial insertion site of AP and results in maximal preexcitation.
- **(2)** Retrograde atrial activation during orthodromic tachycardia and V pacing
  - **(a)** Atrial activation sequence
    - **(i)** Left and right free wall: eccentric
    - **(ii)** Posteroseptal: A_{CSos} earlier than A_{His}
    - **(iii)** Anteroseptal: A_{CSos} later than A_{His}
  - **(b)** Atrial activation sequence when a ventricular premature stimulus is delivered during tachycardia at the time when His is refractory
  - **(c)** The earliest site of atrial activation identifies the site of atrial insertion of an accessory pathway
- **(3)** Relation of local ventricular electrogram to delta: earliest V correlates with ventricular insertion site
- **(4)** Effects of bundle branch block
  - **(a)** Bundle branch block increasing the VA interval and tachycardia cycle length by more than 35 msec followed by ipsilateral free wall accessory pathway
  - **(b)** With septal accessory pathways the increase in VA times is less than 25 msec
  - **(c)** Left anterior fascicular block can increase VA times 15 to 35 msec with left free wall accessory pathway, particularly with a superolateral left-sided accessory pathway
- **(5)** Recording of accessory pathway potential: sharp spike 10 to 30 msec before the onset of the delta wave

6. Diagnosing the presence of multiple accessory pathways
- **a.** Changing antegrade delta waves during sinus rhythm, atrial pacing, atrial fibrillation, and with antiarrhythmic drugs
- **b.** Evidence of multiple routes of retrograde atrial activation
  - **(1)** Changing VA time or activation sequence
  - **(2)** Failure to prolong VA time with ipsilateral bundle branch block
- **c.** Orthodromic tachycardia with antegrade fusion
- **d.** Preexcited tachycardia
  - **(1)** Antegrade conduction over septal accessory pathway
  - **(2)** Antidromic tachycardia faster than orthodromic tachycardia
- **e.** Atypical patterns of preexcitation
- **f.** Mismatch of site of antegrade preexcitation and retrograde atrial activation during AV reentry tachycardia

D. Ventricular tachycardia evaluation
1. Most patients referred for evaluation of ventricular arrhythmia have underlying **coronary artery disease or dilated cardiomyopathy.** The most common reason for performing EPS for these patients is documentation of inducible tachycardia, drug testing, testing the effect and response to antitachycardia pacing, and endocardial mapping to direct attempts at ablation. Rare patients have underlying normal LV function, and those typically have special types of ventricular arrhythmia. In general, however, the most common underlying mechanism is reentry. EPS are generally more reliable in inducing tachycardia and predicting risk among patients with underlying ischemic substrate.
2. An **atrial study** is considered for all patients undergoing evaluation of ventricular tachycardia. This serves three main purposes: diagnosis of underlying advanced conduction system disease, documentation of coexisting SVT, and induction of rare forms of ventricular tachycardia that may be inducible only with atrial pacing.
3. **Programmed ventricular stimulation** is performed as described earlier. If ventricular tachycardia is not induced despite program stimulation from two RV sites (RV apex and outflow tract), repeat stimulation

is performed after isoproterenol infusion. Isoproterenol should not, however, be given to patients with active ischemic heart disease. It is primarily of value to those with exercise- or catecholamine-dependent ventricular tachycardia. LV stimulation is not necessary because RV stimulation techniques have adequate sensitivity and specificity, and the risk of left heart catheterization is avoided. If no ventricular tachycardia is induced with any of these techniques, the arrhythmia is deemed noninducible.

4. **Techniques for terminating induced ventricular tachycardia.** Pacing terminates as many as 85% of instances of induced ventricular tachycardia in the laboratory. Success is more likely to be achieved with slower tachycardia rates (less than 200 beats/min) and in hemodynamically tolerated tachycardia. Other factors predictive of success of pacing include the site of stimulation in relation to the tachycardia zone, ventricular conduction properties, and refractoriness. Pacing also can accelerate tachycardia, an important consideration when antitachycardia pacing is being considered.

5. **Techniques for terminating tachycardia with pacing.** One technique entails use of one or more **progressively earlier premature ventricular stimuli.** The other technique uses **burst pacing** to overdrive the tachycardia but at a greater risk for accelerating it into a hemodynamically unstable arrhythmia. Techniques that can be used if pacing fails include delivery of ultrarapid train stimulation, and synchronized direct current cardioversion.

6. There are a variety of **responses to programmed stimulation.** What is important is the correlation between these responses in different populations of patients and future risk for adverse outcome. For example, induction of single or double bundle branch reentrant beats has no bearing on long-term outcome among persons with normal LV function and is not considered an abnormal finding. Induction of sustained monomorphic ventricular tachycardia, particularly among persons with poor LV function, identifies a subset of patients at high risk for sudden death.

   a. **Sustained monomorphic ventricular tachycardia**

      (1) Induction of sustained monomorphic ventricular tachycardia is the **most important response** and has the highest predictive value. This is particularly true if the induced tachycardia is similar to the clinical arrhythmia in both rate and structure. Patients with easily induced ventricular tachycardia, for example, with single premature beats, have worse outcome than those in whom tachycardia is more difficult to induce. It is important to document reproducibility of ventricular tachycardia during programmed stimulation. Slow, sustained tachycardia, particularly among patients with ischemic substrate, is more reproducible than more rapid tachycardia and among those with nonischemic etiologic factors. Sustained tachycardia has clearly worse prognostic implications than nonsustained tachycardia. There is no agreement on what constitutes an abnormal response among patients with nonsustained tachycardia or whether any therapeutic intervention should be pursued for these patients.

      (2) Among patients with ischemic substrate, programmed stimulation induces sustained monomorphic ventricular tachycardia in as many as 95% of patients with history of clinical sustained ventricular tachycardia, approximately 60% of those with nonsustained ventricular tachycardia, and approximately 50% of patients experiencing sudden cardiac death. Induction of sustained monomorphic ventricular tachycardia in any of the above subsets has very high specificity (more than 90%) for spontaneous clinical ventricular tachycardia and sudden death. Testing at two RV sites increases sensitivity without sacrificing specificity.

    (3) Patients with **nonischemic substrate** are more challenging to evaluate, because EPS are less sensitive and specific. Although patients with inducible sustained monomorphic ventricular tachycardia have a worse prognosis than those in whom tachycardia cannot be induced, the predictive value of abnormal results of EPS is approximately 70% at best. Patients with negative results of EPS are still at high risk for sudden death, even if they have no prior clinical events. The prognosis may be more favorable if inducible tachycardia is suppressed by drugs, but the risk of future events continues to be high. One can never be reassured about the outcome among patients with nonischemic cardiomyopathy using results of EPS.

    (4) BBR tachycardia is a type of ventricular tachycardia with a well-defined macro reentrant circuit. It occurs most often among patients with dilated cardiomyopathy and frequently is symptomatic.

        (a) In the **typical pattern,** the impulse travels antegrade down the right bundle branch, across the interventricular septum, and up the left bundle branch. The tachycardia exhibits a left bundle branch block pattern with a His deflection preceding every QRS complex. In sinus rhythm, the HV interval is abnormally long, and during tachycardia it is at least equal and frequently longer than the baseline HV.

        (b) In rare instances it is difficult to differentiate BBR tachycardia from an SVT with aberration or from a myocardial ventricular tachycardia with retrograde His deflections.

        (c) BBR tachycardia frequently is rapid and exhibits AV dissociation. If cycle length variation takes place, it is important to document where the leading change took place. If HH change takes place before VV change, BBR is likely. A VV change that occurs before HH change and causes variation in the HV interval suggests myocardial ventricular tachycardia. This tachycardia is recurrent and can cause frequent ICD discharges.

        (d) Treatment with **antiarrhythmic agents,** including amiodarone, is not helpful and may lead to stabilization of the reentrant circuit. BBR tachycardia is curable with RF ablation of the right bundle.

b. Polymorphic ventricular tachycardia frequently occurs with high-output stimulation. It also is more likely to occur with increasing numbers of extra stimuli.

    (1) Interpretation of the induction of polymorphic ventricular tachycardia depends on the clinical situation. For example, inducible polymorphic ventricular tachycardia in a survivor of sudden cardiac death is considered extremely important significant. In a patient with ventricular ectopy and normal ventricular function, inducible polymorphic ventricular tachycardia is a nonspecific response.

    (2) Similar interpretation applies to **induced ventricular fibrillation.** If the patient has never had clinical ventricular tachycardia or ventricular fibrillation and has no underlying heart disease, the induced ventricular fibrillation is considered a nonspecific finding that does not warrant therapy.

c. Patients with **hypertrophic cardiomyopathy** represent another subset for whom the predictive value of EPS is problematic. Induction of sustained monomorphic ventricular tachycardia, induction of ventricular fibrillation without aggressive stimulation protocols, or induction of ventricular arrhythmias with atrial pacing or as a result of atrial fibrillation are generally considered to be **poor prognostic signs.** In general, EPS are associated with higher risk to patients with hypertrophic cardiomyopathy, sometimes resulting in intractable ventricular fibrillation.

   d. Summary. It is important to have a thorough understanding of the underlying clinical problem and anatomic substrate to assess the appropriateness of and conclusions drawn from EPS of an individual patient.

     (1) Repetitive responses caused by BBR usually are physiologic, whereas intramyocardial repetitive ventricular responses are abnormal. However, neither of these responses should be used to guide therapy.

     (2) Induced polymorphic ventricular tachycardia and ventricular fibrillation can be considered nonspecific findings or clinically significant depending on the clinical circumstances. However, they should not be used to guide drug therapy in any situation.

     (3) Induced sustained monomorphic ventricular tachycardia identical to the clinical arrhythmia has the highest sensitivity and specificity and has greater importance in predicting outcome.

     (4) Suppression of ventricular tachycardia with drugs constitutes an acceptable and desirable end point. Changing the clinical features of ventricular tachycardia to a hemodynamically tolerated slower arrhythmia is a desirable end point and is predictive of reduction in future events.

     (5) The importance of nonsustained ventricular tachycardia remains controversial. Noninducibility in patients with nonischemic cardiomyopathy or survivors of sudden cardiac death may not provide prediction as accurate as that for patients with underlying ischemic substrate and documented ventricular tachycardia. Therapeutic decisions therefore have be individualized.

7. Mapping of ventricular tachycardia. Mapping of ventricular tachycardia involves identification of the **earliest sites of activation** during tachycardia and detailed outlining of the **tachycardia circuit.** Endocardial mapping has aided in the evaluation of mechanisms of tachycardia and provided the bases for surgical therapy. More recently, mapping has been coupled with RF ablation with high rates of success.

   a. Mapping can be performed with steerable electrode catheters during EPS or can involve introduction of specialized catheters with various configurations designed to compare several simultaneously acquired endocardial electrograms.

   b. For the most part, mapping of ventricular arrhythmias takes place in the left ventricle. However, several types of ventricular tachycardia that originate from the RV outflow tract have been successfully mapped and ablated.

   c. Activation mapping takes place during the tachycardia. The objective is to identify the site of earliest endocardial activation. Because this lengthy process has to take place during tachycardia, it must be hemodynamically tolerable. The earliest activation site corresponds to the exit site of the circuit.

   d. Sites of origin of tachycardia in patients with ischemic heart disease usually are found in the periinfarction zone or in the border of an LV aneurysm. To confirm the site, entrainment from that site is performed. Entrainment involves transient overdrive pacing without terminating the tachycardia. At successful sites, pacing produces QRS morphologic match on all 12 surface leads. The return cycle length after cessation of pacing (the first R-R interval) equals tachycardia cycle length (Fig. 44-10). These two observations imply that depolarizations caused by pacing have the same exit as the tachycardia and that the pacing site is within the circuit.

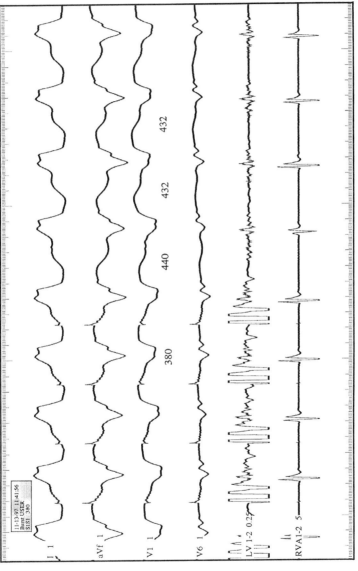

FIG. 44-10. Entrainment of ventricular tachycardia. Pacing at a rate slightly faster (380 msec) than tachycardia cycle length at a site believed to be the isthmus of the tachycardia resulted in concealed entrainment (concealed entrainment) in all 12 leads (only 4 leads are shown here). In addition, the post pacing interval is very close to the tachycardia cycle length, suggesting that the pacing site is within the tachycardia circuit. Application of radio-frequency energy at this site resulted in successful ablation of this tachycardia.

    e. Pace mapping can be used in evaluations of patients with hemo-dynamically intolerable tachycardia. Ventricular pacing is performed at various sites at rates that do not cause hemodynamic instability. The site where pacing results in QRS match with clinical tachycardia ECG findings corresponds to the critical area of the tachycardia circuit.

    f. Mapping can be performed intraoperatively when endocardial resection is considered.

SUGGESTED READINGS

References

1. Zipes DP, DiMarco JP, Gillette PC, et al. Guidelines for clinical intracardiac electrophysiological and catheter ablation procedures: a report of the American College of Cardiology/American Heart Association Task Force on Practice Guidelines (Committee on Clinical Intracardiac Electrophysiological and Catheter Ablation Procedures). *J Am Coll Cardiol* 1995;26:555–573.

2. Josephson ME, Maloney JD, Barold SS, et al. ACC Core Cardiology Training Symposium (COCATS): guidelines for training in adult cardiovascular medicine—training in specialized electrophysiology, cardiac pacing and arrhythmia management. *J Am Coll Cardiol* 1995;25:23–26.

Relevant Book Chapters

Josephson ME. *Clinical cardiac electrophysiology,* 2nd ed. Baltimore: William & Wilkins, 1993.

Vlay SC. *A practical approach to cardiac arrhythmias,* 2nd ed. Boston: Little, Brown, 1996.

Zipes D. *Cardiac EP from cell to bedside.* Philadelphia: Saunders, 1995.

45. CARDIAC PACING

Robert A. Schweikert and Navin Gupta

I. **Introduction.** The indications and technology of cardiac pacing continue to evolve. It is estimated that more than 400,000 pacemakers are implanted each year. As the number and complexity of pacemakers increase, physicians are more likely to encounter patients with pacemakers and contend with the potentially complicated problems they present. It is imperative that a physician caring for a patient who uses a pacemaker understand the basic physiologic and technologic principles of cardiac pacing.

II. **Basic components of cardiac pacemakers**
   A. **Pulse generator**
      1. **Power source (battery).** Lithium-iodine is by far the most common chemical compound used. It has more predictable behavior at the end of life of the battery.
      2. **Circuitry**
         a. **Output circuits** control programmable features of the output pulse, including amplitude and pulse width.
         b. **Sensing circuits** process the intracardiac electrogram, including amplification and filtering of the signal, and provide other functions such as management of external electromagnetic interference. A bandpass filter allows signals of a certain frequency range to be passed while signals of other frequency ranges are blocked or attenuated. Pacemakers use a bandpass filter to differentiate cardiac depolarization signals and repolarization or extracardiac signals.
         c. **Timing circuits** control the pacing intervals and sensing and refractory periods. They may be altered by input from the sensing circuits.
         d. **Telemetry circuits** allow communication between an external programmer and the pulse generator for applications such as pacemaker programming and retrieval of information.
         e. **Microprocessor.** Some pacemakers have computer chips with memory and therefore have enhanced capabilities, such as downloading of new features by means of telemetry and increased storage for diagnostic data.
         f. Sensor circuit for **rate-adaptive pacing**
   B. **Lead system**
      1. **Terminal pin.** The male portion of the proximal lead that connects to the pulse generator.
      2. **Lead body.** Consists of conductors and insulation. The conducting wire connects the stimulating and sensing electrodes to the terminal pin. The lead insulation is most commonly silicone rubber or a polyurethane material.
      3. Stimulating and sensing **electrodes**
      4. **Fixation device**
         a. **Passive fixation.** An attachment mechanism that anchors electrodes to the endocardial trabeculae. These types of leads have a higher rate of early dislodgment but a lower chronic capture threshold than active fixation leads.
         b. **Active fixation.** An attachment mechanism at the lead tip, such as a screw-in electrode, which actively secures the lead to the endocardium. These types of leads have a lower rate of early dislodgment and higher chronic capture threshold than passive fixation leads.
   C. **Lead-heart interface.** Site of energy transfer (pacing) and sensing functions.

III. Polarity. This refers to the electrode configuration of the pacing lead or the configuration of the pulse generator. Polarity may be unipolar or bipolar. Some pacemakers can be programmed to pace in one polarity and sense in another (only if a bipolar lead is present).

    A. Unipolar

        1. Configuration in which the **cathode (negative) is on the lead,** usually the lead tip, and the **anode (positive) is the pacemaker can**

        2. Results in a large sensing antenna

        3. Produces large pacemaker artifact (spikes) on an electrocardiogram (ECG) caused by the proximity of the circuit to ECG electrodes

        4. Advantages. Better sensing of premature ventricular contractions, low-amplitude signals, and shifted axis

        5. Disadvantages

            a. Oversensing of extraneous signals, especially pectoralis muscle activity (myopotentials)

            b. Skeletal muscle stimulation

            c. Large pacer spikes that occur on ECG may obscure native wave structure

    B. Bipolar

        1. Configuration in which the **electrodes are at the stimulating end of the lead**—the cathode (negative) at the distal tip and the anode (positive) at the proximal ring

        2. Smaller sensing antenna

        3. Smaller pacemaker artifact (spikes) on ECG

        4. Advantages

            a. Less myopotential oversensing

            b. Less skeletal muscle stimulation

            c. Smaller pacemaker artifact on ECG does not obscure native wave structure

        5. Disadvantages

            a. More complex lead design is more susceptible to malfunction and failure

            b. Small pacemaker artifact on ECG may be difficult to see

IV. Pacemaker classification. The Inter-Society Commission for Heart Disease Resources/NASPE/BPEG Generic Pacemaker Code (ICHD/NBG Code) is a five-position code developed by the North American Society of Pacing and Electrophysiology (NASPE) and the British Pacing and Electrophysiology Group (BPEG) (Table 45-1).

V. Indications for pacemaker implantation. The American College of Cardiology/American Heart Association Task Force on Practice Guidelines has recently published revised guidelines for pacemaker implantation (Table 45-2).

VI. Physiology of cardiac pacing

    A. Pulse generator output is determined by the output voltage and duration of the stimulating pulse (pulse width). Most implanted cardiac pacemakers work with constant voltage output (as opposed to most temporary cardiac pacemakers, which work with constant current output).

    B. Strength-duration relation. There is an exponential relation between the stimulus amplitude for myocardial stimulation and the pulse width such that there is a **rapidly rising strength-duration curve at pulse widths less than 0.25 msec** and a **flatter curve at pulse widths more than 1.0 msec.**

        1. Rheobase. The **flattened portion of the strength-duration curve** indicating the point at which increasing pulse width is no longer associated with a progressive decrease in stimulus amplitude (voltage) required for myocardial stimulation. In general the rheobase voltage is determined by means of assessing the threshold stimulus voltage at a pulse width of 2.0 msec.

        2. Chronaxie. The threshold pulse width at a stimulus amplitude that is twice the rheobase voltage. The chronaxie pulse duration approximates the point of minimal threshold energy on the strength-duration curve.

Table 45-1. NASPE/BPEG Generic Pacemaker Code

Position	I	II	III	IV	V
Category	Chamber(s) paced	Chamber(s) sensed	Response to sensing	Programmability, rate modulation	Antitachyarrhythmia function(s)
Letter	0 = none	0 = none	0 = none	0 = none	0 = none
	A = atrium	A = atrium	T = triggered	P = simple programmable	P = pacing (anti-tachyarrhythmia)
	V = ventricle	V = ventricle	I = inhibited	M = multiprogrammable	—
	D = dual (A + V)	D = dual (A + V)	D = dual (T + I)	C = communicating	S = shock
	—	—	—	R = rate-adaptive sensor	D = dual (P + S)
Manufacturers' designation only	S = Single (A or V)	S = Single (A or V)	—	—	—

NASPE, North American Society of Pacing and Electrophysiology; *BPEG*, British Pacing and Electrophysiology Group. From Bernstein AD, 1995, with permission.

Table 45-2. Indications for Cardiac Pacing

Indication	Class I	Class II	Class III
Sinus node dysfunction (SND)	1. SND documented in association with symptomatic bradycardia and caused by irreversible factors or essential drug therapy 2. Symptomatic chronotropic incompetence	IIa: No clear association between SND (with heart rate <40 beats/min) and symptoms can be documented IIb: When minimally symptomatic, chronic heart rate <30 beats/min while awake	1. SND with marked sinus bradycardia or pauses but no associated symptoms, including those caused by long-term drug therapy 2. SND in patients with symptoms suggestive of bradycardia that are clearly documented as not associated with a slow heart rate 3. SND with symptomatic bradycardia due to nonessential drug therapy

Acquired atrioventricular (AV) block	1. Third-degree AV block at any anatomic level associated with any one of the following conditions:
	  a. Bradycardia with symptoms presumed to be caused by AV block
	  b. Arrhythmias and other medical conditions that necessitate use of drugs that cause symptomatic bradycardia
	  c. Documented periods of asystole ≥ 3.0 sec or any escape rate < 40 beats/min in awake patients without symptoms
		IIa:
		1. Asymptomatic third-degree AV block at any anatomic site with average awake ventricular rates ≥ 40 beats/min
		2. Asymptomatic type II second-degree AV block
		3. Asymptomatic type I second-degree AV block at intra- or infra-His levels found incidentally at electrophysiologic study performed for other indications
		4. First-degree AV block with symptoms suggestive of pacemaker syndrome and documented alleviation of symptoms with temporary AV pacing
			1. Asymptomatic 1° AV block
			2. Asymptomatic type I 2° AV block at the supra-His (AV node) level or not known to be intra- or infra-Hisian
			3. AV block expected to resolve and unlikely to recur (e.g., drug toxicity, Lyme disease)

continued

591

Table 45-2. *continued*

Indication	Class I	Class II	Class III
	d. After catheter ablation of the AV junction e. Postoperative AV block that is not expected to resolve f. Neuromuscular diseases with AV block such as myotonic muscular dystrophy, Kearns-Sayre syndrome, Erb's atrophy (limb-girdle), and peroneal muscular dystrophy 2. Second-degree AV block regardless of type or site of block with associated symptomatic bradycardia	IIb: Marked first-degree AV block (>0.30 sec) in patients with left ventricular dysfunction and symptoms of congestive heart failure in whom shorter AV interval results in hemodynamic improvement, presumably by decreasing left atrial filling pressure	
Post–myocardial infarction	1. Persistent second-degree AV block in the His-Purkinje system with bilateral bundle branch block or third-degree AV block within or below the His-Purkinje system after acute myocardial infarction 2. Transient advanced (second or third degree) infranodal AV block and associated bundle branch block. If the site of block is uncertain, an electrophysiologic study may be necessary 3. Persistent and symptomatic second- or third-degree AV block	IIa: None IIb: 1. Persistent second- or third-degree AV block at the AV node level	1. Transient AV block without intraventricular conduction defect 2. Transient AV block in the presence of isolated left anterior fascicular block 3. Acquired left anterior fascicular block in the absence of AV block 4. Persistent first-degree AV block in the presence of bundle branch block that is old or age indeterminate

Chronic bifascicular and trifascicular Block	1. Intermittent third-degree AV block 2. Type II second-degree AV block	IIa: 1. Syncope not proved to be caused by AV block when other likely causes have been excluded, specifically ventricular tachycardia (VT) 2. HV interval >100 msec 3. Pacing induced block below the His' bundle that is not physiologic IIb: None
Carotid sinus hypersensitivity (Carotid sinus irritability) and neurally mediated syncope	1. Recurrent syncope caused by carotid sinus stimulation; minimal carotid sinus pressure induces ventricular asystole longer than 3 sec in the absence of any medication that depresses the sinus node or AV conduction	IIa: 1. Recurrent syncope without clear, provocative events and with a hypersensitive cardioinhibitory response 2. Syncope of unexplained origin when major abnormalities of sinus node function or AV conduction are discovered or provoked in electrophysiologic studies IIb: Neurally mediated syncope with marked bradycardia reproduced by a head-up tilt with or without isoproterenol and other provocative maneuvers	1. A hyperactive cardioinhibitory response to carotid sinus stimulation in the absence of symptoms 2. A hyperactive cardioinhibitory response to carotid sinus stimulation in the absence of symptoms 3. A hyperactive cardioinhibitory response to carotid sinus stimulation in the presence of vague symptoms such as dizziness, lightheadedness, or both 4. Recurrent syncope, lightheadedness, or dizziness in the absence of a hyperactive cardioinhibitory response 5. Situational vasovagal syncope in which avoidance behavior is effective

continued

Table 45-2. *continued*

Indication	Class I	Class II	Class III
Termination of tachyarrhythmias	1. Symptomatic recurrent supraventricular tachycardia (SVT) that is reproducibly terminated by pacing after drugs and catheter ablation fail to control the arrhythmia or produce intolerable side effects 2. Symptomatic recurrent sustained VT as part of an automatic defibrillator system	IIa: None IIb: 1. Recurrent SVT or atrial flutter that is reproducibly terminated by pacing as an alternative to drug therapy or ablation	1. Tachycardias frequently accelerated or converted to fibrillation by pacing 2. The presence of accessory pathways with the capacity for rapid anterograde conduction whether or not the pathways participate in the mechanism of the tachycardia
Prevention of tachycardia	Sustained pause-dependent VT with or without prolonged QT in which the efficacy of pacing is thoroughly documented	IIa: High risk with congenital long QT syndrome IIb: 1. AV reentrant or AV node reentrant SVT not responsive to medical or ablative therapy 2. Prevention of symptomatic, drug-refractory, recurrent atrial fibrillation	1. Frequent or complex ventricular ectopic activity without sustained VT in the absence of the long QT syndrome 2. Long QT syndrome of reversible causes

Class I, Conditions for which there is evidence or general agreement that pacing is beneficial, useful, and effective; *Class II*, conditions for which there is conflicting evidence or a divergence of opinion about the usefulness or efficacy of pacing; *IIa*, weight of evidence or opinion is in favor of usefulness or efficacy; *IIb*, usefulness or efficacy is less well established with evidence or opinion; *Class III*, conditions for which there is evidence or general agreement that pacing is not useful or effective and in some cases may be harmful.
From Gregoratos G, 1998, with permission.

C. **Safety margins**
   1. **Voltage.** The voltage output is programmed to a level that is approximately twice the capture (stimulation) threshold for a 2:1 output safety margin.
   2. **Pulse width.** The pulse duration is programmed to a level approximately three times the pulse-width capture threshold for a 3:1 output safety margin. The typical range for pulse width is 0.2 1.0 msec.

D. **Temporal changes in stimulation threshold.** The stimulation threshold typically rises within 24 hours after implantation of a permanent pacemaker lead. The threshold peaks 1 to 2 weeks after implantation. It gradually declines and plateaus approximately 6 weeks after implantation at a level less than the acute peak but greater than the level measured at implantation. The absolute value of the temporal changes in stimulation thresholds varies among individuals and between various types of electrodes.

VII. **Pacemaker timing cycles and intervals**

A. A pacemaker can be thought of as a series of timing circuits. An understanding of how these timing circuits interact can facilitate analysis of pacemaker rhythms. The timing circuit runs until the cycle is completed or until it is reset. Completion of a timing cycle causes release of a pacing output or the initiation of another timing cycle. Figure 45-1 illustrates the basic timing cycles and intervals for a dual-chamber pacemaker. The basic terms and abbreviations used for the pacemaker timing cycles and refractory periods are defined in the glossary (**XVI.**).

B. **Base rate behavior**
   1. **Single-chamber pacemakers** have a timing circuit that is either inhibited (reset) by a sensed native heartbeat or completes its cycle with a stimulus output.
   2. **Dual-chamber pacemakers** are somewhat more complex and incorporate more timing circuits. Figure 45-1 illustrates the timing cycles of a dual-chamber pacemaker in DDD mode. In general base rate (lower rate) pacing for dual-chamber pacemakers involves two timing circuits, as follows:
      a. The first timing circuit is the interval from a ventricular sensed or paced event to an atrial paced event (**atrial escape interval [AEI]**).
      b. The second timing circuit is the interval from an atrial sensed or paced event to a ventricular paced event (**AV interval [AVI]**). An atrial sensed event that occurs before the AEI is complete terminates that interval and initiation of the AVI.
   3. The response of a dual-chamber pacemaker to a sensed ventricular signal varies among manufacturers. Some pacemakers have a ventricle-based timing system and others have an atrium-based timing system.
      a. **Ventricle-based timing.** In this type of pacemaker timing system, the AEI is fixed. A ventricular sensed event during the AEI resets the timing circuit. A ventricular sensed event during an AVI terminates that interval and initiates the AEI.
      b. **Atrium-based timing.** In this type of pacemaker timing system, the AA interval is fixed. A ventricular sensed event during the AEI will reset the AA timing circuit and add the programmed AVI. A ventricular sensed event during the AVI will inhibit a ventricular output but will not alter the AA interval.
   4. **Interpretation of pacemaker rhythm** that has ventricular sensed beats requires knowledge of the type of timing system the pacemaker uses. Ventricle-based and atrium-based timing systems both are analyzed by means of measuring backward from an atrium-paced event. The **point of ventricular sensing** for a **ventricle-based** timing system is the point before the atrial-paced event that is equal to the AEI. For an **atrium-based timing system,** the measurement before the atrium-paced event is the point that is equal to the AA interval. Knowledge of these principles allows one to evaluate the ventricular sensing of a

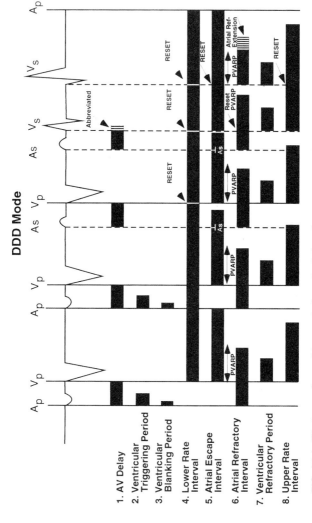

FIG. 45-1. Timing cycles and intervals for a dual-chamber pacemaker. See text for discussion. Modified from Barold SS, 1988, with permission.

DDD Mode

1. AV Delay
2. Ventricular Triggering Period
3. Ventricular Blanking Period
4. Lower Rate Interval
5. Atrial Escape Interval
6. Atrial Refractory Interval
7. Ventricular Refractory Period
8. Upper Rate Interval

A_p V_p A_p V_p As V_p As V_s V_s A_p

PVARP

PVARP

As

PVARP

RESET

RESET

As

RESET

Abbreviated

RESET

RESET

Reset PVARP

RESET

Atrial Ref-Extension

PVARP

given pacemaker. Some pacemakers have incorporated modifications of these systems that take advantage of features of both timing systems (e.g., a pacemaker with an atrium-based timing system may behave as a ventricle-based timing system).

C. Upper rate behavior
1. As sinus rate accelerates, the sensed atrial events terminate the AEI and initiate the AVI. The result is **P-wave synchronous ventricular pacing** (unless the PR interval is shorter than the PV interval, in which case pacing is fully inhibited).
2. The maximum atrial rate that a dual-chamber pacemaker can sense is determined by the **total atrial refractory period (TARP).** The TARP comprises the AVI and the postventricular atrial refractory period (PVARP). When the native atrial intervals become shorter than the TARP as the sinus rate accelerates, some atrial events are not sensed. An abrupt, fixed block occurs as the pacemaker only intermittently senses the P waves. Symptoms may occur as the rate drops precipitously.
3. **Maximum tracking rate interval (MTRI)** or upper rate limit (URL) is an additional timing circuit designed to avoid abrupt block at upper pacing rates.
   a. The MTRI Works in conjunction with the AVI to determine the highest ventricular pacing rate that can be achieved in response to atrial sensed events.
   b. A sensed atrial event initiates the AVI and the MTRI. If the AVI completes its cycle and the MTRI also has completed its cycle, ventricular output occurs at the programmed AV interval. If the AVI completes its cycle and the MTRI has not completed its cycle, ventricular output is delayed until the MTRI has timed out. This prolongs the PV interval and allows continued tracking of the atrial rate. However, the longer PV interval also places ventricular output closer to the following P wave. If the sinus rate accelerates to a sufficient rate, the delayed ventricular output may cause the following P wave to fall within the PVARP and not be sensed. The result is an intermittent dropped beat and a pause similar to the Wenckebach phenomenon. Newer pacemakers may incorporate features designed to limit the degree of fixed block at the upper rate limit, such as rate smoothing (adjustment of the AEI as PV interval changes) and rate-responsive AV delay. However, fixed block at the upper rate limit may still occur, particularly if the device is suboptimally programmed.

VIII. Rate-adaptive pacing
A. The primary goal of rate-adaptive pacing is to **emulate the function of the sinus node** for patients with chronotropic incompetence or atrial arrhythmias that preclude reliable sensing of native sinoatrial rhythm.
B. Primary **components** of rate-adaptive pacemaker system
1. A **sensor** located in the pacing lead or pacemaker itself that detects a physical or physiologic value that is directly or indirectly related to metabolic demand.
2. **Rate-modulating circuitry** within the pacemaker that contains an algorithm that translates a change in the sensed parameter to a change in pacing rate.
3. Algorithm **programming capability** such that a physician can make adjustments to accommodate the heart rate requirements of the individual patient.
C. **Basic technical categories of pacemaker sensors** (Table 45-3). **Motion sensors** are most commonly used because of their simplicity, speed of response, and compatibility with standard unipolar and bipolar pacing leads. Other sensors are more physiologically correct but may necessitate use of technically complex pacing leads. Of the physiologic sensors, only the minute ventilation type is widely available.

IX. Automatic mode switching

A. Definition. Automatic mode switching is the programmable response of a dual-chamber pacemaker during an atrial tachyarrhythmia designed to avoid nonphysiologic ventricular pacing caused by atrial tracking.

B. The device switches from DDD mode to a VVI mode, usually with a gradual reduction in pacing rate. The device switches back to the DDD mode after atrial tachyarrhythmia resolves.

X. Pacemaker implantation: pertinent issues for the physician

A. Preoperative issues. Several issues must be addressed in the care of a patient scheduled for routine pacemaker implantation.

    1. History and physical examination. Attention is given to any findings that may affect the site and approach for pacemaker implantation, such as the patient's hand dominance (pacemakers usually implanted on side opposite the dominant hand), presence of congenital abnormalities (e.g., anomalous venous drainage), presence of central venous lines, presence of tricuspid valve disease, and whether the patient has undergone valve surgery.

    2. Informed consent (risks, benefits and alternatives)

    3. Preprocedure data

        a. Posteroanterior and lateral chest radiograph

        b. 12-lead ECG

        c. Blood tests: serum electrolytes, complete blood cell count, creatinine, and prothrombin and partial thromboplastin times

    4. Medications

        a. Warfarin is discontinued at least 3 days before the procedure. Admission to the hospital for intravenous **heparin** administration is considered if the risk of discontinuation of anticoagulation is high. Heparin may be discontinued 4 to 6 hours before the procedure.

        b. Dosage of oral hypoglycemic agents or insulin may have to be adjusted.

    5. Patient preparation

        a. The patient takes **nothing by mouth** for at least 6 to 8 hours before the procedure. Intravenous hydration may be indicated.

        b. A peripheral intravenous catheter is particularly helpful if placed in the arm ipsilateral to the proposed pacemaker site so that a venogram can be obtained in the event of difficulty with venous access during pacemaker implantation.

        c. The patient is **shaved and washed** with povidone-iodine solution in the area from above the nipple line to the angle of the jaw and from sternum to axillary line on the side of the implantation site.

        d. Antibiotic prophylaxis before pacemaker implantation is controversial, and various prospective studies have provided conflicting information. Some centers have advocated antibiotic prophylaxis with an agent active against staphylococcus for patients at high risk for endocarditis, such as patients with prosthetic valves or complex congenital heart disease, or for redo procedures, prolonged or potentially contaminated procedures. Other centers use antibiotic prophylaxis routinely.

B. Postoperative issues

    1. General recommendations. Most patients are admitted for overnight observation by means of telemetry after pacemaker implantation.

    2. Posteroanterior and lateral **chest radiographs** are obtained to document the position of the pacemaker leads and connection of the terminal pins to the pulse generator. The radiograph also is examined for evidence of pneumothorax, pericardial effusion, or pleural effusion.

    3. Resuming anticoagulation. Intravenous heparin may be resumed 8 to 12 hours after the procedure with avoidance of a heparin bolus. Warfarin may be reinstituted as early as the evening after the procedure. Anticoagulation is not aggressive in the early postimplantation period because of risk for the development of pacemaker pocket hematoma.

Table 45-3. Sensors in rate-responsive pacing

Methods	Physiologic Measurements	How it works	Advantages	Disadvantages
Impedance sensing	Respiratory rate Minute ventilation Stroke volume	Impedance plethysmography	Highly physiologic Highly proportional to metabolic demand	Delayed response Susceptible to electrode motion artifact
Ventricular evoked response Output pulse sensing	Evoked QT interval (stim-T interval)	Reflects catecholamines	More physiologic	Requires ventricular pacing
Vibration, acceleration, gravitation, motion sensing	Body movement	Piezoelectric element	Rapid response No special lead needed	Nonphysiologic and nonspecific Late plateau response
Special sensors on pacing electrode	Central venous temperature[a] dp/dt[b] Mixed venous oxygen saturation[b]	Thermistor Piezoelectric element Optical sensor	More physiologic	Complex lead

[a] No longer produced, although still in use in Japan (dp/dt, ratio of change in pressure to change in time).
[b] Available only in clinical trials.
Modified from Lau C, 1995, with permission.

4. Pacemaker evaluation

  a. Evaluation in the pacemaker clinic before discharge includes assessment of pacing and sensing thresholds and of lead impedance. The pacemaker is programmed to optimize hemodynamic values and minimize battery expenditure.

  b. Capture thresholds are expected to rise over the first 2 to 6 weeks after implantation. The pacemaker is programmed with an adequate safety margin to account for these changes.

  c. Rate adaptation for activity-sensing pacemakers may be programmed according to informal (e.g., hallway walking) or formal (e.g., treadmill) exercise testing.

5. Discharge planning

  a. Discharge instructions usually include patient education regarding the recognition of pacemaker pocket complications such as signs of infection, bleeding, or hematoma. The patient is generally advised to avoid heavy lifting or vigorous activity (especially forceful abduction) with the arm ipsilateral to the implantation site.

  b. The patient is provided with literature regarding the pacemaker, including a wallet card identifying the manufacturer of the pacemaker and leads, model numbers, and serial numbers.

  c. The patient may be provided with and instructed in the use of a transtelephonic monitoring system for remote evaluation of the pacemaker.

  d. Endocarditis prophylaxis is not recommended for patients with pacemakers according to American Heart Association guidelines.

XI. Common pacemaker problems

A. Acute complications of pacemaker implantation

1. Pneumothorax (hemothorax)

  a. This complication may be asymptomatic and detected only on a chest radiograph. The diagnosis is considered for a patient with dyspnea or pleuritic chest pain after implantation.

  b. A small pneumothorax may resolve without intervention. However, severe symptoms, a pneumothorax greater than 10%, or expanding or persistent pneumothorax often necessitate placement of a chest tube.

2. Pacemaker pocket hematoma

  a. This is one of the most common complications of pacemaker implantation and often is caused by small-vessel venous bleeding inside the pacemaker pocket. Bleeding also may arise from arterial vessels or retrograde flow of venous blood along the pacemaker leads into the pocket.

  b. Signs and symptoms include pain, swelling, and sometimes bleeding at the pocket site.

  c. Small hematomas may be managed conservatively with elevation (head of bed 45 degrees or more) and analgesics. Larger or expanding hematomas may necessitate use of a pressure dressing. The patient is positioned on the side contralateral to the pacemaker site. Large hematomas may compromise the integrity of the incision site and cause dehiscence. The patient may need urgent surgical exploration and hematoma evacuation in the electrophysiologic studies laboratory or operating room.

  d. Percutaneous insertion of a needle to drain a hematoma increases risk for infection and is to be avoided.

3. Cardiac or central venous perforation. Perforation may cause pericardial effusion and cardiac tamponade. It is suspected when a patient has chest pain, pericardial friction rub, or hypotension after pacemaker implantation. A chest radiograph may reveal an enlarged cardiac silhouette or an extracardiac lead tip. A change in paced ventricular morphologic features, particularly a right bundle branch pattern, may indicate

migration of the ventricular lead. A patient in hemodynamically unstable condition who has tamponade may need urgent pericardiocentesis and drainage of the effusion.

4. **Diaphragmatic stimulation.** Stimulation of the **left diaphragm** may occur with a pacing lead at the right ventricular apex, particularly at high pacing outputs. The possibility of **cardiac perforation** is considered. Stimulation of the **right diaphragm** may be caused by stimulation of the right phrenic nerve by a displaced atrial lead. Reduction in the pacemaker output voltage or lead repositioning may be necessary.

5. **Local muscular stimulation** may occur with a unipolar pacemaker configuration, particularly if the pulse generator is positioned upside down within the pocket (anode directly in contact with the pectoralis muscle). Fracture of a pacing lead may cause leakage of current into the surrounding tissue and local muscle stimulation.

6. **Pacemaker malfunction**
   a. The pulse generator may be defective or be damaged at the time of implantation (e.g., by electrocautery or direct-current defibrillation).
   b. Improper fixation of the terminal pins of the pacing leads into the pulse generator (e.g., loose set screws) may cause complete or intermittent pacemaker malfunction.

7. **Lead dislodgment or damage**
   a. Pacing leads may become dislodged soon after implantation before the lead has a chance to become fixed through clotting and fibrosis. Lead dislodgment may be suspected if noncapture and under- or oversensing is detected at telemetry or on an ECG. It is confirmed by means of chest radiography or formal pacemaker testing.
   b. The lead may be damaged at the time of implantation, for example through forceful handling or excessively tight retention sutures.
   c. Damage to a lead may change impedance. A break in the insulation of the lead causes low impedance, whereas fracture of the lead conductor causes high impedance.

B. **Chronic complications of pacemaker implantation**
   1. **Pacemaker system infection**
      a. The reported incidence of pacemaker infection is 0% to 19%. The infection may involve only the pacemaker pocket or the entire system with subsequent life-threatening sepsis. There is a higher incidence with repeat operations (e.g., pulse generator replacement). Causative organisms tend to be skin flora such as *Staphylococcus* species.
      b. Treatment includes intravenous antibiotics; however, antibiotic therapy rarely eradicates the infection unless the pacemaker system is removed. The timing of system removal depends on the clinical status of the patient. Prolonged delays, however, are to be avoided.
   2. **Intravascular thrombosis or obstruction**
      a. Initial treatment may include heat and upper extremity elevation. Symptomatic thrombosis of the subclavian or axillary veins may necessitate anticoagulation or systemic thrombolytic therapy. Subsequent therapy may include aspirin or warfarin.
      b. Superior vena caval stenosis or occlusion may necessitate percutaneous balloon dilation or surgical consultation for consideration of repair.
   3. **Twiddler syndrome** is a situation in which a patient, perhaps unwittingly, turns the pacemaker within the pocket. The leads may become twisted and cause excessive traction on the leads and withdrawal from the heart.

XII. **Pacemaker system malfunction**

A. In the evaluation of a patient with suspected pacemaker malfunction, it is important to **interpret the ECG carefully.** Intracardiac tracings obtained by means of telemetric communication with the pacemaker ideally are used for interpretation. **Pacing artifacts or spikes** are a high-frequency signal and often are filtered out by newer digital surface ECG machines. Pacing artifacts from bipolar leads also are smaller and more difficult to see than artifacts from unipolar leads. It may be necessary to record multiple leads or use an older analog recorder to clearly see the pacing artifact. **Pseudo-malfunction** occurs when recording and digital artifacts are misinterpreted. A systematic approach to the ECG of patients who use pacemakers helps to determine the appropriateness of pacing.

B. **General evaluation for possible pacemaker malfunction**
   1. If a recent pacemaker interrogation is available, **review the programmed values** for the pacemaker, particularly the mode, base rate, upper rate limit, intervals, and the presence of other features such as automatic mode switching.
   2. Obtain a **12-lead ECG** and evaluate the following:
      a. Determine whether **pacing stimulus artifacts** are present. If they are, determine whether the appropriate chambers are captured.
      b. If pacing stimulus artifacts are absent: Is **native depolarization** present that is properly timed to explain the absence?
      c. Evaluate **native beats** in relation to paced complexes: Are native beats appropriately sensed?
      d. Evaluate the **timing cycles of a dual-chamber pacemaker** by means of measuring backward from an atrial paced event (see **VII.B.3.**).

C. Patients with pacemaker system malfunction generally exhibit absence of a pacing stimulus artifact, failure to capture, or failure to sense.
   1. **Failure of pacemaker stimulus output.** A differential of the more common causes of pauses during a paced rhythm follows. Application of a **magnet** over the pacemaker should cause asynchronous pacing. If the pauses resolve with application of the magnet, the diagnosis of oversensing is most likely. If the pauses do not resolve, one of the other causes is considered.
      a. **Pulse generator failure**
      b. **Lead failure**
         (1) Lead failure can be caused by loosening of the set screw or terminal pin disconnection, lead conductor failure, or lead insulation failure.
         (2) Suspicion of lead malfunction prompts **chest radiography.** The radiograph may reveal that the terminal pin is not situated properly within the header of the pulse generator or demonstrate a defect in the lead insulation or conductor coil. A substantial increase in lead impedance suggests lead conductor failure. A significant decrease in lead impedance suggests lead insulation failure.
      c. **Oversensing**
         (1) Electromagnetic interference (EMI)
         (2) Myopotentials
         (3) Cross talk
         (4) T-wave oversensing
      d. **Pseudomalfunction**
         (1) Absence of bipolar spike
         (2) Normal pacing functions such as hysteresis or automatic mode switching
   2. **Failure to capture**
      a. **Elevated capture threshold**
         (1) Electrolyte disturbance (e.g., hyperkalemia, acidemia)
         (2) Antiarrhythmic drugs (particularly class IC agents such as flecainide)
         (3) Myocardial fibrosis (e.g., cardiomyopathy, myocardial infarction)

b. Lead malfunction
   (1) Lead fracture. A break in the lead insulation usually decreases impedance, whereas a break in the conductor increases impedance.
   (2) Lead dislodgment or perforation may change paced morphologic features, especially a change from left bundle to right bundle branch structure.

c. Exit block is failure of the pacing output at the distal electrode to stimulate adjacent myocardium. This is often caused by the inflammatory reaction that occurs at the pacemaker lead tip at the time of implantation. It occurs in approximately 5% of cases and may be managed with systemic steroids. Some pacing leads have steroid-eluting electrodes designed to minimize the degree of inflammation at the electrode tip and decrease the incidence of exit block.

d. Latency is the delay between the delivery of an output pulse and the onset of electric systole, as occurs with severe electrolyte disturbances.

e. Pseudomalfunction
   (1) Artifact
   (2) Refractory periods

3. Failure to sense
   a. Lead dislodgment usually is accompanied by failure to capture (see **XII.C.2.**).
   b. Lead insulation failure (see **XII. C.1.b.**)
   c. Inadequate endocardial signal
   d. Change in electrogram
      (1) Transient changes caused by electrolyte or acid-base disturbance
      (2) Permanent changes caused by myocardial infarction or cardiomyopathy
   e. Ectopic beats
   f. Pulse generator failure (sensing circuits)
   g. Functional undersensing, which is undersensing that is caused by normal pacemaker function, such as refractory periods, blanking periods, or safety pacing

D. Other pacemaker malfunctions
   1. Pacemaker syndrome is signs and symptoms caused by inadequate timing of atrial and ventricular contractions. Pacemaker syndrome is commonly caused by retrograde ventriculoatrial (VA) conduction, which causes atrial contraction against closed mitral and tricuspid valves. Pacemaker syndrome also may occur during exercise-induced atrial arrhythmia caused by loss of AV synchrony when a device with an automatic mode-switching feature converts to VVI pacing.

   2. Pacemaker-mediated tachycardia (PMT) is paced tachycardia sustained by the continued active participation of the pacemaker in the rhythm. The resultant wide-complex (paced) tachycardia may appear, at first glance, to be ventricular tachycardia, especially for pacemakers with bipolar leads; the pacing artifact may be difficult to discern on an ECG tracing.
      a. One form of PMT is the rapid ventricular pacing that occurs as a dual-chamber pacemaker attempts to track the rapid atrial rate during an atrial tachyarrhythmia.
      b. Another form of PMT occurs when there is oversensing in the atrial channel, such as myopotentials.
      c. Endless-loop tachycardia (ELT) is a form of PMT in which a repetitive sequence of sensing of retrograde atrial activity triggers a ventricular paced beat at the end of the MTRI. ELT needs a trigger for initiation, which may be any event that causes AV dissociation and

allows retrograde (VA) conduction to occur after a native or paced ventricular beat. The trigger may be a premature ventricular contraction, atrial undersensing, atrial oversensing, or atrial noncapture. ELT is sustained until there is VA block. Application of a magnet over the pacemaker terminates ELT. The most reliable way to prevent ELT is to program the PVARP to a value that exceeds the VA conduction interval. Some pacemakers have PMT or ELT recognition and termination algorithms designed to prevent or terminate PMT and ELT.

XIII. Common issues for the patient with a pacemaker
A. Surgical patients (any operation)
1. Pertinent **history** is obtained and a **physical examination** is performed. The patient undergoes a **pacemaker evaluation** to assess the programmed values, pacing and sensing thresholds, and lead impedance.
2. The **degree of pacemaker dependence** is determined. A patient who depends on a pacemaker needs to have temporary pacing equipment readily available.
3. If the **operative field** is in the area near the pacemaker, the rate response feature of the pacemaker is deactivated to avoid inappropriate rapid pacing caused by vibrations or pressure transmitted to the pulse generator.
4. **Electrocautery** may cause temporary inhibition of pacemaker output because of oversensing of the EMI. Electrocautery is used sparingly and in short bursts. The cautery electrode is placed at a distance from the pacemaker site.
5. The **pacemaker is reevaluated postoperatively** for any sign of malfunction, the presence of a reset mode, and any change in lead threshold or impedance values. A **chest radiograph** is obtained after cardiac operations to check for lead damage or dislodgment.

B. EMI in the hospital environment
1. **Magnetic resonance imaging (MRI).** The magnetic field generated by the electromagnet and the radiofrequency signal produced to modulate the magnetic field for MRI may cause torque forces or malfunction for cardiac pacemakers. Modern pacemakers contain fewer ferromagnetic components than previous pacemakers do, so torque forces become less common. The magnetic forces may close the pacemaker reed switch and cause asynchronous pacing. The radiofrequency signal may inhibit pacing, cause rapid pacing, or cause reversion to reset mode. Unipolar pacemakers are more susceptible to interference from MRI. In general **MRI is avoided** in the care of patients with pacemakers unless it is considered absolutely necessary.
2. **Extracorporeal shock-wave lithotripsy (ESWL)**
   a. ESWL is a treatment for renal calculi that involves production of focused hydraulic shock waves from an underwater spark gap. The spark gap or shock waves can interfere with or damage a pacemaker.
   b. A patient with a pacemaker may undergo ESWL, but the pulse generator must be as far as possible from the focal point of the lithotripsy shock waves.
   c. Activity-based rate-adaptation pacemakers with piezoelectric crystals may be damaged by shock waves, and the shock waves may cause oversensing and subsequent nonphysiologic rapid pacing rates. Such pacemakers are reprogrammed with the rate-adaptive feature deactivated before the procedure. If a pacemaker with a piezoelectric crystal is located in the abdomen, ESWL is not to be performed.
   d. Shock waves may be misinterpreted as atrial activity; therefore dual-chamber pacemakers are programmed to VVI mode to avoid rapid ventricular pacing.
   e. A cardiologist experienced in pacemaker management must be available during the ESWL procedure.

3. **Radiation therapy**
   a. Diagnostic radiation does not interfere with cardiac pacemakers. Therapeutic radiation therapy to the thorax such as that used for breast or lung cancer may cause interference or cumulative damage.
   b. Damage to the integrated circuitry of the pacemaker is caused by leakage currents between the insulated parts. This damage is directly related to the cumulative radiation dose.
   c. The pacemaker is assessed before and after a treatment session. ECG monitoring is recommended for patients who are pacemaker dependent. The pulse generator must be shielded from the ionizing radiation or moved to another site if necessary.
4. **Cardiac monitors** that inject current into a patient's body for measurement of minute ventilation may interfere with pacemakers that work by means of minute ventilation for rate adaptation.
5. **Transcutaneous electric nerve stimulation (TENS)** is a method used for relief of acute and chronic neuromuscular pain. It involves placement of electrodes on the skin over the region of interest that are connected to a pulse generator. TENS is believed to be safe for patients with bipolar pacemakers. Patients with unipolar pacemakers may need a reduction in sensitivity.
6. **Dental equipment.** Some types of dental equipment may cause pacemaker inhibition, particularly for unipolar pacemakers. Vibrations may increase the pacing rate of activity-sensing rate-adaptive pacemakers.
7. **Cardioversion or defibrillation**
   a. The shock from direct current (DC) cardioversion or defibrillation may damage the pulse generator or cause the device being reset. If direct current cardioversion or defibrillation is necessary, the patch electrodes are positioned as far from the pulse generator as possible.
   b. A pacemaker evaluation is performed after the procedure.
8. **Electroconvulsive therapy (ECT)**
   a. ECT is a technique for the management of certain psychiatric disorders and generally does not interfere with pacemaker function.
   b. The patient undergoes a pacemaker evaluation before and after each ECT session. ECG monitoring during the session is prudent. Seizure activity during the procedure may produce myopotential inhibition of unipolar pacemakers.
9. **Diathermy** is therapeutic application of electric current to the skin and may cause pacemaker interference or damage if applied to the region near the pulse generator.
10. **Electrocautery** (see **XIII.A. 4.**)

C. **Environmental EMI**
   1. **Cellular telephones** may interfere with cardiac pacemakers while transmitting or receiving calls. Patients with pacemakers are advised not to carry cellular telephones near the pacemaker site (e.g., shirt pocket) and to hold the telephone to the contralateral ear during use.
   2. **Electronic article surveillance** is a type of antitheft system that consists of a gate that produces an electromagnetic field through which people must walk. The field may cause pacemaker interference, primarily inhibition of pacemaker output. Patients with unipolar dual-chamber pacemakers are particularly susceptible to interference from electronic article surveillance systems.
   3. **Industrial electric equipment** includes devices, such as arc welders, that may generate strong electric fields. The strength of the electric field varies among types of equipment and if sufficiently strong may interfere with unipolar pacemakers. Patients may require individual environmental testing to assure safety.

4. **Microwave ovens.** Because of better sealing of microwave ovens and improved shielding of pulse generators, interference with pacemakers by microwave ovens is no longer considered to be a serious problem.

5. **Metal detectors.** Although the metal detectors in public places such as airports may be set off because of detection of a pacemaker, there generally is no appreciable interference with pacemaker function.

6. **High-voltage power lines** and **electric substations** may cause inhibition or asynchronous pacing in unipolar pacemakers if the patient is quite close to the electric field. At usual public distances from such areas there usually is no pacemaker interference.

XIV. **Cardiac pacing: clinical trials**

A. Numerous clinical trials, mostly small and nonrandomized, have been performed with regard to exercise capacity and quality of life for various pacemaker modes, chambers paced, rate-adaptive pacing, and types of sensors.

B. Clinical trials have firmly established the superiority of rate-adaptive (VVIR) over fixed-rate ventricular pacing (VVI) with regard to quality of life and exercise performance.

C. A number of clinical trials (most of them small and nonrandomized) have demonstrated that physiologic pacing (maintenance of AV synchrony with VDD or DDD mode) improves exercise capacity and quality of life compared with fixed-rate pacing (e.g., VVI mode).

D. Data conflict regarding the benefit of dual-chamber pacing over rate-adaptive ventricular pacing. Some studies have shown that dual-chamber pacing does not increase exercise performance compared with rate-adaptive ventricular pacing (i.e., rate adaptation is likely more important than AV synchrony with regard to exercise performance). However, other studies have demonstrated the superiority of physiologic pacing. Patients with normal sinus node function may benefit from use of a dual-chamber pacemaker because ventricular pacing may cause pacemaker syndrome or an increased incidence of atrial arrhythmias. It is still unclear whether there is a benefit to rate-adaptive dual-chamber pacing (DDDR) over simple dual-chamber pacing (DDD).

E. Some of the larger-scale, randomized studies of cardiac pacing are summarized as follows:

1. Pacemaker Selection in the Elderly trial (**PASE**). A single blind, randomized, controlled trial of ventricular pacing versus dual-chamber pacing involving 407 patients older than 65 years. The primary end point was quality of life with follow-up periods as long as 30 months. Quality of life improved with pacemaker implantation. Patients with sinus node dysfunction, but not atrioventricular block, had significantly better quality of life with dual-chamber pacing compared with ventricular pacing (1).

2. UK Pacing and Cardiovascular Events (**UKPACE**) trial. Ongoing randomized trial comparing VVI(R) versus DDD pacing involving 2,000 patients with high-grade AV block. The primary end point is total mortality rate (2).

3. Canadian Trial of Physiologic Pacing (**CTOPP**). Ongoing randomized trial of VVI(R) versus AAI(R) or DDD(R) involving 2,450 patients undergoing pacemaker implantation. The primary end point is total mortality rate.

4. Mode Selection Trial in Sinus Node Dysfunction (**MOST**). Ongoing randomized trial of VVIR versus DDDR pacing involving 2,000 patients with sinus node dysfunction. The primary end point is total mortality and stroke rates.

5. Pacemaker Atrial Tachycardia Trial (**Pac-A-Tach**). Randomized trial comparing the effect of DDDR versus VVIR pacing modes on the incidence of atrial tachyarrhythmias involving 202 patients with sick sinus syndrome and symptomatic atrial tachyarrhythmias. A second randomization to antiarrhythmic drug (sotalol or quinidine) or no antiarrhythmic drug is examining the effect of antiarrhythmic therapy for suppression of atrial tachyarrhythmias for each pacing mode. Enroll-

ment was completed in October 1996, and 2-year follow-up data collection was completed in October 1998.

6. Systematic Trial of Pacing to prevent Atrial Fibrillation (**STOP-AF**). Ongoing randomized trial of VVI(R) versus DDD(R) or AAI(R) involving approximately 300 patients with sinus node dysfunction to determine the effect of pacing mode on the incidence of recurrent atrial fibrillation (3).

7. Rate Modulated Pacing and Quality of Life (**RAMP**) trial. Ongoing randomized trial comparing DDD versus DDDR pacing involving 400 patients who need dual-chamber pacemakers. The primary end point is quality of life.

XV. Future directions
A. Sensor technology
1. Advances in physiologic sensors and rate-adaptation algorithms.
2. Multiple sensors for more physiologic pacing. For example, a desirable sensor combination has been an activity sensor, which typically has a more rapid response, and another sensor such as minute ventilation, which typically has a more delayed but workload-proportional response.
3. Sensor blending, which is the relative contribution of each sensor during each phase of activity and may be programmable.
4. Sensor cross checking, in which the sensor is used to determine whether an increase in intrinsic atrial rate is appropriate. If the sensor does not confirm activity and the pacemaker senses an increased atrial rate, the pacemaker uses the sensor to dictate the appropriate heart rate. Pacemakers with multiple sensors can be used to detect intersensor disagreement and thereby avoid inappropriately rapid pacing caused by a false-positive response of one sensor.

B. Advances in pulse generator and lead system technology to provide more reliability and safety at acceptable costs
C. Support for large-scale, randomized clinical trials examining quality of life and total mortality for various pacemaker systems in specific patient populations must continue.

XVI. Glossary: basic terminology of cardiac pacing
A. **Anode.** The positive pole. The anode of a unipolar pacing system is the pulse generator case. The anode of a bipolar pacing system is the proximal ring electrode of the pacing lead.

B. **Capture.** The effective cardiac depolarization resulting from a pacing stimulus.

C. **Cardiac stimulation threshold.** The minimum amount of electric energy needed to consistently depolarize cardiac tissue through a given electrode. This threshold changes with time after implantation (acute, subacute and chronic). Measured in milliamperes (mA).

D. **Cathode.** The negative pole. The cathode of a unipolar pacing system is the electrode at the distal portion of the pacing lead. The cathode of a bipolar pacing system is the distal tip electrode of the pacing lead.

E. **Cross talk.** In dual-chamber pacing systems, the inappropriate detection (sensing) of an event or signal in one chamber by the sense amplifier of the other chamber (usually inhibition of a ventricular output pulse caused by ventricular channel detection of an atrial output pulse).

F. **Elective replacement interval (ERI),** also called elective replacement time (ERT) or recommended replacement time (RRT). The indicator that shows the pulse generator has reached the point in its service life at which system failure is likely to occur within 3 to 6 months. The ERI indicator for a pacemaker varies among models and manufacturers but is usually indicated by a change in pacing rate, mode, or function. Pacemaker manufacturers generally recommend pulse generator replacement when the ERI is identified. (*Note:* ERI/ERT and EOL indicators for various pacemaker models are published in a handbook that should be available in the pacemaker clinic.)

G. **Electromagnetic interference (EMI).** Electric signals from noncardiac or nonphysiologic sources that may affect pacemaker function.

H. End of life (EOL). The depletion of battery power for the pulse generator. The end-of-life indicator for a pacemaker varies among models and manufacturers but usually is a decrease in magnet-related pacing rate to a certain percentage of the beginning-of-life rate. There also may be a change in pacemaker mode (e.g., from DDD to VVI). Telemetry of the cell impedance of the pulse generator provides information regarding the status of battery power for pacemakers with such a feature. Pacemaker manufacturers generally recommend urgent replacement of the pulse generator if the EOL of a device is identified. (*Note:* ERI/ERT and EOL indicators for various pacemaker models are published in a handbook that should be available in the pacemaker clinic.)

I. Fusion. The condition that results when pacemaker output occurs at the same time as an intrinsic event and both contribute to cardiac depolarization. The morphologic features of the fused beat resemble those of both paced and intrinsic events.

J. Impedance (Z). Total resistance to the flow of current through a conductor. For pacemaker systems, this includes resistance produced by electronic components and body tissues. Temporal changes in pacing impedance usually include decreasing impedance over the first 1 to 2 weeks after implantation followed by an increase in impedance to a level somewhat higher than the impedance at the time of implantation. Serial measurements of pacing impedance may be useful for the assessment of lead integrity.

K. Magnet mode. The response of a pacemaker when a magnetic field of sufficient strength is applied and closes the reed switch of the pulse generator. The pulse generator paces at a predetermined rate and mode, which varies among pacemaker models and manufacturers. Generally, the mode is asynchronous pacing. Magnet mode can be used to assess pacemaker function and battery status (see *elective replacement interval* and *end of life*).

L. Noncapture. The absence of cardiac depolarization after a pacing stimulus.

M. Ohm's law: $V = I \times R$
   1. Voltage (V). The difference in potential energy between two points, measured in millivolts (mV).
   2. Current (I). The rate of transfer or the flow of electricity, measured in milliamperes (mA).
   3. Resistance (R). The opposition to the flow of electric current through a material, measured in ohms (Ω).

N. Output. The output of a pacemaker is determined by the voltage and pulse width.

O. Pacemaker-mediated tachycardia (PMT). Sudden onset of a sustained ventricular paced rhythm at the maximum tracking rate of the pacemaker. PMT is sustained by continued active participation of the pacemaker in the tachycardia circuit.

P. Pacing interval. The interval between two consecutive paced events, measured in milliseconds (msec).

Q. Pseudofusion. The condition in which an intrinsic event occurs before the pacemaker output is delivered so that the pacemaker output does not contribute to cardiac depolarization. The morphologic features of the pseudofusion beat resemble those of the intrinsic event.

R. Pseudopseudofusion. The condition that occurs when a premature ventricular contraction that resembles the ventricular paced complex follows an atrial output spike.

S. Pulse width. The measurement in milliseconds (msec) of the pacemaker output spike (also called *pulse duration*).

T. Reed switch. A switch within the pulse generator that closes when a magnetic field of sufficient strength is applied to it (such as a ring or doughnut magnet or a programming head). The pacemaker converts to magnet mode.

U. Sensing. The ability of a pacemaker to recognize native cardiac signals. Refers to the amplitude of the signal measured in millivolts (mV) needed for the pacemaker to detect the signal. Higher numbers reflect less sensitivity; lower numbers reflect more sensitivity.

1. **Oversensing.** Sensing inappropriate cardiac or extracardiac signals and responding to them as if they were appropriate native sensed events. Oversensing causes underpacing.
2. **Undersensing.** Failure to recognize and respond appropriately to cardiac signals. Undersensing results in overpacing.

V. **60,000 rule.** Converts rate (beats/min) to interval (msec) and vice versa. There are 60,000 msec in 1 minute.

$$60{,}000 \div \text{rate (beats/min)} = \text{interval (msec)}$$

$$60{,}000 \div \text{interval (ms)} = \text{rate (beats/min)}$$

XVII. Cardiac pacing: timing cycles and refractory periods

A. **P,** native atrial depolarization
B. **A,** atrial paced event
C. **R,** native ventricular depolarization
D. **V,** ventricular paced event
E. **AV,** atrioventricular sequential pacing
F. **AVI, atrioventricular pacing interval** (also called AV delay). In dual-chamber pacing, the period between an atrial sensed or paced event and a ventricular paced event (usually programmable).
G. **Absolute refractory period.** The period following a sensed or paced event during which the sense amplifier is unresponsive to incoming signals.
H. **Relative refractory period.** A noise-sampling period that follows the absolute refractory period during which some incoming signals (generally signals in the frequency range of interference) are monitored with the sense amplifier. Sensed signals during this period may cause the initiation of a new refractory period but do not reset the timing circuit.
I. **ARP, atrial refractory period.** The atrial timing cycle during which the atrial sense amplifier is unresponsive to incoming signals. For single-chamber atrial pacing modes, the atrial refractory period is initiated by an atrial sensed or paced event. For dual-chamber pacing modes, the AV interval and postventricular atrial refractory period (PVARP) determine the total atrial refractory period (TARP). TARP = AVI – PVARP.
J. **VRP, ventricular refractory period.** The timing cycle initiated by a ventricular sensed or paced event during which the ventricular sense amplifier is unresponsive to incoming signals. This is not the same as the ventricular blanking period.
K. **Blanking period.** An interval (usually 12 to 125 msec) initiated by an output pulse during which the sense amplifier is temporarily disabled. In dual-chamber pacing, the blanking period is designed to prevent inappropriate detection of signals from the other chamber (cross talk). For example, an atrial sensed or paced event initiates a ventricular blanking period during which the ventricular sense amplifier is temporarily disabled.
L. **CDW, cross talk detection window.** In dual-chamber pacing, a timing cycle (usually 51 to 150 msec) immediately after the ventricular blanking period during which a ventricular sensed event is considered to be cross talk but causes a triggered ventricular output at the end of an abbreviated AV interval (safety pacing).
M. **AEI, atrial escape interval.** For atrial single-chamber pacing systems, the period from a sensed atrial event to the next atrial paced event. For dual-chamber pacing systems, the period initiated by a ventricular sensed or paced event and ending with the next atrial paced event.
N. **LRL, lower rate limit** (also called *base rate* or *minimum rate*). The rate at which the pacemaker paces in the absence of sensed intrinsic events (generally programmable in most pacemakers).
O. **MTR, maximum tracking rate** (also called *upper rate limit* [URL]). A programmable value for dual-chamber pacemaker sensing and tracking modes

that designates the highest ventricular pacing rate that can be achieved in response to atrial sensed events with 1:1 AV synchrony at the programmed AV delay.

P. MSR, maximum sensor rate. A programmable value in rate-adaptive pacemaker systems that designates the highest pacing rate that can be achieved in response to a sensor input. MSR may be programmed independently of MTR.

Q. RRAVD, rate-responsive atrioventricular delay. A programmable feature of some dual-chamber pacing systems that progressively shortens the PV or AV interval as sinus or sensor-driven atrial rate increases. This is designed to provide a more physiologically correct AVI at higher heart rates and allow tracking of higher atrial rates (a shorter AVI decreases the TARP) and thereby lessen risk for a fixed-block upper rate response.

SUGGESTED READINGS

References

1. Lamas GA, Orav EJ, Stambler BS, et al. Quality of life and clinical outcomes in elderly patients treated with ventricular pacing as compared with dual-chamber pacing: Pacemaker Selection in the Elderly Investigators. *N Engl J Med* 1998;338: 1097–1104.
2. Toff WD, Skehan JD, De Bono DP, Camm AJ. The United Kingdom pacing and cardiovascular events (UKPACE) trial: United Kingdom Pacing and Cardiovascular Events. *Heart* 1997;78:221–223.
3. Charles RG, McComb JM. Systematic trial of pacing to prevent atrial fibrillation (STOP-AF). *Heart* 1997;78:224–25.

Landmark Articles

Lamas GA, Orav EJ, Stambler BS, et al. Quality of life and clinical outcomes in elderly patients treated with ventricular pacing as compared with dual-chamber pacing: Pacemaker Selection in the Elderly Investigators. *N Engl J Med* 1998;338: 1097–1104.

Toff WD, Skehan JD, De Bono DP, Camm AJ. The United Kingdom pacing and cardiovascular events (UKPACE) trial: United Kingdom Pacing and Cardiovascular Events. *Heart* 1997;78:221–223.

Key Reviews

Barold SS, Barold HS. Contemporary issues in rate-adaptive pacing. *Clin Cardiol* 1997;20:726–729.

Barold SS, Falkoff MD, Ung LS, Heinle RA. All dual-chamber pacemakers function in the DDD mode. *Am Heart J* 1988;115:1353–1362.

Bernstein AD, Camm AJ, Fletcher RD, et al. The NASPE/BPEG generic pacemaker code for antibradyarrhythmia and adaptive-rate pacing and antitachyarrhythmia devices. *Pacing Clin Electrophysiol* 1987;10:794–799.

Glikson M, Espinosa RE, Hayes DL. Expanding indications for permanent pacemakers. *Ann Intern Med* 1995;123:443–451.

Gregoratos G, Cheitlin MD, Conill A, et al. ACC/AHA guidelines for implantation of cardiac pacemakers and antiarrhythmia devices: a report of the American College of Cardiology/American Heart Association Task Force on Practice Guidelines (Committee on Pacemaker Implantation). *J Am Coll Cardiol* 1998;31:1175–1209.

Relevant Book Chapters

Barold S. The fourth decade of cardiac pacing: hemodynamic, electrophysiological, and clinical considerations in the selection of the optimal pacemaker. In: Zipes DP, ed. *Cardiac electrophysiology: from cell to bedside,* 2nd ed. Philadelphia: WB Saunders, 1995:1366–92.

Barold SS, Zipes DP. Cardiac pacemakers and antiarrhythmic devices. In: Braunwald E, ed. *Heart disease: a textbook of cardiovascular medicine,* 5th ed. Philadelphia: W B Saunders, 1997:705–741.

Bernstein AD, Parsonnet V. Pacemaker and defibrillator codes. In: Ellenbogen KA, Kay GN, Wilkoff BL, eds. *Clinical cardiac pacing.* Philadelphia: WB Saunders, 1995:279–283.

Ellenbogen KA, ed. *Cardiac pacing,* 2nd ed. Cambridge, UK: Blackwell, 1996.

Ellenbogen KA, Kay GN, Wilkoff BL, eds. *Clinical cardiac pacing.* Philadelphia: WB Saunders, 1995.

Hayes DL. Pacemakers. In: Topol EJ, ed. *Textbook of cardiovascular medicine.* Philadelphia: Lippincott–Raven, 1998:1879–1911.

Lau C, Camm AJ. Overview of ideal sensor characteristics. In: Ellenbogen KA, Kay GN, Wilkoff BL, eds. *Clinical cardiac pacing.* Philadelphia: WB Saunders, 1995:141–66.

46. ANTITACHYCARDIA DEVICES

Ralph S. Augostini

I. **Introduction**

  A. The modern **implantable cardioverter-defibrillator (ICD)** is a multi-functional, multiprogrammable electronic device designed to abort life-threatening arrhythmias. It is programmed to automatically detect and treat episodes of **ventricular tachycardia (VT), ventricular fibrillation (VF), or bradycardia.** Current ICDs have the programming capability of delivering multi-tiered therapies, which may include a combination of **antitachycardia pacing (ATP), cardioversion, or defibrillation.** Some devices also have extensive **bradycardia functions,** which may include **rate-responsive pacing, dual-chamber pacing, and automatic mode switch function.** Multiple clinical trials have demonstrated the efficacy of ICDs to accurately **detect and treat sudden cardiac death.** Two recent prospective randomized clinical trials have demonstrated an **overall mortality benefit of ICD implantation versus medical therapy** in select patient populations at risk for hemodynamically unstable VT.

  B. The development of the ICD closely followed the successful use of external defibrillation to terminate life-threatening ventricular arrhythmias in the intensive care unit setting. The concept of an ICD was first introduced in 1972. First-generation devices were nonprogrammable and provided only the basic function of defibrillation. The early ICD required a thoracotomy approach for placement of an epicardial lead system. The size of the pulse generator limited placement to an abdominal site. Subsequent advancements in electronic technology over the past 20 years have drastically reduced the size of the pulse generator yet improved the programmability and diagnostic data stored within the device. An improved understanding of VF, defibrillation, and cardiac pacing have resulted in the development of biphasic shock waveforms and transvenous pace/defibrillation lead systems that preclude the need for epicardial patches. As a result, modern ICDs are much smaller devices with expansive programming capability placed via a transvenous approach.

  C. The ICD system is similar to a pacemaker in that it incorporates the microprocessor, memory, capacitors, and energy source in a pulse generator that attaches to a lead system interfacing with the heart. New implants are almost exclusively implanted transvenously with the pulse generator placed in a left pectoral location much like a conventional pacemaker. Most systems now incorporate a single right ventricular coil with a hot-can active pulse generator or combined right ventricular coil, superior vena cava coil, and active pulse generator can. The "hot can" serves as an active lead within the shocking configuration. Ventricular sensing and pacing are achieved through two "dedicated bipolar" electrodes at the tip of the right ventricular lead (tip/ring) or via "integrated bipolar" electrodes that incorporate a single right ventricular electrode with the right ventricular coil (tip/coil).

II. **Indications**

  A. An ICD system is indicated for patients who are at **high risk of sudden cardiac death due to ventricular arrhythmias.** The combined American College of Cardiology (ACC)/American Heart Association (AHA) Task Force has most recently published updated guidelines for implantation of cardiac pacemakers and antiarrhythmia devices in 1998. Although it has been updated with several large prospective randomized trials, it recognizes the ongoing evolution of ICD indications and remains liberal in its guidelines. Current indications for ICD implantation are summarized in Table 46-1.

Table 46-1. Criteria for ICD implantation

(A) INDICATIONS

CLASS I
1. Cardiac arrest due to VF or VT not due to a transient or reversible cause
2. Spontaneous sustained VT
3. Syncope of undetermined origin with clinically relevant, hemodynamically significant sustained VT or VF induced at electrophysiologic study when drug therapy is ineffective, not tolerated, or not preferred
4. Nonsustained VT with coronary disease, prior MI, LV dysfunction, and inducible VF or sustained VT at electrophysiologic study that is not suppressible by a class I antiarrhythmic drug

CLASS II
1. Cardiac arrest presumed to be due to VF when electrophysiologic testing is precluded by other medical conditions
2. Severe symptoms attributable to sustained ventricular tachyarrhythmias while awaiting cardiac transplantation
3. Familial or inherited conditions with a high risk for life-threatening ventricular tachyarrhythmias such as long QT syndrome or hypertrophic cardiomyopathy
4. Nonsustained VT with coronary artery disease, prior MI, and LV dysfunction, and inducible sustained VT or VF at electrophysiologic study
5. Recurrent syncope of undetermined etiology in the presence of ventricular dysfunction and inducible ventricular arrhythmias at electrophysiologic study when other causes of syncope have been excluded

(B) CONTRAINDICATIONS

CLASS III
1. Syncope of undetermined cause in a patient without inducible ventricular tachyarrhythmias
2. Incessant VT or VF
3. VF or VT resulting from arrhythmias amenable to surgical or catheter ablations e.g., atrial arrhythmias associated with the Wolff-Parkinson-White syndrome, right ventricular outflow tract VT, idiopathic left ventricular tachycardia, or fascicular VT
4. Ventricular tachyarrhythmias due to transient or reversible disorder (e.g., acute MI, electrolyte imbalance, drugs, trauma)
5. Significant psychiatric illnesses that may be aggravated by device implantation or may preclude systematic follow-up
6. Terminal illnesses with projected life expectance ≤6 months
7. Patients with coronary artery disease with LV dysfunction and prolonged QRS duration in the absence of spontaneous or inducible sustained or nonsustained VT who are undergoing coronary bypass surgery
8. NYHA class IV drug refractory congestive heart failure in patients who are not candidates for cardiac transplantation

VT, ventricular tachycardia; VF, ventricular fibrillation; MI, myocardial infarction; LV, left ventricular; EPS, electrophysiologic study; NSVT, nonsustained ventricular tachycardia; ICD, implantable cardioverter-defibrillator.
Adapted with permission from *ACC/AHA Guidelines for Implantation of Cardiac Pacemakers and Antiarrhythmia Devices.*

  B. As with any expensive invasive therapy, **candidates for ICD implantation should be carefully screened** for appropriateness of the prescribed therapy. The **patient should be educated regarding** the implantation, maintenance, and follow-up of an implantable device. A **thorough discussion** of potential therapies including ATP, low-energy cardioversion, and shock defibrillation should ensue. The **candidate should be allowed to**

make an informed choice prior to implantation of a device. Additionally, as devices incorporate expanded pacemaker capabilities, it will be important to choose the appropriate device for the patient.

III. **Contraindications.** Implantation of an ICD is contraindicated in any patient who has a remedial cause of ventricular arrhythmia such as **acute myocardial infarction, myocardial ischemia, electrolyte imbalance, drug toxicity, hypoxia, or sepsis.** Transient ventricular tachyarrhythmias secondary to electrocution or drowning are not indications for ICD placement. Patients with **incessant ventricular arrhythmias** should not receive an ICD. Additionally, an ICD is contraindicated in any patient with **recurrent syncope of undetermined cause without inducible ventricular tachyarrhythmias** (see Table 46-1).

IV. **Implantation**

A. ICD implantation has evolved into a well-tolerated procedure using the transvenous approach. Many physicians have switched to conscious sedation rather than general anesthesia during implantation and testing procedures. The risks involved with implantation are similar to those of pacemaker insertion. **Operative risks** include **acceleration of arrhythmias, air embolism, bleeding, deep vein thrombosis, hemothorax, infection, myocardial damage, pneumothorax, vascular/cardiac perforation, tamponade, thromboemboli, and death.** The overall mortality rate is less than 1%. **Late complications** include **chronic nerve damage, erosion, extrusion, fluid accumulation, infection, formation of hematomas/cysts, keloids, lead migration, lead dislodgment, and venous occlusion.** Due to the nature of the procedure, a **separate standby external pacemaker/defibrillator** should be immediately available for rescue therapy should the implanted device fail to appropriately treat an arrhythmia.

B. Currently, available devices are small enough to allow almost exclusive use of left pectoral placement. A right pectoral or epicardial system may be necessary in a patient who has an existing left-sided pacemaker or if the patient has undergone prior pectoral surgery (e. g., mastectomy). For patients with high defibrillation thresholds, additional lead placement such as a subcutaneous array or patch may be necessary. Epicardial patch placement is generally reserved for patients who have failed to meet implant criteria with a transvenous lead system or if there has been prior bilateral pectoral surgery. For pectoral implants, a single 2- to 3-in. incision is made transversely below the clavicle or over the deltopectoral groove. Transvenous lead placement is achieved through a subclavian vein puncture or cephalic vein cutdown. An "extrathoracic" subclavian vein puncture or cephalic vein cutdown for access may lead to decreased lead failure attributed to subclavian crush injury. The lead is advanced to the right ventricular apex under fluoroscopic guidance where the tip is secured via an active fixation screw or embedded in the trabeculae with passive fixation times. If there is already a pacemaker lead in the right ventricular apex, then septal placement of the lead tip is chosen. Ideally, the lead tips are placed at maximal distance from each other to avoid device–device interactions. Additionally, septal placement is sometimes necessary to secure a passive fixation lead when there is a smooth right ventricular apex.

C. The lead is tested for pace/sense thresholds utilizing an external high-voltage system analyzer or pacing system analyzer (PSA). In general, an acute pacing threshold of 2 V or less, R-wave amplitude of 5 mV or more, and lead impedance within the accepted range of the manufacturer (typically 300 to 1,200 ohm) are necessary to meet implant criteria. The lead is secured within the pocket with a suture sleeve tie-down. If the device utilizes an atrial lead, then it is deployed at this time. The lead is attached to the pulse generator and the system is placed either in a submuscular or subcutaneous pocket. The pulse generator should be placed with the logo "up" toward the skin and excess lead coiled posteriorly to maximize the ability to communicate with an external programming wand. The device is then interrogated to assure appropriate communication. Pace/sense thresholds are again tested. Capture of a real-time electrogram (EGM) may identify signal noise in the shock-sensing leads.

D. Defibrillation testing may be achieved either through a high-voltage system analyzer or through device-based testing. Most manufacturers recommend a synchronized sinus test shock to assess the integrity of the device/ lead system prior to induction of VF. This is achieved by delivery of a low-energy (less than 2 J) synchronized shock delivered on the QRS complex. This low-energy test allows assessment of appropriate sensing as well as shock impedance (typically 35 to 90 ohm). Following this test, VF is induced with ultrafast burst pacing (30-millisecond intervals), shock on T wave, or application of alternating current (AC). Appropriate ICD detection and effective therapy are verified. Typically, a step-down protocol is incorporated to determine the defibrillation threshold. Two successful therapies that are 10 J less than or equal to the maximal output of the device are required to meet implant criteria. In general, this approach identifies the level of energy (typically 5 to 15 J) required to achieve a 50% to 75% success rate of defibrillation. Defibrillation therapy is then programmed at a level equal to or 10 J over the defibrillation threshold. Rarely, a patient may require the addition of a shocking coil in the superior vena cava, subcutaneous patch, or subcutaneous array to achieve an adequate safety margin.

V. Device replacement

A. Pulse generator replacement represents a vulnerable period for the ICD/lead system. A fourfold increased risk of infection has been reported with ICD pulse generator replacement. In the past, manufacturers have had multiple-lead models of variable pin lengths and diameters. Beginning in 1991 they adopted the 3.2-mm international pace/sense standard (IS-1) and 3.2-mm defibrillation standard (DF-1). Prior to an attempted device replacement, assessment of the chronic lead models should be performed to verify that the appropriate replacement header or adapters are available at the time of surgery.

B. Leads may be inadvertently damaged during exploration of the pocket or during the exchange of pulse generators. **Intra-operative assessment of lead function is imperative** prior to introducing the replacement generator to the operative field. **Replacement of a pace/sense or defibrillation lead may be** necessary and require the use of a different device header. Replacement of an abdominal device should be coordinated with a surgeon who is capable of tunneling a new transvenous lead to the abdominal pocket.

VI. Tachycardia detection and therapy

A. The ICD senses the intracardiac EGM signal via the implanted ventricular sensing electrodes. The determination of a ventricular arrhythmia is recognition of VV intervals that fall within the programmed detection rate and duration criteria. Each VV interval falling inside a therapy zone increments the ICD event counters. If the device reaches a specified number of intervals to detect programmed by the physician, then the ICD will deliver the prescribed therapy. After delivery of therapy, the device either confirms termination of the episode or meets criteria for redetection and the next programmed therapy is delivered. The ICD automatically adjusts its sensitivity thresholds following sensed and paced events through an autogain mechanism. This allows the device to automatically adjust its sensitivity during tachycardia episode in response to the changing amplitude of the ventricular signal. For example, the autogain may rapidly increase sensitivity to detect small-amplitude V signals during VF. This function serves to adapt the ICD to alterations in ventricular signal rather than interpreting no signal and begin pacing. This auto gain feature also allows the device to reduce the incidence of T-wave oversensing as well as cross-chamber sensing, particularly with paced events.

B. Atrioventricular (AV) sequential devices incorporate programmable dual-chamber supraventricular criteria to exclude treatment of supraventricular tachyarrhythmias from inappropriate detection of VT or to identify concurrent VT and supraventricular tachycardia. Single-chamber ventricular devices with morphology discrimination use changes in the morphology of the ventricular sensed EGM as compared to baseline to exclude treatment of supraventricular tachyarrhythmias.

C. Most devices allow for programming of several tachycardia zones. The VT zone is programmed with a lower detection cutoff that would include any clinical VT events. Ideally, the cutoff rate for detection of tachycardia should be above the patient's maximal heart rate to avoid therapy for sinus tachycardia. **Antitachycardia pacing** schemes with burst pacing, ramp pacing, and interburst decrement are all currently available features. **Burst pacing** sequences consist of a set of ventricular pulses delivered at equal intervals to treat VT. **Ramp pacing** consists of a set of ventricular pulses delivered at decreasing intervals to treat VT. Following a failed ATP attempt, **interburst decrement** allows a more aggressive shortening of the intervals during either a burst or ramp attempt. The first pulse of a burst or ramp sequence (S_1) is delivered at a calculated percentage of the tachycardia cycle length. The S_1 percentage cycle lengths, number of pulses, interburst decrement, and number of ATP attempts are all programmable features. Additionally, cardioversion therapy (1 to 34 J) can be programmed in a VT zone. All VT zones have a programmable time limit on episode duration at which point the device defaults to the next zone. Also, if a tachycardia is accelerated to a faster arrhythmia, then the ICD will deliver the therapy appropriate for the rate of the accelerated tachycardia.

D. **Successful ICD treatment of VF can only occur with defibrillation therapy.** All devices are programmed with a VF zone due to the risk of acceleration with ATP or cardioversion. Because of the hemodynamic instability seen with fast VT or VF, the device is typically programmed to treat any sustained episode with intervals of 300 milliseconds or less (heart rate 200 bpm or higher) with defibrillation therapy. The device should be programmed with at least a 10-J safety margin over the defibrillation threshold observed either at implant or during follow-up testing. Up to six additional shocks may be programmed with maximal outputs programmed at the second or third shock and onward.

VII. **Bradycardia detection and therapy**

A. All currently available ICDs provide basic VVI pacing with separate programmable postshock lower rate limit and output. Some dual-chamber devices have been introduced with an atrial lead for diagnostic use only or for AV synchronized pacing. These devices allow multiple programmable pacing modes including DDDR, DDD, DDIR, DDI, AAIR, AAI, VVIR, and VVI. These expanded pacing modes have obviated the need for a separate dual-chamber pacemaker that is sometimes necessary in the chronically ill patients who typically receive ICDs. Additionally, they will likely be shown to reduce the incidence of inappropriate shocks attributed to supraventricular tachycardia.

B. In AV-synchronized devices, the ICD continues to sense tachyarrhythmias in both chambers regardless of the programmed bradycardia pacing mode. To maintain proper sensing, both atrial and ventricular sensing thresholds are adjusted with autogain. The ICD has multiple blanking periods to avoid postpacing polarization, T-wave oversensing, and cross-talk between chambers. To avoid undersensing of tachyarrhythmias, short cross-chamber blanking periods after paced events and no cross-chamber blanking after sensed events are necessary. The AV synchronous devices have programmable refractory periods available for bradycardia functions, but these refractory periods do not affect tachyarrhythmia detection.

VIII. **Magnet function**

A. Confusion abounds concerning the function of a magnet with ICDs. The pulse generator contains a reed switch that is closed when a magnet is placed over the device. Closure of the reed switch prevents delivery of tachyarrhythmia therapy. Unlike pacemakers, **bradycardia pacing is not affected by the use of a magnet in ICDs.** Normal device therapy resumes when the magnet is removed and the reed switch opens.

B. One manufacturer, Cardiac Pacemakers, Inc./Guidant (St. Paul, MN.) has developed two expanded functions during magnet application. In addition to the inhibition of tachyarrhythmia therapy, magnet application can be used to determine the tachycardia mode of the ICD. If a continuous tone is heard, then the tachycardia mode is programmed "off" (off, storage-only, or monitor-only modes). Alternatively, if a series of intermittent tones (synchronized to the R wave) are heard, then the tachycardia mode is programmed "on" and the device will deliver therapy once the magnet is removed and detection is met. A second additional magnet feature is the change of tachycardia mode with magnet. If this feature is programmed "on," the application of a magnet for more than 30 seconds will change the tachycardia mode. If the device is programmed "off" or "monitor-only" (continuous tone), then the device will be programmed "on" (intermittent tone). If the ICD is programmed "on" (intermittent tone), application of a magnet for more than 30 seconds will program the device "off" (continuous tone). If the device is programmed to storage mode, then application of a magnet has no effect on tachycardia mode and a continuous tone will be heard.

IX. **Device–device interaction**

A. Advancements in ICD pacing technology have resulted in the availability of many of the same features found in premium pacemakers. However, many patients have older-generation devices with only basic backup pacing functions. Also, there are a large number of patients who have separate ICD and pacemaker systems. **Device–device interaction remains a significant issue when multiple-lead systems/devices are used.** When a new lead is placed, the lead should be positioned as far from the other leads as possible (at least 2 cm). A dedicated bipolar sensing lead is preferred to minimize the potential of far-field oversensing of the alternate pacing lead.

B. During the implant procedure, **the devices should be tested for device–device interaction.** To simulate a worst case scenario, the pacemaker is programmed in a unipolar configuration at high output. The real-time ICD electrogram and marker channels are observed for oversensing of the pacemaker output resulting in double counting of the paced QRS complex. This may lead to an inappropriate ICD discharge. Defibrillation testing is performed with the pacemaker programmed to DOO/VOO at high output to verify appropriate VF detection and therapy. Pacing stimuli may lead to ICD undersensing of VT/VF with interpretation of the pacing artifact as "sinus rhythm" and failure to recognize the underlying arrhythmia. In addition, the ICD may affect the pacemaker by resetting the pacemaker pulse generator with a high-voltage shock. The pacemaker is programmed with the sensor "on" during an ICD high-output defibrillation test. The pacemaker is subsequently interrogated to verify appropriate communication and programmed mode. **Whenever multiple devices are present and inappropriate ICD discharges are suspected, electrophysiology lab testing for device–device interaction is warranted.** Device–device interaction should also be considered when a patient presents with resetting of the programmed mode, output configuration, or failure of communication with the device.

X. **Managing and following patients**

A. In the United States, **patient registration and tracking is mandated by the government.** Once registered, a patient receives a permanent **identification card** to carry at all times. A **Medic Alert** is strongly encouraged. Manufacturer guidelines suggest that patients should **follow up every 1 to 4 months** depending on clinical status. They should be advised they are likely to receive therapies. At the follow-up visitation, a history of symptoms that might suggest tachyarrhythmias should be obtained. The diagnostic and episode data should be reviewed. Current devices also include stored episode EGMs to allow review of aborted shocks as well as delivered therapies. Device pacing and sensing thresholds should be obtained. **There are no specific guidelines for follow-up testing of ICD defibrillation function.** In general, patients experiencing device activation should be evaluated shortly after the event to assess for safe and appropriate device function. Practice patterns vary widely regarding empiric device programming and electrophysiologic testing of modified ICD programming. Operation of a motor vehicle should be avoided for a minimum of 3 months and preferably 6 months following a symptomatic arrhythmic event.

B. In general, **ICD pulse generators have 3- to 6-year longevity depending on usage.** The programmer allows evaluation of battery status. As the device approaches the elective replacement interval, follow-up visits should be intensified. In general, **once the device reaches the elective replacement interval, it operates normally for at least 3 months** depending on frequency of therapy. Capacitor deformation occurs during periods when no shocks are delivered and results in longer charge times as well as decreased battery longevity. Current ICDs perform an automatic capacitor reformation that charges the capacitors and delivers the energy to an internal test load. This function improves subsequent charge times and battery longevity. Capacitor reformations should be conducted manually every 3 to 6 months if not automatically conducted.

C. Typically, 40% of patients receive a therapy within the first year after implant and 10% per year thereafter. After a patient experiences a first therapy, he or she should seek medical attention for assessment of the appropriateness of the therapy. **If multiple ICD discharges are experienced, medical attention should be sought emergently.** Failure to discriminate between ventricular and supraventricular rhythms is the most common reason for inappropriate shocks. Indeed, up to 40% of shocks are delivered inappropriately for supraventricular rhythms. Irregular VV intervals with a variability greater than 30 milliseconds suggests a supraventricular tachycardia such as atrial fibrillation. Rate stability is a commonly used enhancement to improve the appropriateness of device therapy seen in atrial fibrillation with a rapid ventricular response.

D. Therapy occurring during physical exertion noted to have gradually increasing heart rates and gradually decreasing VV intervals suggests sinus tachycardia. Therapy is likely not appropriate in this setting. Ideally, the cutoff rate for detection of tachyarrhythmias should be greater than the patient's maximal heart rate. In many cases, the VT rate falls within the patient's achievable sinus rate. Programmable enhancements such as sudden onset and sustained high rate can allow sinus tachycardia overlap into the VT zone without delivery of an inappropriate shock. Additional enhancements such as morphology discrimination of the ventricular EGM as well as the introduction of dual chamber devices with timing intervals, marker channels, and mode switching capabilities are likely to improve the specificity of device therapy.

E. In the event of multiple ICD discharges, a magnet can be used to inhibit ICD therapy so that the underlying rhythm can be appropriately assessed and treated. The device should be interrogated as soon as possible to assess ICD function and facilitate diagnosis. If a supraventricular tachycardia is present, then it should be managed as medically appropriate. For patient comfort, the magnet should be left in place to inhibit ICD therapy until the device can be reprogrammed or the supraventricular tachycardia is terminated. If VF is present, the device is assumed inoperable and cardiopulmonary resuscitation with external defibrillation should be applied.

XI. **Electromagnetic interference.** Patients should be counseled to **avoid sources of electromagnetic interference** because such interference may cause the pulse generator to become inhibited and either fail to deliver appropriate therapy or deliver inappropriate therapy. Potential sources of electromagnetic interference include industrial transformers, radiofrequency transmitters such as radar, therapeutic diathermy equipment, arc welding equipment, toy radiotransmitters, antitheft devices, and magnetic security wands. The safe use of medical technologies such as electrosurgery, lithotripsy, external defibrillation, and ionizing radiation can be accomplished by deactivating the device prior to the event. Shielding of the device is also appropriate when possible. The device should be evaluated for appropriate operation following exposure. Magnetic resonance imaging is contraindicated. Recent reports of interference created by cellular phones may be related to either a magnetic field from within the phone or the radiofrequency signal generated by the phone. It is suggested that if an ICD patient wishes to use a cellular phone, it should be held to the ear opposite the device and carried at least 6 to 12 in. away from the pulse generator.

XII. **Future.** It is likely that the indication and role of ICD implantation will continue to evolve. Several studies are currently underway to assess the expanded use of prophylactic ICDs for primary prevention of sudden cardiac death in selected patient populations. Improvements in electronic technology will continue to expand programming capabilities of these devices while reducing their size. Internal atrial defibrillation therapies for atrial fibrillation as well as other supraventricular arrhythmias are currently in clinical trials. Multisite pacing protocols have been initiated to improve the hemodynamic function in patients with co-existent congestive heart failure. Continuous hemodynamic monitoring with the addition of sensors resulting in automatic changes in dual-chamber pacing to improve cardiac function are in the near future. Suggested future directives will incorporate alternative pacing algorithms to suppress foci of automaticity as well as overdrive suppression of reentrant circuits involved in the generation of tachycardias. Automatic pharmacologic infusion therapy commanded by the device has been suggested.

SUGGESTED READINGS
Landmark Articles

Lown B, Axelrod P Implanted standby defibrillators. *Circulation* 1972;46:637–639.

Mirowski M, Reid PR, Mower MM, et al. Termination of ventricular arrhythmias with an implanted automatic defibrillator in human beings. *N Engl J Med* 1980;303: 322–324.

Pinski SL, Trohman RG. Implantable cardioverter-defibrillators: Implications for the non-electrophysiologist. *Ann Intern Med* 1995; 122:770–777.

Moss AJ, Hall WJ, Cannom DS, et al. Improved survival with an implanted defibrillator in patients with coronary disease at high risk for ventricular arrhythmias. *N Engl J Med* 1996;335:1933–1940.

Antiarrhythmics Versus Implantable Defibrillators (AVID) Investigators. A comparison of antiarrhythmic drug therapy with implantable defibrillators in patients resuscitated from near-fatal ventricular arrhythmias. *N Engl J Med* 1997;337: 1576–1583.

Bigger JT Jr. Prophylactic use of implanted cardiac defibrillators in patients at high risk for ventricular arrhythmias after coronary-artery bypass graft surgery. *N Engl J Med* 1997; 337:1569–1575.

Key Reviews

Dreifus LS, Fisch C, Griffin JC, et al. Guidelines for implantation of cardiac pacemakers and antiarrhythmia devices: a report of the American College of Cardiology/American Heart Association Task Force on Assessment of Diagnostic and Therapeutic Cardiovascular Procedures (Committee on Pacemaker Implantation). *Circulation* 1991;84:455–467.

Relevant Book Chapters

Pinski SL, Chen PS. Implantable cardioverter-defibrillators. In: Topol EJ, ed. *Textbook of cardiovascular medicine*. Philadelphia: Lippincott-Raven Publishers, 1998: 1913–1931.

Pinski SL, Simmons TW, Maloney JD. Troubleshooting antitachycardia pacing in patients with defibrillators. In: Estes NAM, Wang P, Manolis A, eds. *Implantable cardioverter-defibrillators: a comprehensive textbook*. New York: Marcel Dekker, 1994:445–477.

47. HEAD-UPRIGHT, TILT TABLE TESTING

Stavros G. Maragos

I. **Introduction**
   A. **Syncope** is defined as a **transient loss of consciousness and postural tone followed by spontaneous recovery.** This is a relatively common complaint, accounting for approximately 3% of emergency department visits and 6% of hospital admissions annually. Often despite extensive diagnostic testing, an etiology for syncope cannot be identified in up to 50% of cases. **Vasovagal syncope,** also known as **neurocardiogenic syncope,** is thought to underlie approximately 40% of syncopal episodes, depending on the age and prevalence of cardiac disease in the population examined.
   B. Over the past two decades, head-upright tilt table testing has become a widely accepted and effective component in the clinical evaluation of patients presenting with syncopal symptoms. Vasovagal syncope can be provoked by raising susceptible individuals upright on a tilt table with or without the concurrent administration of pharmacologic provocative agents. There is substantial agreement that head-upright tilt table testing is an acceptably accurate technique for providing diagnostic evidence for the vasovagal etiology of the syncopal episodes. As such, algorithms for the diagnostic evaluation of syncope have been modified to incorporate earlier use of tilt table testing, resulting in significant potential savings in terms of costs, time to diagnosis, and patient convenience.
II. **Evolution of head-upright tilt table testing.** Since the 1950's, head-upright tilt table testing has been employed to study the effect of postural influences on heart rate and blood pressure regulation. Serendipity led to the observation that during testing certain individuals (often with a clinical history of vasovagal syncope) would develop profound hypotension accompanied by varying degrees of bradyarrhythmia, culminating in syncope. Over the past decade, tilt table testing has been employed as a diagnostic tool in recurrent syncope, with various tilt-testing protocols undergoing extensive validation.
III. **Indications for head-upright tilt table testing**
   A. Head-upright tilt table testing should be the **initial diagnostic test** in the syncopal evaluation after a negative history, physical examination, and routine electrocardiogram (ECG) for patients whose symptoms are consistent with, but not entirely typical of, vasovagal syncope or have experienced repeated unexplained episodes. If the syncopal episode was devoid of the classic clinical features or occurred in a high-risk occupation, tilt table testing is useful to definitively establish the diagnosis and guide therapy. If pharmacologic therapy is appropriate to prevent recurrence of syncope, tilt table testing may be useful in guiding treatment. Table 47-1 outlines the indications for tilt table testing according to the American College of Cardiology guidelines (1). **Severe left ventricular outflow tract obstruction, critical mitral stenosis, critical proximal coronary artery stenosis, or critical cerebrovascular stenosis** are all considered relative contraindications to tilt table testing.
   B. However, **patients with a history typical for vasovagal syncope should have the diagnosis established on a clinical basis.** Common triggers include a stressful event or prolonged standing in the setting volume depletion, physical deconditioning, and states of heightened vagal tone. Characteristic premonitory symptoms often precede vasovagal syncope **including weakness, nausea, diaphoresis, yawning, and generalized warmth.**
   C. Patients whose history is not suggestive of vasovagal syncope should undergo diagnostic evaluation guided by findings in the history and physical exam

Table 47-1. Tilt table testing for evaluation of syncope: summary of principal indications

---

Tilt table testing is warranted:
- Recurrent syncope or single syncopal episode in a high-risk patient, whether or not the medical history is suggestive of neurally mediated (vasovagal) origin, and
  1. No evidence of structural cardiovascular disease

  or

  2. Structural cardiovascular disease is present, but other causes of syncope have been excluded by appropriate testing
- Further evaluation of patients in whom an apparent cause has been established (e.g., asystole, atrioventricular block), but in whom demonstration of susceptibility to neurally mediated syncope would affect treatment plans
- Part of the evaluation of exercise-induced or exercise-associated syncope

Reasonable differences of opinion exist regarding utility of tilt table testing:
- Differentiating convulsive syncope from seizures
- Evaluating patients (especially the elderly) with recurrent unexplained falls
- Assessing recurrent dizziness or presyncope
- Evaluating unexplained syncope in the setting of peripheral neuropathies or dysautonomias
- Follow-up evaluation to assess therapy of neurally mediated syncope

Tilt table testing not warranted:
- Single syncopal episode; without injury and not in a high-risk setting with clear-cut vasovagal clinical features
- Syncope in which an alternative specific cause has been established and in which additional demonstration of a neurally mediated susceptibility would not alter treatment plans

Potential emerging indications
- Recurrent idiopathic vertigo
- Recurrent transient ischemic attacks
- Chronic fatigue syndrome
- Sudden infant death syndrome

From Benditt DG, 1996, with permission.

and ECG. In the appropriate setting, electrophysiologic studies, echocardiography, and neurologic evaluation may be indicated. However, the indiscriminate use of such tests as diagnostic screens is both cost-ineffective and carries a low diagnostic yield.

IV. **Current head-upright tilt table testing protocol**
  A. The past two decades have witnessed the evolution of **multiple protocols for head-upright tilt table testing.** Methodologic variations center on the **degree and duration of tilt** as well as the **use of certain pharmacologic agents.** Table 47-2 outlines the recommendations from the **American College of Cardiology Expert Consensus Document** regarding tilt table testing technique.
  B. At some centers, protocols emphasize a "washout period" during which patients are weaned off nonessential medications prior to testing. In contrast, we have found that many medications promote vasovagal reactions (e.g., diuretics effecting hypovolemia) and thus we prefer not to discontinue these medications for extended periods prior to tilt testing. In the presence of a **positive test** (see Section VI of this chapter), **repeat study following the discontinuation of suspected medications** may be warranted.
  C. To minimize the effects of chronobiologic variation, any **repeat testing should be performed at similar times** of day. **Continuous monitoring of blood pressure and surface ECG** is essential, as is **reliable venous**

Table 47-2. Tilt table testing technique: summary of principal recommendations

Topic	Recommendation
Laboratory	• Quiet, dim lighting, comfortable temperature
Patient	• 20–45 min supine equilibration period
Recordings	• Fasting overnight or for several hours before
Table	procedure
Tilt angle	• Parenteral fluid replacement
Tilt duration	• Follow-up studies should be at similar times
Pharmacologic provocation	of day
Supervision	• Minimum of three ECG leads continuously
Pediatrics	recorded
	• Beat-to-beat blood pressure recordings using the least intrusive means (might not be feasible in children)
	• Foot board support
	• Smooth, rapid transitions (up and down)
	• 60–80 degrees acceptable
	• 70 degrees becoming most common
	• Initial drug-free tilt 30–45 min
	• Pharmacologic provocation—depends on agent
	• Isoproterenol (infusion preferred)
	• Nitroglycerin
	• Edrophonium
	• Nurse or laboratory technician experienced in tilt-table technique and cardiovascular laboratory procedures
	• Physician in attendance or in proximity and immediately available
	• Presents special problems
	• Tilt duration less certain
	• Blood pressure recording by sphygmomanometer is common

From Benditt DG, 1996, with permission.

access. **Noninvasive blood pressure monitors** are preferred, as these avoid the confounding vagal reactions that can accompany arterial puncture and catheterization.

D. Following an equilibration period of 20 to 40 minutes many laboratories begin with intermediate angles of tilt, from 15 to 45 degrees, to exclude severe orthostatic hypotension as a cause for syncope. Next, 60 to 80 degrees of tilt is sustained for 20 to 40 minutes. Full expression of the vasovagal process, culminating in syncope, is essential prior to returning the patient to supine position.

E. **Pharmacologic interventions** are reserved for a second stage if the initial drug-free tilt test is nondiagnostic. Isoproterenol is often used for this purpose, infused in graded doses ranging from 1 to 5 μg/minute at 60 degrees of tilt with 5 minutes supine between dose escalations. Other, less validated provocative pharmacologic agents include nitroglycerin and edrophonium. Pharmacologic provocation may enhance the sensitivity of tilt table testing for patients susceptible to vasovagal syncope, but at the cost of reduced specificity.

V. Pathophysiology

    A. Mammalian evolution has developed intricate autonomic adaptations to upright posture, thus minimizing changes in cerebral perfusion pressure across a broad range of positions and intravascular volumes. With standing,

300 to 800 cm³ of blood shifts from the thorax to the dependent extremities, producing an immediate reduction in ventricular filling volumes and mean arterial pressure. **This volume displacement can be provoked or may occur spontaneously in susceptible individuals.** In response to hypotension, **baroreceptors in the aortic arch and carotid sinuses reflexively decrease afferent signals to the brain's vasomotor center, resulting in a heightened catecholamine state** characterized by increasing heart rate and vasomotor tone.

B. In parallel fashion, the heart functions as a pressure sensory organ due to the activity of C fibers in the inferoposterior walls of the left ventricle. These receptors are stimulated by stretch or pressure (Bezold-Jarisch reflex) and carry impulses from the heart to the vasomotor center via vagal afferents. These C fibers can paradoxically misinterpret an underfilled, hypercontractile ventricle for extreme hypertension, consequently decreasing sympathetic output from the brain and leaving unopposed vagal tone. In susceptible individuals, **this imbalance of autonomic regulation can result in varying degrees of arteriolar vasodilatation and bradycardia,** producing hypotension and syncope.

C. The **head-upright tilt table test exploits any propensity for vasovagal syncope** by eliminating the component of venous return contributed by active contraction of the leg musculature and thus maximizing venous pooling. Observations of characteristic increases in circulating catecholamine levels prior to syncope in susceptible individuals prompted the incorporation of pharmacologic agents such as isoproterenol into tilt table testing protocols. This β-receptor agonist augments the vigor of myocardial contraction via a β₁-receptor effect and reduces peripheral arteriolar tone via a β₂-receptor effect. It is thought that isoproterenol augments positive tilt responses by enhancing the hemodynamic effects that initiate the Bezold-Jarisch reflex.

VI. **Abnormal responses to head-upright tilt table testing.** Table 47-3 defines some of the hemodynamic responses during tilt table testing. A description of the more common categories of abnormal responses to head-upright tilt table testing is given below. The treatment of these conditions is discussed in Chapter 22.

A. **Vasovagal response.** The classic vasovagal response is characterized by two observations: **a sudden drop in mean arterial pressure followed by a decrease in heart rate.** The vasodepressor response (hypotension due to peripheral vasodilatation) and the cardioinhibitory response (bradycardia or transient asystole) may manifest to differing degrees among individuals. **Vasovagal syncope may thus present predominantly as vasodepressor, cardioinhibitory, or mixed.** Rarely, **prolonged asystole may be encountered, necessitating intravenous atropine or transient cardiopulmonary resuscitation.** Full and rapid recovery is the rule, however. In the moments preceding a positive vasovagal response, **many patients**

Table 47-3. Tilt-table testing: hemodynamic parameters

Heart rate response
    Normal: Increase of 10–15 bpm or 10–15% above baseline
    Blunted (chronotropic incompetence): Minimal heart rate change ± 5 bpm
    Exaggerated: Increase >20 bpm or >30% above baseline
    Cardioinhibitory: Abrupt decrease in heart rate and/or AV conduction (>20 bpm)
Blood pressure response
    Normal: Decrease in SBP 0–20 mm Hg, increase in DBP ±10 mm Hg
    Orthostatic hypotension: Gradual drop in SBP >30 mm Hg, DBP >10 mm Hg
    Vasodepressor response: Abrupt decrease in blood pressure independent of
      heart rate

SBP, systolic blood pressure; DBP, diastolic blood pressure; AV, atrioventricular.
Modified from Maloney JD, 1997, with permission.

report typical premonitory symptoms such as nausea, diaphoresis, or warmth.

B. **Orthostatic response.** Although not vasovagal in etiology, orthostatic responses may be elicited by the tilt table testing protocol. These are defined by a gradual drop in systolic blood pressure of 30 mm Hg or more in the setting of sinus tachycardia and without a "vagal" prodrome.

C. **Dysautonomic responses.** A **gradual decrease in blood pressure leading to syncope** is observed. Often, there is a **clinical history of autonomic dysregulation** including constipation, diaphoresis, and thermal intolerance. The postural orthostatic tachycardia syndrome denotes a mild form of autonomic dysfunction whereby tachycardia is unable to compensate for diminished peripheral vascular resistance.

D. **Psychosomatic response.** Patients experience an **apparent loss of consciousness** in the absence of hypotension or bradyarrhythmia, and with normal findings of cerebral blood flow on transcranial Doppler ultrasonography. An underlying psychiatric disorder is postulated.

E. **Cerebral syncope.** A rare cause of **loss of consciousness** is cerebral syncope associated with decreased cerebral blood flow as measured by transcranial Doppler. This occurs in the absence of hypotension or bradycardia and is thought to be a manifestation of disordered cerebral vasoregulation.

VII. **Accuracy of head-upright tilt table testing**

A. **Sensitivity and specificity.** Studies suggest that tilt table testing performed at tilt angles of 60 to 70 degrees, and without pharmacologic provocation, has a specificity of 80% to 90% (10% to 20% false-positive responses in patients not clinically prone to neurally mediated syncopal episodes). Isoproterenol infusion will variably increase sensitivity at the cost of decreased specificity depending on the dose regimen and angle of tilt. The sensitivity of head-upright tilt table testing has been reported to range from 32% to 85% (1).

B. **Reproducibility.** The reproducibility of tilt table testing with current protocols is reported to be 65% to 85%. As such, 15% to 35% of initially "positive" responses will revert to negative on repeat testing, mandating caution in the assessment of the efficacy of various therapeutic interventions (1).

VIII. **Conclusions.** Head-upright tilt table testing has become the effective gold standard among available diagnostic studies in the evaluation of syncope due to vasovagal syndrome and other disturbances of autonomic tone. It is instrumental in establishing a diagnosis in the absence of a classic clinical history and in guiding therapy for vasovagal syncope. However, neither tilt table testing nor other diagnostic modalities are substitutes for sound clinical judgment in the diagnostic evaluation of syncope of unknown origin.

SUGGESTED READINGS

References

1. Benditt DG, Ferguson DW, Grubb BP, et al. Tilt table testing for assessing syncope. *J Am Coll Cardiol* 1996;28:263–275.
2. Maloney JD, Martin RC, Zhu DWX. Tilt table testing as a tool of the invasive cardiac electrophysiologist. In: Singer I, ed. *Interventional electrophysiology.* Baltimore: Williams & Wilkins, 1997:79–130.

Key Reviews

Benditt DG, Ferguson DW, Grubb BP, et al. Tilt table testing for assessing syncope. *J Am Coll Cardiol* 1996;28:263–275.

Calkins H, Byrne M, Morady F, et al. The economic burden of unrecognized vasodepressor syncope. *Am J Med* 1993;95:473–479.

Grubb BP, Temesy-Armos P, Hahn H, Elliott L. Utility of upright tilt table testing in the evaluation and management of syncope of unknown origin. *Am J Med* 1991;90:6–10.

Kosinsky D, Grubb BP, Temesy-Armos P. Pathophysiological aspects of neurocardiogenic syncope; current concepts and new perspectives. *Pacing Clin Electrophysiol* 1995;18:716–724.

Relevant Book Chapters

Benditt DG, Lurie KG, Adler SW, Sakaguchi S. Rationale and methodology of head-up tilt table testing for evaluation of neurally mediated (cardioneurogenic) syncope. In: Zipes DP, Jalife J, eds. *Cardiac electrophysiology: from cell to bedside,* 2nd ed. Philadelphia: WB Saunders, 1995:1115–1129.

Jaeger FJ, Fouad-Tarazi FM, Castle LW. Carotid sinus hypersensitivity and neurally mediated syncope. In: Ellenbogen KA, Kay N, Wilkoff BL, eds. *Clinical cardiac pacing.* Philadelphia: WB Saunders, 1995:333–352.

Maloney JD, Martin RC, Zhu DWX. Tilt table testing as a tool of the invasive cardiac electrophysiologist. In: Singer I, ed. *Interventional electrophysiology.* Baltimore: Williams & Wilkins, 1997:79–130.

SECTION XII. MISCELLANEOUS CONDITIONS

Steven P. Marso

48. INFECTIVE ENDOCARDITIS

Mark Murphy

I. **Introduction**
   A. Infective endocarditis (IE) is **an infection of the endothelial surface of the heart.** It is seen macroscopically as a vegetation. The condition is **always fatal if untreated and continues to cause significant morbidity and mortality** despite modern medical and surgical treatment. The clinical diagnosis is based on multiple elements.
   B. An estimated 10,000 to 15,000 new cases of IE are diagnosed each year in the United States. The incidence of IE has remained constant over time with notable demographic and microbiologic shifts. There has been an increase in the median age (50% are over 54 years), the male-to-female ratio (2.5:1), the number of acute cases, prosthetic valve infections, cases associated with injection drug use, and cases due to gram-negative and fungal infections (although these are still rare), with a slight decrease in the number of cases due to streptococcal species.

II. **Clinical presentation.** Symptoms of IE usually start within 2 weeks of the initiating bacteremia.
   A. **Signs and symptoms.** The clinical spectrum of IE ranges from subacute symptoms to fulminant congestive heart failure with severe valvular regurgitation.
      1. The **hallmarks of IE are fever and a new murmur** (over 85%). However, fever may be absent in the elderly and the uremic population. Murmurs may be absent with right-sided or mural infection.
      2. The patient may complain nonspecifically of fatigue; shortness of breath and arthralgias and/or myalgias are seen in 25% to 45% of cases.
   B. **Physical findings**
      1. **Congestive heart failure** has occurred in up to 55% of cases in the past and tends to be more common in those with aortic valve disease (75%) compared to those with mitral (50%) or tricuspid (19%) valve involvement.
      2. **Neurologic findings** may include clinically apparent cerebral emboli (20%), encephalopathy (10%), mycotic aneurysm leak (less than 5%), meningitis or brain abscess (less than 5%).
      3. Physical findings reflecting **other embolic or immune complex phenomena** associated with IE may be detected such as **petechiae** involving conjunctival, buccal, or palatal surfaces (20% to 40%); **splinter hemorrhages,** dark red linear streaks in the nail bed (10% to 30%); **Osler's nodes,** small tender nodules on the finger pad or toe pad (10% to 25%); **Janeway lesions,** small (less than 5 mm), flat, irregular, nontender red spots, found on the palms and soles, that blanch with pressure (less than 5%); **clubbing** (10% to 20%); **arterial embolism,** including limb ischemia, renal infarction, or myocardial infarction (25% to 45%); **splenomegaly** (25% to 60%); and **Roth's spots,** oval retinal hemorrhages with a clear center (less than 5%).
      4. A formal **fundoscopic examination** should be routine in all patients with suspected or documented fungal IE. It may reveal **chorioretinitis or endophthalmitis.**
      5. Subacute IE tends to have more classical immune complex physical signs because of its relative chronicity.
      6. Typical **valvular involvement** in cases involving injection drug use is tricuspid (78% of cases), mitral (24%), and aortic (8%). Pulmonary emboli that are often septic occur in 75% of injection drug abusers with tricuspid IE.

Table 48-1. Frequency or organisms causing infective endocarditis

Organism	NVE (%)	IDU (%)	Early PVE (%)	Late PVE (%)
Streptococci	60–80	15–20	5	35
Viridans streptococcus	30–40	15	<5	25
S. bovis	15	<5	<5	<5
Enterococci	5–18	2	<5	6
Staphylococci	25	50	50	30
Coagulase-positive	23	50	20	10
Coagulase-negative	<5	<5	30	20
Gram-negative (aerobes)	<5	5	20	10
Fungi	<5	5	10	5
Culture-negative	5–10	<5	<5	<5

NVE, native valve endocarditis; IDU, intravenous drug use; PVE, prosthetic valve endocarditis.
Modified from Alexander RW, 1998, with permission, from Excerpta Medica, Inc.

    7. The clinical distinction between **acute and subacute bacterial endocarditis** is still useful. The former is usually associated with organisms of high pathogenicity (e.g., *Staphylococcus aureus*), and the latter is associated with organisms of low pathogenicity (e.g., *Streptococcus viridans*).

    8. Of note, drugs, thrombophlebitis, sterile embolization, and abscess must be considered in the **differential diagnosis** of fever.

III. Etiology. Table 48-1 presents the various etiologies.

  A. Of patients with IE, **70% to 75% have preexisting cardiac abnormalities,** recognized or unrecognized. Rheumatic heart disease as a substrate for IE is decreasing, with congenital heart disease underlying 6% to 24% of cases of IE. **Mitral valve prolapse with regurgitation and degenerative valvular disease are the leading cardiac conditions** underlying IE in adults.

  B. Native valve endocarditis

    1. The most common microorganisms that cause native valve IE in adults (Table 48-2A) **are viridans streptococcus species,** *S. aureus, Streptococcus bovis,* enterococci, as well as the HACEK group (*Haemophilus, Actinobacillus, Cardiobacterium, Eikenella,* and *Kingella*) (3%). The HACEK group includes fastidious gram-negative organisms that may be considered part of the normal flora of the upper respiratory tract. *Streptococcus bovis* is associated with colonic polyps and colonic cancer.

    2. Right-sided IE in patients using intravenous drugs is usually due to *S. aureus*(60%), and despite the virulence of this organism, the disease tends to be less severe (mortality rates of 2% to 6%) than left-sided IE.

    3. IE from *Pseudomonas aeruginosa* **is both destructive and poorly responsive to antibiotic therapy, and as a result many patients require surgery.**

Table 48-2a. Duke criteria: definite pathologic diagnosis

A. *Microorganisms,* as demonstrated by culture or histology in
    Vegetation
    Vegetation that has embolized
    Intracardiac abscess
B. *Pathologic lesions:* vegetation or intracardiac abscess present, confirmed by histology showing active endocarditis

Modified from Durack DT, 1994, with permission.

    4. Other members of the Enterobacteriaceae *(Escherichia coli, Salmo-nella, Klebsiella, Enterobacter, Proteus, Serratia, Citrobacter, Shigella,* and *Yersinia)* are implicated in sporadic cases of IE.

    5. Streptococcus pneumonia accounts for 1% to 3% of native valve IE, and it may present as part of the "Austrian" triad which also includes pneumococcal pneumonia and meningitis. Alcoholics are typically affected, and mortality is high (30% to 50%). Therapy should be managed in consultation with an infectious disease specialist due to the increasing resistance of pneumococci to penicillin and other antimicrobials.

C. Prosthetic valve endocarditis (PVE). This has increased to account for 10% to 20% of all cases of IE in developed countries. The greatest risk appears to be during the first 6 months after valve implantation.

    1. Prosthetic valve endocarditis occurring within 2 months of surgery (early PVE) is likely to represent nosocomial infection with a predominance of coagulase-negative staphylococci.

    2. The microbiology of PVE with an onset more than 2 months after surgery (late PVE) reflects the pathogens of native valve IE and is most commonly caused by streptococcal species, whereas coagulase-negative staphylococci cause less than 20% of infections in this period. Fungi cause 10% to 15% of PVE cases with a mortality that is higher than that of bacterial PVE. Establishing the diagnosis of fungal PVE can be difficult due to the low yield from blood cultures. *Corynebacterium* species and other coryneform bacteria, often called diphtheroids, are commensals on the skin. Although often contaminants in blood cultures, diphtheroids in multiple cultures cannot be ignored. They are an important cause of PVE occurring in the initial year after surgery (5%).

D. Culture-negative endocarditis. The incidence is about 5% to 10% and may result from prior antibiotic therapy (most common), fastidious or slow-growing organisms (e.g., fungi, HACEK, anaerobes, *Legionella, Chlamydia psittaci, Coxiella, Brucella, Bartonella,* and nutritionally deficient streptococci) or nonbacterial endocarditis (Libman-Sacks, marantic, antiphospholipid syndrome).

E. Fungal endocarditis *(Candida* and *Aspergillus).* This usually occurs in association with **prosthetic valves, indwelling intravascular hardware, immunosuppression, or injection drug use.**

IV. Pathophysiology. The first step in the pathogenesis of a vegetation is the formation of a nonbacterial thrombotic endocarditis, which can result from endothelial injury or a hypercoagulable state.

A. The endothelium is typically injured by one of three hemodynamic mechanisms: a high-velocity jet, flow across a narrow orifice at high velocity, or flow going from a high- to a low-pressure chamber.

B. As a result, vegetations form at characteristic sites of injury, such as along the line of closure of a valve leaflet or the site of impact of a regurgitant jet.

C. Bacteremia is the event that converts nonbacterial thrombotic endocarditis to IE. *Staphylococcus aureus* **may affect normal valves as is often the case with injected drug use.**

V. Laboratory examination

A. Blood tests

    1. Findings usually include a **modest leukocytosis** and a slightly higher or lower **platelet count,** along with other markers of acute infection (e.g., **normochromic normocytic anemia, elevated erythrocyte sedimentation rate,** C-reactive protein, hypergammaglobulinemia, or elevated rheumatoid factor).

    2. Decreased complement and an elevated blood urea nitrogen or creatinine may reflect renal dysfunction from an immune complex glomerulonephritis or drug toxicity.

    3. Blood cultures are critical in the diagnosis and management of IE. Deterioration can be rapid in the acute setting and **therapy should not be delayed for more than 2 to 3 hours while cultures are obtained.**

    a. Three sets of cultures should be drawn over a period of 24 hours at three different venipuncture sites prior to initiation of antimicrobial therapy, clinical condition allowing. Each set should include two flasks: one containing an aerobic medium, and the other an anaerobic medium into which at least 10 mL of blood should be placed.

    b. Intravascular infection leads to continuous bacteremia; therefore, **blood cultures can be obtained in the absence of fever spikes.**

    c. The laboratory should be alerted if **culture-negative IE or a fastidious infecting agent** is suspected, as it may be necessary to enhance the culture medium or prolong the incubation period. For example, the HACEK group (see III.B.1) needs prolonged incubation of up to 21 days. In cases of culture-negative IE, serology for *Brucella, Legionella, Coxiella,* or psittacosis may be useful.

B. Urinalysis. Microhematuria with or without proteinuria may be seen.

C. ECG. All patients with suspected IE should have an ECG.

    1. It may reveal **conduction disturbances** reflecting intramyocardial extension of infection, ranging from a prolonged PR interval to complete heart block (especially with PVE).

    2. Evidence of a new **atrioventricular block** is quite specific for an aortic ring abscess.

    3. Myocardial infarction due to embolization of a vegetation occurs occasionally.

D. Chest x-ray

    1. It may reveal **congestive heart failure or pleural effusions.**

    2. Right-sided IE may cause **nonspecific infiltrates** due to multiple septic pulmonary emboli.

VI. Diagnostic testing

A. Echocardiography. The specificity of echocardiography for the diagnosis of IE is impaired because vegetations occasionally cannot be distinguished from noninfectious lesions such as myxomatous degeneration, thrombus, or pannus. Furthermore, it is not possible to distinguish acute from chronic vegetations.

    1. All patients in whom IE is suspected should have a baseline transthoracic echocardiogram (TTE) to determine the size and location of vegetations, to explore the possibility of complications (e.g., aortic annular ring abscess), and to define underlying cardiac abnormalities (e.g., ventricular dysfunction or valvular abnormalities).

    2. If IE is suspected and the TTE is negative, a transesophageal echocardiogram (TEE) should be strongly considered, as it is much more sensitive (82% to 94%) than TTE (60% to 75%) in detecting vegetations.

        a. A negative TEE is strong evidence against IE in a patient with an equivocal syndrome, especially when mitral valve infection is suspected, but the negative finding does not rule out the diagnosis.

        b. Myocardial abscesses are more reliably detected by TEE (87% sensitive) versus TTE (28% sensitive). Because of acoustic shadowing in the setting of PVE, **TEE is superior** (82% sensitive) to TTE (36% sensitive) in the detection of vegetations.

B. Cinefluoroscopy. If the clinical condition allows, the patient should undergo left heart catheterization with selective coronary angiography if there is a suspicion of obstructive coronary disease. The abnormal rocking motion of a dehisced prosthetic valve may be noted on fluoroscopy.

C. Central nervous system (CNS) imaging. Computed tomography, magnetic resonance imaging, or cerebral angiography should be considered in the patient who has sustained a CNS complication, such as embolic infarct, intracranial bleed, mycotic aneurysm, and in the patient with persistent headaches.

D. Body imaging. Computed tomography or magnetic resonance imaging may be useful in the detection of metastatic infection.

VII. Duke criteria. Given the nonspecific findings in IE, the diagnosis is often difficult. Therefore, criteria have been developed to aid in clinical diagnosis, of which the widely used Duke criteria are the most recent. These criteria are unique in that they include echocardiographic data and consider IDU as a risk factor for the development of IE. Consequently, the Duke criteria are more sensitive in patients with negative blood cultures and right-sided IE than are older criteria. They have not been validated in PVE.

A. The criteria are broken into **definite** (pathologic or clinical), **possible,** and **rejected** diagnostic groups.

B. For a **definite pathologic diagnosis,** either (A or B) of the pathologic findings listed in Table 2a are sufficient.

C. For a **definite clinical diagnosis** (Table 2b), two major criteria, or one major and three minor, or five minor criteria are needed.

D. The **possible diagnostic** group has findings consistent with IE, but they fall short of **"definite"** and do not fall into the **"rejected"** group.

E. For a **rejected diagnosis,** there is a firm alternative diagnosis for clinical manifestations or resolution of clinical manifestations, with antibiotics for 4 days or less, or no pathologic evidence of IE at surgery or autopsy, after antibiotic therapy for 4 days or less.

VIII. Therapy

A. Medical therapy

1. **Principles of therapy.** Antibiotic regimens are necessarily bactericidal, and infectious disease consultation should be obtained early. **Measures of antibiotic effectiveness** are minimum inhibitory concentration (MIC) of antibiotic required to inhibit growth, minimum bactericidal concentration (MBC) of an antibiotic required to kill an organism, and serum bactericidal titer (SBT), which is the highest dilution of a patient's serum that kills 99.9% of an inoculum. **The SBT is clinically helpful when treating unusual organisms, when using unusual antibiotic regimens, or when treatment is failing.** The MIC and MBC are rarely measured in current clinical practice; however, currently recommended antimicrobial regimens are based on their values for specific organisms, and these regimens should be closely followed.

   a. **Penicillin acts synergistically with an aminoglycoside** and high-level aminoglycoside resistance represents the most common and grave obstacle to optimal therapy for enterococcal endocarditis.

   b. Renal function is an important consideration when using **aminoglycosides or vancomycin** and they should be dosed according to estimated creatinine clearance. The doses outlined below are for normal renal function. A vancomycin dose should not exceed 2 g per 24 hours unless serum levels are monitored.

   c. Anticoagulation does not prevent embolization related to IE. In fact, **simultaneous treatment with penicillin and heparin** increases the risk of fatal intracerebral hemorrhage. Warfarin may be given safely during the treatment of patients with PVE; however, a short-acting agent is needed immediately preoperatively and the risk-to-benefit ratio of heparin should be carefully considered on a patient-to-patient basis.

2. **Empiric treatment of IE is often started and continued until the etiologic organism is identified** and the antibiotic sensitivities are known. Occasionally, empiric therapy is administered as a therapeutic trial to help confirm a diagnosis. Empiric therapy for subacute IE consists of ampicillin and gentamicin per the standard regimen for enterococcal endocarditis (Table 3b) with nafcillin, 12 g/24 hours IV in 6 divided doses, added for acute IE. Vancomycin per standard dosing for enterococcal IE is added instead of nafcillin if methicillin-resistant *S. aureus* (MRSA) is suspected, if the patient is penicillin-allergic, or if

Table 48-2b. Duke criteria: definite clinical diagnosis

MAJOR CLINICAL CRITERIA

1. Positive blood culture results for infective endocarditis
    A. Typical microorganisms (in two or more cultures)
       • Viridans streptococcus
       • *S. bovis*
       • HACEK group
       • Community-acquired *Staphylococcus aureus* or enterococci, in the absence of a primary focus
    B. Persistently positive blood culture
       • Recovery of a microorganism consistent with IE from blood cultures drawn more than 12 hr apart

                              or

       • Recovery of a microorganism consistent with IE from all of three or a majority of four or more separate blood cultures, with the first and last drawn at least 1 hr apart
2. Evidence of endocardial involvement
    A. Positive echocardiogram
       • Oscillating intracardiac mass, on valve or supporting structures, or in the path of regurgitant jets or on implanted material, in the absence of an alternative anatomic explanation

                              or

       • Abscess

                              or

       • New partial dehiscence of prosthetic valve

                              or

    B. New valvular regurgitation (increase or change in preexisting murmur not sufficient)

MINOR CLINICAL CRITERIA

1. Predisposition:
    • Predisposing heart condition
    • I.D.U. (Injection drug use)
2. Fever over 38.0°C (100.4°F)
3. Vascular phenomena:
    • Major arterial emboli
    • Septic pulmonary infarcts
    • Mycotic aneurysm
    • Intracranial hemorrhage
    • Conjunctival hemorrhages
    • Janeway lesions
4. Immunologic phenomena:
    • Glomerulonephritis
    • Osler's nodes
    • Roth's spots
    • Rheumatoid factor
5. Microbiologic evidence
    • Positive blood culture but not meeting major criteria
    • Serologic evidence of active infection with organism consistent with infective endocarditis
6. Echocardiogram consistent with infective endocarditis but not meeting major criteria

HACEK, Hemophilus, Actinobacillus, Cardiobacterium, Eikenella, Kingella; IE, infective endocarditis; IDU, injection drug use. Modified from Durack DT, 1994, with permission from Excerpta Medica, Inc.

prosthetic valves are involved. Unless clinical or epidemiologic clues suggest an etiology, treatment for culture-negative IE is the same.

3. Antibiotic therapy **after surgery** is discussed in the surgical therapy section, VIII.C.6.

4. Medical therapies for **specific organisms** are displayed in Tables 48-3A to 48-3F).

5. **Fungal IE.** When fungal IE is diagnosed, the standard of care involves a **combined medical/surgical approach.**

   a. The mainstay of antifungal drug therapy is amphotericin B with or without flucytosine.

      (1) Amphotericin B is infused in 5% dextrose over 2 to 4 hours at a dose of 0.5 mg/kg daily.

      (2) The main **toxicity of amphotericin B** is renal dysfunction; liposomal preparations may be less nephrotoxic.

Table 48-3a. Therapies for native valve infective endocarditis, due to penicillin-susceptible viridans streptococcus or *S. bovis*

Medication	Dosage	Duration of therapy
Penicillin G	12–18 million U/24 hr continuously IV or in 6 divided doses	4 wk
Ceftriaxone	2 g once daily IV or IM	4 wk
Penicillin G *plus* gentamicin *or*, if penicillin-allergic:	12–18 million U/24 hr continuously IV or in 6 divided doses 1 mg/kg IV or IM every 8 hr	2 wk[a]
Vancomycin	30 mg/per 24 hr in 2 divided doses	4 wk

[a] For relatively resistant viridans streptococcus or *S. bovis,* penicillin G dosing is extended to 4 weeks.
IV, intravenous; IM, intramuscular. Modified from Wilson WR, 1995, with permission of the American Medical Association.

Table 48-3b. Standard therapies for susceptible enterococci, for resistant and nutritionally variant viridans streptococcus infective endocarditis, and for prosthetic valve endocarditis due to viridans streptococcus or *S. bovis*

Medication	Dosage	Duration of therapy
Penicillin G *plus* gentamicin *or*	18–30 million U/24 hr continuously IV or in 6 divided doses 1 mg/kg IV or IM every 8 hr	4–6 wk[a]
Ampicillin *plus* gentamicin *or*, if penicillin-allergic:	12 g/24 hr continuously IV or in 6 divided doses 1 mg/kg IV or IM every 8 hr	4–6 wk[a]
Vancomycin *plus* gentamicin	30 mg/kg per 24 hr in 2 divided doses 1 mg/kg IV or IM every 8 hr	4–6 wk[a]

[a] Four-week therapy is recommended for patients with symptoms less than 3 months in duration; 6-week therapy is recommended for patients with symptoms longer than 3 months in duration.
IV, intravenous; IM, intramuscular. Modified from Wilson WR, 1995, with permission of the American Medical Association.

Table 48-3c. Therapies for infective endocarditis due to methicillin-sensitive staphyloccocus in the absence of prosthetic material

Medication	Dosage	Duration of therapy
Nafcillin or oxacillin *plus*	2 g IV every 4 hr	4–6 wk
optional gentamicin *or*	1 mg/kg IV or IM every 8 hr	3–5 d
Cefazolin *plus*	2 g IV every 8 hr	4–6 wk
optional gentamicin *or*, if penicillin-allergic	1 mg/kg IV or IM every 8 hr	3–5 d
Vancomycin[a]	30 mg/kg per 24 hr in 2 divided doses	4–6 wk

[a] Recommended for methicillin-resistant staphylococcus.
IV, intravenous; IM, intramuscular. Modified from Wilson WR, 1995, with permission of the American Medical Association.

Table 48-3d. Therapy for infective endocarditis due to methicillin-sensitive staphylococcus in the presence of prosthetic material

Medication	Dosage	Duration of therapy
Nafcillin[a] or oxacillin	2 g IV every 4 hr	>6 wk
plus rifampin	300 mg orally every 8 hr	>6 wk
plus gentamicin	1 mg/kg IV or IM every 8 hr	2 wk

[a] For methicillin-resistant staphylococcus or for the penicillin-allergic patient, vancomycin, 30 mg/kg per 24 hr IV in two divided doses, is substituted for nafcillin.
IV, intravenous; IM, intramuscular. Modified from Wilson WR, 1995, with permission of the American Medical Association.

Table 48-3e. Therapy for infective endocarditis due to HACEK microorganisms.

Medication	Dosage	Duration of therapy
Ceftriaxone[a] *or*	2 g once daily IV or IM	4 wk
ampicillin *plus*	12 g/24 hr continuously or IV in 6 divided doses	
Gentamicin	1 mg/kg IV or IM every 8 hr	4 wk

[a] The third-generation cephalosporins should be considered the drugs of choice. Length of therapy for prosthetic valve infective endocarditis should be 6 weeks. For patients unable to tolerate β-lactam therapy, the HACEK group are susceptible in vitro to trimethoprim-sulfamethoxazole, fluoroquinolones, and aztreonam. Modified from Wilson WR, 1995, with permission of the American Medical Association.

Table 48-3f. Therapy for Pseudomonas aeruginosa and other gram-negative bacilli (Enterobacteriaceae)[a]

Extended-spectrum penicillin (ticarcillin or piperacillin)
    or third-generation cephalosporin
    or imipenem
plus aminoglycoside

[a] Combination therapy is recommended. The final choice of antibiotic therapy is to be made after sensitivity results are available.

      (3) The primary **toxicity of flucytosine** is bone marrow suppression; for this reason flucytosine blood levels may be useful during therapy.
- **b.** After 1 to 2 weeks at full doses of amphotericin B, surgery should probably be performed. Valve replacement is necessary for fungal IE.
- **c. Long-term oral suppressive therapy** with antifungal agents such as fluconazole or itraconazole is considered necessary by many to prevent relapse.

B. Surgical therapy (Table 48-4)
1. The **fundamental principles** of operative procedures for IE involve debridement of infected tissue, extensive removal of all nonviable tissue, and secure reconstruction of the involved area. Valve competence should be restored with repair of any additional defects under cover of appropriate antibiotic therapy.
2. **Congestive heart failure is the most common indication** for surgery in IE, with 90% of all deaths occurring from congestive heart failure.
3. **Prosthetic valve endocarditis likely needs a combined medical/surgical approach.**
4. **Patients with CNS infarcts or bleeds.** Special attention must be paid to the presurgical candidate who may have had a CNS infarct or bleed, as large doses of heparin are required for a cardiopulmonary bypass. A conservative surgical approach to patients who have sustained a CNS embolic infarct should be to delay surgery for at least 4 and ideally 10 postinfarction days, and for those who have sustained an intracranial hemorrhage for at least 21 days. Some patients may need early surgery in spite of a recent stroke if they are at high risk of recurrent emboli. **If a mycotic aneurysm is found, the timing of surgery should be reconsidered, and prostheses that require postoperative anticoagulation should be avoided.**
5. Metastatic infection usually related to *S. aureus* must be drained if accessible.
6. The optimal duration of **antibiotic therapy after surgery** for IE is not known.
   - **a.** For **native valve IE** caused by relatively antibiotic-resistant organisms with negative cultures of operative specimens, preoperative plus postoperative antibiotic therapy should at least equal a full course of recommended treatment.
   - **b.** For patients with **positive intraoperative cultures,** a full course of therapy should be given postoperatively.
   - **c. Patients with prosthetic valves undergoing surgery for IE should be treated conservatively** and receive a full course of antibiotics postoperatively when organisms are seen in resected material.

Table 48-4. Surgical Indications

CLEAR INDICATIONS

Uncontrolled congestive heart failure due to valve dysfunction
Unstable prosthesis
Uncontrolled/uncontrollable infection (e.g., by fungi or resistant enterococci)
Relapse of prosthetic valve endocarditis after optimal therapy
Recurrent emboli

RELATIVE INDICATIONS

Perivalvular extension of infection (fistula/abscess)
S. aureus endocarditis
Relapse of native valve endocarditis after optimal antimicrobial therapy
Culture-negative endocarditis with persistent unexplained fever (>10 days)
Large vegetations (>10 mm in diameter) with risk of embolization

---

Modified from Braunwald E, 1997, with permission.

IX. Complications

A. Table 48-5 lists the various complications of IE.

B. **Valve ring abscess** is a noteworthy complication of PVE, seen with mechanical and bioprosthetic valves. Infection in the sutures used to secure the sewing ring to the periannular tissue may result in dehiscence of the valve. The clinical finding of a new perivalvular leak in a patient with PVE is worrisome for a valve ring abscess.

C. Extension of a valve abscess beyond the valve ring may result in **myocardial abscess, septal perforation, or purulent pericarditis,** which are complications likely **needing surgery.**

X. Response to therapy.
While a shrinking vegetation during antimicrobial therapy suggests therapeutic success, vegetations may persist unchanged in the face of microbiologic cure. Significant enlargement of a vegetation during treatment indicates possible treatment failure and constitutes a relative indication for surgery.

A. **Blood cultures** should be obtained during therapy for IE to ensure eradication of the organism (see V.A.3).

B. Defervescence usually follows 3 to 7 days of successful antimicrobial therapy, and **persistent or recurrent fever may be a manifestation of therapeutic failure.**

C. Relapses, should they occur, usually manifest themselves clinically within 4 weeks and can be confirmed by blood cultures (see V.A.3). **About 10% of patients have additional episodes** of IE months or years later.

D. The **frequency of emboli falls rapidly after 1 to 2 weeks of antibiotic therapy,** and the risk is felt to be greater in the setting of large vegetations (larger than 10 mm in diameter) and specific infections (fungi, HACEK, and *Streptococcus agalactiae*).

E. Medical management is successful in many patients with IE; however, surgery is required in about 25% of cases.

XI. Prognosis.
The overall mortality of IE is around 30%. **Large vegetations may carry a poorer prognosis.** Notably, the mortality rates in early PVE (40% to 80%) are much higher than in late disease (20% to 40%). **Prognosis is related to bacterial virulence.** The course of *S. aureus* IE is typically fulminant with mortality rates of up to 40%. The presence of the factors in Table 48-6 should trigger an early and aggressive management plan.

XII. Prophylaxis.
Because IE may occur in spite of appropriate antibiotic prophylaxis, the practitioner should **maintain a high index of suspicion in the at-risk patient regarding clinical signs of infection** following dental or other procedures. The at-risk individual should be counseled and advised to carry a card with current prophylaxis recommendations.

Table 48-5. Complications

Cardiac complications
    Congestive heart failure (leading cause of death)
    Abscess (pericardial, aortic annular, or myocardial)
    Conduction abnormalities (due to invasive disease)
    Coronary embolism
    Mycotic aneurysm (often clinically silent)
    Valvular regurgitaton (cusp/leaflet flail or perforation)
    Valvular stenosis
    Prosthetic dehiscence
    Septal perforation (vertricular septal defect)
Extracardiac complications
    Systemic embolism (stroke, renal infarct, splenic infarct, or ischemic limb)
    Mycotic aneurysm
    Abscess
    Immune complex deposition (glomerulonephritis)

Table 48-6. Factors and complications that predispose to a poor outcome

Congestive heart failure (leading adverse prognostic factor)
Nonstreptococcal disease
Aortic valve involvement
Infection on a prosthetic valve
Older age
Abscess formation
HIV with CD4 count <200
Delayed diagnosis
CNS or coronary embolization
Recurrent infective endocarditis

HIV, human immunodeficiency virus; CNS, central nervous system.

   A. In deciding the need for antibiotic prophylaxis, two factors must be considered, namely, the risk of the valve lesion (Table 48-7a) and the type of procedure to be performed (Table 48-7b). Prophylaxis is advised when the combination of the underlying cardiac condition and the procedure seems to pose substantial risk of IE.

   B. Therapy may need to be individualized in a given clinical setting, and **high-risk cardiac patients** (see Table 48-7a) **may need to be prophylaxed prior to low-risk procedures.**

   C. Rates of bacteremia are highest for events that traumatize the oral mucosa, followed by those that traumatize the genitourinary tract. The frequency of bacteremia is relatively low for gastrointestinal diagnostic procedures.

Table 48-7a. Risk of infective endocarditis associated with preexisting cardiac disorders

PROPHYLAXIS FOR ENDOCARDITIS RECOMMENDED

HIGH-RISK CARDIAC CONDITION
Prosthetic heart valves
Previous infective endocarditis
Cyanotic congenital heart disease (single ventricle states, transposition of the great arteries, tetralogy of Fallot)
Surgically constructed systemic-pulmonary shunts (e.g., Blalock shunt)

INTERMEDIATE-RISK CARDIAC CONDITION
Mitral valve prolapse with regurgitation
Acquired valvular dysfunction (e.g., rheumatic heart disease)
Hypertrophic cardiomyopathy
Most congenital cardiac malformations (other than those listed above and below)

PROPHYLAXIS NOT RECOMMENDED

LOW-RISK CARDIAC CONDITION (RISK NO GREATER THAN GENERAL POPULATION)
Mitral valve prolapse without regurgitation[a]
Trivial valvular regurgitation on echocardiography without structural abnormality (except mitral valve prolapse)
Isolated atrial septal defect
Atherosclerotic plaque
Coronary disease or previous coronary artery bypass surgery
Cardiac pacemakers or defibrillators
Previous Kawasaki's disease or rheumatic fever without valvular dysfunction
Surgically repaired intracardiac lesions, with minimal or no hemodynamic abnormality more than 6 months after operation
Innocent heart murmur

[a] See XII.H.2 for further details. Modified from Dajani AS, 1997, with permission.

Table 48-7b. Recommendations for prophylaxis in dental or surgical procedures

PROPHYLAXIS RECOMMENDED FOR HIGH AND MEDIUM RISK CARDIAC CONDITION

OROPHARYNGEAL PROCEDURES
Dental procedures known to induce gingival or mucosal bleeding
Tonsillectomy and/or adenoidectomy
Bronchoscopy with a rigid bronchoscope

GASTROINTESTINAL PROCEDURES[a]
Surgical operations that involve intestinal mucosa
Sclerotherapy for esophageal varices
Esophageal stricture dilatation
Biliary surgery
Endoscopic biliary cannulation with biliary obstruction

GENITOURINARY PROCEDURES
Cystoscopy
Urethral dilatation
Prostate surgery

MISCELLANEOUS
Incision and drainage of infected tissue

PROPHYLAXIS NOT RECOMMENDED

OROPHARYNGEAL
Dental procedures not likely to induce gingival bleeding
Injection of local intraoral anesthetic (except intraligamentary injections)
Shedding of primary teeth
Tympanostomy tube insertion
Endotracheal intubation
Bronchoscopy with a flexible bronchoscope with or without biopsy[b]

GASTROINTESTINAL PROCEDURES[b]
Transesophageal echocardiography
Endoscopy with or without gastrointestinal biopsy

GENITOURINARY PROCEDURES
Postoperative suture removal
Cesarean section
Vaginal hysterectomy or uncomplicated vaginal delivery[b]
Circumcision
Specific procedures in the absence of infection, including:
    Urethral catheterization
    Dilatation and curettage
    Therapeutic abortion
    Sterilization procedures
    Insertion or removal of intrauterine device

CARDIAC PROCEDURES
Cardiac catheterization or balloon angioplasty
Implanted stents, pacemakers, or defibrillators

[a] Prophylaxis is recommended for high-risk but is optional for medium-risk cardiac conditions.
[b] Prophylaxis is optional for high-risk cardiac conditions. Modified from Dajani AS, 1997, with permission.

D. Endocarditis prophylaxis following **dental or oral procedures** is primarily directed against viridans streptococcus; following **genitourinary and gastrointestinal surgery** it is primarily directed against enterococci.

E. Local measures such as application of chlorhexidine (15 mL, rinse for 30 seconds) to the gums prior to a **dental procedure** as an adjunct to antibiotic prophylaxis may be used in patients who are at high risk and/or have poor dental hygiene. Edentulous patients may develop bacteremia from ulcers caused by ill-fitting dentures. It is recognized that unanticipated oral bleeding may occur on some occasions, and in such an event, evidence from animal models suggests that antimicrobial prophylaxis administered within 2 hours of the procedure provides effective prophylaxis.

F. If an unanticipated bacteremia is suspected during **vaginal delivery,** intravenous antibiotics can be administered at that time.

G. **Incision and drainage** or other procedures involving infected tissue may result in bacteremia. For nonoral soft tissue infections, an antistaphylococcal penicillin or first-generation cephalosporin is an appropriate choice of prophylaxis. For urinary tract infection, agents active against gram-negative bacilli are advisable.

H. **Prophylaxis regimens** are displayed in Table 48-7c.

1. Many **cardiac surgical patients** receive antibiotic prophylaxis, primarily directed against *S. aureus*. A first-generation cephalosporin is commonly used, but the choice of antibiotic should be influenced by the antibiotic susceptibility patterns at each hospital. Prophylaxis should be started immediately before the procedure, repeated during prolonged procedures, and continued for no more than 24 hours. A careful preop-

Table 48-7c. Prophylactic regimens

Clinical situation	Antibiotic	Dose
FOR DENTAL, ORAL, RESPIRATORY TRACT, OR ESOPHAGEAL PROCEDURES		
Standard prophylaxis	Amoxicillin	2 g PO 1 hr before procedure
Unable to take oral medications	Ampicillin	2 g IV or IM within 30 min before procedure
Penicillin allergy	Clindamycin *or*	600 mg PO 1 hr before procedure
	cephalexin *or* cephadroxil *or*	2 g PO 1 hr before procedure
	azithromycin *or* clarithromycin	500 mg 1 hr before procedure
FOR GENITOURINARY/GASTROINTESTINAL (EXCLUDING ESOPHAGEAL) PROCEDURES		
High-risk patients	Ampicillin *plus*	2 g IM or IV
	gentamicin (within 30 min of starting procedure) *followed by*	1.5 mg/kg IV or IM (not to exceed 120 mg)
	ampicillin *or*	1 g IM or IV
	amoxil (6 hr later)	1 g PO
High-risk patients allergic to penicillin	Vancomycin *plus*	1 g IV over 1–2 hr
	gentamicin (within 30 min of starting procedure)	1.5 mg/kg IV or IM (not to exceed 120 mg)
Moderate-risk patients	Amoxicillin *or*	2 g PO 1 hr before procedure
	ampicillin	2 g IV or IM within 30 min of starting procedure
Moderate-risk patients allergic to penicillin	Vancomycin	1 g IV over 1–2 hr completed within 30 min of starting the procedure

PO, per oral; IV, intravenous; IM, intramuscular. Modified from Dajani AS, 1997, with permission.

erative dental evaluation is recommended so that, whenever possible, required dental treatment can be completed before valvular cardiac surgery.

2. **Antibiotic prophylaxis for mitral valve prolapse with or without regurgitation** has been a controversial issue in recent times; current guidelines have sought to clarify this issue. Normal valves with normal motion often have minimal regurgitation and this does not appear to increase the risk of endocarditis. However, patients with prolapsing valves who have regurgitation, even if only detectable by Doppler, should receive prophylactic antibiotics. In patients of any age, myxomatous mitral valve degeneration with regurgitation is an indication for antibiotic prophylaxis. Men older than 45 years with mitral valve prolapse but without a consistent systolic murmur may warrant prophylaxis, even in the absence of resting regurgitation. Patients with thickened mitral values that do not leak on resting examination often develop regurgitation with exercise and thus may warrant prophylaxis.

XIII. Controversies
A. Therapy
1. **Short courses of antibiotics** (2 weeks) have shown some efficacy in the injection drug use population, as have oral antibiotics in the same population.
2. **Correct timing of surgery** is the most difficult and critical decision in the management of IE and a balance is needed between medical stabilization and timely surgery.
3. **Valve repair** is a reasonable option for mitral, tricuspid, and, less often, aortic IE in which the infection has been controlled. The choice between mechanical, bioprosthetic, and biologic devices may be made according to the usual criteria. However, there is some evidence that a homograft or even a pulmonary autograft is less likely to be followed by recurrent infection than either a xenograft or a mechanical valve.

B. Prophylaxis
1. Most transplant physicians categorize **patients after cardiac transplantation** as being at moderate risk for endocarditis secondary to continuous immunosuppression and the tendency to develop acquired valvular dysfunction (tricuspid regurgitation from endocardial biopsy).
2. **Noncoronary vascular grafts** may merit antibiotic prophylaxis for the first 6 months after implantation.
3. **Pneumococcal vaccination** should be considered for all patients with prosthetic heart valves.

SUGGESTED READINGS
Landmark Articles

Dajani AS, Taubert KA, Wilson W, et al. Prevention of bacterial endocarditis: recommendations by the American Heart Association. *Circulation* 1997;96:358–366.

Durack DT. Prevention of infective endocarditis. *N Engl J Med* 1995;332:38–44.

Durack DT, Lukes AS, Bright DK. New criteria for diagnosis of infective endocarditis: utilisation of specific echocardiographic findings. *Am J Med* 1994;96:200–209.

Von Reyn CF, Levy BS, Arbeit RD, Friedland G, Crumpacker CS. Infective endocarditis: an analysis based on strict case definitions. *Ann Intern Med* 1981;94: 505–518.

Wilson WR, Karchmer AW, Dajani AS, et al. Antibiotic treatment of adults with infective endocarditis due to streptococci, enterococci, staphylococci, and HACEK microorganisms. *JAMA* 1995;274:1706–1713.

Key Reviews

Child JS, ed. Diagnosis and management of infective endocarditis. *Cardiol Clin North Am* 1996;14.

Farmer JA, Torre G. Endocarditis. *Curr Opin Cardiol* 1997;12:123–130.

Relevant Book Chapters

Alexander RW, Schlant RC, Fuster V, eds. *Hurst's the heart.* New York: McGraw-Hill, 1998:2205–2239.

Baue A, Geha AS, Hammond GL, Laks H, Naunheim KS, eds. *Glenn's thoracic and cardiovascular surgery,* 6th ed. Norwalk, CT: Appleton & Lange, 1996:1915–1930.

Braunwald E, ed. *Heart disease: a textbook of cardiovascular medicine,* 5th ed. Philadelphia: WB Saunders, 1997:1077–1104.

Fauci AS, ed. *Harrison's principles of internal medicine,* 14th ed. New York: McGraw-Hill, 1998:785–791.

Mandell GL, Bennett JE, Dolin R, eds. *Principles and practice of infectious diseases,* 4th ed. New York: Churchill-Livingstone, 1995:740–799.

Otto C. *The practice of clinical echocardiography.* Philadelphia: WB Saunders, 1997: 389–403.

Topol EJ, ed. *Textbook of cardiovascular medicine.* Philadelphia: Lippincott-Raven Publishers, 1998:607–637.

49. RHEUMATIC FEVER

Simone Nader

I. **Introduction.** Classified as a connective tissue or collagen vascular disease, rheumatic fever (RF) is the **leading cause of acquired heart disease in children and young adults.**

   A. The incidence of RF and prevalence of rheumatic heart disease **varies substantially among different countries.** Since the first half of this century, there has been a gradual decline in the incidence of RF in the United States, Japan, and most European countries. In many developing countries the incidence of acute RF approaches or exceeds 100 per 100,000, whereas in the Unites States it is estimated to be less than 2 per 100,000.

   B. Rheumatic fever is more common among populations at high risk for streptococcal pharyngitis, such as military recruits, those in close contact with school age children, and persons of low socioeconomic status. It occurs commonly between the ages of 5 and 18 years and is rare before age 5. Rheumatic fever affects both sexes equally, except for Sydenham's chorea, which is more prevalent in females after puberty.

II. **Clinical presentation.** The clinical manifestations of RF **develop after a silent period of approximately 3 weeks following a tonsillopharyngitis caused by a group A streptococcal (GAS) infection.** The patient initially presents with a sudden onset of constitutional symptoms such as fever, malaise, weight loss, and pallor. The **acute phase of RF is characterized by an exudative and proliferative inflammatory process** involving collagen fibrils. **Multiple organ systems** such as the dermis, central nervous system, synovium, as well as the heart, may be involved. In addition, manifestations may include serositis and involvement of the lungs, kidneys, and central nervous system.

   A. **Diagnostic criteria**

      1. The **Jones criteria,** updated in 1992, are designed to aid in the diagnosis of the first episode of RF. Rheumatic fever can be diagnosed when a **previous upper airway infection with GAS is detected in conjunction with either two major manifestations, or one major and two minor manifestations.** Major manifestations include arthritis, carditis, chorea, erythema marginatum, and subcutaneous nodules. Minor manifestations include fever, arthralgias, high C-reactive protein, high erythrocyte sedimentation rate or prolonged PR interval on electrocardiogram (ECG).

      2. In some circumstances, the **diagnosis of RF can be made without strict adherence to Jones criteria,** as in cases of indolent carditis or isolated cases of chorea when other causes have been excluded.

   B. **Major manifestations**

      1. **Carditis.** This is the most serious and is often regarded as the most specific manifestation of RF, affecting 41% to 83% of patients. It can be defined as pancarditis affecting the endocardium, myocardium, and pericardium.

         a. Cardiac involvement **ranges from an asymptomatic presentation to progressive congestive heart failure and death.**

         b. The main clinical manifestations include **increased heart rate, murmurs, cardiomegaly, rhythm disturbances, pericardial friction rub, and heart failure.**

         c. **Congestive heart failure is rare in the acute phase;** if present, it usually results from myocarditis.

         d. The **most characteristic component of rheumatic carditis is a valvulitis (endocarditis) involving the mitral and aortic valves.**

            (1) **Mitral insufficiency is the hallmark of rheumatic carditis,** whereas aortic insufficiency is less common and is usually associated with mitral insufficiency.

    (2) **The acute mitral valve regurgitation produces an apical systolic murmur** that may be accompanied by a middiastolic Carey Coombs murmur of relative mitral stenosis (a high-pitch early diastolic murmur that varies from day to day). The right-sided valves are rarely involved.

    e. Pericarditis may cause chest pain, friction rubs, and distant heart sounds but is commonly clinically silent.

  2. Arthritis. This is the **most common manifestation of RF but is least specific.** It is present in around 80% of the patients and has been described as **painful, asymmetric, migratory, and transient; it involves large joints,** such as knees, ankles, elbows, wrists, and shoulders. It is **more common in older patients.** It improves markedly with the use of salicylates within 48 hours of treatment. Monoarthritis, oligoarthritis, and involvement of small joints of the extremities are less common. However, arthritis of the first metatarsophalangeal joint, enthesopathy, and axial involvement, especially of the cervical spine, have also been reported. The **arthritis of RF is benign and self-limiting** (lasting 2 to 3 weeks) and does not result in permanent sequelae. Inflammatory changes without signs of infection are seen in the joint fluid.

  3. Sydenham's chorea. Also known as Saint Vitus's dance or chorea minor, this **extrapyramidal disorder is characterized by purposeless and involuntary movements** of face and limbs, muscular hypotonia, and emotional lability.

    a. Initial manifestations include difficulty in writing, talking, or walking. Handwriting may deteriorate; speech may change to an explosive and halting tone; and the patient may become uncoordinated and easily frustrated.

    b. Symptoms tend to be more evident when the patient is under stress or awake and usually disappear during sleeping.

    c. Sydenham's chorea is a **delayed manifestation of RF,** usually appearing 3 months or more after an upper airway infection; it is often the sole manifestation of acute RF. Chorea has been reported in up to 30% of the patients; most cases tend to follow a benign course with complete resolution of the symptoms in 2 to 3 months, although cases of persisting symptoms of more than 2 years have been reported.

    d. It is important to **differentiate the symptoms of Sydenham's chorea from tics, athetosis, conversion reactions, hyperkinesia, and behavioral abnormalities.**

  4. Subcutaneous nodules. These are usually 0.5- to 2-cm-long, **firm, painless, and freely mobile nodules that can be isolated or found in clusters** over the extensor surfaces of joints (knees, elbows, and wrists), bony prominences, tendons, dorsum of foot, occipital region, and cervical processes. They are seen in up to 20% of patients with RF and last for a few days. The skin overlying the nodules is freely mobile and does not have signs of discoloration or inflammation.

  5. Erythema marginatum. This is an **evanescent macular rash,** erythematous, with a pale center of irregular shape. It is **usually nonpruritic and tends to disappear after a few days.** It is highly specific, occurring in less than 5% of patients, and is obvious only in fair-skinned individuals. The lesions vary in size and affect mainly the trunk, abdomen, and inner aspect of arms and thighs, but not the face. The rash may be induced by application of heat; its presence is **suggestive of coexisting carditis.**

C. Minor manifestations. Fever and arthralgias are common but nonspecific findings of RF that can be used to support the diagnosis of RF when only a single major manifestation is present.

  1. Fever is encountered during the acute phase of the disease and does not follow a specific pattern.

  2. Arthralgia is defined as pain in one or more large joints without objective findings of inflammation on physical examination.

3. **Other clinical manifestations** of RF include **abdominal pain, epistaxis, acute glomerulonephritis, rheumatic pneumonitis, hematuria, and encephalitis.** These are not included as a diagnostic criteria for the diagnosis of RF.

III. **Etiology and pathophysiology**

A. The association between tonsillopharyngitis-scarlet fever epidemics and acute RF in the 1930s, the findings of high levels of antistreptolysin O (ASO) in sera of patients with RF, and the confirmation of antibiotics as an efficient mode of prophylaxis of RF provide **strong evidence that GAS is the agent causing initial and recurrent attacks of RF.**

1. **Acute RF might not be caused directly by the bacteria but through an immunologic mechanism.** Supporting evidence includes its onset approximately 3 weeks following an upper respiratory tract infection, its rarity before age 5 when the immune system is still not fully developed, and the cross-reactivity between streptococcal cellular antigens and proteins present in human connective tissue.

   a. The most important antigenic structures (M, T, and R proteins) are localized in the external layer of the cell wall of the bacteria.

   b. The M protein is not only responsible for type-specific immunity; it also has a powerful antiphagocytic action and is classically regarded as a marker of streptococcal rheumatogenic potential. Patients with acute RF possess high levels of antibodies targeted against this protein. Specific M serotypes of GAS have long been recognized to be strong stimulators of a robust immune response and are associated with an increased risk for developing RF.

2. In epidemics of streptococcal pharyngitis, it is estimated that approximately 3% of untreated individuals will go on to develop RF. However, recurrence of RF is seen in about 50% of patients with a prior history of RF. For endemic GAS pharynsial infections, the incidence of RF is much less common.

B. Numerous epidemiologic studies favor a **familial and even genetic predisposition.** A monoclonal antibody to B-cell alloantigen (D8/17) is almost universally detected in patients with RF, whereas this antibody is present in less than 14% of the general population. In addition, susceptibility to RF has also been linked with D-related human leukocyte antigen (HLA-DR) 1, 2, 3, and 4 haplotypes. These genetic markers may be useful in the future to identify individuals susceptible to acute RF.

IV. **Laboratory examination and diagnostic testing.** The diagnosis of RF is a clinical diagnosis because there is no single laboratory study that is diagnostic of RF.

A. **Supporting evidence of antecedent GAS infection can be obtained through cultures or serum antistreptococcal antibodies test.**

1. Neither throat culture nor rapid antigen tests, if positive, differentiate between recent infection associated with RF and chronic carriage of pharyngeal GAS.

2. **Antistreptolysin O is the most commonly available test.**

   a. Elevated or rising ASO titers provide solid evidence for recent GAS infection. A greater than twofold rise in ASO titers compared with convalescent titers is diagnostic.

   b. **Specificity.** An ASO titer can be increased in rheumatoid arthritis, Takayasu's arteritis, and Schönlein-Henoch purpura, as well as in healthy children.

3. **The probability of detecting a previous GAS infection can be increased** by obtaining repeated ASO tests or by looking for antibodies to other streptococcal antigens such as antideoxyribonuclease B (anti-DNAase B), antihyaluronidase, antistreptokinase, and anti–nicotinamide adenine dinucleosidase (anti-NADase).

4. **A slide agglutination test** is commercially available and measures antibodies to several streptococcal antigens. Although this test is simple to perform, it is **not well standardized and is not very repro-**

ducible. Therefore, it is **not recommended** as a definitive test to detect preceding GAS infection.

B. **Biopsies**
1. **Aschoff's nodules in the proliferative stage are considered pathognomonic of rheumatic carditis.** It is encountered in 30% to 40% of biopsies from patients with primary or recurrent episodes of RF. They are most often found in the interventricular septum, the wall of the left ventricle, or the left atrial appendage.
2. **The histological findings of endocarditis** include edema and cellular infiltration of valvular tissue. Hyaline degeneration of the affected valve results in the formation of verrucae at its edge, preventing the normal leaflet coaptation. If the inflammatory process persists, fibrosis and calcification subsequently develop, leading to valvular stenosis.
3. **Endomyocardial biopsy** does not help in diagnosing first attacks of rheumatic carditis. It is **useful in distinguishing between chronic inactive rheumatic heart disease from acute rheumatic carditis.**

C. **Other blood tests**
1. As in any inflammatory process, **leukocytosis, thrombocytosis, hypochromic or normochromic anemia** can be observed.
2. **The favored tests to measure acute phase response are erythrocyte sedimentation rate and C-reactive protein.** Although these tests are nonspecific, they may be helpful monitoring the inflammatory activity of the disease. These levels are **almost always elevated during the acute phase of RF in patients with arthritis and polyarthritis, and are usually normal in patients with chorea.** The erythrocyte sedimentation rate may be elevated in patients with anemia and may be suppressed in patients with congestive heart failure, whereas C-reactive protein is unaffected by these diseases.

D. **X-rays.** Chest radiography may identify an increased cardiac size, an increased pulmonary vasculature, or pulmonary edema.

E. **Electrocardiogram and echocardiogram.** In patients **where carditis is subtle and signs of valvular involvement may be mild or transient, a baseline echocardiogram and electrocardiogram** should be obtained.
1. The most common finding in the **electrocardiogram** is the presence of **P-R prolongation and sinus tachycardia.** Myocarditis may prolong QT interval. In cases of pericarditis, low-voltage QRS complexes and ST-segment changes in the precordial leads can be observed.
2. At the present time there is **insufficient information to allow the use of echocardiography to document valvular regurgitation without accompanying auscultatory findings** as the sole criterion for valvulitis in acute RF. Involvement of mitral and aortic valves and the chordae of mitral valve are characteristic.

V. **Therapy.** It is generally recommended that **patients with suspected RF be admitted for close observation and work-up.**
A. **Arthritis.** Antiinflammatory medications are generally recommended for 3 weeks for symptomatic relief.
1. **Pain resolves within 24 hours of starting therapy with salicylates.**
2. **If pain persists** after salicylate treatment, the **diagnosis of RF is questionable.**
3. The **recommended dose** of salicylate is 100 mg/kg per day, given in 4 to 5 divided doses. For optimal antiinflammatory effect, a serum salicylate level of 20 mg% is adequate.
4. **Toxic effects such as anorexia, nausea, vomiting, and tinnitus** should be avoided.
5. **For patients who cannot tolerate salicylates, nonsteroid antiinflammatory drugs (NSAIDs)** can be tried. However, there is no evidence that NSAIDs are more effective than salicylates. As with salicylates, the improvement is prompt.

B. Carditis
  1. **Strenuous physical activity should be avoided.**
  2. **Congestive heart failure should be treated** with appropriate therapy.
  3. **In patients with significant cardiac involvement, corticosteroids are preferred** over salicylates. The **recommended dose** of corticosteroid is 1 to 2 mg/kg per day, (maximum of 60 mg/day). Salicylate or steroid therapy does not affect the course or natural history of the disease; therefore, the **duration of antiinflammatory therapy** is somewhat arbitrary and is **guided by the severity of disease and response to therapy.** Commonly, therapy is needed for 1 month in patients with relatively mild cardiac involvement. Therapy should be **continued until there is sufficient clinical and laboratory evidence of disease inactivity.**
  4. After cessation of antiinflammatory agents, relapse—the reappearance of mild symptoms—may occur. **The gradual reduction in steroid doses is important to avoid relapses.** If **symptoms are mild, they usually subside without specific treatment.** For **severe symptoms,** treatment with salicylates can be tried before restarting corticosteroids. Use of **salicylates** (75 mg/kg per day) **while tapering corticosteroids** may reduce the likelihood of a relapse.

C. Sydenham's chorea. Although this was once thought to have a benign, self-limiting course, it is recognized today that some patients develop significant morbidity.
  1. **Treatment with haloperidol or valproate is recommended by some investigators.** Haloperidol is used in an initial dose of 0.5 to 1 mg/day and 0.5 mg is added every 3 days for maximum effect or until a maximum dose of 5 mg/day is attained. Sodium valproate (15 to 20 mg/kg per day) is also effective.
  2. In resistant cases, plasmapheresis, intravenous immunoglobulin, reserpine, and perphenazine have also been tried.
  3. **Steroidal therapy is generally not effective** in Sydenham's chorea.

VI. Prevention. See Table 49-1.

A. Primary prevention. The most important step in the treatment of RF is the eradication of GAS infection, thus avoiding chronic and repetitive exposure of antigenic streptococcal components to the host immune system.
  1. **Early therapy is advisable** because it reduces both morbidity and the period of infectivity. Although throat cultures are rarely positive for GAS at the time of onset of RF, studies have shown that antimicrobial therapy, even when started 9 days after the onset of acute streptococcal pharyngitis, is still effective in preventing primary attacks of RF.
  2. **Penicillin** is the agent of choice primarily for its narrow spectrum of activity, longstanding proven efficacy, and low cost.
    a. Best results are achieved with a **single intramuscular dose of penicillin G benzathine.** An intramuscular regimen is preferred in patients unlikely to complete a 10-day course of oral therapy or for patients with personal or family history of RF or rheumatic heart disease. This preparation is painful; **preparations that contain procaine penicillin are less painful.**
    b. When **compared with the intramuscular regimen, the oral regimen has several disadvantages,** such as lower compliance due to its longer duration, more complicated dosage schedules, drug interactions, and, more importantly, socioeconomic factors. The oral antibiotic of choice is penicillin V (phenoxymethyl penicillin) (see Table 49-1 for dosage information). A broader spectrum penicillin such as amoxicillin offers no microbiologic advantage over penicillin.
  3. **Patients allergic to penicillin**
    a. **Oral erythromycin** can be used. The recommended dosage is erythromycin estolate or erythromycin ethyl succinate for 10 days. The maximal dose of erythromycin is 1 g/day.
    b. Although uncommon in the United States, **strains resistant to erythromycin** have been found in some areas of the world and

TABLE 49-1. Prevention or rheumatic fever

PRIMARY PREVENTION

Drug	Dosage	Via	Duration
Benzathine (penicillin G)	600,000 units (≤27 kg)	IM	Once
	1,200,000 units (≥27 kg)	IM	Once
	or		
Penicillin V (children)	250 mg (2–3 times/d)	Oral	10 d
Penicillin V (adolescents and adults)	500 mg (2–3 times/d)	Oral	10 d
PENICILLIN-ALLERGIC PATIENTS			
Erythromycin ethyl succinate	40 mg/kg/d (2–4 times/day up to 1 g/d)	Oral	10 d
Erythromycin estolate	20–40 mg/kg/d (2–4 times/day up to 1 g/d)	Oral	10 d

SECONDARY PREVENTION

Drug	Dosage	Via	Interval
Benzathine (penicillin G)	1.2 million Units	IM	3–4 wk
	or		
Penicillin V	250 mg	Oral	bid
	or		
Sulfadiazine	0.5 g (≤27 kg)	Oral	qd
	1.0 g (>27 kg)	Oral	qd
PENICILLIN- AND SULFADIAZINE-ALLERGIC PATIENTS			
Erythromycin	250 mg	Oral	bid

IM, intramuscular.
Adapted from Dajani AS, 1997, with permission.

have resulted in treatment failures. The new **macrolides, such as azithromycin,** have the advantage of a shorter treatment duration (5 days) and fewer gastrointestinal side effects. These can be used as a second line of therapy for patients 16 years of age or older with GAS pharyngitis. The recommended dosage is 500 mg as a single dose on the first day followed by 250 mg once daily for 4 days.

    c. Another alternative regimen for penicillin-allergic patients is a **10-day course with an oral cephalosporin.** First-generation cephalosporin with a narrower spectrum of action (cefadroxil or cephalexin) is preferable to the broader spectrum antibiotics such as cefaclor, cefuroxime, cefixime, and cefpodoxime. Several reports support the evidence that a 10-day course with oral cephalosporin is superior to 10 days of oral penicillin and a 5-day course with selected oral cephalosporins is comparable to a 10-day course of oral penicillin for eradication of GAS.

    d. Sulfa-derived antibiotics (sulfonamides, trimethoprim) do not eradicate GAS in patients with pharyngitis, and tetracyclines should be avoided because of high prevalence of resistant strains.

B. Secondary prevention. Prophylaxis for preventing recurrences should **start as soon as RF or rheumatic heart disease is diagnosed.**

    1. Penicillin in doses of 600,000 IU (patient's weight less than 27 kg) to 1.2 million IU (patient's weight over 27 kg) every 4 weeks is the recommended regimen in most circumstances. The interval is reduced to 3 weeks for individuals at high risk for developing acute RF or living in endemic areas.

TABLE 49-2. Duration of therapy for secondary prevention of rheumatic fever

Disease state	Duration of therapy
RF + carditis + residual valvular disease	At least 10 years post episode and at least until age 40. Lifelong prophylaxis may be required.
RF + carditis without valvular disease	10 years or beyond adulthood, whichever is longer.
RF without carditis	5 years or until age of 21, whichever is longer.

RF, rheumatic fever.
Adapted from Dajani AS, 1997, with permission.

2. **The duration** of prophylaxis depends on the individual situation. Table 49-2 provides additional information.
   a. Prophylaxis of **recurrent RF in patients without cardiac** manifestations should be continued for 5 years after the last RF attack or up to age 21 years, whichever is longer.
   b. For **patients with RF and carditis but no residual valvular disease,** prophylaxis should extend for a period of 10 years or well into adulthood.
   c. Long-term antibiotic prophylaxis is recommended in **patients with valvular heart disease.**
3. The success of **oral prophylaxis** depends on the patient's understanding and adherence to prescribed regimen. Oral agents are **more appropriate for patients at lower risk for rheumatic recurrences.** Some favor switching patients to oral prophylaxis when they have reached late adolescence or young adulthood and have remained free of rheumatic attacks for at least 5 years.
   a. The preferred oral medication is penicillin V.
   b. For **patients with true or suspected allergy to penicillin, sulfadiazine** can be used (see Table 49-1). **Erythromycin** is an alternative.
   c. It is important to keep in mind that even with optimal patient adherence the **risk of recurrence is higher with oral than with an intramuscular prophylactic regimen.**
C. **Prophylaxis for bacterial endocarditis**
   1. In addition to the antibiotic regimens used for the prevention of recurrences of acute RF, **short-term antibiotic prophylaxis for the prevention of bacterial endocarditis prior to surgical and dental procedures is recommended in patients with rheumatic valvular heart disease** (see Chapter 48).
   2. Antibiotic prophylaxis is **not indicated for patients without evidence of valvular involvement.**

SUGGESTED READINGS
Landmark Articles
Bisno AL. Group A streptococcal infections and acute rheumatic fever. *N Engl J Med* 1991;325:783–793.
Dajani AS, Ayoub E, Bierman FZ, et al. Guidelines for the diagnosis of rheumatic fever: Jones criteria. Updated 1993. *Circulation* 1993;87:302–307.

Key Reviews
Stollerman GH. Rheumatic fever. *Lancet* 1997;349: 935–942.
da Silva NA, de Faria Pereira BA. Acute rheumatic fever. *Pediatr Rheumatol* 1997;23: 545–568.

Relevant Book Chapter
Dajani AS. Rheumatic fever. In: Braunwald E, ed. *Heart disease: a textbook of cardiovascular medicine,* 5th ed. Philadelphia: WB Saunders, 1997:1769–1775.

SECTION XIII. PROCEDURES

Deepak L. Bhatt and Stephen G. Ellis

50. RIGHT HEART CATHETERIZATION

Leslie Cho

I. **Introduction.** Since 1970, right heart catheterization has been an integral part of cardiology. It has led to a new understanding of physiology and has helped to diagnose and manage patients. However, recent controversy surrounding the use of pulmonary artery (PA) catheterization has led to some confusion. It is still the gold standard in hemodynamic monitoring and crucial in the diagnosis and treatment of critically ill patients.

II. **Indications**
   A. **Acute myocardial infarction.** Complicated by hypotension, congestive heart failure, sinus tachycardia, right ventricular infarct, or mechanical complications, such as ventricular septal defect (VSD), pericardial tamponade, or acute mitral regurgitation.
   B. **Assess volume status** in patients for whom physical signs may be unreliable.
   C. **Severe left ventricular failure.** To guide inotropic, diuretic, and afterload reduction management.
   D. **Differentiate between various shock states** (e.g., cardiogenic, septic, or hypovolemic shock).
   E. **Cardiac tamponade.** Although echocardiography is the test of choice, PA catheterization can be used when echo is not readily available or there is concern about recurrence.
   F. **Differentiate between constrictive and restrictive cardiac physiology.**
   G. **Severe pulmonary hypertension.**
   H. **High-risk cardiac patients during pre-, intra-, and postoperative periods.** A PA catheter is used during all cardiac surgeries.
   I. **Severe adult respiratory distress syndrome.** A PA catheter is used during positive end-expiratory pressure (PEEP) trials to assess cardiac outputs (COs).

III. **Contraindications.** There are no absolute contraindications but only relative ones such as profound coagulopathy international normalized ratio greater than 2 or platelet count less than 20,000 to 50,000. Left bundle branch block is a relative contraindication since one of the risks of a PA catheter is right bundle branch block. Temporary pacing availability should be present when inserting a PA catheter in these patients.

IV. **Technique**
   A. **Introducer insertion.** It is important to obtain informed consent from the patient. Table 50-1 lists the major complications of PA catheterization. The patient is **prepped and draped** in sterile fashion. The patient should be draped from head to toe during the catheter insertion. Multiple sites can be used for introducer placement; however, **a site that can be compressed, such as the internal jugular (IJ) vein, is preferred.**
      1. The **IJ vein** (Fig. 50-1) has multiple advantages such as compressibility and minimal risk of pneumothorax. The disadvantages are the ease of carotid artery puncture and limited neck mobility for patients. The IJ can be entered via an anterior or posterior approach. The right side is preferred because the vein runs a direct path to the right atrium. It is easier to access the IJ if the patient is in a Trendelenberg position. The anterior approach uses the triangle created by the two heads of the sternocleidomastoid muscle and the clavicle. Be sure to always keep your finger on the carotid artery and retract it medially. Insert the needle at the apex of the triangle and advance pointing to the ipsilateral nipple at a 45-degree angle. The vein can usually be found 3 to 5 cm from the skin surface and should be found with a finder needle (20-gauge) prior to using the large-bore catheter (16-gauge) needle. If the vein is not found

Table 50-1. Complications of right heart catheterization

Related to the introducer	Related to the catheter passage	Related to the catheter
Arterial puncture	Arrhythmia (*PVC*, NSVT, VF), complete heart block, RBBB	Thrombosis
Pneumothorax	Coiling	PA rupture
Nerve injury	Valve trauma	PA infection
Horner's syndrome	PA perforation	Infection
		Balloon rupture

PVC, premature ventricular contraction; NSVT, nonsustained ventricular tachycardia; VF, ventricular fibrillation; RBBB, right bundle branch block.

or the patient has poor anatomic landmarks, ultrasound guidance may be used. Also, lift the patient's neck to better visualize landmarks or switch sites. Once the IJ is accessed, use the catheter-over-guidewire approach. The guidewire minimizes damage to the vessel. Never force the guidewire. If you are having difficulty threading the wire, reattach the syringe and attempt to aspirate venous blood. The posterior approach minimizes the risk of carotid artery puncture. First, the external jugular vein is located and the IJ is accessed 1 cm superior to the point where the external jugular vein crosses the lateral edge of the sternocleidomastoid muscle. Another posterior approach is to puncture along the posterior edge of the sternocleidomastoid muscle, two fingerwidths above the clavicle. The needle should be pointing toward the posterior aspect of the upper portion of the manubrium sterni.

2. **The subclavian vein** (Fig. 50-1) is associated with greater patient comfort and ease of insertion. However, there is an increased risk of pneumothorax and subclavian artery cannulation, especially in patients on

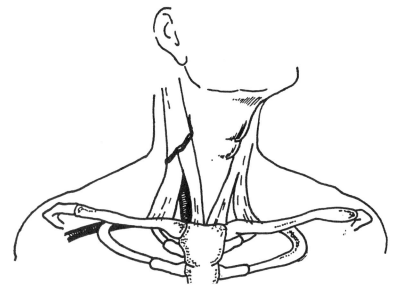

FIG. 50-1. Neck anatomy.

respirators or with coronary obstructive pulmonary disease. The vein lies just under the clavicle at the insertion site for the clavicular head of the sternocleidomastoid muscle. This is where the vein should be entered. The artery lies just beneath the anterior scalene muscle, which is just below the subclavian vein. The lung is underneath the artery. A rolled-up towel can be placed between the shoulder blades to better define landmarks and separate vein from pleura. There are two approaches to cannulating the subclavian vein, infraclavicular and supraclavicular. The infraclavicular approach is used more frequently. The needle is inserted under the clavicle at about 1-cm lateral to the sternocleidomastoid muscle insertion. The needle is then advanced horizontally, nearly parallel to the clavicle. In the supraclavicular approach, the vein is entered from above. The muscle and the clavicle will form an angle and the needle is inserted at this point at a 45-degree angle. The vein should be located no deeper than 2 cm below the skin surface. If you are not sure you are in the vein before dilating, transduce pressure through the needle or obtain a blood gas sample to differentiate between vein and artery.

3. **The femoral vein and other sites** have several advantages including the ease of insertion, easy compressibility, and no risk of pneumothorax. The disadvantages are patient immobility, risk of infection, thrombosis, difficulty floating the Swan-Ganz catheter, and risk of femoral artery puncture. First, palpate the femoral artery at the inguinal ligament. The femoral vein is located 2 cm medially and 2 cm below the femoral artery. In some patients, the vein may lie closer to the artery. The Valsalva maneuver may be used to access the vein. Rarely, venous cutdown is necessary, in which case right basilic and right median cubital veins are used. However, due to venospasm, and difficulty with catheter insertion and threading, the antecubital route is reserved for those who have failed other routes.

B. **Pulmonary artery catheter insertion**
1. After the sheath is placed, the PA catheter can be inserted. Always test the balloon, flush the ports, and make sure the catheter is properly calibrated. After the PA catheter is tested, insert it through the protective sterile covering and then through the sheath. Fluoroscopic guidance and/or pressure tracing can be used during PA catheter insertion. It should advance easily. If not, do not force the catheter but make sure your sheath is in the correct place and properly flushed. Once the catheter has been inserted 15 to 20 cm or after the right atrial tracing is seen, inflate the balloon and advance across the tricuspid valve. The right ventricular tracing will be visualized next, followed by the PA tracing and then, finally, the pulmonary capillary wedge pressure (PCWP) tracing (see Fig. 50-2). Not infrequently, the right ventricular tracing is accompanied by a few premature ventricular ectopic beats. In general, the PA tracing should be reached within 50 to 55 cm if the catheter is advanced from IJ or subclavian or 65 to 70 cm if inserted via a femoral or an arm approach. Once the PCWP is obtained, deflate the balloon and obtain the wedge pressure again by inflating the balloon with 1.5 cm^3 of air. If the PCWP tracing is obtained even when the balloon is deflated or with less than 1.5 cm^3 of air, the catheter is too far advanced and needs to be pulled back. Always monitor pressure wave form when inflating balloon-tipped catheters to immediately identify "overwedging." The likelihood of PA rupture and infarction is directly proportional to catheter being overwedged; PCWP should be read in end-expiration.
2. It is much easier to float the catheter from the right IJ or either SC vein. From the femoral vein it is slightly more difficult. Often, the femoral PA catheter needs to be inserted under fluoroscopic guidance, or an S-shaped femoral swan can be used. When using fluoroscopy, the camera should be in the anteroposterior position and the balloon should be inflated under fluoroscopy. Lastly, check the catheter placement and check for pneu-

mothorax after the procedure with a chest x-ray. Catheter placement may be difficult in patients with low CO, severe tricuspid regurgitation, pulmonary hypertension, or a dilated right atrium or right ventricle.

3. Catheter advancement may be facilitated by a deep inspiration or, in more difficult cases, by a 0. 021-Fr guidewire. The wire is placed inside the distal lumen of the catheter, which improves the stiffness and makes the catheter easier to manipulate. Place a hemostat on the end of the guidewire so that the guidewire is not lost. Advancing the catheter from the femoral vein may be difficult. We recommend using fluoroscopy and an 0.021-Fr guidewire.

V. Complications (Table 50-1)

VI. Troubleshooting (Table 50-2)

VII. Waveforms (Fig. 50-2).

A. **Right atrial systole** occurs after the P wave on electrocardiogram (ECG) produces the a wave. Atrial relaxation, the x descent, occurs with a decline in pressure. The tricuspid valve closure produces a slight upward deflection during the x descent and is known as the c wave. The c wave follows the a wave by the PR interval. The v wave occurs near the end of the T wave and marks atrial filling. Finally, the y descent marks the opening of tricuspid valve with emptying of the atrium. In the normal right atrium, the peak a wave is greater than the peak v wave.

B. **Right ventricular systole** follows the QRS complex of the ECG. With ventricular relaxation, the pressure declines. During the continuous filling from the right atrium, a small a wave is produced that marks the atrial contraction and occurs after the P wave and just before the QRS. End diastole occurs after the a wave. The peak systolic and end-diastolic measurements are used for right ventricular pressures.

C. The **normal pulmonary arterial pressure** consists of a ventricular systole, which corresponds to right ventricular systole and follows the QRS complex. During the relaxation period, pulmonic valve closure produces the incisura, a notch during the decline in pressure. The trough of the pressure decline marks diastole. Pulmonic arterial systolic pressure, end-diastolic pressure, and mean pressure are recorded.

D. The **PCWP tracing** is a transmitted left atrial pressure (LAP). The waveforms are similar to a RAP (RAP) tracing with the a wave corresponding to left atrial systole, the x descent to relaxation, the v wave to filling, and the y descent to emptying. However, the v wave is greater than the a wave in the

Table 50-2. Troubleshooting in right heart catheterization

Problems	Solutions
Arrhythmia	Catheter may be in the RVOT. Pull the catheter back or advance forward.
No PCWP tracing	Catheter tip is usually not far advanced, balloon has ruptured, or the catheter is coiled in the right ventricle. Use fluoroscopy.
Continuous PCWP tracing	Balloon is inflated or the catheter is too far advanced.
Abnormal tracing	Catheter is up against a vessel wall or is too far advanced.
Damped tracing	Caused by either kinked tubing, air or thrombus in the catheter, or catheter up against the vessel wall. Flush and withdraw the catheter.
Change in pressure tracing	Improper calibration, change in patient position or catheter location.

PCWP, pulmonary capillary wedge pressure; RVOT, right ventricular outflow tract.

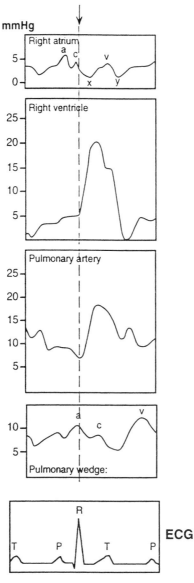

FIG. 50-2. Waveforms.

left atrium and the c wave is not seen due to transmission through pulmonary vasculature. Mean PCWP, a-wave pressure, and v-wave pressure are recorded.

VIII. Pitfalls of the PA catheter. The PA catheter remains the gold standard in monitoring hemodynamics; however, proper interpretation of its data is essential. The data are useless unless the catheter is calibrated correctly. The wedge pressure is an accurate measure of left ventricular filling pressure except in pulmonary venoocclusive disease; mitral stenosis and left atrial myxoma where PCWP equals LAP but LAP does not correspond to left ventricular end-diastolic pressure

(LVEDP); in mitral regurgitation where LAP is greater than LVEDP; in acute aortic insufficiency and noncompliant ventricle where LVEDP is greater than LAP; and in severe respiratory failure with high PEEP. Also, the thermodilution method to assess CO is accurate in most cases except in patients with severe tricuspid regurgitation, intracardiac shunts, in the presence of catheter thrombus, and in low CO. Always measure hemodynamics with the patient in the same position and make sure the catheter is properly calibrated and aligned.

IX. Cardiac output
A. Measurement via thermodilution technique:
1. Prefill syringes with 10 mL of room temperature indicator; then cap the syringe.
2. Check the position of the catheter. Make sure you can obtain the PCWP tracing with 1.5 cc of air and not less.
3. Inject the content of the syringe five separate times. Discard the highest and lowest values and take the mean measurement of the remaining three values.
B. Calculation of CO using the Fick equation:
1. Obtain patient weight in kg.
2. Draw arterial blood gas to obtain oxygen saturation ($AO_2\%$).
3. Draw blood gas from the distal lumen from the PA catheter ($VO_2\%$).
4. Draw hemoglobin.
5. $CO = Wt \times 3 \text{ mL/kg} / [(AO_2\% - VO_2\%) \times 1.36 \times Hgb \times 10]$
6. Oxygen consumption can be measured from a metabolic hood or a Douglas bag. It can also be estimated as 3 mL O_2/kg.

X. Clinical scenarios (see Table 50-4)
A. **Shock** (Table 50-3). Four classes of shock are characterized: hypovolemic, cardiogenic, septic, and anaphylactic. Hypovolemic shock is due to severe decrease in venous return and ventricular preload caused by hemorrhage, dehydration, increased positive intrathoracic pressure, and depressed vasomotor tone. Hemodynamic data consist of decreased blood pressure (BP), CO, PCWP, and increased systemic vascular resistance (SVR). Cardiogenic shock results from failure of the cardiac pump from a change in loading conditions (decrease in preload due to tamponade or increase in preload due to VSD), contractility (acute ischemia or infarction), or an abrupt increase in afterload. Low BP and CO but high PCWP and SVR characterize cardiogenic shock due to left ventricular dysfunction. Predominant elevation of RAP is indicative of right ventricular failure and isolated elevation of the PCWP is indicative of left ventricular failure. Hemodynamics of septic shock are low BP, PCWP, and SVR but high CO. Low BP, PCWP, SVR and low CO characterize the late phase of septic shock. Finally, not much is known about anaphylactic shock. However, there is a hyperkinetic phase characterized by low SVR with high CO and a hypokinetic phase later on that is dominated by profound hypovolemia with decreased CO.
B. **Right ventricular failure** (Fig. 50-3, Table 50-4) may be due to right ventricle infarction, severe pulmonary hypertension, pulmonary embolism, or increased preload due to left-to-right shunt. Right ventricle infarct (Fig. 50-3) produces increased RAP and right ventricular end-diastolic pressure and low CO and BP. Because the right ventricle dilates and becomes less distensible, a

Table 50-3. Interpreting data in right heart catheterization

	Blood pressure	PCWP	CO	SVR
Septic	Low	Low	High	Low
Cardiogenic	Low	High	Low	High
Hypovolemic	Low	Low	Low	High

PCWP, pulmonary capillary wedge pressure; CO, cardiac output; SVR, systemic vascular resistance.

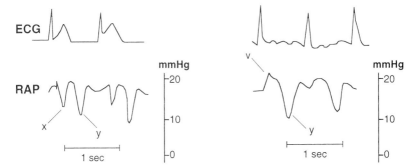

FIG. 50-3. Right ventricular infarction without tricuspid regurgitation (*left*); right ventricular infarction with tricuspid regurgitation (*right*).

dip-and-plateau pattern on the RVP tracing is seen. In the right atrial tracing, there is a steep y descent. With severe tricuspid regurgitation and right ventricle infarction, the dip-and-plateau pattern is lost. Blunted x descent, prominent v wave, and steep y descent are seen.

C. **Acute mitral regurgitation** (Fig. 50-4) may be due to papillary muscle dysfunction or rupture; the left atrium is subjected to increased pressure. Regurgitation produces a large v-wave tracing that occurs after the T wave on ECG. A v-wave pressure that is twice the value of PCWP is considered to be abnormal. In chronic mitral regurgitation, v wave may be modest in amplitude due to chronic atrial dilatation. Other causes for prominent v waves are severe tricuspid regurgitation and VSD.

D. **Tricuspid regurgitation.** The right atrium systolic wave may resemble the right ventricle tracing. There is increased right atrial and right ventricular end-diastolic pressure, blunted x descent, prominent v wave, and steep y descent.

E. **Cardiac tamponade** (Fig. 50-5). The classic hallmark of tamponade is equalization of pressure where RAP = right ventricle pressure = PCWP. The right atrial waveform is characterized by a deep x descent and absent y descent (due to lack of rapid ventricular filling at the beginning of diastole). Also, RAP, right ventricular pressure, and PCWP are increased.

F. **Constrictive pericarditis** (Fig. 50-6) is characterized by brisk ventricular filling during early diastole and limited ventricular filling during late dias-

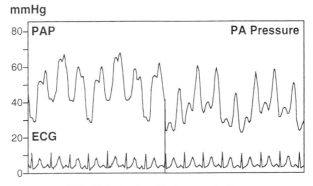

FIG. 50-4. Acute mitral regurgitation.

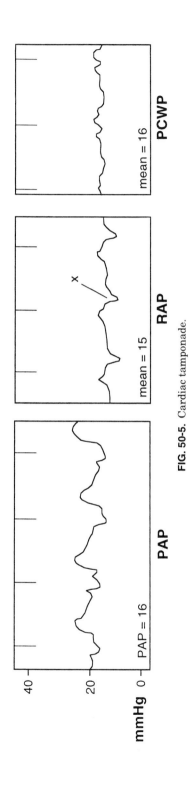

FIG. 50-5. Cardiac tamponade.

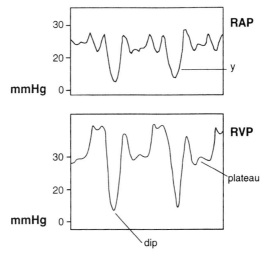

FIG. 50-6. Constrictive pericarditis.

tole. The restriction results in the elevation and equalization of right and left end-diastolic ventricular pressures. The dip-and-plateau waveform is seen in constrictive pericarditis as well as restrictive cardiomyopathy, right ventricular infarct, and massive pulmonary embolism.

G. **Massive pulmonary embolism.** There is ventricularization of the PA waveform with rapid end-systolic descent and a hardly visible or absent dicrotic notch due to obstruction in the PA.

H. **Restrictive cardiomyopathy** due to impaired diastolic filling includes a heterogeneous group of illnesses, such as hemochromatosis, amyloidosis, endomyocardial fibrosis, etc. There is prominent y descent but the dip-and-plateau waveform is less pronounced due to pandiastolic hindrance to ventricular filling (see Table 50-5).

XI. **Formulas** (see Table 50-6)

Cardiac output by Fick equation (CO L/minute) = [Wt × 3 mL/kg] / [($AO_2\%$ – $VO_2\%$) × 1.36 × Hgb × 10]

Cardiac index (CI L/minute per m²): CI = CO/BSA BSA = body surface area

Stroke volume (SV mL/beat): SV = CO/HR HR = heart rate

Pulmonary arteriolar resistance (PAR, dynes.second.cm⁻⁵):

PAR = mean PAP – mean PCWP/CO × 80

PAP = pulmonary arterial pressure

Systemic vascular resistance (SVR, dynes.second.cm⁻⁵):

SVR = (mean SAP – mean RAP)/CO × 80

SAP = systemic arterial pressure RAP = right atrial pressure

Also, 125 mL/minute per m² can be used as O_2 consumption estimate.

CI = 125 mL/minute per m²/O_2 content.

O_2 content = saturation difference × 1.36 × hemoglobin × 10

XII. **Intracardiac shunt.** Intracardiac shunt can be evaluated by using a PA catheter and performing a saturation "run." Blood samples are obtained from the pulmonary artery and regions of the right ventricular, right atrial, and superior vena cava and inferior vena cava. With the catheter positioned in the pulmonary artery, CO by Fick is obtained. While the operator manipulates and pulls the catheter back under fluoroscopic and pressure control, the blood sample from each location is aspirated. Pulmonary venous blood sample is collected by inflating the balloon and then aspirating. A left-to right shunt is suggested

Table 50-4. Clinical scenarios in right heart catheterization

Clinical scenarios	Data	Tracing
RV infarct	↑RA ↓CO ↓BP RA > PCWP Steep y descent Square root sign (RV diastolic dip and plateau)	Fig. 50-3
Acute mitral regurgitation	↑PCWP, prominent V wave	Fig. 50-4
Acute VSD	Oxygen saturation step up from RA to PA	
Noncardiac pulmonary edema	Normal PCWP	
Massive pulmonary embolism	↓BP ↓CO ↑PA and normal PCWP	
Pulmonary hypertension	↑RA ↑RV ↑PA and normal PCWP. PA and RV systolic pressure may reach systemic levels	
Tamponade	Equalization of pressure RA = RV = PCWP ↑RA ↑RV ↑PCWP Paradoxic pulse, blunted y descent, prominent x descent on RA tracing	Fig. 50-5
Constrictive pericarditis	↑RA ↑PCWP Dip and plateau in RV pressure M- or W-shaped jugular venous pressure	Fig. 50-6
Tricuspid regurgitation	↑RA ↑RVEDP Blunted x descent, prominent V wave, steep y descent, and ventricularization of RA pressure	

RV, right ventricular; VSD, ventricular septal defect; RA, right atrial; CO, cardiac output; BP, blood pressure; PCWP, pulmonary capillary wedge pressure; EDP, end-diastolic pressure.

when a step-up, or increase, of oxygen saturation exceeds that of a proximal compartment by more than 7% in the case of atrial shunt or more than 5% in ventricular or great vessel shunts.

Normally, the effective pulmonary blood flow is equal to the systemic blood flow. However with a left-to-right shunt, pulmonary blood flow is equal to systemic blood flow plus shunt flow. In right-to-left shunt, the effective pulmonary blood flow is decreased by the amount of shunt. The shunt fraction is the ratio of pulmonary to systemic flow, Q_p/Q_s, where Q_p is pulmonary flow and Q_s is systemic

Table 50-5. Differentiating diastolic dysfunction

	Constrictive pericarditis	RV infarct	Tamponade	Restrictive cardiac disease
Pulsus paradoxus	Rare	Occasional	Frequent	Rare
RA waveforms	Prominent y descent	Prominent y descent	Prominent x descent	Prominent y descent
Equalization of diastolic pressure	Frequent	Frequent	Frequent	Rare
Dip and plateau	Frequent	Frequent	Absent	Frequent

RA, right atrial; RV, right ventricular.

Table 50-6. Normal values and formulas

Right atrium		0–8 mm Hg
Right ventricle		15–30/0–8 mm Hg
PA		15–30/3–12 mm Hg
PCWP		6–12 mm Hg
CO		4–8 L/min
CI	CO/body surface area	2.8–4.2 L/min/m^2
SV	CO/HR	40–120 cm^3/beat
SVR	(MAP – CVP) × 80/CO	770–1,500 dynes sec/cm^2
PVR	(PAP – PCWP) × 80/CO	20–120 dynes sec/cm^2
Fick CO	$wt \times 3\ mL/kg$	4–8 L/min
	(AO$_2$ – VO$_2$) × 1.36 × Hgb × 10	
SVR	(MAP – CVP) × 80/CO	770–1,500 dynes sec/cm^2
Shunt fraction	Q_p/Q_s	>2.0 Large defect
		1.5–2.0 Small defect
		<1.5 Right to left

PA, pulmonary artery; PCWP, pulmonary capillary wedge pressure; CO, cardiac output; CI, cardiac index; SV, stroke volume; SVR, systemic vascular resistance; PVR, pulmonary vascular resistance; HR, heart rate; MAP, mean arterial pressure; CVP, central venous pressure; PAP, pulmonary arterial pressure; AO$_2$, arterial oxygen; VO$_2$, venous oxygen; Hgb, hemoglobin.

flow. For atrial septal defect, the mixed venous oxygen content is computed as the sum of three times the superior vena cava plus one time the inferior vena cava oxygen content divided by 4.

A. **Calculation for left-to-right shunt**
  1. Shunt fraction = Q_p/Q_s
  2. Q_p = systemic flow – shunt flow = O$_2$ consumption/10 × (pulmonary vein – PA O$_2$ difference)
  3. Q_s = O$_2$ consumption/10 × (arterial – mixed venous O$_2$ difference)
  4. Simplified calculation using saturation only:
     Q_p/Q_s= (arterial sat. – mixed venous sat.)/(pulmonary vein sat. – pulmonary artery sat.).
     In right-to-left shunt, systemic flow is oxygen consumption divided by arterial oxygen content minus pulmonary arterial oxygen content. Pulmonary blood flow is calculated by oxygen consumption divided by pulmonary vein oxygen content minus pulmonary arterial content. A shunt fraction ratio of greater than 1.5 often necessitates closure.

B. **Calculation of aortic valve area** (AVA)
  1. Planimeter five aortic–left ventricular gradients and average the area (Fig. 50-7).
  2. Measure systolic ejection periods (SEP) and average the values.
  3. Convert planimeter area to mean systolic pressure gradient:

     Mean valve gradient (MVG) = area × scale factor/SEP

  4. Compute aortic valve flow using $\dfrac{1000 \times \text{cardiac output}}{\text{HR} \times \text{SEP}}$
  5. Compute valve area =
     valve flow/$K \times C \times \sqrt{\text{peak LV pressure} - \text{peak aortic pressure}}$
     using the Gorlin formula where K = 44.3 and C is an empirical constant that is 1 for semilunar valves and tricuspid valve and 0.85 for mitral valve.
  6. Simplified AVA =
     $\dfrac{\text{CO}}{\sqrt{\text{gradient}}}$ [gradient = peak LV pressure – peak aortic pressure].
     This quick formula for valve area differs from the Gorlin formula by 18% ± 13% in patients with bradycardia or tachycardia. If the heart rate is above 90 this number should be divided by 1.35.

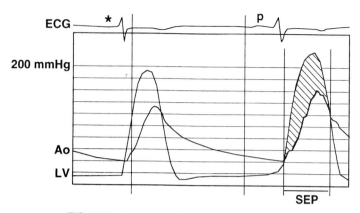

FIG. 50-7. Aortic and left ventricular waveform.

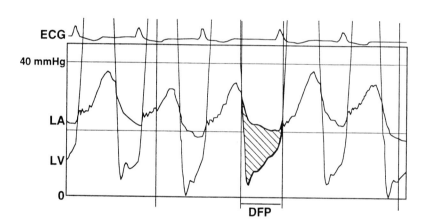

FIG. 50-8. Left ventricular and pulmonary capillary waveform.

C. Calculation of mitral valve area

1. Planimeter five left ventricular-pulmonary capillary wedge areas (Fig. 50-8).
2. Measure diastolic filling period (DFP).
3. Convert planimetered area to mean diastolic pressure gradient (MVG) where MVG = area × scale factor/DFP
4. Compute mitral valve flow using $\dfrac{1000 \times \text{cardiac output}}{\text{HR} \times \text{DFP}}$
5. Compute mitral valve area using the Gorlin formula where mitral valve flow is divided by $44.3 \times 0.85 \times \sqrt{\text{diastolic pressure difference}}$

SUGGESTED READINGS

Landmark Articles
Chatterjee K, Swan HJ, Ganz W, et al. Use of a balloon-tipped flotation electrode catheter for cardiac monitoring. *Am J Cardiol* 1975;36:56–61.

Segal J, Pearl RG, Ford AJ Jr, et al. Instantaneous and continuous cardiac output obtained with a Doppler pulmonary artery catheter. *J Am Coll Cardiol* 1989;13: 1382–1392.

Swan HJ, Ganz W, Forrester J, et al. Catheterization of the heart in man with use of a flow-directed balloon-tipped catheter. *N Engl J Med* 1970:283:447–451.

Key Reviews

Amin DK, Shah PK, Swan HJ. The Swan-Ganz catheter: choosing and using the equipment. *J Crit Illness* 1986;1:24–32.

Amin DK, Shah PK, Swan HJ. The Swan-Ganz catheter: tips on interpreting results. *J Crit Illness* 1986;1:32–38.

Mueller HS, Chatterjee K, Davis KB, et al. Present use of bedside right heart catheterization in patients with cardiac disease. *J Am Coll Cardiol* 1998;32:840–864.

Swan HJ, Shah PK. The rationale for bedside hemodynamic monitoring. *J Crit Illness* 1986;1:39–45.

Relevant Book Chapters

Kern MJ. *The cardiac catheterization handbook,* 2nd ed. St. Louis: Mosby–Year Book, 1995.

Marini J. *The ICU book.* Baltimore: Williams & Wilkins, 1987.

Perret C, Tagan D, Feihl F, Marini JJ. *The pulmonary artery catheter in critical care: a concise handbook.* Cambridge (Mass.): Blackwell Science, 1996.

51. TEMPORARY TRANSVENOUS PACING

Debabrata Mukherjee

I. **Indications**
   A. **Acute myocardial infarction.** Indications for temporary pacing in this setting include development of a new right bundle branch block with either left axis (left anterior hemiblock) or right axis deviation (left posterior hemiblock), new left bundle branch block (LBBB) with first-degree atrioventricular (AV) block, alternating left and right bundle branch block, Mobitz type II block, and complete heart block. Another indication is right ventricular infarction and bradyarrythmias. Patients with right ventricular infarction and loss of AV synchrony will benefit from AV sequential pacing.
   B. **Bradycardia.** Temporary pacing is indicated in patients with hemodynamically significant bradycardia. Reversible causes such as digitalis, antiarrhythmic agents, and electrolyte disturbances such as hyperkalemia should be determined and reversed.
   C. **Termination of tachycardias (overdrive pacing).** Temporary pacing is indicated for overdrive pacing and termination of atrial flutter (type 1 with long excitable gap), supraventricular tachycardia due to AV nodal reentry, and sustained monomorphic ventricular tachycardia.
   D. **Bridge to permanent pacing.** Temporary pacing may be used as a bridge to permanent pacing in patients with complete heart block, high-grade second-degree block, severe sinus node dysfunction, and asystole.
   E. **Ventricular tachycardia.** Temporary pacing is indicated in patients with bradycardia-dependent ventricular tachycardia and recurrent tachyarrythmias secondary to long QT syndrome.
   F. **Myocarditis (such as Lyme disease) with heart block.**
   G. **Prophylactic.** Prophylactic temporary pacing is indicated in patients with LBBB undergoing right heart catheterization and/or myocardial biopsy, rotablation of the right coronary artery as it supplies the AV node in 90% of individuals, and cardioversion in patients with the sick sinus syndrome.
II. **Contraindications**
   A. Poor vascular access
   B. Bleeding disorders or anticoagulant therapy. If the international normalized ratio is greater than 1.8 and platelets are less than 50,000, they need to be corrected prior to elective placement of a transvenous pacer.
III. **Patient preparation**
   A. **Informed consent** should be obtained for the procedure. However, if the patient is hemodynamically unstable due to a cardiac arrhythmia that could be improved with a pacemaker, this procedure is indicated emergently.
   B. If the procedure is elective, peripheral intravenous access should be obtained prior to the start of the procedure.
   C. The procedure should be performed in a monitored setting that is equipped for cardiopulmonary resuscitation and has fluoroscopy available.
IV. **Technique**
   A. **Sites.** Preferred sites for pacemaker insertion are the **subclavian and internal jugular veins.** However, if a permanent pacemaker will eventually be inserted, the left subclavian site should not be used for temporary pacing if the patient is right-handed. The right subclavian vein should be avoided for temporary pacing if the patient is left-handed. The easiest access in the catheterization lab is usually the femoral vein.
   B. **Position.** The patient should be placed supine in bed. The patient may be placed in the Trendelenberg position for internal jugular and subclavian vein cannulation.

C. Placement

1. A 5-Fr venous sheath is inserted into one of the central veins and 5-Fr pacing catheters are used. The pacing catheter is advanced under fluoroscopy near the right ventricular apex for ventricular pacing and to the right atrial appendage for atrial pacing. The catheter is advanced to the tricuspid valve and turned either clockwise or counterclockwise to direct the tip anteriorly. An attempt is made to cross the valve directly. If unsuccessful, gentle pressure is applied and the catheter is torqued, allowing the middle portion to prolapse across the valve into the right ventricle. If the tricuspid valve is difficult to traverse, it may be possible to enter the right ventricle by looping the tip of the catheter against the lateral atrial wall and then rotating the loop medially against the atrial septum with the catheter tip just above the tricuspid valve. Another option is increasing the tip bend prior to attempting to traverse the right ventricle. Once the catheter has entered the right ventricle, it is rotated so that the tip points inferiorly to the apex with minimal movement in systole. Some degree of buckling is acceptable; however, excessive buckling increases the risk of perforation. Ideally, the pacemaker tip should be near the apex of the right ventricle. The ideal catheter placement site is on the diaphragmatic surface or "floor" of the right ventricle anywhere between its midpoint and its apex. The floor of the more proximal ventricle is a second choice. The true apex is not a good choice for placement of the catheter tip. The paced ECG from this location usually shows a LBBB pattern with left axis deviation. Ventricular pacing can also be done with the tip in the right ventricular outflow tract if the catheter cannot be placed on the floor of the right ventricle in a stable position. The pacer tip is considerably less stable at this site compared to the right ventricle floor and is more likely to be displaced. Pacing from this location will show a LBBB pattern with an inferior axis. The threshold may be higher with the tip in the right ventricular outflow tract.

2. For atrial pacing the right atrium is the easiest chamber to reach and pace, but stable position is usually found in the right atrial appendage. For atrial pacing a 5-Fr J-tipped atrial pacing catheter is used. The atrial appendage is directed anteriorly above the tricuspid annulus and multiple planes are frequently helpful in verifying location. (The catheter appears as a "J" in the left anterior oblique projection as an "L" in the right anterior oblique projection.)

3. Both atrial and ventricular pacing may be performed by placing the catheter in the coronary sinus. The coronary sinus in its proximal portion courses along the left atrium. Ventricular pacing may be achieved by positioning the catheter in a great cardiac vein off the coronary sinus. The threshold in the coronary sinus is frequently high, but sometimes it may be a more stable location than the atrial appendage. Post–heart surgery patients often may have had their right atrial appendage resected, and steerable electrophysiologic pacing catheters may be useful in such patients.

D. Testing.
Once a catheter is in a stable position, threshold testing should be performed. The distal electrode on the pacing catheter is used as the cathode and connects with the negative terminal, and the ring is used as the anode and connects with the positive terminal of the generator. The pacing catheter is attached via a cable to the pacemaker generator. Pacing is started at a rate 10 to 20 beats faster than the intrinsic rate with 5-mA output. If capture is not seen at this point, the catheter needs to be repositioned. Once capture is seen, the output is slowly decreased until loss of capture is seen. The lowest capturing current is the pacing threshold. If the catheter is in good position, the threshold should be less than 1 mA. Pacing output should be three times the threshold, but pacing is usually performed at a minimum of 3 mA (even if three times the threshold is less than 3 mA). This is because minor dislodgment can cause major changes in threshold and adds a safety margin. To determine sensing, the sensing setting is gradually

decreased (increased millivolts) until asynchronous pacing seen. This is the sensing threshold. The pacer is set at twice the sensing threshold. For dual-chamber pacing, the AV interval will need to be programmed. A default of 150 milliseconds is frequently used, but the optimal AV delay may be different in individual patients. Patients with diastolic ventricular dysfunction may need longer AV delay for ventricular filling. In patients with marginal cardiac reserve, obtaining cardiac output measurements at various AV intervals and heart rates may help determine the optimum AV interval and heart rate.

    E. Tachycardia termination. Reentrant tachyarrhythmias may be pace-terminated. This involves pacing the chamber in which the reentrant circuit exists. Overdrive pacing is initiated at 10 to 15 beats faster than the tachycardia. Pacing is done for several captured beats up to 10 to 15 seconds and then abruptly stopped. If tachycardia persists, the pacing rate is sequentially increased by 10 beats and pacing repeated. The major complication of this technique is conversion to a faster or unstable rhythm. The advantage is post-tachycardia pauses can be treated with pacing if necessary and direct current cardioversion may be avoided.

V. Chest x-ray
    A. Postprocedure chest x-ray needs to be evaluated for pneumothorax.
    B. For right ventricular apex pacing, the electrode tip should be located to the left of the spine, and directed inferiorly and anteriorly.
    C. For pacing through the coronary sinus, the tip is to the left of the spine, directed posteriorly and superiorly.

VI. Pacer care
    A. Check the catheter insertion site daily for signs of infection and apply a new sterile dressing.
    B. Obtain a daily 12-lead surface ECG.
    C. Check pacemaker function daily by determining the sensing and pacing threshold, and check the underlying rhythm daily by decreasing the pacing rate gradually to "off." Abrupt termination in pacing may increase the risk of long pauses.

VII. Complications
    A. Related to **central venous access** such as pneumothorax, hemothorax, air embolism, thrombosis.
    B. Cardiac arrhythmias such as premature ventricular contractions (PVC), premature atrial contractions (PAC), ventricular tachycardia, right bundle branch block.
    C. Myocardial perforation with cardiac tamponade. The unipolar recording from the tip normally shows pronounced ST elevation compared to the proximal electrode. ST depression from the tip is associated with perforation.
    D. Pacemaker dysfunction with generator failure, over- or undersensing, electrode displacement with failure to capture.
    E. Complete heart block in patients with preexisting LBBB due to catheter irritation of the right bundle.

VIII. Transcutaneous pacing. Transcutaneous ventricular pacing involves placement of large-surface-area, high-impedance electrodes (Zoll pads) on the anterior and posterior chest walls. It usually requires long pulse widths (20 to 40 milliseconds) and high outputs of up to 100 to 200 mA. Transcutaneous pacing may be useful when transvenous pacing is contraindicated and in code situations. It avoids the complications associated with transvenous pacers such as pneumothorax, right ventricle perforation, infection, bleeding, and venous thrombosis. The major drawbacks are failure to capture and patient discomfort.

SUGGESTED READINGS
Relevant Book Chapters

Barold SS, Zipes DP. Cardiac pacemakers and antiarrhythmic devices. In: Braunwald E, ed. *Heart disease: a textbook of cardiovascular medicine,* 5th ed. Philadelphia: WB Saunders, 1997:705–731.

Deligonul U, Kern MJ, Serota H, Roth R. Angiographic data. In: Kern MJ, ed. *The cardiac catheterization handbook.* St. Louis: Mosby–Year Book, 1991:309–313.

Fletcher RD, Wish M, Alexander EP. Temporary cardiac pacing. In: Schlant RC, Wayne Alexander R, O'Rourke RA, Roberts R, Sonnenblick EH, eds. *Hurst's the heart: arteries and veins,* 8th ed. New York: McGraw-Hill, 1994:807–813.

Keim S. Temporary pacing. In: Uretsky BF, ed.*Cardiac catheterization: concepts, techniques and applications.* Boston: Blackwell Scientific, 1997:618–629.

52. PERICARDIOCENTESIS

Tom A. Grady and Deepak L. Bhatt

I. **Indications**
  A. **Cardiac Tamponade**
    1. **Hypotension** resulting from a pericardial effusion is an absolute indication for pericardiocentesis. The physiologic effect of pericardial effusions should be thought of as a continuum ranging from effusions with mild hemodynamic involvement, which are often asymptomatic, to effusions that impair diastolic filling leading to hemodynamic compromise and eventual circulatory collapse.
    2. **Fluid accumulation** within the finite pericardial space increases the intrapericardial pressure, which is then transmitted to all four cardiac chambers, increasing their pressure during both systole and diastole. The rate at which the intrapericardial pressure rises and impinges on cardiac hemodynamics depends on several factors, including:
      a. **Volume of the effusion**
      b. **Rate of fluid accumulation within the pericardial space**
      c. **Distensibility of the pericardium**
      d. **Volume status** of the patient
      e. **Intrapulmonary pressures,** as positive airway pressure will be transmitted to the intrapericardial cavity and have a detrimental effect on cardiac hemodynamics
  B. **Pericardial effusion of uncertain etiology.** When there is doubt as to the cause of an effusion, if it is large enough to be safely approached by a percutaneous route, pericardiocentesis should be performed.
II. **Contraindications.** In the case of symptomatic cardiac tamponade, prompt removal of the effusion is essential; pericardiocentesis or placement of a pericardial window via a surgical approach should be performed. In elective cases, when the effusion is not compromising cardiac hemodynamics, elective pericardiocentesis should be deferred in the following situations:
  A. **Infection.** The presence of an underlying infection at the entry site where the pericardiocentesis needle is to be introduced should be avoided.
  B. **Pulmonary disease.** Significant pulmonary pathology may lead to respiratory collapse if there is an inadvertent pneumothorax during pericardiocentesis.
  C. **Hemodynamic instability.** Hemodynamic instability not resulting from a pericardial effusion, such as septic shock or hypovolemia, is not an indication for drainage of the effusion. In these situations, a pulmonary artery catheter and echocardiographic Doppler flow data can be useful in sorting out the underlying etiology of the hypotension.
  D. **Anticoagulation.** With an international normalized ratio greater than 1.8, infusion of fresh frozen plasma prior to or at the time of pericardiocentesis should be considered.
  E. **Thrombocytopenia.** A platelet count less than 50,000, with evidence of bleeding, or a platelet count of less than 20,000 is a relative contraindication. Platelet transfusion prior to or at the time of pericardiocentesis should be considered.
  F. **Trauma.** Acute traumatic hemopericardium, in which blood enters the pericardial space as rapidly as it can be aspirated, requires immediate surgical exploration of the mediastinum. In this way, repair of the cause of the effusion can be performed and the mediastinum can be examined for further evidence of injury.
  G. **Aortic dissection.** Tamponade secondary to an aortic dissection is best treated surgically, as pericardiocentesis can extend the dissection and accelerate bleeding into the pericardial space.

H. **Small or posteriorly located effusions.** Due to their small size, pericardial effusions judged to be less than 200 cm³ are technically difficult to drain percutaneously. In addition, posteriorly located effusions due to their position behind the heart are difficult to approach via a percutaneous route. In these cases, echocardiographic guidance is of value in locating the effusion and guiding the approach.

I. **Loculated effusions.** Clot, as demonstrated by the presence of fibrinous stranding on echocardiography, is difficult to drain percutaneously. This is often the case with postoperative effusions.

J. **Purulent effusions.** In order to permit extensive drainage of the effusion and to obtain serology as well as cultures, surgical drainage is preferred. In addition, the majority of purulent effusions are loculated and are difficult to drain due to the viscosity of the pericardial fluid. Moreover, the risk of spreading the infection to other mediastinal structures is increased when the percutaneous approach is used to drain a purulent pericardial effusion.

K. **Suspected malignant effusion.** If it is highly likely that an effusion is malignant based on the clinical setting, consideration should be given for initial surgical drainage and placement of a pericardial window.

III. **Patient preparation**

A. If possible, pericardiocentesis should be performed in a procedure laboratory where fluoroscopic and hemodynamic monitoring is available. A physician with experience in pericardiocentesis and hemodynamic interpretation should be present to either conduct or supervise the procedure. The procedure should be thoroughly explained to the patient and family. Informed consent should be obtained and documented in the medical record.

B. Prior to an elective procedure, a **pulmonary artery catheter** should be placed. With the aid of a properly positioned pulmonary artery catheter, cardiac hemodynamics can be accurately recorded and monitored. Hemodynamic support during the preparation of the patient may include administration of intravenous fluids.

1. Before the procedure, the patient's blood should be typed and cross-matched.

2. **Two-dimensional echocardiography** is of value in guiding pericardiocentesis. Anatomic structures of the heart, along with location, size, and diameter of the pericardial effusion, and hemodynamic information, can be obtained.

3. The lung is effectively avoided with an **echo-guided approach.**

4. **Fluoroscopy** is particularly useful in confirming the position of the guidewire.

C. The patient's head and thorax are tilted up 30 to 45 degrees. Positioning pillows underneath the patient's neck and torso aids in patient comfort and facilitates the pooling of the effusion caudally. Echocardiography helps in deciding on the anatomic approach. By using the subxyphoid approach, the tract of the needle is extrapleural and avoids the coronary and internal mammary vessels. Other approaches can include the fourth and fifth intercostal space along the left sternal border, and the apical approach along the fifth and sixth intercostal space, along the left axillary line.

IV. **TECHNIQUE**

A. **Anesthesia.** Once the anatomic approach has been selected, the skin is shaved, cleansed, and prepared in aseptic fashion. A sterile field surrounding the entrance site is established. The subcutaneous tissue is anesthetized with a local anesthetic such as 1% lidocaine. If the subxyphoid approach is used, one infiltrates the area where the xyphoid process and left costal margin meet, first with a 25-gauge needle and then with a 21-gauge needle. If the apical or parasternal approach is used, then the periosteum of the superior margin of the rib below where the needle is to be inserted is anesthetized.

B. **Entering the pericardial space**

1. An 18-gauge Cook needle is attached via a three-way stopcock to a hand-held syringe containing 1% lidocaine. In very obese patients, the longer

needle that is supplied with most pericardiocentesis kits can be used; the authors do not routinely use this longer needle, as more difficulties are encountered in directing its course. If one wishes to record intrapericardial pressures, one port of the stopcock can be connected to fluid-filled transducer tubing. The transducer tubing is then attached to a calibration system, which will record the pressure waveform. Remember to balance and zero the system prior to starting the procedure. For electrocardiogram (ECG)–guided pericardiocentesis, the metal hub of the needle can be attached by a sterile connector to the V lead of an ECG machine; the limb leads of the ECG machine are attached to the patient in the usual manner. The ECG-guided approach adds little when echocardiographic guidance is also utilized.

    2. With the **subxyphoid approach,** the tip of the Cook needle is directed posteriorly and toward the patient's left shoulder. The needle is then advanced, with approximately a 30-degree angulation to the plane of the body, just underneath the junction of the xyphoid process and left costal margin. As the needle is gradually advanced, the operator gently attempts to aspirate fluid. The needle is advanced until pericardial fluid is aspirated; sometimes the pericardium is felt to give. Inject small amounts of lidocaine as the needle is slowly advanced to ensure needle patency. Puncture of pericardium can be painful; additional lidocaine can be injected.

    3. When the **apical approach** is used, echocardiography is necessary to locate the effusion. The distance from chest wall to the effusion should be measured echocardiographically and the needle should be marked with a hemostat (the ruler on the handle of a scalpel blade can be used). Once the location of the effusion has been determined, the tip of the needle is oriented toward the right shoulder. The intercostal space used for needle insertion will be determined by the location of the pericardial effusion, but in most instances, the intercostal space between the fifth and sixth rib is used. The needle is then advanced until the tip of the needle comes in contact with the upper margin of the sixth rib. At this point, the tip of the needle is advanced over the sixth rib until pericardial fluid is aspirated.

    4. If **ECG monitoring** is in place, ST-segment elevation or premature ventricular contractions (PVC) may appear on the ECG, indicating that the needle has reached the epicardium; PR segment elevation and premature atrial contractions (PAC) can be seen with atrial puncture. If this occurs, the needle is gradually withdrawn while aspirating so that the needle lies within the pericardial space and the ECG changes resolve. If fluid cannot be freely aspirated, then the needle is gradually withdrawn avoiding all unnecessary motion; the needle is then flushed and the procedure repeated.

C. Confirming needle position

    1. If one is unsure as to whether the needle is in the atrium, ventricle, or pericardial space, a few milliliters of contrast dye can be injected under fluoroscopic observation.

    2. **Echo contrast,** using agitated saline, can be injected to determine the position of the tip of the needle. To perform an echo contrast study, a three-way stopcock is connected to two 10-mL syringes. The third port of the three-way stopcock is then connected to an intravenous line, which is attached to the patient. With the arrow on the three-way stopcock turned away from the patient, the saline is agitated in the two syringes. Once the saline is agitated to create small bubbles, the arrow on the three-way stopcock is turned toward the patient's port and injected. When the contrast medium swirls and disappears, the needle is within a cardiac chamber. If, however, the appearance of the contrast remains within the space where the needle is located, it is in the pericardial space. If pressure monitoring is available, the pericardial catheter pressure waveform can be transduced to differentiate pericardial from ventricular pressure. When the needle is in the pericardial free space, pericardial and right atrial pressures have similar waveforms and, with tamponade, will be equal. If bloody fluid is aspirated, remember that pericardial fluid does not clot quickly. Also, when a drop of pericardial fluid is placed on a piece of gauze, it spreads as a central red spot surrounded by a pale halo.

D. Pericardial catheter placement

1. When advancing the needle, remember to monitor pulse oximetry, heart rate, and blood pressure. A sudden drop in blood pressure or an increase in heart rate may be a clue that the hub of the needle is in a cardiac chamber. A drop in the oxygen saturation or the patient complaining of sharp pleuritic pain or back/shoulder pain may indicate the development of a pneumothorax.

2. Once in the pericardial free space, a soft, floppy-tip guidewire is advanced through the pericardiocentesis needle. The guidewire is advanced until the tip of the guidewire is within the pericardial space as confirmed by either fluoroscopy or echocardiography. The needle is then withdrawn, always keeping the stiff end of the guidewire tethered.

3. After the needle has been withdrawn, a small nick is made in the skin with a no. 11 scalpel, and a soft no. 5- or 6-Fr dilator is advanced over the guidewire. The dilator serves to widen the entrance site where the needle was placed so that the pericardial catheter can be easily advanced. Once the entrance site is dilated, the dilator is gently removed over the guidewire.

4. A tapered, large-bore, 6- or 7-Fr catheter with multiple side holes and a distal hole is advanced over the guidewire. Some operators favor use of a pigtail catheter. Once the catheter is properly positioned, the guidewire is removed. A few milliliters of pericardial fluid are then aspirated from the catheter. If pericardial fluid is not aspirated, the catheter can be gently rotated or slightly withdrawn, as the distal end of the catheter may be obstructed. If using a transducer, the catheter can be connected to the transducer tubing and intrapericardial pressures can be recorded.

5. **Relief of tamponade** is signaled by a nearly immediate increase in systolic blood pressure and pulse pressure, along with a decrease in right atrial pressure. Usually, removal of 50 to 100 cm^3 of pericardial fluid is sufficient to create a noticeable improvement in hemodynamics; in contradistinction, removal of this amount of fluid from an intracardiac chamber should cause further deterioration. If there is no improvement, unexpected loculation of the effusion or an effusive-constrictive process should be considered.

E. Diagnostic studies. After recording intrapericardial pressures, the transducer tubing can be disconnected. When the etiology of the pericardial effusion is uncertain, pericardial fluid samples should be sent for relevant serologic analysis. The following studies should be considered: protein, amylase, lactate dehydrogenase, glucose, cholesterol, cell count (hematocrit as well as white blood cell count with a differential), and bacteriologic culture for aerobic/anaerobic bacteria, tuberculosis, parasites, fungi, viral studies, as well as special stains (including Gram, fungal, and acid-fast). Approximately 100 mL of fluid should be collected in a heparinized container for cytologic examination, though larger quantities will increase the yield.

F. Fluid drainage. Once the appropriate studies have been obtained, the remaining pericardial fluid can be drained by manual syringe aspiration. Very large effusions can be drained by connecting the proximal portion of intravenous tubing to the distal end of the pericardial catheter. The distal end of the intravenous tubing will have a 16-gauge needle attached to it and this needle can be inserted into a vacuum bottle. Free flow of pericardial fluid should then occur into the vacuum bottle. Sometimes the pull of the vacuum bottle will cause the tubing to collapse and flow to cease; it is then necessary to revert to manual suction. When no further fluid can be aspirated or drained, a clinical and hemodynamic reassessment of the patient should be made. If the catheter is to be removed, it is withdrawn gently. Once removed, pressure is applied over the entrance site until hemostasis is achieved. A sterile dressing should then be applied.

G. Postprocedural care

1. When reaccumulation of pericardial fluid occurs, it is desirable to leave the pericardial catheter in place for several hours to permit repeat aspiration of fluid. If this is the case, the pericardial catheter should be securely sutured and attached via a three-way stopcock to a closed drainage system. The pericardial catheter should be aspirated every 4 to 6 hours and flushed with saline. Pericardial drainage volumes should be recorded and the catheter removed when the drainage is less than 30 mL/24 hours; a follow-up echo is also recommended before removing the catheter. Because of the risk of infection, the pericardial catheter should be removed within 48 to 72 hours of placement. If still draining more than 30 mL/24 hours after 72 hours, the option of placing of a pericardial window via a surgical approach should be considered.

2. Following the pericardiocentesis, patients should be observed for 24 hours in an intensive care setting, monitoring for reaccumulation of the effusion and clinical evidence of cardiac tamponade. A chest x-ray should be obtained to exclude the presence of a pneumothorax. The chest x-ray will also allow comparison of the postprocedure cardiac silhouette with the preprocedure cardiac silhouette.

H. Sclerotherapy. In certain situations, instillation of a nonabsorbable corticosteroid, antineoplastic agent, or sclerosing agent can be performed via the pericardial catheter. If a sclerosing agent is to be used, doxycycline and bleomycin are most commonly used. The technique for use of sclerosing agents varies but usually involves delivering the sclerosing agent in 30 to 50 mL of saline with 5 mL of 1% to 2% lidocaine as an anesthetic. The sclerosing agent is allowed to remain within the pericardial space for 1 to 2 hours. The pericardial space is then drained so that apposition of the visceral and parietal surfaces can occur. The goal is to obliterate the pericardial space. This procedure is repeated until drainage is less than 50 to 75 mL/day. As the process can be quite painful, adequate analgesia is mandatory. Sclerotherapy has an effusion-free success rate of approximately 75%. Survival for patients with a malignant effusion is only 3.1 ± 2.8 months.

I. Percutaneous balloon pericardiotomy. Percutaneous balloon pericardiotomy (PBP) uses a balloon-dilating catheter to create a pericardial window and is a therapeutic option for patients with advanced malignancy and limited life expectancy. Only physicians with interventional cardiology training and extensive experience with pericardiocentesis should attempt PBP. The success rate of PBP is approximately 85%.

V. Complications. The technical difficulty of pericardiocentesis varies according to the location and size of the pericardial fluid. The risk decreases and the likelihood of success increases with increasing size of the effusion. The risks and possible complications of pericardiocentesis include:

A. Death. Most series studying the complication rate of pericardiocentesis prior to 1990 and the advent of echocardiography reported a procedure complication rate of approximately 10% with a mortality rate of 2% to 4%. However, with the widespread use of echocardiography to document the size and location of the effusion, the complication rate has declined to the order of 2% to 3% with a mortality rate of less than 1%.

B. Infection. This risk is minimized by proper sterile technique. However, infection of the pericardial space can be catastrophic.

C. Pneumothorax. Echo guidance minimizes the risk of pneumothorax.

D. Cardiac laceration can lead to hemopericardium, resultant tamponade, and death. This is much less likely with the apical approach, as puncture of the thick-walled left ventricle is better tolerated than puncture of the right ventricle by the subxyphoid approach.

E. Acute pulmonary edema. Sudden ventricular dilatation can occur if tamponade is decompressed too quickly, especially if vigorous volume resuscitation has also been employed. Instead, the drainage of fluid should occur over about 20 minutes.

F. Artery laceration. Coronary, pericardial, or internal mammary artery laceration may occur. The left parasternal approach risks puncture of the left internal mammary artery and left anterior descending artery. The mammary artery runs 1 to 2.5 cm lateral to the sternal border; thus puncture at this location should be avoided.

G. Peritoneal puncture. Puncture of the peritoneal cavity or abdominal viscera can occur with the subxyphoid route. This is much more likely with the presence of a large amount of ascites. Echocardiography or fluoroscopy can minimize this possibility.

H. Arrhythmias. Vasovagal bradyarrhythmias can occur at the time of pericardial puncture. Atrial or ventricular arrhythmias can occur with cardiac chamber puncture.

SUGGESTED READINGS

Key Reviews
Tsang TSM, Freeman WK, Sinak LJ, Seward JB. Echocardiographically guided pericardiocentesis: evolution and state-of-the-art technique. *Mayo Clin Proc* 1998;73: 647–652.

Relevant Book Chapters
Brockman RG, Ziskind AA. Pericardiocentesis and associated treatment of pericardial effusion. In: Brown DL, ed. *Cardiac intensive care.* Philadelphia: WB Saunders, 1998:657–663.

Klein AL, Scalia GM. Diseases of the pericardium, restrictive cardiomyopathy and diastolic dysfunction. In: Topol EJ, ed. *Comprehensive cardiovascular medicine.* Philadelphia: Lippincott-Raven Publishers, 1998:707–715.

Lorell BH, Grossman W. Profiles in constrictive pericarditis, restrictive cardiomyopathy, and cardiac tamponade. In: Baim DS, Grossman W, eds. *Cardiac catheterization, angiography and intervention.* Baltimore: Williams & Wilkins, 1996:807–817.

Lorell BH. Pericardial diseases. In: Braunwald EB, ed. *Heart disease: a textbook of cardiovascular medicine.* Philadelphia: WB Saunders, 1997: 1485–1496.

Tilkian AG, Daily EK. Pericardiocentesis and drainage. In: Cardiovascular procedures: diagnostic techniques and therapeutic procedures. St. Louis: Mosby–Year Book, 1986:231–256.

53. CARDIOVERSION

JoAnne Micale Foody and Gregory Kidwell

I. **Introduction.** Electrical countershock is a rapid method of terminating most cardiac arrhythmias. It successfully converts both supraventricular and ventricular tachycardias by depolarizing a critical mass of myocardium, thereby allowing establishment of a normal rhythm. External cardiac defibrillation for ventricular fibrillation is an emergency procedure and the only successful form of treatment.

II. **Cardioversion** describes the means by which electrical countershock is used to terminate cardiac arrhythmias other than ventricular defibrillation. **Defibrillation** is the process of electrically depolarizing a critical mass of myocardium in an effort to terminate ventricular fibrillation. Basic strategies apply for the performance of a successful cardioversion or defibrillation.

III. **Indications and contraindications for defibrillation and cardioversion**

A. Electrical therapy for cardiac arrhythmias can be **emergent or elective.** Defibrillation, or the termination of ventricular fibrillation, is indicated, with rare exception, in the presence of ventricular fibrillation. Defibrillation is contraindicated in patients who have clearly established a desire not to be resuscitated. Cardioversion may be performed on an urgent or emergent basis if an arrhythmia results in hemodynamic instability or is associated with severe symptoms. For elective cardioversion, the likelihood of obtaining and maintaining normal sinus rhythm must be weighed against the potential risks of the procedure.

B. **Indications for electrical cardioversion** can be grouped based on consensus into **class I indications, in which consensus exists** for cardioversion, or **class II indications, in which controversy exists** with respect to the necessity and utility of the procedure (Table 53-1). Contraindications for cardioversion include atrial or atrial appendage thrombi.

IV. **Patient preparation**

A. **Informed consent**

B. In patients on **digoxin,** levels are recommended only if there is a question of digitalis toxicity.

C. **NPO for 6 to 8 hours** prior to elective procedure.

D. **Anticoagulants** may be administered prior to procedure

E. For atrial fibrillation or atrial flutter, **antiarrhythmic drugs** should be started 24 to 48 hours prior to the procedure.

F. **Intravenous line**

G. **Continuous ECG monitoring**

H. **Oxygen and equipment for intubation** and mechanical ventilation if required.

I. **Paddles/patches** should be positioned with the anterior paddle to the right sternum at the level of the third or fourth intercostal space and the second paddle just outside the cardiac apex or posteriorly at the left infrascapular region.

J. **Sedation.** Amnesia induced by means of intravenous diazepam (Valium), midazolam (Versed), or one of the short-acting barbiturates such as thiopental sodium (Pentothal) or methohexital sodium (Brevital) should be administered (Table 53-2).

V. **Sedation.** Ideally, an anesthesiologist or respiratory technician should be available to manage the airway and sedation. Initial sedation can be accomplished through a variety of medications including short-acting barbiturates or benzodiazepines such as diazepam, the latter also being an amnestic agent (Table 53-2). Blood pressure should be monitored throughout the anesthesia and 100% oxygen should be administered via a face mask. Just prior to cardioversion,

Table 53-1. Indications for cardioversion

Class I	Emergency cardioversion of any arrhythmia resulting in:	Hemodynamic instability Myocardial ischemia Congestive heart failure
	Ventricular tachycardia atrial fibrillation/flutter	Hemodynamic compromise Rapid ventricular response Symptomatic intolerance
	Supraventricular arrhythmias (wide or narrow)	Hemodynamic instability
Class II		
	Atrial fibrillation/flutter with *caution* in:	Asymptomatic arrhythmia Atrial fibrillation with a slow ventricular response
	Sick sinus syndrome or conduction system disease	May require temporary pacemaker

an intravenous agent is given for the final sedation and amnesia. Although there has been extensive experience with intravenous diazepam, the recent trend has been to move toward short-acting agents such as midazolam, sodium methohexital, or propofol. Normally, at the time of cardioversion, a patient should not be responsive to simple verbal stimuli to assure that there is no recollection of the cardioversion upon recovery. (See Table 53-2 for dosing of different agents.)

VI. Technique

A. Energy output and selection

1. The energy output (in watts-seconds or joules) is determined by the power (volts multiplied by amperes) and duration of the impulse. The energy output can be selected by the operator and varies between 10 and 360 J (Table 53-3). Energy selection of successful cardioversion requires knowledge of the variable effecting energy delivery. This depends on two factors: the energy output and transthoracic impedance. Impedance is dependent on the patient's body habitus and the connection between the defibrillator and the patient.

2. For emergency defibrillation, 200 J is initially used. If this is unsuccessful, the energy is increased to 300 J; thereafter, the use of the maximum possible output (360 J) is appropriate. Recent studies indicate

Table 53-2. Commonly used sedatives

Generic name	Brand name	Route of administration	Elimination ($t_{1/2}$ min)	Dose
Diazepam	Valium	Parenteral: 5 mg/mL	43 ± 13	2–20 mg
Midazolam	Versed	Parenteral: 1 and 5 mg/mL	1.9 ± 0.6	1–5 mg
Lorazepam	Ativan	Parenteral: 2 and 4 mg/mL	14 ± 5	2 mg or 0.44 mg/kg
Propofol	Diprivan	Parenteral: 0.5–0.1 mg/kg	5 ± 2.5	25–50 mg
Thiopental Sodium	Pentothal	Parenteral: 3–5 mg/kg	10 ± 5	150–300 mg
Methohexital Sodium	Brevital	Parenteral: 0.25–1 mg/kg	5 ± 2.5	30–100 mg

Table 53-3. Arrhythmias, energy selection, and synchronization

Arrhythmia	Energy output (Js)	Synchronization
Ventricular fibrillation		
Initial	200	No
Subsequent	300	No
	360 (maximum)	No
Atrial fibrillation		
Initial	100	Yes
Subsequent	200, 300, 360	Yes
Atrial flutter		
Initial	20–50	Yes
Subsequent	100	Yes
	200	Yes
Atrial tachycardia		
Initial	50	Yes
Subsequent	100	Yes
	200 (maximum)	Yes
Ventricular tachycardia		
Initial	100	Yes
Subsequent	200, 300, 360	Yes

that excess current may produce myocardial injury and possibly hinder resuscitation.

3. A damped sinusoidal waveform has been the most widely use waveform to deliver current in transthoracic defibrillation. However, more recently biphasic and multipulse shocks have been reported to be superior for transthoracic defibrillation in animals and humans. The apparent ability of this waveform to achieve equivalent defibrillation efficacy at lower energy thresholds has permitted the introduction of smaller and lighter defibrillators for prehospital use suitable for more widespread community use. Additional studies of biphasic as well as multiphasic multipathway waveforms will require further clinical evaluation.

B. **Synchronization.** The principle danger of transthoracic elective cardioversion is the provocation of ventricular fibrillation. To avoid delivery of a shock during the vulnerable period, which may cause ventricular fibrillation, all defibrillators have a control mechanism that allows synchronization of the electrical shock on the R wave of the electrocardiogram (ECG). Synchronization must be used for cardioversion of all arrhythmias except ventricular fibrillation. If inadvertently placed in synchronized mode, a defibrillator may fail to discharge during ventricular fibrillation because it may not detect an ECG deflection large enough to allow synchronization.

C. **Electrode position.** Electrical defibrillation and cardioversion are accomplished by delivering an adequate current density of electrical waveform through the abnormally functioning myocardium. In order to maximize the amount of myocardial mass that is defibrillated or cardioverted, correct placement of the defibrillation electrodes is very important. For most emergency defibrillations, the recommended electrode placement is the anterior apical position with one electrode placed anteriorly under the right clavicle just to the right of the sternum and the other at the level of the left nipple in the midaxillary line. Incorrect placement of electrodes may result in failure to defibrillate.

D. In elective cardioversions, the anteroposterior electrode position is generally the most effective for cardioversion of atrial fibrillation. The right anterior–left posterior position or the sternal posterior position may be more effective in atrial fibrillation due to an atrial septal defect or a diffuse cardiomyopathy.

VII. Cardioversion of specific arrhythmias

A. Ventricular tachycardia. Cardioversion is the primary method used to terminate monomorphic ventricular tachycardia. The energy required for conversion is typically 100 J and the success rate is approximately 95% to 100%. Lower energy levels are occasionally effective; however, even synchronized, lower energies have the potential to convert the rhythm to ventricular fibrillation. A synchronized countershock should be used to terminate ventricular tachycardia, with three exceptions: (1) in an extreme emergency with rapid compromise and insufficient time for synchronization; (2) in digitalis toxicity–induced ventricular tachycardia where pacing may be safer; or (3) incessantly recurrent ventricular tachycardia when overdrive pace termination may be safer and more readily repeated. Polymorphic ventricular tachycardia should be treated as ventricular fibrillation.

B. Atrial fibrillation

1. In the general population, atrial fibrillation is the most common indication for cardioversion. Sinus rhythm improves cardiac output in most patients. This is particularly true in patients with noncompliant ventricles, severe left ventricular dysfunction, or mitral stenosis. Factors influencing the success of cardioversion of atrial fibrillation include:

   Duration of arrhythmia
   Degree of atrial fibrosis
   Atrial size

2. Echo studies suggest that a left atrial size greater than 4.5 cm is associated with a high (20% to 25%) risk of recurrent atrial fibrillation. However, this is not at contradiction to direct current (DC) cardioversion. Cardioversion is more likely to be complicated by systemic emboli in patients with atrial fibrillation of more than 48 to 72 hours duration and these patients require anticoagulation or transesophageal echocardiography to document the absence of left atrial thrombus prior to cardioversion.

3. Atrial fibrillation is routinely cardioverted in circumstances that result in:

   Hemodynamic compromise
   Ischemia
   Congestive heart failure
   Difficulty in controlling the ventricular response
   Idiopathic atrial fibrillation of less than 1 year's duration
   Embolic episodes

C. Atrial flutter. This is a regular atrial rhythm most evident on the surface ECG as a sawtooth appearance of the baseline in the inferior leads. Atrial flutter has been divided into type 1 (classic) in which the atrial rate is in the range of 200 to 300 complexes per minute and type II in which the rate is 320 to 430 complexes per minute. Type 1 atrial flutter can often be converted to sinus rhythm with rapid atrial pacing, whereas type 2 cannot. Cardioversion remains the treatment of choice for terminating atrial flutter. Success rates range from 75% to 100%. The typical energy requirements for conversion of atrial flutter are low (25 to 50 J). Although anticoagulation is not currently required for cardioversion of atrial flutter in all cases, it should be considered in patients with longstanding tachycardia, poor left ventricular function, left atrial enlargement, or mitral stenosis.

D. Supraventricular tachycardia. Medications such as adenosine or verapamil are generally successful in the termination of supraventricular tachycardia with success rates of 75% to 80%. In instances where these rhythms cannot be terminated or pose a substantial risk to the patient, cardioversion is the treatment of choice.

E. **Wolff-Parkinson-White syndrome.** Atrial fibrillation in patients with Wolff-Parkinson-White syndrome can be associated with 1:1 conduction over the accessory pathway leading to a ventricular response that may be extremely rapid (occasionally more than 300 bpm). Patients with a preexcited RR interval of less than 250 milliseconds are known to be at particularly high risk of ventricular fibrillation. Digoxin and verapamil may exacerbate the condition by blocking normal conduction via the AV node while providing even more rapid conduction down the accessory pathway. If there is hemodynamic instability, prompt electrical cardioversion is the treatment of choice. If the patient remains hemodynamically stable, intravenous procainamide is the drug of choice for rate control and chemical cardioversion.

VIII. **Special considerations**

   A. **Anticoagulation.** In hemodynamically unstable patients or in patients with significant ischemia due to arrhythmia, time may not warrant the consideration of anticoagulation. However, in other instances, patients are routinely anticoagulated prior to pharmacologic or electrical cardioversion.

   If a patient is hemodynamically stable and not hospitalized, the patient is given oral anticoagulation for 3 to 4 weeks prior to elective cardioversion. If hospitalization is required for other reasons and if cardioversion is appropriate, 2 days of heparin therapy before and 1 day of heparin post cardioversion is recommended. Transesophageal echocardiography is performed sometime during the 2 days of heparin therapy to rule out an intraatrial thrombus. In general, unless the atrial fibrillation is of very recent onset in a patient with an otherwise structurally normal heart, or the patient has a transesophageal echocardiogram showing no left atrial or left atrial appendage clot, it is recommended that all patients undergoing either chemical or electrical cardioversion be anticoagulated.

   Anticoagulation is recommended for 3 weeks prior to cardioversion of atrial fibrillation, for at least 4 weeks after cardioversion, and, if the patient is heparinized, an overlap of heparin and warfarin for at least 72 hours.

   B. **Cardioversion and digitalis.** Cardioversion of patients on digitalis remains controversial. Early reports suggested that toxic doses of ouabain increased the risk of ventricular fibrillation following DC cardioversion. Nonetheless, cardioversion can be performed safely in patients receiving digitalis. If there is a question of digitalis toxicity, it is generally recommended that lower energy levels be utilized. If increased ectopy is noted at any energy level, prophylactic lidocaine should be administered.

   C. **Cardioversion during pregnancy.** Synchronized, DC cardioversion has been performed successfully in all trimesters of pregnancy without untoward effects on the mother or fetus.

IX. **Complications of cardioversion.** Cardioversion is safe and highly effective. With proper technique, adequate sedation, and routine monitoring, few complications exist. The following are potential complications.

   A. Respiratory compromise and/or aspiration might occur.

   B. Cardiac output decreases after cardioversion of atrial fibrillation in more than a third of patients, and the decrease may last a week. A gradual increase in cardiac output then occurs over the next several weeks. The increase is caused by the return of left atrial mechanical activity as the atrial myopathy of chronic atrial fibrillation subsides.

   C. Acute pulmonary edema is rare; 50% of cases occur within 3 hours of cardioversion, with a mortality of 18%. The reduced cardiac performance after cardioversion most likely results from the combination of heart disease and cardiac depressant effects of anesthetic drugs used. Pulmonary and/or coronary artery emboli and the resumption of right atrial mechanical activity before left atrial mechanical activity may be additional factors in the pathogenesis of pulmonary edema after cardioversion.

   D. Embolization and anticoagulation. Patients should be adequately anticoagulated prior to elective cardioversion. Anticoagulant therapy should be continued for a month or longer prior to cardioversion of atrial fibrillation. If this is not possible or contraindicated, transesophageal echocardiography may be useful to exclude the existence of a left atrial thrombus prior to cardioversion. In emergent circumstances this is often not feasible. In general, the risk of embolization with emergent cardioversion is 1:500.

E. Myocardial injury during cardioversion. As electrical current passes through the myocardium, damage to myocardial tissues might occur. However, this is rarely clinically evident.

F. Prophylactic temporary pacemaker insertion may be required prior to cardioversion in patients with sick sinus syndrome or severe conduction system disease.

SUGGESTED READINGS

Key Reviews

Arnold AZ, Mick MJ, Maurek RP, Loop, FD, Trohman, RG. Role of prophylactic anticoagulation for direct current cardioversion in patients with atrial flutter or fibrillation. *J Am Coll Cardiol* 1992;19:851–855.

Bardy GH, Marchlinsky FE, Sharma AD, et al. Multicenter comparison of truncated biphasic shocks and standard damped sinusoidal waveform monophasic shocks for transthoracic ventricular defibrillation. *Circulation* 1996;94:2507–2514.

Black IW, Fatkin D, Sagar KP, et al. Exclusion of atrial thrombus by transesophageal echocardiography does not preclude embolism after cardioversion of atrial fibrillation. A multicenter study. *Circulation* 1994;89:2509–2513.

Greene HL, DiMarco JP, Kudenchuk PJ, et al. Comparison of monophasic and biphasic pulse waveforms for transthoracic cardioversion. *Am J Cardiol* 1995;75:1135–1139.

Lown B, Amaringham R, Neuman J. New method for terminating cardiac arrhythmias: used of synchronized capacitor discharge. *JAMA* 1962;182:548–555.

Standards and guidelines for cardiopulmonary resuscitation and emergency cardiac care. *JAMA* 1986;255:2942–2943.

54. ENDOMYOCARDIAL BIOPSY

Milind Shah

I. **Indications and contraindications.** The indications for right ventricular and left ventricular endomyocardial biopsy are listed in Table 54-1, of which **monitoring of cardiac transplant rejection and anthracycline toxicity,** as well as **diagnosing some forms of myocarditis,** are the only definitive reasons to perform this procedure. Left ventricular biopsy is very uncommon. Relative contraindications are listed in Table 54-2.

II. **Patient preparation.** As with any other procedure, **patient education** and **informed consent** are necessary. A small dose of **midazolam** is sometimes necessary. Monitoring of **heart rate, blood pressure, electrocardiogram (ECG), and pulse oximetry** are necessary. Positioning of the patient depends on the approach, i.e., internal jugular (most common) or femoral vein. Different maneuvers like Valsalva, leg elevation with a wedge, and Trendelenberg position increase central venous pressure and can be helpful in obtaining venous access. Imaging modalities include fluoroscopy or echocardiography (the latter for bedside procedures, pregnant patients, heterotopic heart transplant recipients, or if a specific site needs to be biopsied).

III. **Devices**

   A. **Sheath.** Standard (10-cm) short sheath (8 or 9 Fr) is needed for the right internal jugular (IJ) approach. The intermediate length (45 cm and 8 Fr) sheath is good to use from left IJ or right subclavian to straighten venous angulations. For femoral approach, an 85-cm-long sheath with 94-cm-long dilator is used. Two curves are available at the tip: 7-cm for dilated right atrium or transplanted hearts and 5-cm right coronary or "Tampa Bay"–type guiding catheters (8 Fr, internal diameter 0.078-in.) can also be substituted for the long sheaths. The Tampa Bay catheter has a 7-cm curve followed by a 1.1-cm distal angulated tip segment, providing more stability in the ventricle.

   B. **Bioptome.** There are two basic types of bioptome: (1) Independent, i. e., does not require sheath for positioning; and (2) flexible, i. e., requires sheath for positioning. Resterilizable and reusable bioptomes are widely used, but disposable bioptomes are also available. For IJ and SC approaches, 50-cm-long bioptomes are used, whereas for femoral use the bioptomes are available in 95- to 105-cm length. The selection of the size of bioptome (5.4 to 9 Fr) depends on the access site as well as the inner diameter of the sheath (see Table 54-3).

IV. **Technique.** Right ventricular endomyocardial biopsies can be performed from either right or left internal jugular, subclavian, or femoral veins. If necessary, a left ventricular endomyocardial biopsy can be obtained via the femoral artery approach. Direct left ventricular needle biopsy from the cardiac apex has been abandoned because of the high complication rate.

   A. **Right ventricular biopsy**

      1. **Internal jugular vein approach.** After standard preparation and local anesthesia with 1% lidocaine, the required anatomic landmarks (see Chapter 50) are identified. A vein-localizing pilot puncture is sometimes made with a 22-gauge needle. The same directions, the right internal jugular vein is punctured with the larger bore 18-gauge (Cook) needle and an 8-Fr short sheath is introduced using standard technique. The bioptome, with jaws closed, is advanced under fluoroscopic or echocardiographic guidance across the atrial suture line (in allografts) until its tip lies against the lower third of the lateral right atrial wall. It is then rotated gently counterclockwise and is simultaneously advanced into the right ventricular cavity (see Fig. 54-1). Rotation is continued until the catheter reaches the apical half of the right ventricle and the

Table 54-1. Indications

RV BIOPSY
1. Monitoring of cardiac allograft rejection
2. Diagnosis and staging of anthracycline toxicity
3. Diagnosis of myocarditis
4. Diagnoses of select secondary cardiomyopathies (e.g., sarcoidosis, amyloidosis, hemochromatosis, glycogen storage disease, Fabry's disease)
5. Diagnosis of restrictive versus constrictive myocardial disease
6. Unexplained life-threatening ventricular arrhythmias

LV BIOPSY
1. Failed or nondiagnostic RV biopsy
2. Diseases with selective LV involvement (i.e., endomyocardial fibrosis, scleroderma, left heart radiation, and endocardial fibroelastosis of infants and newborns)

RV, right ventricular; LV, left ventricular.

handle clamp points posterior. At this point the tip of the bioptome rests on the interventricular septum. The position is confirmed by lack of further advancement, generation of premature ventricular contractions, and fluoroscopy findings of bioptome going across the spine and its tip lying below the upper margin of the left hemidiaphragm. Generation of premature atrial contractions should be of concern and a bite is not taken unless atrial tissue is desired. If there is any doubt about the position, the bioptome is withdrawn and the same process is repeated with confirmation in at least two fluoroscopic views (30 degrees right anterior oblique and 60 degrees left anterior oblique). Once in the desired position, the bioptome is withdrawn about 1 cm, and is advanced again after the jaws have been opened. When it touches the endocardium, the jaws are closed and 2 to 3 seconds are allowed for severing the tissue before the bioptome is withdrawn with its jaws closed. A small tug is often felt while withdrawing, but excessive tugging and multiple premature ventricular contractions should prompt consideration of another pass. Usually three to seven biopsy specimens are obtained to reduce sampling error. For

Table 54-2. Relative contraindications

1. Coagulopathy
   a. INR > 1.5
   b. Platelet count < 100,000
2. RA or RV thrombus
3. Any prior surgery or procedure affecting passage to RV (i.e., SVC or IVC interruption), Mustard or Senning procedures for TGA, mechanical tricuspid prosthesis, and sometimes venous filters for thromboembolism (if femoral route)
4. Significant right-to-left shunt is a relative contraindication because of risk of paradoxic embolism (air or thrombus)
5. Recent MI leading to possible thinning of myocardium of the ventricle being biopsied
6. Profound hemodynamic compromise
7. Severe tachycardia

INR, international normalized ratio; RA, right atrial; RV, right ventricular; SVC, superior vena cava; IVC, inferior vena cava; TGA, xxx; MI, myocardial infarction.

Table 54-3. Bioptomes

(A) INDEPENDENT

1. The **Sakakibara-Konno** Bioptome: Stiff shaft with two large cutting cups, requires "cut-down." Reusable. Not used in USA.
2. The **Kawai** Bioptome: Requires a removable stylet. Highly flexible tip that can be deflected up to 40 degrees in one direction and up to 10 degrees in opposite direction, providing good maneuverability. Reusable. Can be used for RV or LV, but not popular in USA.
3. The **Stanford-Scholten** Bioptome: Two hemispheric cutting jaws of which one can be opened and the other is fixed. Adjustable nuts for setting the force of cutting jaw. Distal curve of the catheter varies between 45 and 90 degrees depending on whether the clamp is locked on first or second click. Distal curve lies in the same plane as the handle of the clamp to facilitate orientation. Can be reused for more than 50 procedures without the need for sharpening or service. Very popular in USA.
4. The **Fehling** Bioptome: Scissors action cutting jaws. Reusable. Popular in USA.

(B) FLEXIBLE

1. The **King's** Bioptome: Scissors action cutting jaws. Handle's thumb ring is pushed in to open the jaws. Reusable. Widely used in Europe.
2. The **Stanford LV** Bioptome: Similar design as mentioned above, but longer with smaller diameter. Reusable.
3. The **Cordis** Bioptome: Scissors action cutting jaws, stainless steel wire coil with flexible shaft and formable tip, spring-loaded three-ring plastic handle that controls the jaws. Disposable.

frozen section, one extra sample is needed. Once the procedure is completed, the venous sheath is removed and hemostasis achieved. Patients are observed for about an hour before discharge to home.

Because of the unusual orientation of the donor heart in heterotopic heart transplant patients, special precautions are listed in Table 54-4.

2. Femoral vein approach. After standard preparation and local anesthesia with 1% lidocaine, the required anatomic landmarks (see Chapter 50) are identified. Right (more common) or left femoral vein is punctured with a no. 18 (Cook) needle and 0.038-in. guidewire is advanced up to the right atrium. A long (85-cm) 7-Fr sheath with dilator (larger 7-cm curve used for transplant recipients) is advanced over the wire and on entering right atrium the dilator is withdrawn. Tricuspid valve is crossed with the help of the wire (a balloon-tipped catheter can also be used) and the sheath is advanced into the right ventricle. The pressure tracing as well as fluoroscopy (posteroanterior and 60-degree left anterior oblique views) are used to confirm position pointing toward the interventricular septum. The side port of the sheath is connected to a slow continuous intravenous infusion to prevent clot formation inside the sheath. A long (100-cm) floppy-shaft bioptome is used to acquire samples. The remaining details of the procedure are the same as mentioned earlier in IV.A.1.

3. Subclavian vein approach. After standard preparation and local anesthesia with 1% lidocaine, the required anatomic landmarks (see

Table 54-4. Heterotopic heart transplant: special precautions

1. Donor right atrium is in right hemithorax.
2. A radiopaque ring may mark the connection of donor and recipient atria.
3. Both fluoroscopy and echocardiography are used for procedure guidance.

Chapter 50) are identified. The subclavian vein is punctured using an 18-gauge (Cook) needle followed by insertion of an intermediate length (45-cm) 8-Fr sheath. The sheath is advanced over a 0.035-in. wire, across the tricuspid valve into the right ventricle. The pressure tracing as well as fluoroscopy (posteroanterior and 60-degree left anterior oblique views) are used to confirm position pointing toward the inter-ventricular septum. The side port of the sheath is connected to a slow continuous intravenous infusion to prevent clot formation inside the sheath. The standard length (50-cm), flexible shaft bioptomes are used to acquire samples. The remaining details of the procedure are the same as mentioned earlier in IV:A.1.

B. Left ventricular biopsy

1. Femoral arterial approach. After standard preparation and local anesthesia with 1% lidocaine, the required anatomic landmarks (see Chapter 56) are identified. Right (more common) or left femoral artery is punctured with an 18-gauge (Cook) needle and 0.035-in. exchange length guidewire is advanced up to the ascending aorta. An 8-Fr, long (90-cm) curved Teflon sheath with dilator is introduced and advanced to the descending thoracic aorta and the dilator is removed. A regular length 7-Fr pigtail catheter is advanced over the wire, and the aortic valve is crossed in the conventional way. The sheath is then advanced into the left ventricular cavity by sliding over the pigtail catheter. The tip of the sheath is directed distal to the mitral apparatus, away from thinner posterobasal wall. The pigtail catheter is removed, the position of the sheath reconfirmed (fluoroscopy and pressure tracings) and, 5, 000 U heparin given intravenously prior to insertion of the bioptome. Stanford left ventricular bioptome (6 Fr, 100 cm) is then advanced and biopsy samples are collected in the same fashion as mentioned earlier. Heparin is not reversed with protamine at the end of the procedure to minimize thrombus formation at the biopsy sites. Catheters must frequently be flushed during the procedure.

V. Complications

A. Mortality. Endomyocardial biopsy can be performed safely with only 0.05% procedure-related mortality as reported in a worldwide survey of more than 6,000 procedures published in 1980.

B. Cardiac perforation and tamponade. The reported incidence of cardiac perforation is 0.3% to 0.5% and can rapidly result in tamponade. The risk can be minimized by carefully monitoring catheter position, gentle catheter advancement, monitoring symptoms of chest pain, and hemodynamic data. In recently transplanted patients, the atrial suture line also poses a higher risk for perforation. Patients with suspected perforation should be closely monitored for 10 to 15 minutes. Echocardiography as well as fluoroscopy (loss of motion of right atrium or left ventricle) can confirm the diagnosis.

C. Thromboembolism. Right-sided thromboembolism is possible but rare. Using a sheath with a back bleed valve and aspirating air prior to inserting the bioptome minimizes the chance of air embolism. Cerebral embolization during left ventricular biopsy can be minimized by heparinization as mentioned earlier.

D. Arrhythmia. Various atrial and ventricular arrhythmias are possible but are generally transient, and can be avoided with a careful approach. Brady-arrhythmic episodes in heart transplant patients respond only to β_1 stimulants and not to atropine. The incidence of sustained malignant ventricular arrhythmia is about 0.8%, and poking the endocardial surface with the closed bioptome head can terminate sustained ventricular tachycardia not abating on withdrawal of catheter.

E. Bundle branch block. This can be transient or permanent, but can be prevented by cautious technique and confirmation of bioptome position before taking a sample.

F. **Tricuspid valve (or mitral valve for left ventricular biopsy) dysfunction.** The bioptome can damage the chordae or papillary muscle and produce significant valvular regurgitation, but this can be avoided by careful confirmation of bioptome position prior to sampling.

G. **Damage to vena cava, coronary sinus, hepatic vein, and coronary arteries.** Gentle advancement of bioptome and position confirmation with different fluoroscopic views can minimize these complications. Occasionally, a deeper bite with the bioptome can resect a branch of coronary artery and create coronary artery to right ventricular fistula, which most of the time is of no clinical significance. If the catheter inadvertently enters the pleural space or mediastinum, emergent surgery will most likely be needed.

H. **Local complications.** Hematoma, local infection, injury to lung (pneumothorax, incidence 0.9%) and nerve (recurrent laryngeal palsy and Horner's syndrome) are possible but rare while achieving vascular access. Careful identification of anatomic landmarks can reduce that risk. Transient recurrent laryngeal nerve palsy due to local anesthetic effect is possible but passes without any residual deficit.

SUGGESTED READINGS
Relevant Book Chapters
Baim D, Grossman W. *Cardiac catheterization, angiography, and intervention,* 5th ed. Baltimore: Williams & Wilkins, 1996:407–420.
Kern M. *The cardiac catheterization handbook,* 2nd ed. St. Louis: Mosby–Year:Book, 1995:422–429.

55. INTRAAORTIC BALLOON COUNTERPULSATION

Matthew T. Roe

I. **Introduction.** Intraaortic balloon counterpulsation (IABC) is needed to **support hemodynamics** in cardiogenic shock and to **relieve medically refractory ischemia** in patients with severe coronary disease. The duration of support with an intraaortic balloon pump (IABP) is usually short since multiple complications can develop in patients treated with IABC. Therefore, patients considered for IABC should be carefully selected and should be closely monitored while the balloon catheter is in place.

II. **Indications**
   A. **Cardiogenic shock**
      1. **Bridge to revascularization.** Intraaortic balloon counterpulsation provides temporary hemodynamic stabilization for patients with cardiogenic shock caused by acute myocardial infarction (MI) to allow for attempted revascularization. Hospital survival rates for cardiogenic shock with balloon pump support alone, without revascularization, are poor (5% to 20%). Early revascularization with percutaneous transluminal coronary angioplasty (PTCA) improves survival rates in cardiogenic shock caused by acute MI.
         a. In the Global Utilization of Streptokinase and Tissue Plasminogen Activator for Occluded Coronary Arteries (GUSTO I) trial comparing fibrinolytic regimens for acute ST-elevation MI, percutaneous transluminal coronary angioplasty (PTCA) was the only factor associated with a lower 30-day mortality rate in 2,972 patients with cardiogenic shock (1).
         b. Additionally, early placement of an IABP in this cohort of patients was also associated with lower 30-day and 1-year mortality rates (2).
      2. **Bridge to a tertiary center.** Thrombolytic therapy alone in patients with cardiogenic shock is less successful than mechanical reperfusion. However, the addition of IABC to thrombolysis can improve outcomes in patients with cardiogenic shock. In 46 patients with acute MI and cardiogenic shock treated at community hospitals without angioplasty capabilities, simultaneous treatment with thrombolysis and IABC was associated with an improved 1-year survival rate (67% versus 32%) and successful transfer to a tertiary facility for revascularization when thrombolysis failed (3).
   B. **Refractory unstable angina.** Patients with severe coronary disease who have refractory ischemia or hemodynamic instability show **dramatic improvement** when IABC is used prior to revascularization. The 1994 Agency for Health Care Policy and Research clinical practice guidelines for unstable angina recommend IABC for high-risk, medically refractory unstable angina patients as a bridge to stabilize the patient before emergent percutaneous revascularization or coronary artery bypass grafting (CABG) (4).
   C. **Acute MI catheter-based reperfusion.** The **benefits** of IABC for patients with acute MI without cardiogenic shock treated with catheter-based reperfusion are **uncertain.**
      1. In a randomized trial of 182 hemodynamically stable patients who underwent direct PTCA for acute MI, prophylactic IABC for 2 days after the procedure reduced recurrent ischemia and reocclusion of the infarct-related artery but had no effect on survival or reinfarction (5).
      2. In the PAMI II (Primary Angioplasty in Myocardial Infarction II) trial, 437 high-risk patients (age greater than 70 years, multivessel coronary disease, reduced ejection fraction, vein graft disease, or persistent ventricular arrhythmias) treated with direct PTCA for acute MI were randomized to ±1 to 2 days of IABC after PTCA (6). Patients treated with

IABC had a slight reduction in recurrent ischemia but had no reduction in mortality, reinfarction, or infarct-related artery reocclusion. Thus, hemodynamically stable patients with acute MI treated with catheter-based reperfusion are not likely to benefit from IABP support after the intervention.

D. **High-risk percutaneous revascularization.** Patients at high risk for complications during percutaneous revascularization include those with unprotected left main coronary disease, left ventricular dysfunction (ejection fraction less than 40%), the target vessel supplying more than 40% of the myocardial territory, or severe congestive heart failure (CHF). In patients with one or more of these risk factors, periprocedural mortality increases twofold to sixfold when standard PTCA is used. Placement of an IABP in these high-risk patients affords the operator a longer duration of ischemia during balloon inflation before CHF and hypotension develop.

1. In a review of studies in which IABC was used during high-risk PTCA, successful revascularization was accomplished in 86% to 100% of patients, in-hospital mortality rates were 6% to 19%, and rates of MI and cases requiring emergent CABG were 0% to 6%. Additionally, high-risk patients treated with rotational coronary atherectomy were shown to have less procedural hypotension and better procedural success when IABC was used.

2. While there are no specific recommendations for when to use IABC during high-risk coronary interventions, improved percutaneous revascularization techniques with coronary stents and adjunctive glycoprotein IIb/IIIa receptor antagonists have reduced the need for prophylactic IABP placement in high-risk patients.

E. **End-stage cardiomyopathy/bridge to cardiac transplantation.** An IABP improves cardiac output and lowers filling pressures in patients with dilated and ischemic cardiomyopathy and can be used for long-term support prior to cardiac transplantation.

1. **Disadvantages** of prolonged IABP support in patients awaiting cardiac transplantation include a high risk of infection and the need for continuous bed rest.

2. However, with improved inotropic therapy and implantable left ventricular assist devices for patients awaiting cardiac transplantation, IABC is now used less commonly for prolonged mechanical support in patients with end-stage cardiomyopathy.

F. **Support during noncardiac surgery.** Patients with severe coronary disease, recent MI, and severe left ventricular dysfunction are at high risk for cardiac complications when they undergo noncardiac surgery. Case reports have demonstrated that high-risk patients are stabilized hemodynamically and have acceptable postoperative outcomes when prophylactic IABP support is utilized during and after noncardiac surgical procedures.

G. **Mechanical complications of acute MI. Acute mitral regurgitation** and **ventricular septal defect** are devastating complications of acute MI and frequently cause rapid deterioration progressing to cardiogenic shock. An IABP should be placed prior to surgical repair in patients with hemodynamically significant mitral regurgitation or ventricular septal defect after an MI.

H. **Decompensated aortic stenosis** can be managed with temporary IABP support to improve the stroke volume and reduce the transvalvular gradient prior to aortic valve replacement. However, since aortic insufficiency is often associated with aortic stenosis, careful monitoring of patients with aortic stenosis early after initiation of IABC is recommended to ensure that aortic insufficiency is not worsened by the balloon pump.

I. **Refractory ventricular arrhythmias.** Incessant ventricular tachycardia compromises left ventricular filling, reduces stroke volume, and causes or worsens ischemia. Intraaortic balloon counterpulsation improved hemodynamics, lessened ischemia, and controlled refractory ventricular arrhythmias in 86% of patients in a large case series.

J. Weaning from cardiopulmonary bypass/postoperative pump failure. Patients with severe left ventricular dysfunction or those with prolonged runs on cardiopulmonary bypass can be difficult to wean from bypass after open heart surgery due to stunned myocardium from prolonged cardioplegic arrest. For these patients IABP support improves hemodynamics and facilitates weaning from cardiopulmonary bypass.

III. Contraindications

A. Aortic dissection. Any type of aortic dissection precludes IABP use due to the potential of the balloon catheter to extend the dissection and to worsen ischemia of a peripheral vascular bed that may be involved by the dissection.

B. Abdominal or thoracic aneurysm. Using IABP with an abdominal or thoracic aneurysm can precipitate an acute aortic dissection, dislodgment of atheroemboli, or aortic rupture, so the presence of an aneurysm is an **absolute contraindication** to IABP use.

C. Severe peripheral vascular disease

1. The majority of the complications of IABC are from vascular insufficiency in the accessed leg due to the **large size of the balloon sheath and catheter and the concomitant presence of peripheral vascular disease** in patients who typically need IABC. The IABP catheters range in size between 8.5 Fr and 10. 5 Fr, and sheaths are sized between 9 Fr and 11 Fr.

2. **Limb ischemia and threatened limb viability** can result when peripheral perfusion is compromised by the balloon catheter and sheath. The IABP catheter can be inserted without a sheath to reduce the diameter of obstruction in the iliac vessels, but in patients with tortuous aortoiliac vessels, sheathless IABP insertion can be difficult (see V.C).

3. Severe peripheral vascular disease thus is relative contraindication to IABP insertion, depending on the necessity of IABP support and the degree of vascular compromise.

D. Descending aortic and peripheral vascular grafts

1. **Prosthetic descending aortic grafts and iliofemoral vascular grafts** are relative contraindications to IABC. Consultation with a vascular surgeon is recommended before attempting balloon pump insertion in these patients.

2. **Iliac artery stents** are not an absolute contraindication to IABP placement but passage of the guidewire and balloon catheter through the stent must be performed under direct fluoroscopic vision.

E. Coagulopathy or contraindication to heparin

1. The balloon catheter is thrombogenic, and intravenous heparin is commonly given while the IABP is in place to prevent thrombi from developing on the balloon surface. Patients with a contraindication to heparin, such as those with prior heparin-induced thrombocytopenia, can be **anticoagulated with alternative agents** like hirudin derivatives or low molecular weight heparin analogs.

2. After cardiac surgery, heparin can be avoided due to the increased risk of intrathoracic bleeding, but IABP support in such patients is usually of short duration. In nonsurgical patients, if an anticoagulant cannot be given or if a severe coagulopathy exists that could precipitate bleeding at the access site, IABC is discouraged but could safely be undertaken for a short period of time.

F. Moderate to severe aortic insufficiency. By inflating during diastole, the IABP can worsen aortic insufficiency when blood is displaced to the proximal aorta. No consensus exists as to what degree of aortic insufficiency absolutely contraindicates IABP use. Therefore, **careful monitoring** of patients with aortic insufficiency who absolutely need IABP support is recommended.

IV. Hemodynamics of balloon pump function

A. Decreased afterload

1. As systole begins, the intraaortic balloon rapidly deflates and creates negative pressure in the aorta, which reduces afterload and improves

forward flow from the left ventricle. Afterload reduction occurs because the aortic end-diastolic pressure is reduced, and this results in an increase in cardiac output of approximately 20% and a decrease in the mean pulmonary capillary wedge pressure of approximately 20%.

2. The **overall hemodynamic benefit** of IABP appears to be a reduction in left ventricular wall stress from decreased filling pressures and decreased afterload, which in turn improves stroke volume and cardiac output (Figs. 55-1 and 55-2).

B. Augmented coronary perfusion

1. When the balloon inflates during diastole, it displaces blood to the proximal aorta and augments aortic diastolic pressure and, thus, coronary perfusion pressure. The augmentation of coronary perfusion pressure is more dramatic when systemic hypotension is present (Figs. 55-1 and 55-2).

2. Doppler flow studies have demonstrated that peak coronary flow velocity is increased with IABP support, but there is no improvement in coronary flow past critical coronary stenoses (unless the obstructions are first relieved with percutaneous revascularization). Also, collateral coronary flow does not increase with IABP support. Thus, with severe, non-revascularized coronary disease, IABP relieves ischemia more through decreased left ventricular wall stress and decreased myocardial oxygen demand than through increased coronary perfusion.

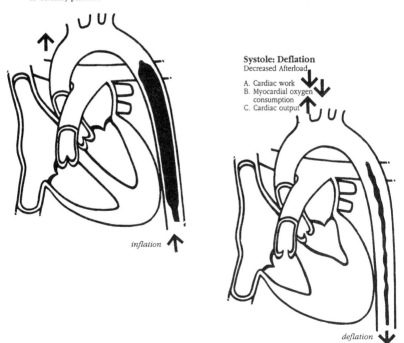

Diastole: Inflation
Augmentation of
Diastolic Pressure

A. Coronary perfusion

inflation

Systole: Deflation
Decreased Afterload

A. Cardiac work
B. Myocardial oxygen
consumption
C. Cardiac output

deflation

FIG. 55-1. By inflating during diastole, the intraaortic balloon pump increases coronary perfusion. Deflation of the balloon at the onset of systole decreases myocardial wall stress and oxygen demand and increases cardiac output. Courtesy of Datascope Corp.

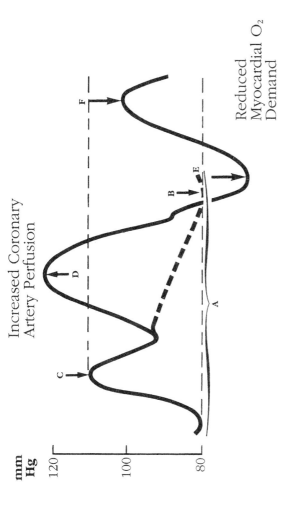

mm
Hg

120

100

80

Increased Coronary
Artery Perfusion

Reduced
Myocardial O₂
Demand

A. **One Complete Cardiac Cycle**
B. **Unassisted Aortic End Diastolic Pressure**
C. **Unassisted Systolic Pressure**
D. **Diastolic Augmentation**
E. **Assisted Aortic End Diastolic Pressure**
F. **Reduced Systolic Pressure**

FIG. 55-2. Proper timing of balloon function occurs when the balloon inflates on the downslope of the systolic pressure waveform and deflates before the onset of the next systolic waveform. The IABP inflation in diastole increases diastolic pressure to improve coronary artery perfusion and to increase mean arterial pressure. Additionally, aortic end-diastolic pressure is reduced when the balloon deflates in end diastole to lower afterload and myocardial oxygen demand. Courtesy of Datascope Corp.

691

V. Insertion technique/patient evaluation and monitoring

A. Balloon sizing is based on a patient's height. Three common balloon sizes are available: 50 cm^3 for patients over 6 ft tall; 40 cm^3 for patients between 5 ft 4 in. and 6 ft, and 34 cm^3 for patients under 5 ft 4 in. Balloon length and diameter increases with each larger size. The 40-cm^3 balloon is most commonly used, whereas the 50-cm^3 balloon is rarely used because the balloon is too long for most patients.

B. Evaluating peripheral vasculature. Proximal and distal pulses are assessed in both legs, and ankle/brachial indices (ABIs) can also be determined. The leg with the strongest pulses and/or the best ABI score should be chosen for access.

C. Insertion technique

1. **Gaining access/sheath insertion.** The leg chosen for access should be shaved and prepped with antiseptic solution from the umbilicus to the knee. After infiltration with a local anesthetic, the femoral artery is accessed with an 18-gauge introducer needle and a 0.030-in. × 145-cm J-tipped guidewire is advanced through the needle to the aortic arch under **fluoroscopy.** A smaller 5-Fr dilator is first inserted over the wire to dilate the subcutaneous tissues. Then the sheath, loaded with a larger dilator that is 1 Fr smaller than the sheath, is inserted over the guidewire. The guidewire should be left in place in the aortic arch.

2. **Balloon insertion.** The sheaths are sized between 9 Fr and 11 Fr and are 6 to 11 in. long, and the balloon catheter is sized between 8.5 Fr and 10.5 Fr. The most common sheath used is 10 Fr, with a 9.5-Fr balloon. The prewrapped balloon is inserted over the guidewire and is advanced until the proximal tip is positioned 1 cm below the left subclavian artery and 2 cm below the carina. The guidewire is then removed, and the distal tip of the balloon is visualized under fluoroscopy to ensure that it is out of the sheath.

3. **Insertion without fluoroscopy.** Fluoroscopic guidance is recommended for placement of the IABP, but if fluoroscopy is unavailable, the distance from the angle of Louis to the umbilicus and then to the common femoral artery insertion site is measured to determine the approximate distance the balloon must be advanced.

4. **Surgical insertion**

   a. Occasionally, balloon pumps can be inserted surgically **by directly exposing the common femoral artery** or by suturing a 6- to 12-mm prosthetic graft end-to-side to the femoral artery to provide a conduit for the catheter. Distal limb ischemia is reduced with these methods, but grafts must be removed surgically and the femoral artery has to be directly repaired after IABP removal when surgical access is used.

   b. Balloon pumps can also be inserted directly into the ascending or thoracic aorta **during open heart surgery.**

5. **Difficulties with access.** If passage of the guidewire is difficult, a 5-Fr sheath can be placed in the common femoral artery and contrast medium can be injected through the sheath or through a pigtail catheter to define the iliofemoral anatomy.

   a. If severe iliac or femoral artery obstructions are demonstrated, the balloon can be inserted on the contralateral side, the obstructions can be treated with peripheral angioplasty and stenting prior to balloon insertion, or the procedure can be aborted.

   b. If severe obstruction or aneurysmal dilatation of the distal abdominal aorta is demonstrated, the balloon catheter should not be inserted.

6. **Sheathless insertion.** In patients with peripheral vascular disease, the balloon catheter can be inserted without a sheath, directly over the guidewire, after appropriate dilation of the subcutaneous tissue. Retrospective reviews have shown that lower limb ischemia is reduced with this technique. However, a sheathless balloon catheter cannot be repo-

sitioned once it is placed and has a greater potential to become infected from skin flora than a sheathed balloon catheter. Smaller size balloon catheters and stiffer guidewires are being developed to aid in sheathless insertion.

7. Tortuous iliofemoral vessels

  a. When the tortuosity of the iliofemoral vessels prevents passage of the 0.030-in. guidewire supplied in the IABP kit, a 0.035-in. Wholey wire can be used to traverse the tortuous vessels. A long (45 or 60 cm) flexible sheath is then placed in the descending aorta past the tortuous iliac vessels.

  b. A superstiff 0.038-in. wire is then exchanged through the sheath. The 11-in. IABP sheath is inserted over the superstiff wire, which provides more support for placement of the less flexible IABP sheath. The superstiff wire is then exchanged for the 0.030-in. standard IABP wire through the sheath, and the balloon catheter is inserted over this wire into the proper position.

D. Initial setup

  1. After insertion, the helium gas line of the balloon catheter is connected to the IABP console and the central lumen of the catheter is attached to an arterial pressure monitor device on the console with pressure tubing, after allowing the line to back-bleed.

  2. Balloon autoinflation is initiated from the console, the arterial line attached to the central lumen of the catheter is flushed, and the initial IABP inflation is at 1:2 (per cardiac cycle) while the timing is adjusted (see Section VI of this chapter).

  3. Balloon inflation is then observed under fluoroscopy to ensure that the balloon is completely out of the sheath. If the balloon is found to be kinked or not inflating fully, it should be repositioned by pulling the sheath back a few inches, or the balloon can be manually inflated.

  4. Finally, the sheath and balloon catheter are sutured in place, dressed using sterile technique, and the inflation is changed to 1:1.

E. Monitoring

  1. A chest x-ray is immediately obtained after IABP placement to verify the catheter position, even if fluoroscopic guidance has been used.

  2. Intravenous heparin is started once the balloon and sheath are secure to maintain the activated partial thromboplastin time (aPTT) at 50 to 70 seconds.

  3. Daily chest x-rays are recommended while the IABP is in place to check the position of the catheter. If the catheter needs to be repositioned, it can be manipulated through a sterile plastic sleeve that is placed over the part of the catheter that extrudes from the sheath.

  4. Daily hemoglobin and platelet counts are followed to monitor for hemolysis and thrombocytopenia.

F. Care of the patient with an IABP

  1. The patient should be kept supine in bed, and peripheral pulses are regularly evaluated.

  2. The accessed leg should be secured to prevent inadvertent movement by the patient.

  3. Prophylactic antibiotics are not recommended while the IABP is in place.

  4. Blood samples generally should not be obtained from the central lumen of the IABP because the risk of clotting the lumen is increased, and air or small thrombi can be injected through the central lumen during flushing of the tubing after blood withdrawal.

VI. Balloon pump triggering and timing

  A. Triggering. Balloon pump inflation can be triggered by the surface electrocardiogram (ECG), the arterial pressure waveform, a paced rhythm, or an internal asynchronous mode.

1. Preferably, the surface ECG is used to trigger IABP inflation, which is appropriately delayed after the R wave to begin at the time in the cardiac cycle when the aortic valve closes (dicrotic notch).
2. If the IABP fails to trigger properly from the surface ECG, change the lead being evaluated, check surface electrode placement, or increase the QRS gain on the console monitor.
3. For patients with poor surface ECG tracings, the balloon can be triggered from the central arterial pressure waveform. Pacing spikes should be used to trigger the balloon in patients who are 100% paced.
4. When the patient is arresting or when the other triggering mechanisms are not working correctly, an internal asynchronous mode can be used to trigger the balloon to inflate at a regular interval.

B. **Timing.** Ideal balloon pump timing occurs when the balloon inflates on the downslope of the systolic pressure waveform before the dicrotic notch and deflates prior to the onset of the next systolic pressure waveform (see Fig. 55-2). Timing is usually adjusted manually but can be automatically adjusted by internal algorithms programmed into the console.

1. **Early inflation** (Fig. 55-3) is inflation of the IABP prior to aortic valve closure (dicrotic notch).
   a. There is premature closure of the aortic valve with increased afterload, left ventricular wall stress, and myocardial oxygen demand. Stroke volume is decreased.
   b. It is corrected by delaying inflation until after aortic valve closure.
2. **Late inflation** (Fig. 55-4) is inflation of the IABP well after closure of the aortic valve.
   a. There is diminished diastolic pressure augmentation and suboptimal coronary perfusion.
   b. It is corrected by adjusting inflation to occur just prior to the dicrotic notch.
3. **Early deflation** (Fig. 55-5) is deflation of the IABP before isovolumic left ventricular contraction.
   a. There is suboptimal diastolic augmentation, coronary perfusion, and afterload reduction, which then causes increased myocardial oxygen demand.

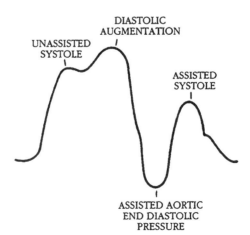

FIG. 55-3. With early balloon inflation, the aortic valve closes prematurely and left ventricular wall stress and myocardial oxygen demand are increased. Courtesy of Datascope Corp.

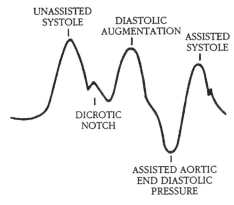

FIG. 55-4. With late balloon inflation, there is suboptimal augmentation of diastolic aortic pressure and coronary perfusion. Courtesy of Datascope Corp.

    b. It is corrected by delaying deflation until just before the onset of systole.
  4. Late deflation (Fig. 55-6) is deflation of the IABP after the onset of systole.
    a. There is impaired left ventricular emptying, increased afterload and preload, increased myocardial oxygen consumption, and reduced stroke volume.
    b. It is corrected by adjusting deflation to occur just before the onset of systole.
  5. During arrhythmias. Adequate augmentation with the balloon pump is difficult to achieve with tachyarrhythmias. When heart rates approach 150 beats per minute, there is insufficient time for the helium gas to shuttle in and out of the balloon with each inflation. With rapid atrial fibrillation, variable systolic pressure waveforms caused by inadequate left ventricular filling and rapid pulse rates make augmentation especially

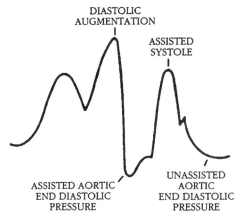

FIG. 55-5. With early balloon deflation, there is suboptimal augmentation of coronary perfusion and afterload reduction. Courtesy of Datascope Corp.

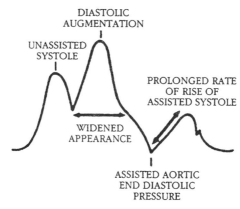

DIASTOLIC
AUGMENTATION

UNASSISTED
SYSTOLE

PROLONGED RATE
OF RISE OF
ASSISTED SYSTOLE

WIDENED
APPEARANCE

ASSISTED AORTIC
END DIASTOLIC
PRESSURE

FIG. 55-6. With late balloon deflation, there is no afterload reduction and myocardial oxygen consumption is increased. Courtesy of Datascope Corp.

difficult. Adjusting balloon inflation to 1:2 can sometimes improve augmentation with tachyarrhythmias.

C. Troubleshooting. In the situation of **console alarms,** there may be:

   1. Loose connections in the gas drive line or arterial pressure tubing.

   2. Blood in the tubing. If blood is detected in the gas drive lumen, put the balloon catheter on standby and evaluate for balloon rupture or entrapment (see VII).

   3. Poor augmentation

     a. Adjust the timing.

     b. Change the triggering mechanism (see VI.A).

     c. Evaluate inflation/deflation of the balloon and the catheter position under fluoroscopy to look for balloon kinking.

     d. If the IABP is thought to be positioned in a false lumen of the aorta due to poor augmentation, 10 to 20 cm^3 of contrast media can be injected through the central lumen of the catheter to evaluate the position under fluoroscopy.

VII. Complications

A. Vascular. Common vascular complications of IABP use include limb ischemia, hematoma around the access site, and bleeding from the access site. Rates of vascular complications vary from 5% to 20%, depending on the patient populations studied. Diabetes, female sex, preexisting peripheral vascular disease, history of smoking, and catheter size are all independent risk factors that are strongly associated with the development of ischemic vascular complications from IABP use.

   1. Ischemia

     a. If ischemia develops in the accessed leg, the balloon catheter and sheath should be removed and hemostasis obtained at the access site.

     b. If ischemia is still present, then consultation with a vascular surgeon is indicated. Surgical intervention for ischemic limbs caused by IABP catheters includes thrombectomy, surgical bypass grafts, and, rarely, amputation.

   2. Bleeding

     a. Bleeding around the access site develops in 1% to 5% of patients treated with IABP and is usually controlled with prolonged manual pressure at the access site.

     b. Hematomas that develop at the access site may require transfusion of blood products and, occasionally, direct arterial repair.

    c. Pseudoaneurysms after IABP removal are rare but often require surgical correction.

B. Infection. Infectious complications are rare and include access site infections, catheter infections, and bacteremia. No studies have addressed how frequently balloon catheters become infected and how frequently they need to be changed to limit infectious complications.

C. Balloon rupture should be considered if blood is detected in the gas drive line lumen or if balloon augmentation ceases.

    1. Small leaks in the balloon can develop from damage to the balloon surface caused by inflation against calcified aortic plaques. Rates of balloon leak can be as high as 4.2%.

    2. Potential complications for the patient include helium gas embolism and balloon entrapment when blood leaks into the balloon, clots, and prevents adequate deflation of the balloon for removal.

    3. Use of standard size balloons (40 cm^3) in patients under 170 cm tall has been shown to be associated with balloon rupture and is thought to be caused by damage to the balloon when inflation occurs in the smaller and more plaque-laden distal abdominal aorta. Thus, a 34-cm^3 balloon should be used in patients under 170 cm tall.

D. Balloon entrapment occurs when balloon rupture causes a clot to form within the balloon to prevent deflation during removal. When resistance is encountered during balloon catheter removal, balloon entrapment should be considered and fluoroscopy immediately carried out to assess the position of the retained catheter.

    1. Management of balloon entrapment usually involves surgical extraction because forceful removal of a partially deflated balloon catheter could cause serious vascular injury.

    2. Case reports have documented successful lysis of clots within the balloon by instilling thrombolytic agents through the gas drive lumen of the IABP catheter. The balloons were deflated after clot lysis, and the catheters were successfully removed.

E. Red blood cell and platelet destruction. Due to the shear forces of the balloon catheter, hemolytic anemia and mild thrombocytopenia can occur during IABP support. Daily hemoglobin and platelet values should be checked. Platelet counts below 50,000 are unlikely to be caused by the IABP, and alternative causes should be investigated.

F. Other complications. Rare complications of IABP use include acute renal failure, mesenteric ischemia, and paraplegia from plaque embolization to or thrombosis of the renal, mesenteric, or spinal arteries, respectively. Aortic dissections and aortic perforations rarely occur and usually happen during insertion.

VIII. Removal of the IABP catheter

A. Weaning. Whether IABC needs to be weaned before the balloon catheter is removed depends on multiple factors, including the duration of support, the hemodynamic status of the patient, and left ventricular function.

    1. The usual practice is to change IABP inflation to 1:2 for a few hours and then to 1:3 while closely monitoring the patient's hemodynamics.

    2. At the same time, intravenous inotropic drugs are used to simulate the IABP's hemodynamic effects. Dobutamine or milrinone is used to maintain an adequate cardiac output, while nitroprusside is used to replace the afterload reduction provided by the IABP.

    3. If weaning is tolerated hemodynamically, the balloon can then be removed.

B. Withdrawal of the balloon catheter and sheath

    1. Intravenous heparin should be discontinued for at least 4 hours prior to removal of the catheter. The activated coagulation time (ACT) is checked until it falls below 150 seconds.

    2. Percutaneously placed catheters can then be removed manually, but surgically placed catheters need to be removed with direct arterial repair.

3. To begin removal of the balloon catheter, the balloon is changed to standby and the gas drive line is disconnected. Then, the balloon catheter is pulled back until resistance is met, indicating that the catheter is in the sheath. The sheath and the balloon catheter are then withdrawn together as a unit, but excessive force should never be applied.

C. Hemostasis

  1. After the balloon is withdrawn, the puncture site is allowed to bleed back for 1 to 2 seconds while holding pressure distal to the puncture site to evacuate proximal thrombi.

  2. Then, manual pressure is applied proximal to the puncture site and back-bleeding is again done to evacuate distal thrombi.

  3. Manual pressure is then applied for 30 to 45 minutes over the puncture site until adequate hemostasis is achieved.

  4. A compressive dressing is applied thereafter.

D. Monitoring during IABP removal

  1. During the application of manual pressure to the puncture site, the distal pulses in the leg should be continually assessed and pressure should be adjusted to maintain adequate distal perfusion.

  2. The patient should be confined to strict bed rest for 6 to 12 hours after the catheter and sheath have been removed, and the leg should be periodically assessed for signs of ischemia.

IX. Changing the IABP catheter

A. Reasons for changing the IABP

  1. When patients require prolonged IABP support, some clinicians change the catheter and sheath every 4 to 5 days to prevent infectious complications, but there is no consensus regarding this dilemma.

  2. Other reasons for changing the IABP include balloon entrapment and rupture, kinking of the catheter or sheath, which prevents adequate balloon inflation, or fevers, which could indicate bacteremia from a line infection.

B. Simultaneous change. In patients who are critically dependent on IABP support and who need the IABP changed for one of the above reasons, the catheter and sheath need to be changed simultaneously with placement of a new IABP.

  1. Contralateral femoral artery

    a. When the contralateral femoral artery can be used, it is accessed and the sheath is placed. A guidewire is then positioned in the aortic arch while the old balloon is on standby.

    b. Counterpulsation is reinitiated, and the new balloon catheter is prepared and readied for use.

    c. The old balloon is then deflated and quickly withdrawn, while the new balloon catheter is placed over the guidewire from the contralateral femoral artery. This technique limits the period without IABP support during the change to less than 30 seconds.

    d. Anticoagulation can safely be discontinued before and after a simultaneous change to aid achieving hemostasis at the old access site.

  2. Same femoral artery

    a. When the contralateral femoral artery cannot be used, the old catheter and sheath must be removed and changed under direct vision.

    b. The accessed femoral artery is exposed surgically, and a purse-string suture is placed around the preexisting sheath.

    c. The old sheath is then removed and tension is applied to the suture for hemostasis.

      (1) The small dilator in the catheter package is directly inserted into the previous puncture site, and the guidewire is advanced to the aortic arch through it.

      (2) The sheath is advanced over the guidewire into the proper position, and the purse-string suture is tied down.

(3) The balloon catheter is then inserted via the sheath, and the soft tissue and skin incision are closed with sutures.

d. In emergency situations, the preexisting sheath can be rewired and a new balloon catheter inserted through the old sheath, but infectious complications are high with this approach.

SELECTED READINGS

References

1. Holmes DR Jr, Bates ER, Kleinman NS, et al. Contemporary reperfusion therapy for cardiogenic shock: the GUSTO-I trial experience. *J Am Coll Cardiol* 1995;26: 668–674.
2. Anderson RD, Ohman EM, Holmes DR Jr, et al. Use of intraaortic balloon counterpulsation in patients presenting with cardiogenic shock: observations from the GUSTO-I study. *J Am Coll Cardiol* 1997; 30:708–715.
3. Kovack PJ, Rasak MA, Bates ER, et al. Thrombolysis plus aortic counterpulsation: improved survival in patients who present to community hospitals with cardiogenic shock. *J Am Coll Cardiol* 1997; 29: 1454–1458.
4. Braunwald EG, Mark DB, Jones RH, et al. Unstable angina: diagnosis and management. Clinical Practice Guideline No. 10. AHCPR Publication No. 94-0602. Rockville, MD: Agency for Health Care Policy Research and the National Heart, Lung, and Blood Institute, Public Health Service, US Department of Health and Human Services, May 1994.
5. Ohman EM, George BS, White CJ, et al. Use of aortic counterpulsation to improve sustained coronary artery patency during acute myocardial infarction: results of a randomized trial. *Circulation* 1994;90:792–799.
6. Stone GW, Marsalese D, Brodie BR, et al. A prospective, randomized evaluation of prophylactic intraaortic balloon counterpulsation in high-risk patients with acute myocardial infarction treated with primary angioplasty. *J Am Coll Cardiol* 1997;29: 1459–1467.

Landmark Articles

Ohman EM, George BS, White CJ, et al. Use of aortic counterpulsation to improve sustained coronary artery patency during acute myocardial infarction. *Circulation* 1994;90:792–799.

Patel JJ, Kopisyansky C, Boston B, et al. Prospective evaluation of complications associated with percutaneous intraaortic balloon counterpulsation. *Am J Cardiol* 1995;76: 1205–1207.

Stone GW, Marsalese D, Brodie BR, et al. A prospective, randomized evaluation of prophylactic intraaortic balloon counterpulsation in high risk patients with acute myocardial infarction treated with primary angioplasty. *J Am Coll Cardiol* 1997;29: 1459–1467.

Key Reviews

Aguirre FV, Kern MJ, Bach R, et al. Intraaortic balloon pump support during high-risk coronary angioplasty. *Cardiology* 1994; 84: 175–186.

Kantrowitz A, Cardona RR, Freed PS. Percutaneous intra-aortic balloon counterpulsation. *Crit Care Clin* 1992; 8:819–837.

Kern MJ. Intra-aortic balloon counterpulsation. *Coronary Artery Dis* 1991;2:649–660.

Mueller HS. Role of intra-aortic counterpulsation in cardiogenic shock and acute myocardial infarction. *Cardiology* 1994;84:168–174.

Relevant Book Chapters

Aroesty JM, Shawl FA. Circulatory assist devices. In: Baim D, Grossman W, eds. *Cardiac catheterization, angiography, and intervention,* 5th ed. Baltimore: Williams & Wilkins, 1996:421–435.

Maccioli GA, ed. *Intra-aortic balloon pump therapy.* Baltimore: Williams & Wilkins, 1997.

56. LEFT HEART CATHETERIZATION

Deepak L. Bhatt

I. **Introduction.** In 1958, Dr. Mason Sones and his colleagues at the Cleveland Clinic performed the first selective coronary arteriogram. Since then, left heart catheterization (LHC) has become a crucial part of diagnostic cardiology. Over 1.5 million cardiac catheterizations are performed yearly in the United States. Despite the advent of other imaging modalities, coronary arteriography remains the clinical gold standard for determining the presence of significant coronary artery disease (CAD).

Left heart catheterization is an invasive procedure with serious attendant risks (1). To be competent in LHC, at a minimum, a cardiologist-in-training must perform 300 catheterizations, serving as primary operator on 200. If in a training phase, the operator must be supervised by a cardiologist who is already competent in the procedure. Of note, there is often a tendency, once a lesion is noted on coronary arteriography, to proceed with percutaneous intervention. Therefore, before performing a LHC, there should already be a plan of how to use the information that is obtained.

II. **Indications.** The American College of Cardiology along with the American Heart Association (ACC/AHA) have categorized reasonable indications for LHC as class I, when there is consensus that LHC is indicated, or class II, when there is no consensus that LHC is indicated but nonetheless the procedure is frequently performed.

A. **Acute myocardial infarction (MI).** Left heart catheterization is given a class II indication for routine use in acute MI. It can be used with the goal of performing primary angioplasty for patients with acute ST-elevation MI. The role of LHC in stable patients with NQWMI (Non-Q-wave MI) is controversial (class II), though the author's preference is to proceed with LHC. Left heart catheterization is strongly indicated (class I) in the patient with postinfarction complications such as recurrent ischemia or mechanical complications of MI; LHC is given a class II indication for postinfarction complications such as congestive heart failure, cardiogenic shock, and ventricular arrhythmias, though the authors feel that LHC is strongly indicated in these circumstances. Patients with persistent pain or unresolved ECG changes after thrombolytic therapy are also class I candidates for LHC. Routine LHC soon after thrombolytic therapy in a patient who appears to have clinically reperfused is a class II indication. Patients with significant angina after an MI or with a positive stress test are class I candidates for LHC; mild angina after an MI is designated as class II.

B. **Unstable angina.** Left heart catheterization is given a class I indication in the patient with refractory unstable angina that cannot be controlled by medical therapy. Its role in unstable angina that can be medically controlled is controversial. Suspected Prinzmetal's angina is a class I indication for LHC.

C. **Chronic stable angina.** Left heart catheterization is given a class I indication in chronic stable angina for patients whose angina is poorly controlled by medicines or who are intolerant of antianginal medications.

D. **Abnormal stress test.** A stress test that is positive at a low work load (6.5 METS) or that is classified as high risk is a class I indication for LHC. An ST depression of 2 mm, especially in multiple leads or persisting into recovery 6 minutes, an ST elevation of 2 mm in leads without Q waves, a drop in blood pressure of more than 10 mm Hg with exercise, or development of ventricular tachycardia with exercise constitutes a high-risk stress test. A high-risk stress test on a concomitant imaging modality showing left ventricle dilatation, a drop in EF (ejection fraction) 10%, or multiple areas of ischemia is a class I indication for catheterization. These indications hold true even if the patient is asymptomatic. Positive stress tests without high-risk criteria are class II indications for LHC.

E. Ventricular arrhythmia. A history of sustained ventricular tachycardia or sudden cardiac death, if there is no obvious metabolic cause, is considered a class I indication for LHC, as an alternative to initial stress testing, in order to search for significant CAD.

F. Left ventricular dysfunction. Left heart catheterization can provide an estimate of left ventricular function and regional wall motion. Left ventricular dysfunction of unknown etiology, with EF less than 40%, is a class I indication for LHC to rule out CAD.

G. Valvular heart disease. Left heart catheterization can be performed to assess the severity of outflow tract obstruction (aortic stenosis, hypertrophic obstructive cardiomyopathy). It can also help quantify aortic and mitral regurgitation (MR). With the advancements in Doppler and color echocardiography, the major role of cardiac catheterization is to provide confirmatory data and to rule out CAD requiring surgery. Left heart catheterization has a class I indication in patients requiring valve surgery who have angina or an abnormal ECG. Most centers perform LHC before valve surgery for men above age 40 and women above age 50 to rule out clinically silent CAD. Younger patients may require LHC, if cardiac risk factors are present.

H. Preoperative. Left heart catheterization is performed before ascending aortic aneurysm surgery or some cases of ascending aortic dissection surgery. It is also performed on patients with congenital heart disease to evaluate lesions such as ventricular septal defects and to rule out concomitant coronary anomalies or atherosclerotic disease, if symptomatic. In patients with angina or a positive stress test who are to undergo major vascular surgery, LHC is given a class I indication, but in the case of planned major surgery other than vascular surgery, LHC is given a class II indication.

III. Contraindications. The following are relative contraindications to performing an LHC.

A. Coagulopathy. Coagulopathy must be corrected prior to elective catheterization. The usual recommendation for patients on warfarin (Coumadin) is to discontinue it 3 nights before the procedure. In elective cases, an international normalized ratio less than 1.8 is a cutoff that is often used. If the patient is heparinized, this is usually stopped 2 hours before the procedure. A platelet count less than 50,000 substantially increases the risk of bleeding. After thrombolytic therapy, bleeding is more likely and elective catheterization is best deferred. However, if the indication for the procedure is urgent, it is possible to proceed with caution, with blood products ready for support as needed. Antecedent glycoprotein IIb/IIIa therapy poses much less of a risk. Body habitus is also a factor in deciding what level of anticoagulation is acceptable before a catheterization. Obesity increases the chances of bleeding (if multiple attempts at access are needed) and makes bleeding that occurs more difficult to detect. Finally, the availability of closure devices makes it possible to seal the artery after the procedure. While the first-generation closure devices allow earlier ambulation, the second-generation closure devices will probably decrease bleeding.

B. Renal failure. A rising creatinine is generally a reason to defer elective cardiac catheterization. In a patient on dialysis, catheterization is generally timed immediately after the dialysis. In a patient with stable but moderately severe renal failure, catheterization may be performed with an awareness of the increased risk of needing dialysis.

C. Dye allergy. A history of allergy to previous contrast administration should be sought. While an allergy to shellfish and seafood has been linked to contrast reactions in some studies, other studies dispute such a relationship. Individuals with a history of asthma or atopy are at increased risk of contrast allergies. Management of patients with a history of dye allergy is described below.

D. Infection. Active infection is a reason to defer elective cardiac catheterization. Local skin infection at the site of the potential puncture is also undesirable. Fungal infection in groin creases should be treated before elective cardiac catheterization via the femoral approach; this is a particular concern in obese patients.

E. Laboratory abnormalities: anemia, electrolyte imbalances. Severe anemia, hypo- or hyperkalemia should be corrected before the elective procedure. In the presence of digitalis toxicity, elective catheterization is best deferred.

F. Decompensated heart failure. Severe heart failure raises the risks of cardiac catheterization. It is best to optimize medical therapy before elective catheterization. At a minimum, the patient should be able to lie supine without respiratory insufficiency.

G. Severe peripheral vascular disease. Symptoms of claudication warrant careful assessment of pulses. An inadequate lower extremity pulse favors an upper extremity approach. A synthetic vascular graft that is older than 6 months is not a strict contraindication to catheterization, but special care should be taken in gaining access, as well as hemostasis. The risk of embolization of friable atheroma or thrombus is heightened, however, and this risk increases with the age of the graft.

H. Abdominal aortic aneurysm. Presence of an abdominal aortic aneurysm (AAA) requires special care during a cardiac catheterization (see below). An arm approach obviates the need to cross the AAA altogether.

I. Uncontrolled severe hypertension. Blood pressure should be controlled before elective cardiac catheterization to maximize the safety of the procedure. In particular, severe bleeding can occur at the access site after sheath removal if the patient is very hypertensive, especially above 180/100 mm Hg.

IV. Patient preparation

A. Informed consent. A detailed discussion with the patient (and family) should outline the indication for the procedure, as well as the alternative treatment and diagnostic options. Specific mention of the serious risks of complications, such as death, MI, stroke, and kidney failure, must be made (see complications listed below). The possible need for emergency coronary artery bypass graft (CABG) should be noted. The risk of serious complications should be individualized. Informed consent should be documented in the medical record.

B. Medications. If percutaneous coronary intervention is likely, pretreatment with aspirin 325 mg by mouth (PO) should be given before the catheterization, as it has been shown to improve outcomes with angioplasty. If stenting is a strong possibility, clopidogrel 300 mg PO should be given as a loading dose prior to the procedure. Metformin should be stopped at the time of the procedure, although the risk of lactic acidosis is extremely low in a patient with normal creatinine.

C. Education. Patients should be warned that they might feel a hot sensation lasting about 30 seconds due to the injection of ionic contrast dye. Some patients may also feel nauseated. Patients should be specifically instructed to cough when they hear anyone in the room say "cough." This maneuver helps dye-induced bradycardia resolve more quickly.

D. Equipment. Before performing a cardiac catheterization, it is essential to ensure that the monitoring equipment is fully functional. Continuous ECG monitoring of heart rate, rhythm, and ST segments, an automated blood pressure cuff, and continuous pulse oximetry are mandatory. Resuscitation equipment should be tested and ready. In particular, defibrillators and intubation trays must be next to the patient. If a long procedure is anticipated, many operators prefer placement of a Foley or Texas urinary catheter. Before actually beginning the procedure, the fluoroscopy and cine equipment should be tested by taking a picture of the patient's nameplate. The usual frame rate of cine film is set at 30 frames/second; 60 frames/second can be useful for tachycardiac patients. In addition, the table should move freely to the level of the patient's groin.

E. Contrast dye

1. **Choice of contrast.** Ionic contrast dye is used during most cardiac catheterizations. In certain circumstances, low osmolar nonionic dye, which is ten times as expensive as ionic dye, can be used (2). The indications for nonionic dye vary greatly between institutions. The literature supports that nonionic dye produces less left ventricular dysfunction, bradycardia, and hypotension, as well as less nausea and emesis. Thus, it is useful in cases of suspected left main stenosis, severe left ventricular dysfunction, and severe aortic stenosis. Other indications for nonionic dye are severe renal dysfunction and a reported allergy to contrast dye. However, no reduction in acute renal failure or anaphylactoid reaction has been conclusively demonstrated with the use of nonionic dye. There is evidence that nonionic contrast is more thrombogenic than ionic contrast. Therefore, it should be used with caution in patients with acute coronary syndromes. Whenever nonionic contrast is used, 5 IU of heparin per cubic centimeter of contrast should be added.

2. **Dye allergy**

   a. **Premedication.** If a patient reports an allergy to contrast dye or a history of prior anaphylactoid reaction, it is customary to premedicate with prednisone 40 mg PO q6h × 4 doses or with hydrocortisone 100 mg intravenously (IV) × 1 at least 6 hours before the procedure, and with cimetidine (Tagamet) 400 mg IV × 1 and diphenhydramine (Benadryl) 50 mg IV × 1. With a history of possible life-threatening dye allergies, it is also prudent to administer small quantities of dye (1 cm^3) and observe for a few minutes before proceeding.

   b. **Treatment.** If a patient develops signs of an allergic reaction, treatment should be prompt. If signs such as hives or rash develop, treatment with diphenhydramine is usually sufficient. Hydrocortisone is also often given, though its effects would not be manifest for several hours. In cases of oropharyngeal edema, bronchospasm, or hypotension, 0.3 cm^3 of 1:1,000 epinephrine should be administered subcutaneously. With refractory symptoms, 10 µg/minute of IV epinephrine can be administered until symptoms abate.

   c. **Latex allergy** has become increasingly recognized as a clinical entity, especially in patients who are health care workers. True latex allergy can include urticaria, angioedema, laryngospasm, bronchospasm, and anaphylaxis. If a patient describes a possible latex allergy, allergy testing, including skin testing and RAST (rapid antigen serum testing), should be considered. Patients with latex allergy should be scheduled as the first case of the day in order to avoid latex dust from prior procedures. Written protocols outlining materials to be avoided should be strictly followed. A cart with latex-free items should be made available. The sheath is a source of latex exposure. Therefore, a sheathless approach involving catheter exchanges over a wire is preferred.

   d. **Sedation.** Commonly used sedatives include the benzodiazepines midazolam 1 to 2 mg IV or lorazepam 1 to 2 mg IV. Some operators use fentanyl 25 mg IV or morphine 1 to 2 mg IV for pain relief. Diphenhydramine 25 or 50 mg IV can also be used for sedation. Continuous pulse oximetry should be followed to ensure that sedation has not been excessive.

   e. **Radiation safety.** Radiation poses a threat to lab personnel; therefore, every effort should be made to decrease exposure. The source is scatter from the x-ray beam originating under the table. Lead aprons (with at least 0.5-mm-thickness lead lining) and thyroid collars are mandatory to minimize radiation exposure. Leaded eyeglasses should also be considered. In addition, radiation badges are worn inside the lead apron and outside the thyroid collar to monitor cumulative radiation exposure. A leaded acrylic shield should be utilized between the patient and the operator closest to the patient. Standing further from the table also reduces radiation exposure by the inverse square of the distance. A number of additional steps can be taken to minimize radiation to both the operator and patient. Fluoroscopy and, in particular, cine time should be minimized. The image intensifier should be positioned as close as possible to the patient to reduce radiation scatter. To decrease radiation, higher magnification should be used judiciously. "Coning down" on a region of interest with the use of collimators can also reduce the amount of radiation, as can the use of lung field collimators. Right anterior oblique (RAO) views produce less radiation scatter for the operator than do left anterior oblique (LAO) views. Higher cine frame rates increase radiation exposure; use of 30 frames/second produces less radiation exposure than use of 60 frames/second. In the rare situation that a pregnant patient needs catheterization, a lead apron should be placed over the abdomen. This precaution should also be taken for premenopausal women.

V. Access site

A. Femoral artery. Femoral artery cannulation is the most common form of arterial access for cardiac catheterization (Fig. 56-1) The patient is first positioned appropriately, with the knees about 12 in. apart. The table should allow enough movement to perform fluoroscopy of the groin. Anatomic landmarks are then identified. The inguinal ligament is located. Then the femoral pulse is palpated approximately 2 cm (finger breadths) below the inguinal ligament; this marks the site of arterial access. Alternatively, fluoroscopy can be used to locate the femoral head. The entry point on the skin is located over the inferior border of the femoral head. Care must be taken not to enter the artery above the inguinal ligament, as this increases the chance of retroperitoneal bleeding. Arterial entry that is too low must also be avoided, as this can lead to pseudoaneurysm or arteriovenous fistula formation. Once the site of entry has been identified (and marked, if so desired), the area is cleaned with povidone-iodine (Betadine) and surgically draped. Local anesthesia is given slowly (it hurts less when delivered slowly), while the clinician observes the heart rate monitor and watches for signs of a vagal reaction (nausea, lightheadedness, yawning). The usual choice is procaine 1%. A subcutaneous wheal is raised with about 3 cm^3 using a 25-gauge needle. Next, an additional 6 to 10 cm^3 is delivered to the deeper tissues with a 22-gauge needle. In patients with an allergy to ester-type anesthetics, lidocaine 2% can be used. Once the site is anesthetized, an 18-gauge Cook needle is inserted into the artery. Upon nearing the artery, a side-to-side motion of the needle indicates a position either medial or lateral to the artery. Up-and-down motion indicates correct positioning. In addition, when the needle is above the artery, it transmits the arterial pulsation to the fingertips. Once brisk arterial blood return is established, a 0.035-in. J-tipped 45-cm guidewire is inserted, the needle is withdrawn, and an arterial sheath with a dilator is placed over the wire. Then the wire and dilator are removed. The sheath is then flushed with saline. A 6-Fr sheath is generally used for diagnostic catheterizations in the United States, though 4-Fr sheaths are often used in Europe. An 8-Fr sheath is used for acute cases or planned interventions. A 5-Fr sheath is preferred over larger sheaths for patients with peripheral vascular disease.

B. Arm approach. In certain patients it may be desirable to perform the catheterization via a brachial or radial route, for which specialized equipment is available. Percutaneous brachial or radial access is similar to the femoral approach described above. In addition, a surgical cut-down can be

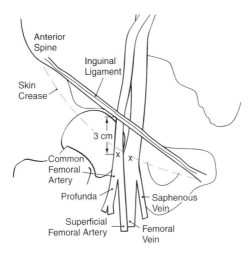

FIG. 56-1. Landmarks for right femoral artery puncture. From Baim DS, 1996, with permission.

performed to enter the brachial or radial arteries under direct visualization. For a left arm approach, Judkins catheters are adequate. For a right arm approach, Amplatz or multipurpose catheters are used, although it may be difficult to engage a left internal mammary artery (LIMA) graft from the right arm; a specially designed brachial internal mammary artery catheter is available for the latter purpose. In rare circumstances, an axillary approach can be used, though the rate of neurovascular complications is higher.

C. **Special situations.** In patients with prosthetic femoral grafts, it is preferable to use a dilator first before placing the sheath to prevent the sheath from kinking as it passes through the graft. This technique is also useful in obese patients. If a synthetic graft is old, fluoroscopy can be performed to see if the graft is heavily calcified—a sign that it may not seal well after sheath removal. In patients with tortuous or diseased vessels, a Wholey wire or Terumo Glidewire™ can be used to get catheters up the aorta. If marked iliac tortuosity is present and causes inability to torque catheters, a long sheath can be used to straighten out the iliac vessel. At times, a stiffer wire (such as an Amplatz wire) can provide better support to advance catheters. In patients with a AAA for whom a femoral approach is chosen, exchange wires should be used for every change of catheter. Use of a softer wire (such as a Wholey wire) can prove less traumatic to the vessel, as can using a JR4 to direct the guidewire.

VI. **Technique**
   A. **Engaging the vessel**
      1. **Left coronary artery (LCA).** Catheters are flushed with heparinized saline and passed through the sheath over a J-tipped guidewire. Using fluoroscopic guidance in the LAO projection, the left main coronary artery is cannulated, typically with a Judkins L4. The catheter tip should be coaxial to the left main coronary artery, meaning that its tip should not be touching the upper wall of the left main coronary artery. In a small person, a Judkins L3.5 catheter can be used. In a larger person or a person with a dilated aorta, a JL5 or even a larger JL6 can be used. If the catheter does not engage the left main ostium easily, a slight clockwise or more often a counterclockwise rotation of the catheter hub may help. With the JL catheters, unless the aorta is dilated and provides

no hinge point for the JL catheter, counterclockwise rotation moves the catheter tip anteriorly and clockwise rotation moves it posteriorly.

Care should be taken to prevent the catheter from too deeply engaging ("deep-seating") the left main coronary artery. The pressure waveform must be observed for **damping** (a decrease in the systolic pressure) or **ventricularization** (when the waveform looks like a ventricular pressure tracing), both of which indicate a need to pull the catheter back and also raise the possibility of significant left main coronary artery disease. An adequate amount of dye reflux should be seen, unless ostial disease is present. If significant left main coronary artery disease is suspected, a cusp view (with the catheter placed in the left sinus of Valsalva) can be taken. Injection of contrast should be gentle and pressure gradually increased ("ramping"). Enough contrast should be injected to opacify the entire coronary artery and ensure reflux into the aorta (usually about 8 cm³ for the LCA). Injection force should be forceful enough to prevent "streaming," the inadequate opacification of coronary arteries that can create the illusion of stenoses. Care should be taken to inspect the injection syringe for air bubbles before each injection and to hold the syringe upright while injecting.

2. **Right coronary artery (RCA).** Catheterization of the RCA is similar to that of the left, except that a Judkins R4 is advanced into the right coronary cusp, again in the LAO projection. The RCA is usually located anteriorly in the right sinus, in a position that is lower than the LCA ostium. As the catheter is slowly pulled back 2 cm above the aortic valve, it is rotated clockwise, causing it to engage. With the JR catheter, clockwise rotation moves the catheter anteriorly. In addition, clockwise rotation can cause the catheter to dip downward. Thus, it may be necessary to apply backward traction on the catheter as it is being rotated clockwise. Sometimes it is necessary to repeat the clockwise rotation at different levels in order to engage the right coronary ostium. If the JR4 does not easily engage the RCA or if the pressure dampens, ostial disease, spasm, selective intubation of the conus (which arises separately 50% of the time), or anatomic variation in the direction of the proximal RCA should be suspected. A cusp view can be taken to clarify these situations. Care should be taken to avoid subselectively intubating the conus branch.

If difficulty is encountered in engaging the RCA because of the orientation of the ostium, a 3DR or a No Torque Right catheter can be useful. Both catheters are designed to be placed above the aortic valve and pulled back without torquing maneuvers. An Amplatz or multipurpose catheter can be useful for an upwardly angled ostium. An anterior or posterior origin can often be engaged with an Amplatz catheter. The most common cause of an incomplete LHC is a high and anterior RCA. In order to locate its ostium, less clockwise torque should be applied to the catheter, so that it faces more anteriorly, and the catheter can then search for the ostium superior to the usual location. Less dye is needed to opacify the RCA than the LCA; overinjection can cause ventricular fibrillation. Sometimes, if a catheter is tenuously engaged, particularly in the right coronary ostium, a deep breath can dislodge it and should be avoided.

3. **Left internal mammary artery.** Catheterization of the LIMA is done either in the posteroanterior or shallow LAO projection. First, the catheter (usually a JR4 catheter or a LIMA catheter) is positioned by pulling it back in the aorta while applying counterclockwise torque until it enters the left subclavian artery. At this point many operators will obtain an angiogram of the left subclavian artery to rule out a stenosis proximal to the LIMA and to give a hint of the angle of take-off of the LIMA. Next, the wire (J-tipped guidewire or Wholey wire) is advanced into the subclavian artery. Next, the catheter is advanced

over the wire into the subclavian, the wire is removed, and the catheter is slowly pulled back with a slight counterclockwise rotation until it engages the ostium of the LIMA. Movements around the ostium must be gentle to reduce the risk of dissection of the vessel; frequent test injections are helpful. In addition, if a 6-Fr sheath is in place, switching to a 5-Fr catheter will likely be less traumatic to the ostium of the LIMA. Turning the head to the left or right and pulling the arm caudally are maneuvers that can help engage the LIMA. If the ostium points downward at a sharp angle, the LIMA catheter is more likely to engage it selectively. The special LIMA catheter provides a slightly different angulation. It is best to use nonionic contrast to minimize the pain caused by ionic dye running through the arteries of the chest wall. If the ostium cannot be engaged successfully, a nonselective angiogram can be taken with the tip of the catheter as close to the ostium as possible. A blood pressure cuff should be inflated above systolic pressure in the left arm to facilitate dye movement down the LIMA.

4. **Right internal mammary artery (RIMA).** Catheterization of the RIMA is similar to that of the LIMA. The catheter (either JR4 or LIMA) is placed in the brachiocephalic trunk by pulling back in the aorta while applying counterclockwise rotation. The wire is advanced into the right subclavian artery. Care must be taken to avoid the right carotid artery. The wire is removed and the catheter is pulled back until it engages the ostium of the RIMA.

5. **Saphenous vein grafts (SVGs).** Catheterization of SVGs depends on the specific type of graft. The grafts are by necessity anastomosed to the anterior surface of the aorta. The orientation of SVGs from caudal to cranial is usually: RCA, left anterior descending coronary artery (LAD), diagonal branches of LAD, and marginal branches of left circumflex artery (LCX). In the LAO view, grafts to the RCA usually point to the patient's right, whereas grafts to the left system are usually oriented more to the patient's left. It is the practice of some surgeons to place circular graft markers around the ostia of the vein grafts on the outer surface of the aorta. In the steep LAO projection, the catheter tip should extend beyond the plane of these markers, if the catheter is truly engaged in a vein graft. Injections into presumed vein graft stumps should be forceful to ensure that the graft is truly occluded, as opposed to poor opacification from a tenuously engaged catheter. Review of the operative note is mandatory before a catheterization in order to know where grafts were placed. In particular, it should be noted whether any LIMA or RIMA grafts are in situ or free (attached to the aorta). A previous catheterization, if done, should be reviewed. Particular attention should be paid to the location of the grafts. The relative relationship to surgical clips should be noted, as this will save time and effort in finding grafts during the catheterization. If a graft cannot be found or a stump identified during a catheterization, an aortogram should be performed (see VI.E below).

   a. **SVG to RCA.** Engaging this graft can be as simple as pulling back on the JR4 as it sits in the ostium to the RCA while in the LAO projection. Often this graft has a steep downward orientation from the aorta. In this situation, a multipurpose catheter can be useful to engage the graft. The multipurpose catheter can enter deeply into the graft if not handled carefully. Alternatively, a right bypass catheter or a right modified Amplatz catheter can be useful to engage the RCA graft.

   b. **SVG to LAD.** The graft to the LAD is most easily engaged in the RAO view. To engage this graft, it is necessary to withdraw the catheter from the SVG to the RCA by pulling back. If the catheter does not fall into place, clockwise rotation of the JR4 at an area cranial to the SVG to RCA graft ostium will locate the LAD graft. It may be necessary to move the catheter up and down along the anterior surface of the aorta several times. Left bypass, left Amplatz, and multipurpose catheters are all alternative catheters that can be used. A similar clockwise rotation to move the catheter tip along the anterior aortic surface is necessary.

c. **SVG to LCX.** To engage this graft, it is necessary to withdraw the catheter from the SVG to the LAD by pulling back, while remaining in the RAO projection. If the catheter does not fall into place, clockwise rotation of the JR4 at an area cranial to the SVG to LAD graft ostium will locate the LCX graft. The technique is otherwise similar to that for engaging the graft to the LAD.

B. **Imaging the vessels**

1. **Normal coronary anatomy.** The left main coronary artery originates from the left coronary cusp. It usually bifurcates into a LAD and a LCX, though it sometimes trifurcates to include a ramus intermedius. The LAD courses along the anterior interventricular groove, supplying numerous septal perforators to the septum, and a variable number of diagonal branches to the anterolateral wall of the left ventricle, and usually continues to the apex. The LCX courses along the left atrioventricular (AV) groove, providing a variable number of marginal branches to supply the lateral wall. In some institutions the first marginal branch is called the high lateral branch of the circumflex, with subsequent branches called lateral or posterolateral branches, depending on their destination. The LCX continues in the AV groove for a variable distance. In patients in whom the LCX is dominant (see below), the LCX reaches the posterior interventricular groove and gives rise to a posterior descending artery (PDA) branch.

   The RCA originates from the right coronary cusp and courses along the right AV groove, providing atrial branches (to the right atrium) and marginal branches (to the right ventricle). A conus branch originates as the first branch from the proximal RCA to supply the right ventricular outflow tract; about half of the time, this branch has an ostium that is separate from the RCA ostium. It is usually unnecessary to visualize a separate conus branch, unless collaterals to the LAD are suspected. The RCA gives off a branch to the sinus node about 60% of the time (otherwise a left atrial branch of the LCX serves this function). The first major branch the distal RCA gives off is the PDA, in a right dominant system. **Dominance** refers to which artery gives off a PDA and supplies the posterior part of the heart. In about 85% of patients, this will be the RCA; in 7% the RCA and LCX will be codominant; and in another 8% the LCX will be dominant. The PDA courses along the inferior interventricular groove, providing septal perforators to supply the inferior septum. After giving off a PDA, the RCA continues as a posterolateral segment supplying a variable number of posterior ventricular branches. From this posterolateral segment, the RCA usually (90% of the time) provides a branch to supply the AV node.

2. **Basic principles.** Several views of the coronary arteries are required to prevent excessive overlap of vessel segments and to delineate the severity of stenoses. A general principle that is useful is that in an RAO view the spine is on the left of the screen, whereas in an LAO view the spine is on the right of the screen. Cranial views bring the silhouette of the diaphragm into the field of view. The diagonal and obtuse marginal branches tend to move in synchrony, since they supply the lateral aspect of the heart, whereas the LAD is located on the anterior portion of the heart. The AV continuation of the LCX lies in the AV groove and (in patients in sinus rhythm) has an "atrial kick" to it. This sort of atrial kick can also be seen in atrial branches from either the LCX or RCA. In the RAO view, a diagonal branch, and not the LAD itself, usually lies on the heart border. In the LAO view, the LAD runs along the border of

the heart silhouette, not the diagonal branches. Caudal angulation tends to move posterior vessels (such as the posterolateral branches of the RCA or the obtuse marginal branches of the LCX) inferiorly. Cranial angulation tends to move posterior vessels superiorly.

Patients should be instructed to take in a deep breath and hold it before most views for the purpose of moving the diaphragm out of the way. The RAO cranial view can be done at end expiration, in order to facilitate the splaying out of the diagonals from the LAD, or at end inspiration to view the proximal LCX. The LAO caudal can be done at end expiration to visualize the left main and ostial LAD, or at end inspiration to view the LCX. Panning motion should be smooth and slow. It is best to wait for two to three systolic cycles and focus on proximal vessels before panning down the length of the artery of interest. It is important to pan to look for collaterals.

3. **Different views (Figs. 56-2–56-8)**
   a. **Left coronary artery.** There is wide variation in the sequence of views obtained. Many operators start with a posteroanterior view and focus on the left main coronary artery, sometimes with a coned-down view to improve resolution. The problem with a pure posteroanterior view is that there is significant overlap with the spine. Therefore, a little bit of RAO angulation ("shallow RAO") can be used to get the coronaries off the spine. A steeper amount of RAO provides greater separation of the LAD from the LCX. A slight amount of caudal angulation can be used to decrease the foreshortening of the proximal circumflex in the straight RAO view and to place the diagonals below the LAD. Thus, a **20 degree RAO, 20 degree caudal** is often the first view, displaying the entire left coronary system. This view also provides a good view of the proximal LCX and of the origin of a ramus intermedius branch, if present. The contour collimator (called the wedge or shield) should be moved to the upper right of the screen. A **30 degree RAO, 25 degree cranial** view can be used to separate the diagonals from the LAD, placing them above the LAD. The wedge should be placed in the upper right of the screen. A **PA with 40 degree cranial** angulation can be useful in viewing the mid-and distal portions of the LAD. The **45 degree LAO, 30 degree cranial**

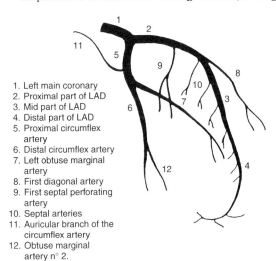

1. Left main coronary
2. Proximal part of LAD
3. Mid part of LAD
4. Distal part of LAD
5. Proximal circumflex artery
6. Distal circumflex artery
7. Left obtuse marginal artery
8. First diagonal artery
9. First septal perforating artery
10. Septal arteries
11. Auricular branch of the circumflex artery
12. Obtuse marginal artery n° 2.

FIG. 56-2. Posteroanterior view of left coronary artery. Modified from Kern MJ, 1995, with permission.

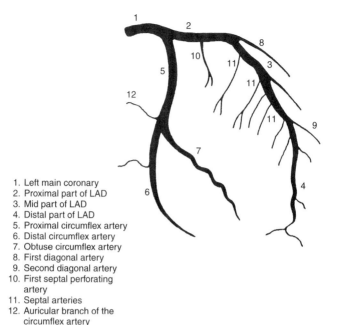

1. Left main coronary
2. Proximal part of LAD
3. Mid part of LAD
4. Distal part of LAD
5. Proximal circumflex artery
6. Distal circumflex artery
7. Obtuse circumflex artery
8. First diagonal artery
9. Second diagonal artery
10. First septal perforating artery
11. Septal arteries
12. Auricular branch of the circumflex artery

FIG. 56-3. Right anterior oblique caudal view of left coronary artery. Modified from Kern MJ, 1995, with permission.

view is good for separating the LAD from its diagonal branches, especially for vertically oriented hearts. There should be enough LAO angulation to get the LAD off the spine. This view can also be good for a left-sided PDA branch. Steeper degrees of LAO further separate the LAD from the LCX and can get the LCX off the spine, but can also cause the origins of the diagonals to overlap the LAD and cause the

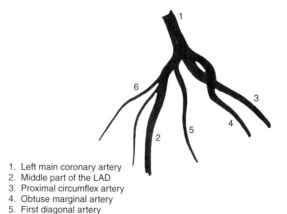

1. Left main coronary artery
2. Middle part of the LAD
3. Proximal circumflex artery
4. Obtuse marginal artery
5. First diagonal artery
6. Septal perforating artery

FIG. 56-4. Left anterior oblique cranial view of left coronary artery. Modified from Kern MJ, 1995, with permission.

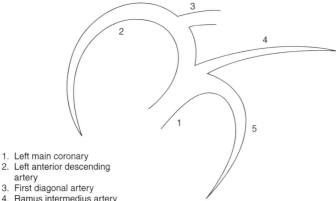

1. Left main coronary
2. Left anterior descending
   artery
3. First diagonal artery
4. Ramus intermedius artery
5. Left circumflex artery

FIG. 56-5. Left anterior oblique caudal view of left coronary artery. Modified from Boucher RA, 1988, with permission.

distal LAD to overlap the diaphragm. The **45 degree LAO, 30 degree caudal** (the "spider" view) is useful for looking at the left main coronary artery and the proximal origin of the LCX. The proximal LAD is also seen, but is foreshortened, unless the heart is horizontal in orientation. There must be enough LAO to get the cardiac silhouette off the spine. There is usually no need for a wedge, as it increases the haziness of this view further. Minimal to no panning is required. The **lateral** view provides delineation of the mid-LAD. In addition, the distal LAD does not overlap diaphragm and the LCX is

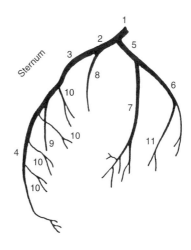

1. Left main coronary artery
2. Proximal part of LAD
3. Middle part of LAD
4. Distal part of LAD
5. Proximal circumflex artery
6. Distal circumflex artery
7. Obtuse marginal artery
8. First diagonal artery
9. Second diagonal artery
10. Septal arteries
11. Obtuse marginal artery n° 2

FIG. 56-6. Left lateral view of left coronary artery. Modified from Kern MJ, 1995, with permission.

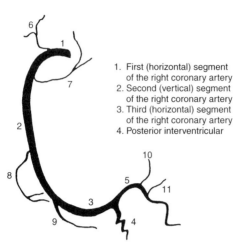

FIG. 56-7. Left anterior oblique view of right coronary artery. Modified from Kern MJ, 1995, with permission.

1. First (horizontal) segment of the right coronary artery
2. Second (vertical) segment of the right coronary artery
3. Third (horizontal) segment of the right coronary artery
4. Posterior interventricular
5. Retroventricular artery
6. Conus branch
7. Artery of the sinus node
8. Right ventricular artery
9. Right marginal artery
10. Artery of the A-V node
11. Diaphragmatic artery

off the spine. The patient's hands should be placed behind the head for the lateral view. The shield should be placed above the course of the LAD. Panning involves dropping the table height and moving the table cranially. The **PA with 30 degree caudal** angulation provides a good view of the LCX.

b. **Right coronary artery.** The RCA is usually viewed in LAO and RAO views. The **30 degree RAO** provides a good view of the proximal

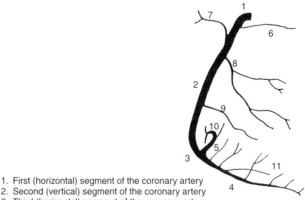

1. First (horizontal) segment of the coronary artery
2. Second (vertical) segment of the coronary artery
3. Third (horizontal) segment of the coronary artery
4. Posterior descending artery
5. Retroventricular artery
6. Conus branch
7. Artery of the sinus node
8. Right ventricular artery
9. Right marginal artery
10. Artery of the A-V node
11. Inferior septal arteries

FIG. 56-8. Right anterior oblique view of right coronary artery. Modified from Kern MJ, 1995, with permission.

and mid-RCA and also of the PDA, which is laid out lengthwise. Cranial angulation can help separate the PDA from the distal vessel. The **40 degree LAO** view provides a good view of the proximal and mid-RCA, and if cranial angulation is added, a good view of the posterolateral arteries. The **PA with 30 degree cranial** can provide a useful view of the origins of the PDA and posterolateral branches. The lateral view of the RCA can provide a good view of the mid-RCA. In the RAO view, the right atrium and ventricle are separated by the RCA in the AV groove. Thus, atrial branches will be directed toward the atrium and marginal branches will be directed toward the ventricle.

c. **Bypass grafts.** For grafts, an LAO and an RAO view are required to visualize the body of the graft. Additional views are dictated by the grafted vessel. A particularly useful view for the LIMA-LAD anastomosis is the lateral view; cranial LAO and cranial RAO views can also be useful. The graft to the diagonal can be visualized in the cranial LAO and cranial RAO views. The graft to the marginal branch can be seen in the RAO and lateral views. The graft to the distal RCA can be visualized in the cranial LAO and lateral views.

4. **Congenital coronary anomalies.** Coronary artery anomalies should be suspected if there is an absent coronary artery and a large area of myocardium that appears nonperfused (3). The most common anomaly is an absent left main coronary artery trunk, in which the LAD and LCX have separate ostia (incidence 0.47%). If the LAD is first cannulated, the LCX can be engaged with a clockwise rotation; sometimes one size larger catheter (JL5) is needed. Likewise, if the LCX is first cannulated, counterclockwise rotation, perhaps with a size smaller catheter (a JL3.5), is needed to engage the LAD. The next most common anomaly is the LCX originating from the right sinus of Valsalva (0.45%). The next most common anomaly is the RCA originating from the ascending aorta above the sinus of Valsalva (0.18%). The RCA originating from the left sinus of Valsalva is the next most common anomaly, originating superior and anterior to the left main (0.13%).

The origin of the left main artery from the right sinus is even less common (0.02%), but can result in sudden death if the left main artery passes between the aorta and the pulmonary artery (extremely rare). The left main artery can also pass into the ventricular septum (most common), anterior to the pulmonary artery or posterior to the aorta. The 30 degree RAO view can help define the relationship between the coronary artery and the great vessels. If the course is septal, septal perforators can be seen originating from the left main.

The other coronary anomalies occur much less frequently. The Amplatz (left or right, depending on the cusp of origin) and multipurpose catheters are especially useful to cannulate anomalous coronary arteries.

Though not truly a congenital anomaly, every angiographer should be aware of **myocardial bridging.** This is an apparent narrowing of a coronary artery (usually the mid-LAD) that is present only during systole. There have been reports of bridging involving the diagonal branches of the LAD, the marginal branches of the LCX, and the distal RCA. Since the majority of coronary blood flow occurs during diastole, myocardial bridges are rarely pathologic, but there have been patients treated with CABG and, more recently, stenting. Nitroglycerin, by dilating epicardial vessels, can make bridging seem even more pronounced. A phenomenon similar to bridging can occur in hypertrophic obstructive cardiomyopathy, in which septal perforators from the LAD can become obliterated during systole,

5. **Quantification of coronary stenosis.** It is important to always obtain at least two perpendicular views of each coronary artery lesion. A single view, or even multiple views, can miss an eccentric lesion. Severity of a

lesion is based on percent diameter stenosis compared to a "normal" reference segment. Lesions are generally classified as severe if 70% or more are in the LAD, LCX, and RCA or 50% are in the left main artery. In measuring the size of vessels and stenoses, it is useful to note that a 6-Fr catheter has an external diameter of 2 mm. Formal quantitative coronary angiography or use of calipers can improve the measurement of coronary artery stenoses. Quantitative coronary angiography decreases the inter- and intra-observer variability of grading stenosis severity. The minimal luminal diameter in the most severe view correlates best with perfusion imaging; minimum luminal diameters less than 1.2 to 1.5 mm in proximal vessels typically reduce hyperemic flow.

6. **Limitations of coronary angiography.** Sometimes the severity of a lesion is difficult to gage based on visual angiographic estimates alone, particularly in the presence of diffuse disease. Angiography only provides an outline of the lumen, the so-called "luminogram." In addition, the angiogram can underestimate the presence of atheroma because of outward remodeling of the arterial wall (the Glagov phenomenon). Furthermore, angiography can only visualize arteries greater than 200 μm in diameter. The physiologic importance of 40% to 70% stenoses cannot be determined by angiography alone and flow limitation should be demonstrated before percutaneous intervention. Techniques such as intravascular ultrasound and the Doppler pressure wire (see Chapter 57) can aid in determining whether ambiguous lesions on angiography are significant.

C. **Crossing the aortic valve**
   1. **Normal aortic valve.** The pigtail catheter is most commonly used to cross native aortic valves. Tissue valves can also be crossed, but crossing mechanical valves (e.g., St. Jude, Björk-Shiley, Medtronic-Hall) risks catheter entrapment and is best avoided. The catheter should be made to loop above the aortic valve. Pulling back very slowly, the catheter should give, and can then be rapidly advanced into the left ventricle during systole. If the patient takes a deep breath and holds it while the pigtail catheter is being unlooped, this can facilitate the passage of the catheter into the left ventricle. Sometimes the guidewire itself may be useful in crossing the valve, in which case the catheter is simply advanced over the guidewire into the left ventricle. A single operator can cross the aortic valve without assistance, but if two operators are present, one can move the catheter and change its orientation while the other moves the wire back and forth. The pressure in the left ventricle is recorded continuously; the catheter is pulled back into the aorta in a single motion to determine the aortic pressure, and the pullback pressure gradient can be calculated.
   2. **Aortic stenosis.** In more severe cases of aortic stenosis, difficulty may be encountered in passing any catheter across the aortic valve. In this circumstance a 0.038-in. straight-tipped wire can be used to cross the valve. If this method is elected, a 5,000-U bolus of heparin is recommended by some operators. The timer should be started, and no more than 3 to 4 minutes should be allowed per attempt at crossing. Between each attempt the wire should be withdrawn and wiped, blood aspirated and discarded, and the catheter flushed. Special care must be used during this maneuver to avoid perforating the aortic cusps or potentially dissecting often the coronary ostia. If a 6-Fr sheath is used, a 5-Fr pigtail catheter often provides the right angle for wire passage; in addition, simultaneous aortic and femoral pressures can be recorded and compared to the left ventricular pressure simultaneously using two transducers. A JR4 or AL1 catheter can also provide the correct orientation for wire passage across the aortic valve. The combination of a Feldman catheter and Rosen wire is an alternative approach to cross stenotic aortic valves. Another way to determine the pressure gradient is to use a

double-lumen pigtail catheter and measure the left ventricular and aortic pressures simultaneously. Chapter 50 on right heart catheterization and hemodynamic measurements discusses the method to calculate the aortic gradient.

D. Left ventriculography

1. Setting up the view. The pigtail catheter (commonly the angled version) is positioned in the midcavity of the left ventricle. The pigtail should look like a "6" in the RAO projection. If the pigtail twists with each beat, this indicates it is caught in the mitral valve apparatus and needs to be repositioned. The monitor should be observed for ectopy. Once a stable rhythm is present, ventriculography can proceed. First, the left ventricular end-diastolic pressure (LVEDP) should be measured on a 40 scale. In patients with an elevated LVEDP (>25 mm Hg), a left ventriculogram is generally contraindicated. If the decision to proceed with the left ventriculogram is made, sublingual nitroglycerin should first be given to lower the LVEDP. With more moderate degrees of left ventricular dysfunction, non-ionic dye, which is less of a myocardial depressant, can be used. Digital subtraction can be used instead of cinefluoroscopy to obtain the left ventriculogram. This allows a smaller amount of contrast to be used. With digital subtraction, the view needs to be carefully centered because panning is not possible. **The left ventriculogram is best avoided in patients with critical aortic stenosis, significant left main artery disease, or severe left ventricle dysfunction.**

2. Views. The **30 degree RAO** view is used to look at overall left ventricular function. In particular, the anterior, apical, and inferior walls can be assessed (see Fig. 56-9). Some operators routinely pan to the LIMA to see if it is patent in patients who might require CABG. The RAO view is also useful to assess mitral leaflet prolapse and MR. The LAO cranial view can also assess MR and avoids overlap of the aorta with the left atrium that occurs in the RAO view. **Mitral regurgitation** can be graded on a scale of 1 to 4; 1 represents trace MR, with mild left atrial opacification that clears with one beat; 2 represents a mild to moderate degree of opacification, though less than the left ventricle; 3 represents moderate to severe opacification of the left atrium equal to the left ventricle; and 4 represents complete opacification of the left atrium greater

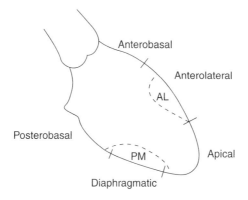

RAO

FIG. 56-9. Thirty-degree right anterior oblique view of the left ventricle. Modified from Tilkian, 1986, with permission.

than the left ventricle. Panning toward the left atrium may be needed if MR is present. The catheter itself can cause MR if it is caught in the mitral valve apparatus or if it induces premature ventricular contractions. The correlation between angiographic and echocardiographic MR is excellent. The **60 degree LAO** projection allows evaluation of the septum and the posterior and lateral walls (see Fig. 56-10). Ventricular septal defects are best identified in the LAO projection with slight cranial angulation. If biplane imaging capability exists, RAO and LAO views of the left ventricle can be obtained simultaneously.

3. **Settings.** For a ventriculogram, the flow injector can be set at a rate of 10 to 15 cm^3/second for a total volume of about 35 to 50 cm^3, with a rate rise of 0.4 (to minimize ectopy and to keep the catheter from moving abruptly), and a pressure of 600. The exact settings will vary depending on the size of the heart and the need to limit contrast.

E. **Aortography.** Aortography is usually performed in the LAO position, with the catheter about 2 cm above the aortic leaflets. Compared to a ventriculogram, a larger volume of contrast is needed to opacify the aorta. The flow injector is set to a higher total volume than for the left ventriculogram, usually about 60 cm^3 at 20 to 25 cm^3/second. No rate rise is necessary (other than to keep smaller size catheters from moving) and a pressure limit of 600 is used. **Aortic insufficiency** can be identified with a grading system similar to that for MR; 1 represents trace aortic insufficiency that clears from the left ventricle with each beat; 2 represents mild left ventricular opacification that takes more than one beat to clear; 3 represents moderate left ventricular opacification equal to the aortic root; and 4 represents complete opacification of the left ventricle greater than the aortic root. Diseases of the aorta such as aneurysms or dissection can also be identified. An aortogram can also aid in nonselective visualization of anomalous coronary arteries or grafts that are difficult to engage. However, the absence of filling of a bypass graft on aortography does not exclude its presence. The aorta needs to be well and heavily opacified to ensure that grafts are seen.

An aortogram can be performed with the pigtail catheter placed in the descending aorta slightly above the level of the origins of the renal arteries (the L1 vertebral body) to rule out **renal artery stenosis.** A JR4 can be

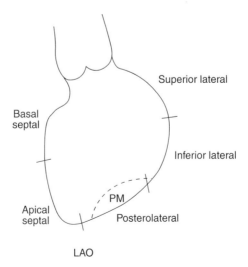

FIG. 56-10. Sixty-degree left anterior oblique view of the left ventricle. Modified from Tilkian, 1986, with permission.

used to obtain selective renal arteriograms by turning the tip of the catheter so that it points to either the left or right in the posteroanterior view. The catheter is then pulled gradually back when it is in the vicinity of the renal artery ostia until it engages. Digital acquisition should be used.

Carotid angiography is sometimes necessary to confirm the degree of carotid artery stenosis seen on a noninvasive study. A variety of catheters (the Headhunter and Newton series) can be used to selectively cannulate the common carotid artery. These catheters are advanced to the aortic arch over a guidewire and pulled back to engage the artery of interest. A Newton 5 can be used to engage the right common carotid artery and a Newton 2, with its smaller curve, can be used to engage the left common carotid artery. There is a 0.5% to 1% risk of stroke with this procedure. Digital acquisition and use of nonionic contrast are mandatory.

F. **Provocative testing.** In patients in whom coronary artery spasm is suspected, IV methylergonovine can be given to provoke spasm (4). Once significant angiographic stenosis has been ruled out, 0.05 mg of IV methylergonovine is administered. If the patient develops his or her typical chest pain or ST elevation on ECG monitoring, the coronary arteries are catheterized immediately. The ECG changes can help determine which coronary artery to cannulate first. If there are no ECG changes or chest pain, the right coronary (which is statistically more likely to have spasm) and then the left coronary should be recatheterized 5 minutes after the methylergonovine has been administered. A positive response consists of a focal area of spasm that is relieved by intracoronary nitroglycerin (a usual dose of 100 to 200 µg). Diffuse spasm can be physiologic and is also treated with nitroglycerin and verapamil (also 100 to 200 µg). Since the half-life of methylergonovine is longer than that of SL nitroglycerin, it is important to realize that spasm can recur after a dose of nitroglycerin. If the initial dose of methylergonovine does not provoke a response, an additional dose of 0.2 mg can be given a few minutes after the first. Alternatively, some operators prefer giving a single dose of 0.2 mg.

VII. **Postcatheterization care**

A. **Sheath removal.** The sheath is removed once the procedure is complete. Adequate local anesthesia should be reinjected if the previously given amount has lost its efficacy. After the sheath is removed, hemostasis is generally obtained with direct manual pressure of the fingertips over the pulse, without sterile gauze to obscure the view. Pressure is held for approximately 20 minutes (about 3 minutes for each French size) until there is no bleeding. In patients who have coagulopathy, poorly controlled hypertension, or aortic regurgitation with a wide pulse pressure, a longer duration of pressure is necessary. Care must be taken to intermittently allow adequate blood flow to the distal extremity. It is therefore best to be able to directly visualize the extremity to assess its color. If both arterial and venous sheaths are present, it is best to remove the venous sheath first and obtain hemostasis before removing the arterial sheath. In patients with severe aortic stenosis or significant left main coronary artery disease, lab personnel should be prepared to rapidly treat a vagal episode, which can be life threatening in these situations. Adequate administration of anesthesia before removal of the sheath decreases the chance of a vagal reaction.

Bed rest is generally required for 6 hours after a femoral sheath is removed, though some operators require 1 hour for each French size. In fact, 2.5 hours is a sufficient period of bed rest for 5-Fr sheaths. Two hours of keeping the arm straight is necessary after a brachial or radial procedure. During the postprocedure observation period it is necessary to monitor heart rate, temperature, blood pressure, urine output, distal pulses, and the access site (for pain, bleeding, or hematoma). The use of sandbags placed over the groin site is discouraged. Before discharge it is best to have the patient ambulate under observation. Specific discharge instructions should include the possibility of late access-site bleeding and the need to hold pressure and call for emergency help.

Intravenous fluids are often given after a cardiac catheterization. The osmotic load of the contrast dye can cause a large diuresis. Intravenous fluids (e.g., normal saline at 100 cm³/hour for several hours) can prevent volume depletion. Care should be used in patients with a history of congestive heart failure, in whom liberal IV fluids could contribute to pulmonary edema.

  B. **Compression/closure devices.** The **FemoStop** is a pneumatic compression device that can be used for holding pressure in cases of prolonged bleeding. The **C clamp** is a mechanical clamp that can also be used for holding prolonged pressure. If either of these methods is employed, direct supervision of the patient is still required.

  The 8-Fr **Angio-Seal** hemostatic puncture closure device is a method that can be used to obtain hemostasis in an uncomplicated femoral procedure if an 8-Fr or smaller sheath was used. A biodegradable collagen plug is deployed to the femoral artery puncture site using a guidewire and special sheath. No manual pressure is required and ambulation can begin after 1 hour. The **Perclose Techstar** is a percutaneous vascular suture device that allows immediate ambulation (of course, after the effects of any sedation given during the procedure have worn off). Prior to its use, a 35 degree RAO view of the right femoral artery should be taken to ensure that the sheath has been placed above the femoral artery bifurcation. The device is currently available in 6-, 8-, or 10-Fr sizes. The **Vasoseal** is a collagen plug that is placed over the femoral artery puncture site. It comes in several sizes; in order to determine the appropriate size, it is necessary to place a depth marker on the needle during the initial arterial puncture. Ambulation can begin 1 hour after placement. The Angio-Seal device is generally preferred over the other devices due to its ease of use and general reliability. Other improved devices are likely to be available in the near future.

VIII. **Complications**
  A. **Death.** There is a 0.1% risk of death from LHC. This risk is substantially higher in patients undergoing urgent catheterization for acute coronary syndromes. In addition, patients with left main coronary artery disease, severe aortic stenosis, or severe left ventricular dysfunction are known to be patient subgroups with a particularly increased risk. Advanced age increases the risk of death.

  B. **Myocardial infarction.** There is a 0.05% risk of MI from LHC. Myocardial infarction can result from coronary dissection, disruption of a preexisting atheromatous plaque, a large air embolus, or a thrombus. Patients with acute coronary syndromes have a higher risk of MI.

  C. **Stroke.** Stroke occurs in 0.05% of catheterizations. There is a risk of stroke from an inadvertent air embolus or thrombus. Presence of aortic atheroma is a risk factor for embolic complications. Dislodgment of atheromatous debris in the aorta can lead to a stroke. This risk can be minimized by use of 260-cm exchange wires for catheter changes in patients with known severe aortic disease.

  D. **Coronary artery dissection.** Engagement of the coronary arteries can rarely cause dissection. It is most often due to injection of contrast through a catheter that is not coaxial to the coronary artery, causing rupture of a preexisting plaque, or placement of the catheter too deeply into the coronary artery (so-called deep-throating). Particular caution should be used with Amplatz catheters. In cases of left main coronary artery dissection, a stent can be placed emergently and the patient can be placed on peripheral cardiopulmonary support until the surgical team can be mobilized.

  E. **Coronary artery spasm.** Engagement of the coronary arteries, in particular the RCA, can cause spasm. This is best treated with withdrawal of the catheter. Subsequent reengagement and administration of intracoronary nitroglycerin (100 to 200 µg) may also be necessary for more rapid resolution of spasm.

  F. **Renal failure.** Contrast dye can precipitate renal failure in any patient, although certain patients (elevated creatinine, diabetes, proteinuria, dehydration) are at higher risk. Adequate prehydration with normal saline can decrease this risk. The best way to minimize contrast-induced renal failure is limiting the amount of dye used. Using less than 30 cm^3 of contrast dye dramatically reduces the incidence of renal failure in even the highest risk patients (5). Biplane cineangiography can maximize the amount of information obtained with each view.

G. **Emergency coronary artery bypass graft.** There is a risk of needing emergency CABG as a complication of the catheterization (e.g., dissection of the left main coronary artery). There is also the possibility of identification of critical disease, such as severe left main coronary artery disease, that may prompt emergency CABG as the most expedient treatment.

H. **Arrhythmias.** A risk of ventricular fibrillation (0.5%) exists with catheterization. This rhythm is treated with electrical defibrillation. Overinjection of contrast into the RCA in particular can cause ventricular fibrillation. Contrast dye (less so nonionic dye) can cause transient bradycardia, best dealt with by having the patient cough and by minimizing the amount of dye injected with each angiogram.

I. **Heart failure.** The osmotic load of contrast dye can put a patient with diminished cardiac or renal function into overt pulmonary edema. In patients with severe cardiac or renal disease, injection of contrast should be limited and use of nonionic, low-osmolar dye should be considered.

J. **Vagal reaction.** If a patient develops hypotension and/or bradycardia, a vagal reaction should be considered. It is common to see this when local anesthetic is being administered or when the sheath is being removed. Atropine 1 mg IV should be ready and given in these situations. Adequate anesthesia can help prevent such reactions. In a patient with severe aortic stenosis or left main coronary artery disease, a vagal reaction can start a downward spiral that leads to death. Levophed (about 10 μg) should always be ready and used immediately in such cases of hypotension.

K. **Vascular**

   1. **Femoral.** Pseudoaneurysms, arteriovenous fistulas, arterial thrombosis, and peripheral emboli are possible vascular complications. Careful technique can minimize these events. In particular, paying attention to puncture location and obtaining adequate hemostasis after sheath removal are the best ways to decrease vascular complications. For example, the smaller sheaths (5-Fr) are preferable in patients with significant peripheral vascular disease. Frequent aspiration and discarding of blood from the arterial sheath, followed by gentle flushing, is useful. If an attempted cannulation is unsuccessful but an arterial puncture has been made, the needle should be withdrawn and adequate manual pressure held (about 5 minutes). If an inadvertent venous puncture has been made, the needle should be removed and pressure held (for about 3 minutes). Proceeding directly to arterial puncture without removing the needle and holding pressure increases the chance of arteriovenous fistula formation. If a venous puncture is planned, it should be made lower than the arterial puncture site. Bruits should be auscultated both before and after the procedure. A new bruit may indicate a vascular complication. **Ultrasound** is an essential part of the management of groin complications. If there is a large pseudoaneurysm present, surgery may be required after a trial of ultrasound-guided compression. Small pseudoaneurysms (less than 2 cm) tend to close spontaneously but should be followed by serial ultrasound examinations. An arteriovenous fistula that does not close spontaneously in 2 to 4 weeks requires surgical repair.

   2. **Brachial/radial.** When using an upper extremity approach, blood pressure should first be checked in both arms. If there is a difference between arms, peripheral vascular disease should be suspected and the side with the higher blood pressure should be used. For a radial approach, an Allen test must be performed to assess the patency of col-

lateral ulnar circulation. There is a higher rate of vascular complications such as thrombosis with the upper extremity approach in comparison to the femoral approach.

L. Bleeding. Access site bleeding can be significant. If there is a great deal of oozing around the sheath, it can be exchanged for a sheath one French size larger. Adequate manual pressure is usually sufficient to stop bleeding after sheath removal. It is typical practice to check the activated clotting time on patients who had been on heparin prior to the procedure and only proceed with sheath removal if the clotting time is below 160. Some institutions use protamine (1 mg per 100 U heparin) to reverse heparinization, but this exposes the patient to the potential for allergic reactions to protamine (namely, hypotension). Even more concerning is **retroperitoneal bleeding.** If a patient complains of severe back pain after a catheterization, this should be considered. An unexpected drop in hemoglobin after a catheterization should also raise this possibility. Obese patients, in particular, can have a major bleed without obvious external signs. The test to diagnose a retroperitoneal bleed is a noncontrast computed tomography scan.

M. Infection. There is a risk of infection, as with any invasive procedure. This risk can be minimized with proper attention to sterile technique. There is usually no need for prophylactic antibiotics. However, some operators do give antibiotics after use of a percutaneous vascular suture device in patients who are at elevated risk for infection, such as obese or diabetic patients. Endocarditis prophylaxis for patients with valvular heart disease or prosthetic valves is unnecessary.

N. Neuropathy. There is a slight risk of damage to the femoral nerve from inadvertent puncture. Femoral hematoma (or retroperitoneal bleeding) can also cause compromise of the femoral nerve. Function usually improves with time but can take several months.

O. Allergy. As discussed above, contrast dye can cause adverse reactions, ranging from hives to anaphylaxis. Severe anaphylactoid reactions to contrast dye occur in about 0. 1% of cases. Local anesthetic can also cause problems due to specific allergies to the amide or ester component, or to the preservative. A variety of agents are available. Procaine (an ester agent), lidocaine (an amide agent), and bupivacaine (a preservative-free amide agent) are three alternatives.

SUGGESTED READINGS
References
1. Pepine CJ. ACC/AHA Guidelines for cardiac catheterization and cardiac catheterization laboratories. ACC/AHA Ad Hoc Task Force on Cardiac Catheterization. *J Am Coll Cardiol* 1991;18:1149–1182.
2. Matthai WH, Kussmal WG, Krol J, Goin JE, Schwartz JS, Hirshfeld JW. A comparison of low- with high-osmolar contrast agents in cardiac angiography: identification of criteria for selective use. *Circulation* 1994;89:291–301.
3. Yamanaka O, Hobbs RE. Coronary artery anomalies in 126,595 patients undergoing coronary arteriography. *Catheter Cardiovasc Diagn* 1990;21:28–40.
4. Heupler FA, Proudfit WL, Razavi M, Shirey EK, Greenstreet R, Sheldon WC. Ergonovine maleate provocative test for coronary arterial spasm. *Am J Cardiol* 1978;41:631–640.
5. Manske CL, Sprafka JM, Strony JT, Wang Y. Contrast nephropathy in azotemic diabetic patients undergoing coronary angiography. *Am J Med* 1990;89:615–620.

Key Review
Boucher RA, Myler RK, Clark DA, Stertzer SH. Coronary angiography and angioplasty. *Catheter Cardiovasc Diagn* 1988;14:269–285.

Relevant Book Chapters
Baim DS, Grossman W. *Cardiac catheterization, angiography, and intervention,* 5th ed. Baltimore: Williams & Wilkins, 1996:183–218.

Baum S. *Abram's angiography,* 4th ed. Boston: Little, Brown and Company, 1997: 241–252.

Ellis SG. Coronary angiography. In: Fuster V, Ross R, Topol E, eds. *Atherosclerosis and coronary artery disease,* Vol. 2. Philadelphia: Lippincott-Raven Publishers, 1996: 1433–1450.

Green CE. *Coronary cinematography.* Philadelphia: Lippincott-Raven Publishers, 1996:39–68.

Kern MJ. *The cardiac catheterization handbook,* 2nd ed. St. Louis: Mosby–Year Book, 1995:266–375.

Pepine CJ. Coronary angiography and cardiac catheterization. In: Topol EJ, ed. *Textbook of cardiovascular medicine.* Philadelphia: Lippincott-Raven Publishers, 1998: 1935–1976.

Tilkian AG, Daily EK. *Cardiovascular procedures: diagnostic techniques and therapeutic procedures.* St. Louis: Mosby, 1986:117–151.

57. INTERVENTIONAL CARDIOLOGY

Walter A. Tan and Stephen G. Ellis

I. **Introduction.** The number of percutaneous coronary interventions (PCIs) is projected to be greater than 750,000 in the United States alone by the year 2000. At many centers more than 50% of patients receive at least one stent. Recently, there have been important advances with respect to periprocedure platelet inhibition in decreasing postprocedural clinical events.

II. **Indications.** The ideal candidate for PCI has the following characteristics: (a) **symptomatic with viable myocardium;** (b) anticipated **high likelihood of death, myocardial infarction (MI), or significant symptoms** if left untreated; (c) **low risk for adverse events.** For those who do not fulfill these criteria, careful judgment must be exercised in reassessing the benefit-to-risk ratio in conjunction with the patient and his or her family.

III. **Contraindications.** Significant and active **bleeding** that precludes anticoagulation is an absolute contraindication for PCI. Relative contraindications are **bleeding diathesis, coronary anatomy that is unsuitable** or carries prohibitive risks (including chronic total occlusion, diffuse distal disease, and most cases of **left main trunk (LMT) stenosis), repeated multivessel restenoses,** or **terminal illness** with poor short term prospects.

IV. **Revascularization strategy.** When revascularization is indicated, the choice between percutaneous as opposed to surgical modalities is determined by many factors. There is equivalence in mortality and MI at 5 years between the strategies of **multivessel percutaneous transluminal coronary angioplasty (PTCA) and coronary artery bypass graft (CABG)** (1). In the Bypass Angioplasty Revascularization Investigation (BARI) trial, the CABG arm was more invasive and slightly more costly, but only 8% had a repeat revascularization rate over the subsequent 5 years. In the balloon angioplasty arm, incremental procedures were more common, with approximately half of the cases coming back for repeat revascularization (PCI or CABG), most within a year of the index procedure (7 of 10 were PCI). Whether these data remain applicable in the modern PCI era is questionable. In the Evaluation of Platelet IIb/IIIa Inhibitor for Stenting (EPISTENT) trial, stenting and abciximab decreased the 6-month target vessel evascularization (TVR) rate to 8.7% (2).

At present, **PCI is considered the superior alternative** in patients with severe comorbidities (such as age or severe coronary obstructive pulmonary disease) that make the risk of surgery prohibitive or for persistently symptomatic patients with single-vessel disease. For those patients who fall between these two extremes, Table 57-1 addresses other determinants that should be taken into consideration in deciding on revascularization strategies.

A. **Myocardial infarction with ST elevation**
  1. **Primary angioplasty**
     a. Current reevaluation of direct angioplasty compared with fibrinolytic therapy for MI with ST elevation has shown better results with regard to death (4.7% versus 6.7%) and death/MI (7.8% versus 11.6%) by pooled analysis of the larger trials. This is presumed to be predominantly a result of restoration of TIMI grade 3 flow (TIMI is Thrombolysis in Myocardial Infarction trial) in almost twice the proportion of patients in the PTCA as compared to fibrinolytic arm, along with a lower occurrence of strokes (0% versus 2.8%, $p = .003$). However, these outcomes were attained in early selected series that did not use accelerated tissue plasminogen activator (atPA), and in the context of highly dedicated operators and catheterization laboratories that were logistically geared to expedited revascularization. Less dramatic outcome differences were evident from the Global

Table 57-1. PCI vs. surgery: special considerations that determine mode of revascularization

Favor PCI	Favor CABG
• Single, double, or triple vessel disease with suitable anatomy, especially if LV function is normal	• Multiple-vessel disease characteristics that are unfavorable for PCI; LMT, chronic occlusions or 3-vessel severe proximal disease with nonfocal stenosis
• Acute MI with or without cardiogenic shock	• Concomitant valvular, aortic root, or congenital heart disease that will require surgery
• Prior sternotomy, especially if recent	• Severe LV dysfunction with multi-vessel disease
• Severe comorbidity (e.g., COPD) that makes risk for surgery prohibitive	• Multivessel restenosis (especially diffuse in-stent) or repeated restenosis of proximal single-vessel disease
• Limited life expectancy but requires palliative therapy for symptomatic CAD	• Possibly longstanding or insulin-dependent diabetes mellitus, especially if with abnormal LV
• No more available bypass conduits	• Strong patient preference to avoid repeat revascularizations

PCI, percutaneous coronary intervention; CABG, coronary artery bypass graft; LV, left ventricular; LMT, XXX; MI, myocardial infarction; COPD, coronary occlusive pulmonary disease; CAD, coronary artery disease.

Use of Strategies to Open Occluded Coronary Arteries (GUSTO IIb) trial, the largest randomized controlled trial (RCT) to examine this issue, showing a smaller difference in a composite 30-day end point of death, reinfarction, and disabling stroke (9.6% versus 13.7%, odds ratio = 0.67, p = 0.033) (3). This was corroborated by the community-based Myocardial Infarction Triage and Intervention Investigators (MITI) Registry, which consisted of a cohort of 12,331 consecutive patients with acute MI. Surprisingly, there was no significant difference in mortality between the two treatment groups even within the high-risk subsets of patients. Hence, it appears that real-world conditions diminish the incremental benefits of direct PTCA. However the addition of abciximab to direct PTCA decreased the death and MI rates by 40% in the ReoPro in Acute MI and Primary PTCA Organization and Randomized Trial (RAPPORT) (4).
b. The key to benefit is **prompt reperfusion,** and the key to prompt reperfusion is decisiveness. Institutional consensus protocols may help to alleviate the problem of delays to therapy. Table 57-2 outlines the advantages and disadvantages of each approach. The strategy of direct percutaneous intervention is favored in the following circumstances:

1. In a setting of experienced operators, expedited catheterization lab services (door-to-balloon time of less than 60 minutes), and ready access to emergency bypass surgery.
2. Patients presenting with MI who are not eligible for fibrinolytic therapy.
3. Patients who are at high risk for stroke (cerebrovascular accident or neurosurgical procedure within previous 6 months, severe uncontrolled hypertension with systolic blood pressure

Table 57-2. Comparison of invasive versus medical reperfusion strategies in the management of acute myocardial infarction

Characteristics	Direct PCI	Thrombolytic Rx
Time to initation of Rx	+	+++
TIMI grade 3 flow achieved	++++	++
Availability	–	+++
Applicability: Proportion of patients eligible	+++	+
Elderly	+++	+
History of bleeding or recent surgery	++	–
Threatened renal failure	–	+++
History of CABG	++	+
Presence of shock state	+	±
Early prognostication	+++	NA
Recurrent ischemia	+++	+
Late patency	+++	++

Legend (semiquantitative estimates of benefit as compared to no therapy):
++++   extremely favorable
 +++   highly favorable
  ++   moderately favorable
   +   mildly favorable
   ±   equivocal benefit
   –   no benefit or unfavorable
PCI, percutaneous coronary intervention; TIMI, Thrombolysis in Myocardial Infarction; CABG, coronary artery bypass graft; NA, not applicable.

greater than 180 mm Hg, or MI accompanied by head trauma such as in a motor vehicular accident).

4. Cardiogenic shock.

2. **Primary stenting.** Primary stenting may improve the results of catheter-based reperfusion. However, results of prospective RCT are forthcoming.

3. **Rescue angioplasty.** Up to 26% of patients who have received thrombolysis for MI fail to achieve patency by 180 minutes post therapy (TIMI grade 2 or 3 flow). The merits of early fallback mechanical reperfusion were examined in the Randomized Comparison of Rescue Angioplasty (RESCUE) trial where 151 patients with failed lytic therapy for anterior wall MI within 8 hours of chest pain were randomized between rescue PTCA versus routine therapy. Patency was reestablished in 92% of patients in the intervention arm. Thirty-day exercise left ventricular ejection fraction (LVEF) and the composite of death or severe heart failure were improved in the rescue PTCA arm. These benefits have not been established for an infarct-related artery with less than TIMI 2 flow, and studies from the pre-glycoprotein (GP) IIb/IIIa era in fact suggest possible harm with attempted intervention in infarct-related arteries with TIMI 3 flow.

Patients with **persistent chest pain or ST-segment elevation 2 hours after lytic therapy should be considered for rescue intervention,** especially in the following situations: (a) Killip class III or IV status; (b) new left bundle branch block or more than 2 mm ST elevation involving in excess of four electrocardiogram (ECG) leads; (c) large inferior MI (as evidenced by right ventricular involvement, concurrent anterior ST elevation, or atrioventricular block); (d) anterior wall MI with less than 70% resolution of ST elevation; and (e) poor cardiac reserve due to prior MIs.

4. **Delayed (secondary) angioplasty.** There are those who advocate a conservative approach across the board, reserving catheterization only

for recurrent symptoms or documented ischemia after MI. This viewpoint is primarily based on data from TIMI 2 and SWIFT (Should We Intervene Following Thrombolysis?) trials, which suggested limited benefit from early percutaneous revascularization. However, these studies are severely limited because of the late application of revascularization, outdated interventional practices, and suboptimal antiplatelet regimens.

An aggressive approach is to perform angiography for all MI patients for purposes of risk stratification, as well as PCI with adjunctive abciximab therapy if indicated. The alternative conservative approach would be to catheterize patients only if they develop post-MI pain, congestive heart failure, sustained ventricular tachycardia, or have a positive pre-discharge stress test.

5. **Cardiogenic shock.** Cardiogenic shock represents a very-high-risk situation that carries an in-hospital mortality of up to 80%. **Intraaortic balloon pump (IABP) support** is an important and effective maneuver to help stabilize the patient, with anticipated hemodynamic effects that include an augmentation of systemic pressure despite a decrease in afterload, thereby sparing the myocardium from further increased metabolic demands. However, IABP therapy alone has not been shown to alter outcome.

The current practice is to send patients with cardiogenic shock for **emergency catheterization and revascularization.** Patients will likely require both mechanical (IABP) and pharmacologic (intravenous inotropes) support.

Care must be taken to **rule out quickly other important etiologies** that can compose up to 15% of this population: (a) right ventricular infarction, (b) mechanical complications of MI (ventricular septal defect, acute mitral regurgitation (MR), or cardiac rupture), (c) significant blood loss related to the use of anticoagulation and fibrinolytic therapy, (d) sepsis, (e) pulmonary embolism, (f) hypovolemia from overdiuresis, (g) hemo-/pneumothorax from central lines, (h) drug-related, or (i) other concomitant diagnosis such as hypertrophic obstructive cardiomyopathy.

B. **Acute coronary syndromes (unstable angina and non-ST segment MI).** The **high-risk** patients include (a) prolonged rest pain (more than 20 minutes); (b) presence of S_3, a new MR murmur, pulmonary edema, or other manifestations of hemodynamic instability; (c) presence of dynamic ST charges greater than 1 mm; (d) a positive creatine kinase MB (CK-MB) or troponin assay; and (e) presence of severe left ventricular dysfunction. The **intermediate risk** subgroup consists of patients older than 65 years, or patients with such features as new onset class III or IV angina, nocturnal angina, rest angina relieved with nitroglycerin, and angina with T-wave changes, Q waves, or resting ST depression less than 1 mm in multiple leads.

Along with aggressive medical therapy, a strategy of early angiography is preferred for these patients. If PCI is indicated, there is evidence that events can be mitigated by adjunctive use of GPIIb/IIIa inhibitors (Table 57-3). The largest RCT to examine this question was Platelet Glycoprotein IIb/IIIa in Unstable Angina: Receptor Suppression Using Integrilin Therapy (PURSUIT), an international study utilizing eptifibatide in a study population of 10,498 patients. Only a modest benefit was seen, with a 9.6% relative risk reduction (RRR) in 30-day death or MI (14.2% versus 15.7%, $p = .04$) at the cost of slight excess bleeding. In contrast, there was a 23% RRR in the subgroup of 4,358 North American patients (16.2% versus 12.4%; $p = .006$), who underwent significantly more revascularization than their foreign counterparts. This suggests that maximal benefit from these platelet inhibitors may be most evident in the setting of coronary interventions.

It is difficult to discern how the results from the Veterans Affairs Non-Q-Wave Infarction Strategies in Hospital (VANQWISH) trial should impact contemporary practice. This RCT compared routine angiography with possible revascularization versus a conservative approach and found no mortality difference at 23 months. The applicability of this study is questionable given

Table 57-3. Randomized clinical trials of platelet GPIIb/IIIa receptor antagonists in the setting of percutaneous coronary intervention

Patient population	Trial	N	% death + MI (at 1 month)		% major bleeding		6 mo. repeat revascularization	
			Control	IIbIIIa	Control	IIbIIIa	Control	IIbIIIa
Hi risk (evolving MI, severe or high-risk comorphology)	EPIC	2099	10.3	6.9	7.0	$14.0^{a,*}$	20.2 / 21.3	$15.4^{a,b}$ / $13.5^{a,c}$
RESTORE (Tirofiban)		2139	6.4	5.0	2.1	2.4	17.1^{PCI} / 6.8^{CABG}	15.7 / 5.5
Acute MI with ST elevation undergoing primary PTCA	RAPPORT	483	5.8	4.6	9.5	16.6*	21.9	20.7
Refractory UA	CAPTURE	1265	9.0	4.8*	3.8	1.9*	24.9	25.4
All comers: 50% UA, 29% stable angina	EPILOG	2792	9.1	3.8*	3.1	2.7	19.4	18.7
All comers: 38% UA, 59% elective cases	IMPACT II (Eptifibatide)	4010	8.6	6.9	4.8	5.2	—	—
All comers: 57% UA, 43% stable angina	EPISTENT (only stent groups compared)	1603	7.8	3.0*	2.2	1.5	10.6	8.7

[a] Abciximab bolus + infusion group (as opposed to bolus only).

[b] Acute coronary syndromes subgroup ($N = 288$).

[c] Stable angina subgroup ($N = 408$).

* $p \leq 0.05$.

CAPTURE, Chimeric 7E3 AntiPlatelet in Unstable Angina Refractory to Standard Treatment; EPIC, Evaluation of 7E3 for the Prevention of Ischemic Complications; EPILOG, Evaluation in PTCA to Improve Long-term Outcome with Abciximab GP IIb/IIIa Blockade; EPISTENT, Stent Substudy of the EPILOG Trial; IMPACT, Integrilin to Minimize Platelet Aggregation and Coronary Thrombosis; RAPPORT, ReoPro in Acute MI and Primary PTCA Organization and Randomized Trial; RESTORE, Randomized Efficacy Study of Tirofiban for Outcomes and Restenosis; MI, myocardial infarction; PCI, percutaneous coronary intervention; UA, unstable angina.

the high surgical mortality rate, lack of stents and antiplatelet adjuncts for PCI, and inclusion of MI patients who received fibrinolytic therapy (5).

C. Chronic stable angina. While PCI has not yet been shown to improve survival or attenuate the incidence of MI, its utility in attenuating symptoms is established. RITA 2 (Randomized Intervention Treatment of Angina 2) is the largest RCT comparing PCI against medical therapy for angina, with a median follow-up of 2.7 years (6). The study population had a representative case mix: 46% had abnormal left ventricular function, 53% had multivessel disease, and 53% had class 2 or worse angina. Percutaneous coronary intervention was successful in 93% of cases, and only 9% of patients received stents. The primary end point of death or MI was higher in the PCI group: 6.3% versus 3.3% ($p = .02$). After hospital discharge, 23% of the medical group eventually required revascularization as compared to 11% for the PCI group. Similar to the results seen in the ACME (A Comparison of Angioplasty with Medical Therapy in the Treatment of Single-Vessel Coronary Disease) trial (7), there was greater symptomatic improvement and improved exercise time in patients who received PCI.

Therefore, at the present time, candidates for revascularization include failed medical therapy, severely impaired lifestyle, a large area of jeopardized myocardium on stress imaging, and the presence of ventricular tachyarrhythmias or moderate to severe left ventricular dysfunction.

D. Silent ischemia. It is not entirely clear as to how to approach these patients given the paucity of data and the problem of detecting silent ischemia. A reasonable approach is to revascularize patients with diabetes mellitus, poor exercise tolerance, a history of coronary artery disease or angina, abnormal left ventricular function, or a finding of substantial jeopardized myocardium on noninvasive testing.

V. Complications

A. Acute complications. There has been a consistent downtrend for complications in PCI (Table 57-4), primarily due to the advent of stents, better antiplatelet regimens, improved technique and effective adjunctive medical therapy.

1. The current incidence of **cardiac mortality** is around 1.0%. However, in high-risk subsets such as unprotected LMT or left main equivalent, PCI still has in-hospital mortality rate of more than 10%.

2. The incidence of **periprocedural Q-wave MI and emergency CABG** has also decreased steadily to 0.4% and approximately 1.0%, respectively. For each of these adverse outcomes, a complication rate of under 0.5% is the benchmark for which operators with a typical case mix should aim.

3. A significant proportion of **periprocedural MACE** (major adverse clinical events) can be attributed to acute vessel closure. The majority of such episodes typically occur during or within 6 hours after the procedure. Predictors include unstable angina presentation, suboptimal anticoagulation, and complex lesion morphology. Dissections and thrombi are the most common underlying mechanisms. Stenting is a particularly suitable remedy for dissections with compromised flow, whereas GPIIb/IIIa blockade probably prevents or attenuates thrombus formation. Episodes of abrupt closure that are promptly and successfully treated without CK elevation have no apparent long-term sequelae. In circumstances where there is persistent occlusion, emergent CABG should be considered if there is ongoing ischemia, hemodynamic instability, or a large region of jeopardized myocardium.

4. The previously rare complications of **coronary perforation and cardiac tamponade** have been observed with increased frequency in the context of aggressive anticoagulation and ablative [rotablator directional atherectomy (DCA) and excimer laser coronary angioplasty (ELCA)] technologies (8). The overall incidence is 0.5%, with an incidence of about 1% for atherectomy devices and 0.1% for standalone PTCA. A larger balloon-to-artery ratio (more than 1.19) is associated

Table 57-4. Percutaneous intervention at the Cleveland Clinic Foundation: patient characteristics, results, and complications

Factor	1993	1994	1995	1996	1997
Patients (no.)	1,841	1,969	2,023	2,158	2,118
Multivessel disease (%)	60.1	62.0	63.5	64.4	65.1
Mean number of arteries treated per patient ($\pm$ standard deviation)	1.55 ± 0.85	1.52 ± 0.85	1.51 ± 0.85	1.60 ± 0.88	1.63 ± 0.92
Average AHA/ACC score (A=1, B_1=2, B_2=3, C=4)	2.78	2.61	2.57	2.52	2.48
Mean age ($\pm$ standard deviation)	62 ± 11	62 ± 11	63 ± 11	63 ± 11	63 ± 11
LVEF $\leq 35\%$ (%)	7.9	8.1	8.7	8.4	11.7
History of prior CABG (%)	33.4	29.9	30.3	29.1	28.8
Presence of diabetes mellitus (%)	25.4	26.0	25.3	27.1	26.9
Acute coronary syndrome presentation (%)	76.0	72.5	65.0	70.1	80.9
Abciximab therapy (%)	0	0	9.9	25.6	32.5
Stent (%): Elective	5.3	5.4	27.9	54.3	62.3
Bail-out	1.7	2.1	4.9	5.6	2.4
Rotational atherectomy (%)	12.2	21.0	20.9	17.1	19.2
All-site procedural success (%)	89.5	91.6	92.8	91.8	92.2
Death (%): Cardiac	1.0	1.3	1.1	1.2	0.9
Noncardiac	0.6	0.7	0.3	0.2	0.4
Emergency CABG (%)	1.7	1.7	0.9	0.9	1.1
Q-wave MI (%)	1.5	1.4	0.3	0.2	0.4
NonQ MI (3$\times$ upper limit of CK MB) (%)	5.1	5.8	6.2	5.7	5.1
Patients receiving blood transfusions (%)	10.3	8.0	6.3	5.0	5.5

AHA/ACC, American Heart Association/American College of Cardiology; LVEF, left ventricular ejection fraction; CABG, coronary artery bypass graft; MI, myocardial infarction; CKMB, creatine kinase MB.

with a slight increase in the risk of perforation. Death or MI occurs in more than half of these cases where extravasated contrast is observed. It is noteworthy that instances of delayed tamponade have been described up to 24 hours post intervention.

When a perforation is detected, platelet antagonists should be stopped and reversed while immediate local tamponade is performed. This is accomplished by a 10- to 20-minute balloon inflation at 2 to 4 atm across the perforation. If this is not successful, a more prolonged inflation (up to 45 minutes) should be applied, possibly with a perfusion balloon to maintain distal flow. No further heparin should be given, but reversal with protamine is done only in cases of free contrast extravasation, since some anticoagulation is still required to prevent vessel thrombosis. Afterward a pulmonary arterial catheter should be inserted for monitoring, and the patient should be admitted to the cardiac intensive care unit with serial echocardiograms performed. If balloon tamponade fails, the patient should be typed and crossed for blood, a surgeon should be notified promptly and percardiocentesis performed expeditiously. On occasions where the perforation involves an end artery (e.g., tip of the posterior descending artery or diagonal artery), local hemostasis may be attained by deployment of new generation embolic coils (Bernstein coils or "liquid metal").

5. Judging by the frequency of postprocedural CK elevations even in the absence of acute closure, the incidence of **intracoronary embolization** is probably underestimated. Up to 8% of patients have a CK release more than three times the upper limit of normal, which has been linked to an increased long-term mortality in several retrospective series. This phenomenon is more typically encountered in degenerated vein graft interventions, complex lesions, and highly thrombogenic milieus such as in acute MI. It is mitigated by the use of GPIIb/IIIa inhibitors.

6. Significant **bleeding,** usually from the arterial access site, has diminished in spite of increased usage of antiplatelet regimes. A variety of factors have probably contributed to this: reduced anticoagulation regimens, more vigilant monitoring of activated clotting time (ACT) and activated partial thromboplastin time (aPTT) levels, smaller and more trackable devices, earlier sheath removal, and avoiding routine venous sheath placement.

B. **Long-term failure: the problem of restenosis.** The Achilles heel of PCI is the relatively high restenosis rates (Table 57-5). Although this rarely manifests as death (1%/year) or MI (2.5%/year), the morbidity and cost of recurrent angina and repeat revascularization and hospitalization remain substantial.

1. The **mechanism** of restenosis consists of arterial contracture (recoil) and a tissue hyperplastic response to injury. Lumen loss is predominantly due to vessel recoil for PTCA and neointimal hyperplasia for stented vessels.

2. The **incidence** of restenosis ranges from 16% to 74% depending on a variety of factors, including the clinical presentation and lesion characteristics. Typically, 80% of restenosis will be declared within 3 months of PTCA, and almost all cases will have accrued by 6 months post PTCA. It is also noteworthy that close to 4 of 10 patients who remain asymptomatic actually have clinically silent restenosis (9).

3. It is likewise important to bear in mind that **not all symptoms after PCI are attributable to restenosis.** Symptom persistence/recurrence within the first month are more typical for incomplete revascularization, and those after 6 months were almost always secondary to new lesions.

4. Despite intensive investigations in this field, the ability to predict which individual patient will develop restenosis remains severely limited. Characteristics that are associated with increased risk are diabetes mel-

Table 57-5.   Rates of restenosis and MACE from selected large clinical trials

Device/ procedure	Setting/patient population	Year	N	Restenosis (%)	1 year MACE (%)
Stent (heparin-coated PS)	*Benestent II:* 12% DM; no AMI, 42% UA; 59% B2, 0.5% C, 28% calcified, de novo lesions, mean lesion length ~8.5 mm		414	16[†]	16
PTCA		95–96	413	30	22
Rotablator (high-speed)	*ERBAC:* 16% DM; no AMI, 17% UA; 64% B2, 13% C, 40% calcified, mean lesion length ~11 mm		231	57	46
ELCA		91–93	232	59	48
PTCA			222	51	37*
DCA (7-F cutters)	*BOAT:* 14% DM; no AMI, ~71% UA; ~5% 6% thrombus, ostial, 9% bifurcation, 18% calcified, 26% with lesion length > 10 mm		497	31*	21
PTCA		94–95	492	40	25

* $0.001 < p < 0.05$; [†] $p < 0.001$.
BOAT, Balloon versus Optimal Atherectomy Trial; ERBAC, Excimer Laser, Rotablator and Balloon Angioplasty Comparison; PS, Palmaz-Schatz; PTCA, percutaneous transluminal coronary angioplasty; ELCA, excimer laser coronary angioplasty; DCA, directional coronary atherectomy; DM, diastolic murmur; AMI, acute myocardial infarction; UA, unstable angina; MACE, major adverse cardiac event.

litus, history of restenosis, unstable angina presentation, chronic total occlusions, long lesion length (more than 10 mm), vessel involved [saphenous vein graft (SVG) disease > left anterior descending artery > right coronary artery or circumflex artery], small vessel diameter (under 3.0 mm), ostial lesions, and suboptimal postprocedural percent stenosis or minimal luminal diameter.

   5. There is no good preventive therapy for restenosis. Stenting attenuates restenosis rates compared with PTCA (see Table 57-5). Radiation therapy is an emerging modality for this problem.

 C. **Risk stratification by vessel and lesion characteristics.** The American College of Cardiology/American Heart Association (ACC/AHA) score is a three-level classification system for lesion morphology to predict success of PTCA (Table 57-6). This was estimated to be greater than 85% for type A lesions, 60% to 85% for type B lesions, and less than 60% for type C lesions, with a corresponding increasing gradient of acute complications. However, even with meticulous scrutiny, preprocedural coronary lesion morphology

Table 57-6.   American College of Cardiology/American Heart Association lesion morphology score

TYPE A LESIONS (SUCCESS >85%; COMPLICATION ≤ 2%)	
Discrete (<10 mm length)	Little or no calcification
Concentric	Less than totally occlusive
Readily accessible	Nonostial in location
Nonangulated segment, <45 degrees	No major branch involvement
Smooth contour	Absence of thrombus
TYPE B LESIONS (MODERATE SUCCESS 60 TO 85%; COMPLICATIONS 10%)	
Tubular (10–20 mm length)	Moderate to heavy calcification
Eccentric	Total occlusion <3 months old
Moderate tortuosity of proximal segment	Ostial in location
Moderately angulated segment, >45 degrees, <90 degrees	Bifurcation lesions requiring double guidewires
Irregular contour	Some thrombus present
TYPE C LESIONS (LOW SUCCESS, <60%; COMPLICATIONS 20%)	
Diffuse (>2 cm length)	Total occlusions >3 months old
Excessive tortuosity of proximal segment	Inability to protect major side branches
Extremely angulated segments (>90 degree) lesions	Degenerated vein grafts with friable lesions

Modified from Ryan TJ, 1988.

(coupled with left ventricular function and modified ACC/AHA morphology scoring) can only account for 9% of the variance in complication risk (10). Furthermore, this scheme was devised during the prestent era and is considered to be outdated. Nevertheless, specific lesion characteristics such as presence of thrombus, occlusion, aged vein grafts, type C and some type B characteristics still retain some predictive capacity.

1. **Thrombus** can be found in up to 40% of patients referred to the catheterization lab for acute coronary syndromes and is one of the strongest angiographic predictors of adverse events. Within the context of PCI, the incidences of acute closure, distal embolization, and no-reflow phenomenon are all increased, and recognition of thrombus should prompt the use of platelet GPIIb/IIIa inhibitor. A high degree of suspicion must therefore be maintained, since angiography has poor sensitivity for thrombi detection, although specificity may be adequate.

2. The attrition rate of **SVG**s is 15% to 20% by 1 year, 1% to 2% per year up to 6 years, and up to 4% per year thereafter. The management of the degenerated SVG (defined as very diffuse disease spanning at least half of the graft's length) is a challenging task. Reasonable acute success rates are attainable but restenosis rates of up to 60% have been reported. The Saphenous Vein De Novo Trial (SAVED) investigators trial likewise demonstrated an absence of restenosis attenuation upon randomized comparison of Palmaz-Schatz (PS) stenting to PTCA for discrete SVG disease (37% versus 46%; p = NS). Nonetheless, there were short-term advantages with regard to superior angiographic outcomes and a reduction in major cardiac events (TVR and non-Q MI) with stenting. Abciximab has not been shown to improve outcome, perhaps because of the nature of the emboli (cholesterol debris). Devices to prevent embolization are under investigation.

3. **Long and diffuse lesions** have been markers for acute complications and poor long-term results. It is difficult to sort out the contribution of this feature per se because long lesions by nature tend to overlap with bifurcating, angulated, or small-caliber segments and contain more plaque. There is a significantly higher incidence of angiographic resteno-

sis for lesions greater than 15 mm in length or with vessel reference diameters smaller than 2.5 mm. Preliminary data do suggest that features such as presence of diabetes and small vessel size may potentiate any adverse impact that might accompany long lesions.

4. The **chronically occluded artery** presents a special challenge to the interventionalist and may be encountered in as many as a third of patients referred to angiography. Poor acute procedural success rates (approximately 65%) have been reported, and predictors of failure are occlusion of more than 3 months duration, absence of antegrade flow, angiographically abrupt lesion appearance, and the presence of bridging collaterals. Restenosis rates were 74% for the PTCA arm of the Stenting in Chronic Coronary Occlusion (SICCO) study, compared to 32% in stented patients, with corresponding TVR rates of 42% and 22%.

5. **Unprotected left main coronary stenosis PCI** is still controversial because of the high attrition rates: in-hospital mortality of 69% and 11% for patients presenting with and without acute MI, respectively, and 1-year mortality of up to 10.7% unheralded deaths. These statistics argue for circumspect application of PCI to this subgroup of patients until further understanding of the causes of death becomes available.

VI. Device overview
A. Interventional devices

1. **Balloons** are used in almost all cases, sometimes as sole therapy, but mostly as secondary therapy in conjunction with other devices, to pre- or postdilate lesions, and to deliver stents. However, even by the early 1990s, conventional balloon angioplasty was still associated with a high incidence of abrupt closure, emergency bypass, and 6-month TVR. The introduction of **stents** has relegated the strategy of stand alone PTCA to less than 25% of today's cases. However, modern day PTCA is associated with improved rates of target lesion revascularization (13.8% to 19.7%). It has been postulated that these trends may be attributable to more aggressive balloon sizing and dilatations with the availability of backup stenting. Given the cost of stents to the health care system and the relative intractability of diffuse in-stent restenosis, coupled with the margin of safety that platelet GPIIb/IIIa inhibitors offer, a strategy of provisional stenting for select low-risk lesions may obtain equivalent outcome. A preliminary report from optimal coronary balloon angioplasty with provisional stenting versus primary stent (OCBAS) trial supports this viewpoint.

2. **Intracoronary stents** have revolutionized interventional practice in the 1990s. Of the 750,000 coronary interventions projected for the United States in the year 2000, close to 70% will involve at least one stent. Multiple stent designs and materials are available with varying degrees of radiopacity and ease of delivery. No stent has convincingly demonstrated improved restenosis rates compared with the others.

   a. **Advantages.** Stents have increased procedural success rates, even for lesions that previously would have been rated to be unfavorable for conventional balloon angioplasty. They have played a key role in decreasing the need for emergency CABG to around 1.0% (see Table 57-4). They are also estimated to decrease restenosis and the need for TVR at 6-month follow-up by 5 to 6 patients per 100 treated in Balloon-Expandable-Stent Trial (BENESTENT) type lesions (11). Combination therapy with GPIIb/IIIa inhibitors offers even greater benefit. Data from the EPISTENT trial revealed improved 6-month death/MI/TVR rates in the stent–abciximab group compared with the stent–placebo group: 13% versus 18.3%, $p = .003$.

   b. **Disadvantages**

      (1) **Generalizability.** It has been estimated that only about 20% of the cases encountered in practice would meet BENESTENT criteria, which required patients to have stable angina due to

a de novo lesion under 15 mm in length in a vessel greater than 3 mm in diameter that supplied normal myocardium (11). Although EPISTENT and other recent trials have shown broader applicability (2), there remains a substantial proportion of lesions that are either inaccessible (those in severely tortuous or calcified vessels) or not recommended for stenting (small and diffusely diseased vessels).

   (2) **Cost.** Worldwide, stent sales are projected to exceed $3 billion in the year 2000. In some countries, CABG is the cheaper alternative when more than two stents are required for a procedure.

c. **Complications**

   (1) **Subacute thrombosis** must always be in the differential diagnosis of recurrent chest pain occurring within 3 weeks of stent implantation. This problem has diminished from approximately 3.6% to 0.6% due to a better antiplatelet regimen (aspirin and ticlopidine) (12) and improved stent deployment. However, there is a retreat from high-pressure balloon inflations as preliminary reports show little difference in MACE and restenosis between mean pressures of 17 atm versus 11 atm inflations.

   (2) **In-stent restenosis,** especially when diffuse, can be very difficult to manage. Predictors include presence of diabetes, long lesions, suboptimal deployment, multiple sequential stents, and small vessel caliber.

   (3) Attempts at stenting less optimal targets (eg., small tortuous vessel, angulated or heavily calcified lesion, and the like) have occasionally resulted in **forced deployment into more proximal vessel segments, or stent embolization typically to peripheral vessels.** The former confers an unplanned risk of restenosis to non–target vessel segments, whereas adverse sequelae with the latter have been exceedingly rare.

   (4) **Thrombotic thrombocytopenic purpura (TTP)** has been reported with the use of ticlopidin.

   (5) Rarely, injudiciously placed multiple stents may present an obstacle to future bypass grafting to that vessel.

3. **Percutaneous transluminal rotational atherectomy** employs an intracoronary drill and has earned its niche by allowing treatment of undilatable fibrocalcific lesions. This procedure can be useful in lesions with severe superficial calcium, ostial and bifurcation stenosis, diffusely diseased vessels, chronic total occlusions, and in-stent restenosis. However, several RCTs comparing it with balloon angioplasty have not shown any benefit with regard to long-term restenosis rates or MACE (see Table 57-5). Its specific utility might be to open an otherwise refractory lesion to allow stent deployment for more enduring results, but this remains to be proven.

   Adequate operator training and experience is critical to help avoid potentially devastating complications such as vessel perforation, cardiac tamponade, complete heart block, or no-reflow phenomenon. Increased frequencies of low-grade chest pressure and slightly higher CK levels postprocedurally have also been noted.

4. **Other devices. Directional atherectomy** was the first catheter-based device approved after coronary balloons, but its use decreased dramatically after early RCT reports of excess deaths and MI at 1 year and high rates of embolization of debris in vein graft interventions. **Excimer laser coronary angioplasty** has been associated with a higher rate of transient vessel closure, perforation, emergency surgery, and possibly restenosis. It is used rarely for refractory in-stent restenosis. The **Angiojet** (Possis Medical Inc., Minneapolis, MN.) is a suction device that was envisioned for removing thrombus. It is undergoing clinical evaluation and has been observed to provoke significant bradycar-

dia that requires temporary pacing. The **Acolysis** (Angiosonics, USA) device utilizes ultrasound energy to dissolve thrombus and is currently being investigated for clinical use.

B. **Therapeutic adjuncts**

1. **Radiation-based therapy** was associated with a striking reduction of angiographic restenosis (from 54% to 17%) in a double-blind placebo-controlled randomized trial utilizing a catheter-based gamma source plus stenting in 55 patients with restenosis (13). For de novo lesions, lower-than-expected restenosis rates were seen with the application of adjunctive catheter-delivered β radiation, allowing for reduced treatment time and operator exposure. Several RCTs involving coronary arteries will be available soon. It appears that the desired dose falls between 800 to 3,000 cGy, as low doses can actually provoke cellular proliferation, while higher doses carry the risk of vessel wall injury that could result in perforation and pseudoaneurysm formation. Less penetrating β emitters (liquid-filled balloon catheter or impregnated stents) may be easier to handle in the catheterization laboratory and are also under evaluation. However, failures have been reported because of radiation dose tail-off, with consequent induction of cellular proliferation in the segments just beyond the stent edges. The long-term safety of this modality still must be confirmed.

2. In high-risk situations, a 5-Fr **temporary pacemaker wire** is inserted via a femoral vein and typically set on backup mode. These include anticipated bradycardia unresponsive to IV atropine, especially in the patient who has marginal hemodynamic reserve, or when significant debulking is planned such as with the rotablator in the arterial territory supplying the atrioventricular node.

3. **Prophylactic intraaortic balloon counterpulsation** should be considered for patients with cardiogenic shock or severe decompensated heart failure, and in interventions involving the sole remaining conduit or unprotected left main artery. The operator should always anticipate the possible need for adjunctive or rescue IABP counterpulsation in high-risk patients. In certain situations, having ready arterial access (i.e., a 5-Fr arterial sheath in the opposite groin) might be prudent. Complications as reported in a placebo-controlled RCT utilizing an IABP in the setting of acute MI included vascular repair or thrombectomy (5% versus 2%), severe bleeding (2% versus 1%), and a mean blood transfusion rate of 1.3 versus 0.9 units.

4. **Percutaneous cardiopulmonary bypass support (CPS)** provides systemic perfusion to vital organs such as the brain and kidneys independent of status of ventricular function or cardiac rhythm (e.g., asystole or incessant ventricular tachycardia) and therefore serves as a valuable last resort. To provide optimal benefit, CPS must be applied within 15 to 20 minutes of hemodynamic collapse. It is important to realize that CPS does not provide the afterload reduction that IABP counterpulsation affords, nor does it spare the myocardium from ischemia due to the effects of vessel closure.

C. **Diagnostic adjuncts**

1. **Imaging modalities**

a. **Intravascular ultrasound (IVUS)** is an important complementary imaging tool that generates a cross-sectional tomographic assessment of both the lumen and, in contrast to angiography, also the vessel wall. It is considered the gold standard for measurement of vessel dimensions such as normal reference diameter, vessel cross-sectional area (CSA), and minimal luminal diameter. This technology has provided valuable insights into vessel wall anatomy and physiology, and device-specific responses to injury. In clinical practice, IVUS has been helpful in the evaluation of indeterminate lesions, hazy angiographic appearance, or for apparent LMT disease.

Studies with first-generation stents have repeatedly proven the incremental value of IVUS in optimizing stent deployment (14). As many as half of all stents are "suboptimally" deployed in spite of a 0% or less residual stenosis measurement based on quantitative coronary angiography. There is also no question that IVUS allows for more elegant device selection and sizing (e.g., more precise balloon to artery sizing, or use of rotablator for unsuspected near-circumferential vessel calcification). However, definitive proof is still forthcoming whether or not IVUS can modify long-term clinical outcomes to justify the time and expense it entails.

    b. Angioscopy has special utility in differentiating thrombus from dissection. With angioscopy as the gold standard, thrombus has been shown to be angiographically silent in as many as 48.3% of cases and manifests itself as haziness in 21.3%, a filling defect in 15%, and a hanging defect in 15% of cases. Currently, angioscopy is used only for research applications.

2. Physiologic assessment of the coronary lesion can be very helpful in assessing lesions of intermediate angiographic severity, an in-laboratory stress test that will permit objective decision making about the need for PCI.

    a. Coronary flow reserve (CFR) and myocardial fractional flow reserve (FFR) utilize intracoronary Doppler flow velocities or pressures after hyperemic challenge with adenosine. Coronary flow reserve takes the ratio of hyperemic to baseline flow, with the cutoff of more than 2.0 demonstrated to have good correlation with normal perfusion. The Doppler Endpoints Balloon Angioplasty Trial Europe (DEBATE) study showed that a post angioplasty CFR of more than 2.5, in conjunction with a residual stenosis of less than 35%, has modest predictive value for stand alone balloon angioplasty for midterm outcomes. Coronary flow reserve has been hampered by its sensitivity to abnormalities in the myocardial resistance vessels imposed by left ventricular hypertrophy, ischemia, or impaired left ventricular function. Taking the ratio of CFR between diseased and nondiseased vessel (relative CFR) may overcome this limitation, but further validation is needed.

    b. Fractional flow reserve is less variable than CFR during altered hemodynamic conditions. It is the ratio of the distal pressure versus that proximal to the stenosis after adenosine infusion. An FFR less than 0.75 indicates significant stenosis, and an FFR greater than 0.9 is a criterion for an adequate result post PCI (15).

    c. Translesional pressure gradient is less frequently used, mainly because it requires the use of a 2.2-Fr Tracker catheter, which may decrease the lesional cross-sectional area further, consequently overestimating stenosis severity in vessels less than 2.5 mm in diameter. Under ideal conditions, a translesional gradient of less than 15 mm Hg is indicative of less significant stenosis.

3. Pulmonary artery (PA) catheters are not commonly used since direct assessment of left ventricular end-diastolic pressure is feasible during left heart catheterization, and in consideration of minimizing vessel punctures. However, **PA catheters are inserted in high-risk situations** where an on-line measure of filling pressures is advisable. This applies to patients with severe and decompensated heart failure or valvular stenosis, or PCI to a sole remaining conduit or unprotected LMT with low cardiac reserve. A PA catheter may also be considered if a complicated postinterventional course requiring attentive hemodynamic management is anticipated, or for expectant management of cases of coronary perforation.

VII. Adjunctive pharmacologic therapy

    A. Heparin. Adequate periprocedural anticoagulation is critical for optimal PCI outcome. Heparin catalyzes the effect of antithrombin III on coagulative proteinases such as factors II, XII, XI, IX, X and tissue factor VIIa. An ACT level of more than 300 seconds on the HemoTec (Medtronic Inc., Minneapolis, MN.)

system (approximately equivalent to 350 seconds on the Hemochron [International Technidyne Corp., Edison, N.J.] system) appears to be a safe range for avoiding acute vessel closure that is due to thrombus formation (16). In general, an initial IV heparin bolus of 100 µg/kg is adequate to achieve target ACT in most instances, with additional doses titrated according to the ACT level. Patients with acute coronary syndromes typically have slightly higher heparin requirements to attain the same ACT levels. Dose adjustment is necessary if GPIIb/IIIa antagonists are used concurrently (see below).

The **duration of therapy** is dependent on the setting. In the context of primary PCI for acute MI, postprocedural heparin should probably be continued for 48 hours. In the elective setting, no further heparin post procedure is required unless there is a suboptimal result, residual thrombus, or dissection. In these circumstances, it might be prudent to continue the infusion for at least an additional 12 to 24 hours if a GPIIb/IIIa antagonist is not used.

B. Direct thrombin inhibitors. The advantages these agents have over heparin are efficacy against clot-bound thrombin, resistance to inactivation by platelet factor 4 and thrombospondin, and nondependence on antithrombin III pathways. The practical advantage of direct antithrombins is their more predictable and consistent anticoagulant effect compared to heparin, decreasing the need for serial blood level monitoring. Unfortunately, cost and ease of reversal remain problems.

1. **Hirudin** is the best studied agent in this class. In randomized comparisons to heparin for acute coronary syndromes, there was a statistically significant reduction in death and MI at 30 days in the GUSTO IIb trial, and equivalence as an adjunct to fibrinolytic therapy for acute MI in the TIMI 9B trial. The rates of bleeding were similar among treatment groups in both trials.

   In the context of PCI, **Hirulog,** a synthetic analog of hirudin, was observed to reduce the broad composite endpoint of death, MI, abrupt closure, repeat revascularization, and the need for IABP therapy in patients with postinfarction angina but not for unstable angina. The bleeding rate was significantly lower for the Hirulog group.

   The current recommended dosage of hirudin is a 0.2-µg bolus followed by 0.1 µg/kg per hour infusion to maintain an aPTT of 50 to 75 seconds. The specific niche of hirudin at this time is as a proven alternative to heparin in cases of heparin-induced thrombocytopenia.

2. In contrast to unfractionated heparins (UHs), **low molecular weight heparins (LMWHs)** have high activity against factor Xa as well as thrombin, superb bioavailability, and a lower tendency to cause osteoporosis and thrombocytopenia. Several RCTs have validated their equivalence and possible superiority to UH in terms of efficacy and safety under a variety of circumstances including acute MI, non-Q-wave MI, unstable angina, silent ischemia, PCI with or without stenting, and venous thrombosis. The efficacy of LMWHs has been demonstrated up to 1 year in patients with acute coronary syndromes.

   Enoxaparin is given subcutaneously 1 mg/kg every 12 hours for acute coronary syndromes (as opposed to 30 mg every 12 hours for deep venous thrombosis prophylaxis). ACT or aPTT monitoring is not useful, and protamine can only reverse its anti–factor Xa effect by a maximum of 60%.

C. Platelet GPIIb/IIIa receptor antagonists

1. **Background.** Antagonists to the platelet GPIIb/IIIa receptor have been proven to have a mitigating role for periprocedural adverse events (17). There are up to 80,000 copies of these integrins on the platelet cell surface, serving as ligands for fibrinogen crosslinkage, the final common pathway for platelet aggregation and thrombus formation even under arterial shear stress conditions.

2. **Benefits.** To date, more than 30,000 patients have been enrolled in 12 RCTs evaluating GPIIb/IIIa antagonists in the context of acute coronary syndromes, and half of these trials have involved PCI (see Table 57-3).

Pooled data from the five RCTs using abciximab demonstrated a 5.2% absolute reduction in 30-day rates of death, MI, and urgent revascularization. This advantage is maintained through to 6 months, but there is no attenuation of the target revascularization rate. In addition, these benefits are consistent across all subsets of patients and are independent of the percutaneous device used.

There is also a probable synergism conferred by these agents when used as an adjunct to direct PTCA for acute MI. RAPPORT, a 483-patient RCT, suggested benefit in terms of 30-day composite end points (5.8% versus 11.2%; $p = .03$), but at the cost of a significant rate of major bleeding in the abciximab arm (16.6% versus 9.5%; $p = .02$). These findings await further refinement by several ongoing large multicenter RCTs.

Put into perspective, the combination abciximab with stenting can potentially prevent 7 deaths, 51 MIs (including 2 Q-wave and 43 large non-Q-wave MIs), 10 urgent and 20 elective revascularization procedures per 1,000 patients treated. Ad hoc ("rescue") utilization of abciximab for thrombus or dissection is an attractive option from the standpoint of cost effectiveness. There are currently conflicting data, and this strategy will need validation in a randomized trial.

3. The main trade-offs, aside from **cost**, are **bleeding and thrombocytopenia. Ongoing bleeding** is an absolute contraindication, while relative contraindications include recent CVA; known intracranial neoplasm, aneurysm or arteriovenous malformation; systolic blood pressure higher than 180 or diastolic blood pressure higher than 100 mm Hg; known hemorrhagic diathesis; and recent major surgery. Additional precautions include the avoidance of central venous or arterial lines. Early sheath removal is encouraged and may be performed once ACT levels reach 140 seconds or lower.

Thrombocytopenia has been observed in 1% to 5% of patients, but the true incidence is probably lower, since these estimates were against a background of heparin therapy which itself carries immunogenic properties. Adverse clinical events can be avoided with serial monitoring of platelets at 2 and 24 hours after abciximab bolus with timely discontinuation of the drug. Platelet transfusions are required only if active bleeding is present or for threatened bleeding with a platelet count of less than 20,000. Readministration of abciximab has not been associated with diminished efficacy or increased rates of thrombocytopenia.

4. **Current recommended doses for abciximab** include a preprocedural IV bolus of 0.25 mg/kg body weight followed by an IV infusion of 0.125 µg/kg per minute for 12 hours. The target ACT is 201 to 250 seconds, which is usually achieved by giving heparin at a lower initial bolus dose of 50 µg/kg IV. For patients who already arrive at the catheterization laboratory on heparin, an ACT should be drawn with further anticoagulation titrated accordingly. Abciximab typically raises the ACT an additional 30 to 50 seconds.

5. **Reversal.** Should a patient require emergent surgery, the following should be done: (a) Stop the abciximab infusion. (b) Draw blood for type and cross. (c) Give two pooled units of platelet transfusion (at least 5 to 6 platelet concentrates/pool), if possible 20 to 30 minutes after drug cessation. This reverses platelet receptor blockade to less than 50%, thus normalizing all biochemical parameters of platelet aggregation and coagulation. (d) Notify the anesthesiologist to anticipate a lower intraoperative heparin requirement.

D. **Adenosine 5-diphosphate (ADP) antagonists.** Ticlopidine and clopidogrel are thienopyridine derivatives that block ADP-mediated platelet aggregation without affecting the cyclooxygenase pathway.

1. **Ticlopidine** was first used extensively for cerebrovascular disease where its superiority to aspirin (ASA) has been proven, along with an apparently comparable safety profile. The widely used regimen is ticlopidine 500 mg PO loading dose at least 3 days pre-PCI whenever possi-

ble, based on anticipated near-maximal antiplatelet effect by 4 days. If the patient receives stents, the maintenance dose is 250 mg b.i.d. for 2 to 3 weeks with lifelong ASA which has also been shown to be an effective pharmacologic adjunct to stenting to prevent subacute thrombosis. However there is a <1% incidence of significant neutropenia, typically within the first 3 months of therapy. In addition, a recent report has associated this drug with life-threatening TTP which is unpredictable in spite of platelet surveillance every 2 weeks, and has also been documented to occur with less than a week's course of therapy.

2. **Clopidogrel** is an alternative agent that is being increasingly used. Evidence for its efficacy and safety comes from the Clopidogrel Versus Aspirin in Patients at Risk of Ischemic Events (CAPRIE) trial. This involved 19,000 patients with recent MI or ischemic stroke, and symptomatic peripheral vascular disease randomized to clopidogrel 75 mg/day versus ASA 325 mg/day. There was a modest reduction in overall vascular events, but no difference in the subgroup of recent MI patients (18). More importantly, follow-up of these patients up to 3 years has not uncovered any excess incidence of TTP. Although data are lacking for clopidogrel as an adjunct to stenting, it may serve as a reasonable alternative given the concerns with ticlopidine. The recommended loading dose is 300 mg PO (preferably at least 2 hours prior to PCI based on anticipated near-maximal antiplatelet effect by 2 hours), followed by 75 mg/day for a month if the patient receives stents, along with lifelong ASA therapy.

VIII. **Operator characteristics.** Several studies have indicated an inverse association between operator and institutional volume with complication rates. The 1998 ACC/AHA guidelines for PTCA recommended the maintenance of an annual procedural volume of more than 75 cases per operator and an annual hospital case load of more than 400 patients, barring a few exceptions. Percutaneous coronary intervention should be done only in settings where there is ready on-site access to emergency cardiac surgery. Finally, the guidelines call for each center to have an institutional review mechanism for credentialing and quality maintenance (19).

The mandate of the interventionalist includes following through with aggressive secondary prevention after the procedure. The window of patient suggestibility during and after PCI is an opportune time to impress on the patient the urgency of modifying his or her lifestyle.

IX. **Other catheter-based therapies for the heart**
   A. **Valvuloplasty**
      1. **Percutaneous mitral valvuloplasty**
         a. **Background. Percutaneous mitral valvuloplasty (PMV)** has emerged as the therapy of choice for suitable candidates afflicted with mitral stenosis (MS) and has been proven to be as effective, safe, and durable (up to 7 years follow-up), when compared to both closed and open mitral commissurotomy (20). It must be kept in mind, however, that these results were obtained from Indian and Tunisian study populations that tend to consist of younger patients with more pliable valves that have less calcification.
         b. The **key indication** for PMV is the presence of lifestyle-limiting symptoms. Exceptions to this rule are as follows: (i) anticipated difficulty for the pregnant patient; (ii) patients with severe MS who require major extracardiac surgery; and (iii) patients with a previous history of systemic embolism who are at high risk for a recurrent event. Absolute contraindications are left atrial thrombus and severe MR. Severe calcification, severe fusion of submitral apparatus, and valvular disease that require open heart surgery constitute relative contraindications.
         c. The **acute results** of PMV on selected patients from different series has been a doubling of the valve area, a slight increase in cardiac

index, a marked decrease in left atrial pressure, and a decrease in pulmonary arterial pressure and resistance. Exercise capacity can be anticipated to improve following these hemodynamic changes.

d. **Major procedural complications** include a 1.4% incidence of in-hospital mortality (commonly related to cardiac perforation or tamponade), less than 2% stroke or transient ischemic attack, less than 4% severe MR, and 1% mitral valve surgery. These may be attenuated by meticulous technique, transesophageal echocardiographic guidance, and a stepwise approach with interval echo interrogation for MR. The incidence of significant atrial septal defect as a consequence of transseptal puncture and balloon crossing is much less common with current lower profile equipment. Other complications attendant to the practice of catheterization also apply.

e. **Patient preparation** should include a **thorough evaluation of all cardiac valves** and assessment of other potential causes of pulmonary hypertension. A **transesophageal echocardiogram** should be obtained to screen for left atrial or left atrial appendage thrombus. **Coumadin must be discontinued 3 to 4 days prior to PMV.** The patient who is at high risk for systemic embolism should be hospitalized to receive interim heparin coverage as international normalized ratio levels decline.

2. **Balloon aortic valvuloplasty**

a. **Indication.** The treatment for calcific aortic stenosis (AS) is aortic valve replacement, and balloon aortic valvuloplasty (BAV) should only be considered for patients who are not surgical candidates. The rare indications for BAV are (i) as bailout for acutely decompensated AS requiring prolonged IABP support, mechanical ventilation, or pressor support; or in the context of acute MI; (ii) as palliation for severe and refractory symptoms in a patient who is not a surgical candidate or has limited longevity due to a comorbidity; (iii) as a bridge procedure during pregnancy, or (iv) for the high surgical risk patient with severe comorbidities (e.g., coronary obstructive pulmonary disease) who requires major noncardiac surgery.

b. The **typical result** as reported from several series is an increase in aortic valve area from 0.5 to 0.6 cm² to 0.9 cm², with a modest improvement in cardiac output. BAV offers an improved quality of life for the short term. However, the process of elastic recoil may begin as early as hours post BAV, with progressive fibrosis and ossification leading to an almost 100% restenosis rate by 1 year.

c. **Procedural complications** include cerebrovascular events (1% to 2%), severe aortic insufficiency (less than 1%), and sudden hemodynamic collapse due to aortic rupture, cardiac perforation, acute MI, or left ventricular perforation (less than 1%). The most common complication is injury to the femoral artery (10% to 15%). The in-hospital mortality rate ranges from 3.5% to 13.5%, a reflection of the case mix of severely ill patients.

B. **Percutaneous transluminal septal myocardial ablation for hypertrophic obstructive cardiomyopathy.** This investigational technique employs selective intracoronary injection of alcohol into the proximal septal perforators (from the left anterior descending or, rarely, diagonal or circumflex arteries). The objective is to reduce myocardial septal thickening by means of myocardial infarction.

In the largest published case series (n = 100) involving percutaneous transluminal septal myocardial ablation, 85% of patients had a more than 50% early reduction in left ventricular outflow tract gradient, and 11% developed heart block requiring a permanent pacemaker. At 3 months, 39% and 45% had complete and more than 50% resolution of left ventricular outflow tract gradients, respectively. There was also a mean improvement of 1.67 points in terms of New York Heart Association functional class status. There were

2 deaths (1 ventricular fibrillation, 1 pulmonary embolism) and several refractory cases that have required a repeat procedure targeting a separate septal perforator artery. It remains to be seen as to whether this procedure will turn out to be a viable option for one of the heterogeneous subsets of this relatively rare disease.

C. **Percutaneous transluminal myocardial revascularization.** Surgical and percutaneous laser myocardial revascularization therapy for symptomatic patients poorly suited for CABG or PCI is currently undergoing evaluation. Initial nonblinded surgical RCTs suggest a possible mortality benefit (as an adjunct to CABG) and improvements in New York Heart Association class and angina. Angiogenesis and local denervation are probable mechanisms as channel patency is not long term. Durability, possibility of placebo effect, and high perioperative mortality in unstable patients remain concerns. Several percutaneous transluminal myocardial revascularization systems are being evaluated with phase II trials.

D. **Percutaneous balloon pericardiotomy.** This technique involves balloon dilatation via a percutaneous subxiphoid approach to create a pericardial window of approximately 1.5 to 2 cm in diameter to allow fluid drainage into the pleural space. It is an important option for cancer patients with anticipated short life expectancy who present with impending cardiac tamponade.

E. **Local delivery: drugs, genes, and coated stents**
   1. The relative success of the local application of mechanical therapies to coronary lesions has encouraged parallel research in local drug delivery. By confining an agent to the lesion site, greater local concentrations can be achieved with reduced potential for systemic toxicity. While several agents have shown promise in animal models of restenosis, to date no drug (heparin, LMWH, c-myc antisense oligonucleotides, etc.) has shown benefit in humans.
   2. In contrast, the feasibility of site-specific gene transfection to induce therapeutic angiogenesis has been shown in a landmark case series. Patients with rest pain due to peripheral vascular ischemia were treated with naked cDNA encoding for vascular endothelial growth factor impregnated into hydrogel-coated balloons. Amelioration of pain and hemodynamic deficit was documented in some patients, and limb salvage was observed in one (21). However, remote cutaneous spider angiomata have been observed in some of these patients, and concerns remain regarding the potential hazards of ectopic neovascular formation and permissive effects on neoplastic proliferation. Clinical trials involving coronary arteries and SVGs are under way.
   3. **Special stents.** There is also nascent technology involving polymers such as polyamine-dextran sulfate coating to allow drug impregnation of stents. Such a stent with covalently bound heparin was evaluated in BENESTENT II (see also Table 57-5) with favorable results (11).

      Radioactive stents are undergoing clinical evaluation (see VI.B), but there has been difficulty in ensuring uniform lesion dosimetry to avoid a penumbra effect. Nonetheless, this entire field of research holds the promise of yielding safer targeted therapies for both de novo and restenotic disease.

X. **Appendix: Procedure overview.** Only general principles will be discussed here to provide the noninterventionalist a conceptual understanding of procedure. For details and specific instructions, we refer the reader to the suggested references at the end of this chapter.

A. **Approaches.** Arterial access has been traditionally obtained via the femoral arteries. This provides a relatively large conduit through which a wide range of equipment can be passed rapidly and safely, allowing the operator strategic flexibility should a critical situation arise (e.g., urgent need for IABP or CPS). The current generation of balloons and stents allows for easier brachial and radial approaches. These offer the advantage of patient convenience and earlier ambulation, but do not allow a wide margin of error and can sometimes be more uncomfortable to the patient. The latter approaches are particularly useful for the patient who cannot tolerate a supine position due to respiratory or musculoskeletal problems, or for the rare occasion when warfarin anticoagulation cannot be reversed in time for an urgent procedure.

B. Equipment

　1. Eight French sheaths and guide catheters are typically used at present, although 6- and 7-Fr systems are occasionally employed. The general principles of cardiac catheterization apply with additional caution required because of the potential for greater harm that larger equipment and intracoronary manipulations bring. Guide catheters should be chosen that provide coaxiality to the vessel and adequate support to pass the wire, balloons, or stents. The specific situation dictates which catheter feature is important. For instance, if a small guide catheter (6-Fr) is used, an acutely angled primary or secondary curve may become an impediment to smooth stent passage and is therefore best avoided.

　2. Guidewires are the means by which coronary vessels are accessed and serve as the rail over which all other devices travel. Extreme care must be taken not to lose wire position once the wire tip is optimally situated beyond the target lesion, as this can sometimes spell the difference between success or failure. To inadvertently pull it out may mean loss of access to a vessel that has dissected or closed. Allowing it to migrate forward risks vessel perturbation or, worse, perforation.

　　Wires range from very soft, soft, intermediate, stiff, to extra stiff. The latter are useful for difficult lesions or total occlusions, and provide a good rail over which to advance balloons and stents. However, a key principle of wire deployment is to avoid endothelial disruption and therefore softer tipped wires should be used whenever possible. These may also be better at negotiating tortuous vessels.

　　Guidewires typically come in 0.014-in. diameters, except for the rotablator wire, which is 0.009 in. Two lengths are available: short (about 180 cm) and exchange (about 300 cm) lengths. The former is ideal for monorail (as opposed to over-the-wire) systems wherein the guidewire exits the balloon catheter near its leading end, thus allowing for ease of manipulation and obviating the need for an assistant. However, this can become inconvenient when there is a need to take out the wire to change the tip configuration. The option of leaving a balloon inside the target vessel to hold ground already gained is not available. Exchange length guidewires offer direct wire control at all times, but the length sometimes makes wire management a cumbersome task and requires an assistant.

C. Vessel sizing. Current optimal technique designed to minimize restenosis requires an attempt to reduce lesions to less than 30% quantitative coronary angiography (QCA) or less than 20% (visual estimate) stenosis. However, aggressive oversizing of devices increases the risk of major complications and provocation of neointimal hyperplasia. The possibility of restenosis wherever the device is applied must be remembered. Hence, therapy should be reserved for those lesions whose natural history is predicted to be worse than the risk for restenosis.

SUGGESTED READINGS

References

1. Anonymous. Comparison of coronary bypass surgery with angioplasty in patients with multivessel disease. The Bypass Angioplasty Revascularization Investigation (BARI) Investigators [published erratum appears in *N Engl J Med* 1997;336:147]. *N Engl J Med* 1996;335:217–225.
2. Anonymous. Randomised placebo-controlled and balloon-angioplasty-controlled trial to assess safety of coronary stenting with use of platelet glycoprotein-IIb/IIIa blockade. The EPISTENT Investigators. Evaluation of Platelet IIb/IIIa Inhibitor for Stenting. *Lancet* 1998;352:87–92.

3. Anonymous. A clinical trial comparing primary coronary angioplasty with tissue plasminogen activator for acute myocardial infarction. The Global Use of Strategies to Open Occluded Coronary Arteries in Acute Coronary Syndromes (GUSTO IIb) Angioplasty Substudy Investigators [published erratum appears in *N Engl J Med* 1997;337:287]. *N Engl J Med* 1997;336:1621–1628.

4. Brener SJ, Barr LA, Burchenal JEB, et al. A randomized, placebo-controlled trial of platelet glycoprotein IIb/IIIa blockade with primary angioplasty for acute myocardial infarction. *Circulation* 1998;98:734–741.

5. Boden WE, O'Rourke RA, Crawford MH, et al. Outcomes in patients with acute non-Q-wave myocardial infarction randomly assigned to an invasive as compared with a conservative management strategy. Veterans Affairs Non-Q-Wave Infarction Strategies in Hospital (VANQWISH) Trial Investigators. *N Engl J Med* 1998;338:1785–1792.

6. Anonymous. Coronary angioplasty versus medical therapy for angina: the second Randomised Intervention Treatment of Angina (RITA-2) trial. RITA-2 trial participants. *Lancet* 1997;350:461–468.

7. Parisi AF, Folland ED, Hartigan P. A comparison of angioplasty with medical therapy in the treatment of single-vessel coronary artery disease. Veterans Affairs ACME Investigators. *N Engl J Med* 1992;326:10–16.

8. Ellis SG, Ajluni S, Arnold AZ, et al. Increased coronary perforation in the new device era. Incidence, classification, management, and outcome. *Circulation* 1994;90:2725–2730.

9. Nobuyoshi M, Kimura T, Nosaka H, et al. Restenosis after successful percutaneous transluminal coronary angioplasty: serial angiographic follow-up of 229 patients. *J Am Coll Cardiol* 1988;12:616–623.

10. Ellis SG. Coronary lesions at increased risk. *American Heart Journal* 1995;130: 643–6.

11. Serruys PW, Emanuelsson H, van der Giessen W, et al. Heparin-coated Palmaz-Schatz stents in human coronary arteries. Early outcome of the Benestent-II Pilot Study. *Circulation* 1996;93:412–422.

12. Schomig A, Neumann FJ, Kastrati A, et al. A randomized comparison of antiplatelet and anticoagulant therapy after the placement of coronary-artery stents [see comments]. *N Engl J Med* 1996;334:1084–1089.

13. Teirstein PS, Massullo V, Jani S, et al. Catheter-based radiotherapy to inhibit restenosis after coronary stenting. *N Engl J Med* 1997;336:1697–1703.

14. Colombo A, Hall P, Nakamura S, et al. Intracoronary stenting without anticoagulation accomplished with intravascular ultrasound guidance. *Circulation* 1995; 91:1676–1688.

15. Pijls NH, De Bruyne B, Peels K, et al. Measurement of fractional flow reserve to assess the functional severity of coronary artery stenoses. *N Engl J Med* 1996;334:1703–1708.

16. Ferguson JJ, Dougherty KG, Gaos CM, Bush HS, Marsh KC, Leachman DR. Relation between procedural activated coagulation time and outcome after percutaneous transluminal coronary angioplasty. *J Am Coll Cardiol* 1994;23:1061–1065.

17. Anonymous. Randomised placebo-controlled trial of abciximab before and during coronary intervention in refractory unstable angina: the CAPTURE Study [published erratum appears in *Lancet* 1997;350(9079):744]. *Lancet* 1997;349: 1429–1435.

18. Anonymous. A randomised, blinded, trial of clopidogrel versus aspirin in patients at risk of ischaemic events (CAPRIE). CAPRIE Steering Committee. *Lancet* 1996;348:1329–1339.

19. Hirshfeld JW Jr, Ellis SG, Faxon DP. Recommendations for the assessment and maintenance of proficiency in coronary interventional procedures: statement of the American College of Cardiology. *J Am Coll Cardiol* 1998;31:722–743.

20. Reyes VP, Raju BS, Wynne J, et al. Percutaneous balloon valvuloplasty compared with open surgical commissurotomy for mitral stenosis. *N Engl J Med* 1994;331:961–967.

21. Isner JM, Pieczek A, Schainfeld R, et al. Clinical evidence of angiogenesis after arterial gene transfer of phVEGF165 in patient with ischaemic limb. *Lancet* 1996; 348:370–374.

Key Reviews
Ryan TJ, et al. Guidelines for PTCA: A report of the ACC/AHA Task Force on Assessment of diagnostic and therapeutic cardiovascular procedures. *J Am Coll Cardiol* 1988;12:529–545.

Relevant Book Chapters
Ellis SG, Holmes DR, eds. Evaluating stenosis stenting: QCA, coronary flow reserve and IVUS. In *Strategic approaches in coronary intervention,* 2nd ed. Baltimore: Lippincott Williams & Wilkins, (in press).
Freed M, Grines C, Safian RD, eds. *The new manual of interventional cardiology.* Birmingham, MI: Physicians Press, 1998:459–580.
Kern MJ, Deligonul U, eds. *The interventional cardiac catheterization handbook.* St. Louis: Mosby, 1996:13–45, 50–77.
Topol EJ, ed. *Textbook of interventional cardiology,* 3rd ed. Philadelphia: WB Saunders, 1998:3–51, 78–123, 147–162, 379–415, 821–838, 921–928.

58. TRANSTHORACIC ECHOCARDIOGRAPHY

Steve Lin and Guy Armstrong

I. **Introduction.** Transthoracic echocardiography is a reliable and versatile tool for the assessment of cardiac structure, function, and pathophysiology.

II. **Indications.** Common indications and corresponding aims of the echocardiographic evaluation are listed in Table 58-1.

A. **Transducer selection.** The adult echocardiographic examination typically begins with a 2.5- to 3.5-MHz phased array transducer. Lower frequency transducers have less attenuation and greater penetration of tissue. With increasing frequency, there is less depth penetration but greater spatial resolution of the image. In a thin individual or a pediatric patient, a 3.0- to 5.0-MHz transducer usually provides adequate penetration. Harmonic imaging is a recent innovation that improves image quality by receiving at twice the transmitting frequency (typically send at 1.8 MHz, receive at 3.6 MHz). For optimum two-dimensional (2D) resolution, select the highest frequency transducer that provides adequate far-field penetration. For the Doppler examination, modern transducers use a lower frequency transducer to record high velocities. The Pedoff probe is a continuous wave, nonimaging probe (typical frequency 1.8 MHz) used mainly to detect higher velocity profiles and confirm velocities obtained by other imaging methods.

B. **ECG lead placement.** The ECG lead placement allows identification of arrhythmias and timing of cardiac events during the echocardiographic examination. The three-lead system is most commonly used. It is important that irregular beats be identified and excluded from analysis. For example, a postectopic beat will falsely increase the 2D assessment of ejection fraction and Doppler assessment of transaortic gradient. In general, any Doppler index requires the average of at least three measurements. For patients in atrial fibrillation, 7 to 10 beats should be averaged.

C. **2D image acquisition**

1. **Patient and probe positioning.** The probe can be held with the right or left hand depending on the patient side one chooses to scan from. Standard imaging planes are illustrated in Figs. 58-1–58-6. The patient should be in the left lateral decubitus position as this brings the heart into contact with the chest wall. The left arm is extended behind the head to permit access to the apical and parasternal windows.

   a. **Parasternal windows.** The parasternal long axis view is acquired with the ridge of the transducer pointing toward the patient's right shoulder. Angling the beam toward the right hip brings the right ventricular inflow into view. Angling the beam toward the right shoulder allows evaluation of the right ventricular outflow tract. The probe is then turned 90 degrees clockwise from the parasternal long-axis view to obtain the parasternal short-axis view. Imaging of the left ventricular apex is acquired by tilting the beam towards the point of maximal impulse and as the transducer is angled back along the cardiac long axis, sequential cross-sectional views of the left ventricular cavity toward the base are obtained. Chamber dimensions are measured from the trailing echo of the proximal structure to the leading echo of the distal structure. Reference dimensions of the various cardiac chambers are listed in Table 58-2.

   b. **Apical window.** The transducer is placed in the mid-axillary line with the transducer ridge pointing toward the patient's left to obtain the four-chamber view. The left ventricular apex is aligned in the middle of the screen sector by sliding the transducer medially. The ultrasound beam is angled anteriorly to obtain the five-chamber

Table 58-1. Common indications and corresponding aims of echocardiographic evaluation

Indications	Echocardiographic evaluation
Valvular heart disease	Valvular morphology, regurgitation, and stenosis. Ventricular size and function.
Infective endocarditis	Vegetation, abscess, fistula, and valvular pathology.
Coronary artery disease	Wall motion abnormalities and ventricular function. Ischemic complications.
Congestive heart failure	Systolic and diastolic function, chamber size, endomyocardial appearance, and wall motion abnormalities. Valvular pathology.
Pericardial disease	Pericardial effusion, thickening, and calcification. Right ventricular size and function. Respiratory variations in mitral valve and hepatic vein inflow. Respiratory effects on inferior vena cava diameter.
Cardiac tamponade	Pericardial effusion. Right ventricular collapse. Respiratory variations in mitral valve and hepatic vein inflow. Respiratory effects on inferior vena cava diameter.
Ascending aortic pathology	Aneurysm, atheroma, intramural hematoma, and dissection. Aortic valve pathology.
Pulmonary hypertension	Right ventricular systolic pressure. Right and left ventricular function. Tricuspid, pulmonary, and mitral valve pathology. Interatrial shunt. Respiratory effects on inferior vena cava diameter.
Systemic hypertension	Left ventricular function, wall thickness, and wall motion abnormalities. Coarctation.
Embolic disease	Left atrial and ventricular thrombus. Mitral valve pathology. Aortic atheroma. Left ventricular function. Interatrial shunt.
Arrhythmias	Left atrial and ventricular thrombus. Ventricular size and function. Atrial dimensions and mitral valve pathology.
Syncope	Left ventricular outflow obstruction. Aortic and mitral valvular pathology. Left ventricular function and wall motion abnormalities. Congenital anomalies.
Cardiac trauma	Ascending aortic dissection and aneurysm. Cardiac tamponade.
Congenital heart disease	Congenital anomaly and shunt calculation.
Critically ill	Wall motion abnormalities and ventricular function. Valvular pathology. Pericardial effusion and tamponade. Right-to-left shunt. Volume status.

view or posteriorly to visualize the coronary sinus. From the four-chamber view, the probe is rotated counterclockwise to acquire the two-chamber view and further counterclockwise to the apical long-axis view.

  c. **Subcostal windows.** The patient is supine with knees flexed to relax the abdominal muscles. The transducer is moved to the subxyphoid position with the ridge pointing toward the patient's right. The subcostal view is particularly helpful for evaluation of right heart structures. The ultrasound beam can be angled anteriorly to assess the interatrial septum or posteriorly for the tricuspid valve. Turning the probe 90 degrees clockwise allows a short-axis examination of the left ventricle. When the probe is turned 90 degrees counterclockwise, the

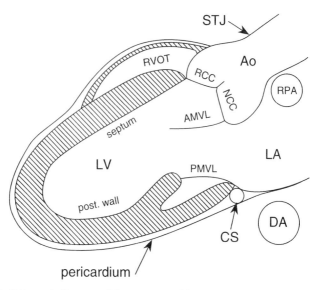

FIG. 58-1. Schematic diagram of the parasternal long-axis view in diastole. AML, anterior mitral leaflet; Ao, aorta; CS, coronary sinus; DA, descending aorta; LA, left atrium; LV, left ventricle; NCC, noncoronary cusp; PML, posterior mitral leaflet; PW, posterior wall; RCC, right coronary cusp; RPA, right pulmonary artery; RVOT, right ventricular outflow tract; STJ, sinotubular junction. From Otto CM, 1995, with permission.

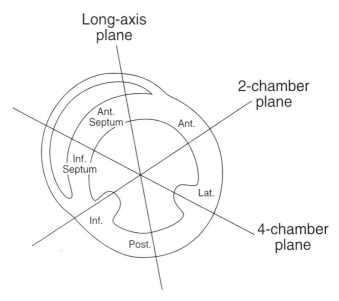

FIG. 58-2. Schematic diagram of the parasternal short-axis view at the level of papillary muscles. Ant. Septum, anterior septum; Ant., anterior wall; Inf. Septum, inferior septum; Inf., inferior wall; Lat., lateral wall; Post., posterior wall. From Otto CM, 1995, with permission.

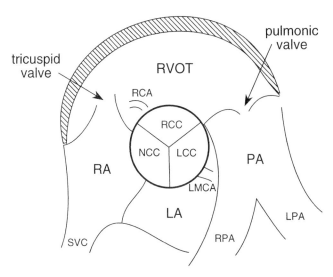

FIG. 58-3. Schematic diagram of the parasternal short-axis view at the aortic valve level. LA, left atrium; LCC, left coronary cusp; LMT, left main trunk; LPA, left pulmonary artery; NCC, non-coronary cusp; PA, pulmonary artery; PV, pulmonary valve; RA, right atrium; RCA, right coronary artery; RCC, right coronary cusp; RPA, right pulmonary artery; RVOT, right ventricular outflow tract; SVC, superior vena cava; TV, tricuspid valve. From Otto CM, 1995, with permission.

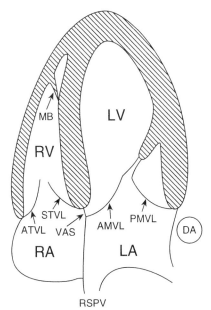

FIG. 58-4. Schematic diagram of the apical four-chamber view. AML, anterior mitral leaflet; ATL, anterior tricuspid leaflet; DA, descending aorta; PML, posterior mitral leaflet; LA, left atrium; LV, left ventricle; MB, moderator band; RA, right atrium; RUPV, right upper pulmonary vein; RV, right ventricle; STL, septal tricuspid leaflet. From Otto CM, 1995, with permission.

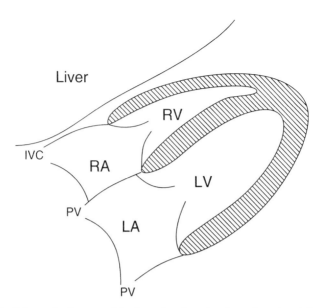

FIG. 58-5. Schematic diagram of the four-chamber view from the subcostal approach. IVC, inferior vena cava; LA, left atrium; LV, left ventricle; RA, right atrium; RV, right ventricle. From Otto CM, 1995, with permission.

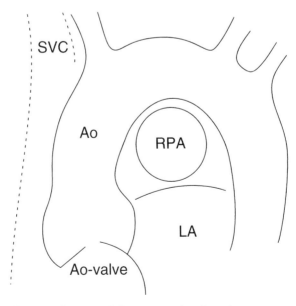

FIG. 58-6. Schematic diagram of the aorta and right pulmonary artery from the suprasternal notch window. Ao, aorta; AV, aortic valve; LA, left atrium; RPA, right pulmonary artery; SVC, superior vena cava. From Otto CM, 1995, with permission.

Table 58-2. Reference cardiac chamber dimensions in adults

Echocardiographic view	Reference range (cm)
Apical four-chamber	
Left ventricle ED major	6.3–9.5
Left ventricle ED minor	3.7–5.8
Left ventricle ES minor	2.8–4.7
Right ventricle major	5.5–9.1
Right ventricle minor	2.6–4.3
Parasternal long axis	
Left ventricle ED	3.5–5.7
Left ventricle ES	2.3–4.0
Right ventricle ED	1.9–3.8
Aortic root ED	2.0–3.7
Left atrium ES	1.9–4.0
Septum ED	0.6–1.1
Posterior wall left ventricle ED	0.6–1.1
Parasternal short-axis papillary muscle level	
Left ventricle ED	3.5–5.7
Left ventricle ES	2.6–4.8

ED, end diastole, peak of R wave; ES, end systole, the maximal downward excursion of the anteroseptum.

hepatic vein and inferior vena cava come into view. From this position, angling the beam perpendicular to the patient will visualize the descending aorta. When the examination is compromised by body habitus or other factors (e. g., surgical drains and dressings), the subcostal window may provide the only accessible window.

d. **Suprasternal and paraspinal windows.** The aortic arch is best visualized from the suprasternal notch position with the ridge pointing cephalad. The neck is extended during the suprasternal notch examination. The right parasternal window can be helpful in evaluating the ascending aorta and the interatrial septum. These images are acquired with the patient in the right lateral decubitus position. Less commonly used, the right paraspinal window with the patient in the prone position can detect descending aortic dissection and confirm fluid as pericardial or pleural.

e. **Off-axis windows.** In certain scenarios, enhanced visualization and Doppler interrogation of cardiac structures may be obtained using off-axis imaging views. For example, optimal interrogation of the tricuspid regurgitant flow can often be obtained from an off-axis apical four-chamber view as the transducer slides medially to minimize the angle between the ultrasound beam and the regurgitant velocity vector. For greater visualization of the proximal aorta, the evaluation of the ascending aortic dissection from the parasternal long-axis window may require shifting the transducer to a higher intercostal space.

f. **Helpful tips.** Subtle movements of the transducer will produce the optimal view once the imaging window is located. Full expiration to decrease lung volume, except in the subcostal views, improves visualization by shifting the heart closer to the transducer. Zoom in on the structure of interest and confirm findings with alternative views or Doppler evaluation. Harmonic imaging may significantly improve image quality in technically difficult views. Finally, consider subcostal imaging for challenging thoracic windows. The entire short-axis and four-chamber views may be obtained from this window.

When transthoracic echocardiography is unable to provide adequate resolution of cardiac structures or flow profiles to answer the clinical question, transesophageal echocardiography examination should be considered. The transesophageal window, however, does not invariably give better information. It is usually not better than transthoracic imaging for visualization of the left ventricular apex (e.g., for mural thrombus) or for Doppler assessment of aortic stenosis, pulmonary stenosis, and tricuspid regurgitation.

D. Contrast echocardiography. Contrast echocardiography is performed typically by a rapid bolus injection of 10 mL of agitated normal saline solution through an arm vein. Agitation is obtained by exchanging the solution between two syringes interconnected by a three-way stopcock before intravenous injection. An interatrial shunt is diagnosed if the echo contrast appeared in the left atrium within three cardiac cycles after its appearance in the right atrium, either spontaneously or after a cough or Valsalva release. Intrapulmonary shunt is differentiated from an interatrial shunt by a delayed appearance of contrast bubble in the left atrium. Visualization of the spectral Doppler display of tricuspid regurgitation can also be enhanced using agitated saline contrast.

Modern contrast agents comprising a mixture of sonicated albumin and perfluorocarbons can transit the pulmonary capillary bed and therefore opacify the left heart and coronary circulation. Current active research in contrast echocardiography includes its application for endocardial border enhancement, myocardial perfusion, and ultrasound-guided drug delivery.

1. **Machine settings.** To obtain the best images and accurate Doppler information, it is important to optimize the machine settings during different parts of the examination.

   a. **Time gain compensation.** These controls differentially amplify the echo signals returning from different depths to compensate for attenuation of the ultrasound beam with increasing distance from the transducer. The general guideline for initial time gain compensation setting is in the midrange with slightly lower gain in the near field and higher settings in the far field to compensate for attenuation of the beam with increasing depth.

   b. **Depth.** Start with the greatest depth to get an overview, then decrease the depth to include all of the target structure. A depth of 16 cm is usually adequate for the apical window and 12 cm for parasternal imaging. Increasing depth will decrease frame rate, which reduces temporal resolution.

   c. **Transmit gain.** Transmit gain adjusts the transducer's power output. The gain control should be initially set high and then adjusted downward. Setting the power too low results in inadequate returning signals and poor image quality, while setting it too high results in image white-out.

   d. **Compress.** The compress setting is also known as dynamic range. It converts the range of returning echo intensities, which may vary a billion fold in intensity, into 100 to 200 visual shades of brightness or the "gray scale." Increasing the compress will "soften" the image and allow identification of lower level signals. Typically, as the compress is increased, the gain should be decreased to maximize the spectrum of the gray scale.

   e. **Focus (or Position).** The focus is shifted to focus the ultrasound beam to the depth of interest to maximize spatial resolution. This is especially important when imaging near-field structures (e.g., looking for an apical left ventricular thrombus from the apical windows). When adjusted proximally, however, distal structures may appear blurred as the ultrasound beams scatter.

   f. **Persistence.** Temporal averaging of the latest frame with the previous frames to produce a smooth or less noisy display. Fast-moving cardiac structures (e.g., valve leaflets) may appear blurred if the persistence is set above low.

2. **Imaging artifacts**

a. **Acoustic shadowing.** Highly reflective structures block transmission of ultrasound to distal structures, causing these far-field structures to be poorly imaged (e.g., a mechanical mitral prosthesis prevents good visualization of the left atrium from the apical window).

b. **Reverberation.** Echo signals originating from two strong reflectors and resulting in multiple parallel images of target object in the far field (e.g., pacing leads in the right ventricle or calcified ascending aorta). May be eliminated by changing the angle, depth, or transducer frequency.

c. **Refraction.** Side-by-side double image resulting from ultrasound deflection as it passes through a tissue layer proximal to the structure of interest.

d. **Beam width artifact.** Strong reflectors at the edge of central beam superimposed on structure in the central zone even though signal intensity falls off at the edge of the beam. This limits lateral resolution.

e. **Range ambiguity.** Echo signals from earlier pulse cycle reach transducer on the next receiving cycle due to re-reflection, resulting in deep structures appearing closer to the transducer than actual location or appearance of an anatomically unexpected echo.

f. **Side lobe artifacts.** In addition to the central beam, transducers produce side lobes 10 to 30 degrees off axis. Any echoes returning from structures in these peripheral beams are displayed as if they arose from targets within the main beam. Thus strong reflectors may be imaged by these low intensity side lobes and displayed in an erroneous position on the screen, a major source of "clutter" in cardiac cavities. Harmonic echoes have much lower intensity side lobes, with a resulting reduction in side lobe artifacts in the image.

E. **M-Mode echocardiography.** Despite the increasing emphasis on 2D imaging, the M-mode display remains an integral and complementary element of the transthoracic examination. The M-mode cursor is guided by 2D imaging to identify the structure of interest. The image is displayed like a graph, with time on the x axis and distance from the transducer on the y axis. Although limited by its single scan line, its high sampling rate allows for accurate evaluation of rapidly moving valvular structures and endocardium. Measurements acquired during the M-mode examination are obtained from the leading echo of the proximal structure to the leading echo of the distal structure. M-Mode echocardiography is especially useful for systolic anterior motion of anterior mitral leaflet, diastolic collapse of the right ventricle, and identification of artifacts. Combinations of M-mode with color Doppler imaging are also useful for estimation of aortic regurgitant jet width and evaluation of ventricular filling patterns.

F. **Doppler echocardiography**

1. **Doppler principles.** Doppler interrogation typically measures velocity of red blood cells; however, newer machines are able to measure myocardial motion as well. The Doppler images are more complex because they contain velocity, as well as the spatial and temporal elements present in the 2D imaging. Generally, an increase in one factor results in a reduction in one of the others. The Doppler principle states that sound frequency increases as the sound source moves toward the observer and decreases as the source moves away. The change in frequency between the transmitted sound and the reflected sound is termed the Doppler shift. The Doppler equation relates the component of velocity parallel to the ultrasound beam to the Doppler shift:

$$\text{Velocity} = (F_d \times c) / (2 \times F_t \times \text{Cos } \theta)$$

Table 58-3. Reference Doppler velocities

Doppler measurements	Range (m/sec)
Tricuspid valve	0.3–0.7
Pulmonary valve	0.6–0.9
Aortic valve	1.0–1.7
E-wave mitral valve	
<50 yrs.	.72±.14
>50 yrs.	.62±.14
A-wave mitral valve	0.4–0.7
<50 yrs.	.40±.10
>50 yrs.	.59±.14

where F_d is Doppler frequency shift, F_t is transducer frequency, c is velocity of sound in tissue (1.56 m/second), and θ is angle between the transmitted ultrasound beam transmitted and the velocity direction.

The angle should be less than 20 degrees, so that the true flow velocity is underestimated by less than 6%. Adhering to this requirement frequently results in off-axis or unusual 2D images; the best transducer position for Doppler interrogation is usually slightly different from the optimal position for 2D images. Reference Doppler velocities in the adult examination are shown in Table 58-3.

2. **Pulsed wave and continuous wave Doppler**
   a. In the pulsed wave mode, a single crystal sends and receives short bursts of ultrasonic beams at a specific pulse repetition frequency and location. The ultrasound is reflected from the moving blood cell at a selected location and received by the same crystal. The maximum velocity that can be determined by the pulsed wave Doppler is the Nyquist (or aliasing) velocity. This appears as wrap around on the time-based pulsed wave display where the velocities above the Nyquist limit appear to be going in the opposite direction. Shifting the Doppler baseline up or down can double the maximal unambiguous velocity, which typically is less than 2 m/second. Higher velocities can also be recorded without aliasing as the sample volume is moved closer to the transducer. The relationships of Nyquist velocity, depth, and transducer frequency are given by the equation:

$$V_N = 60/f_0 d$$

where V_N is Nyquist velocity with maximal baseline shift (m/second), f_0 is transducer frequency (MHz), and d is depth (cm).
   b. The continuous wave Doppler has two crystals, one sending and the other receiving continuously. The maximal frequency shift that can be recorded by continuous wave Doppler is not limited by the pulse repetition frequency (PRF) or the Nyquist phenomenon. Unlike pulsed wave Doppler, continuous wave Doppler measures the maximal velocity along the ultrasound beam. It is especially suited for recording high velocities because there is no aliasing. Continuous wave Doppler, however, is limited by the range ambiguity or the inability to identify those structures along the beam path that are responsible for the velocity measured. In general, continuous wave Doppler is used to assess high-velocity flow and pulsed wave Doppler to measure low-velocity flow in specific areas. Clinical applications of pulsed wave versus continuous wave Doppler are listed in Table 58-4.
3. **Color flow imaging.** Color flow imaging codes blood velocity as color shades; generally red represents flow toward the transducer and blue

Table 58-4. Clinical applications of pulsed versus continuous wave Doppler

Pulse wave	Continuous wave
Diastolic filling parameters	Dynamic LVOT gradient
Location of flow disturbance	dp/dt
LVOT velocity and TVI	Peak flow velocity and TVI
Mitral inflow velocity	Pressure half-time
Pulmonary and hepatic vein velocity	Pulmonary systolic pressure
	Transvalvular gradient
	Regurgitant volume

LVOT, left ventricular outflow tract; TVI, time velocity integral; dp/dt, index of the rate of left ventricular pressure rise. Modified from Oh JK, 1994, with permission.

represents flow away. Lighter shades represent higher velocities as displayed by the on-screen color map. When the flow velocity is higher than the Nyquist limit (indicated on the color map), color aliasing occurs (depicted as a mosaic mixture of red, blue, and white). Like 2D imaging, color Doppler spatial resolution is higher axial to the beam than lateral. For example, the parasternal long-axis width of the aortic regurgitant jet in the left ventricular output tract (LVOT) correlates with severity, but the jet width in the apical view (lateral to the beam) is an unreliable guide to the degree of regurgitation.

To estimate velocity along a given scan line, the instrument compares the phase change from two successive pulses. For acceptable velocity resolution, several (typically eight) pulses must be compared, limiting the image frame rate. The maximum number of pulses that can be emitted in one second is the pulse repetition frequency, determined by the velocity of sound in tissue and the depth of the color sector:

$$PRF = c/2d$$

where c is velocity of sound in tissue (1.56 m/second) and d is depth (cm).

A full sector color map is the summation of color Doppler data from each scan line. The number of times per second this process can be repeated in a given frame equals the frame rate. Typically the narrowest sector width is selected to maximize the pulses per scan line and frame rate for optimum resolution. The line density (i.e., the number of scan lines per sector) is determined by the ultrasound machine. The quality of the color Doppler data displayed is influenced primarily by the number of pulses per scan line and the line density. Factors are directly related to the PRF, but inversely related to one another by the relationship:

$$PRF = (Frames/second) \times (scan\ lines/frame) \times (pulses/scan\ line)$$

For a given PRF, the frame rate can be increased and the color quality can be improved (as the number of pulses per scan line increases) by narrowing the sector width. Modern machines are capable of parallel processing, whereby multiple scan lines are analyzed for each ultrasound pulse, thus allowing higher frame rates at any given sector width and depth. General principles of color Doppler evaluation of a high versus low velocity jet are summarized in Table 58-5.

4. Factors affecting Doppler image

  a. Machine settings

    (1) Transducer frequency. The net effect of increasing transducer frequency depends on the opposing effects of (a) depth attenuation and loss of signal strength which decreases area of

Table 58-5. Recommendations for color Doppler interrogation

High-velocity jet (e.g., mitral regurgitation)	Low-velocity flow (e.g., venous flow or proximal flow convergence)
Maximize Nyquist velocity: • Low frequency transducer • Minimize imaging depth	Maximize low velocity sensitivity: • High frequency transducer • Reduce PRF by lowering the velocity scale • Increase number of pulses per scan line
Maximize frame rate: • Narrow sector width • Minimize imaging depth	Maximize frame rate: • Narrow sector width • Minimize imaging depth Maximize gain: • Avoid artifacts

flow disturbance, (b) higher Doppler shift and lower aliasing velocity tending to increase area of color flow disturbance. Thus transesophageal echocardiography generally produces larger areas of flow disturbance despite the higher frequency transducer because of less attenuation occurring at the shallow depth settings used for transesophageal echocardiography.

(2) **Depth setting.** Minimizing the depth setting to encompass only the region of interest will maximize the PRF and frame rate. For a given depth setting the Nyquist or aliasing velocity (which is related to the PRF) can be adjusted. For imaging regurgitant flow it should be set at about 45 to 60 cm/second. Higher Nyquist limits will reduce the area of color flow disturbance. Lower limits are used to enlarge the region of proximal flow convergence for analysis of regurgitant flow.

(3) **Gain.** Adjust the color gain until just before the noise appears in the color. Increased color gain will increase the size of color flow disturbance. Conversely, 2D gain should be decreased during the color Doppler examination; this will increase color flow disturbance because each pixel is assigned to either 2D or color. Modern machines also have a tissue priority control. If a pixel has both color and 2D signals assigned, the user-defined tissue priority will determine whether color or 2D is displayed. For pulsed wave and continuous wave Doppler, start with a high gain setting until the desired signal is appreciated. The gain is decreased until noise and clutter are adequately suppressed.

(4) **Baseline.** Used primarily for unwrapping aliased signals. Generally leave it in the middle of the color bar, but it can be adjusted to maximize the velocity that can be displayed with pulsed wave or color Doppler. This is also useful for highlighting a specific velocity as in proximal convergence analysis.

(5) **Wall filter.** Excludes low-velocity, high-amplitude signals from myocardial motion. If set too high it will tend to decrease the color flow disturbance. A typical initial setting is 400 Hz. The wall filter should be minimized during analysis of the proximal flow convergence region to avoid overestimation of low velocities. That is, set low for pulse-wave and high for continuous-wave Doppler.

(6) **Beam width.** Especially important with pulsed wave and continuous wave Doppler. As the ultrasound beam propagates it spreads out. For example, when sampling pulmonary venous flow with pulse Doppler from the apical view, the sample vol-

ume may be at 16 cm depth and the ultrasound beam may be over 1 cm in width. This can lead to the detection of aortic flow, which is displayed as if it arose along the beam axis (from the pulmonary vein).

(7) **Gate length or sample size.** This is the size of the pulsed wave Doppler sampling region. It is usually set at 3 to 5 mm. Increasing the size will give a less noisy signal but may pick up spurious signals from other areas.

(8) **Scale.** Controls the range of Doppler velocities displayed. As the velocity scale increases, the velocity limits increase and the displayed waveform size decreases.

(9) **Compress.** For pulsed wave and continuous wave Doppler, it adjusts the gray scale, which controls image softness. Decrease the compress to enhance the edges of the spectral envelope. Increase the compress to enhance the various velocities displayed within the Doppler spectrum. Set at 30 dB or higher initially.

(10) **Reject.** For pulsed wave and continuous wave Doppler, it removes low-amplitude signals ("noise") from the spectral display. The reject control is initially set at a low level (20% to 40% maximum) to allow the display of a wide range of signals. The reject is then increased to remove signals that obscure the image.

b. **Imaging factors**

(1) **Interrogation angle.** Each color pixel represents the component of velocity parallel to the ultrasound beam. This is related to the true flow velocity by the cosine of the angle between the blood flow and the interrogating ultrasound beam. Thus, from the suprasternal notch, flow in the ascending aorta appears red, in the descending aorta blue, and in the arch black (no flow detected) due to the different intercept angles of the ultrasound beam with blood flow.

(2) **Attenuation** [see also II.F.4.a(1)]. Loss of signal strength due to too high a transducer frequency for the required depth will result in a reduced area of color flow disturbance (e.g., imaging for valvular regurgitation from the transgastric window).

(3) **Acoustic shadowing** (see also under II.C). Loss of signal strength due to a proximal reflector of ultrasound (e.g., a mechanical prosthetic valve preventing apical imaging of mitral regurgitant jet in the left atrium).

c. **Hemodynamic factors**

(1) **Flow volume.** Increasing regurgitant volume results in an increased area of color flow disturbance, and this is the basis for the common practice of judging the severity of valvular regurgitation by the size of the color jet. However, as outlined in this chapter, many other hemodynamic and machine factors affect the color flow appearance. Thus it is important to include other factors in the assessment of regurgitation, such as ventricular and atrial size, the morphologic appearance of the valve, the width of the color jet at its narrowest point (vena contracta), and analysis of the proximal flow convergence region.

(2) **Driving pressure.** Increased pressure gradient across a regurgitant orifice will result in increased color flow disturbance in the receiving chamber. Color jet size is closely related to jet momentum, given by flow rate multiplied by jet velocity.

(3) **Chamber constraint.** Impingement of a regurgitant jet against walls of the receiving chamber will decrease the size of the color disturbance (Coanda effect). For example, severe but eccentric mitral regurgitation may have a very small area of

color flow disturbance because the jet spreads out as a thin layer over the constraining left atrial wall.

F. Doppler echocardiographic applications

1. **Bernoulli equation.** The Bernoulli equation allows measurement of relative pressure differences across valves, shunts, and outflow tract obstruction. In its complete form, the Bernoulli equation is too complex for routine clinical use:

$$\Delta P = 1/2\rho \, (V_2^2 - V_1^2) + \int_1^2 (dv/dt) \, ds + R(v)$$

Convective flow   Viscous
acceleration   acceleration   resistance

where V_2 is velocity distal to an obstruction and V_1 is velocity proximal to an obstruction. Blood density is constant ($1/2\rho \cong 4$, with P in mm Hg and V in m/second). In most clinical settings, flow acceleration and viscous friction are negligible. The equation can thus be simplified as:

Peak instantaneous pressure gradient $= 4 \times (V_2^2 - V_1^2)$.

If $V_1 \leq 1.0$ m/second, the equation is further simplified to:

Peak instantaneous pressure gradient $= 4 \times V^2$
(simplified Bernoulli equation)

The simplified Bernoulli equation is unreliable when: (a) V_1 is greater than 1.0 m/second, which occurs in serial lesions (subvalvular and valvular stenosis) and mixed stenosis with regurgitation; (b) viscous resistance becomes significant in the evaluation of long stenoses (e.g., tunnel-like ventricular septal defect, coarctation, and coronary artery disease); (c) when the inertial term (flow acceleration) is not negligible, as for flow through normal valves.

2. **Continuity equation.** The continuity equation is an application of the principle of conservation of mass, which states that flow across a conduit of varying diameter is equal at all points. This equation is especially useful in the assessment of stenotic aortic valve area that cannot be accurately planimetered from the transthoracic window.

Stroke volume $= A_1 \times TVI_1 = A_2 \times TVI_2$

where time velocity integral (TVI) represents the sum of velocities during a cardiac cycle.

For flow immediately in series (e.g., LVOT and aortic valve) the equation can be simplified as:

Flow $= A_1 \times V_1 = A_2 \times V_2$

In the case of the aortic valve:

$$\text{Area}_{\text{aortic valve}} = \text{Area}_{\text{LVOT}} \times TVI_{\text{LVOT}}/TVI_{\text{aortic valve}} <> \text{Area}_{\text{aortic valve}}$$
$$= (\text{diameter}_{\text{LVOT}})^2 \times 0.785 \times TVI_{\text{LVOT}}/TVI_{\text{aortic valve}}$$

3. **Proximal isovelocity surface area.** The proximal isovelocity surface area (PISA) method is another application of the principle of conservation of mass and is based on the phenomenon that flow accelerates proximal to a narrowed orifice. This is illustrated by the acceleration of water in the tub before it enters the drain pipe. Color Doppler demonstrates this acceleration proximal to the regurgitant surface as a series of concentric colored ("isovelocity") hemispheres. Blood at each hemisphere has an identical velocity that can be determined from the color

velocity map. The PISA method can be used to calculate the mitral valve area, quantifying mitral regurgitation and flow across a ventricular septal defect.

The surface area of a hemisphere is $2\pi r^2$ where r is the radius of the hemisphere.

Flow can be determined by:

Flow = $\text{Area}_{\text{shell}} \times V_{\text{Shell}}$

Flow = $2\pi r^2 \times V_{\text{aliasing velocity}}$.

Effective regurgitant orifice area (ERO) = flow/V_{max}, where V_{max} is the peak continuous wave velocity of the regurgitant jet.

Regurgitant volume = ERO × TVI.

SUGGESTED READINGS
Key Reviews
Edwards WD, Tajik AJ, Seward JB. Standard nomenclature and anatomic basis for regional tomographic analysis of the heart. *Mayo Clin Proc* 1981;56:479–497.
Nishimura RA, Tajik AJ. Quantitative hemodynamics by Doppler echocardiography: a noninvasive alternative to cardiac catheterization. *Prog Cardiovasc Dis* 1994;36: 309–42.

Relevant Books Chapters
Feigenbaum H. *Echocardiography,* 5th ed. Philadelphia: Lea & Febiger, 1993:1–59.
Hewlett-Packard SONOS 1000 Ultrasound Imaging System Users Guide, Vols. 1 and 2.
Oh JK, Seward JB, Tajik AJ. *The echo manual.* Boston: Little, Brown and Company, 1994:7–22.
Otto CM, Pearlman AS. *Otto and Pearlman's textbook of clinical echocardiography.* Philadelphia: WB Saunders, 1995:21–64.
Topol EJ. *Comprehensive cardiovascular medicine: principles of imaging.* Philadelphia: Lippincott-Raven Publishers, 1998:1441–1476.
Weyman A. *Principles and practice of echocardiography,* 2nd ed. Philadelphia: Lea & Febiger, 1994:3–28.

59. TRANSESOPHAGEAL ECHOCARDIOGRAPHY

Maran Thamilarasan

I. **Indications.** In general, transesophageal echocardiography (TEE) is performed when there is a clinical question for which the information obtained by transthoracic echocardiography (TTE) does not provide a sufficient answer. This may be to better define pathology that has been identified by TTE or to obtain images when transthoracic images are inadequate. The close position of the esophagus to the heart allows for improved visualization of many cardiac structures, particularly those that are posteriorly located. In addition, higher frequency probes can be used given the shorter distance between the probe and the heart, further enhancing resolution.

Indications for varying diagnoses and clinical situations are listed in Table 59-1. Specific indications include (a) examination to rule out a cardiac source of embolus and (b) assessment of valves for endocarditis and accompanying complications (such as abscess). The assessment of native and prosthetic valvular function, in terms of degree and mechanism of regurgitation or stenosis, is a common indication for TEE. Acoustic shadowing by prosthetic valves poses less of a problem for TEE than it does for TTE. Congenital cardiovascular abnormalities, as well as tumors and masses, can also be well delineated by TEE. The ability to assess the ascending, arch, and descending aorta has enabled TEE to play an important role in the diagnosis of aortic dissection, aneurysms, and atheroma. Assessment of atrial pathology and function has become an increasingly important role for TEE, particularly prior to cardioversion for atrial fibrillation and atrial flutter.

Transesophageal echocardiography has come to play an important role in the operating room. This is particularly true in cardiothoracic surgery, where TEE can be used to assess the mechanism of valvular abnormalities and subsequently evaluate the efficacy of repair or replacement. Transesophageal echocardiography can be used to guide the location of the aortic cross-clamp, so that segments with severe atheromatous involvement can be avoided, thereby reducing the risk of embolization. In addition, TEE can provide an assessment of left ventricular function and regional wall motion. This can be valuable in noncardiac surgery as well, to assess left ventricular function during the operation. Transesophageal echocardiography is also used during percutaneous interventional procedures, such as during valvuloplasty or atrial septal defect closure, to help guide catheter position and evaluate the success and complications of the procedure.

II. **Contraindications.**

A. There are few **absolute** contraindications to the performance of TEE (Table 59-2). These include the **presence of pharyngeal or esophageal obstruction, active upper gastrointestinal bleeding,** and **suspected or known perforated viscus.** If there is instability of the cervical vertebrae, then the exam cannot be performed.

B. **Relative** contraindications include the **presence of esophageal varices** and **suspected esophageal diverticulum.** In these cases, it is prudent to obtain gastrointestinal evaluation prior to proceeding, if the study must be performed. Severe cervical arthritis, in which patients may have difficulty with neck flexion, may make it difficult to pass the probe. Oropharyngeal pathology, anatomic distortion, or extreme muscle weakness can likewise make it difficult to proceed with the examination.

C. **Severe cardiopulmonary disease** is not a contraindication to evaluation by TEE (on the contrary, it is often in these patients that critical information needs to be obtained), but the operator must be particularly careful to minimize any stress on the patient. This is particularly true in **suspected aortic dissection,** where any sudden increase in blood pressure caused by patient

Table 59-1. Indications in specific conditions and clinical situations

Indication	Clinical conditions
Inadequate TTE images	Obesity, chest wall deformity, pulmonary disease
Native valve disease	Mechanism of regurgitation, valve planimetry
Prosthetic valve disease	Periprosthetic leaks, thrombus, pannus, vegetations, valve dehiscence
Endocarditis	Valvular vegetations, ring abscess, fistulas, vegetations on indwelling catheters
Aortic disease	Dissection, intramural hematoma, aneurysm, atheroma
Source of embolus	Thrombus, atheroma, patent foramen ovale, valve strands, mass, vegetation
Atrial function	Atrial or appendage thrombus, spontaneous echo contrast, appendage flow velocities
Pericardial disease	Pericardial thickness, masses, effusion
Interatrial septum	Patent foramen ovale, ASD
Coronary disease	Complications of acute MI: ventricular septal defect, papillary muscle dysfunction or rupture, pseudoaneurysm, aneurysm
Congenital cardiac disease	ASD, VSD, anomalous pulmonary venous drainage, coarctation, arterial switch, fistulas
Cardiothoracic surgical OR	Mechanism of valvular disease, success of repair or replacement, LV wall motion abnormalities, guidance for aortic cross-clamp: avoiding areas of severe atheroma, postop complications (SAM, dissection)
General surgical OR	Assess LV function
Catheterization lab	Guide catheter position during valvuloplasty, ASD closure, evaluate success of these procedures
Miscellaneous	Proximal pulmonary embolism, masses or tumors, unexplained hypotension in the ICU; to look for any pathology described above

TTE, transthoracic echocardiography; OR, operating room; MI, myocardial infarction; ASD, atrial septal defect; VSD, ventricular septal defect; LV, left ventricular; SAM, systolic anterior motion; ICU, intensive care unit.

discomfort could result in extension of the dissection. In cases where there is **respiratory instability,** endotracheal intubation with assisted ventilation should be considered prior to the procedure. Patients who are **hypotensive** may not be able to receive sedative agents, which could lead to further hemodynamic compromise. In these patients, the examination may need to be performed with topical anesthesia alone. This is obviously much more difficult for the patient, and TEE should be done only if critical information not obtainable by other methods is needed.

D. Given the invasive nature of the procedure, prudence must be observed in patients who are prone to **bleeding.** The procedure is commonly performed on patients who are anticoagulated, such as in those with atrial arrhythmias prior to cardioversion. However, there is increased risk in those who are over-anticoagulated. Though no set guidelines exist, it would seem advisable to **delay the exam if possible in patients with an international normalized ratio greater than 5 or a partial thromboplastin time greater than 100 seconds. Thrombocytopenia** may also increase the risk, particularly with platelet counts less than $50,000/mm^3$. The TEE can still be

Table 59-2. Transesophageal echocardiography contraindications

---

Absolute
> Esophageal or pharyngeal obstruction
> Suspected or known perforated viscus
> Gastrointestinal bleeding that has not been evaluated
> Instability of cervical vertebrae
> Uncooperative patient

Relative
> Esophageal varices or diverticula
> Cervical arthritis
> Oropharyngeal distortion
> Bleeding diathesis or over-anticoagulation

---

performed if needed, as the absolute risk still remains low, but meticulous attention must be paid during esophageal intubation.

E. **Esophageal infections,** such as those that occur in the context of human immunodeficiency virus (HIV), do not necessarily represent contraindications to the procedure. **Patient discomfort** due to the presence of the probe in the esophagus may preclude the examination. Universal precautions should be followed (as they should for any patient). Some operators prefer to use a protective disposable sheath, which can be placed over the TEE probe during the exam and subsequently discarded. Image quality may be somewhat compromised by this method. The standard disinfectants used to clean the probe will inactivate HIV.

F. A patient who is very uncooperative is at significant risk for complications from the procedure, and consideration should be given to aborting the TEE.

III. **Personnel.** The American Society of Echocardiography has proposed the following guidelines for operators who wish to perform TEE: (a) as background, interpretation of a minimum of 300 transthoracic echocardiograms; (b) a minimum of 25 esophageal intubations under the guidance of a gastroenterologist or a skilled transesophageal echocardiographer; and (c) a minimum of 50 TEE examinations during training. Furthermore, operators should perform a minimum of 50 to 75 TEE examinations yearly to maintain competency.

The presence of a skilled assistant is invaluable during the procedure. The assistant should be either a sonographer or a registered nurse. The role of the assistant is to monitor vital signs during the procedure, to ensure proper suctioning of oropharyngeal secretions, and to administer medications.

IV. **Equipment.** Necessary equipment is listed in Table 59-3.

V. **The transesophageal probe.** The probe is a modification of the standard gastroscope, with transducers in place of the fiberoptics. The conventional rotary controls with inner and outer dials are present. The inner dial typically guides anteflexion and retroflexion, whereas the outer dial controls medial and lateral movement of the tip. A locking mechanism is present, which must not be in effect when the probe is advanced or withdrawn, as esophageal trauma may result. The multiplane probe (see below) also has a lever control to guide rotation. Use of a biplane probe (see below) will require switching between the transverse and longitudinal planes by a control switch on the echo machine. Advancement and withdrawal of the probe, rotation of the probe about its long axis, and the manipulations available using the above rotary controls constitute the means by which specific images can be obtained (diagramed in Fig. 59-1).

VI. **Patient preparation** (Table 59-4). The patient should have had nothing by mouth (NPO) for at least 4 hours prior to the procedure. Possible contraindications should be ruled out by asking for a history of odynophagia or dysphagia. It is important to be aware of any history of radiation therapy to the mediastinum or cervical region, which may have resulted in stricture formation.

Table 59-3. Equipment for transesophageal echocardiography

1. Echo machine and probe (calibrate prior to intubation)
2. Sphygmomanometer
3. ECG rhythm monitor
4. Pulse oximeter
5. Supplemental oxygen
6. Wall suction with Yankauer
7. Intravenous lines and tubing
8. Topical anesthetic agents
9. Sedative medications
10. Bite block
11. Gloves and goggles
12. Emergency equipment
    a. Drugs (e.g., atropine, epinephrine, narcan, flumazenil, lidocaine)
    b. Defibrillator
    c. Intubation supplies

The extent of prior workup for any history of gastrointestinal bleeding must be reviewed. Appropriate inquiries should be made with regard to allergies and prior tolerance of sedative medications. It should be ensured that the patient understands the procedure and indications before proceeding.

VII. Step-by-step guide to the examination
   A. The patient's **dentures,** if present, should be removed.
   B. An intravenous (IV) line should be inserted to allow for administration of medications and saline contrast for study.

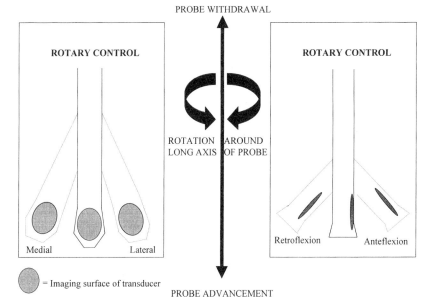

FIG. 59-1. Specific images can be obtained by advancement and withdrawal of the probe, rotation of the probe about its long axis, and by the manipulations that are possible using rotary controls.

Table 59-4. Preparation for transesophageal echocardiography

Patient must have had nothing by mouth (NPO) for at least 4 hr prior to the TEE
Assess for possible contraindications:
    History of odynophagia or dysphagia
    History of mediastinal or cervical radiation that might have resulted in stric-
      ture formation
    History of and workup for gastrointestinal bleeding
Allergies to and previous tolerance of sedative medications
Patient understanding of procedure and indications
Informed consent of patient

  C. The need for **antibiotic prophylaxis** should be considered. The American
     Heart Association does not recommend routine antibiotic prophylaxis for
     endoscopy. The reported incidence of transient bacteremia with endoscopy
     (without biopsy) is no higher than the contamination rates reported with
     blood cultures. If the patient has a prosthetic heart valve, a prior history of
     endocarditis, or poor dentition, then one might wish to consider optional pro-
     phylaxis. At the Cleveland Clinic Foundation, we rarely give antibiotic
     prophylaxis. Obviously, if the indication for the TEE is to look for evidence
     for endocarditis, then blood cultures must be drawn prior to administration
     of any antibiotics.
  D. A **blood pressure cuff** should be placed on the patient's arm.
  E. **ECG leads** should be applied and hooked up to the telemetry monitor.
  F. A **pulse oximeter** is applied to the patient's finger or ear.
  G. A **nasal cannula** is applied so that supplemental oxygen can be given as
     needed.
  H. While sitting up, the patient is asked to swallow **viscous 2% lidocaine** for
     topical anesthesia. **Cetacaine spray (10%) or xylocaine spray (4%)** is
     also used for this purpose. Begin by spraying the posterior tongue and hard
     palate. With each application, spray farther back into the posterior pharynx.
     The **gag reflex** should be checked (with tongue depressor or using gloved
     finger) and **topical anesthesia** applied until the reflex is dulled. By visu-
     alizing the area being sprayed, inadvertent spraying of the vocal cord and
     resultant laryngospasm can be avoided. Some operators advocate the use of
     drying agents to minimize oropharyngeal secretions (such as subcutaneous
     atropine or glycopyrrolate). We generally have not found a need for use of
     such agents, which can cause an increase in heart rate.
  I. Have the patient lie down on the left side (left lateral decubitus position),
     facing the echo machine (alternatively, the patient can lie on the right side,
     with the machine on the right), with neck flexed. Transesophageal echocar-
     diography can be performed with the patient sitting, but it is easier in the
     lateral position.
  J. **Midazolam** is the preferred agent for sedation, having the benefit of a short
     half-life. It also produces an antegrade amnestic effect. Typically, give IV
     doses of 0.5 mg every 3 to 5 minutes until adequate sedation is achieved (the
     goal is to reduce anxiety, but sufficient self-ventilation must be maintained,
     and patient should remain capable of following commands, e.g., swallowing
     when needed). Check pulse oximetry and blood pressure before each dose.
     Meperidine is also given as sedation (typically given 12.5 to 25 mg IV per
     dose). Meperidine possesses an analgesic effect, and helps to suppress the
     gag reflex as well. Again, **check vital signs before each dose. Fentanyl**
     can also be used for sedation (typically 25 µg IV per dose), and may be bet-
     ter tolerated in patients with poor left ventricular function, with low blood
     pressure, or with renal impairment. Additional doses of these sedatives and
     anxiolytics may be administered during the procedure if needed.

K. With adequate sedation and topical anesthesia (diminution of gag reflex), **begin probe insertion.** There are two approaches that are generally used. The first is the **digital technique,** which is especially useful with the larger size multiplane probe. With this method, the bite guard is inserted onto the shaft of the probe, such that after esophageal intubation the bite guard can be moved into place. The distal end of the probe is lubricated. The imaging surface of the transducer is placed toward the tongue. The tip of the transducer is placed under the index finger, and is slowly guided downward and posterior to the hypopharynx. At this point the patient is asked to swallow, and gentle pressure is applied with the other hand to guide the probe down. Swallowing will result in relaxation of the upper esophageal sphincter. If resistance is met, stop, let patient relax, and reattempt or redirect as needed. Using the finger as a guide will help center the probe into the region of the hypopharynx over the esophagus and avoid the lateral recesses.

An **alternative method is to use the rotary controls on the TEE probe** to guide the intubation. The bite guard is inserted first. The probe is inserted through the bite guard, and gentle anteflexion is applied as the probe is passed over the back of the tongue. The probe is then returned to the neutral position, or with slight retroflexion, as it is passed down into the esophagus. The patient is asked to swallow as the probe is advanced past the upper esophageal sphincter. The operator is still able to guide the probe if needed by insertion of a finger around the side of the bite guard.

Patients will often gag as the probe enters the upper esophagus (even with adequate anesthesia); however, patients generally find it more comfortable once the probe has passed beyond this point (usually at 25 cm, past the level of the carina). The probe should be advanced to approximately 30 to 40 cm (midesophageal level).

In intubated patients, it is important to **secure the endotracheal tube firmly to one side of the mouth** to prevent dislodgment and inadvertent extubation. Direct visualization with a laryngoscope may be needed. **Sedation** is equally important in these patients, and given the tendency for partially sedated patients to bite on their tubes, a **paralyzing agent** is often required. Intubation in the supine position is not a problem, as the airway is protected. Other catheters in the esophagus, such as feeding tubes or nasogastric tubes, might have to be removed prior to the procedure; they may become interposed between the esophagus and the TEE probe, interfering with the images. If left in, these tubes may become dislodged by the TEE probe, and tube position should be reconfirmed after the echo examination.

For patients with tracheostomies, some operators will carefully and gently deflate the cuff to facilitate probe insertion.

VIII. **Imaging.** Transesophageal echocardiography technology has undergone much evolution, from the initial monoplane views to the current multiplane probes. Monoplane TEE provides for images in the horizontal plane only, perpendicular to the shaft of the endoscope. Longitudinal relationships among cardiac structures are difficult to appreciate. With biplane TEE, the orthogonal longitudinal plane can also be obtained, in addition to the planes provided for by the monoplane probe. Some systems having two transducers require repositioning when switch between transducers is made. Others have biplane phased array to allow for scanning from a single transducer position. Either system requires much manipulation to obtain off-axis views, making the exam more difficult, as well as causing more discomfort for the patient. With multiplane TEE, the transducer array can be rotated to produce a continuum of transverse and longitudinal images from a single probe position. It is easier to obtain intermediate and off-axis images between the primary imaging planes, requiring less probe manipulation, flexion, and extension than with the biplane system. There is increased sensitivity for detection of small abnormalities, such as left atrial appendage thrombi or vegetations, and for detecting periprosthetic leaks and aortic dissection.

Table 59-5. Biplane transesophageal echocardiography

	Transverse	Longitudinal
Transgastric (typically at 35–40 cm)	Short-axis view of the left ventricle, at level of papillary muscles and mitral valve. Short axis of right ventricle.	Two-chamber view of the left atrium, left ventricle, mitral valve. Can be rotated for two-chamber view of right atrium, right ventricle, tricuspid valve
Midesophageal (typically at 30–35 cm)	Four-chamber view, with or without left ventricular outflow tract.	Two-chamber view of left atrium, left ventricle, left atrial appendage, mitral valve
Upper esophageal (typically at 25–30 cm)	Short-axis view of aortic valve, right ventricular outflow tract. With manipulation of probe, proximal coronary arteries, pulmonary veins, left atrial appendage, superior vena cava, ascending aorta, and atrial septum	Long-axis views of ascending aorta. With probe rotation, right ventricular outflow tract, main pulmonary artery
Aorta	Short-axis view of the thoracic aorta and long-axis view of the aortic arch	Long-axis view of the aortic arch. Short-axis view of the arch and some of the great vessels; particularly the left subclavian artery can be seen

A. **Basic views.** The TEE exam tends to be more goal-directed than the transthoracic examination, as there may be time constraints imposed by how long the patient can tolerate the presence of the esophageal probe. Initial views should focus on the question at hand, but it is still important to perform a comprehensive and thorough examination. Some operators prefer to start with the transgastric views and work back, whereas others start with the upper esophageal views. The order is not important, as long as the operator develops a consistent approach.

The probe may inadvertently rotate during insertion and may need initial manipulation prior to commencement of the examination. The left atrium should be seen at the center of the screen. If the aorta is seen (which is posterior to the esophagus), then the probe must be rotated anteriorly. Air in the esophagus, which is interposed between the probe and the heart, may affect image quality. This generally lessens as the exam progresses (from ongoing peristaltic activity in the esophagus). Similarly, the presence of a hiatal hernia may compromise image quality.

Views obtained from multiplane TEE will be described first. These views are described in terms of degrees of rotation that are required to obtain particular images. At each transducer location, start array at 0 degrees and rotate to 180 degrees at 5- to 15-degree increments to obtain a complete sweep. The standard horizontal plane is designated as 0 degrees. At around 45 degrees, short-axis views are obtained. Ninety degrees is defined as the longitudinal plane, while at around 135 degrees the long-axis cardiac views are obtained. At 180 degrees, a mirror image view of the standard horizontal plane is obtained. Given the variable anatomic relationships between structures, the degree of probe manipulation required to obtain the standard views will vary from patient to patient.

1. **Transgastric views**
   a. **Proximal** (Fig. 59-2A). These are images obtained from the fundus of the stomach. A cross-sectional view of the left and right ventricles is obtained at 0 degrees. By rotating the shaft of the endoscope to center the left ventricle in the field of view, serial short-axis ("dough-nut") views of the left ventricle can be obtained. Anteflexion of the probe will give rise to basal views, with the mitral and tricuspid valves seen in cross section. With the transducer in a more neutral position, mid- and apical short-axis views will be obtained.

   At 80 to 100 degrees, a two-chamber view of left atrium (with appendage) and left ventricle (anterior and inferior walls of left ventricle, mitral leaflets, papillary muscles) will be obtained. At 120 degrees plus, a long-axis outflow tract view with aortic valve and ascending aorta will be visualized. The anteroseptal and posterior walls of left ventricle are seen. Depending on the alignment with the transducer, this view may be useful in obtaining velocities across the aortic valve.

   Bringing the array back to 0 degrees and rotating the shaft of endoscope to center the right ventricle in view will allow for interrogation of the right-sided structures (Fig. 59-2B). At 30 to 60 degrees, the three leaflets of the tricuspid valve are visualized (anterior leaflet at bottom, posterior leaflet on top, and septal leaflet to the right). At around 70 to 80 degrees, the right ventricular inflow tract view (superior vena cava, tricuspid valve with anterior and posterior leaflets) is obtained. At 90 to 100 degrees, the right ventricular outflow and pulmonary valve become visible also. At 110 to 130 degrees, the two-chamber view of the right ventricle and right atrium can be seen. By rotating to 130 to 150 degrees, the papillary muscles and chordae supporting the tricuspid valve are further delineated.

   b. **Deep Transgastric.** The probe is advanced further into the stomach with the tip anteflexed. At 0 degrees, a foreshortened five-chamber view is obtained. This view allows for Doppler interrogation of the aortic valve and left ventricular outflow tract. By rotating the multiplane array, different segments of the left ventricle apex can be visualized in the search for thrombus or aneurysm.

2. **Lower and middle esophagus** (Fig. 59-3A, B). With the array at 0 degrees, a four-chamber view is obtained (some retroflexion of the probe is needed for a true four-chamber view, as with anteflexion one will see portions of the left ventricular outflow tract and aortic valve). This view is similar to an inverted transthoracic apical four-chamber view. Keeping the left atrium and left ventricle in the center of the view field, rotation of the array will allow for a thorough evaluation of the left-sided structures. Doppler interrogation of mitral inflow is generally performed with the array at 0 to 30 degrees. Skillful maneuvers as the array is rotated   to 90 degrees will allow for interrogation of both leaflets of the mitral valve, including the specific scallops of the posterior leaflet. Rotation of the array to 90 to 110 degrees reveals the two-chamber view (left atrium/left ventricle), with the anterior and inferior walls of the left ventricle visualized. The left atrial appendage and left upper pulmonary vein are also seen. Long-axis views of the left ventricular outflow tract, aortic valve (right and non-coronary cusps), and proximal ascending aorta are obtained by rotation to 120–140 degrees. The anterior mitral leaflet is particularly well seen in these views. This complete sweep will allow for full delineation of the extent of mitral regurgitation.

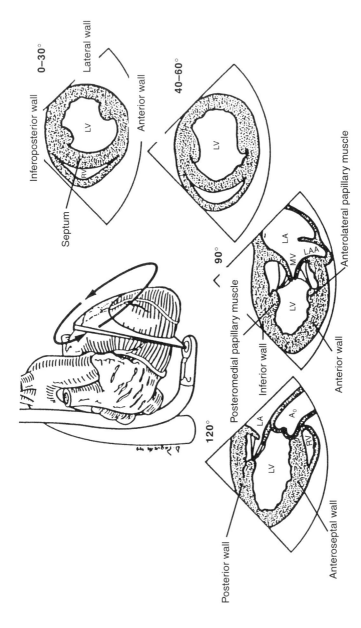

FIG. 59-2A. Schematic diagram showing representative multiplane transesophageal echocardiography sections of the left heart from the proximal transgastric location. Ao, aorta; LA, left atrium; LV, left ventricle; RA, right atrium; RV, right ventricle; SVC, superior vena cava; LAA, left atrial appendage; MV, mitral valve. Modified from Roelandt JRTC, 1996, with permission.

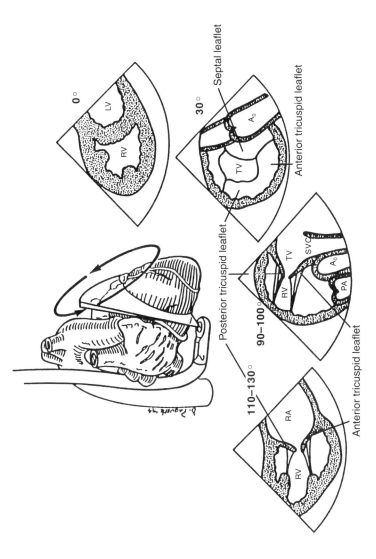

FIG. 59-2B. Schematic of images from a transgastric, multiplane sweep through the right ventricle. LV, left ventricle; RA, right atrium; RV, right ventricle; TV, tricuspid valve; SVC, superior vena cava; PA, pulmonary artery; Ao, aorta. Modified from Roelandt JRTC, 1996, with permission.

0°

30°

Septal leaflet

Anterior tricuspid leaflet

Posterior tricuspid leaflet

90–100°

110–130°

Anterior tricuspid leaflet

LV

RV

TV

Ao

RV

TV

SVC

Ao

PA

RA

RV

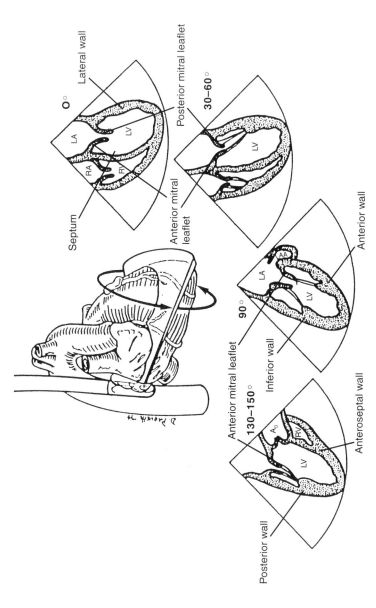

FIG. 59-3A. Schematic diagram showing some representative sections of the left heart that can be obtained with multiplane transesophageal echocardiography from the lower and middle esophagus. Ao, aorta; LA, left atrium; LAA, left atrial appendage; LV, left ventricle; RA, right atrium; RV, right ventricle. Modified from Roelandt JRTC, 1996, with permission.

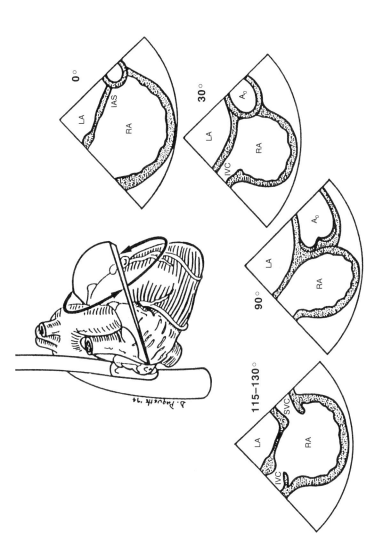

FIG. 59-3B. Schematic diagram showing representative multiplane transesophageal echocardiography sections of the atria and interatrial septum that can be obtained from the lower-middle esophagus. Ao, aorta; IVC, inferior vena cava; LA, left atrium; RA, right atrium; SVC, superior vena cava; IAS, interatrial septum. Modified from Roelandt JRTC, 1996, with permission.

Similar views of right-sided structures can also be obtained. At 0 degrees (in the four-chamber view as described above), the septal and anterior leaflets of the tricuspid valve are seen. The endoscope is then rotated to bring the interatrial septum and the right atrium to the center of view (some withdrawal or advancement of probe may be necessary to optimize visualization of the interatrial septum). By rotation of the multiplane array, the interatrial septum and fossa ovalis can be thoroughly examined for evidence for a patent foramen ovale and atrial septal defect. Agitated saline contrast can be given intravenously at this time to look for evidence of shunting. At approximately 100 degrees, the superior vena cava and inferior vena cava can be seen entering the right atrium, and the right atrial appendage can also be seen. This is a good view to evaluate for anomalous pulmonary venous drainage into the right atrium or superior vena cava, or a sinus venosus atrial septal defect. Further rotation will allow for assessment of the right pulmonary veins.

3. **Upper esophagus (30 cm)—base of the heart** (Fig. 59-4A). With the array at 0 degrees, a five-chamber cross-sectional view of the left atrium, left ventricle, right atrium, right ventricle, and aortic valve is obtained. At 40–60 degrees, the three leaflets of the aortic valve become visible (right coronary cusp at bottom of screen, noncoronary cusp on top and to the left, left coronary cusp on the right). Planimetry of the aortic valve orifice is often possible in this view. Subtle in and out movements will allow for visualization of the proximal coronaries. The left atrial appendage is also seen in this view (zooming in on the atrial appendage, with subsequent rotation of the array will allow for inspection for thrombus). At 60 to 100 degrees, the tricuspid valve and right ventricular outflow tract/pulmonic valve become visible. At 120 degrees, long-axis images of the left ventricular outflow tract, aortic valve (non- and right coronary cusps), and proximal ascending aorta are seen. Withdrawal of the probe will allow for visualization of more segments of the ascending aorta. With the probe withdrawn further into the upper esophagus (Fig. 59-4B), the pulmonary artery and its bifurcation can be visualized (from 0 to 45 degrees).

4. **Aorta.** Counterclockwise rotation of the endoscope brings the aorta into view. Typically the probe is advanced beyond the diaphragm and then slowly pulled back, following the aorta back to the arch. Rotation of the probe is required to keep the aorta in view in the center of the screen. At the level of the diaphragm, the aorta is posterior to the esophagus. In the midesophagus, the aorta is medial, whereas the ascending aorta and arch lie anterior to the esophagus. At 0 degrees, the aorta is seen as a circular structure. Long-axis images (at 100 to 130 degrees) can provide further information as needed at selected intervals. At the arch, the aorta is curved in front of the esophagus, presenting a sausage-shaped structure with the probe at 0 degrees. Gentle clockwise rotation will follow the arch back to the ascending aorta. The ascending aorta is visualized in the longitudinal planes as discussed with the other views. Multiplane TEE has reduced the so-called blind spot of the ascending aorta (where the trachea is interposed between the esophagus and aorta, an area that poses a problem for horizontal plane imaging).

B. **Biplane probe.** There are times in which a biplane probe may be used. It is a smaller probe, so it may be beneficial to use in certain cases when there might be difficulty in esophageal intubation with the multiplane probe. The basic biplane views are summarized in Table 59-5. By manipulating the probe via rotation about the long axis and use of the rotary controls, intermediate and off-axis images besides the standard transverse and longitudinal views described above can be obtained. Through hands-on experience, the operator will come to be familiar with these maneuvers.

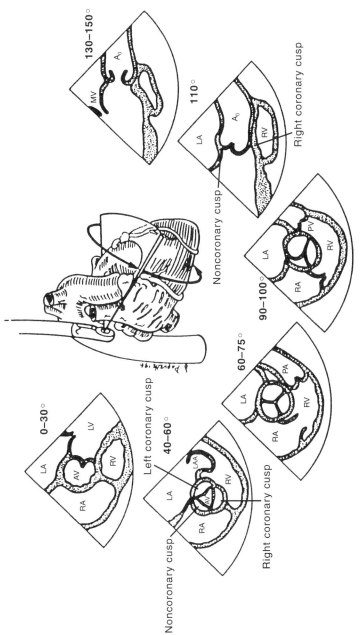

FIG. 59-4A. Schematic representation of selected multiplane transesophageal echocardiography views of the aorta and aortic valve from the upper esophagus. Ao, aorta; LA, left atrium; LV, left ventricle; RA, right atrium; RV, right ventricle; PA, pulmonary artery; PV, pulmonary valve; LAA, left atrial appendage; MV, mitral valve. Modified from Roelandt, JRTC, 1996, with permission.

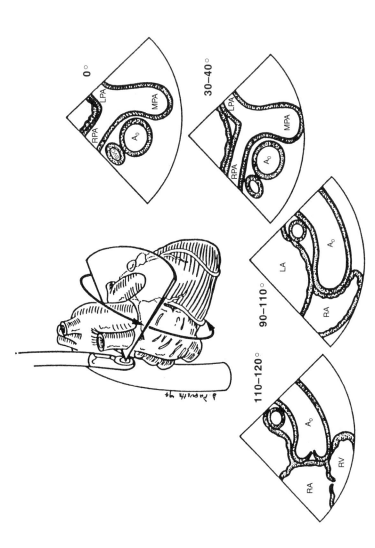

FIG. 59-4B. Schematic of some of the multiplane transesophageal echocardiography views of the aorta and pulmonary artery that can be obtained from the upper esophagus. Ao, aorta; LA, left atrium; LPA, left pulmonary artery; PA, main pulmonary artery; RA, right atrium; RPA, right pulmonary artery; RV, right ventricle; SVC, superior vena cava. Modified from Roelandt, JRTC, 1996, with permission.

IX. **Patient recovery.** The patient's NPO status should be maintained until there is return of the gag reflex. When the patient does commence oral intake, he or she should initially take a small sip of ice water. If it does not feel cold, then there is still some topical anesthetic effect present. Until this is dissipated, the patient should refrain from any hot drinks to avoid scalding. Appropriate precautions should be followed if sedatives were used, as the effects persist for several hours. Patients might have dizziness and orthostatic symptoms for up to several hours later, and should be instructed to sit or lie down if this occurs. Patients should not drive or operate any heavy equipment until the next day.

X. **Probe care.** Following use, the probe should be cleaned with soap, water, and an enzymatic solution to remove saliva. The nonimmersible parts of the probe, such as the handle and rotary controls, should be cleaned with alcohol. Afterward the probe should be soaked in a glutaraldehyde solution for a minimum of 20 minutes and a maximum of several hours to eliminate bacteria. The probe should not soak in this solution overnight. It can then be rinsed with water and air-dried. The probe should be inspected closely for any tears or perforations.

XI. **Complications.** In reported series, the incidence of major and minor complications is 2% to 3%, with the vast majority being minor complications. Major complications (death, esophageal perforation, significant arrhythmias, congestive heart failure, and aspiration) occur with a frequency of 0.3% percent, with a reported mortality of less than 0.01%. Reported minor complications include transient hypotension, hypertension (particularly with agitation), hypoxia, and arrhythmias (such as sustained ventricular tachycardia, nonsustained ventricular tachycardia, and transient atrioventricular block). Methemoglobinemia has been rarely reported due to the anesthetic spray and should be considered if cyanosis occurs. Other complications of intubation include tracheal intubation, laryngospasm, and vocal cord paralysis. Sore throat is not uncommon after the procedure and may persist for a day. Anaphylaxis and other allergic reactions can occur due to the medications used.

XII. **Pitfalls.** The improved resolution and anatomic detail provided by TEE, as compared with transthoracic echocardiography, is what makes it such a powerful diagnostic tool. However, this can also lead to misinterpretation of normal structures. Trabeculations in the atrial appendage can be mistaken for thrombi, and lipomatous hypertrophy of the interatrial septum can be incorrectly labeled as a mass, as can the eustachian valve. The transverse and oblique sinuses can be mistaken for abscess cavities. Off-axis images may create the appearance of a mass on the aortic valve when one of the cusps is cut obliquely (examination in other views and planes will help to clarify this). The lungs can give rise to reverberation artifacts, which can erroneously be diagnosed as dissection flaps (presence in nonanatomic planes, lack of disruption of color Doppler of blood flow, and crossing of normal anatomy all favor diagnosis of artifact).

These pitfalls are best minimized by the experience of the operator, but variations in anatomy may provide diagnostic dilemmas for even the most skilled echocardiographer.

SUGGESTED READINGS

Key Reviews

Foster E, Redberg RF, Schiller NB. Transesophageal echocardiography: indications and technical considerations. *Cardiology Clin* 1993;11:355–360.

Schneider AT, Hsu TL, Scwartz SL, Pandian NG. Single, biplane, multiplane and three-dimensional transesophageal echocardiography: echocardiographic-anatomic correlations. *Cardiol Clin* 1993;11:361–387.

Khanderia BK, Tajik AJ, Seward JB. Multiplane transesophageal echocardiography: examination technique, anatomic correlations and image orientation. *Crit Care Clin* 1996;12:203–233.

Khanderia BK, Seward JB, Tajik AJ. Critical appraisal of transesophageal echocardiography: limitations and pitfalls. *Crit Care Clin* 1996;12:235–251.

Relevant Book Chapters

Griffin BP. Transesophageal echocardiography. In: Topol EJ, ed. *Textbook of cardiovascular medicine.* Philadelphia: Lippincott-Raven Publishers, 1998:1337–1366.

Freeman WK, Seward JB, Tajik AJ. Multiplane transesophageal echocardiography. In: *Transesophageal echocardiography.* Boston: Little, Brown and Company, 1994.

Roelandt JRTC, Pandian NG, eds. *Multiplane transesophageal echocardiography.* New York: Churchill Livingstone, 199:15–68.

Appendix: Drug Index

Michael A. Militello, Cardiology Clinical Pharmacist
The Cleveland Clinic Foundation

This appendix includes most of the available cardiovascular drugs used in clinical practice. The information is arranged in two simultaneous schemes: alphabetically according to drug class and by therapeutic class. Each entry contains the brand and generic name of a drug; usual starting dose and maximal dose where available; mechanism of action; indications both labeled and unlabeled; side effects occurring in more than 1% of the population or, if less than 1%, those that are considered potentially life threatening; and, finally, comments. The table includes some drug interactions; however, this information is not complete. It is important to realize that many of the medications used cardiovascularly and noncardiovascularly have significant drug interactions and one should be aware of these when prescribing any new medication.

ADRENERGIC ANTAGONISTS—PERIPHERAL					
Drug	Dose	Mechanism of action	Indication	Side effects	Comments
Guanadrel (Hylorel)	Initial oral: 5 mg twice daily Maximum: 150 mg/d	Inhibits peripheral adrenergic neurons by initially decreasing the release of norepinephrine and then causing depletion of neuronal norepinephrine	Labeled: Hypertension	- Orthostatic hypotension - Edema (see comments) - Depression - Diarrhea - Drowsiness/fatigue - Dry mouth - Angina - Sexual dysfunction	- Contraindicated in patients with pheochromocytoma, CHF, and patients on MAOIs - Significant sodium and water retention occurs - Use with caution in patients with peptic ulcer disease, renal dysfunction, and asthma - Discontinue 2–3 days prior to surgery because of risk of cardiovascular collapse during anesthesia induction - Exaggerated response to vasopressors
Guanethidine (Ismelin)	Initial oral: 10 mg daily Maximum: 300 mg/d		Labeled: Hypertension	- Orthostatic hypotension - Edema (see comments) - Depression - Diarrhea (may be severe) - Drowsiness/fatigue - Dry mouth - Angina - Sexual dysfunction	- Contraindicated in patients with pheochromocytoma, CHF, and patients on MAOIs - Exaggerated response to exogenous administered vasopressors - May aggravate asthma - Significant sodium and water retention occurs - Do not increase doses more frequently than 5–7 days - High incidence of severe depression
Reserpine (various)	Initial oral: 0.1–0.5 mg daily Maximum: 0.25 mg/d (see comments)	Binds to central and peripheral adrenergic neurons destroying storage vesicles for norepinephrine and dopamine thus decreasing sympathetic outflow	Labeled: Hypertension, Psychotic states (decrease agitation of patients in psychotic states)	- Depression (see comment) - Drowsiness - Nasal congestion - Nausea/vomiting/ abdominal cramps - ↑ gastric acid production - Edema (see comment) - Sexual dysfunction	- Rarely used because of high incidence of side effects - Significant sodium and water retention occurs - Use cautiously in patients with: depression, peptic ulcer disease, renal dysfunction, and gallstones

α-ADRENERGIC AGONIST—CENTRAL

Drug	Dose	Mechanism of action	Indication	Side effects	Comments
General information		Centrally acting α_2-agonist $\downarrow$'s sympathetic outflow		- Sedation - Dry mouth - Hypotension - Dizziness - Sexual dysfunction - Bradycardia - Nausea - Headache	- Abrupt withdrawal will cause rebound hypertension - Rebound hypertension can be severe with concurrent administration of β-blockers
Clonidine (Catapres) (Catapres-TTS)	Initial oral: 0.1 mg 2 times daily Maximum: 2.4 mg/d Transdermal patch TTS 1–0.1 mg/24 h TTS-2–0.2 mg/24 h TTS-3–0.3 mg/24 h	See general information for α-adrenergic agonist	Labeled: Hypertension Unlabeled: Hypertensive urgencies, alcohol and opiate withdrawal, smoking cessation, Tourette's syndrome	- See general information for α-adrenergic agonist - Depression	- CrCl < 10 mL/min reduce dose by 25–50% - When initiating a patch in a patient on clonidine full oral doses must be given the first day, then 1/2 dose the second day and then 1/2 of the second day's dose on the third day then discontinue PO - Patches are replaced weekly - 15% of patients develop contact dermatitis with patches
Guanfacine (Tenex)	Initial oral: 1 mg daily Maximum: 2 mg/d	See general information for α-adrenergic agonist	Labeled: Hypertension Unlabeled: Opiate withdrawal, migraine headache prophylaxis	- See general information for α-adrenergic agonist - Constipation	- Risk of rebound hypertension usually less severe because of long half-life

continued

α-ADRENERGIC AGONIST—CENTRAL (*continued*)

Drug	Dose	Mechanism of action	Indication	Side effects	Comments
Guanabenz (Wytensin)	Initial oral: 4 mg twice daily Maximum: 32 mg/daily	See general information for α-adrenergic agonist	Labeled: Hypertension	- See general information for α-adrenergic agonist - Muscular weakness	
Methyldopa (Aldomet) Methyldopate HCl	Initial oral: 250 mg 2–4 times daily Maximum: 2000 mg/d IV: 250 mg 3–4 times daily up to 1,000 mg 4 times daily	See general information for α-adrenergic agonist	Labeled: Hypertension, hypertensive emergency (IV only)	- See general information for α-adrenergic agonist - Peripheral edema - Hemolytic anemia - Drug fever - Depression - Nightmares - Hepatocellular injury - Anxiety	- Positive Coombs test 10–20% of patients within 6–12 mo - Hemolytic anemia <1% - SLE-like syndrome - Hepatitis is rare - Measure Coombs test at baseline, 6 and 12 mo

α_1-ADRENERGIC ANTAGONIST

Drug	Dose	Mechanism of action	Indication	Side effects	Comments
General information		Peripherally acting α_1- receptor antagonist		- Orthostatic hypotension - Dizziness - Lightheadedness - Drowsiness - Headache - Dry mouth - Malaise	- Give first dose and increased doses at bedtime to limit orthostatic hypotension
Doxazosin (Cardura)	Initial oral: 1 mg daily Maximum: 16 mg daily	See general information for alpha adrenergic antagonist	Labeled: Hypertension	See general information for α-adrenergic antagonist	- Doses >4 mg daily will ↑ risk of orthostatic hypotension
Phentolamine (Regitine)	Hypertensive crisis: 5–20 mg IV push every 1–2 hr Pheochromocytoma diagnosis: 5 mg IV Extravasation: see comments	Competitive nonselective α-adrenergic antagonist having similar affinities for α_1- and α_2-receptors	Labeled: Hypertensive crisis in patients with pheochromocytoma, diagnosis of pheochromocytoma, treatment of skin necrosis in patients with norepinepherine extravasation	- Hypotension - Tachycardia - Arrhythmias - Angina - Nausea/vomiting/diarrhea - Exacerbates peptic ulcer disease - Nasal congestion - Flushing	- Very short duration with a half-life 19 minutes - May be used to treat extravasation of dopamine and epinephrine - Disulfiram reaction may occur - Has + inotropic and chronotropic effects - Extravasation: 5–10 mg diluted in 10 mL of normal saline. Phentolamine is injected in multiple sites around the area of extravasation with 27- to 30-gauge needles changing the needle after each injection. This should be done within 12 hr of extravasation. Skin color should return to normal within 1 hr if treament was effective

continued

α_1-ADRENERGIC ANTAGONIST (*continued*)

Drug	Dose	Mechanism of action	Indication	Side effects	Comments
Prazosin (Minipress)	Initial oral: 1 mg 2–3 times daily Maximum: 20 mg/d	See general information for α-adrenergic antagonist	Labeled: Hypertension Unlabeled: Raynaud's syndrome, benign prostatic hypertrophy, CHF	See general information for α-adrenergic antagonist	- Few patients benefit from doses >40 mg/d
Terazosin (Hytrin)	Initial oral: 1 mg daily Maximum: 20 mg/d	See general information for α-adrenergic antagonist	Labeled: Hypertension, benign prostatic hypertrophy	See general information for α-adrenergic antagonist	

ANGIOTENSIN-CONVERTING ENZYME INHIBITORS					
Drug	Dose	Mechanism of action	Indication	Side effects	Comments
General Information		Inhibits the conversion of angiotensin I to angiotensin II by blocking ACE		- Cough - Acute renal failure - Angioedema - Hyperkalemia - Proteinuria - Hypotension - Headache - Rash - Neutropenia/ agranulocytosis - Dizziness	- Angioedema is rare and may occur at any time during therapy; however, usually occurs with first dose - Severe hypotension seen in patients who are volume-depleted - Contraindicated in pregnancy and bilateral renal artery stenosis or unilateral renal artery stenosis in patients with solitary kidney - Neutropenia and/or agranulocytosis has been reported with many ACE-I - Hematologic abnormalities usually associated collagen vascular disorders, higher doses, and renal dysfunction
Benazepril (Lotensin)	Initial oral: 10 mg daily (see comments) Maximum: 80 mg daily	See general ACE-I information	Labeled: Hypertension	See general ACE-I information	- May need to use twice daily - Use lower doses with renal insufficiency
Captopril (Capoten)	Initial oral: 6.25–12.5 2–3 times daily (see comments) Maximum: 150–450 mg/d	See general ACE-I information	Labeled: Hypertension, heart failure, treatment of left ventricular dysfunction post MI, diabetic nephropathy	- See general ACE-I information - Neutropenia/ agranulocytosis - Abnormal taste	- Most patients do not have an increased response to doses greater than 100 mg 3 times daily - Not a prodrug - Reduce dose in patients with renal dysfunction - Food decreases extent of absorption - Target dosage for heart failure: 50 mg 3 times daily

continued

ANGIOTENSIN-CONVERTING ENZYME INHIBITORS (*continued*)

Drug	Dose	Mechanism of action	Indication	Side effects	Comments
Enalapril (Vasotec)	Initial oral: 2.5 mg 1–2 times daily (see comments) Maximum: 40 mg/d divided doses IV: 0.625–1.25 mg every 6 hr given over 5 min	See general ACE-I information	Labeled: Hypertension, heart failure (symptomatic and asymptomatic)	- See general ACE-I information - Neutropenia/ agranulocytosis - Abnormal taste	- Reduce dose in patients with renal dysfunction - Target dosage for heart failure: 10 mg 2 times daily
Fosinopril (Monopril)	Initial oral: 10 mg daily (see comments) Maximum: 80 mg/d divided doses	See general ACE-I information	Labeled: Hypertension and heart failure	- See general ACE-I information - Neutropenia/ agranulocytosis - Abnormal taste	
Lisinopril (Zestril/ Prinivil)	Initial oral: 2.5 mg daily (see comments) Maximum: 40 mg/d	See general ACE-I information	Labeled: Hypertension, heart failure, and post MI	- See general ACE-I information - Neutropenia	- Not a prodrug - Reduce dose in patients with renal failure - Target dosage for heart failure: 20 mg daily

Drug	Dosing		Indications	Adverse Effects	Comments
Moexipril (Univasc)	Initial oral: 7.5 mg daily (see comments) Maximum: 30 mg/d divided doses	See general ACE-I information	Labeled: Hypertension	- See general ACE-I information - Abnormal taste - Neutropenia	- Food decreases extent of absorption - Reduce dose in patients with renal dysfunction
Quinapril (Accupril)	Initial oral: 10 mg daily (see comments) Maximum: 80 mg/d	See general ACE-I information	Labeled: Hypertension and heart failure	- See general ACE-I information - Neutropenia/agranulocytosis	- Reduce dose in patients with renal dysfunction - Target dosage for heart failure: 20 mg 2 times daily
Ramipril (Altace)	Initial oral: 2.5 mg daily (see comments) Maximum: 10 mg/d divided doses	See general ACE-I information	Labeled: Hypertension, and symptomatic heart failure post MI	- See general ACE-I information - Neutropenia/agranulocytosis	- Reduce dose in patients with renal dysfunction
Trandolapril (Mavik)	Initial oral: 1–2 mg daily (see comments) Maximum: 8 mg/d divided doses	See general ACE-I information	Labeled: Hypertension	- See general ACE-I information	- Reduce dose in patients with hepatic and renal dysfunction

ANGIOTENSIN II RECEPTOR BLOCKERS					
Drug	Dose	Mechanism of action	Indication	Side effects	Comments
General information		Selectively binds to the angiotensin II (AT1) receptor in vascular smooth muscle and in the adrenal cortex thus inhibiting the effects of angiotensin II		- Hypotension - Dizziness - Headache	- Use smaller initial doses in patients on diuretics or suspected volume depletion - Use with caution in patients with renal artery stenosis and patients with renal dysfunction - Contraindicated in pregnancy
Irbesartan (Avapro)	Initial oral: 150 mg daily Maximum: 300 mg daily	See general information for angiotensin II receptor blocker	Labeled: Hypertension Unlabeled: CHF in patients intolerant to ACE-I	See general information for angiotensin II receptor blockers	- See general information for angiotensin II receptor blockers - Adverse effects were greater with placebo in clinical trials than with irbesartan
Losartan (Cozaar)	Initial oral: 50 mg daily Maximum: 100 mg daily	See general information for angiotensin II receptor blocker	Labeled: Hypertension Unlabeled: CHF in patients intolerant to ACE-I	- See general information for angiotensin II receptor blockers - Hyperkalemia - Diarrhea - Dyspepsia - Insomnia	- See general information for angiotensin II receptor blockers - Angioedema has been reported with losartan - Hepatotoxicity has been reported - Reduce dose in patients with hepatic dysfunction - E-3174 metabolite is 40 times as potent as losartan
Valsartan (Diovan)	Initial oral: 80 mg daily Maximum: 320 mg daily	See general information for angiotensin II receptor blocker	Labeled: Hypertension Unlabeled: CHF in patients intolerant to ACE-I	- See general information for angiotensin II receptor blockers - Neutropenia has been reported	- See general information for angiotensin II receptor blockers - Hepatotoxicity has been reported - Initiate therapy with lower doses in patients with hepatic dysfunction and in patients with CrCl < 20–30 mL/min

ANTIARRHYTHMICS

Drug	Dose	Mechanism of action	Indication	Side effects	Comments
Class Ia		Decrease phase 0 depolarization rate and slow intracardiac conduction and prolong refractory period. Effects are associated with sodium and potassium channel blockade.		- Proarrhythmic - Torsades de pointes	- ECG effects: Prolongs QRS, QT, and (±) PR
Quinidine (Various)	Initial oral: 200–400 mg every 6–8 hr	See general information for class Ia	Labeled: atrial fibrillation and flutter, ventricular arrhythmias	- Diarrhea - Nausea/vomiting/abdominal cramping - Rash - Hypotension - Fever - Cinchonism: tinnitus, blurred vision, headache and/or delirium - Platelet-mediated thrombocytopenia - Lupus-like syndrome	- May produce hypotension secondary to a-blocking activity - IV not recommended because of hypotension - Vagolytic effect may enhance AV nodal conduction - Each salt form has varying degrees of quinidine base: sulfate (83%), gluconate (62%), and polygalaturnate (60%) - Quinidine will ↑ digoxin levels and enhance warfarin's effect - Amiodarone ↑'s quinidine levels - Therapeutic range 2–6 mg/L

continued

ANTIARRHYTHMICS (continued)

Drug	Dose	Mechanism of action	Indication	Side effects	Comments
Procainamide (Pronestyl, Procan)	Initial oral: 50 mg/kg/d (normal renal function) *Immediate release:* give every 3–4 hr *Sustained release:* give every 6–8 hr *Procanbid:* give every 12 hr Maximum: 9 g/d IV: Loading dose 14–17 mg/kg up to 1,500 mg infuse at 20 mg/min Maintenance: 2–4 mg/min	See general information for class Ia	Labeled: ventricular arrhythmias Unlabeled: atrial arrhythmias	- Drug-induced SLE - GI symptoms - Hypotension (IV) - Rash - Insomnia/confusion - Chemical hepatitis (rare) - Myopathy - Agranulocytosis	- 50–85% of patients develop (+) ANA and 30–50% will develop symptoms of SLE - Adjust dose in patients with renal dysfunction - 50% eliminated renally - Hepatic elimination by acetylation: there are slow and fast acetylators - Slow acetylators are at higher risk for developing drug induced SLE: fever, arthralgia, rash, pericarditis, and pleuritis - Heart block, bradycardia, and asystole may occur - Therapeutic range: procainamide 4–10 mg/L; NAPA < 20 mg/L

Drug	Dosage	Mechanism of action	Indications	Adverse effects	Comments
Disopyramide (Norpace)	Initial oral load: 300–400 mg Maintenance: 100–200 mg every 6 hr for immediate release 200–400 mg every 12 hr for sustained release Maximum: 1.6 g/d	See general information for class Ia	Labeled: Ventricular arrhythmias Unlabeled: Atrial arrhythmias	- Dry mouth - Urinary retention - Constipation - Blurred vision - Hypotension - Nausea/vomiting - Heart block - Hypoglycemia - Nervousness	- Anticholinergic adverse effects limit its usefulness - Signficant negative inotropic activity and may be useful in patients with hypertrophic obstructive cardiomyopathy - Adjust dosage in patients with CHF, renal insufficiency, hepatic disease, and the elderly - May speed AV nodal conduction secondary to vagolytic effects - Therapeutic range 2–6 mg/L
Class Ib		Decrease phase 0 depolarization rate and slow intracardiac conduction. Moderate sodium channel blocking activity. Shorten action potential duration and refractory period in ventricular tissue.		- Drowsiness - Slurred speech (perioral numbness) - Confusion/ disorientation - Seizures - Paresthesias - Coma - Proarrhythmic - Tremor	- CNS side effects usually occur at levels > 5 mg/L: seizures, coma, pyschosis, tinnitus, tremor - ECG effects: no significant effects

continued

Drug	Dose	Mechanism of action	Indication	Side effects	Comments
Lidocaine (Xylocaine)	IV: Loading dose: 1–1.5 mg/kg given over 2 min repeat every 5–10 min to a maximum of 3 mg/kg. Maintanence: 1–4 mg/min	See general information for class Ib antiarrhythmics	Labeled: Acute treatment of ventricular arrhythmias	- See general information for class Ib - Cardiac depression (with high levels) - Tinnitus - Bradycardia/asystole	- Metabolized in the liver and is dependent on liver blood flow - Use lower maintanance doses in patients with heart failure and liver disease - Levels should be monitored with infusions lasting greater than 24 hr and signs and symptoms of toxicity - Acute phase reactant α_1-acid glycoprotein binds to lidocaine and total lidocaine levels may be high with normal free lidocaine levels. - Half-life may double after 24–48 hr of continuous infusions - Therapeutic levels: 1.5–5 mg/L
Mexilitine (Mexitil)	Initial oral: 400 mg one time then 200–300 mg every 8 hr Maximum: 1200 mg/d	See general information for Class Ib antiarrhythmics	Labeled: Ventricular arrhythmias Unlabeled: Reducing pain associated with diabetic neuropathy	- See general information for class Ib - Nausea/vomiting/anorexia - Thrombocytopenia (rare) - AV block	- CNS side effects similar to lidocaine - Should be given with food to decrease GI side effects - 40% of patients complain of minor CNS side effects - Commonly used with other antiarrhythmics - Reduce dose in patients with hepatic disease and CHF - Reduced dosages may be required in patients with CrCl < 10 mL/min - Therapeutic levels: 0.5–2 mg/L
Tocainide (Tonocard)	Initial oral: 400 mg every 8–12 hr	See general information for Class Ib antiarrhythmics	Labeled: Ventricular arrhythmias Unlabeled: Treatment of myotonic dystrophy, and	- See general information for class Ib - Arthralgia - Agranulocytosis - Aplastic Anemia	- Reduce dose in patients with severe liver disease and renal disease - Agranulocytosis, aplastic anemia, and interstitial pneumonitis rarely occur, but tocainide is rarely used because of this

Drug	Dose	Mechanism	Indications	Side effects	Comments
	Maximum: 2,400 mg/d		trigeminal neuralgia	- Thrombocytopenia - Hepatic granulomas - Interstitial Pneumonitis	- Therapeutic levels: 3–10 mg/L
Class Ic General information		Decrease phase 0 depolarization rate and slow intracardiac conduction velocity to the greatest degree. Most potent sodium channel blockers		- Bradycardia - Heart block - Proarrhythmic - Worsen heart failure - Dizziness	- ECG effects: Prolong PR interval and QRS complex; little to no effect on QT interval - Generally avoided in patients with structural heart disease due to increased mortality - May worsen heart failure
Flecainide (Tambocor)	Initial oral: 50 mg every 12 hr Maximum: 300 mg/d	See general information for class Ic	Labeled: Paroxsysmal atrial fibrillation and flutter, paroxsysmal supraventricular tachycardias (AVNRT), ventricular arrhythmias (see comments)	- See general information for class Ic - Significant (-) inotropy - Blurred vision - Headache - GI upset - Neutropenia	- Increases threshold for electrical defibrillation - Reduce dose in patients with heart failure, liver disease, or renal insufficiency - Therapeutic drug levels: 0.2–1 mg/L
Propafenone (Rythmol)	Initial oral: 150 mg every 8 hr Maximum: 1200 mg/d	See general information for class Ic	Labeled: Ventricular arrhythmias Unlabeled: Supraventricular arrhythmias	- See general information for class Ic - Metallic/bitter taste - Headache - GI upset - Cholestatic jaundice (rare)	- Exhibits β-blocking activity, therefore may worsen asthma or obstructive lung disease - Reduce dose in patients with hepatic disease - Therapeutic drug levels not established

continued

ANTIARRHYTHMICS (continued)

Drug	Dose	Mechanism of action	Indication	Side effects	Comments
Class I mixed Moricizine (Ethmozine)	Initial oral: 200 mg every 8 hr Maximum: 300 mg every 8 hr	See general information for class Ib and Ic	Labeled: Ventricular arrhythmias	- See general information for class Ic	- Reduce dose in patients with hepatic disease or renal insufficiency - Therapeutic drug levels not established
Class II β-Blockers	See β-Blockers	See β-Blockers	See β-Blockers	See β-Blockers	See β-Blockers - ECG effects: Prolongs PR interval and sinus bradycardia
Class III Amiodarone (Cordarone)	Oral loading: 800–1,600 mg/d for 1–3 wk; then 600–800 mg/d for 4 wk Oral maintenance: 100–400 mg daily IV: Initial 150 mg over 10 min then 1 mg/min for 6 hr; then 0.5 mg/min f 10 l	Potassium channel blocker, sodium channel blocker, β-blocker activity, and calcium channel blocking activity	Labeled: Ventricular arrhythmias Unlabeled: Atrial arrhythmias	- Hyper-/hypothyroidism - Chemical hepatitis - Pulmonary fibrosis - Bradycardia - Heart block - Proarrhythmic - Torsades de pointes (rare) - Peripheral neuropathy - Tremor - Blue-gray skin discoloration - Photosensitivity - Corneal microdeposits - GI upset	- ECG effect: Sinus bradycardia, prolong PR interval, QRS complex, and QT interval - IV administration may cause hypotension secondary to amiodarone's vasodilating effects as well as solubilizing agent Tween-80 - Long half-life range 25–53 d - Adverse effects may be prolonged after discontinuation due to long half-life - GI upset limits large oral doses - Desethylamiodarone active metabolite - Use lowest possible maintenance dose to limit toxicity - IV concentrations of > 2mg/mL may cause phlebitis and should be administered by central venous catheter - Therapeutic drug levels: 1–2 mg/L

Bretylium (Bretylol)	IV 5 mg/kg IV push in an unconscious patient if no response then give 10 mg/kg If patient is conscious then give above doses as a 10-min infusion Maintenance: 1–2 mg/min	Exact mechanism unknown, however, initially causes release of norepinephrine from sympathetic nerve terminals and accumulates in these nerve terminals thus preventing further release of norepinephrine; with direct inhibition of potassium channels	Labeled: Life-threatening ventricular arrhythmias	- Hpertension then hypotension - Nausea - Severe vomiting - Retching - Diarrhea - Flushing - Dyspnea - Diaphoresis - Nasal congestion - Irritating to veins	- ECG effect: Sinus bradycardia - Initially blood pressure and heart rate will increase, then there is a fall in blood pressure - Patients receiving bretylium have ↑ sensitivity to catecholamines - Therapeutic drug levels not established
Ibutilide (Corvert)	IV Patients > 60 kg 1mg infused over 10 min followed by another 1 mg infusion over 10 min if patient did not convert to NSR Patients < 60 kg give 0.01 mg/kg in the same fashion as above	- Increase sodium influx - May block potassium channels - Exact mechanism is controversial	Labeled: Conversion of atrial fibrillation or flutter	- Very proarrhythmic - 1.7% risk of inducing a ventricular arrhythmia requiring D/C cardioversion - Torsades de pointes - AV block	- ECG effect: Prolongs QT interval - Patients must be off all medications that prolong the QT interval for at least 5 half-lives prior to receiving ibutilide - Monitor patient for at least four hours or until QT interval normalizes whichever is longer - Correct serum magnesium and potassium levels prior to initiating therapy - Therapeutic drug levels not useful

continued

ANTIARRHYTHMICS (continued)					
Drug	Dose	Mechanism of action	Indication	Side effects	Comments
Sotalol (Betapace)	Initial oral: 80 mg every 12 hr (see comments) Maximum: 640 mg/d	Potassium channel blocker and β-blocker	Labeled: Ventricular arrhythmias Unlabeled: Atrial fibrillation	- See general information for β-blockers - Proarrhythmic - Torsades de pointes	- ECG effect: Sinus bradycardia, prolongs QT and PR interval - See general information for β-blockers - Reduce dose in patients with renal dysfunction - High incidence of proarrhythmic effect - maintain QT interval to <550 ms - Therapeutic drug levels: not clinically useful
Class IV General information		Prolong AV nodal refractory period			- ECG effects: Prolongs PR interval and sinus bradycardia - Avoid in patients with WPW and atrial fibrillation
Diltiazem (Cardizem)	IV: Loading dose: 0.15–0.25 mg/kg given over 2 min; if no response in 5–10 min then 0.35 mg/kg over 2 min (see diltiazem under calcium channel blockers for oral dosing) Maintenance:	See general information for class IV antiarrhythmics	See diltiazem under calcium channel blockers	See diltiazem under calcium channel blockers	See diltiazem under calcium channel blockers

Verapamil (Various)	See calcium channel blockers	See general information for class IV antiarrhythmics	See verapamil under calcium channel blockers	See verapamil under calcium channel blockers	See verapamil under calcium channel blockers
Others					
Adenosine (Adenocard)	IV: 6 mg rapid IV push if no response 12 mg rapid IV push if no response may repeat once	α_1-Receptor agonist leading to depression of AV nodal conduction, and SA node firing	Labeled: Conversion of paroxysmal supraventricular tachycardia	- Facial flushing - Shortness of breath - Chest pressure - Nausea - Arrhythmias - May provoke bronchospasm in asthmatic patients	- Doses should be given at most proximal point - Follow each dose with a 10- to 20-mL normal saline flush - May decrease dose if giving through a central catheter - Half-life about 9 sec - Patients taking methylxanthine may not respond - May produce transient asystole
Digoxin (Lanoxin)	IV: Load: 10–15 µg/kg: 50% given initially then 25% in 6 h and 25% 6 h after second dose (see comments) Maintenance: 0.0625–0.5 mg daily dependent on renal function and patient size	↑ AV nodal refractory period secondary to ↑ in vagal tone and sympathetic withdrawal	Labeled: Heart failure, slows ventricular response in patients with atrial fibrillation/flutter, and paroxysmal atrial tachycardia	- Bradycardia - AV block - Anorexia - Nausea - Diarrhea - Abdominal pain - Blurred vision - Yellow-green halo around light - Confusion	- ECG effects: Prolongs PR interval, depresses ST segment, and flattens T-wave - Use lower loading doses in the elderly and patients with uremia - Bioavailability of oral tablets is 70% therefore patients may require less if given IV digoxin - Many of the side effects are signs of digoxin toxicity - Effects are diminished with increased sympathetic tone - Therapeutic drug levels: 1–2 ng/mL - Toxicity may be seen in patients with therapeutic levels

ANTICOAGULANTS

Direct thrombin inhibitor

Drug	Dose	Mechanism of action	Indication	Side effects	Comments
Bivalirudin (Hirulog)	Investi-gational protocols	Directly binds to thrombin inacti-vating its activity	Investigational for acute coronary syndromes, and DVT prophylaxis	See lepirudin	- Available as investigational use
Lepirudin (rDNA) (Refludan)	IV Loading dose: 0.4 mg/kg over 15–20 sec then 0.15 mg/kg/hr (see comments)	Directly binds to thrombin inacti-vating its activity	Labeled: Anticoagu-lation in patients with heparin induced thrombo-cytopenia and associated throm-boembolic disease	- Bleeding - Abnormal liver function - Rash - Cough/bronchospasm/dyspnea	- Monitor aPTT to goal of 1.5–2.5 above control - Reduce dose in patients with CrCl < 60 mL/min or serum creatinine > 1.5 mg/dL (refer to package insert); avoid continuous infusion when CrCl <15 mL/min - No reversal agent bleeding complications - Expensive $500–700/d
Heparin (various)	Various dosing regimens	Binds to antithrom-bin III increasing its ability to inac-tivate thrombin, as well as acti-vated factors IX, X, XI, XII	Labeled: Treatment and prophylaxis of venous and arterial thrombo-sis	- Bleeding - Thrombocytopenia (see comments) - Elevated AST/ALT - Osteoporosis (long term therapy)	- Heparin induced thrombocytopenia occurs in two forms, antibody-mediated and non-antibody-mediated - 10–15% of patients will have lower platelet count - 1–3% of those with heparin associated throm-bocytopenia will go on to develop antibody-mediated HIT

Heparinoid

Drug	Dose	Mechanism of action	Indication	Side effects	Comments
Danaparoid (Organan)	DVT Prophy-laxis:	Potentiates antitrombin III activity which is	Labeled: Prophy-laxis of postoper-ative deep vein	- Bleeding - Thrombocytopenia - Hyperkalemia	- 5–10 % cross reactivity to heparin induced thrombocytopenia in vitro

750 U every 12 hr by subcutaneous injection Unlabeled use for HIT: Bolus dose < 60 kg–1,500 U 60–74 kg–2,250 U 75–90 kg–3,000 U > 90 kg–3,750 U Then 400 U/hr for 4 hr then 300 U/hr for 4 hr then 150–200 U/hr using antifactor Xa levels maintaining a range of 0.5–0.8 antifactor Xa U/mL. (see comments)	responsible for its anti-factor Xa activity	thrombosis in patients undergoing elective hip replacement Unlabeled: Anticoagulant in patients with heparin induced thrombocytopenia and associated thromboembolic disease	- Discomfort at injection site	- Use with caution in patients with CrCl < 20 mL/min - Monitor antifactor Xa levels in patients with renal dysfunction - Bleeding rates similar to those seen with unfractionated heparin - Calibration curve needs to be specific for danaparoid; LMWH calibration curves are not accurate

continued

ANTICOAGULANTS (*continued*)

(LMWH)

Drug	Dose	Mechanism of action	Indication	Side effects	Comments
General information		Antifactor Xa activity greater than antithrombin activity; however each LMWH has different degrees of antifactor Xa/IIa ratios		- Bleeding - Thrombocytopenia - Rash - Hematoma at injection site - Fever	- Each LMWH has a different anti-factor Xa:IIa ratio and are not considered interchangeable - LMWH produce less heparin induced thrombocytopenia - Patients with heparin induced thrombocytopenia secondary to unfractionated heparin have a high cross-reactivity to LMWH 50–80%
Ardeparin (Normiflo)	DVT Prophylaxis for knee replacement surgery: 50 U/kg subcutaneously every 12 hr	See general information for LMWH	Labeled: Deep vein thrombosis prophylaxis after knee replacement	See general information for LMWH	- Lowest anti-factor Xa:IIa ratio - Use with caution in patients with renal failure
Dalteparin (Fragmin)	DVT Prophylaxis for high risk abdominal surgery: 2,500 IU subcutaneously every 12 hr	See general information for LMWH	Labeled: Prophylaxis against deep vein thrombosis in high risk patients undergoing abdominal surgery	See general information for LMWH	- Renal elimination primary route elimination

	Dosage		Indications	Adverse reactions	Comments
Enoxaparin (Lovenox)	*DVT Prophylaxis:* Hip or knee replacement surgery: 30 mg SC every 12 hr; Abdominal surgery: 40 mg SC daily; *Unstable angina:* 1 mg/kg SC every 12 hr	See general information for LMWH	Labeled: Deep vein thrombosis prophylaxis in patients undergoing knee or hip replacement, and abdominal surgery, unstable angina	See general information for LMWH	- Highest anti-factor Xa:IIa ratio - May need to adjust dose in renal failure; elimination is primarily renal but no recommendations from the manufacturer have been established
Oral Anticoagulants					
General information		Indirect acting anticoagulants by altering the synthesis of coagulation factors II, VII, IX, X, by interfering with vitamin K utilization		- Bleeding - Skin necrosis - Purple toe syndrome - Dermatitis - Cholesterol microembolization - Alopecia	- Avoid large initial doses to reduce risk of hemorrhage and necrosis secondary to the initial decrease in proteins C and S - Maintain INR between 2–3 for most indications except for mechanical heart valves where the range is 2.5–3.5 - Contraindications: Pregnancy, severe uncontrolled hypertension, unreliable patients, hemorrhage tendencies - Besides PT/INR Monitor for evidence of bleeding or bruising and hemoglobin and hematocrit

continued

ANTICOAGULANTS (*continued*)

Drug	Dose	Mechanism of action	Indication	Side effects	Comments
Warfarin (Coumadin)	Initial oral: See comments	See general information for oral anticoagulants	Labeled: Treatment and prophylaxis: of deep vein thrombosis and pulmonary embolism, thromboembolic complications of atrial fibrillation and cardiac valve replacement, and reduce the risk of death, recurrent MI and thromboembolic events after MI	See general information for oral anticoagulants	- Initiation of warfarin therapy is variable; however, 5–10 mg daily is typical - Patients with malabsorption syndromes may require higher doses of warfarin - Numerous drug–drug and food–drug interactions
Dicumarol (Dicoumarol)	Initial oral: See comments	See general information for oral anticoagulants	Labeled: See Warfarin	See general information for oral anticoagulants	- Doses range from 20 to 200 mg daily - Rarely used

β-ADRENERGIC ANTAGONIST					
Drug	Dose	Mechanism of action	Indication	Side effects	Comments
General information		β-Receptor blockade		- Bradycardia - Bronchospasm in predisposed patients - CHF exacerbation - Dizziness - Fatigue - Depression - Sleep disturbances - Hypotension - Sexual dysfunction - Dyslipidemia	- Contraindications: Bradycardia, > 1st degree heart block, cardiogenic shock, acute heart failure, asthma or severe bronchospastic lung disease - β-Blockers possess a high degree of interpatient variability between dose and effect - $β_1$-Selective β-blockers lose selectivity with high doses - Abrupt withdrawal of β-blockers may cause rebound hypertension, precipitate angina in patients with CAD - β-Blockers blunt hypoglycemic reactions - β-Blockers have produced profound hypertension in patients abruptly withdrawing from clonidine
Acebutolol (Sectral)	Initial oral: 200 mg 1–2 times daily Maximum: 1200 mg/d	$β_1$-Selective adrenergic blocker with intrinsic sympathomimetic and membrane stabilizing activity	Labeled: Hypertension and ventricular premature complexes	- See general information for β-blockers	- Resting heart rate will be increased because of ISA
Atenolol (Tenormin)	Initial oral: 25 mg daily (see comments) Maximum: 200 mg daily	$β_1$-Selective adrenergic blocker	Labeled: Hypertension, angina pectoris, and MI Unlabeled: Supraventricular arrhythmias, ventricular	- See general information for β-blockers	- Adjust dose in patients with renal dysfunction - Lower incidence of CNS adverse effects because of low penetration into CNS

continued

Drug	Dose	Mechanism of action	Indication	Side effects	Comments
	IV (see comments): Acute MI 5 mg IV over 5 min then repeated in 10 min then start oral therapy		arrhythmias, migraine headache prophylaxis, alcohol withdrawal anxiety, esophageal varices rebleeding		
Betaxolol (Kerlone)	Initial oral: 10 mg daily Maximum: 40 mg daily	β_1-Selective adrenergic blocker with intrinsic sympathomimetic activity	Labeled: Hypertension	- See general information for β-blockers	- Usually seen as eye drops - Systemic effects may be seen with ophthalmic administration
Bisoprolol (Zebeta)	Initial oral: 2.5–5 mg daily Maximum: 20 mg daily	β_1-Selective adrenergic blocker	Labeled: Hypertension Unlabeled: Angina pectoris, supraventricular arrhythmias, ventricular premature complexes	- See general information for β-blockers	- Adjust dose in patients with renal dysfunction
Carteolol (Cartrol)	Initial oral: 2.5 mg daily Maximum: 10 mg daily	Nonselective β-adrenergic blocker with intrinsic sympathomimetic activity	Labeled: Hypertension Unlabeled: Angina pectoris	- See general information for β-blockers	- Adjust dose in patients with renal dysfunction

Drug	Classification	Dosing	Indications	Side Effects	Comments
Esmolol (Brevibloc)	β_1-Selective adrenergic blocker	IV: Loading dose 500 µg/kg over 1 min. Maintenance dose: 25–300 µg/kg/min. Titrate by 25–50 µg/kg/min every 5–10 min some patients may need a second 500 µg/kg load during titration phase	Labeled: Supraventricular arrhythmias and sinus tachycardia. Unlabeled: Angina pectoris and as adjunctive therapy for acute aortic dissection	- See general information for β-blockers - Nausea - Vomiting - Inflammation and induration at injection site commonly occurs	- Half-life = 9 min - Metabolized in blood by red blood cell esterases to active and inactive metabolites. - Active metabolites may accumulate in patients with significant renal impairment - Extravasation may cause skin necrosis - IV concentrations should not exceed 10 mg/mL
Metoprolol (Lopressor)	β_1-Selective adrenergic blocker	Initial Oral: 25–50 mg 2 times daily. Maximum: 450 mg/d. IV: Acute MI 5 mg IV every 2 min for 3 doses	Labeled: Hypertension, angina pectoris, and myocardial infarction. Unlabeled: Ventricular arrhythmias, supraventricular arrhythmias, migraine prophylaxis, essential	- See general information for β-blockers	

continued

Drug	Dose	Mechanism of action	Indication	Side effects	Comments
			tremor, aggressive behavior, antipsychotic-induced akathisia, stable congestive heart failure		
Nadolol (Corgard)	Initial oral: 40 mg daily Maximum: 320 mg daily	Nonselective β-adrenergic blocker	Labeled: Hypertension and angina pectoris Unlabeled: Ventricular arrhythmias, migraine prophylaxis, essential tremor, lithium induced tremor, Parkinson's tremor, aggressive behavior, antipsychotic-induced akathisia, esophageal varices rebleeding, anxiety, ↓ intraocular pressure	- See general information for β-blockers	- Adjust dose in patients with renal dysfunction

Drug	Dose	Classification	Indications		Comments
Penbutolol (Levatol)	Initial oral: 20 mg daily Maximum: 80 mg daily	Nonselective β-adrenergic blocker with intrinsic sympathomimetic activity	Labeled: Hypertension	- See general information for β-blockers	- High lipid solubility leads to increased CNS penetration and depression - Systemic effects may be seen with ophthalmic administration
Pindolol (Visken)	Initial oral: 5 mg twice daily Maximum: 60 mg daily	Nonselective β-adrenergic blocker with intrinsic sympathomimetic and membrane stabilizing activity	Labeled: Hypertension Unlabeled: Ventricular arrhythmias, anxiety, antipsychotic-induced akathisia	- See general information for β-blockers	- Adjust dose in patients with severe renal and/or hepatic dysfunction
Pr...dol	Initial oral: 10 mg 3–4 times daily Maximum: 480 mg/d ... V (see comments): ... mg slow push ... min ... every ... o a ... m	Non-selective β-adrenergic blocker with membrane stabilizing activity	Labeled: Hypertension, angina pectoris, supraventricular and ventricular arrhythmias, digitalis-induced tachyarrhythmias, MI, pheochromocytoma, migraine prophylaxis, hypertrophic obstructive cardiomyopathy, essential tremor	- See general information for β-blockers	- IV dose is much smaller than oral dose because of high first-pass effect - Oral dosage form available as immediate release, sustained release formulation and oral solution - High lipid solubility leads to increased CNS penetration and depression. - Adjust dosage downward in patients with liver dysfunction and in geriatric patients

continued

Drug	Dose	Mechanism of action	Indication	Side effects	Comments
			Unlabeled: Alcohol withdrawal, esophageal varices rebleeding, anxiety, acute panic disorders, thyrotoxicosis		
...ol (...ocadren)	Initial oral: 10 mg twice daily Maximum: 60 mg/d	Non-selective β-adrenergic blocker	Labeled: Hypertension, ventricular arrhythmias, MI, glaucoma Unlabeled: Migraine prophylaxis, essential tremor, anxiety	- See general information for β-blockers	- Systemic effects may be seen with ophthalmic administration

β-α ANTAGONISTS					
Drug	Dose	Mechanism of action	Indication	Side effects	Comments
Carvedilol (Coreg)	Initial oral: CHF: 3.125 mg 2 times daily (see comments) HTN: 6.25 mg 2 times daily Maximum: CHF: 50 mg 2 times daily HTN: 50 mg/d	Nonselective β-adenergic blocker and $α_1$-adenergic blocker	Labeled: Mild to moderate (NYHA Class II–III) heart failure, essential hypertension	- See general information for β-blockers	- Patients with CHF should be started on carvedilol only after stabilization on ACE-I, diuretics, and/or digitalis - CHF: dose should be titrated no sooner than every 2 weeks to maximally tolerated doses. Patients weighing <85 kg maximum dose is 25 mg 2 times daily
Labetalol (Normodyne/ Trandate)	Initial oral: 100 mg twice daily Maximum: 2,400 mg/d IV dosing: *Multiple injection method* 20 mg IV push over 2 minutes may repeat every 10 minutes to a cumulative dose of 300 mg *Intermittent infusion method* Initiate dose at 2 mg/min until satisfactory response then discontinue infusion. Maximum of 300 mg. May repeat when blood pressure begins to rise	Nonselective β-adrenergic blocker and $α_1$-adrenergic blocker	Labeled: Hypertension Unlabeled: Hypertensive crisis, pheochromocytoma, acute aortic dissection, clonidine withdrawal hypertension	- See general information for β-blocker	- May be effective as a single agent in patients with acute aortic dissection. - IV labetalol has 7:1 β- to- α activity whereas oral labetalol has 3:1 β-to-α activity - Because of long half-life labetalol is not recommended as a continuous infusion

CALCIUM CHANNEL BLOCKERS

Dihydropyridine

Drug	Dose	Mechanism of action	Indication	Side effects	Comments
General information		Blocks calcium channels in vascular smooth muscle producing vasodilatation of peripheral and coronary arteries. Reflex ↑ in sympathetic tone negates the effects on SA and AV nodal conduction		- Peripheral edema - Flushing - Headache - Dizziness - Rash - Hypotension - Reflex tachycardia	- Currently it is no longer recommended to use immediate release dihydropyridine calcium channel blockers to acutely lower blood pressure due to potential for inducing stroke and MI. Also, large doses of short acting calcium channel blockers *may* increase risk of MI. - Calcium channel blockers have many drug interactions because of hepatic metabolism
Amlodipine (Norvasc)	Initial oral: 2.5 mg daily Maximum: 10 mg/d	See general information for dihydropyridine calcium channel blockers	Labeled: Hypertension and stable and vasospastic angina	See general information for dihydropyridine calcium channel blockers	- Reduce dose in patients with hepatic dysfunction
Felodipine (Plendil)	Initial oral: 5 mg daily Maximum: 40 mg/d	See general information for dihydropyridine calcium channel blockers	Labeled: Hypertension	See general information for dihydropyridine calcium channel blockers	- Reduce dose in patients with hepatic dysfunction - Grapefruit juice increases bioavailability and should be avoided
Isradipine (DynaCirc)	Initial oral: 2.5 mg 2 times daily Maximum: 20 mg/d	See general information for dihydropyridine calcium channel blockers	Labeled: Hypertension	See general information for dihydropyridine calcium channel blockers	- Doses greater than 10 mg daily add no benefit

Drug	Dose	Mechanism	Indications	Adverse effects	Special considerations
(Cardene) IV Initiate infusion at 5 mg/hr ↑ by 2.5 mg/hr every 15 minutes to a maximum of 15 mg/hr	20 mg three times daily Maximum: 120 mg/d	...mation for dihydropyridine calcium channel blockers	...tension (immediate and sustained release and IV) and stable angina (immediate release only)	...tion for dihydropyridine calcium channel blockers	hepatic dysfunction
Nifedipine (Procardia, Adalat)	Initial oral: 10 mg 3 times daily Maximum: 180 mg/d (see comments)	See general information for dihydropyridine calcium channel blockers	Labeled: Hypertension and vasospastic angina (sustained release only) Unlabeled: Migraine headache prophylaxis, primary pulmonary hypertension, lower esophageal sphincter spasm	See general information for dihydropyridine calcium channel blockers - Gingival hyperplasia (rare)	- Reduce dose in patients with cirrhosis - Grapefruit juice increases bioavailability and should be avoided
Nisoldipine (Sular)	Initial oral: 20 mg daily Maximum: 60 mg/d	See general information for dihydropyridine calcium channel blockers	Labeled: Hypertension	See general information for dihydropyridine calcium channel blockers	- Grapefruit and high-fat meals increase bioavailability and should be avoided - Reduce dose in patients with hepatic dysfunction
Benzothiazepine					
Diltiazem (Cardizem, Dilacor)	Initial oral: 30 mg 3 times daily Maximum: 360 mg/d	Calcium channel blockade produces vasodilatation of coronary and peripheral	Labeled: Hypertension angina and supraventricular arrhythmias	- Negative inotropic - Headache - Flushing - Dizziness - Edema	- Avoid in patients with WPW and concurrent atrial fibrillation - Consider reduced doses in patients with hepatic dysfunction

continued

CALCIUM CHANNEL BLOCKERS (*continued*)

Drug	Dose	Mechanism of action	Indication	Side effects	Comments
	(See diltiazem under antiarrhythmics for IV dosing)	arteries as well as ↓ heart rate and prolonging AV nodal conduction.		- Bradycardia - AV block - Hypotension	
Diphenylalkylamine					
Verapamil (Calan, Isoptin)	Initial oral: 80 mg 3 times daily Maximum: 480 mg/d	Calcium channel blockade produces vasodilatation of coronary and peripheral arteries as well as ↓ heart rate and prolonging AV nodal conduction.	Labeled: Hypertension, angina, supraventricular arrhythmias Unlabeled: Migraine and cluster headache prophylaxis, exercise-induced asthma, hypertrophic obstructive cardiomyopathy, nocturnal leg cramps	- Negative inotropic - Constipation - Hypotension - Bradycardia - AV block	- Avoid in patients with WPW and concurrent atrial fibrillation - Consider reduced doses in patients with hepatic dysfunction

Miscellaneous

Bepridil (Vascor)	Initial oral: 200 mg daily Maximum: 400 mg/d	Type 4 calcium channel blocker and has properties similar to typical calcium channel blockers and may inhibit fast sodium channels	Labeled: Stable angina	- Dizziness - Headache - Nausea/dyspepsia/ abdominal pain/ anorexia - Weakness - Bradycardia - Nervousness - Diarrhea - Torsades de pointes	- Causes QT prolongation - Many patients cannot tolerate side effects - Reserved for patients who are either intolerant or maximized to other antianginals - Data are lacking for dosage adjustments in patients with hepatic dysfunction

DIURETICS						
Drug	Dose	Mechanism of action	Indication	Side effects	Comments	
Loop						
General information		Block chloride reabsorption in the ascending loop of Henle, sodium and water, then follow	See individual agent	- ↓ Serum electrolytes: K, Cl, Mg, Ca, Phosphate, Na - Ototoxicity - Tinnitis - Hyperuricemia - Hyperglycemia - Rash - Azotemia - Dyslipidemia	- Loop diuretics gain access to the lumen of the nephron by organic acid pump and do not rely on glomerular filtration - Overdiuresis may cause a hypochloremic metabolic alkalosis - Additive ototoxic effects when loop diuretics are added to other ototoxic drugs	
Bumetanide (Bumex)	Initial oral: 0.5 mg 1–2 times daily Maximum: 10 mg daily IV: 0.5–1 mg to a maximum of 10 mg daily	See general information for loop diuretic	Labeled: Edema	- See general information for loop diuretic	- Onset 10–30 min - IV Furosemide/bumetanide ratio is 40:1 - IV/PO conversion 1:1 - IV doses up to 0.5–1 mg should be given over 1–2 min - IV doses 3–5 mg should be given over 10 min - IV doses >5 mg should be infused at 0.25 mg/min to reduce risk of ototoxicity - Continuous infusions of bumetanide have been used - Contains a sulfhydryl group and patients allergic to sulfonamides may cross-react	
Ethacrynic acid (Edecrin)	Initial oral: 50 mg daily Maximum: 400 mg daily	See general information for loop diuretic	Labeled: Edema	- See general information for loop diuretic	- Onset within 30 minutes - Safest alternative in patients allergic to bumetanide, furosemide, torsemide, or thiazides because contains no sulfhydryl group.	

	IV: 50 mg or 0.5–1 mg/kg to a maximum of 100 mg daily infused over several minutes			- 50 mg of IV ethacrynic acid ~ 35 mg furosemide ~ 1 mg bumetanide - Give IV doses slowly to limit ototoxicity
Furosemide (Lasix)	Initial oral: 20 mg 1–3 times daily Maximum: 480 mg/d (see comments) IV: Variable Doses > 200 mg should be infused at 4 mg/min	See general information for loop diuretic	Labeled: Edema and hypertension Unlabeled: Hypercalcemia	- See general information for loop diuretic	- To limit ototoxicity doses > 160 mg should be infused at 4 mg/min - IV/PO conversion 1:2 - Bioavailability may be decreased in patients with CHF - IV Furosemide/bumetanide ratio is 40:1
Torsemide (Demadex)	Initial oral: 5 mg/d Maximum: 200 mg/d IV: Highly variable Give IV doses over 2 min	See general information for loop diuretic	Labeled: Edema and hypertension	- See general information for loop diuretic	- 5–10 mg torsemide ~ 20 mg IV furosemide - IV/PO conversion 1:1 - Bioavailability similar in healthy individuals when compared to patients with CHF

continued

Drug	Dose	Mechanism of action	Indication	Side effects	Comments
Thiazide and like diuretics					
General information		Interfere with sodium ion transport in the distal convoluted tubule with chloride and water excretion being enhanced	Labeled: Edema and hypertension Unlabeled: Diabetes insipidus, prophylaxis of renal calculus associated with hypercalcemia	- $\downarrow$ in serum electrolytes: K, Mg, Cl, Na - $\uparrow$ Calcium and uric acid levels - Dehydration - Rash - Hypersensitivity reactions - Dyslipidemia - Hyperglycemia - Hematologic abnormalities (rare) - Photosensitivity	- Thiazides are not effective in patients with CrCl < 30 mL/min - Patients allergic to sulfonamide-derived drugs may be allergic to thiazide diuretics - Recommended first-line therapy for hypertension - Synergistic diuresis when added to loop diuretics
Chlorothiazide (Diuril)	Initial oral: 500 mg 1–2 times daily Maximum: 2,000 mg/d IV: 250–1,000 mg 1–2 times daily	See general information for thiazide and thiazide-like diuretics	See general information for thiazide and thiazide-like diuretics	See general information for thiazide and thiazide-like diuretics	- Only thiazide available for IV administration
Chlorthalidone (Hygroton)	Initial oral: 25 mg daily Maximum: 100 mg/d	See general information for thiazide and thiazide-like diuretics	See general information for thiazide and thiazide-like diuretics	See general information for thiazide and thiazide-like diuretics	- Thiazide-like diuretic - Doses >25 mg rarely improve diuresis

Drug	Dosing	Action	Indication	Adverse Effects	Comments
Hydrochloro-thiazide (Hydro-Diuril)	Initial oral: 12.5–25 mg daily Maximum: 50 mg/d	See general information for thiazide and thiazide-like diuretics	See general information for thiazide and thiazide-like diuretics	See general information for thiazide and thiazide-like diuretics	- Thiazide-like diuretics - Does not affect lipid levels
Indapamide (Lozol)	Initial oral: 1.25–2.5 mg daily Maximum: 5 mg/d	See general information for thiazide and thiazide-like diuretics	See general information for thiazide and thiazide-like diuretics	See general information for thiazide and thiazide-like diuretics	
Metolazone (Zaroxolyn)	Initial oral: 2.5–10 mg/d Maximum: 20 mg/d	See general information for thiazide and thiazide-like diuretics	See general information for thiazide and thiazide-like diuretics	See general information for thiazide and thiazide-like diuretics	- Thiazide-like diuretics - May be useful in patients with CrCl < 30 mL/min - Long half-life may cause prolonged diuresis - Hypokalemia may limit duration of therapy

Potassium Sparing

Drug	Dosing	Action	Indication	Adverse Effects	Comments
Amiloride (Midamor)	Initial oral: 5 mg daily Maximum: 20 mg daily	Acts directly on the distal convoluted tubule and collecting ducts to decrease active transport of sodium and potassium	Labeled: adjunctive diuretic to thiazide and loop diuretics Unlabeled: reduce lithium associated polyuria, hyperaldosteronism	- Nausea/vomiting/diarrhea - Headache - Rash - Hyperkalemia - Hyperchloremic metabolic acidosis - Hyponatremia - Gynecomastia - Impotence	- Weak diuretic effect and its use is to help prevent hypokalemia in patients on potassium-wasting diuretics - Use cautiously in patients with renal dysfunction secondary to potential for hyperkalemia

continued

Drug	Dose	Mechanism of action	Indication	Side effects	Comments
DIURETICS (*continued*)					
Spirono-lactone (Aldactone)	Initial oral: 50 mg 1–2 times daily Maximum 400 mg/d	Competitive inhibitor of aldo-sterone in the distal convoluted tubule	Labeled: Primary aldosteronism, edema, hyper-tension, and hypokalemia associated with loop or thiazide diuretics	- Hyperkalemia - Fatigue - Gynecomastia - Sexual dysfunction - Breast tenderness in women - Nausea/vomiting/ diarrhea - Confusion	- Long half-life of metabolites - Use cautiously in patients with renal dysfunc-tion secondary to potentiation of hyperkalemia
Triamterene (Dyrenium)	Initial oral: 50 mg daily Maximum: 300 mg/d	Acts directly on the distal convoluted tubule and col-lecting ducts to decrease active transport of sodium and potassium	Labeled: Edema, and hypokalemia associated with loop or thiazide diuretics	- Rash - Hyperkalemia - Nausea/vomiting/ diarrhea - Hyponatremia - Megaloblastic ane-mia (see comments)	- Use cautiously in patients with renal dysfunc-tion secondary to potentiation of hyperkalemia - May cause metabolic acidosis - Megaloblastic anemia may occur in alcoholic cirrhosis
CARBONIC ANHYDRASE INHIBITORS					
Drug	Dose	Mechanism of action	Indication	Side effects	Comments
Acetazol-amide (Diamox)	Initial oral: 250 mg 1–4 times daily Maintenance: varies IV: 250–500 mg once daily for edema	Carbonic anhydrase inhibitor	Labeled: Edema, centrencephalic epilepsies, glau-coma, acute mountain sickness	- Malaise - Anorexia - Diarrhea - Metallic taste - Depression - Rash - Black stools	- Not useful as a diuretic for long term treat-ment; loses effectiveness within 24–48 hr - Causes a metabolic acidosis - Reduce dose in patients with renal dysfunction - Ineffective when CrCl < 10 mL/min - May be used acutely for metabolic alkalosis induced by loop diuretics

INOTROPIC AGENTS

Drug	Dose	Mechanism of action	Indication	Side effects	Comments
Amrinone (Inocor)	Loading dose: 0.5 mg/kg given over 5 min (see comments) Maintenance dose: 5–15 μg/kg/min	Myocardial cell phosphodiesterase inhibitor which results in an ↑ in intracellular cAMP thus ↑ contractility. It is also a potent vasodilator by direct effects on vascular smooth muscle	Labeled: Short-term management of congestive heart failure	- Thrombocytopenia - Ventricular arrhythmias - Hypotension - Nausea - Hepatotoxicity - Hypersensitivity reactions	- If hypotension occurs during loading dose decrease the rate of administration and give over 15–20 min - Half-life prolonged in patients with heart failure - Thrombocytopenia dose and duration-dependent occurring within 48–72 hr. Reversible upon discontinuation - Consider dosage adjustment in patients with renal failure and liver dysfunction - Long half-life (4–6 hr) may cause prolonged hypotension in patients
Dopamine (Intropin)	1–3 μg/kg/min primarily dopamine effects 5–10 μg/kg/min primarily β effects 10–20 μg/kg/min primarily α effects	Mixed α, β, and dopaminergic agonist	Labeled: Hypotension, shock secondary to cardiogenic, septicemia, and trauma	- Tachycardia - Ventricular arrhythmias - Hypertension - Headache - Nausea	- Dose-dependent effects; lower doses produce an increase in renal blood flow, medium range doses β effects predominate, and higher doses α effects predominate - Central line is recommended - Skin necrosis may occur with extravasation - Short half-life ~ 2 min - Central line required when given by continuous infusion

continued

INOTROPIC AGENTS *(continued)*

Drug	Dose	Mechanism of action	Indication	Side effects	Comments
Dobutamine (Dobutrex)	2.5–20 µg/kg/min	Relatively selective β-receptor agonist	Labeled: Short-term inotropic support in patients with acute cardiac decompensation	- Tachycardia - Hypo-/hypertension - Ventricular arrhythmias - Nausea - Headache - Myocardial ischemia	- Dose-dependent tachycardia - Tachyphylaxis may occur with prolonged administration - Long-term outpatient administration in dependent patients may have an increase in mortality, secondary to ventricular arrhythmias - May be used in combination with phosphodiesterase inhibitors
Epinephrine (Adrenalin)	0.01–0.05 µg/kg/min primarily β effects 0.05–1 µg/kg/min α and β effects	Mixed α and β agonist	Labeled: Ventricular standstill, shock, anaphylaxis	- Tachycardia - Flushing - Hypertension - Restlessness - Exacerbation of narrow-angle glaucoma - Ventricular arrhythmias	- May decrease renal and splanchnic blood flow secondary to vasoconstriction - Increase myocardial oxygen demand - Central line required for continuous infusion - Extravasation may lead to skin necrosis - Short half-life ~ 2 min - Central line required when given by continuous infusion

Drug	Dose	Action	Indications	Side Effects	Comments
Isoproternol (Isuprel)	2–20 μg/kg/min	Nonselective β-receptor agonist	Labeled: Shock, heart block, Adams-Stokes attacks, bronchospasm Unlabeled: Bradycardia until temporary pacing can be accomplished, Torsades de pointes	- Tachycardia - Ventricular arrhythmias - Hypotension - Myocardial ischemia - Mild tremors - Nervousness - Flushing	- Short half-life < 5 min - May worsen myocardial ischemia - More likely to induce arrhythmias than other inotropic agents - May be effective in patients with β-blocker overdose
Milrinone (Primacor)	Loading dose: 50 μg/kg Maintenance dose: 0.375–7.5 μg/kg/min	Myocardial cell phosphodiesterase inhibitor which results in an ↑ in intracellular cAMP thus ↑ contractility. It is also a potent vasodilator by direct effects on vascular smooth muscle	Labeled: Short-term management of CHF	- Hypotension - Ventricular arrhythmias - Supraventricular arrhythmias - Angina - Chest pain - Headache - Tremor - Thrombocytopenia (rare)	- Thrombocytopenia occurs < 1% of patients - Long-term therapy may ↑ mortality secondary to ventricular arrhythmias - May be used in combination with dobutamine because of different mechanism of action - Loading dose may not be needed in patients with severe renal dysfunction - Loading dose may cause hypotension

LIPID LOWERING AGENTS					
Drug	Dose	Mechanism of action	Indication	Side effects	Comments

Bile Acid Resins

Drug	Dose	Mechanism of action	Indication	Side effects	Comments
Cholestyramine (Questran Light)	Initial oral: 4 g 1–2 times daily (anhydrous cholestyramine) Maximum: 24 g/d divided doses (Anhydrous cholestyramine)	Bind intestinal bile acids preventing enterohepatic recycling leading to increased stool elimination of bile acid	Labeled: Hypercholesterolemia and relief partial biliary obstruction pruritus Unlabeled: *Clostridium difficile* toxin binder; adjunct to thyroid and digitalis overdose	- Constipation - Flatulence - Abdominal pain - Bloating - Heartburn - Steatorrhea - Diarrhea - Hypertriglyceridemia	- 4 g of cholestyramine = 5 g of colestipol - Many drug interactions: digoxin, thyroid hormones, warfarin, fat-soluble vitamins, others - Separate from other medications - May raise triglycerides - High rate of noncompliance secondary to taste - No systemic effects
Colestipol (Colestid)	Initial oral: 5 g 1–2 times daily Maximum: Powder 30 g/d divided doses Tablets 16 g/d divided doses	See cholestyramine	Labeled: Hypercholesterolemia Unlabeled: adjunct to digitalis overdose	See cholestyramine	See Cholestyramine

Fibric Acids

Clofibrate (Atromid-S)	Initial oral: 1 g 2 times daily	- Exact mechanism unknown; however, triglyceride and VLDL clearance is increased and ↓ cholesterol synthesis	Labeled: Type III, IV, and V hyperlipidemia	- Nausea - Dyspepsia - Flatulence - Myalgia - ↑ AST/ALT - Renal failure (rare) - Anemia, agranulocytosis, leukopenia	- Rarely used because ↑ risk of cholelithiasis and hepatic malignancy (animal studies) with no substantial cardiovascular benefits - Monitor liver function tests and CBC - Contraindicated in patients with significant hepatic and renal dysfunction, primary biliary cirrhosis, and pregnancy - Reduce dose in patients with renal dysfunction - Enhance effects of warfarin, insulin, and sulfonylureas
Fenofibrate (Tricor)	Initial oral: 67–201 mg/d (three 67-mg capsules)	- Exact mechanism unknown - Inhibits triglyceride synthesis and stimulates catabolism of VLDL	Labeled: Types IV and V hyperlipidemia	- Rash - Gastrointestinal disturbances - ↑ AST/ALT - Arthralgia - Headache - Flu-like symptoms - Dyspepsia	- Combination with an HMG-CoA reductase inhibitor may increase risk of rhabdomyolysis - Contraindicated in patients with severe hepatic and renal disease, and gallbladder disease - Monitor liver function tests - Reduce dose to 67 mg daily if CrCl is < 50 mL/min - May enhance effects of warfarin - Bile acid sequestrants decrease absorption
Gemfibrozil (Lopid)	Initial oral: 600 mg 2 times daily	- Exact mechanism unknown, however there is inhibition of lipolysis and ↓ VLDL levels and ↑ HDL levels	Labeled: Types IV and V hyperlipidemia, and reduces risk of coronary heart disease in type IIb patients	- Dyspepsia - Abdominal pain - Cholelithiasis - Diarrhea - Fatigue - Mild to moderate hyperglycemia - Rash - Hepatotoxicity - Drowsiness/dizziness or blurred vision	- Associated with rhabdomyolysis when given with statins - Occasional hematologic abnormalities - Monitor liver function tests - May enhance warfarin effects

continued

LIPID LOWERING AGENTS (continued)					
Drug	Dose	Mechanism of action	Indication	Side effects	Comments
HMG-CoA Reductase Inhibitors					
General information		Inhibit HMG-CoA, the rate-controlling enzyme for endogenous cholesterol production		- Heartburn/flatulence/nausea - Rash/pruritus - ↑ creatine phosphokinase - Myalgia - Lenticula opacities - Gynecomastia - Hepatotoxicity	- All statins are substrates for cytochrome P450 system 3A4 to different degrees and inhibitors of this enzyme may increase statin levels increasing risk for rhabdomyolysis - Rhabdomyolysis is rare but increases with concomitant administration of cyclosporine, gemfibrozil, niacin, erythromycin, itraconazole, and ketoconazole - May enhance warfarin effects - Monitor: LFT periodically - Statins produce a dose-dependent reduction in LDL
Atorvastatin (Lipitor)	Initial oral: 10 mg/d Maximum: 80 mg/d	See general information for HMG-CoA reductase inhibitors	Labeled: Hypercholesterolemia and mixed lipidemia	See general information for HMG-CoA reductase inhibitors	- Greatest effect on LDL cholesterol and triglycerides
Cerivastatin (Baycol)	Initial oral: 0.3 mg daily Maximum: same	See general information for HMG-CoA reductase inhibitors	Labeled: Hypercholesterolemia, and mixed lipidemia	See general information for HMG-CoA reductase inhibitors	Currently, higher doses are being studied
Fluvastatin (Lescol)	Initial oral: 20–40 mg/d Maximum: 80 mg/d	See general information for HMG-CoA reductase inhibitors	Labeled: Hypercholesterolemia	See general information for HMG-CoA reductase inhibitors	- Weakest effect on LDL

Drug	Dosing	Mechanism	Indication	Adverse Reactions	Comments
Lovastatin (Mevacor)	Initial oral: 10–20 mg daily Maximum: 80 mg/d	See general information for HMG-CoA reductase inhibitors	Labeled: Hypercholesterolemia, and slow the progression of atherosclerosis	See general information for HMG-CoA reductase inhibitors	- Taken with evening meals increase absorption - Studies support use in primary prevention
Pravastatin (Pravachol)	Initial oral: 10–20 mg/d Maximum: 40 mg/d	See general information for HMG-CoA reductase inhibitors	Labeled: Slow progression of atherosclerosis, primary prevention of coronary events, and hypercholesterolemia	See general information for HMG-CoA reductase inhibitors	- Only statin indicated for both primary and secondary prevention
Simvastatin (Zocor)	Initial oral: 5–10 mg/d Maximum: 40 mg/d	See general information for HMG-CoA reductase inhibitors	Labeled: Hypercholesterolemia and coronary heart disease	See general information for HMG-CoA reductase inhibitors	- Studies support use in secondary prevention
Others					
Niacin (nicotinic acid) (various)	Initial oral: 100 mg 2–3 times daily titrated to 3 g/d Maximum: 8 g/d divided doses	- Exact mechanism unknown - Inhibition of lipolysis, reduced LDL and VLDL synthesis and ↑ lipoprotein lipase activity may be involved	Labeled: Vitamin B_3 replacement Unlabeled: Hypercholesterolemia	- Facial flushing - Hyperuricemia - Hyperglycemia - Gastric irritation - Pruritis - Chemical hepatitis	- Sustained release formulations are avoided because of greater risk for hepatotoxicity - Flushing minimized with aspirin - Effective for ↓ TC (total cholesterol), LDL, triglycerides, and ↑ HDL - Food helps ↓ GI intolerance

NITRATES

Drug	Dose	Mechanism of action	Indication	Side effects	Comments
General information		Biotransformation of nitrates releases nitric oxide causing vasodilatation through cAMP. Venous dilatation predominates.		- Headache - Hypotension (large doses) - Flushing - Dizziness - Rash - Nausea - Methemoglobinemia - Reflex tachycardia	- Long-term nitrate use without nitrate-free intervals leads to nitrate tolerance; with loss of hemodynamic and antianginal effects; mechanism is controversial - Tolerance can be limited by providing a nitrate-free interval of 10–12 hr - Headache and postural hypotension usually decrease over several days of therapy - Causes coronary artery dilatation and improves collateral blood flow
Isosorbide dinitrate (Isordil, Sorbitrate)	Initial oral: 10 mg 3 times daily allowing for a 12 hr nitrate free interval Maximum: 40 mg/dose	- See general information for nitrates	Labeled: Prevention of anginal attacks Unlabeled: heart failure when used in combination with hydralazine	- See general information for nitrates	- Used in combination with hydralazine in CHF
Isosorbide Mononitrate (Imdur, Ismo, Monoket)	Initial oral: Immediate release 10–20 mg 2 times daily separated by 7 hr Sustained release: 15–30 mg daily to a maximum	- See general information for nitrates	Labeled: Prevention of anginal attacks	- See general information for nitrates	- Longer half-life may lead to nitrate tolerance if dosed greater than once daily

Drug	Dose		Indications		Comments
Nitroglycerin Paste (Nitrol)	Initial: ½–4 in. every 6 hr holding one dose to allow for a 12-hr nitrate-free interval	- See general information for nitrates	Labeled: Prevention of anginal attacks	- See general information for nitrates	- Inconvenient for long-term therapy secondary to ointment is messy. - Dose absorbed is related to skin surface area in which ointment is applied - Quick onset once applied to skin
Nitroglycerin Patch (Various)	0.2–0.8 mg/hr patch on for 12 hr and off for 12 hr	- See general information for nitrates	Labeled: Prevention of anginal attacks	- See general information for nitrates - Contact dermatitis	- Some patients develop a contact dermatitis with certain patches - Inform patients to rotate patch sites
Nitroglycerin SL (Nitrostat, Nitrolingual spray)	Use as needed for chest pain 0.4 mg every 5 min × 3	- See general information for nitrates	Labeled: Acute treatment or prophylaxis or anginal attacks	- See general information for nitrates	- Each spray delivers 0.4 mg of nitroglycerin - Most common sublingual tablet is 0.4 mg (0.3–0.6 mg) - Effective for acute anginal attacks and prophylaxis of angina for known exertional activities - Tablets start degrading once bottle is opened and if stored correctly should be replaced every 3–6 months
Nitroglycerin IV (Tridil)	IV: 5–10 µg/min initially then increase by 5–10 µg/min every 5–10 min for relief of chest pain	- See general information for nitrates	Labeled: Perioperative hypertension, CHF with acute MI, angina, Unlabeled: Hypertensive crisis; pulmonary hypertension	- See general information for nitrates	- Methemoglobinemia may occur with high doses - May increase intracranial pressure - IV formulation is poorly soluble

PLATELET INHIBITORS

Drug	Dose	Mechanism of action	Indication	Side effects	Comments
Cyclooxygenase inhibitor					
Aspirin	Initial oral: 162–325 mg × 1 Maintenance: 81–325 mg daily	Irreversibly acetylate platelet cyclooxygenase decreasing the formation of thromboxane A_2 from arachidonic acid	Labeled: analgesic, antipyretic, anti-inflammatory, MI, transient ischemic attack, cerebrovascular accident	- Bleeding - Gastric ulceration - Nausea/dyspepsia/ heartburn - Hemolytic anemia - Tinnitus (large doses or overdose)	- Food and enteric coating decreases gastric upset
Glycoprotein IIb/IIIa inhibitors					
Abciximab (Reopro)	PCI: 0.25 mg/kg 10–60 min before intervention immediately followed by 0.125 µg/kg/min (maximum 10 µg/min) for 12 hr Unstable angina with PCI: 0.25 mg/kg starting 18–24 hr	Murine-derived monoclonal antibody Fab fragment to the human GP IIb/IIIa receptor on the platelet surface, inhibiting platelet aggregation	Labeled: PCI and unstable angina when percutaneous coronary intervention is planned within 24 hr	- Bleeding - Thrombocytopenia - Hypersensitivity reactions	- Platelet function returns to normal usually within 48 hr; abciximab can be seen in the circulation bound to platelets for up to 10 days - Data are lacking for readministration of abciximab - Thrombocytopenia is usually transient - Low immunogenicity

Drug	Dosage	Mechanism	Indication	Adverse Effects	Comments
	before PCI, immediately followed by 0.125 µg/kg/min (maximum 10 µg/min), infusion ending 1 hr after intervention				- Typical infusions should continue for 48–72 hr and should be continued for 24 hr after PTCA or atherectomy - All patients should receive aspirin - Most patients in clinical studies also received heparin - Use lower doses in patients with renal dysfunction - Monitor hemoglobin/hematocrit and platelet counts
Eptifibatide (Integrilin)	Acute coronary syndrome: 180 µg/kg bolus followed by 2 µg/kg/min for a maximum of 96 hr (see comments) PCI: 135 µg/kg bolus followed by 0.5 µg/kg/min for 20–24 hr	Heptapeptide antagonist that reversibly inhibits GP IIb/IIIa receptor on the platelet surface, inhibiting platelet aggregation	Labeled: Acute coronary syndromes (unstable angina and non-Q wave MI) with or without percutaneous intervention	- Bleeding - Thrombocytopenia	
Tirofiban (Aggrastat)	Acute Coronary Syndrome:	Nonpeptide antagonist that reversibly inhibits	Acute coronary syndrome in patients who are being	- Bleeding - Thrombocytopenia	- Infusions should continue for 12–24 hr after PTCA or atherectomy continued

PLATELET INHIBITORS (continued)

Drug	Dose	Mechanism of action	Indication	Side effects	Comments
	0.4 µg/kg/min for 30 minutes then 0.1 µg/kg/min for 48 hr. For patients with CrCl < 30 mL/min the dose should be cut in half.	GP IIb/IIIa receptor on the platelet surface inhibiting platelet aggregation	treated medically and those undergoing PTCA or atherectomy		- Heparin and aspirin should be given concomitantly - Monitor hemoglobin/hematocrit and platelet counts
Others					
Clopidogrel (Plavix)	Initial oral: 75 mg daily	Inhibition of adenosine diphosphate–induced platelet aggregation	Labeled: Reduce the risk of MI, stroke, and/or peripheral arterial disease in patients with a completed MI, stroke, and/or peripheral arterial disease Unlabeled: Adjunctive therapy after coronary artery stent placement	- Diarrhea - Headache - Dizziness - Abdominal pain/nausea/dyspepsia - Purpura - Rash	- Most side effects when compared to aspirin in clinical trials were less in the clopidogrel-treated group - Maximal effects are seen 3–7 days after initiation of therapy

Drug	Dosing	Mechanism	Indications	Adverse Effects	Comments
Ticlopidine (Ticlid)	Initial oral: 250 mg twice daily		Labeled: Reduce the risk of thrombotic stroke in patients with completed thrombotic stroke or stroke precursors Unlabeled: Adjunctive therapy for coronary artery stent placement and alternative to aspirin in patients unable to take aspirin	- Diarrhea - Nausea/dyspepsia/vomiting/anorexia - Rash - Neutropenia - Purpura	- Severe neutropenia occurs in 0.8% of patients and has been associated with death - CBC with differential should be measured at baseline and every 2 weeks for the first 3 months of therapy - Patients should be monitored for fevers or other signs of infection - Case reports of thrombotic thrombocytopenic purpura have been reported with ticlopidine - Maximal effects seen 3–7 days after initiation of therapy
Dipyridamole (Persantine)	Initial oral: 25–100 mg 4 times daily IV for stress test: 0.142 mg/kg/min over 4 min (0.57 mg/kg) to a maximum dose of 60 mg	Antiplatelet mechanism not established but related to inhibition of adenosine reuptake phosphodiesterase inhibition, and inhibition of thromboxane A_2 formation Stress testing: Coronary vasodilatation by preventing degradation of adenosine	Labeled: Adjunct to warfarin therapy to prevent postoperative thromboembolic events of cardiac valve and intravenously for stress test	- Exacerbation of angina - Dizziness - Hypotension - Tachycardia - Headache - Rash - GI distress - Dyspnea - Bronchoconstriction	- Methylxanthines antagonize the effects of dipyramidole and should be discontinued from 36–48 hr prior to administration - Aminophylline 50–250 mg over 30–60 sec may be given to reverse dipyramidole effects. - Use with caution in patients with bronchospastic lung disease; may exacerbate asthma

THROMBOLYTICS

Drug	Dose	Mechanism of action	Indication	Side effects	Comments
Alteplase, tpa (Activase)	*Acute MI Accelerated (Front Loaded):* Patients >67 kg total dose = 100 mg 15 mg IV bolus then 50 mg over 30 min then 35 mg over 60 min Patients ≤67 kg total dose < 100 mg 15 mg IV bolus then 0.75 mg/kg (50 mg max) over 30 min then 0.5 mg/kg (35 mg max) over 60 min *Acute ischemic stroke:* 0.9 mg/kg over 60 min with 10% of total dose given over the first minute *Pulmonary Embolism:* 100 mg given over 120 min	rTPA binds to clot bound plasminogen to catalyze conversion to plasmin. The specificity for clot bound plasminogen decreases systemic fibrinolysis	Labeled: Acute MI, pulmonary embolism, and acute ischemic stroke	- Bleeding - Intracranial hemorrhage (0.7%) - Hypotension - Nausea/vomiting - Epistaxis	- Acute MI patients should receive aspirin and heparin during TPA infusion - Pulmonary embolism heparin should be started at the end of the alteplase infusion - TPA is not specific for fresh clot and binds to any clot-bound plasminogen - No antigenicity; therefore may be used without risk of antibody formation - Short half-life about 4 min - Considered superior to streptokinase - Risk of intracranial hemorrhage > streptokinase - Age > 65 years old and weight < 70 kg are independent risk factors for intracranial hemorrhage
Anistreplase- APSAC (Eminase)	Acute MI 30 U IV over 2–5 min	APSAC is an inactive streptokinase/plasminogen complex that in vivo becomes activated by deacylation thus expressing the catalytic	Labeled: Acute MI	- Bleeding - Anaphylactic reactions - Hypotension - Rash - Intracranial hemorrhage	- Heparin offers no advantage to APSAC and increases risks of bleeding - More expensive than streptokinase - Same allergy precautions to streptokinase

Drug	Dose	Action	Indications	Adverse Effects	Comments
		properties of the complex to convert plasminogen to plasmin			
Reteplase, rPA (Retavase)	Acute MI 10 U over 2 min followed by a second 10 U bolus in 30 min	Single-stranded mutant of wild type TPA with similar action to TPA with less high-affinity fibrin binding, but increased potency	Labeled: Acute MI	- Bleeding - Intracranial hemorrhage	
Streptokinase, SK (Streptase)	Acute MI: Intravenous: 1.5 million IU over 60 minutes Intracoronary: 20,000 IU followed by 2,000 IU/min for 60 min (total dose = 140,000 IU) Pulmonary embolism: 250,000 IU given IV over 30 min then 100,000 IU/hr for 24 hr. May continue for 72 hr if DVT suspected DVT: 250,000 IU given IV over 30 min then 100,000 IU/hr for 72 hr Arterial thrombosis or embolism: 250,000 IU given IV over 30 min then 100,000 IU/hr for 24–72 hr	Binds to clot bound and circulating plasminogen; this complex then catalyzes the conversion of plasminogen to plasmin. Not specific for clot bound plasminogen and therefore produces a systemic fibrinolytic state	Labeled: Acute MI, pulmonary embolism, deep vein thrombosis, arterial thrombosis or embolism, occlusion of AV cannulae	- Bleeding - Bronchospasm - Periorbital swelling - Angioedema edema - Anaphylaxis - Hypotension - Rash - Intracranial hemorrhage (0.2%) - Fever - Urticaria	- Should not receive streptokinase if within the last 12 months have received APSAC or streptokinase - Intracranial hemorrhage occurs less often than with alteplase - Heparin usually not given with streptokinase; if needed the heparin is initiated 4 hr after streptokinase infusion without a bolus

continued

THROMBOLYTICS (continued)					
Drug	Dose	Mechanism of action	Indication	Side effects	Comments
	Arteriovenous cannulae occlusion: Instill 250,000 IU in 2 mL of solution into each occluded limb of cannula slowly. Clamp off cannula for 12 hr. After treatment aspirate contents flush with saline and reconnect cannula				
Urokinase (Abbokinase)	Pulmonary embolism: 4400 IU/kg over 10 min then 4,400 IU/kg/hr for 12 hr Intracoronary infusion: 750,000 IU over 2 hr; 6,000 IU/min for 2 hr Catheter occlusion: 5,000 IU in each lumen let dwell for 1–4 h then aspirate: may repeat if first dose does not clear. Large vessel thrombi: 4,400 IU/kg over 10 min: then 4,400 IU/kg/hr for 24–72 hr	Directly activates plasminogen; causes less systemic fibrinolysis than streptokinase	Labeled: Pulmonary embolism, intracoronary administration for coronary artery thrombosis, IV catheter clearance	- Bleeding - Allergic reactions - Fever/chills/rigors	- Less antigenic than streptokinase - Shorter half-life than streptokinase therefore produces less systemic fibrinolysis

VASODILATORS					
Drug	Dose	Mechanism of action	Indication	Side effects	Comments
Diazoxide	IV bolus: 1–3 mg/kg (150 mg max) over 30 seconds (see comments) IV Infusion: 10–30 mg/min up to 5 mg/kg until blood pressure controlled; May repeat every 4–24 hr as needed (see comments)	Direct relaxation of arteriolar smooth muscle	Labeled: Hypertensive emergencies (IV) and hypoglycemia (PO)	- Hypotension - Nausea/vomiting - Dizziness - Hyperglycemia - Edema - Thrombocytopenia - Hirsutism	- Not often used because of unpredictable lowering of blood pressure - Causes hyperglycemia via inhibition of insulin release and decreasing peripheral utilization of glucose - May induce cerebral or myocardial ischemia - Significant sodium and water reabsorption with repeated dosing - Oral therapy may be used for chronic hypoglycemia related to insulin-secreting tumors - IV therapy should not be used for more than 10 days
Hydralazine (Apresoline)	Initial oral: 10–25 mg 3–4 times daily Maximum: 400 mg/d IV: 10–20 mg 4–6 times daily up to 40 mg/dose	Direct relaxation of arteriolar smooth muscle	Labeled: Hypertension (PO), hypertensive emergencies (IV) Unlabeled: Heart failure	- Palpitations - Flushing - Tachycardia - Myocardial ischemia - Headache - Nausea/vomiting/anorexia - Hypotension - Drug-induced SLE - Sodium and water retention	- Hydralazine IV has unpredictable effects and is rarely used for hypertensive emergencies - Long-term use may lead to drug-induced SLE - ↑ intracranial pressure - May ↑ myocardial oxygen demand and potentially causes coronary "steal" phenomena

continued

VASODILATORS (continued)

Drug	Dose	Mechanism of action	Indication	Side effects	Comments
Fenoldopam (Corolpam)	IV: 0.025–0.3 µg/kg/min (see comments)	Dopamine-1 receptor agonist causing smooth muscle relaxation causing vasodilatation and increased renal blood flow	Labeled: Short-term management of hypertensive emergencies and urgencies	- Hypotension - Headache - Flushing - Nausea - Tachycardia - Hypokalemia (rarely)	- Some clinical trials used doses of up to 1.6 µg/kg/min - Most patients respond to 0.1–0.8 µg/kg/min - ↑ renal blood flow, ↑ CrCl in clinical trials - Short half-life of 5–10 minutes - Natriuresis and diuresis can be seen - Very expensive - Blood pressure lowering effects equal to that of nitroprusside - Use with caution in patients with glaucoma - No toxic metabolites
Minoxidil (Loniten)	Initial oral: 2.5–5 mg daily Maximum: 100 mg/d in divided doses	Direct vasodilator with primary effect on arterial smooth muscle	Labeled: Hypertension Unlabeled: Heart failure	- Significant reflex tachycardia - Sodium and water retention - Edema - Weight gain - Hypertrichosis - Breast tenderness - Gynocomastia - Headache	- Use with β-blockers to decrease reflex tachycardia - Sodium and water retention will occur and patients commonly need diuretics

| Nitroprusside (sodium) (Nipride) | IV: 0.3–10 µg/kg/min most patients require 3 µg/kg/min Doses should not exceed 10 µg/kg/min for more than 10 min (see comments) | Direct vasodilatation occurs secondary to the liberation of the nitroso group from the the nitrosocyanide structure. It possesses a balanced effect on both veins and arteries | Labeled: Hypertensive emergencies, and management of acute CHF | - Hypotension
- Thiocynate toxicity
- Cyanide toxicity
- Headache
- Nausea
- Confusion
- Metabolic acidosis | - Doses of 10 µg/kg/min for more than 10 min ↑ the risk of developing cyanide toxicity
- Short half-life of about 3 min
- Patients with hepatic failure at an ↑ risk of developing cyanide toxicity: this is suspected in patients with a metabolic acidosis, venous hyperoxemia, ↑ lactate, air hunger, confusion, seizures, ataxia, and potentially stroke.
- Patients with suspected cyanide toxicity should receive inhaled amyl nitrite while administering 300 mg of IV sodium nitrite, then administer 12.5 mg of IV sodium thiosulfate. If symptoms reappear administer ½ the amount of sodium nitrite and sodium thiosulfate. These modalities shift cyanide conversion to thiocyanate. Cyanide levels are not helpful because it may take up to 5 days to get results
- Thiocynate is a neurotoxin causing confusion, psychosis, lethargy, tinnitus, convulsions, and hyperreflexia. Hemodialysis removes thiocyanate from the blood. Levels are typically not monitored unless infusion of >3 days or when high doses are used, in patients with renal failure. |

VASOPRESSORS					
Drug	Dose	Mechanism of action	Indication	Side effects	Comments
Dopamine (Intropin)	See dopamine under Inotropic agents	Mixed α, β and dopaminergic agonist	See dopamine under Inotropic agents	See dopamine under Inotropic agents	- Initially may see initial vasodilatation then vasoconstriction - Alpha effects are typically seen with doses greater than 10 μg/kg/min - Central line required when given by continuous infusion
Epinephrine (Adrenalin)	See epinephrine under Inotropic agents	Mixed α and β agonist	See epinephrine under Inotropic agents	See epinephrine under Inotropic agents	See epinephrine under Inotropic agents - Lower doses β effects predominate and higher doses α effects predominate - Vasopressor of choice in septic shock - Acidemia may blunt pressor effects - Endotracheal administration in cardiac arrest is 2–2.5 times that of IV - Central line required when given by continuous infusion
Norepinephrine (Levophed)	0.1–3.5 μg/kg/min	Mixed α and β agonist	Hypotension	- Hypertension - Headache - Trembling - Ventricular arrhythmias	- Primary effect is vasoconstriction - Administer by central line - ↓ renal splanchnic, hepatic, and peripheral blood flow due to vasoconstriction - β effects are usually off-set by baroreceptor-mediated vagal stimulation - Central line required when given by continuous infusion
Phenylephrine (Neo-Synephrine)	0.5–15 μg/kg/min	Pure α agonist	Hypotension	- Bradycardia - Hypertension - Myocardial ischemia	- No β effects - Useful in patients with tachycardia from mixed α/β agonists - Administer by central line - Extravasation may cause skin necrosis - Central line required when given by continuous infusion

MISCELLANEOUS AGENTS					
Drug	Dose	Mechanism of action	Indication	Side effects	Comments
Aminocaproic acid (Amicar)	IV: 4–5 g given over 1 hr then 1 g/hr for 8 hr or until bleeding stops	Inhibits activation of plasminogen to plasmin	Labeled: Enhance hemostasis when fibrinolysis contributes to bleeding	- Hypotension - Bradycardia - Rash - Headache - Myopathy - Tinnitus - GI irritation	- Reduce dose by 25% in patients with oliguria or ESRD; accumulates in this patient population - Decreased platelet function - Monitoring: fibrinogen, fibrin split products - Rapid infusions may cause hypotension, bradycardia, and arrhythmias - Randomized data are lacking for counteracting thrombolytics
Digoxin Immune Fab (Digibind)	Dependent on total body stores of digoxin or digitoxin. If the amount of ingested or total body stores is unknown then 20 vials should be administered. Infuse dose over 15–30 min through a 0.22 μm filter	Digoxin immune Fab binds to serum digoxin decreasing free digoxin from binding to receptors	Labeled: Treatment of life-threatening digoxin or digitoxin toxicity	- Anaphylaxis - Serum sickness - Hypokalemia - Erythema at injection site	- Onset within 30 minutes - Many digoxin assays are report inaccurate digoxin levels after digibind therapy - Patients with know allergy to sheep proteins may have an anaphylactic reaction to digibind - Patients with severe renal failure may have a delayed rebound toxicity with digibind therapy - Each vial of digoxin immune Fab binds 0.6 mg of digoxin or digitoxin - No. vials = (dig level [ng/ml] × body weight in kg)/100 for digoxin and 1,000 for digitoxin

continued

MISCELLANEOUS AGENTS (*continued*)

Drug	Dose	Mechanism of action	Indication	Side effects	Comments
Protamine sulfate	Variable: 1 mg binds about 100 U of heparin sodium usual range 25–50 mg Maximum: 50 mg IV once	Protamine is a strong base that complexes with heparin (acid) and forms an inactive stable salt	Labeled: Heparin overdose	- Hypotension (see comments) - Bradycardia (see comments) - Dyspnea - Transient flushing - Hypersensitivity reactions (see comments)	- Rapid onset of action and heparin neutralization occurs within 5 minutes - Hypotension, bradycardia, dyspnea, and flushing may occur with rapid administration - Hypersensitivity reactions including anaphylaxis occurs in < 1% of patients - Patients predisposed to hypersensitivty reactions include: patients allergic to fish, diabetics on insulin containing protamine, and vasectomized males
Vitamin K—Phytonadione (Mephyton, Aqua Mephyton)	Variable: Range 0.5–10 mg sc or IV 2.5–10 mg orally	Replete Vit K stores needed for the formation of blood coagulation factors II, VII, IX, X in the liver	Labeled: Hypoprothrombinemia secondary to coumarin or indandione overdose, antibacterial therapy, malabsorption states and ↓ synthesis, and prophylaxis and treatment of hemorrhage disease of newborns	- Rare hypersensitivity reactions	- Anaphylaxis has occurred in some patients

CHF, Congestive heart failure; MAOI, monoamine oxidase inhibitor; ACE, angiotensin-converting enzyme; SLE, systemic lupus erythematosus; IV, intravenous; GI, gastrointestinal; AV, atrioventricular; ANA, antinuclear antibodies; AVNRT, atrioventricular node reentrant tachycardia; NSR, normal sinus R; SA, sinoatrial; WPW, Wolff-Parkinson-White syndrome; DVT, deep vein thrombosis; HIT, heparin-induced thrombocytopenia; AST, aspartate aminotransferase; ALT, alanine aminotransferase; aPTT, activated partial thromboplastin time; LMWH, low molecular weight heparin; SC, subcutaneous; INR, international normalized ratio; ISA, intrinsic sympathomimetic activity; VLDL, very low density lipoprotein; HDL, high-density lipoprotein; CBC, complete blood count; HMG-CoA β-hydroxy-β-methylglutaryl coenzyme A; LFT, liver function tests; ESRD, end-stage renal disease; PCI, percutaneous coronary intervention; PTCA, percutaneous transluminal coronary angioplasty; TPA, tissue plasminogen activator.

SUBJECT INDEX

AAA. *See* Abdominal aortic aneurysm
Abbokinase. *See* Urokinase
Abciximab (Reopro)
   description, 824–825
   and percutaneous coronary interven-
      tion, 737
   for unstable angina, 31–32
Abdominal aortic aneurysm (AAA),
      336–339
   atherosclerosis and, 336
   clinical course, 336–337
   clinical presentation, 336
   complications during repair, 339
   contraindication in intraortic balloon
      counterpulsation, 689
   contraindication to left heart catheter-
      ization, 702
   diagnostic testing, 337–338
   etiology, 336
   genetics and, 336
   incidence, 336
   male-to-female ratio, 336
   pathophysiology, 336–337
   physical examination, 336
   signs and symptoms, 336
   therapy, 338–339
     intravenous dosing for acute medical
       management, 338
      medical, 338
      percutaneous, 339
      surgical, 339
   ultrasound, 337
Abdominal ultrasound
   in abdominal aortic aneurysms, 337
Accessory pathways
   evaluation, in electrophysiologic stud-
      ies, 580–582
     antidromic AV reentry tachycardia,
      580–581
     common locations, 580
     diagnosing multiple accessory path-
      ways, 582
     localizing, 581–582
     orthodromic AV reentrant tachycar-
      dia, 580
     preexcitation, 580
Accupril (Quinapril)
   description, 783
ACE. *See* Angiotensin-converting enzyme
      inhibitors
Acebutolol (Sectral)
   description, 799
Acetazolamide (Diamox)
   description, 814

ACLS. *See* Advanced cardiac life support
ACME. *See* Angioplasty Compared to
      Medicine study
Acolysis, 733
Activase (Alteplase, tpa)
   description, 828
Acute coronary syndrome, 472
Acute pericarditis, 354–362
Adalat. *See* Nifedipine
Adenocard. *See* Adenosine
Adenosine (Adenocard)
   to assess ischemia, 75
   for atrial flutter, 257
   characteristics, 331
   description, 793
   in electrophysiologic studies, 572
   for emergency management of acute
      tachycardic episodes, 266
   for idiopathic ventricular tachycardia,
      275
   in nuclear imaging, 529
   and percutaneous coronary interven-
      tion, 737–738
   in stable angina, 73
   and stress echocardiography, 539, 542
Adjuvant therapy
   for acute myocardial infarction, 18–21
Adrenalin (Epinephrine)
   description, 816, 834
α-Adrenergic agonists, central
   description, 777–778
α$_1$-Adrenergic agonists
   description, 779–780
Adrenergic agonists, peripheral
   description, 776
Adult respiratory distress syndrome
      (ARDS)
   and right heart catheterization, 653
Advanced cardiac life support (ACLS)
   in sudden cardiac death, 302
AED. *See* Automated external defibrillator
Afterdepolarizations
   delayed, 249
   early, 249
Afterload-reducing agents
   in mitral regurgitation, 201–202,
      204–205
Age
   coronary artery disease in women, 484
   as risk factor, 56
Age-predicted maximum heart rate
      (APMHR)
   in exercise electrocardiographic test-
      ing, 516

Aggrastat. *See* Tirofiban

Alcohol
  toxicity in systolic heart failure, 104, 109

Alcohol septal ablation
  for hypertrophic cardiomyopathy, 137

Aldactone (Spironolactone)
  description, 814

Aldomet (Methyldopa)
  description, 778

Allergies
  as complication of left heart catheterization, 720
  dye, contraindication to left heart catheterization, 701–702

Allograft vasculopathy
  in postoperative cardiac transplantation, 161–163

Altace (Ramipril)
  description, 783

Alteplase, tpa (Activase)
  description, 828

American College of Cardiology
  assessment guidelines after myocardial infarction, 58
  stepwise approach to preoperative cardiac evaluation, 422, 425

American Heart Association
  assessment guidelines after myocardial infarction, 58
  stepwise approach to preoperative cardiac evaluation, 422, 425

Amicar. *See* Aminocaproic acid

Amiloride (Midamor)
  description, 813

Aminocaproic acid (Amicar)
  description, 835

Aminoglycosides
  for infective endocarditis, 633

Amiodarone (Cordarone, Pacerone)
  characteristics, 329
  for chronic heart failure, 113
  description, 790
  for hypertrophic cardiomyopathy, 275
  for restoration and maintenance of sinus rhythm, 254, 256
  for sarcoidosis, 276
  for sudden cardiac death prevention, 303

Amlodipine (Norvasc)
  description, 806
  for stable angina, 84

Amphotericin B
  for infective endocarditis, 635

Amrinone (Inocor)
  description, 815

Amylase
  in postoperative cardiac transplantation, 159

Amyloidosis
  chemotherapy for, 119–120
  diagnosis, 119
  familial, 119

primary, 119
  senile cardiac, 119

Anemia
  contraindication to left heart catheterization, 702
  and high-output heart failure, 142

Anesthesia
  in cardioversion, 676–677
  in pericardiocentesis, 671
  perioperative management, 431
  for transesophageal echocardiography, 762

Angina
  in aortic stenosis, 167, 169–170
  classification, 72
  decubitus, 72
  and left heart catheterization, 700
  nocturnal, 72
  postinfarction, 53
  rebound, 81
  risk prediction, 74, 88
  second-wind, 72
  stable, 71–90
    baseline electrocardiogram, 72
    clinical presentation, 71–72
    chronic, and percutaneous coronary intervention, 727
    controversies, 88–89
    diagnostic testing, 71–78
    indications for coronary angiography, 77
    and left heart catheterization, 700
    physical findings, 73
    risk stratification, 88
    signs and symptoms, 71–72
    therapy, 78–88
  syndrome X, 95–96
  in women, 482

Angiocardiography
  radionuclide, 533
  in tricuspid regurgitation, 228

Angioedema
  as side effect of ACE inhibitors, 110

Angiojet, 733

Angioplasty Compared to Medicine (ACME) study, 86

Angioscopy, 735

Angio-Seal, 718

Angiotensin-converting enzyme (ACE) inhibitors
  for acute myocardial infarction, 20
  in cardiogenic shock, 47
  for chronic heart failure, 109–110, 112
  description, 781–783
  in LV pump failure, 47
  after myocardial infarction, 63
  for stable angina, 85
  for unstable angina, 33

Angiotensin II receptor blockers
  description, 784

Anistreplase-APSAC (Eminase)
  for acute myocardial infarction, 17
  description, 828–829

Annuloaortic ectasia, 340–341
Anode
    definition, in cardiac pacing, 607
Anthracycline
    toxicity in systolic heart failure, 104
Antiarrhythmic drugs, 325–332
    for acute myocardial infarction, 20
    characteristics, 327–331
    for chronic heart failure, 111–113
    classification, 325
    description, 785–793
    future directions, 325
    for mitral regurgitation, 202
    in mitral stenosis, 213
    overview, 325
    for sudden cardiac death, 306
    for syncope, 318
    for unstable angina, 34
Antibiotics
    in aortic regurgitation, 190
    in aortic stenosis, 178
    in Marfan syndrome, 414
    and pacemaker implantation, 598–600
    prophylactic, 178, 190, 394–395, 414
    for unstable angina, 34
    for ventricular septal defects, 394–395
Anticoagulants
    description, 794–798
    oral, 797
Anticoagulation
    for atrial flutter, 257
    cardioversion and, 680
    for chronic heart failure, 112
    contraindication in pericardiocentesis,
        670
    for hyperthyroidism, 143
    in mitral stenosis, 213
    for prosthetic heart valves, 236–237
    in postoperative cardiac transplanta-
        tion, 159
    for thrombosis, 244
    in ventricular aneurysm, 52
Antihypertensive medications, 469–471
Antilymphocyte globulin
    in postoperative cardiac transplanta-
        tion, 161
Antioxidants
    after myocardial infarction, 64
    for stable angina, 85–86
    for women, to prevent coronary artery
        disease, 491–493
Antiplatelet therapy
    for acute myocardial infarction, 5
    after myocardial infarction, 62
    for unstable angina, 30
Antistreptolysin O
    and rheumatic fever, 646
Antitachycardia devices
    bradycardia detection and therapy, 616
    contraindications, 614
    criteria for ICD implantation, 613
    device–device interaction, 617
    device replacement, 615

electromagnetic interference, 618–619
future of, 619
implantation, 614–615
indications, 611–614
magnet function, 616–617
managing patients, 617–618
overview, 612
tachycardia detection and therapy,
    615–616
Antithrombins
    for acute myocardial infarction, 18–19
    direct, 31
    for unstable angina, 30–31
Aorta
    abdominal, 335
    anatomy, 335
    aortic arch, 335
    ascending, 335
    coarctation, 399–401
    descending thoracic, 335
    histology, 335
        adventitia, 335
        intima, 335
        media, 335
    physiology, 335
        elasticity, 335
        systemic vascular resistance, 335
    in transesophageal echocardiography,
        770, 771, 772
Aortic aneurysm
    abdominal (AAA), 336–339
        atherosclerosis and, 336
        clinical course, 336–337
        clinical presentation, 336
        complications during repair, 339
        diagnostic testing, 337–338
        etiology, 336
        genetics and, 336
        incidence, 336
        male-to-female ratio, 336
        pathophysiology, 336–337
        physical examination, 336
        signs and symptoms, 336
        therapy, 338–339
            intravenous dosing for acute med-
                ical management, 338
            medical, 338
            percutaneous, 339
            surgical, 339
    thoracic aortic (TAA)
        clinical course, 341–342
        clinical presentation, 340
        complications, 342
        diagnostic testing, 342
        etiology, 340–341
        incidence, 339–340
        laboratory examination, 340
        pathophysiology, 341–342
        physical examination, 340
            cardiac, 340
            pulmonary, 340
            vascular, 340
        signs and symptoms, 340

Aortic aneurysm (*contd.*)
  therapy, 341–343
    medical, 342
    percutaneous, 342
    surgical, 341–343
  definition, 335
Aortic dissection
  anatomic appearance, 344
  atypical variants of dissection, 351
  classification schemes, 343–344
  clinical presentation, 344–345
  comparison of imaging modalities, 348
  complications, 350
  contraindications
    in intraortic balloon counterpulsa-
      tion, 689
    in pericardiocentesis, 670
  controversies, 351–352
  diagnostic testing, 346–348
  epidemiology, 343
  etiology, 345–346
  and evaluation of chest pain, 452
  and hyptertensive emergencies,
    443–444
  laboratory examination, 345
  myocardial infarction and, 4
  pathophysiology, 345–346
  physical examination, 345
    cardiac, 345
    neurologic, 345
    vascular, 345
  signs and symptoms, 344–345
  therapy, 348–350
    caveats, 348–349
    long-term management, 350
    medical, 349
    percutaneous, 350
    priority of, 348
    surgical, 349–350
    surgical versus medical, 349
Aortic homografts, 232
Aortic insufficiency
  contraindication, in intraortic balloon
    counterpulsation, 689
Aortic regurgitation
  asymptomatic, 192
  clinical presentation, 182
  controversies, 192
  diagnostic testing, 186–190
  etiology, 184, 185
  follow-up care, 192
  laboratory testing, 186
  natural history, 185–186
  pathophysiology, 184–185
  physical findings, 181–184
  sudden death, 186
  therapy, 190–192
Aortic stenosis
  acquired, 169
  clinical presentation, 167
  congenital, 168–169, 171
  controversies, 181
  decompensated, and intraortic balloon
    counterpulsation, 688

  diagnostic testing, 170–177
  etiology, 168–169
  laboratory examination, 170
  and left heart catheterization, 714–715
  natural history, 169–170
  pathophysiology, 169
  physical findings, 167, 168
  preoperative management, 429
  signs and symptoms, 167
  therapy, 177–181
  valve replacement, 179–180
    complications, 180
    mechanical, 180
Aortic valve disease. *See* Aortic regurgi-
    tation; Aortic stenosis
Aortic valve endocarditis
  homografts in, 235
Aortography
  in abdominal aortic aneurysms,
    337–338
  in aortic dissection, 347
  in aortic regurgitation, 190
  in left heart catheterization, 716–717
  in thoracic aortic aneurysm, 342
Apical septal defects, 392
APMHR. *See* Age-predicted maximum
    heart rate
Apolipoproteins, 456
Apresoline. *See* Hydralazine
Aqua Mephyton (Vitamin K)
  description, 836
Arbutamine
  to assess ischemia, 75
  in stable angina, 74
  and stress echocardiography, 539, 541
Arch aneurysm, 342
Ardeparin (Normiflo)
  description, 796
ARDS. *See* Adult respiratory distress syn-
    drome
Argatroban
  for unstable angina, 31
Arrhythmias
  in endomyocardial biopsy, 685
  in exercise electrocardiographic test-
    ing, 511–512, 516
  in left heart catheterization, 719
  management in diastolic heart failure,
    125
  preoperative management, 429
  in postoperative cardiac transplanta-
    tion, 157–158
Arrhythmogenic right ventricular dyspla-
    sia (ARVD), 276
  in isolated right heart failure, 146
  therapy, 148
Arterial examination
  in aortic regurgitation, 183
  in aortic stenosis, 167
Arterial hypoxemia
  in cardiogenic shock, 45
  in LV pump failure, 45
Arterial switch, 416

Arteriovenous fistulas
    and high-output heart failure, 141–143
Arthritis
    and rheumatic fever, 645
        therapy, 647
ARVD. *See* Arrhythmogenic right ventric-
        ular dysplasia
Ascending aneurysm, 342
Aschoff's nodules
    and rheumatic fever, 647
ASDs. *See* Atrial septal defects
Aspergillus infection
    in postoperative cardiac transplanta-
        tion, 162
Aspirin
    for acute myocardial infarction, 5
    for atrial fibrillation, 252
    description, 824
    for embolic stroke, 245
    after myocardial infarction, 62
    for pericarditis, 54
    for post–mocardial infarction peri-
        carditis, 359
    for stable angina, 78
    for unstable angina, 30
    for women, to prevent coronary artery
        disease, 494
Asystole
    clinical presentation, 298
    etiology, 298
    therapy, 298
Atenolol (Tenormin)
    description, 799
Atherectomy
    directional, 733
    percutaneous transluminal rotational,
        730, 733
Atherosclerosis
    and abdominal aortic aneurysms, 336
Atherosclerotic ulcer
    in aortic dissection, 351
Athlete's heart
    in hypertrophic cardiomyopathy, 139
Atorvastatin (Lipitor)
    description, 820
Atrial fibrillation
    in aortic stenosis, 178
    cardioversion and, 679
    and chronic heart failure, 109
    clinical presentation, 250
    diagnostic testing, 251
    differential diagnosis, 250
    etiology, 250–251
    in exercise electrocardiographic
        testing, 511
    and hypertrophic cardiomyopathy, 138
    laboratory evaluation, 251
    pathophysiology, 251
    postoperative, 256
    prosthetic heart valves and, 242
    therapy, 251–256
        control of ventricular response,
            251–252
        sinus rhythm restoration and main-
            tenance, 253–256

        thromboembolic risk management,
            252
Atrial flutter
    cardioversion and, 679
    clinical presentation, 256–257
    diagnosis, 257
    laboratory examination, 257–258
    pathophysiology, 257
    therapy, 258–259
Atrial inflow
    for diastolic heart failure, 123
Atrial pressures
    for diastolic heart failure, 123
Atrial septal defects (ASDs)
    anatomy, 387–388
    clinical presentation, 388
    coronary sinus, 388
    diagnostic testing, 389–390
    embryology, 387
    laboratory examination, 388–389
    life expectancy, 387
    ostium primum, 387
    ostium secundum, 387
    overview, 387
    sinus venosus, 387
    therapy, 390–391
    types, 387–388
Atrial stimulation
    in electrophysiologic studies, 567
Atrial tachycardia
    clinical presentation, 260
    diagnostic testing, 260
    laboratory examination, 260
    subclassifications, 260–261
        automatic atrial, 260–261
        intraatrial reentry, 260
        triggered atrial, 261
Atrioventricular conduction distur-
        bances
    classification, 285–289
        first-degree atrioventricular block,
            285
        second-degree atrioventricular
            block, 285
        third-degree atrioventricular block,
            289
    clinical presentation, 289
    diagnostic testing, 290
        first-degree atrioventricular block,
            290
        second-degree atrioventricular
            block, 290
        third-degree atrioventricular block,
            290
    etiology, 290, 291
    physical findings, 289
    signs and symptoms, 289
    therapy, 290–293
        medical, 290–293
        pacing, 293
Atrioventricular nodal reentrant tachy-
        cardia (AVNRT)
    clinical presentation, 261

Atrioventricular nodal reentrant tachy-
     cardia (AVNRT) (*contd.*)
   diagnosis, 262
   laboratory features, 262
   pathophysiology, 261–262
   therapy, 261–263
Atrioventricular node
   anatomy, 281
Atrioventricular canal-type septal
     defects, 392
Atrioventricular sequential devices
   in ICD transplantation, 615–616
Atromid-S (Clofibrate)
   description, 819
Atropine
   for sinus node dysfunction, 285
   in stable angina, 74
   and stress echocardiography, 541
Auscultation
   in aortic regurgitation, 183–184
   in aortic stenosis, 167–168
   in hypertrophic cardiomyopathy, 130,
     131
   in mitral regurgitation, 194, 195
   in mitral stenosis, 208–209
   in mitral valve prolapse, 205, 206
Automated external defibrillator (AED)
   in sudden cardiac death, 307
Automaticity
   abnormal, 249
   deranged, 249
   normal, 249
Autonomic testing
   in sinus node dysfunction, 284
Avapro (Irbesartan)
   description, 784
AVNRT. *See* Atrioventricular nodal reen-
     trant tachycardia
AV sequential pacing
   in RV pump failure, 49
Azathioprine
   dosage, 159
   drug interactions, 159
   in postoperative cardiac transplanta-
     tion, 158, 159
   side effects, 159
Azithromycin
   for rheumatic fever, 649

Bacterial endocarditis, 650
Balloon angioplasty
   for coarctation of the aorta, 401
   in Tetralogy of Fallot, 405
BARI. *See* Bypass Angioplasty Revascu-
     larization Investigators
β-Adrenergic agonists
   in cardiogenic shock, 47
   in LV pump failure, 47
   in Marfan syndrome, 414
Balke protocol, 509
Batista procedure, 201–203
Baycol (Cerivastatin)
   description, 820

Bayes' theorem, 503, 507
β-Adrenergic antagonists
   description, 799–804
β-α antagonists
   description, 805
β-Blockers
   for abdominal aortic aneurysms,
     338–339
   for acute myocardial infarction, 19–20
   for aortic dissection, 349
   for aortic regurgitation, 191
   for atrial fibrillation, 251
   for chronic heart failure, 111
   contraindications, 63, 135
   in exercise electrocardiographic test-
     ing, 505–506
   for hyperthyroidism, 143
   for hypertrophic cardiomyopathy, 135
   for long QT syndrome, 322
   for mitral regurgitation, 202
   in mitral stenosis, 213
   after myocardial infarction, 61–63
   preoperative management, 430
   as prevention after myocardial infarc-
     tion, 64
   for sinus tachycardia, 250
   for stable angina, 81, 82
   for unstable angina, 33
Benazepril (Lotensin)
   description, 781
Benzodiazepines
   description, 807–808
Bepridil (Vascor)
   description, 809
Bernoulli equation, 756
Betapace. *See* Sotalol
Betaxolol (Kerlone)
   description, 800
Biatrial anastomosis
   in orthotopic transplantation, 157
Bicaval anastomosis
   in orthotopic transplantation, 157
Bicycle
   versus treadmill exercise echocardiog-
     raphy, 538
Bifascicular block, 294
Bile acid resins
   description, 818
Bileaflet tilting disc, 232
Biochemical markers
   in evaluation of chest pain, 448–451
Bioprostheses
   in aortic stenosis, 180
   in tricuspid stenosis, 223
   valves, 231–246
Biopsy
   endomyocardial, 102, 125, 158, 159,
     162, 681–686
   and rheumatic fever, 647
Bioptome
   for endomyocardial biopsy, 682
   types, 684
Bisoprolol (Zebeta)
   description, 800

Bivalirudin (Hirulog)
  description, 794
  for unstable angina, 31
  for percutaneous coronary intervention, 736
Björk-Shiley single tilting-disc, 233, 235
Blalock-Taussig shunt, 416
Bleeding
  as complication of intraortic balloon counterpulsation, 696–697
  as complication of left heart catheterization, 720
  as complication of percutaneous coronary intervention, 729
Blocadren (Timolol)
  description, 804
Blood flow tracers, 534
Blood pressure
  in aortic regurgitation, 181–183
  ambulatory monitoring, 466
  in exercise electrocardiographic testing, 516–517
  measurements in, 465–466
Bradyarrhythmias
  and electrophysiologic studies, 563, 571–574
  preoperative management, 429
  postsurgical, 294
Bradycardia
  detection and therapy, 616
  in ICD transplantation, 616
  and long QT syndrome, 320
  temporary transvenous pacing and, 666
  and Torsades de pointes, 278, 279
Brain death
  in cardiac transplantation, 154–155
Braunwald classification system, 25, 27
Bretylium tosylate (Bretylol)
  characteristics, 330
  description, 791
Bretylol. See Bretylium tosylate
Brevibloc. See Esmolol
Bruce protocol
  advantages, 509
  disadvantages, 509
  modified, 509
Brugada criteria
  in ventricular tachycardia, 267–270
Bumetanide (Bumex)
  description, 810
Bumex. See Bumetanide
Bundle branches
  anatomy, 281
  in endomyocardial biopsy, 685
Bupropion
  for smoking cessation
    after myocardial infarction, 61
    for prevention of cardiovascular disease, 476–477
Burst pacing
  in electrophysiologic studies, 567, 568
Bypass Angioplasty Revascularization Investigators (BARI), 86

CABG. See Coronary artery bypass graft
Caged ball, 231–234
Calan. See Verapamil
Calcium channel blockers
  for acute myocardial infarction, 20
  for atrial fibrillation, 252
  for chronic heart failure, 112
  contraindications, 63–64, 135
  description, 806–809
  for hypertrophic cardiomyopathy, 135, 137
  after myocardial infarction, 63–64
  for sinus tachycardia, 250
  for stable angina, 81, 83–84
  for unstable angina, 33
  for ventricular tachycardia, 271
Capoten. See Captopril
Captopril (Capoten)
  description, 781
  for hypertensive urgencies, 444–445
Capture
  definition, in cardiac pacing, 607
Carbonic anhydrase inhibitors
  description, 814
Carcinoid syndrome
  and pulmonary valve stenosis, 229, 230
  in tricuspid stenosis, 220
Carden (Nicardipine)
  description, 807
Cardiac arrest
  in exercise electrocardiographic testing, 511
Cardiac enzymes
  in unstable angina, 27–28
Cardiac index
  in systolic heart failure, 102
Cardiac monitors
  and pacemaker patients, 605
Cardiac output
  in atrial fibrillation, 253
  and right heart catheterization, 658
  in systolic heart failure, 102
Cardiac pacing
  automatic mode switching, 598
  classification, 589, 590
  clinical trials, 606–607
  complications, 600–602
    cardiac or central venous perforation, 601
    diaphragmatic stimulation, 601
    intravascular thrombosis or obstruction, 601–602
    lead dislodgment or damage, 601
    local muscular stimulation, 601
    pacemaker malfunction, 601
    pacemaker pocket hematoma, 600–601
    pacemaker system infection, 601
    pneumothorax, 600
    Twiddler syndrome, 602
  future of, 607
  glossary of basic cardiac pacing terminology, 607–609
  implantation issues for the physician, 598, 600

Cardiac pacing, implantation issues for the physician, (*contd.*)
  postoperative, 600
  preoperative, 598, 600
  indications for implantation, 589, 591–594
  overview, 588
  pacemaker components, 588
    lead-heart interface, 588
    lead system, 588
    pulse generator, 588
  pacemaker system malfunction, 601–604
  pacemaker timing cycles and intervals, 595–597
    base rate behavior, 595–597
    upper rate behavior, 597
  patient issues, 604–606
    electromagnetic interference, 604–605
    environmental interference, 605–606
    surgery, 604
  physiology, 589, 595
  polarity, 589
    bipolar, 589
    unipolar, 589
  rate-adaptive, 597–598, 599
  timing cycles and refractory periods, 609–610
Cardiac perforation
  in endomyocardial biopsy, 685
  and percutaneous coronary intervention, 727–729
Cardiac risk, in noncardiac surgical procedures
  background, 421
  clinical predictors, 424
  clinical presentation, 421–423
  criteria for estimating risk, 424–425
  diagnostic testing, 425–428
  energy requirements, 423
  functional capacity, 421, 423
  laboratory examination, 423–424
  perioperative management, 431–432
  physical findings, 421, 423
  preoperative evaluation objective, 421
  signs and symptoms, 421
  stepwise approach, 422
  therapy, 428–432
  type of operation, 423
Cardiac rupture
  clinical presentation, 43
  diagnostic testing, 44
  laboratory examination, 44
  pathophysiology, 44
  physical findings, 43
  signs and symptoms, 43
  therapy, 44
Cardiac stimulation threshold
  definition, in cardiac pacing, 607
Cardiac syncope
  electrical, 313
  mechanical, 313
Cardiac tamponade
  in diastolic heart failure, 126–128

  in endomyocardial biopsy, 685
  and percutaneous coronary intervention, 727–729
  in pericarditis, 361, 670
  and right heart catheterization, 653, 659, 660
Cardiac transplantation. *See* Transplantation, cardiac
Cardioactive drugs
  in electrophysiologic studies, 571–572
Cardiogenic shock, 107–109
  causes, 46
  classification, 45
  clinical presentation, 45
  and diabetes mellitus, 472
  diagnostic testing, 46
  etiology, 45
  hemodynamic monitoring, 107
  and intraortic balloon counterpulsation, 687, 725
  laboratory examination, 45–46
  physical findings, 45
  signs and symptoms, 45
  therapy, 46–48
  treatment algorithm, 108
  for ventricular septal defect, 41
Cardiomyopathy
  dilated, 103, 274, 275
  end-stage, and intraortic balloon counterpulsation, 688
  hypertrophic, 275
  ischemic, 103–104
  nonischemic, 546
  peripartum, 103
  preoperative management, 429
  restrictive, 117–120
Cardiomyoplasty
  in heart failure, 152
Cardiopulmonary bypass
  and percutaneous coronary interventions, 734
  weaning, and intraortic balloon counterpulsation, 689
Cardiopulmonary resuscitation (CPR)
  in sudden cardiac death, 302
Cardiovascular risk factors
  diabetes mellitus, 471–474
  economic consequences, 455
  hyperlipidemia, 455–463
  hypertension, 463–471
  morbidity, 455
  mortality, 455
  obesity, 474–475
  overview, 455
  prevention, 455
  sedentary lifestyle, 477–478
  tobacco, 475–477
Cardioversion
  anticoagulation and, 680
  chemical, 253
  complications, 680–681
  contraindications, 676
  description, 676

digitalis and, 680
direct cardiac, 253–255
indications, 676, 677
and pacemaker patients, 255, 605
patient preparation, 676
during pregnancy, 680
sedation, 676–677
of specific arrhythmias, 679–680
   atrial fibrillation, 679
   atrial flutter, 679
   supraventricular tachycardia, 679
   ventricular tachycardia, 679
   Wolff-Parkinson-White syndrome, 680
technique, 677–679
   electrode position, 678–679
   energy output and selection, 677–678
   synchronization, 678
Carditis
   and rheumatic fever, 644–645
   therapy, 648
Cardizem. See Diltiazam
Cardura (Doxazosin)
   description, 779
Carotid angiography
   in left heart catheterization, 717
Carotid artery disease
   preoperative management, 430–431
Carotid sinus hypersensitivity
   diagnostic testing, 300
   etiology, 298, 300
   pathophysiology, 298, 300
   risks, 300
   sites of potential lesions, 298, 300
   therapy, 300
Carotid sinus massage
   in electrophysiologic studies, 574
   in hypersensitivity, 300
   in sinus node dysfunction, 284
Carotid sinus syncope, 313
Carotid sinus syndrome, 298
Carpentier-Edwards valves, 232
Carteolol (Cartrol)
   description, 800
Cartrol. See Carteolol
Carvedilol (Coreg)
   description, 805
Catapres, Catapres TTS (Clonidine)
   description, 777
   for hypertensive urgencies, 445
   for smoking cessation
      after myocardial infarction, 61
      for prevention of cardiovascular disease, 477
Catheter ablation
   for atrial flutter, 261
   for ventricular tachycardia, 271
Catheterization, cardiac
   in aortic regurgitation, 189–190
   in aortic stenosis, 175–177
   assessment after myocardial infarction, 56
   in atrial septal defects, 389–390

in cardiac rupture, 44
in cardiogenic shock, 45
in coarctation of the aorta, 400
compared with stress echocardiography, 547
in constrictive pericarditis, 379–380, 381, 382
diagnostic, 29
for diastolic heart failure, 123
in hypertrophic cardiomyopathy, 133
in isolated right heart failure, 147–148
left heart, 102, 700–721
in LV pump failure, 45
in mitral regurgitation, 199
in mitral stenosis, 212
in patent ductus arteriosus, 397
in pericardial effusion with cardiac compression or cardiac tamponade, 370
in postoperative cardiac transplantation, 159
prosthetic heart valves and, 242
right heart, 102, 147–148, 653–665
in RV pump failure, 49
in systolic heart failure, 102
technique, 175–176
in Tetralogy of Fallot, 404
in tricuspid regurgitation, 228
in tricuspid stenosis, 222
in unstable angina, 29, 35–36
in ventricular septal defects, 394
Catheterization, pulmonary artery
   in papillary muscle rupture, 42
Cathode
   definition, in cardiac pacing, 607
ccTGA. See Congenitally corrected transposition of the great arteries
Central blood volume
   for diastolic heart failure, 125
Central nervous system (CNS)
   imaging, in infective endocarditis, 631–633
Central venous perforation
   as complication of pacemaker implantation, 601
Cephalosporin
   for rheumatic fever, 649
Cerebral syncope
   tilt table testing and, 624
Cerivastatin (Baycol)
   description, 820
Cetacaine
   for transesophageal echocardiography, 762
Chagas' disease
   and cardiomyopathy, 276
Chest pain
   clinical presentation, 446–447
   diagnostic testing, 447–451
      biochemical markers, 448–451
      electrocardiogram, 447–448
      imaging studies, 451
   differentiating cardiac from noncardiac, 447

Chest pain (*contd.*)
  differential diagnosis, 451–452
  etiology, 448
  evaluation and assessment, 445–452
  history, 446
  physical examination, 446–447
  risk factors, 446
CHF. *See* Congestive heart failure
Chlorothiazide (Diuril)
  description, 812
Chlorthalidone (Hygroton)
  description, 812
Cholecystitis, acute
  myocardial infarction and, 4
Cholesterol-altering drugs
  for women, to prevent coronary artery
    disease, 491–492
Cholesterol levels
  in women, 483–484
Cholestyramine (Questran Light)
  description, 818
Chronotropic incompetence
  to induce ischemia, 73
Cineangiography, coronary
  in aortic stenosis, 176
Cinefluoroscopy
  in infective endocarditis, 632
  prosthetic heart valves and, 241–242
Cisapride
  and Torsades de pointes, 278
Clofibrate (Atromid-S)
  description, 819
Clonidine (Catapres, Catapres TTS)
  description, 777
  for hyptertensive urgencies, 445
  for smoking cessation
    after myocardial infarction, 61
    for prevention of cardiovascular dis-
      ease, 477
Clopidogrel (Plavix)
  description, 826
  for embolic stroke, 245
  after myocardial infarction, 62
  and percutaneous coronary interven-
    tion, 738
  for stable angina, 78
  for unstable angina, 30
CMV
  in postoperative cardiac transplanta-
    tion, 162
CNS. *See* Central nervous system
Coagulopathy
  contraindication to left heart catheter-
    ization, 701
Coarctation of the aorta
  anatomy, 399
  clinical presentation, 399–400
  collateral circulation, 399
  diagnostic testing, 400
  embryology, 399
  laboratory examination, 400
  neonatal, 400–401
  overview, 399

physical examination, 399–400
  recurrence, 401
  signs and symptoms, 399
  therapy, 400–401
Cocaine
  myocardial infarction and, 21–22
Colchicine
  for idiopathic pericarditis, 358
  for pericarditis, 54
Colestid. *See* Colestipol
Colestipol (Colestid)
  description, 818
Commissurotomy, closed
  in mitral stenosis, 215
Compression/closure devices
  in left heart catheterization, 718
Computed tomography (CT)
  in abdominal aortic aneurysms, 337
  in aortic dissection, 347
  in pericardial effusion without tam-
    ponade, 366
  prosthetic heart valves and, 242
  for pseudoaneurysm, 45
  in thoracic aortic aneurysm, 342
Conduction disturbances
  preoperative management, 429
  prosthetic heart valves and, 242
Congenital heart disease
  aortic stenosis, 168–169, 171
  atrial septal defect, 387–391
  coarctation of the aorta, 399–401
  congenitally corrected transposition of
    the great arteries, 407–409
  Ebstein's anomaly, 409–412
  and isolated right heart failure, 145
  long QT syndrome, 320–324
  Marfan syndrome, 411–415
  patent ductus arteriosus, 396–398
  postoperative anatomy of adult
    patients with, 415–416
  pulmonary stenosis, and plmonary
    valve stenosis, 229
  Tetralogy of Fallot, 276, 401–406
  therapy, 148
  ventricular septal defect, 39–41,
    391–395
Congenitally corrected transposition of
    the great arteries (ccTGA)
  anatomy, 407, 408
  clinical presentation, 407
  diagnostic evaluation, 408–409
  laboratory examination, 408
  therapy, 409
Congestive heart failure (CHF), 99–114
  classification, 100
  clinical predictors of LV function after
    myocardial infarction, 113
  controversies, 112
  diagnostic testing, 100–103
  etiology, 103–104
  and infective endocarditis, 629
  laboratory evaluation, 99–100
  prognosis, 100

signs and symptoms, 99, 101
treatment, 104–112
Constrictive pericarditis, 361
  clinical presentation, 373
  diagnostic testing, 375–380
  etiology, 374–375
  laboratory examination, 375
  overview, 373
  pathophysiology, 375
  physical findings, 373–374
  and right heart catheterization,
       659–661
  signs and symptoms, 373
  therapy, 380–382
Continuity equation, 756
Contraceptives
  oral, and risk of coronary artery dis-
       ease, 487
Contrast echocardiography, 750–751
Copper 62, 534
Cordarone. See Amiodarone
Coreg (Carvedilol)
  description, 805
Corgard (Nadolol)
  description, 802
Cornell protocol, 509
Corolpam (Fenoldopam)
  description, 832
Coronary angiography
  in cardiac transplantation, 156–157
  to determine cardiac risk in noncar-
       diac operations, 428
  after myocardial infarction, 59
  in papillary muscle rupture, 42
  in stable angina, 76
  in sudden cardiac death, 302
Coronary angioplasty
  preoperative management, 430
Coronary arteries
  congenital, 713
  dissection, in left heart catheteriza-
       tion, 718
  left heart catheterization, 709–713
  spasm, in left heart catheterization,
       718
Coronary artery bypass graft (CABG)
  for acute myocardial infarction, 18
  arterial grafts, 87
  compared with medical treatment, 87
  compared with PTCA, 87–88
  elective, 59–61
  emergency, 18, 59
    in left heart catheterization, 719
  after myocardial infarction, 59–61
  and percutaneous coronary interven-
       tion, 727
  previous, 87
  preoperative management, 430
  for stable angina, 87–88
  venous grafts, 87
Coronary artery disease
  preoperative management, 429–430
  prevention, 455

risk factors
  diabetes mellitus, 471–474
  economic consequences, 455
  hyperlipidemia, 455–463
  hypertension, 463–471
  morbidity, 455
  mortality, 455
  obesity, 474–475
  overview, 455
  prevention, 455
  sedentary lifestyle, 477–478
  tobacco, 475–477
  women and, 481–499
Coronary stenosis
  quantification, 713–714
Coronary syndromes, acute
  and diabetes mellitus, 472
  and interventional cardiology, 725–727
  and sinus node dysfunction, 282
Corridor procedure
  for restoration and maintenance of
       sinus rhythm, 255–256
Corticosteroids
  dosages, 160
  in postoperative cardiac transplanta-
       tion, 160
  side effects, 160
Corvert. See Ibutilide
Cough
  as side effect of ACE inhibitors, 110
Coumadin. See Warfarin sodium
Cozaar (Losartan)
  description, 784
CPR. See Cardiopulmonary resuscitation
Creatine kinase
  in acute myocardial infarction, 4
  in evaluation of chest pain, 449–450
  in unstable angina, 27
Cross talk
  definition, in cardiac pacing, 607
CT. See Computed tomography
Culture-negative endocarditis, 631
Cyclooxygenase inhibitor
  description, 824
Cyclosporine
  dosage, 159
  drug interactions, 160, 161
  in postoperative cardiac transplanta-
       tion, 158, 159–160
  side effects, 159

DADs. See Delayed afterdepolarizations
Daily activities
  after myocardial infarction, 65
Dalteparin (Fragmin)
  description, 796
  for unstable angina, 31
Danaparoid (Organan)
  description, 794–795
Davies' disease, 117–119
DCC. See Direct current cardioversion
Death, 455
  in dual-chamber cardiac pacing,
       306–307

Death (*contd.*)
 during exercise electrocardiographic
  testing, 512
  prevention, 64
 in left heart catheterization, 718
 periocardiocentesis and, 674
 pharmacologic agent prevention of,
  303–304, 305
 in post–myocardial infarction, 64
 randomized trials, 304, 305
 sudden cardiac. *See* Sudden cardiac
  death
DeBakey classification scheme, 343, 344
Defibrillators
 automated external (AED), 307
 dual-chamber pacemaker-, 306–307
 implantable cardioverter-, 323
 and pacemaker patients, 605
 public access, 307
 testing in ICD implantation, 615
Dehiscence, 244–245
Delayed afterdepolarizations (DADs),
 249
Demadex (Torsemide)
 description, 811
Dental equipment
 and pacemaker patients, 605
Dental procedures
 and infective endocarditis, 640–641
Diabetes mellitus
 and acute coronary syndrome, 472
 and acute myocardial infarction, 20
 etiology, 471–472
 after myocardial infarction, 65
 pathophysiology, 471–472
 as predictive factor in coronary artery
  disease, 471–474
 risk factors, 471–473
 risk interventions, 473–474
 and silent ischemia, 92
 therapy, 473–474
 in women, 485
Dialysis
 for uremic pericarditis, 360
Diamox (Acetazolamide)
 description, 814
Diaphragmatic stimulation
 as complication of pacemaker implantation, 601
Diastolic heart failure
 cardiac cycle, 116
 classification, 118
 clinical controversies, 126–128
 clinical presentation, 115–117
 diagnostic testing, 120–125
 Doppler echocardiography, 121, 122
 etiology, 117–120
 hemodynamic parameters, 126
 laboratory examination, 117
 left ventricular inflow velocities, 127
 physical findings, 116–117
 signs and symptoms, 115
 therapy, 125–126
 ventricular pressures, 123, 124

Diastolic murmur
 in aortic regurgitation, 183–184
 in tricuspid stenosis, 220
Diathermy
 and pacemaker patients, 605
Diazoxide
 description, 831
Dicoumarol. *See* Dicumarol
Dicumarol (Dicoumarol)
 description, 798
Diet
 after chronic heart failure, 109
 in prevention of cardiovascular disease, 460, 469
 after stable angina, 88
 for women, to prevent coronary artery
  disease, 490
Digibind (Digoxin-specific Fab fragments), 293
 description, 835
Digitalis
 for atrial fibrillation, 252
 cardioversion and, 680
 interaction with calcium channel
  blockers, 84
 for mitral regurgitation, 202
 in mitral stenosis, 213
 toxicity, 249, 274, 293
Digoxin (Lanoxin)
 for atrial fibrillation, 252
 characteristics, 331
 for chronic heart failure, 110
 description, 793
 dosing, 110
 in exercise electrocardiographic testing, 506
 side effects, 110
Digoxin-specific Fab fragments
  (Digibind), 293
 description, 835
Dihydropyridines
 description, 806–807
 for stable angina, 84
Dilacor. *See* Diltiazem
Dilantin (Phenytoin)
 characteristics, 328
Dilated cardiomyopathy, 103
Diltiazem (Cardizem, Dilacor)
 for atrial flutter, 257
 characteristics, 331
 description, 792, 807–808
 for hypertrophic cardiomyopathy, 135
Diovan (Valsartan)
 description, 784
Diphenylalkylamines
 description, 808
Dipyridamole (Persantine)
 description, 827
 in stable angina, 73
Direct cardiac cardioversion
 for atrial flutter, 259
Direct current cardioversion (DCC),
 251–256

Discordant transposition of the great
    arteries (dTGA), 416
Disopyramide (Norpace)
    characteristics, 327
    for chemical cardioversion of atrial fib-
        rillation, 254–255
    description, 787
Diuretics
    for acute pulmonary edema, 106–107
    in cardiogenic shock, 47, 107
    for chronic heart failure, 111
    description, 810–814
    in LV pump failure, 47
    in mitral regurgitation, 202
Diuril (Chlorothiazide)
    description, 812
Dobutamine (Dobutrex)
    for acute myocardial infarction, 21
    for acute pulmonary edema, 107
    to assess ischemia, 75
    in cardiogenic shock, 47
    description, 816
    echocardiography, 556–557
    in nuclear imaging, 529
    in LV pump failure, 47
    in RV pump failure, 49
    in stable angina, 74
    stress echocardiography, 539, 541
        to determine cardiac risk in noncar-
            diac operations, 427–428
Dobutrex. See Dobutamine
Dopamine (Intropin)
    in cardiogenic shock, 47
    description, 815, 834
    in LV pump failure, 47
Doppler echocardiography
    in aortic regurgitation, 187–189
    clinical applications, 753, 756–757
    color flow imaging, 751–753
    in constrictive pericarditis, 376–378
    factors affecting image, 753–756
    in mitral regurgitation, 197–199
    in mitral stenosis, 210–211
    principles, 751–752
    prosthetic heart valves and, 239–240
    and pulmonary valve stenosis, 229
    pulsed wave and continuous wave, 752
    in stress echocardiography, 537
    and Tetralogy of Fallot, 404
    transthoracic, 751–757
    in tricuspid regurgitation, 226–227
    in tricuspid stenosis, 222
    velocities, 752
Doxazosin (Cardura)
    description, 779
Doxorubicin hydrochloride
    toxicity in systolic heart failure, 104
Dressler's syndrome
    clinical presentation, 55
    late, 55
        clinical presentation, 55
        therapy, 55

post–myocardial infarction pericardi-
        tis and, 359
    therapy, 55
dTGA. See Discordant transposition of
        the great arteries
Dual-chamber pacing
    for hypertrophic cardiomyopathy,
        136–137
    in sudden cardiac death, 306–307
Duchenne's muscular dystrophy
    in systolic heart failure, 104
    in ventricular tachycardia, 275
Duke criteria, 633, 634
Dye
    contraindication to left heart catheter-
        ization, 701–702
DynaCirc (Isradine)
    description, 806
Dypyridamole
    to assess ischemia, 75
    contraindication in nuclear imaging,
        523
    perfusion imaging, to determine car-
        diac risk in noncardiac opera-
        tions, 427
    and stress echocardiography, 539,
        541–542
Dyrenium (Triamterene)
    description, 814
Dysautonomic syndromes, 311–313
    tilt table testing and, 624
Dyslipidemia
    and diabetes mellitus, 472
    in postoperative cardiac transplanta-
        tion, 163
    in women, 483–484
Dysopyramide
    for hypertrophic cardiomyopathy, 135
Dyspnea
    in diastolic heart failure, 115
    in mitral stenosis, 207
    in systolic heart failure, 99

EADs. See Early afterdepolarizations
Eagle criteria, 424–425
Early afterdepolarizations (EADs), 249
Ebstein's anomaly
    anatomy, 410
    clinical presentation, 410
    diagnostic evaluation, 411–412
    laboratory examination, 411
    overview, 409
    physical examination, 410
    signs and symptoms, 410
    treatment, 412
ECG. See Electrocardiography
Echocardiography
    in acute myocardial infarction, 5
    in aortic regurgitation, 186–189
    in aortic stenosis, 170–172
    to assess ischemia, 75
    assessment after myocardial infarc-
        tion, 58
    in atrial fibrillation, 251

Echocardiography (*contd.*)
in atrial septal defects, 389
in cardiac rupture, 44
in cardiogenic shock, 45, 107
in cardiac transplantation, 156, 159
in coarctation of the aorta, 400
in constrictive pericarditis, 375–378
contrast, in transthoracic echocardiography, 750–751
in diastolic heart failure, 120–123, 126
Doppler
in aortic regurgitation, 187–189
clinical applications, 753, 756–757
color flow imaging, 751–753
in constrictive pericarditis, 376–378
factors affecting image, 753–756
in mitral regurgitation, 197–199
in mitral stenosis, 210–211
principles, 751–752
prosthetic heart valves and, 239–240
and pulmonary valve stenosis, 229
pulsed wave and continuous wave,
752
in stress echocardiography, 537
and Tetralogy of Fallot, 404
transthoracic, 751–757
in tricuspid regurgitation, 226–227
in tricuspid stenosis, 222
velocities, 752
in Ebstein's anomaly, 411
in evaluation of chest pain, 451
exercise, compared with stress
echocardiography, 547
in hypertrophic cardiomyopathy, 131
in idiopathic pericarditis, 357
in infective endocarditis, 632
intraoperative, 203
in isolated right heart failure, 147
in LV pump failure, 45
in Marfan syndrome, 412, 414
in mitral regurgitation, 197–198, 203, 204
in mitral stenosis, 210–211
in mitral valve prolapse, 207
M-mode, 751
in aortic regurgitation, 186
in constrictive pericarditis, 376
in transthoracic echocardiography,
751
in papillary muscle rupture, 42
in pericarditis, 54
prosthetic heart valves and, 237–239
for pseudoaneurysm, 45
and pulmonary valve regurgitation,
230–231
and pulmonary valve stenosis, 229
in rheumatic fever, 647
in RV pump failure, 49, 50
in stable angina, 76
in sudden cardiac death, 302
in syncope, 314
in systolic heart failure, 100–102
and Tetralogy of Fallot, 403–404
transesophageal, 40

in tricuspid regurgitation, 224–228
in tricuspid stenosis, 222
in tuberculous pericarditis, 359
two-dimensional echocardiography
in constrictive pericarditis, 376
and myocardial viability, 556–557
dobutamine echocardiography,
556–557
resting echocardiography, 556
in stress echocardiography, 537
in unstable angina, 28
in ventricular aneurysm, 51
in ventricular septal defects, 39–40,
393–394
ECMO systems
contraindications, 152
design, 151
in heart failure, 151–152
indications, 152
ECT. *See* Electroconvulsive therapy
Edecrin (Ethacrynic acid)
description, 810–811
Effusions
contraindication in pericardiocentesis,
671
loculated, 671
malignant, 671
purulent, 671
Ehlers-Danlos syndrome, 345
Eisenmenger syndrome, 395
Elderly
antihypertensive medications, 469–471
hypertension in, 464–465
in hypertrophic cardiomyopathy, 140
triggered atrial tachycardia in, 261
Elective replacement interval (ERI)
definition, in cardiac pacing, 607–608
Electrocardiography (ECG)
ambulatory, to determine cardiac risk
in noncardiac operations, 428
in aortic dissection, 345
in acute myocardial infarction, 5, 7–11,
13
in aortic regurgitation, 186
in aortic stenosis, 170
to assess ischemia, 74
in atrial fibrillation, 251
in atrial septal defects, 388–389
baseline, 72
in cardiac rupture, 44
in coarctation of the aorta, 400
for congenitally corrected transposition of the great arteries, 408
in constrictive pericarditis, 375
to determine cardiac risk in noncardiac operations, 423–424
in diastolic heart failure, 117
in Ebstein's anomaly, 411
in evaluation of chest pain, 447–448
exercise testing and, 503–522
in hypertrophic cardiomyopathy, 131,
132
in idiopathic pericarditis, 354–356
in infective endocarditis, 632

in ischemic ventricular tachycardia, 272, 273
in isolated right heart failure, 146, 147
lead placement in transthoracic echocardiography, 744
in Marfan syndrome, 412
in mitral regurgitation, 196
in mitral stenosis, 213
in mitral valve prolapse, 207
in patent ductus arteriosus, 397
in pericardial effusion without tamponade, 363
in pericardiocentesis, 672
in pericarditis, 54
in rheumatic fever, 647
in RV pump failure, 49
signal-averaged, in syncope, 316
in silent ischemia, 93
in sinoatrial exist block, 282
in sinus arrest, 282
in sinus bradycardia, 282
and sinus node dysfunction, 281–284
in stable angina, 72
in sudden cardiac death, 301, 302
in syncope, 314, 316
in systolic heart failure, 100
and Tetralogy of Fallot, 403
in thoracic aortic aneurysms, 340
in tricuspid regurgitation, 224
in unstable angina, 25, 26
in ventricular aneurysm, 51
in ventricular septal defects, 39, 393
Electrocautery
   and pacemaker patients, 604
Electroconvulsive therapy (ECT)
   and pacemaker patients, 605
Electrolytes
   abnormalities
      in syncope, 318
      in systolic heart failure, 99–100
   imbalance, contraindication to left heart catheterization, 702
   and Torsades de pointes, 278
Electromagnetic interference (EMI)
   definition, in cardiac pacing, 608
   environmental, 605–606
   in the hospital environment, 604–605
   in ICD transplantation, 618–619
Electrophysiologic studies (EPS)
   atrial stimulation, 567
   cardioactive drugs during, 571–572
   equipment and setting, 563–564
   indications, 563
   interpretation of findings, 571–587
      accessory pathways evaluation, 580–582
      bradyarrhythmia evaluation, 571–574
      SVT evaluation, 574–580
      ventricular tachycardia evaluation, 581–587
   overview, 563
   techniques and procedures, 564–567
      access and catheter placement, 564–565

baseline assessment, 565
preprocedure preparation, 564
programmed stimulation, 565–567
ventricular fibrillation, induction, 570
ventricular stimulation, 568–570, 571
Electrophysiologic (EP) testing
   in hypertrophic cardiomyopathy, 138
   in sudden cardiac death, 302
   in syncope, 316–317
      findings, 317
      indications, 317
      limitations and disadvantages, 317
ELT. See Endless-loop tachycardia
Embolic stroke
   and prosthetic heart valves, 245
Embolism
   clinical presentation, 53
   intracoronary, and percutaneous coronary intervention, 729
   in left heart catheterization, 718
   physical findings, 53
   signs and symptoms, 53
   and statins, 463
   therapy, 53–54
   in women, 486
EMI. See Electromagnetic interference
Eminase (Anistreplase-APSAC)
   description, 828–829
Enalapril (Vasotec)
   description, 782
Endless-loop tachycardia (ELT), 604
Endocarditis
   aortic valve, 235
   enterobacteriaceae, 631
   flucytosine and, 637
   fungal, 631
   homografts and, 235
   infective, 629–642
   for mitral regurgitation, 202
   in mitral valve prolapse, 207
   native valve, 630–631
   penicillin and, 633
   prophylaxis, 202, 207
   prosthetic heart valves and, 241–243, 631
   subacute bacterial, 139
   transesophageal echocardiography and, 243
   valve ring abscess and, 638
   vancomycin and, 633
End of life (EOL)
   definition, in cardiac pacing, 608
Endomyocardial biopsy
   complications, 685–686
   contraindications, 682, 683
   devices, 682
   for diastolic heart failure, 125
   indications, 682, 683
   mortality and, 685
   patient preparation, 682
   in postoperative cardiac transplantation, 158, 159, 162
   in systolic heart failure, 102
   technique, 681–685

Endomyocardial biopsy, technique
        (*contd.*)
    left ventricular biopsy, 685
    right ventricular biopsy, 681–685
Endomyocardial fibrosis, 117–119
Enoxaparin (Lovenox)
    description, 797
    for unstable angina, 31
Enterobacteriaceae
    and infective endocarditis, 631
Environment
    and pacemaker patients, 605–606
EOL. *See* End of life
Eosinophilic cardiomyopathy, 119
EP. *See* Electrophysiologic testing
Epinephrine (Adrenalin)
    description, 816, 834
EPS. *See* Electrophysiologic studies
Eptifibatide (Integrilin)
    description, 825
    for unstable angina, 31–32
ERI. *See* Elective replacement interval
Erythema marginatum
    and rheumatic fever, 645
Erythromycin
    for rheumatic fever, 648–649
Esmolol (Brevibloc)
    for atrial flutter, 257
    characteristics, 329
    description, 801
Esophagus
    in transesophageal echocardiography,
        765–770
Estrogen replacement therapy
    contraindications, 497–498
    dosage, 497
    after myocardial infarction, 64
    side effects, 497–498
    for stable angina, 85
    in women, 488, 494–498
ESWL. *See* Extracorporeal shock-wave
        lithotripsy
Ethacrynic acid (Edecrin)
    description, 810–811
Ethambutol
    for tuberculous pericarditis, 359
Ethmozine. *See* Moricizine
Excimer laser coronary angioplasty, 733
Exercise
    after myocardial infarction, 64–65
    to prevent cardiovascular disease, 469,
        487–488
    after stable angina, 88
    women and, 487–488, 491
Exercise echocardiography
    compared with stress echocardiogra-
        phy, 547
Exercise electrocardiographic testing
    advantages, 503
    complications, 509–512
    contraindications, 503, 506
    data
        interpretation, 521
        results, 511–517, 518–520

    death during, 512
    disadvantages, 503
    exercise protocols, 506–509
    guidelines, 504–505
    indications, 503, 504–505
    limitations, 503–504
    patient preparation, 505–506, 507
    positive predictive value (PPV),
        505
    prognosis, 520, 521
    recovery, 521
    sensitivity and specificity, 503, 505
    submaximal, 503
    termination, 517–521
    women and, 503
Exercise stress test
    abnormal, and left heart catheteriza-
        tion, 700–701
    to assess ischemia, 74
    assessment after myocardial infarc-
        tion, 56–58, 65
    in coarctation of the aorta, 400
    to determine cardiac risk in noncar-
        diac operations, 426
    high risk prediction, 74
    to induce ischemia, 73
    nuclear imaging and, 528
    in stress echocardiography, 537–538
    in sudden cardiac death, 302
Exertion, perceived, 516
Extracorporeal shock-wave lithotripsy
        (ESWL)
    and pacemaker patients, 604–605

Family care
    after myocardial infarction, 65
Fascicular blocks
    bifascicular, 294
    electrocardiographic features, 295
    trifascicular, 294, 297
    unifascicular, 294
Fatigue
    in mitral stenosis, 208
FDG, 534
Felodipine (Plendil)
    description, 806
Fenofibrate (Tricor)
    description, 819
Fenoldopam (Corolpam)
    description, 832
Fentanyl
    for transesophageal echocardiogra-
        phy, 762
Fibric acids
    description, 819
Fibrinolysis
    for acute myocardial infarction, 14, 15
Fibrinogen
    cofactors, 480
    etiology, 480
    pathophysiology, 480
    risk reduction, 480
    therapy, 480

Fibrinolytic therapy
    for acute myocardial infarction, 16–17
        contraindications, 16
    for thrombosis, 244
FK-506 (Tacrolimus)
    in postoperative cardiac transplanta-
        tion, 161
Flecainide (Tambocor)
    characteristics, 328
    description, 789
    for chemical cardioversion of atrial fib-
        rillation, 254
Flucytosine
    for infective endocarditis, 637
Fluid administration
    in pericardiocentesis, 673–674
    in RV pump failure, 49
Fluoroscopy
    in intraortic balloon counterpulsation,
        692
Fluvastatin (Lescol)
    description, 820
    in prevention of cardiovascular dis-
        ease, 461
Fontan procedure, 416
Formulas
    and right heart catheterization, 661
Fosinopril (Monopril)
    description, 782
Fragmin (Dalteparin)
    description, 796
    for unstable angina, 31
Functional capacity
    in exercise electrocardiographic test-
        ing, 517
Fungal endocarditis, 631
Furosemide (Lasix)
    description, 811
Fusion
    definition, in cardiac pacing, 608

Gallavardin's phenomenon
    in aortic stenosis, 168
Gemfibrozil (Lopid)
    description, 819
Gene therapy
    for stable angina, 86
Genetics
    and abdominal aortic aneurysms, 336
    counseling
        in Marfan syndrome, 414
    in hypertrophic cardiomyopathy,
        130–131
    and rheumatic fever, 646
Geriatrics
    antihypertensive medications, 469–471
    hypertension in, 464–465
    in hypertrophic cardiomyopathy, 140
    triggered atrial tachycardia in, 261
Glenn procedure, 415–416
Glucose levels
    and diabetes mellitus, 473
    in women, 485

Glycoproteins
    description, 824
    for percutaneous coronary interven-
        tion, 736–737
    for unstable angina, 31–32, 36
Glycosides
    in cardiogenic shock, 47
    in LV pump failure, 47
Goldman criteria, 424, 425
Gorlin formula, 211–213
Graham Steell murmur, 230
Guanabenz (Wytensin)
    description, 778
Guanadrel (Hylorel)
    description, 776
Guanethidine (Ismelin)
    description, 776
Guanfacine (Tenex)
    description, 777
Guidewires
    in percutaneous coronary interven-
        tion, 741

Haloperidol
    for Sydenham's chorea, 648
Hancock II porcine valve, 232
Harrison subclassification of antiarrhyth-
    mic drugs, 325, 326
HCM. See Hypertrophic cardiomyopathy
HDL-C
    after myocardial infarction, 62
    in women, 484
Heart block
    in stable angina, 73–74
Heart failure
    acute, 104–109
    in aortic stenosis, 167
    chronic, 109
    decompensated
        acute, 109
        contraindication to left heart
            catheterization, 702
        hemodynamics-directed protocol for
            therapy, 105
    hemodynamic effects of medications, 48
    high-output, 141–144
    isolated, right, 145–148
    in left heart catheterization, 719
    surgical options, 149–153
        dynamic cardiomyoplasty, 152
        ECMO, 151–152
        left ventriculotomy, partial, 151–153
        mitral annuloplasty, 153
        ventricular assist devices, 149–151
    as symptom of hypertrophic cardiomy-
        opathy, 129
Heart failure syndrome, 99, 101
Heartmate, 150
Heart rate
    management in diastolic heart failure,
        125–126
Hematoma
    as complication of pacemaker implan-
        tation, 600–601

Hemochromatosis
    primary, 120
    secondary, 120
Hemodynamic instability
    contraindication in pericardiocentesis,
        670
Hemodynamic monitoring
    in aortic stenosis, 171–174
    for cardiogenic shock, 107
    perioperative management, 431
    in RV pump failure, 49
Hemolysis, prosthetic heart valves and,
        243–244
    diagnostic testing, 243
    etiology, 243
    laboratory examination, 243
    pathophysiology, 243
    therapy, 243–244
Hemoptysis
    in mitral stenosis, 207
Hemostatis
    in intraortic balloon counterpulsation,
        698
Heparin, low-molecular-weight
    contraindication, in intraortic balloon
        counterpulsation, 689
    for infective endocarditis, 633
    for percutaneous coronary interven-
        tion, 735–736
    for unstable angina, 31, 36
Heparin, unfractionated
    for acute myocardial infarction, 18–19
    for atrial fibrillation, 252
    description, 794
    for embolic complications after
        myocardial infarction, 53
    for hyperthyroidism, 143
    interaction with nitrates, 80
    and pacemaker implantation, 598
    during pregnancy with prosthetic
        heart valves, 237
    for prosthetic heart valves, 236
    for thrombosis, 244
    for unstable angina, 30–31, 36
Heparinoid
    description, 794–795
Hepatic congestion
    in tricuspid stenosis, 220
Heterografts, 232
Hibernation
    and myocardial viability, 550
High-output heart failure
    clinical presentation, 142
    diagnosis, 142
    etiology, 141–144
    physical findings, 142
    symptoms, 142
    treatment, 141–144
Hirudin
    for percutaneous coronary interven-
        tion, 736
    for unstable angina, 31

Hirulog (Bivalirudin)
    description, 794
    for unstable angina, 31
    for percutaneous coronary interven-
        tion, 736
His bundle
    anatomy, 281
HMG CoA reductase inhibitors
    description, 820–821
    in prevention of cardiovascular dis-
        ease, 461–463
    for unstable angina, 33–34
Hoarseness
    in mitral stenosis, 207
Holosystolic murmurs
    in mitral regurgitation, 194
Holter monitoring
    in stable angina, 78
    in syncope, 314–316
    in Tetralogy of Fallot, 404
Home programs
    after myocardial infarction, 65
Homografts
    in aortic stenosis, 180
    in aortic valve endocarditis, 235
Homocysteine
    etiology, 479–480
    laboratory examination, 480
    pathophysiology, 479–480
    risk reduction, 480
    therapy, 480
Hormones
    contraindications, 497–498
    dosage, 497
    after myocardial infarction, 64
    side effects, 497–498
    for stable angina, 85
    in women, 488, 494–498
Hydralazine (Apresoline)
    for chronic heart failure, 110–111
    description, 831
    for hyptertensive emergencies, 442
Hydrochlorothiazide (Hydro-Diuril)
    description, 813
Hydro-Diuril. See Hydrochlorothiazide
Hygroton (Chlorthalidone)
    description, 812
Hylorel (Guanadrel)
    description, 776
Hypercatecholaminemia, 437
    and hyptertensive emergencies, 444
Hyperinsulinemia
    and diabetes mellitus, 473
    management, 474
Hyperlipidemia
    lipid-lowering trials, 456–458
        primary prevention, 457
        regression, 456–457
        secondary prevention, 457–458
        vasoregulation clinical studies, 458
    lipid management, 458–463

guidelines for primary prevention,
458–459
guidelines for secondary prevention,
459–460
types of therapy, 460–463
combination, 461–463
diet, 460
pharmacotherapy, 460–462
physiology, 455–456
as predictive factor in coronary artery
disease, 455
in stable angina, 79
Hypertension
accelerated, 434–435
in aortic dissection, 345
autoregulation, 438
blood pressure
ambulatory monitoring, 466
measurements in, 465–466
classification, 434–436
emergencies, 434–435
pseudoemergencies, 436
urgencies, 435–436
clinical presentation, 436, 465–467
contraindication to left heart catheterization, 702
crisis, 434–436
and diabetes mellitus, 471–473
diagnostic testing, 439
etiology, 436–437, 464
laboratory evaluation, 439, 467
malignant, 434–435
management in diastolic heart failure,
125
after myocardial infarction, 65
pathophysiology, 437–439, 464–465
physical examination, 436, 466–467
postoperative, 163, 437, 444
as predictive factor in coronary artery
disease, 463–471
preoperative management, 429
prognosis, 438–439
risk stratification, 467–468
signs and symptoms, 436
systemic, 434
therapy, 439–445
hypertensive emergencies, 439–444
hypertensive urgencies, 444–445
medical, 469–471
neurologic emergencies, 439
nonpharmacologic, 468–469
in women, 486
Hypertensive encephalopathy, 435
Hyperthyroidism
clinical diagnosis, 143
therapy, 143
Hypertriglyceridemia
and diabetes mellitus, 472
Hypertrophic cardiomyopathy (HCM)
clinical presentation, 129–130
diagnostic testing, 131–135

echocardiography
classification, 133
criteria for diagnosis, 132
electrocardiographic findings, 132
genetic aspects, 130–131
hemodynamics
findings during cardiac catheterization, 133
tracings, 134
management, 135–138
algorithm, 136
pharmacologic therapy, 137
mortality, 130
natural history, 129
physical examination, 130
prevalence, 129
risk stratification for sudden death,
138
signs and symptoms, 129
Hypocalcemia
and Torsades de pointes, 278
Hypokalemia
and Torsades de pointes, 278
Hypomagnesemia
and Torsades de pointes, 278
Hypotension
in aortic dissection, 345
Hytrin (Terazosin)
description, 780

IABC. See Intraaortic balloon counterpulsation
IABP. See Intraaortic balloon pump
Ibuprofen
for idiopathic pericarditis, 357
Ibutilide (Corvert)
characteristics, 330
description, 791
for restoration and maintenance of
sinus rhythm, 254
ICD. See Implantable cardioverter-
defibrillator
Idiopathic degenerative disease
and sinus node dysfunction, 282
Idiopathic fibrosis
and atrioventricular conduction disturbances, 290
Idiopathic pericarditis, 354–358
clinical presentation, 354
diagnostic testing, 354–357
differential diagnosis, 357
electrocardiographic evolution, 355, 356
etiology, 355
laboratory examination, 354–357
physical findings, 354
signs and symptoms, 354
therapy, 357–358
Idiopathic restrictive cardiomyopathy,
117
IE. See Infective endocarditis
Iliofemoral vessels
in intraortic balloon counterpulsation,
693

IMAC trial, 113
Imaging studies. *See also* Computed
    tomography; Echocardiography;
    Magnetic resonance imaging;
    Radiograph, chest; Trans-
    esophageal echocardiography;
    Transthoracic Echocardiography;
    Ultrasonography
  in evaluation of chest pain, 451
  interpretation, in nuclear imaging,
    529–532
  and percutaneous coronary interven-
    tions, 734–735
Imdur (Isosorbide Mononitrate)
  description, 822
Immunosuppressive therapy
  for myocarditis, 113
  in postoperative cardiac transplanta-
    tion, 159–161
Impedance
  definition, in cardiac pacing, 608
Implantable cardiac defibrillator (ICD).
    See also Antitachycardia devices
  for chronic heart failure, 113
  criteria for implantation, 613
  for ventricular tachycardia, 271
Implantable devices
  in sudden cardiac death, 304, 305–306
Implantation. *See also* Pacemakers
  antibiotics and, 598–600
  central venous perforation and, 601
  complications, 601
  criteria for, 613
  defibrillator-cardioverters, 323
  diaphragmatic stimulation and, 601
  hematoma and, 600–601
  heparin for, 598
  heterotopic, 157
  indications for, 589, 591–594
  infection and, 601
  intravascular thrombosis and, 601–602
  issues for the physician, 598–600
  lead system dislodgment or damage, 601
  muscular stimulation and, 601
  orthotopic, 157
  pneumothorax and, 600
  postimplantation management, 151
  prevention, 304–306
  tachycardia and, 615–616
  testing, 615
  Twiddler syndrome and, 602
  in ventricular aneurysm, 52
  ventricular assist devices, 150
  warfarin sodium for, 598
Impulse conduction disorders, 249–250
Impulse formation disorders, 249
Indapamide (Lozol)
  description, 813
Inderal. *See* Propranolol
Indomethacin
  for idiopathic pericarditis, 357
Infection
  as complication of intraaortic balloon
    counterpulsation, 697

  as complication of left heart catheter-
    ization, 720
  as complication of pacemaker implan-
    tation, 601
  contraindication to left heart catheter-
    ization, 702
  contraindication in pericardiocentesis,
    670
  in postoperative cardiac transplanta-
    tion, 162
Infective endocarditis (IE)
  clinical presentation, 629–630
  complications, 638
  controversies, 642
  diagnostic testing, 631–633
  Duke criteria, 633, 634
  etiology, 630–631
  incidence, 629
  laboratory examination, 631–632
  overview, 629
  pathophysiology, 631
  physical findings, 629–630
  prognosis, 638
  prophylaxis, 638–642
  response to therapy, 638
  signs and symptoms, 629
  therapy, 633–637
    medical, 633–637
    surgical, 637
Infundibular hypoplasia
  and Tetralogy of Fallot, 402
Inlet septal defects, 392
Inocor (Amrinone)
  description, 815
Inotropic agents
  for acute myocardial infarction, 21
  for acute pulmonary edema, 107
  for cardiogenic shock, 107
  description, 815–817
  in RV pump failure, 49
Insulin resistance syndrome, 472, 475
Integrilin (Eptifibatide)
  description, 825
  for unstable angina, 31–32
Interventional cardiology
  complications, 727–732, 733
    acute, 727–729
    long-term failure, 729–730
    restenosis, 729–730
    risk stratification by vessel and
      lesion characteristics, 730–732
  contraindications, 722
  device overview, 731–735
    diagnostic adjuncts, 734–735
    interventional devices, 731–733
    therapeutic adjuncts, 734
  indications, 722
  local delivery, 740
  operator characteristics, 738
  pharmacologic therapy, 735–738
  procedure overview, 740–741
    approaches, 740–741
    equipment, 741
    vessel sizing, 741

revascularization strategy, 721–727
    acute coronary syndromes, 725–727
    chronic stable angina, 727
    myocardial infarction with ST eleva-
        tion, 721–725
    silent ischemia, 727
    overview, 722
    percutaneous balloon pericardiotomy,
        740
    percutaneous transluminal myocardial
        revascularization, 740
    percutaneous transluminal septal
        myocardial ablation for hyper-
        trophic obstructive cardiomyopa-
        thy, 739–740
    valvuloplasty, 738–739
Interventional devices, 731–733
    balloons, 732
    stents, 731–733
Intraaortic balloon counterpulsation
    (IABC)
    balloon pump triggering and timing,
        693–696
    for cardiogenic shock, 107
    changing the IABP catheter, 698–699
    complications, 696–697
    contraindications, 689
    hemodynamics of balloon pump func-
        tion, 689–691
    indications, 687–689
    insertion technique, 691–693
    overview, 687
    patient evaluation and monitoring, 693
    removal of the IABP catheter, 697–698
Intraaortic balloon pump (IABP)
    for acute myocardial infarction, 20
    in aortic stenosis, 178–179
    in cardiogenic shock, 47–48, 725
    contraindications in aortic regurgita-
        tion, 191
    in LV pump failure, 47–48
    monitoring, 693
    patient care, 693
    in RV pump failure, 51
    for unstable angina, 35
    for ventricular septal defect, 41
Intracardiac shunt
    and right heart catheterization,
        661–664
Intracardiac signals
    in electrophysiologic studies, 564
Intramural hematoma
    in aortic dissection, 351
Intravascular thrombosis
    as complication of pacemaker implan-
        tation, 601–602
Intravascular ultrasound (IVUS), 77
    and percutaneous coronary interven-
        tions, 734–735
Intraventricular conduction disturbances
    electrocardiographic findings, 294,
        295, 296–297

etiology, 294
    therapy, 294
Intropin. See Dopamine
Ionic contrast media
    and Torsades de pointes, 278
Irbesartan (Avapro)
    description, 784
Iron chelation
    for primary hemochromatosis, 120
Ischemia
    assessment after myocardial infarc-
        tion, 56–58
    clinical presentation, 51–53
    as complication of intraaortic balloon
        counterpulsation, 696
    infarct expansion, 51–53
    management in diastolic heart failure,
        125
    methods to assess, 74–76
    methods to induce, 73–74
    and percutaneous coronary interven-
        tion, 727
    postinfarction angina, 53
    reinfarction, 53
    silent, 78, 91–94, 727
    and stress echocardiography, 543
    therapy, 53
Ischemic cardiomyopathy, 103–104
Ischemic cascade
    in stress echocardiography, 538–539
Ischemic ventricular tachycardia
    accelerated idioventricular rhythm,
        272, 273
    diagnostic testing, 272
    etiology, 271–272
    laboratory examination, 272
    pathophysiology, 271–272
    predictors, 272
Ismelin (Guanethidine)
    description, 776
Ismo (Isosorbide Mononitrate)
    description, 822
Isolation procedure, left atrial
    for restoration and maintenance of
        sinus rhythm, 256
Isoniazid
    for tuberculous pericarditis, 359
Isoproterenol (Isuprel)
    description, 817
    in electrophysiologic studies, 571–572
    for sinus node dysfunction, 285
Isoptin. See Verapamil
Isordil. See Isosorbide
Isosorbide dinitrate (Isordil, Sorbitrate)
    for chronic heart failure, 110–111
    description, 822
Isosorbide Mononitrate (Imdur, Ismo,
    Monoket)
    description, 822
Isotopes
    to assess ischemia, 75–76
    dual imaging, 528
Isovolumic relaxation time (IVRT)
    in diastolic heart failure, 117, 120

Isradipine (DynaCirc)
  description, 806
Isuprel. *See* Isoproterenol
IVRT. *See* Isovolumic relaxation time
IVUS. *See* Intravascular ultrasound

Jantene procedure, 416
Jervell and Lange-Nielsen (JLN) syndrome, 320–321
JLN. *See* Jervell and Lange-Nielsen syndrome
Jones criteria, 644
Junctional rhythms
  clinical presentation, 293
  electrocardiographic findings, 292, 293
  etiology, 293
  therapy, 293–294

Kay-Suzuku caged-disk, 233
Kerlone (Betaxolol)
  description, 800
Killip classification, 45
Kussmaul's sign, 373

Labetalol (Normodyne/Trandate)
  contraindications, 442
  description, 805
  for hyptertensive emergencies, 442
  for hyptertensive urgencies, 445
Lactic acidosis
  in cardiogenic shock, 45
  in LV pump failure, 45
Lamifiban
  for unstable angina, 32, 33
Lanoxin. *See* Digoxin
Laplace's law, 337
Lasix (Furosemide)
  description, 811
LDL. *See* Low-density lipoprotein
Lead system
  in cardiac pacing, 588
  dislodgment or damage, as complication of pacemaker implantation, 601
  lead-heart interface, 588
  replacement in ICD transplantation, 615
Leaflets, 238
Left heart catheterization, 102, 700–721
  complications, 718–720
  contraindications, 701–702
  indications, 700–701
  overview, 700
  patient preparation, 701–704
    contrast dye, 703–704
    education, 702
    equipment, 701–703
    informed consent, 702
    medications, 702
  postcatheterization care, 717–718
  technique, 705–718
    aortography, 716–717
    crossing the aortic valve, 714–715

    engaging the vessel, 705–708, 712
    imaging the vessels, 708–714
    left ventriculography, 715–716
    provocative testing, 717
Left ventricular dysfunction
  and left heart catheterization, 701
Lepirudin (rDNA, Refludan)
  description, 794
Lescol. *See* Fluvastatin
Levatol (Penbutol)
  description, 803
Levophed (Norepinephrine)
  description, 834
Lidocaine (Xylocaine)
  for acute myocardial infarction, 20
  characteristics, 327
  description, 788
  for transesophageal echocardiography, 762
  for ventricular tachycardia, 270
Lifestyle
  fitness and, 478
  modification after myocardial infarction, 65
  modification after stable angina, 88
  sedentary, as predictive factor in coronary artery disease, 477–478
    pathophysiology, 477
    risk reduction, 477–478
Lipase
  in postoperative cardiac transplantation, 159
Lipid-modifying enzymes, 456
Lipids
  and diabetes mellitus, 473–474
  lipid-lowering agents
    description, 818–821
  lipid-lowering trials, 456–458
    primary prevention, 457
    regression, 456–457
    secondary prevention, 457–458
    vasoregulation clinical studies, 458
  management, 458–463
    after myocardial infarction, 61–62
    guidelines for primary prevention, 458–459
    guidelines for secondary prevention, 459–460
    types of therapy, 460–463
      combination, 461–463
      diet, 460
      pharmacotherapy, 460–462
  for stable angina, 79
  for unstable angina, 33–34
Lipitor (Atorvastatin)
  description, 820
Lipoproteins, 455–456
Lisinopril (Zestril/Prinivil)
  description, 782
Liver function tests
  in isolated right heart failure, 147
  in systolic heart failure, 100
Löffler's disease, 119

Long QT syndrome (LQTS), 249, 277
  diagnostic testing, 320, 321
  epidemiology, 320
  molecular biology of, 320–322
  overview, 320
  therapy, 321–323
Loniten (Minoxidil)
  description, 832
Loop recorder
  in syncope, 316
Lopid (Gemfibrozil)
  description, 819
Lopressor. See Metoprolol
Losartan (Cozaar)
  description, 784
Lotensin (Benazepril)
  description, 781
Lovastatin (Mevacor)
  description, 821
  in prevention of cardiovascular dis-
    ease, 461
Lovenox (Enoxaparin)
  description, 797
  for unstable angina, 31
Low-density lipoprotein (LDL), 61–62
  in women, 484
Lozol (Indapamide)
  description, 813
Lp(a)
  pathophysiology, 478–479
  therapy, 479
LQTS. See Long QT syndrome
LV function
  assessment after myocardial infarc-
    tion, 56
LV hypertrophy
  in diastolic heart failure, 117
LV pump failure
  classification, 45
  clinical presentation, 45
  diagnostic testing, 46
  etiology, 45
  laboratory examination, 45–46
  physical findings, 45
  signs and symptoms, 45
  therapy, 46–48
Lyme disease
  temporary transvenous pacing and,
    666

MACE
  and percutaneous coronary interven-
    tion, 727
Macrolides
  for rheumatic fever, 649
Magnesium
  for acute myocardial infarction, 20
Magnet
  function in ICD transplantation,
    616–617
Magnetic resonance imaging (MRI)
  in abdominal aortic aneurysms, 338
  in coarctation of the aorta, 400

  in hypertrophic cardiomyopathy, 133
  in Marfan syndrome, 414
  and pacemaker patients, 604
  in patent ductus arteriosus, 397
  prosthetic heart valves and, 242
  in pericardial effusion without tam-
    ponade, 366
  for pseudoaneurysm, 45
  in Tetralogy of Fallot, 404
  in thoracic aortic aneurysm, 342
Magnetic resonance spectroscopy
  in aortic dissection, 346
  in hypertrophic cardiomyopathy, 133
  in sudden cardiac death, 302
Magnet mode
  definition, in cardiac pacing, 608
Mahaim reentrant tachycardia, 265
Malignant disease
  in postoperative cardiac transplanta-
    tion, 163
Marfan syndrome, 345
  clinical features, 412
  diagnosis, 412
  diagnostic evaluation, 411–414
  differential diagnosis, 414
  laboratory examination, 412
  overview, 412
  physical examination, 412
  pregnancy and, 415
  signs and symptoms, 412
  therapy, 414–415
MASS. See Medicine, Angioplasty or
    Surgery Study
Mavik (Trandolapril)
  description, 783
Maze procedure
  for restoration and maintenance of
    sinus rhythm, 255
Mechanical valves, 231–234
Medic Alert, 617
Medicine, Angioplasty or Surgery Study
    (MASS), 86
Medtronic-Hall valves, 235
Menopause
  coronary artery disease and, 484–485
Meperidine
  for transesophageal echocardiogra-
    phy, 762
Mephyton (Vitamin K)
  description, 836
Metabolic radiopharmaceuticals, 534
Metabolic stress testing
  in systolic heart failure, 101–103
Methyldopa (Aldomet)
  description, 778
Methyldopate HCl
  description, 778
Metolazone (Zaroxolyn)
  description, 813
Metoprolol (Lopressor)
  for atrial flutter, 257
  characteristics, 329
  description, 801

Mevacor. *See* Lovastatin
Mexiletine (Mexitil)
    characteristics, 328
    description, 788
Mexitil. *See* Mexiletine
MI. *See* Myocardial infarction
Mibefradil
    for stable angina, 84
Midamor (Amiloride)
    description, 813
Midazolam
    for transesophageal echocardiography, 762
Milrinone (Primacor)
    for acute pulmonary edema, 107
    in cardiogenic shock, 47
    description, 817
    in LV pump failure, 47
Minipress (Prazosin)
    description, 780
Minoxidil (Loniten)
    description, 832
Mitral annuloplasty
    in heart failure, 153
Mitral regurgitation (MR)
    acute, 200
        medical therapy, 200
        percutaneous therapy, 200
        surgical therapy, 200
    chronic, 194, 200–204
        choice of therapy, 200–201
        medical therapy, 201–202
        postsurgical follow-up care, 204
        surgical therapy, 201–203
    clinical presentation, 194–195
    controversies, 204–205
    diagnostic testing, 197–199
    differential diagnosis, 194–195
    etiology, 195–196
    in hypertrophic cardiomyopathy, 132
    laboratory examination, 196–197
    pathophysiology, 195–196
    physical findings, 194, 195
    and right heart catheterization, 659
    signs and symptoms, 194
    therapy, 199–204
Mitral stenosis
    clinical presentation, 207–209
    controversies, 216–217
    diagnostic testing, 210–213
    etiology, 209
    laboratory examination, 210–213
    pathophysiology, 209–210
    physical findings, 208–209
    preoperative management, 428–429
    signs and symptoms, 207–208
    therapy, 213–216
    valvotomy, 215–216
Mitral valve prolapse
    clinical presentation, 205–206
    diagnostic testing, 207
    etiology, 206
    laboratory examination, 207

    pathophysiology, 206
    physical findings, 205–206
    repair, 276
    signs and symptoms, 205
    therapy, 207
Mitral valve repair
    in mitral regurgitation, 202
    in mitral stenosis, 216
    in mitral valve prolapse, 276
Mitral valve replacement
    for hypertrophic cardiomyopathy, 138
    for mitral regurgitation, 202
    in mitral stenosis, 216
Mitral valvotomy
    in mitral stenosis, 215–216
M-mode echocardiography, 751
    in aortic regurgitation, 186
    in constrictive pericarditis, 376
    in transthoracic echocardiography, 751
Mobitz I atrioventricular block, 289, 290
Mobitz II atrioventricular block, 290, 292
Moexipril (Univasc)
    description, 783
Molecular biology
    and long QT syndrome, 320–322
Monoket (Isosorbide Mononitrate)
    description, 822
Monopril (Fosinopril)
    description, 782
Morbidity. *See* Death
Moricizine (Ethmozine)
    characteristics, 328
    description, 790
    for chemical cardioversion of atrial fibrillation, 255
Mortality
    coronary artery disease and, 455
    and percutaneous coronary intervention, 727
    in women, 482
MR. *See* Mitral regurgitation
MRI. *See* Magnetic resonance imaging
Multifocal atrial tachycardia, 261
Multisystem failure
    ventricular septal defect and, 41
Muromonab-CD-3 (OKT3)
    in postoperative cardiac transplantation, 161
Muscular dystrophy
    Duchenne's, 104, 275
    myotonic, 275
    in systolic heart failure, 104
    in ventricular tachycardia, 275
Muscular septal defects, 392
Muscular stimulation
    as complication of pacemaker implantation, 601
Mustard operation, 416
Mycophenolate mofetil
    in postoperative cardiac transplantation, 161
Myocardial infarction (MI)
    acute, 3–24

and intraortic balloon counterpulsation, 688
and left heart catheterization, 700
and right heart catheterization, 653
atrial fibrillation in, 256
clinical presentation, 3–4
cocaine abuse and, 21–22
complications
of arrhythmia, 52
embolic, 53–54
ischemic, 51–53
mechanical, 4, 39–52
pericarditis, 54–55
diagnostic testing, 5
differential diagnosis, 4
laboratory examination, 4–5
in left heart catheterization, 718
mortality, 6
physical examination, 3–4
post–, 56–67
algorithms for treatment, 57–58
prevention after hospital treatment,
64–65
risk stratification, 56–58
secondary prevention, 61–64
sudden cardiac death prevention, 64
therapy, 58–61
postoperative, 22
risk stratification, 3, 5
signs and symptoms, 3
standard of care, 22
temporary transvenous pacing and,
666
therapy, 5–21
in women, 481–483
Myocardial ischemia
in diastolic heart failure, 117
and hyptertensive emergencies, 444
as symptom of hypertrophic cardiomyopathy, 129
Myocardial laser revascularization
for stable angina, 88
Myocardial perfusion imaging
pharmacologic
to determine cardiac risk in noncardiac operations, 427
stress
to determine cardiac risk in noncardiac operations, 426–427
Myocardial tagging
in hypertrophic cardiomyopathy, 133
Myocardial viability
assessment, 550–557
positron emission tomography,
550–553
single-photon imaging techniques,
553–556
two-dimensional echocardiography,
556–557
choice of imaging technique, 557–558
clinical data, 549
clinical presentation, 549–550
etiology, 550

hibernation, 550
overview, 549
pathophysiology, 550
revascularization procedures, 549
stunning, 549–550
therapy, 558
Myocarditis
acute, 276
immunosuppressive therapy, 113
myocardial infarction and, 4
temporary transvenous pacing and,
666
Myoglobin
in evaluation of chest pain, 450

Naldolol (Corgard)
description, 802
NAPA
characteristics, 327
Native valve endocarditis, 630–631
Naughton protocol, 509
Neonatal coarctation, 400–401
Neoplastic pericarditis
clinical presentation, 360
diagnostic testing, 360
laboratory examination, 360
therapy, 361
Neo-Synephrine (Phenylephrine)
description, 834
Neurally mediated syncope, 311–312
Neurocardiogenic syncope
tilt table testing and, 620
Neuropathy
as complication of left heart catheterization, 720
Niacin (nicotinic acid)
description, 821
Nicardipine (Carden)
description, 807
Nicotine
gum, 476
nasal spray, 476
patch, 476
replacement therapy, 476
smoking cessation after myocardial
infarction, 61
Nifedipine (Procardia, Adalat)
for aortic regurgitation, 190–191
description, 807
for hyptertensive urgencies, 445
Nimodipine
for hyptertensive emergencies, 443
Nipride. See Nitroprusside sodium
Nisoldipine (Sular)
description, 807
Nitrates
description, 821–823
for mitral regurgitation, 202
for stable angina, 79–81
for unstable angina, 33
Nitroglycerin
for acute myocardial infarction, 12
for acute pulmonary edema, 106

Nitroglycerin (*contd.*)
  in cardiogenic shock, 47
  for hyptertensive emergencies,
    442
  IV (Tridil), description, 823
  in LV pump failure, 47
  paste (Nitrol), description, 823
  patch, description, 823
  preoperative management, 430
  SL (Nitrostat, Nitrolingual spray),
    description, 823
Nitroprusside sodium (Nipride)
  in cardiogenic shock, 47
  description, 833
  in LV pump failure, 47
  for ventricular septal defect, 41
Noncapture
  definition, in cardiac pacing, 608
Noncardiac surgery
  support, and intraortic balloon
    counterpulsation, 688
Noncardiovascular syncope, 313–314
Nonischemic ventricular tachycardia,
    271–272
Nonsteroidal anti-inflammatory drugs
    (NSAIDS)
  in idiopathic pericarditis, 357
Noradrenergic drugs
  in weight loss management, 475
    in women, 490
Norepinephrine (Levophed)
  description, 834
Normiflo (Ardeparin)
  description, 796
Normodyne/Trandate. *See* Labetalol
Norpace. *See* Disopyramide
Norvasc (Amlodipine)
  description, 806
  for stable angina, 84
Norwood operation, 415
NSAIDS. *See* Nonsteroidal anti-
    inflammatory drugs
Nuclear imaging
  clinical applications, 531–534
    perfusion analysis, 531–533
    ventricular function assessment,
      533–534
  contraindications, 523
  equipment, 523–524
  image interpretation, 529–532
  imaging protocols, 527–528
    dual isotope, 528
    technetium 99m, 528
    thallium 201, 527–528
  indications, 523
  mechanics and techniques, 524–527
  overview, 523
  PET, 534–535
  stress protocols, 528–529
Nuclear stress testing
  compared with stress echocardiogra-
    phy, 547

Obesity
  pathophysiology, 474–475
  as predictive factor in coronary artery
    disease, 474–475
  therapy, 475
  in women, 486
Obstruction
  in hypertrophic cardiomyopathy, 132
Occluders, 238
Ohm's law
  definition, in cardiac pacing, 608
OPO. *See* Organ procurement organiza-
    tion
Organ procurement organization (OPO),
    156
Orgaran (Danaparoid)
  description, 794–795
Orlistat
  in weight loss management, 475
    in women, 490
Orthopnea
  in systolic heart failure, 99
Orthostatic syncope, 311–313
  tilt table testing and, 624
Orthotopic implantation, 157
Ortner's syndrome, 207
Ostium primum defects, 387
Ostium secundum defects, 387
Output
  definition, in cardiac pacing, 608
Overdrive pacing
  temporary transvenous pacing and,
    666
Oversensing
  definition, in cardiac pacing, 609
Oxygen
  for acute myocardial infarction, 5, 12

PABV. *See* Percutaneous aortic balloon
    valvuloplasty
Pacemaker-defibrillators
  in sudden cardiac death, 306–307
Pacemaker pocket hematoma
  as complication of pacemaker implan-
    tation, 600–601
Pacemakers
  care, 668
  classification, 589
  components, 588
    lead-heart interface, 588
    lead system, 588
    pulse generator, 588
  dual-chamber, 595
  implantation issues for the physician,
    598–600
    postoperative, 600
    preoperative, 598–600
  indications for implantation, 589,
    591–594
  malfunction, 601, 601–604
  -mediated tachycardia, 603–604
    definition, in cardiac pacing, 608
  preoperative management, 429

for restoration and maintenance of
sinus rhythm, 255
rhythm interpretation, 595–597
single-chamber, 595
for syncope, 318
system malfunction, 601–604
timing cycles and intervals, 595–597
base rate behavior, 595–597
upper rate behavior, 597
wires, and percutaneous coronary
interventions, 734
Pacemaker syndrome, 603
Pacerone. *See* Amiodarone
Pacing
antitachycardia, 616
for asystole, 298
for atrial flutter, 259
burst, 567, 568, 616
cardiac
automatic mode switching, 598
classification, 589, 590
clinical trials, 606–607
complications, 600–602
cardiac or central venous perforation, 601
diaphragmatic stimulation, 601
intravascular thrombosis or
obstruction, 601–602
lead dislodgment or damage, 601
local muscular stimulation, 601
pacemaker malfunction, 601
pacemaker pocket hematoma,
600–601
pacemaker system infection, 601
pneumothorax, 600
Twiddler syndrome, 602
future of, 607
glossary of basic cardiac pacing terminology, 607–609
implantation issues for the physician, 598, 600
postoperative, 600
preoperative, 598, 600
indications for implantation, 589,
591–594
for long QT syndrome, 321–323
overview, 588
pacemaker components, 588
lead system, 588
lead-heart interface, 588
pulse generator, 588
pacemaker system malfunction,
601–604
pacemaker timing cycles and intervals, 595–597
base rate behavior, 595–597
upper rate behavior, 597
patient issues, 604–606
electromagnetic interference,
604–605
environmental interference,
605–606
surgery, 604

physiology, 589, 595
polarity, 589
bipolar, 589
unipolar, 589
rate-adaptive, 597–598, 599
timing cycles and refractory periods,
609–610
continuous, in electrophysiologic studies, 567
dual-chamber
for hypertrophic cardiomyopathy,
136–137
for sudden cardiac death, 306–307
indications for permanent, 286–288
interval
definition, in cardiac pacing, 608
for intraventricular conduction disturbances, 294
overdrive, 666
ramp, 616
rapid atrial, 259
in sinus node dysfunction, 285, 293
stimuli, in electrophysiologic studies,
565–566
and stress echocardiography, 539, 542
transcutaneous, 668
transvenous, temporary, 666–669
chest radiography and, 668
complications, 668
contraindications, 666
indications, 666
pacer care, 668
patient preparation, 666
technique, 666–668
Pain
chest, 446–452
in pericarditis, 54
Palpation
in aortic regurgitation, 183
in aortic stenosis, 167
in hypertrophic cardiomyopathy, 130
in mitral regurgitation, 194
in mitral stenosis, 208
Pannus formation
and prosthetic heart valves, 245
Papillary muscle rupture
clinical presentation, 41
diagnostic testing, 42
laboratory examination, 42
pathophysiology, 42
physical findings, 41
prognosis, 43
signs and symptoms, 41
therapy, 41–43
Paraplegia
as complication of aortic dissection,
350
Parchment heart
in isolated right heart failure, 147
Parenchymal disease
in isolated right heart failure, 146
Parenteral medications
for hyptertensive emergencies, 441

Patent ductus arteriosus (PDA)
　anatomy, 396
　clinical presentation, 396–397
　diagnostic testing, 397
　differential diagnosis, 396–397
　embryology, 396
　laboratory examination, 397
　overview, 396
　physical findings, 396
　signs and symptoms, 396
　therapy, 397–398
Patient education
　after myocardial infarction, 64–65
PBP. See Percutaneous balloon pericardiotomy
PCI. See Percutaneous coronary intervention
PDA. See Patent ductus arteriosus
Penbutolol (Levatol)
　description, 803
Penicillin
　for infective endocarditis, 633
　for rheumatic fever, 648, 649–650
Perceived exertion
　in exercise electrocardiographic testing, 516
Perclose Techstar, 718
Percutaneous aortic balloon valvuloplasty (PABV)
　in aortic stenosis, 179, 181
Percutaneous balloon mitral valvuloplasty
　controversy, 216–217
　in mitral stenosis, 213–214
Percutaneous balloon pericardiotomy (PBP), 740
　in pericardial effusion with cardiac compression or cardiac tamponade, 371
　in pericardiocentesis, 674
Percutaneous coronary intervention (PCI)
　for acute myocardial infarction, 14
Percutaneous revascularization
　for abdominal aortic aneurysms, 339
　for acute myocardial infarction, 17–18
　in aortic stenosis, 178–179
　for atrial flutter, 259
　in cardiac rupture, 44
　high-risk, and intraortic balloon counterpulsation, 688
　for long-term management of acute tachycardic episodes, 267
　in papillary muscle rupture, 42
　for unstable angina, 34
　for ventricular septal defect, 41
Percutaneous transluminal coronary angioplasty (PTCA)
　in cardiogenic shock, 48
　in LV pump failure, 48
　after myocardial infarction, 59
　primary, 721–724
　prophylaxis, 734

　secondary, 724–725
　success rates, 731
　for stable angina, 86–87
　for unstable angina, 34
Percutaneous transluminal myocardial revascularization, 740
Percutaneous transluminal rotational atherectomy, 730, 733
Percutaneous transluminal septal myocardial ablation
　for hypertrophic obstructive cardiomyopathy, 739–740
Perfusion analysis, in nuclear imaging, 531–533
　coronary artery disease detection, 532
　myocardial perfusion imaging, 531–533
　risk stratification, 532
Perfusion scintigraphy
　compared with stress echocardiography, 548
Pericardial cysts, 366
Pericardial effusion
　with cardiac compression or cardiac tamponade, 367–371
　　clinical presentation, 367
　　diagnostic testing, 368–370
　　laboratory examination, 368–370
　　pathophysiology, 367–368
　　physical findings, 367
　　signs and symptoms, 367
　　therapy, 370–371
　overview, 363
　in pericardiocentesis, 670
　without tamponade, 363–367
　　clinical presentation, 363
　　diagnostic testing, 363–367
　　etiology, 363, 364–365
　　laboratory examination, 363–367
　　physical findings, 363
　　signs and symptoms, 363
　　therapy, 367
Pericardial fat, 366
Pericardial sclerosis
　for neoplastic pericarditis, 361
Pericardial window
　in pericardial effusion with cardiac compression or cardiac tamponade, 371
Pericardiectomy
　for idiopathic pericarditis, 358
　in pericardial effusion with cardiac compression or cardiac tamponade, 371
　in RV pump failure, 51
　for tuberculous pericarditis, 359
Pericardiocentesis
　in cardiac rupture, 44
　complications, 674–675
　contraindications, 670–671
　death and, 674
　for idiopathic pericarditis, 358
　indications, 670
　infection and, 674

patient preparation, 671
in pericardial effusion with cardiac compression or cardiac tamponade, 370–371
in pericardial effusion without tamponade, 366–367
postprocedural care, 674
technique, 671–674
Pericarditis
acute, 354–362
complications, 361
constrictive, 361
  clinical presentation, 373
  diagnostic testing, 375–380
  etiology, 374–375
  laboratory examination, 375
  overview, 373
  pathophysiology, 375
  physical findings, 373–374
  signs and symptoms, 373
  therapy, 380–382
early, 54–55
  clinical presentation, 54
  diagnostic testing, 54
  etiology, 54
  laboratory examination, 54
  pain, 54
  pathophysiology, 54
  physical findings, 54
  signs and symptoms, 54
  therapy, 54–55
and evaluation of chest pain, 452
follow-up, 361
idiopathic, 354–358
  clinical presentation, 354
  diagnostic testing, 354–357
  differential diagnosis, 357
  electrocardiographic evolution, 355, 356
  etiology, 355
  laboratory examination, 354–357
  physical findings, 354
  signs and symptoms, 354
  therapy, 357–358
late, 55
  clinical presentation, 55
  therapy, 55
myocardial infarction and, 4
neoplastic
  clinical presentation, 360
  diagnostic testing, 360
  laboratory examination, 360
  therapy, 361
post–myocardial infarction
  clinical presentation, 359
  Dressler's syndrome, 359
  etiology, 359
  laboratory examination, 359
  postpericardiotomy syndrome, 360
  therapy, 359
purulent
  clinical presentation, 358
  diagnosis, 358

  etiology, 358
  therapy, 358
recurrent, 361
and rheumatic fever, 645
tuberculous
  clinical presentation, 358
  diagnostic testing, 359
  etiology, 358–359
  laboratory examination, 359
  therapy, 359
uremic
  clinical presentation, 360
  etiology, 360
  therapy, 360
viral, 358
Perimembranous septal defects, 392
Peripartum cardiomyopathy, 103
Permanent atrioventricular junctional reentrant tachycardia, 265
Persantine. See Dipyridamole
PET. See Positron emission tomography
Pharmacologic agents
in prevention of sudden cardiac death, 303–304, 305
Pharmacologic testing
nuclear imaging and, 528–529
in sinus node dysfunction, 284
in sudden cardiac death, 302
tilt table testing and, 622
Pharmacotherapy
in prevention of cardiovascular disease, 460
Phentolamine (Regitine)
description, 779
and hypertensive emergencies, 444
Phenylephrine (Neo-Synephrine)
description, 834
Phenytoin (Dilantin)
characteristics, 328
Phlebotomy
for primary hemochromatosis, 120
Phosphodiesterase inhibitors
in cardiogenic shock, 47
in LV pump failure, 47
Pindolol (Visken)
description, 803
PISA. See Proximal isovelocity surface area
Plaque
rupture, in unstable angina, 28
Platelet glycoprotein IIb/IIIa antagonists
description, 824
for percutaneous coronary intervention, 736–737
for unstable angina, 31–32, 36
Platelet inhibitors
description, 824–827
for stable angina, 78–86
Plavix. See Clonidogrel
Plendil (Felodipine)
description, 806
Pleural effusion, 366

Pneumocystis carinii infection
  in postoperative cardiac transplanta-
    tion, 162
Pneumothorax
  as complication of pacemaker implan-
    tation, 600
Polarity
  in cardiac pacing, 589
Positive predictive value (PPV)
  in exercise electrocardiographic test-
    ing, 505
Positron emission tomography (PET)
  blood flow tracers, 534
  clinical applications, 535
  in hypertrophic cardiomyopathy, 135
  metabolic imaging with SPECT, 534
  metabolic radiopharmaceuticals, 534
  and myocardial viability, 550–553
    assessment of myocardial blood
      flow, 551–552
    assessment of myocardial metabo-
      lism, 550–551
    findings, 551–553
    quantitative perfusion measure-
      ments, 552
    testing procedures, 552
  patterns of perfusion and metabolic
    imaging, 535
  protocols, 534–535
  in silent ischemia, 91–92
Post–myocardial infarction, 56–67
  algorithms for treatment, 57–58
  prevention after hospital treatment,
    64–65
  risk stratification, 56–58
  secondary prevention, 61–64
  sudden cardiac death prevention, 64
  therapy, 58–61
Post–myocardial infarction pericarditis
  clinical presentation, 359
  Dressler's syndrome, 359
  etiology, 359
  laboratory examination, 359
  postpericardiotomy syndrome, 360
  therapy, 359
Postsurgical bradyarrhythmias
  etiology, 294
  therapy, 294
Posttransplantation lymphoproliferative
    disorder (PTLD)
  in postoperative cardiac transplanta-
    tion, 163
Potts shunt, 416
PPV. See Positive predictive value
Pravachol. See Pravastatin
Pravastatin (Pravachol)
  description, 821
  in prevention of cardiovascular dis-
    ease, 461
Prazosin (Minipress)
  description, 780
Prednisone
  for idiopathic pericarditis, 357–358

Preexcitation syndromes
  clinical presentation, 263
  diagnostic testing, 265–266
  etiology, 263
  laboratory examination, 265–266
  pathophysiology, 263–265
  therapy, 266–267
    emergency management, 266
    long-term management, 266–267
    percutaneous therapy, 267
Pregnancy
  aortic dissection and, 345
  cardioversion and, 680
  heparin and, 237
  Marfan syndrome and, 415
  prosthetic heart valves and, 237
Pressure gradients
  in stable angina, 78
Presyncope
  as symptom of hypertrophic cardiomy-
    opathy, 129
Primacor. See Milrinone
Probucol
  for stable angina, 86
Procainamide (Procan SR, Procanbid,
    Pronestyl)
  characteristics, 327
  description, 786
  in electrophysiologic studies, 572
  for emergency management of acute
    tachycardic episodes, 266
  for restoration and maintenance of
    sinus rhythm, 253–254
  for ventricular tachycardia, 270
Procanbid. See Procainamide
Procan SR. See Procainamide
Procardia. See Nifedipine
Pronestyl. See Procainamide
Propafenone (Rythmol)
  characteristics, 329
  description, 789
  for chemical cardioversion of atrial fib-
    rillation, 254
Propranolol (Inderal)
  for atrial tachycardia, 261
  characteristics, 329
  description, 803–804
Prosthetic heart valves
  acoustic characteristics, 238
  anticoagulation therapy, 236–237
    immediate postoperative period, 236
    management in noncardiac surgery,
      236–237
    during pregnancy, 237
  calculations, 240–241
    continuity equation, 240–241
    dimensionless index, 241
    pressure half time, 241
  clinical presentation, 237
  complications, 241–245
  diagnostic testing, 237–239
  Doppler evaluation, 239–242
  dysfunction, 241–245

follow-up post vale surgery, 235–236
laboratory examination, 237–239
patient–prosthesis mismatch, 245
physical findings, 237
regurgitation, 240, 241
selection, 234–235
bioprosthetic valves, 234, 235
clinical factors, 234
homografts, 235
mechanical, 235
valve repair, 234
characteristics favoring, 234
stenosis, 240–241
types, 231–234
bioprosthetic valves, 232, 234, 235
mechanical, 231–234, 235
Prosthetic valve endocarditis (PVE), 631
Protamine sulfate
description, 836
Provocative testing
in aortic stenosis, 176
Proximal isovelocity surface area (PISA),
756–757
Pseudoaneurysm
clinical presentation, 44
diagnostic testing, 44–45
laboratory examination, 44–45
pathophysiology, 44
physical findings, 44
signs and symptoms, 44
therapy, 45
Pseudofusion
definition, in cardiac pacing, 608
Pseudohypotension
in aortic dissection, 345
Pseudopulmonary stenosis, 229
Pseudopseudofusion
definition, in cardiac pacing, 608
Psychosomatic response
tilt table testing and, 624
PTCA. See Percutaneous transluminal
coronary angioplasty
PTLD. See Posttransplantation lymphoproliferative disorder
Public access defibrillation
in sudden cardiac death, 307
Pulmonary arterial pressure
normal, 656
and right heart catheterization, 656
Pulmonary artery hypertension
and pulmonary valve regurgitation,
230
Pulmonary balloon valvuloplasty
in Tetralogy of Fallot, 405
Pulmonary congestion
in mitral regurgitation, 194
Pulmonary disease
contraindication in pericardiocentesis,
670
Pulmonary edema
acute, 105–107
and hyptertensive emergencies, 444
management, 106

Pulmonary embolism
and evaluation of chest pain, 452
myocardial infarction and, 4
and right heart catheterization, 661
Pulmonary valve regurgitation
clinical presentation, 230
diagnostic testing, 230–231
etiology, 230
physical findings, 230
signs and symptoms, 230
therapy, 231
Pulmonary valve stenosis
clinical presentation, 229
diagnostic testing, 229
etiology, 229
physical findings, 229
signs and symptoms, 229
therapy, 230
Pulmonary vascular disease
in isolated right heart failure, 146
Pulse generator
replacement in ICD transplantation, 615
Pulseless electrical activity
definition, 294
emergency intervention, 298
etiology, 298, 299
therapy, 298
Pulse width
definition, in cardiac pacing, 609
Pulsus parvus et tardus
in aortic stenosis, 167
Purulent pericarditis
clinical presentation, 358
diagnosis, 358
etiology, 358
therapy, 358
PVE. See Prosthetic valve endocarditis
Pyridoxine
for tuberculous pericarditis, 359

Quantitative pulmonary flow scans
in Tetralogy of Fallot, 404
QT dispersion
and long QT syndrome, 320
QT syndromes
long, 249, 277, 320–324
Questran Light (Cholestyramine)
description, 818
Quinaglute. See Quinidine
Quinapril (Accupril)
description, 783
Quinidex. See Quinidine
Quinidine (Quinaglute, Quinidex)
characteristics, 327
description, 785
for chemical cardioversion of atrial fibrillation, 255

Radiation therapy
and constrictive pericarditis, 374
and pacemaker patients, 605
and percutaneous coronary interventions, 734

Radiofrequency ablation
    in atrioventricular nodal reentrant
        tachycardia, 261–263
Radiograph, chest
    in aortic dissection, 345
    in aortic regurgitation, 186
    in aortic stenosis, 170
    in atrial septal defects, 389
    for cardiogenic shock, 45
    in coarctation of the aorta, 400
    for congenitally corrected transposi-
        tion of the great arteries, 408
    in constrictive pericarditis, 375
    for diastolic heart failure, 117
    in Ebstein's anomaly, 411
    in infective endocarditis, 632
    in isolated right heart failure, 147
    for LV pump failure, 45
    in Marfan syndrome, 412
    in mitral regurgitation, 197
    in mitral stenosis, 213
    in mitral valve prolapse, 207
    for papillary muscle rupture, 42
    in patent ductus arteriosus, 397
    in pericardial effusion without tam-
        ponade, 363
    for pseudoaneurysm, 44
    and rheumatic fever, 647
    in systolic heart failure, 100
    temporary transvenous pacing and,
        668
    and Tetralogy of Fallot, 403
    in thoracic aortic aneurysms, 340
    in tuberculous pericarditis, 359
    in ventricular aneurysm, 51
    in ventricular septal defects, 393
Radionuclide angiocardiography, 533
Radionuclide perfusion imaging
    in aortic regurgitation, 189
    to assess ischemia, 75–76
    assessment after myocardial infarc-
        tion, 58
    for diastolic heart failure, 123–125
    in evaluation of chest pain, 451
    in hypertrophic cardiomyopathy,
        134–135
    in sudden cardiac death, 302
Radiopharmaceuticals
    to assess ischemia, 75–76
    metabolic, 534
    in nuclear imaging, 524–527
Ramipril (Altace)
    description, 783
Randomized Intervention Tretment of
        Angina trial (RITA-2), 86
Randomized trials
    chronic heart failure, 113
    hypertension, 464–465
    interventional cardiology, 725–727
    lipid-lowering, 456–458
    prevention of coronary artery disease
        in women, 491–494
    stable angina, 86

sudden cardiac death, 304, 305
unstable angina, 35–36
vasoregulation, 458
ventricular tachycardia, 270
Rapamycin
    in postoperative cardiac transplanta-
        tion, 161
Rastelli procedure, 416
Reed switch
    definition, in cardiac pacing, 609
Refludan (Lepirudin)
    description, 794
Regitine. See Phentolamine
Rehabilitation program
    after myocardial infarction, 64–65
Rejection
    in postoperative cardiac transplanta-
        tion, 161–162
        acute cellular, 162
        hyperacute, 162
        vascular (humoral), 162
Renal failure
    in left heart catheterization, 718–719
    contraindication to left heart catheteri-
        zation, 701
Reopro (Abciximab)
    description, 824–825
    and percutaneous coronary interven-
        tion, 737
    for unstable angina, 31–32
Reperfusion
    for acute myocardial infarction, 12, 14
    and intraortic balloon counterpulsa-
        tion, 687–688
Rescue angioplasty, 724
Reserpine
    description, 776
Restenosis
    and percutaneous coronary interven-
        tion, 729–730
Restrictive cardiomyopathies
    in diastolic heart failure, 117–120
    eosinophilic, 119
    idiopathic, 117
    primary, 117–119
    and right heart catheterization, 661
    secondary, 119–120
Retavase. See Reteplase, rPA
Reteplase, rPA (Retavase)
    description, 829
    for acute myocardial infarction, 17
Revascularization
    and myocardial viability, 549
    preoperative management, 429–430
    for stable angina, 86–87
Rheumatic fever
    clinical presentation, 644–646
        diagnostic criteria, 644
        major manifestations, 644–645
        minor manifestations, 645–646
    diagnostic testing, 646–647
    etiology, 646
    incidence, 644

laboratory examination, 646–647
pathophysiology, 646
prevention, 648–650
    primary, 648–649
    secondary, 649–650
therapy, 647–648
Rheumatic heart disease
    and mitral stenosis, 209
    and pulmonary valve stenosis, 229
Rifampin
    for tuberculous pericarditis, 359
Right atrial systole
    and right heart catheterization, 656
Right heart catheterization, 102, 147–148,
    653–665
    acute mitral regurgitation and, 659, 662
    cardiac output, 658
    cardiac tamponade and, 659, 660
    complications, 654, 656
    constrictive pericarditis and, 659–661
    contraindications, 653
    formulas, 661
    indications, 653
    intracardiac shunt, 661–664
    massive pulmonary embolism and, 661
    overview, 653
    PA catheter pitfalls, 657–658
    restrictive cardiomyopathy and, 661,
        552
    right ventricular failure and, 658–659
    shock and, 658
    technique, 653–656
    tricuspid regurgitation and, 659
    troubleshooting, 656
    waveforms, 656–657
Right heart failure
    clinical presentation, 145
    diagnosis, 147–148
    etiology, 145–147
    isolated, 145–148
    laboratory examination, 147
    physical findings, 145
    signs and symptoms, 145, 146
    therapy, 148
Right ventricular infarction
    therapy, 148
Right ventricular failure, 658–659
Right ventricular systole
    and right heart catheterization, 656
RITA-2. See Randomized Intervention
        Treatment of Angina trial
Romano-Ward (RW) syndrome, 321
Ross procedure
    in aortic stenosis, 179–180
Rubidium 82, 534
Rupture
    in abdominal aortic aneurysms, 337
    cardiac, 43–44
    as complication of intraortic balloon
        counterpulsation, 697
    papillary muscle, 41–43
    in thoracic aortic aneurysms, 340,
        341–342

RV assist device
    in RV pump failure, 51
RV infarction
    and isolated right heart failure,
        145–146
RV pump failure
    clinical presentation, 48
    diagnostic testing, 49
    laboratory examination, 49
    pathophysiology, 48–49
    physical findings, 48
    signs and symptoms, 48
    therapy, 49–51
RW. See Romano-Ward syndrome
Rythmol. See Propafenone

60,000 rule
    definition, in cardiac pacing, 609
SACT. See Sinoatrial conduction time
Sarcoidosis, 120
    and ventricular tachycardia, 276
SCD. See Sudden cardiac death
Scleropathy
    in pericardiocentesis, 674
Sectral (Acebutolol)
    description, 799
Sedatives
    in cardioversion, 676–677
Senning operation, 416
Sensing
    definition, in cardiac pacing, 609
Sensor technology, future of, 607
Septal defects
    and isolated right heart failure, 145
Septal myotomymyectomy
    for hypertrophic cardiomyopathy,
        137
Serotonin reuptake inhibitors
    in weight loss management, 475
        in women, 490
Serum studies
    in systolic heart failure, 99–100
Sewing ring, 238–239
Sexual activity
    after myocardial infarction, 65
Sheath
    for endomyocardial biopsy, 682
    in percutaneous coronary interven-
        tion, 741
    removal, in left heart catheterization,
        717–718
Shock
    and right heart catheterization, 658
Shunts
    intracardiac, and right heart catheteri-
        zation, 661–664
    and isolated right heart failure, 145
    left-to-right, 145
    in Tetralogy of Fallot, 404
Sicilian gambit classification of antiar-
        rhythmic drugs, 325, 326
Signal-averaged electrocardiography
    in syncope, 316

Sildenafil
  interaction with nitrates, 80
Silent ischemia, 78, 91–94
  classification, 91
  clinical presentation, 91
  controversies, 93
  diabetes and, 92
  diagnostic testing, 91–92
  management, 91–93
  mechanisms, 92
  prognosis, 93
Simvastatin (Zocor)
  description, 821
  in prevention of cardiovascular disease, 461
Single-leaflet tilting disc, 232, 233
Single-photon imaging techniques
  and myocardial viability, 553–556
    diagnostic accuracy, 555
    limitations, 555
    physiology, 553–554
    rest-redistribution
      after acute myocardial infarction, 554–555
      thallium imaging, 554
    stress-redistribution imaging, 554
    stress-redistribution-reinjection protocol, 554
    technetium 99m sestamibi, 555–556
    thallium quantitation, 555
    thallium scan viability, 555
Single-vessel disease
  in stable angina, 89
Sinoatrial conduction time (SACT)
  in electrophysiologic studies, 567
Sinoatrial node
  anatomy, 281, 282
Sinus node dysfunction
  clinical presentation, 281–284
  diagnostic testing, 284–285
    invasive, 284–285
    noninvasive, 284
  electrocardiographic findings, 282
  etiology, 282, 283
  therapy, 285
Sinus node evaluation
  in electrophysiologic studies, 567
Sinus node recovery time (SNRT)
  in electrophysiologic studies, 567
Sinus node reentry tachycardia
  clinical presentation, 260
  pathophysiology, 260
  therapy, 260
Sinus rhythm
  restoration and maintenance in atrial fibrillation, 253–256
Sinus tachycardia
  clinical presentation, 250
  diagnostic testing, 250
  etiology, 250
  laboratory examination, 250
  pathophysiology, 250
  therapy, 250

Sinus venosus defects, 387
Situational syncope, 312
Skin cancer
  in postoperative cardiac transplantation, 163
Smoking, cessation
  and diabetes mellitus, 473
  and myocardial infarction, 61
  pathophysiology, 476
  as predictive factor in coronary artery disease, 475–477
  risk factor in coronary arter disease, 486–487
  risk reduction for coronary artery disease, 476–477
  and stable angina, 88
  therapy, 476–477
  women and, to prevent coronary artery disease, 493–494
SNRT. See Sinus node recovery time
Social support
  after myocardial infarction, 65
Sodium nitroprusside
  for acute pulmonary edema, 106
  for aortic dissection, 349
  for hyptertensive emergencies, 440, 442
  side effects, 442
Sorbitrate. See Isosorbide
Sotalol (Betapace)
  characteristics, 330
  for chemical cardioversion of atrial fibrillation, 254
  description, 792
  as prophylaxis for postoperative atrial fibrillation, 256
  for sarcoidosis, 276
SPECT, 534
Spironolactone (Aldactone)
  description, 814
Stanford classification scheme, 343, 344
Starr-Edwards caged-ball, 233, 235
Statins
  for unstable angina, 33–34
Stenosis
  in stable angina, 77–78
Stentless porcine bioprosthesis, 232
Stents
  for acute myocardial infarction, 15–16, 724
  primary, 724
  for unstable angina, 34
Steroids
  in postoperative cardiac transplantation, 158
St. Jude's bileaflet tilting-disk, 233, 235
Stomach
  distal, in transesophageal echocardiography, 765
Storage disorders, 120
Strauss method, 567
Streptase. See Streptokinase

Streptococcus pneumonia
  and infective endocarditis, 631
Streptokinase, SK (Streptase)
  for acute myocardial infarction, 16–17,
    19
  description, 829–830
  for thrombosis, 244
Streptomycin
  for tuberculous pericarditis, 359
Stress echocardiography
  in aortic regurgitation, 189
  in aortic stenosis, 174–175
  atrial pacing and, 542
  comparison with other modalities,
    547–548
  contraindications, 539–540
  exercise echocardiography, 540–541,
    543
  indications, 539–540
  interpretation, 541–547
    controversies, 546
    exercise echocardiography, 543
    false-negative results, 545
    false-positive results, 545–546
    nonexercise echocardiography,
      543–545
    prognostic value, 541–543
    subjective findings, 542
  in mitral stenosis, 211
  overview, 537
  pharmacologic stress echocardiogra-
    phy, 541–542
  physiology, 537–539
    exercise stress, 537–539
    nonexercise stress, 539
  technique, 540–542
    equipment, 540
    patient preparation, 540
    performing the test, 540–542
  technology, 537
    image modalities, 537
    image processing and presentation,
      537
Stress testing
  abnormal, and left heart catheteriza-
    tion, 700–701
  assessment after myocardial infarc-
    tion, 56–58
  in coarctation of the aorta, 400
  to determine cardiac risk in noncar-
    diac operations, 426
  indications, 29
  metabolic
    in systolic heart failure, 101–103
  noninvasive, 28–29
  in stable angina, 71–75
  in unstable angina, 28–29
Stroke
  clinical presentation, 53
  intracoronary, and percutaneous coro-
    nary intervention, 729
  in left heart catheterization, 718
  physical findings, 53
  signs and symptoms, 53

and statins, 463
  therapy, 53–54
  in women, 486
Stunning
  and myocardial viability, 549–550
Subacute bacterial endocarditis, 139
Subaortic septal defects, 393
Subcutaneous nodules
  and rheumatic fever, 645
Submaximal exercise electrocardio-
    graphic testing, 503
Subxiphoid pericardiostomy
  for idiopathic pericarditis, 358
  for neoplastic pericarditis, 361
  in pericardial effusion with cardiac
    compression or cardiac tampon-
    ade, 371
Sudden cardiac death (SCD)
  antiarrhythmic drugs and, 306
  in aortic regurgitation, 186
  in aortic stenosis, 170
  automated external defibrillator and
    public access defibrillation, 307
  clinical presentation, 301
  controversies, 306
  diagnostic testing, 301–302
  dual-chamber pacemaker-defibrillators
    and, 306–307
  etiology, 301, 302
  future, 306–307
  and hypertrophic cardiomyopathy, 129
  incidence, 301
  prevention
    antiarrhythmic drugs versus ICDs,
      306
    future, 306
    after myocardial infarction, 64, 135
    primary prevention, 303–305
      identification of individuals at
        risk, 303
      implantable devices, 304–305
      pharmacologic agents, 303
      surgical/percutaneous techniques,
        303–304
    secondary prevention, 305–306
      implantable devices, 305–306
      pharmacologic agents, 305
  prognostic testing, 301–302
  risk stratification, 138
  therapy, acute, 301–303
Sular (Nisoldipine)
  description, 807
Supine bicycle test
  to assess ischemia, 75
Supracristal septal defects, 393
Supraventricular tachyarrhythmias,
    250–267
  atrial fibrillation, 250–256
  atrial flutter, 256–259
  atrial tachycardias, 260–261
  atrioventricular nodal reentrant tachy-
    cardia, 261–263
  multifocal atrial tachycardias, 261
  preexcitation syndromes, 263–267

Supraventricular tachyarrhythmias
  (*contd.*)
  preoperative management, 429
  sinus node entry tachycardia, 259–260
  sinus tachycardia, 250
Supraventricular tachycardia (SVT)
  cardioversion and, 679
  in electrophysiologic studies, 564,
    574–580
    atrial flutter, 580
    baseline, 574
    induced tachycardia
      evaluation, 575–579
      significance, 579
    programmed stimulation, 574–575
Surgical revascularization
  in cardiogenic shock, 48
  in LV pump failure, 48
  in stable angina, 89
  for unstable angina, 34–35
SVT. *See* Supraventricular tachycardia
Sydenham's chorea
  and rheumatic fever, 645
    therapy, 648
    symptoms, 645
Sympathetic cardiac denervation, left
  for long QT syndrome, 323
Syncope
  in aortic stenosis, 167
  cardiac, 313
  carotid sinus, 313
  clinical presentation, 310–314
  diagnostic testing, 314–318
  electrical, 313
  and electrophysiologic studies, 563
  etiology, 311–314
  follow-up, 319
  laboratory examination, 314
  neurally mediated, 311–312
  noncardiovascular, 313–314
  orthostatic, 311–313
  overview, 310
  pathophysiology, 311–314
  physical findings, 310–311
  signs and symptoms, 310, 311, 312
  situational, 312
  as symptom of hypertrophic cardiomy-
    opathy, 129
  tilt table testing and, 620
  treatment, 318–319
    device therapy, 318
    medical, 318
    surgical therapy, 318–319
  unknown/unexplained, 314
Syndrome X, 95–96
  clinical presentation, 95
  diagnostic testing, 95
  differential diagnosis, 95
  etiology, 95
  obesity and, 475
  pathophysiology, 95
  prognosis, 95
  therapy, 95

Systemic-to-pulmonary shunt, 416
  and Tetralogy of Fallot, 403
Systolic heart failure, 99–114
  classification, 100
  clinical predictors of LV function after
    myocardial infarction, 113
  controversies, 112
  diagnostic testing, 100–103
  etiology, 103–104
  laboratory evaluation, 99–100
  prognosis, 100
  signs and symptoms, 99, 101
  treatment, 104–112
Systolic murmur
  in aortic regurgitation, 183

TAA. *See* Thoracic aortic aneurysm
Tachyarrhythmias
  atrial fibrillation, 250–256
  atrial flutter, 256–259
  atrial tachycardias, 260–261
  atrioventricular nodal reentrant tachy-
    cardia (AVNRT), 261–263
  and electrophysiologic studies, 563
  impulse conduction disorders, 249–250
  impulse formation disorders, 249
  multifocal atrial tachycardias, 261
  preexcitation syndromes, 263–267
  sinus node reentry tachycardia,
    259–260
  sinus tachycardia, 250
  supraventricular, 250–267
  ventricular, 267–279
  ventricular fibrillation, 279
  ventricular tachycardia, 267–279
Tachycardia
  detection and therapy, 615
  in ICD implantation, 615–616
Tachycardia-bradycardia syndrome, 284
  indications for pacing, 285
Tacrolimus (FK-506)
  in postoperative cardiac transplanta-
    tion, 161
Tambocor. *See* Flecainide
Tardokinesis, 546
Technetium 99m
  to assess ischemia, 76
  in evaluation of chest pain, 451
  in nuclear imaging, 527, 528
    basic protocols, 528
    factors affecting image quality, 528
    general characteristics, 527
    kinetics, 527
TEE. *See* Transesophageal echocardiog-
    raphy
Tenex (Guanfacine)
  description, 777
Tenormin (Atenolol)
  description, 799
TENS. *See* Transcutaneous electric nerve
    stimulation
Terazosin (Hytrin)
  description, 780

Tetralogy of Fallot
  anatomy, 402
  clinical presentation, 401–403
  diagnostic testing, 403–404
  embryology, 402
  follow-up care, 405–406
  incidence, 402
  in infants, 405
  laboratory examination, 403
  repair, 276
  therapy, 405–406
Thallium 201
  to assess ischemia, 75–76
  in nuclear imaging, 524–526, 527–528
    characteristics, 525–526
    general features, 527
    kinetics, 526
    variations from standard protocol,
      527–528
Thiamine
  deficiency, and high-output heart fail-
    ure, 143
Thiazides
  description, 811–813
Thoracic aortic aneurysm (TAA)
  clinical course, 341–342
  clinical presentation, 340
  complications, 342
  contraindication, in intraortic balloon
    counterpulsation, 689
  diagnostic testing, 342
  etiology, 340–341
  incidence, 339–340
  laboratory examination, 340
  pathophysiology, 341–342
  physical examination, 340
    cardiac, 340
    pulmonary, 340
    vascular, 340
  signs and symptoms, 340
  therapy, 341–343
    medical, 342
    percutaneous, 342
    surgical, 341–343
Thoracotomy
  in cardiac rupture, 44
Thrombin inhibitors
  description, 794
  for percutaneous coronary interven-
    tion, 736
Thrombocytopenia
  contraindication in pericardiocentesis,
    670
  and percutaneous coronary interven-
    tion, 737
Thromboembolism
  in endomyocardial biopsy, 685
Thrombolysis
  bleeding complications, 17
Thrombolytic agents
  for acute myocardial infarction, 14, 15
    contraindications, 15

analysis of trials, 60
  description, 828–830
  for unstable angina, 34
Thrombosis, prosthetic heart valves and,
    244
  diagnostic testing, 244
  laboratory examination, 244
  therapy, 244
Thrombotic thrombocytopenic purpura
    (TTP), 733
Thrombus formation
  and percutaneous coronary interven-
    tion, 731
  in unstable angina, 28
Thyroid
  disorders in systolic heart failure, 104
  status in systolic heart failure, 100
TIAs. See Transient ischemic attacks
Ticlid. See Ticlopidine
Ticlopidine (Ticlid)
  description, 827
  after myocardial infarction, 62
  and percutaneous coronary interven-
    tion, 737–738
  for stable angina, 78
  and thrombotic thrombocytopenic
    purpura, 733
  for unstable angina, 30
Tilt-table testing
  abnormal responses to, 623–624
  accuracy, 624
  evolution, 620
  indications, 620–621
  mechanism, 317
  overview, 620
  pathophysiology, 621–623
  reproducibility, 624
  sensitivity and specificity, 624
  in sinus node dysfunction, 284
  in syncope, 317–318
  testing protocol, 621–622
  upright, 317–318
Time constant of relaxation, 123
TIMI IIIb trial
  for unstable angina, 35
Timolol (Blocadren)
  description, 804
Tirofiban (Aggrastat)
  description, 825–826
  for unstable angina, 32
Tissue typing
  in postoperative cardiac transplanta-
    tion, 159
Tobacco
  and diabetes mellitus, 473
  and myocardial infarction, 61
  pathophysiology, 476
  as predictive factor in coronary artery
    disease, 475–477
  risk factor in coronary arter disease,
    486–487
  risk reduction for coronary artery dis-
    ease, 476–477

Tobacco (*contd.*)
  and stable angina, 88
  therapy, 476–477
  women and, to prevent coronary
      artery disease, 493–494
Tocainide (Tonocard)
  characteristics, 328
  description, 788–789
Tonocard. *See* Tocainide
Torsades de pointes, 249, 277
  drug implications and, 278
  etiology, 278
  therapy, 278–279
Torsemide (Demadex)
  description, 811
Toxins
  in systolic heart failure, 104
Toxoplasma gondii infection
  in postoperative cardiac transplanta-
      tion, 162
tPA
  for acute myocardial infarction, 16
Trandolapril (Mavik)
  description, 783
Transcatheter device closure
  in patent ductus arteriosus, 398
  for ventricular septal defects, 394
Transcutaneous electric nerve stimula-
      tion (TENS)
  and pacemaker patients, 605
Transcutaneous pacing, 668
Transesophageal echocardiography (TEE)
  in aortic dissection, 347
  in aortic regurgitation, 189
  in aortic stenosis, 174
  in atrial fibrillation, 253
  in atrial septal defects, 389
  complications, 773
  contraindications, 758–760
  in endocarditis, 243
  equipment, 760, 761
  examination guide, 761–763
  imaging, 763–772
    basic views, 764–770
      aorta, 770
      lower and middle esophagus, 765,
        768, 769
      transgastric, 765, 766, 767
      upper esophagus, 770, 771, 772
    biplane, 764, 770
  indications, 758, 759
  in mitral stenosis, 214–215
  patient preparation, 760–761, 762
  patient recovery, 773
  personnel, 760
  pitfalls, 773
  probe care, 773
  prosthetic heart valves and, 237–239
  in Tetralogy of Fallot, 404
  in thoracic aortic aneurysm, 342
  and thrombosis, 244
  transesophageal probe, 760, 761

Transient ischemic attacks (TIAs)
  in mitral valve prolapse, 205
Transplantation, cardiac
  complications
    allograft vasculopathy, 161–163
    dyslipidemia, 163
    hypertension, 163
    infection, 162
    malignant disease, 163
    postoperative, 157–158
    rejection, 161–162
    tricuspid regurgitation, 163
  coronary angiography and, 156–157
  death and, 164
  donor, 154–156
    care of, 155–156
    criteria, 154–155
    exclusion criteria, 155
    matching with recipient, 155
  echocardiography and, 156
  for hypertrophic cardiomyopathy,
      135–136
  immunosuppressive agents, 159–161
  indications, 154
  management
    long-term, 159
    postoperative, 158–159
  outcomes, 163–164
  recipient
    hospitalization, 163
    physiologic concerns, 157
  risk factors, 164
  status listings, 155
  surgical techniques, 157
    heterotopic implantation, 157
    orthotopic implantation, 157
Transthoracic echocardiography (TTE)
  in aortic dissection, 347
  contrast, 750–751
  Doppler, 751–757
  ECG lead placement, 744
  indications, 744, 745
  M-mode, 751
  in patent ductus arteriosus, 397
  in pericardial effusion with cardiac
      compression or cardiac tampon-
      ade, 368–370
  in pericardial effusion without tam-
      ponade, 365–366
  in thoracic aortic aneurysm, 342
  transducer selection, 744
  two-dimensional image acquisition,
      744–750
Transvenous pacing, temporary, 666–669
  chest radiography and, 668
  complications, 668
  contraindications, 666
  indications, 666
  pacer care, 668
  patient preparation, 666
  technique, 666–668
Trauma
  contraindication in pericardiocentesis,
      670

Travel
  after myocardial infarction, 65
Treadmill, 540
  versus bicycle exercise echocardiography, 538
Triamterene (Dyrenium)
  description, 814
Tricor (Fenofibrate)
  description, 819
Tricuspid regurgitation
  clinical presentation, 223–224
  etiology, 224, 225
  laboratory examination, 224–228
  in mitral regurgitation, 195
  pathophysiology, 224
  physical findings, 223–224
  in postoperative cardiac transplantation, 163
  and right heart catheterization, 659
  signs and symptoms, 223
  therapy, 228
Tricuspid stenosis
  carcinoid syndrome and, 220
  clinical presentation, 220
  diagnosis, 222
  diagnostic testing, 221–222
  etiology, 220–221
  laboratory examination, 221–222
  pathophysiology, 220–221
  physical findings, 220
  signs and symptoms, 220
  therapy, 221–223
Trifascicular block, 294, 297
Triglycerides
  after myocardial infarction, 62
  and women, to prevent coronary artery disease, 484–485
Troponins
  in acute myocardial infarction, 4–5
  in evaluation of chest pain, 450–451
  in unstable angina, 27–28
Trypanosoma cruzi
  and cardiomyopathy, 276
TTE. See Transthoracic echocardiography
TTP. See Thrombotic thrombocytopenic purpura
Tuberculous pericarditis
  clinical presentation, 358
  diagnostic testing, 359
  etiology, 358–359
  laboratory examination, 359
  therapy, 359
T-wave alternans
  and long QT syndrome, 320
T-wave morphology
  and long QT syndrome, 320, 322
Twiddler syndrome
  as complication of pacemaker implantation, 602
Two-dimensional echocardiography
  in constrictive pericarditis, 376
  and myocardial viability, 556–557

dobutamine echocardiography, 556–557
  resting echocardiography, 556
  in stress echocardiography, 537

UA. See Unstable angina
Uhl's anomaly
  in isolated right heart failure, 147
  therapy, 148
Ulcer, atherosclerotic
  in aortic dissection, 351
Ultrasonography
  in abdominal aortic aneurysms, 337
  intravascular, 77, 734–735
  in stable angina, 77
Undersensing
  definition, in cardiac pacing, 609
Unifascicular block, 294
Univasc (Moexipril)
  description, 783
Unstable angina (UA)
  clinical presentation, 25–26
  controversies, 35–36
  demographics, 25–26
  diagnostic testing, 28–29
  etiology, 28
  follow-up, 36
  laboratory examination, 26–28
  and left heart catheterization, 700
  physical findings, 26
  refractory, and intraortic balloon counterpulsation, 687
  risk factors, 25, 26
  signs and symptoms, 26
  therapy, 29–35, 36
Uremic pericarditis
  clinical presentation, 360
  etiology, 360
  therapy, 360
Urokinase (Abbokinase)
  description, 830
  for thrombosis, 244

VADs. See Ventricular assist devices
Vagal reaction
  in left heart catheterization, 719
Valproate
  for Sydenham's chorea, 648
Valsartan (Diovan)
  description, 784
Valve replacement
  in aortic stenosis, 179–180
  complications, 180
  mechanical, 180
Valve ring abscess
  and infective endocarditis, 638
Valve sounds
  in aortic regurgitation, 184
Valvular abnormalities
  and isolated right heart failure, 145
Valvular disorders
  and left heart catheterization, 701

Valvular disorders (*contd.*)
  preoperative management, 428–429
  in systolic heart failure, 104
Valvuloplasty, 738–739
  balloon aortic, 739
  percutaneous mitral, 738–739
Vancomycin
  for infective endocarditis, 633
VANQWISH. *See* Veterans Affairs Non-Q-
    Wave Infarction Strategies in Hos-
    pital trial
Vascor (Bepridil)
  description, 809
Vascular disease
  contraindication in intraortic balloon
    counterpulsation, 689
  contraindication to left heart catheteri-
    zation, 702
  in left heart catheterization, 719–720
Vascular endothelial growth factor
    (VEGF)
  for stable angina, 86
Vascular grafts
  contraindication, in intraortic balloon
    counterpulsation, 689
Vasodilator therapy
  for aortic dissection, 350
  in aortic stenosis, 178
    dosing, 178
    indications, 178
  in cardiogenic shock, 45, 107
  drugs, description, 831–833
  in LV pump failure, 45
  in papillary muscle rupture, 42
  in ventricular septal defect, 41
Vasopressors
  in cardiogenic shock, 47
  description, 834
  in LV pump failure, 47
Vasoregulation
  clinical studies, 458
Vasoseal, 718
Vasotec (Enalapril)
  description, 782
Vasovagal syncope
  tilt table testing and, 620, 623–624
Vaughan Williams classification of antiar-
    rhythmic drugs, 325, 326
VEGF. *See* Vascular endothelial growth
    factor
Veins
  femoral, 655
  IJ, 653–654
  in right heart catheterization, 653–655
  subclavian, 654–655
Ventricular aneurysm
  acute, 51
  chronic, 51
  clinical presentation, 51
  diagnostic testing, 51
  pathophysiology, 51
  physical findings, 51
  therapy, 51–52

Ventricular arrhythmias
  and left heart catheterization, 701
  preoperative management, 429
  refractory, and intraortic balloon
    counterpulsation, 688
Ventricular assist devices (VADs)
  for cardiogenic shock, 107–108
  centrifugal, 149–150
  choice of, 150
  complications, 149–150, 151
    embolic, 151
    infection, 151
    malignant arrhythmias, 151
    perioperative bleeding, 151
  contraindications, 149
  external, 149
  in heart failure, 149–151
  Heartmate, 150
  hemopumps, 149
  implantable, 150
  indications, 149
  left ventricular assist (LVAD), 150–151
  postimplantation management, 151
  pulsatile, 150
  right ventricular assist (RVAD), 151
  surgical approach, 150–151
Ventricular fibrillation
  course of disease, 279
  in electrophysiologic studies, 570
  in exercise electrocardiographic test-
    ing, 511
  induction, 570
Ventricular function, assessment in
    nuclear imaging, 533–534
  ECG-gated perfusion imaging, 533–534
  gated blood-pool imaging, 533
  radionuclide angiocardiography, 533
Ventricular inflow
  for diastolic heart failure, 120–123
Ventricular pressures
  for diastolic heart failure, 123
Ventricular septal defect (VSD)
  anatomy, 391–393
  apical, 39–40, 392
  associated lesions, 393
  atrioventricular canal-type, 392
  basal, 39
  clinical presentation, 39, 393
  diagnostic testing, 39–40, 393–394
  differential diagnosis, 393
  embryology, 392
  histopathology, 39
  inlet, 392
  laboratory examination, 39–40, 393
  mortality rate, 41
  muscular, 392
  natural history, 392
  overview, 392
  perimembranous, 392
  physical findings, 39, 393
  right heart catheterization, 40
  signs and symptoms, 39, 393

subaortic, 393
supracristal, 393
therapy, 40–41, 394–395
types, 391–394
Ventricular stimulation
in electrophysiologic studies, 568–570, 571
Ventricular tachycardia (VT)
arrhythmogenic right ventricular dysplasia and, 276
cardiomyopathy and, 275
cardioversion and, 679
clinical presentation, 267
differential diagnosis, 267–270
drug-induced, 274
evaluation, in electrophysiologic studies, 581–587
atrial study, 582
coronary artery disease, 582
dilated cardiomyopathy, 582
mapping, 585–587
programmed ventricular stimulation, 581–583
responses to programmed stimulation, 583–585
techniques for terminating tachycardia with pacing, 583
in exercise electrocardiographic testing, 511
idiopathic, 274–275
inflammatory and infectious conditions and, 276
long QT syndrome and, 277
muscular dystrophies and, 275
nonsustained, 267
prevention and prophylactic treatment, 270–271
repetitive monomorphic, 275
structural abnormalities and, 276
temporary transvenous pacing and, 666
therapy, 270
types, 271–279
ischemic, 271–272
nonischemic, 271–277
torsades de point, 277–279
Wolff-Parkinson-White syndrome and, 276
Ventriculectomy, partial left
echocardiographic findings, 152
as experimental procedure, 153
patient selection criteria, 152
postoperative medical management, 152
surgical approach, 152
survival, 151–153
Ventriculography
in hypertrophic cardiomyopathy, 133
left
in left heart catheterization, 715–716
in mitral regurgitation, 199
Venturi effect, 132

Verapamil (Calan, Isoptin)
for atrial flutter, 257
characteristics, 330
description, 793, 808
for emergency management of acute tachycardic episodes, 266
for hypertrophic cardiomyopathy, 135
for stable angina, 84
Veterans Affairs Non-Q-Wave Infarction Strategies in Hospital trial (VAN-QWISH)
for unstable angina, 35–36, 725–727
Viability assessment
in systolic heart failure, 102
Viral pericarditis, 358
Visken (Pindolol)
description, 803
Vitamin A
for stable angina, 85–86
Vitamin C
for stable angina, 86
Vitamin E
for prevention of coronary artery disease in women, 493
for stable angina, 85
Vitamin K–Phytonadione (Mephyton, Aqua Mephyton)
description, 836
VSD. See Ventricular septal defect
VT. See Ventricular tachycardia

Warfarin sodium (Coumadin)
for atrial fibrillation, 252
for chronic heart failure, 112
description, 798
for embolic complications after myocardial infarction, 53
for hyperthyroidism, 143
after myocardial infarction, 62
and pacemaker implantation, 598
for prosthetic heart valves, 236
for stable angina, 78–79
for thrombosis, 244
in ventricular aneurysm, 52
Waterson shunt, 416
Waveforms
and right heart catheterization, 656–657
Weight
reduction after myocardial infarction, 65
reduction to prevent cardiovascular disease, 468
and women, to prevent coronary artery disease, 490–491
Windows, in transthoracic echocardiography, 744–749
apical, 744–745
off-axis, 749
paraspinal, 749
parasternal, 744
subcostal, 745–749
suprasternal, 749

Wolff-Parkinson-White syndrome
  and atrial fibrillation, 256
  cardioversion and, 680
  and preexcitation syndromes, 263–265
  and ventricular tachycardia, 276
Women
  coronary artery disease and, 481–499
    age and, 484
    angina pectoris and, 482
    cholesterol and dyslipidemia,
      483–484
    clinical presentation, 481–483
    contraceptives,@I1:oral, 487
    diabetes mellitus and blood glucose,
      485
    estrogen levels, 488
    HDL-C and, 484
    hypertension and stroke, 486
    LDL-C and, 484
    menopause and, 484–485
    mortality, 482
    myocardial infarction and, 481–483
    obesity, 486
    physical activity, 487–488
    prevention
      antioxidant therapy, 491–493
      aspirin therapy, 494
      cholesterol-altering drugs,
        491–492
      diet, 490
      estrogen therapy, 494–498
      exercise, 491
      primary, 488–489
      secondary, 489
      smoking cessation, 493–494
      weight management, 490–491
    psychosocial aspects, 488
    risk factors, 482, 483–488
      modification, 488–498
      smoking, 486–487
      triglycerides and, 484–485
  estrogen replacement therapy, 488,
    494–498
    contraindications, 497–498
    dosage, 497
    after myocardial infarction, 64
    side effects, 497–498
    for stable angina, 85
  exercise electrocardiographic testing
    in, 503
  pregnancy
    aortic dissection and, 345
    cardioversion and, 680
    Marfan syndrome and, 415
    prosthetic heart valves and, 237
  stroke and, 486
Wytensin (Guanabenz)
  description, 778

X-ray. See Radiograph
Xylocaine. See Lidocaine

Yamaguchi's apical hypertrophic cardiomyopathy, 139–140

Zaroxolyn (Metolazone)
  description, 813
Zebeta (Bisoprolol)
  description, 800
Zestril/Prinivil (Lisinopril)
  description, 782
Zocor. See Simvastatin

greeno
Hose job #3